P.W. Dettmer

Technology Research.

The Esophageal Mucosa

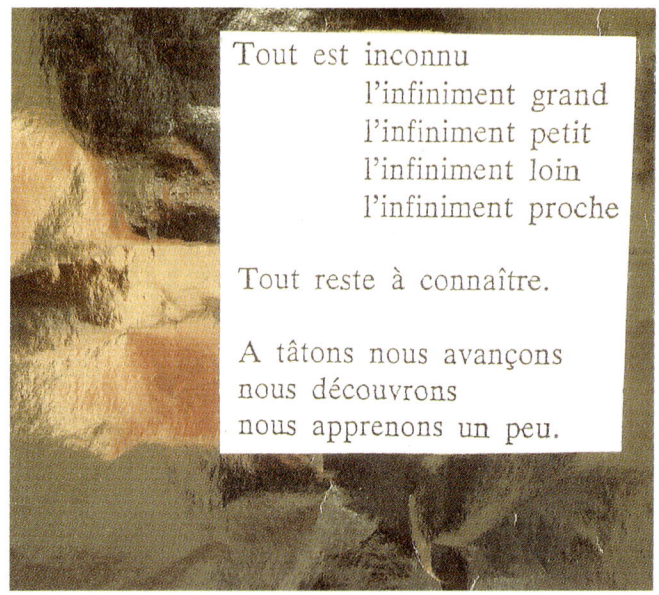

Tout est inconnu
    l'infiniment grand
    l'infiniment petit
    l'infiniment loin
    l'infiniment proche

Tout reste à connaître.

A tâtons nous avançons
nous découvrons
nous apprenons un peu.

Federico Mayor
Aguafuertes

Monsieur Federico Mayor,
    Directeur Général de l'U.N.E.S.C.O.,
Monsieur Adnan Badran,
    Directeur Général Adjoint pour les Sciences,
Monsieur Eiji Hattori,
    Conseiller auprès du Directeur Général
    et mon ami proche depuis si longtemps

Je vous ai rencontrés longuement lors de l'élaboration du 4ème Congrès de l'O.E.S.O.

Vous m'avez rendue facile l'exposition que je vous ai faite de toutes les particularités de la démarche scientifique de notre Groupe.

Et vous avez fait en sorte d'éclairer cette activité polydisciplinaire internationale de la lumière prestigieuse de votre Organisme, en acceptant que cette manifestation se tienne dans le cadre emblématique du siège de l'U.N.E.S.C.O., à Paris.

De 45 pays, tous les membres de l'O.E.S.O. vous sont reconnaissants de cette faveur qu'ils savent exceptionnelle. En leur nom, en tant que Directeur Scientifique de l'O.E.S.O., je vous adresse l'expression motivée de notre gratitude vraie.

En mon nom personnel, j'y ajoute celle de mon enthousiasme pour la manière dont vous rendez concrètes les valeurs que vous représentez.

Robert Giuli

Mr Federico Mayor,
Director General of U.N.E.S.C.O.,
Mr Adnan Badran,
Deputy Director General,
Assistant Director General for Science,
Mr Eiji Hattori,
Advisor to the Director General,
and my very close friend for such a long time,

I had lengthy encounters with you at the time of the planning of the O.E.S.O. Congress.

You made the presentation of all the specific scientific goals of our Group easy.

And you enhanced the international polydisciplinary activity of our endeavor with the prestigious light of your Organization, by accepting that this event take place in the emblematic Headquarters of U.N.E.S.C.O., in Paris.

Originating from 45 different countries, all the members of O.E.S.O. are grateful to you for this favor that they recognize as exceptional.

On their behalf, as Scientific Director of O.E.S.O., may I genuinely express my profound appreciation.

And, on my personal behalf, may I also add the expression of my enthusiasm for the way in which you implement the values that you stand for.

Robert Giuli

O. E. S. O.

Organisation internationale d'Etudes Statistiques pour les maladies de l'Œsophage
International Organization for Statistical Studies on Diseases of the Esophagus

Assistance Publique — Hôpitaux de Paris

Université Paris 7 — Faculté Xavier-Bichat

R. Giuli,

G.N.J. Tytgat, T.R. DeMeester, J.P. Galmiche
(Eds)

The Esophageal Mucosa

300 questions — 300 answers

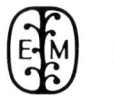 1994

ELSEVIER

Amsterdam – Lausanne – New York – Oxford – Shannon – Tokyo

International Congress Series No. 1052
ISBN 0 444 81753 0

This book is printed on acid-free paper.

Published by:
Elsevier Science B.V.
P.O. Box 211
1000 AE Amsterdam
The Netherlands

In order to ensure rapid publication this volume was prepared using a method of electronic text processing known as Optical Character Recognition (OCR). Scientific accuracy and consistency of style were handled by the author. Time did not allow for the usual extensive editing process of the Publisher.

Printed in the Netherlands

Editors

Robert Giuli, MD, FACS, FCCP
Professor of Surgery
University of Paris 7
Service de Chirurgie Digestive
Hôpital Beaujon
100 boulevard du Général Leclerc
92110 Clichy, Paris, France

Guido N.J. Tytgat, MD
Professor of Medicine
Professor of Gastroenterology
University of Amsterdam
Department of Gastroenterology-Hepatology
Academic Medical Center
Meibergdreef 9
1105 AZ Amsterdam, The Netherlands

Tom R. DeMeester, MD, FACS, FCCP
Professor of Surgery
University of Southern California
Chairman of the Department of Surgery
USC Healthcare Consultation Center
1510 San Pablo Street, Suite 514
Los Angeles, CA 90033-4612, U.S.A.

Jean-Paul Galmiche, MD
Professor of Gastroenterology
University of Nantes
Service d'Hépatologie et Gastro-Entérologie
Hôpital Guillaume et René Laënnec
B.P. 1005
44035 Nantes Cedex 01, France

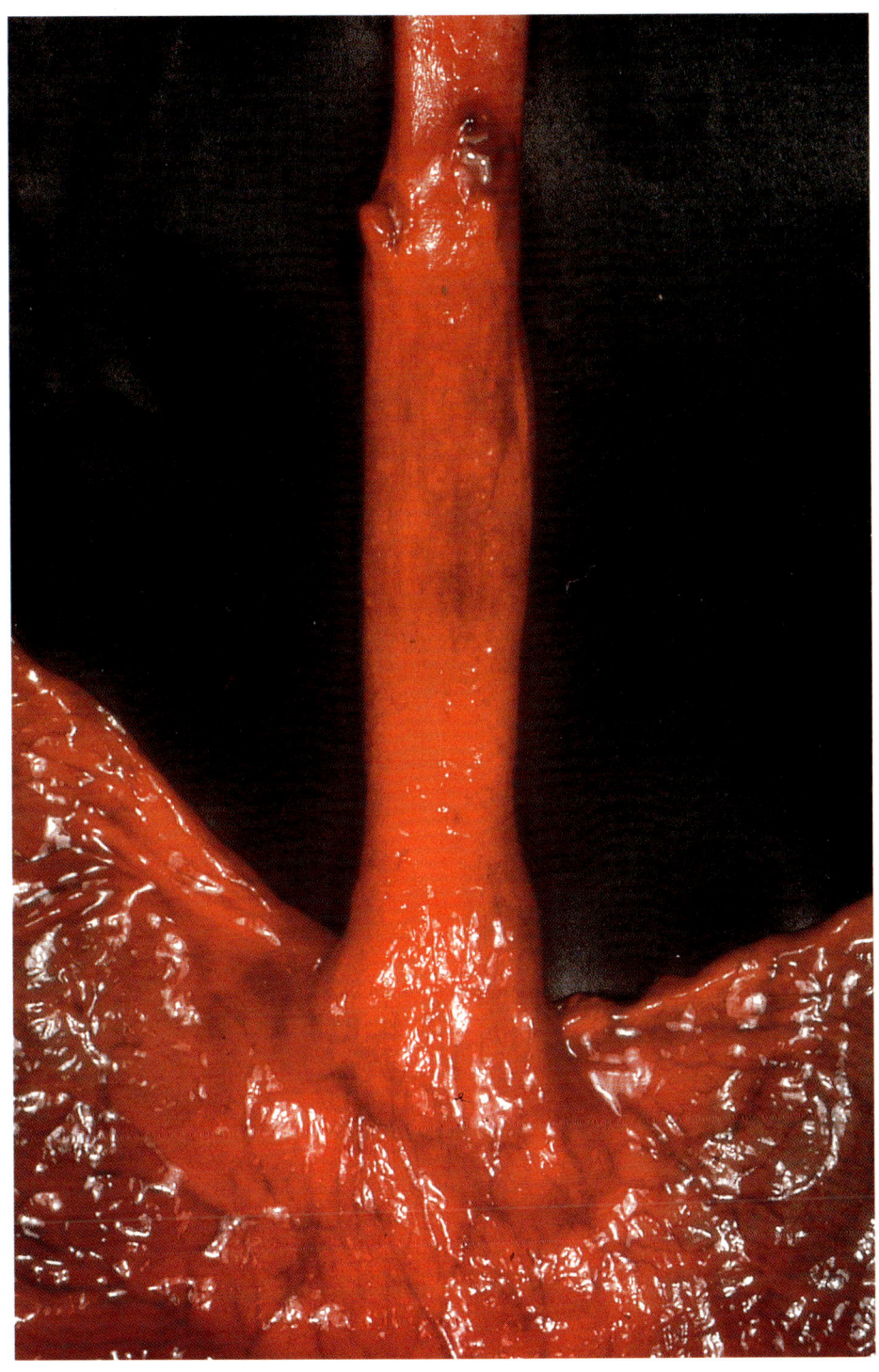

Avant-Propos

Cet ouvrage est fait de trois cents questions importantes qui concernent '*la muqueuse oesophagienne*'.

Le procédé qui a été mis en oeuvre pour mettre au point toutes ces questions, comme leurs réponses sous la forme d'articles scientifiques ou de présentations orales, rendent évidentes aussi bien les opinions concordantes que les divergences,

et aujourd'hui, cet ouvrage exhaustif que l'on doit au Professeur Giuli et aux spécialistes internationaux de la discipline, offre une approche nouvelle et un utile enrichissement des connaissances, à la fois pour ceux qui y ont participé et pour tous les autres qui vont le lire.

En médecine, la vérification concrète d'une idée repose certes sur le résultat d'un essai prospectif randomisé, mais il est clair qu'une telle démarche ne saurait être envisagée pour la plupart des réflexions élaborées par le chercheur ou le clinicien.

La méthodologie de consensus qui a été mise en oeuvre dans ce livre projette la lumière sur tel point précis de notre démarche clinique, et permettra d'orienter les travaux de recherche dans ce domaine important.

Melvin Schapiro

Foreword

This text addresses three hundred important questions that relate to the '*Esophageal Mucosa*'.

The exercise that was used to develop the questions, the written and oral presentations that addressed the controversial and consensus opinions about the answers,

and now this compilation by Professor Giuli and the international experts, is a novel and valuable learning experience for both participants and readers.

Documentation of concepts in medicine is usually dependent upon the prospective randomized trial. That this cannot be accomplished for a majority of basic and clinical concepts is apparent.

The consensus methodology that appears in this book serves to focus our clinical activities, and is valuable for the further design of research studies in this important area.

Melvin Schapiro, MD, FACP, FACG

Clinical Professor of Medicine
Center for Health Sciences
University of California at Los Angeles
President of the 10th World Congresses of Gastroenterology

Introduction

Cet ouvrage est le quatrième d'une série qui a été inaugurée en 1984, à la suite du premier Congrès mondial de l'O.E.S.O.

Le pari était là, lorsque j'avais pensé — c'était un peu une aventure — de les réunir tous, tous les spécialistes de toutes les disciplines concernant un seul et même organe, pour répondre à une démarche qui ne leur était pas familière: je ne leur demandais pas une conférence, ni une mise au point exhaustive sur un sujet, ni une communication qu'ils auraient choisie.

Non. Je leur proposais une démarche originale et plus difficile: il s'agissait pour chacun, spécialiste incontesté de haute réputation, d'accepter de *ne pas* faire état de sa propre expérience, mais de se servir de tout ce qu'elle représentait pour rechercher, et trouver, les éléments, d'une synthèse *élective* sur un seul point extrêmement précis, extrêmement limité, qui faisait la matière d'une seule et brève question.

Pour ce quatrième Congrès mondial de l'O.E.S.O. comme pour les trois premiers, lorsque j'ai élaboré les 300 questions relevant du thème unique qui était cette fois 'la muqueuse oesophagienne', j'ai pensé, pour répondre à chacune d'elles, à un ami personnel, ou encore à une personnalité que je ne connaissais pas encore, mais dont les travaux m'avaient impressionné.

C'est là que les membres du Comité Scientifique de l'O.E.S.O. ont joué tout leur rôle, et combien primordial, pour peaufiner la forme des questions, leur but, leur portée, ou suggérer un nom particulièrement approprié pour apporter sa réponse.

Et ainsi, d'autres personnalités ont été contactées pour participer à cet ouvrage.

C'est cet enthousiasme collectif qui a rendu possible et qui a bâti ce livre: comme à l'occasion du Congrès, chacun a joué le jeu difficile qui lui était demandé, et a fourni sa part originale et essentielle à l'élaboration de cette sorte d'encyclopédie qui couvre maintenant un chapitre passionnant de l'oesophagologie.

*

Je remercie chacun d'eux.
Je sais gré à chacun de tout ce qu'il nous a apporté.
Je suis fier de la présence de Guido Tytgat, Tom DeMeester et Jean-Paul Galmiche à mes côtés comme co-éditeurs de ce quatrième volume: ils lui apportent leur réputation, et tout ce que signifie leur exceptionnelle valeur scientifique.
Ils sont aussi mes amis, et ils ont su m'aider à chaque pas de l'élaboration difficile du Congrès prestigieux qui a été à l'origine de cet ouvrage.

Introduction

This book is the fourth in a series of publications, inaugurated in 1984 after the first World Congress of O.E.S.O.

It was a wager of the most challenging and venturesome sort, when I first imagined that it would be possible to bring together all of these specialists, from all disciplines, concerning one single organ, to participate in an approach that they were not familiar with. I sought not a conference and I asked neither for an exhaustive commentary, nor a paper that they would have chosen themselves.

No! I proposed an original and more difficult procedure: each one, an indisputable specialist of high reputation, was asked to agree *not to* report on his or her very own experience, but rather to make use of this experience to seek, and find, the elements of an *elective* synthesis on an extremely precise and limited point, granting the material for a response to a single and most specific question.

For this Fourth O.E.S.O. World Congress, as for the first three, at the time when I was devising the 300 questions focusing on the specific theme, which this time was 'The Esophageal Mucosa', to answer each question, I thought to ask either a personal friend, or even a known author whom I had maybe never met, but whose work had impressed me.

It was then that the members of the Permanent Scientific Committee of O.E.S.O. fulfilled their role, and how prominent indeed it was, to polish the terminology of the questions and widen their potential scope, or to suggest a more appropriate contributor.

And in this way, other valuable specialists were contacted to participate.

This collective enthusiasm has made the elaboration of this book possible, as it significantly contributed to the smooth and original functioning of the Congress: everyone fully played the challenging game asked of them, and offered a unique and essential part to construct this kind of encyclopedia that now covers a fascinating area of esophagology.

*

I thank each one of them.

I am grateful to each one for all that was given towards this effort.

I am proud to have Guido Tytgat, Tom DeMeester, and Jean-Paul Galmiche with me as co-editors of this fourth volume: they bestow upon it their vast reputations, and all that their exceptional importance represents to the scientific world.

They are also very close friends, who have known how to help me efficiently in each step of the laborious preparation of the Congress that was at the origin of this book.

Et c'est le privilège du Directeur Scientifique de l'O.E.S.O. de savoir que ce train polydisciplinaire, rempli de projets d'avenir, est maintenant lancé à toute allure, poussé par la force enthousiaste de chacun, et qu'il ira loin, pour visiter des zones fascinantes encore mal explorées de notre belle et difficile spécialité.

Robert Giuli

Très à part, parce que sa participation a été unique, je desire rendre un hommage particulier à Michèle Liégeon.

Collaboratrice attentive, à l'intelligence claire, à l'enthousiasme communicatif, douée d'une méticulosité inégalable dans la quête de la perfection, elle a contribué d'une manière exceptionnellement efficace à donner à cet ouvrage, comme aux précédents, certaines des qualités que le lecteur saura j'espère lui trouver.

And it is a privilege for the Scientific Director of O.E.S.O. to watch this polydisciplinary locomotive, charged with future projects, now running at full speed driven by the ardent force in each of us, and to know that it will go far in finding fascinating areas yet to be explored in our splendid and complex specialty.

R. Giuli, MD, FACS
Professor of Surgery
Scientific Director of O.E.S.O.

Very much apart, because her participation has been exceptionally remarkable, I would like to pay particular tribute to Michèle Liégeon.

An attentive and precious assistant, keenly intelligent, communicatively enthusiastic, endowed with matchless meticulousness in her quest for excellence, she has been outstandingly efficient in giving this volume, as the preceding ones, a certain perfection that, I hope, the reader will easily perceive.

Préface

Le quatrième Congrès de l'O.E.S.O., consacré à la muqueuse oesophagienne et ses affections, s'est tenu en septembre 1993 dans les installations prestigieuses du siège de l'U.N.E.S.C.O. à Paris, avec toutes les possibilités exceptionnelles qu'il offre pour la tenue de réunions internationales et de confrontations scientifiques satellites variées.

Les qualités extraordinaires du Professeur Robert Giuli, son talent, ses capacités, son énergie et celle de son équipe à laquelle j'associe les siens, ont été les garants de l'organisation parfaite du 4ème Congrès O.E.S.O., qui fut le plus important de ceux qu'il avait jusqu'alors organisés.

Une telle manifestation est certainement la seule de ce type dans la communauté scientifique, à réunir les meilleurs du monde dans toutes les disciplines, pour concentrer tout leur intérêt exclusivement sur l'oesophage et ses affections. Egalement parfaitement unique est la formule du Congrès O.E.S.O., fondée sur une série de questions garantissant que toutes les différentes facettes des connaissances d'aujourd'hui seront l'objet d'une complète exploration en profondeur, avec une rigueur et une méticulosité incomparables qu'il serait impossible d'espérer d'une formule différente, et qui ne sont d'ailleurs pratiquement jamais atteintes lors des Congrès scientifiques habituels.

C'est vrai que, plus importantes que tout, porteuses d'un agrément nouveau et d'un enrichissement pour l'esprit, sont les différences existant entre les points de vue et les mises en exergue particulières effectuées dans des disciplines différentes. C'est peut-être au travers de ces divergences de pensée, exprimées et discutées dans une atmosphère toujours amicale, que se cache le vrai secret du succès de cette rencontre internationale.

Toutes les disciplines ont été l'objet d'une même exploration acharnée, à la flamme d'une même chandelle, mais chacune sous un angle de vue très légèrement différent. Et du mélange de tous ces aspects variés d'un même problème, résulte une approche encore plus approfondie de sa compréhension.

*

Le *leitmotiv* du Congrès O.E.S.O. 1993 était la muqueuse oesophagienne et sa pathologie, couverte dans le sens large du terme: les mécanismes à l'origine de son inflammation — ceux de la maladie du reflux — ceux de sa transformation métaplasique en muqueuse cylindrique — ou encore ceux qui sont à l'origine de sa sténose fibreuse sous ses différents aspects, avec toutes les approches thérapeutiques qui en découlent.

Preface

The Fourth O.E.S.O. Congress, centered on the esophageal mucosa and its diseases, took place in September 1993 in the splendid surroundings of the U.N.E.S.C.O. headquarters in Paris, with prestigious facilities for round-table international discussions and various satellite scientific activities.

The extraordinarily talented, capable and energetic qualities of Professor Robert Giuli and his supporting team, including his family, guaranteed perfect organization of this fourth O.E.S.O. meeting, which was the largest held so far.

This event is truly unique in the scientific world, because it gathers the world's best in all disciplines, with focused attention on the esophagus and its diseases. Also truly unique is the structure of the O.E.S.O. Congresses, which are centered upon a series of key questions ensuring that every aspect of current knowledge and wisdom is explored with an unrivaled degree of depth and thoroughness which otherwise would be impossible, and which is almost never reached at standard scientific meetings.

Indeed, most important, refreshing and thought-provoking are the differences in views and emphases between the various disciplines. Perhaps it is through these discrepancies, discussed in a very friendly atmosphere, that the true secret of success of this worldwide encounter is hidden.

All disciplines were looking and struggling with the same burning candle, but were watching from slightly different angles of perception. Integration of all these various aspects of the same problem creates a greater depth of understanding.

*

The *leitmotif* of the 1993 O.E.S.O. meeting was the esophageal mucosa and its diseases. This can be interpreted broadly, and covers aspects including: mechanisms leading to inflammation; mechanisms related to reflux disease; mechanisms leading to metaplastic change in columnar metaplasia; facts or features leading to fibrotic stricturing and the subsequent therapeutic approaches.

Comme des ouvertures latérales sur le tronc commun de ce thème, ont été en même temps organisés de nombreux symposia satellites et ateliers. Pour n'en citer que quelques uns : les meilleures indications de la pH-métrie oesophagienne — les altérations moléculaires de la muqueuse dysplasique — le rôle des prokinétiques en oesophagologie — les perspectives de la thérapeutique acido-suppressive à long terme — les aspects socio-économiques de la maladie du reflux, etc.

*

Aussi unique en son genre que le Congrès, est le livre qui lui fait suite, en conservant la même formule générale d'une série de questions dont les réponses sont fournies par les meilleurs spécialistes du monde dans le domaine. Outre les questions traitées et discutées oralement lors du Congrès, de nombreuses autres ont été ajoutées, pour être bien sûr qu'aucun aspect particulier du sujet traité n'aura été laissé dans l'ombre.

Le lecteur perspicace percevra d'emblée combien un tel ouvrage correspond réellement à la meilleure et la plus moderne *'bible de l'oesophagologie'* : c'est un trésor encyclopédique de renseignements qu'il contient, et que ne peut offrir aujourd'hui aucun autre ouvrage sur l'oesophage.

Comme j'y ai déjà insisté, la puissance de son contenu tient à l'approche polydisciplinaire du thème, et à la dimension complète de l'analyse effectuée. Sans le moindre doute, c'est un livre qui doit demeurer sur le bureau même — ou au moins à portée de main — de tous ceux qui sont impliqués dans la pathologie de l'oesophage, qu'ils soient chercheurs de laboratoire, électrophysiologistes, histopathologistes, économistes de la Santé, pédiatres, ou enfin, et ce ne sont pas les moins concernés, les gastro-entérologues et les chirurgiens de leurs équipes.

Je souhaite à ce volume tout le succès qu'il mérite.
Et puis, je suis fier de féliciter Robert Giuli et son équipe, en premier lieu Michèle Liégeon, pour la tâche redoutable qu'ils ont entreprise et si bien réussie, de publier un tel monument.
Ils méritent toute notre reconnaissance et notre admiration.

*

Dès maintenant, nous attendons avec impatience le prochain Congrès O.E.S.O. de 1996, qui se déroulera dans le même ensemble prestigieux de l'U.N.E.S.C.O.
Il sera principalement consacré au sphincter inférieur de l'oesophage et ses affections.

Si l'on considère le succès du Congrès 1993, il est aisé de comprendre pourquoi tout ce que l'on en attend déjà se situe à un niveau particulièrement élevé.

Guido N.J. Tytgat

Branching sideways from that main stem of the *leitmotif* were several high quality satellite symposia and workshops. Just to name a few: the optimal use of pH monitoring in the esophagus; the molecular alteration in the metaplastic dysplastic mucosa; the role of prokinetics in esophagology; the possible achievements with long-term pronounced acid suppressive therapy; the health economic aspects of gastroesophageal reflux disease, etc.

*

Equally unique as the meeting itself, is the ensuing book which follows the same overall format, that is, a sequence of questions thoroughly answered by world-leading experts in the field. In addition to the questions directly discussed at the meeting, many others were added, to guarantee that no aspect relevant to the topic would be left uncovered.

The astute reader will readily appreciate that this edition really does correspond to the updated '*bible in esophagology*': an encyclopedic wealth of information is present in this book, which cannot be found in any other textbook on the esophagus.

As already stressed, the strength of the contents of this handbook resides in the multidisciplinary approach and the thoroughness of the analysis. Beyond any doubt, this book should be on the desk or at handreach of everybody involved in esophageal disease, be it the basic researcher, the electrophysiologist, the histopathologist, the health economist, the pediatrician and, last but not least, the gastroenterologist and his surgical teammates.

I wish this book well and every possible success.

Moreover, I take pride in congratulating Professor Robert Giuli and his team, especially Michèle Liégeon, for a formidable task, very well done indeed, in editing this monumental work.

They deserve all our credit and admiration.

*

We are now already looking forward to the O.E.S.O. Congress scheduled to take place in 1996, in the same prominent setting of U.N.E.S.C.O.

It will mainly concentrate on the lower esophageal sphincter and its diseases.

Based on the success of the 1993 meeting, it is easy to understand why the expectations are very high.

G.N.J. Tytgat, MD
Professor of Gastroenterology
President of Honor of O.E.S.O.

Préface

'*La muqueuse oesophagienne, 300 questions — 300 réponses*' est un livre unique dans sa forme, fait de réponses courtes et ponctuelles à toute une symphonie de questions portant sur la muqueuse oesophagienne.

Il faut applaudir à la menée à bien de cette démarche qui a consisté à décortiquer efficacement et complètement, par une série de questions exactement focalisées, tout ce que l'on sait sur la muqueuse oesophagienne. Cet ouvrage nous livre des pensées d'avant-garde sur les lésions de la muqueuse oesophagienne liées au reflux, et les mystères de sa métaplasie en muqueuse dite de Barrett, cette forme particulière de cicatrisation avec sa tendance à évoluer vers la dysplasie.

L'impact de ce livre lui est donné par toutes ces ouvertures qu'il offre sur les avancées les plus pointues de nos connaissances actuelles: je veux dire les domaines dans lesquels il reste encore plus à connaître que ce qui est déjà connu.

Présentée sous une forme et dans une structure traditionnelles, une telle entreprise aurait eu toutes chances d'aboutir à un ouvrage d'opinions particulières plus que de faits précis, mais c'est là que cette formule de questions-réponses a apporté, comme conséquence obligée, concision et densité en place de développements académiques et subjectifs.

Toutes ces réponses sont fournies par un ensemble de plus de 200 spécialistes de renom dans des disciplines très diverses, procurant ainsi un souffle général qui permet de faire apparaître des dénominateurs communs aux différents problèmes, et d'éviter ainsi de laisser la vérité dans un flou lié à des contraintes de marché, ou l'exposé d'idées fausses sous la plume irréfutable de très hautes autorités.

Cet ouvrage est sans conteste le meilleur que Robert Giuli, Directeur Scientifique de l'O.E.S.O., a realisé.

La formule originale qu'il a mise au point, peaufinée maintenant au long de 16 années et au fil de ses trois précédents ouvrages, a abouti à un art achevé d'offrir au lecteur une analyse complète, plaisante, et parfaitement scientifique du thème traité.

Mes collaborateurs m'ont subtilisé ces trois premiers ouvrages, et je sais qu'ils vont faire de même avec celui-ci.

Lisez le, cachez le donc, si vous espérez le conserver. C'est vrai qu'il vaut ça!

Tom R. DeMeester

Preface

'*The Esophageal Mucosa, 300 Questions — 300 Answers*' is a unique publication that consists of short, pithy answers to a symphony of questions on the esophageal mucosa.

It was an applaudable task to unravel efficiently and thoroughly, by a series of well-focused questions, what is known about the esophageal mucosa. The book conveys frontier thoughts on reflux induced mucosal injury, and the mystery of Barrett's metaplasia, a peculiar form of healing with a tendency to undergo dysplastic change. As such, the book is an exhaustive reference for practitioners and scientists interested in esophageal disease.

The strength of the book is its emphasis on the frontiers of knowledge; that is, the areas where there is still more to be known than that which is currently understood.

Under a common structural format, this could result in a book of opinions rather than of facts; but the question and answer format ensures brevity and content, rather than an editorial response.

The answers are drawn from a pool of more than 200 reputed specialists from different disciplines. This provides a breadth of response that allows common denominators regarding specific issues to emerge, thus avoiding the suppression of truth by economic pressures, or erroneous concepts espoused by the compelling lips of outspoken personalities.

This issue is clearly the best that Professor Robert Giuli, the Scientific Director of O.E.S.O., has produced.

His original format, refined over the past 16 years and three previous issues, has emerged as an art of presenting a thorough, entertaining yet scientific examination of a theme.

My research fellows have confiscated his previous issues, and I suspect that they will do the same with this one.

Read it and hide it, if you expect to retain it. It's that good.

T.R. DeMeester, MD, FACS
Professor of Surgery
President of Honor of O.E.S.O.

Préface

C'est maintenant devenu une tradition qu'un ouvrage fasse suite à chaque Congrès O.E.S.O.

Après le précédent qui portait sur les troubles moteurs de l'oesophage, le 4è Congrès, tenu à Paris en septembre 1993, était consacré à la muqueuse oesophagienne.

Il faut exprimer à Robert Giuli nos félicitations pour l'énorme somme de travail qu'il a investie et l'énergie impressionnante qu'il a déployée pour coordonner les compétences différentes mais complémentaires nécessaires au succès complet de cet événement, aussi bien dans sa portée scientifique que dans ses aspects d'agrément.

Au premier abord, l'oesophage n'est qu'un simple organe creux, qui ne semble servir qu'à assurer le passage des aliments depuis la bouche vers l'estomac. En fait, l'oesophage est le siège de très nombreux troubles moteurs, inflammatoires, ou encore d'affections néoplasiques, dont la complexité est tout aussi grande que celle des affections des portions sous-jacentes du tube digestif.

Pour couvrir une pathologie d'une telle diversité, une liste de questions, établie longtemps à l'avance, a été proposée aux plus grands spécialistes du monde de la physiologie, de la gastroentérologie, de l'anatomo-pathologie, de la pharmacologie et de la chirurgie oesophagienne, pour leur apporter une réponse aussi concise et focalisée que possible.

Quels sont les responsables de l'agression de la muqueuse oesophagienne? Comment leur résiste-t-elle? Pourquoi une cicatrisation de type cylindrique apparaît-elle? Quels sont les meilleurs et les plus précoces marqueurs de l'évolution vers les stades de dysplasie et de cancer? Quelles sont les méthodes les mieux appropriées pour surveiller ces malades et traiter les lésions néoplasiques développées sur une muqueuse de ce type?

Telles sont quelques unes des 300 questions discutées en septembre dernier et dont les réponses structurées composent aujourd'hui ce livre.

Il est conçu selon la même formule que celle qui a été adoptée pour les trois premiers ouvrages de cette série, et suit fidèlement la conception originale et le déroulement du Congrès lui-même.

En l'ouvrant à n'importe quelle page, le lecteur y trouvera d'emblée la réponse qu'il recherche et l'opinion autorisée qui lui importe.

Il faut espérer que l'intérêt de ce livre sera le même pour les lecteurs non spécialistes que pour les 'oesophagologues' confirmés qui pourront y trouver des approfondissements utiles à propos de certaines questions spécifiques. L'approche polydisciplinaire adoptée rend possible de réunir un amas de connaissances qu'il serait difficile de rassembler à partir de sources éparpillées.

Preface

It has now become a tradition that a book be published ensuing the O.E.S.O. Congresses.

Following the previous meeting on esophageal motor disorders, the fourth Congress, held in Paris in September 1993, was devoted to the esophageal mucosa.

Robert Giuli is to be congratulated for the huge amount of work and the impressive energy deployed in coordinating all the different but complementary activities which led to a very successful scientific and social event.

At first glance, the esophagus seems a simple, hollow organ. Its only apparent function is to ensure the passage of nutrients from the mouth to the stomach. In fact, the esophagus is the site of various motor, inflammatory and neoplastic disorders, whose complexity is in no way inferior to those of the lower portions of the gastrointestinal tract.

To respond to this diversity, a list of questions was prepared long in advance, and the world's leading specialists in physiology, gastroenterology, pathology, pharmacology and esophageal surgery were invited to give as concise and precise answers as possible:

What are the factors that attack the epithelial mucosa? How does it resist? Why does a glandular type of healing take place? What are the most accurate and earliest markers of the evolution toward dysplasia and cancer? What are the best methods of surveillance and treatment of neoplastic lesions developed on this type of mucosa?

These are amongst the 300 questions debated last September, and which are now discussed in this book.

The volume is organized in a format which was already adopted in the three previous ones in this series, and which strictly follows the original concept and the format of the Congress itself.

By opening the book at any page, the reader will find at once the answer he needs and the authoritative opinion he is looking for.

It is hoped that this book will be useful for both nonspecialist readers, and to well confirmed 'esophagologists' who may find deeper insights into some specific questions. This multidisciplinary approach makes it possible to include much of the information usually difficult to collect from scattered sources.

Nous sommes profondément reconnaissants à tous les auteurs, spécialistes de haute réputation venant de 20 pays, sans la participation et la ponctualité desquels un tel livre n'aurait jamais pu être réalisé.

En tant que Secrétaire Général de ce Congrès, j'ai ressenti un privilège rare et vécu une expérience extrêmement enrichissante d'avoir été, avec nos Présidents G. Tytgat et T. DeMeester, aux côtés de Robert Giuli dans l'organisation d'un événement scientifique de cette importance, en même temps que d'une extraordinaire manifestation d'amitié.

Jean-Paul Galmiche

We are extremely grateful to all the authors, who are well recognized experts from over 20 countries. Without their contribution and punctuality, this book would never have gone to press.

As the Secretary General, it has been a rare privilege and an extremely rewarding experience, along with our Presidents G. Tytgat and T. DeMeester, to serve with Robert Giuli in the organization of this important scientific event, as well as an extraordinary manifestation of friendship.

Jean-Paul Galmiche
Professor of Gastroenterology

Contents

Squamous mucosa and reflux

Anatomy-Physiology

What is the relationship between anatomic variants of the hiatus and the efficiency of the antireflux barrier?

How can one determine the function of the valve of the diaphragm
– in the normal individual?
– in cases of hiatus hernia?

What are the characteristics of the normal blood supply of the esophagus?

When is the esophageal mucosa normal?

What is basically wrong with the LES in reflux disease?

Is there a disorder of esophageal clearance in cases of hiatus hernia?

What information can be given by recording of evoked potentials of the esophagus?

Reflux and mucosa

Mucosal protective agents

Endoscopy

xl

xliv

The dysplastic mucosa

The adenocarcinomatous mucosa

Senior Contributors

L.M.A. AKKERMANS
Department of Experimental Surgery, University Hospital, Utrecht, The Netherlands

A.P. ALBINO, PhD
Head of Laboratory of Mammalian Cell Transformation, Memorial-Sloan-Kettering Cancer Center, New York, USA

N.K. ALTORKI, MD
Associate Professor of Surgery, Division of Cardiothoracic Surgery, New York Hospital Cornell Medical Center, New York, USA

D. ANTONIOLI, MD
Department of Pathology, Beth Israel Hospital, Harvard Medical School, Boston, Massachusetts, USA

H.D. APPELMAN, MD
Professor of Pathology, Department of Pathology, University of Michigan Hospitals, Ann Arbor, Michigan, USA

D. ARMSTRONG, MA, MRCP (UK), FRCP (C)
Intestinal Disease Research Unit, McMaster University, Hamilton, Ontario, Canada

H. ASTE
Department of Gastroenterology, Endoscopy Unit, Ospedale San Martino, Genova, Italy

S. ATTWOOD, MCR, FRCS, FRCSI
Department of Clinical Surgery, St. James's Hospital, Dublin, Ireland

J. BANCEWICZ, FRCS, FRCSI
Reader in Surgery, University of Manchester, Hope Hospital, Salford, United Kingdom

J.-Ph. BARBIER
Professor of Gastroenterology, Hepatology-Gastroenterology, Hôpital Laënnec, Paris, France

R. BARDINI
Department of Surgery, University of Padova, Padova, Italy

C.M. BATE, MD
Department of Gastroenterology, Royal Albert Edward Infirmary, Wigan, United Kingdom

P. BECHI, MD
Associate Professor of Surgery, Surgical Clinic 3, University of Florence, Florence, Italy

J.R. BENNETT, MD
Gastro-Intestinal Unit, Hull Royal Infirmary, Hull, United Kingdom

L.H. BERNSTEIN, PhD
Professor and Scientific Director of the Cancer Surveillance Program, Department of Preventive Medicine, USC School of Medicine, Los Angeles, California, USA

M.A. BIGARD
Professor of Gastroenterology, Hepatology-Gastroenterology, CHU Nancy - Hôpitaux de Brabois, Vandoeuvre, France

W.V. BOGOMOLETZ
Anatomy-Pathology-Cytology, Institut Jean Godinot, Reims, France

E. BOLLSCHWEILLER, MD, PhD
Surgery Clinic, Klinikum Rechts der Isar, Technical University of Munich, Munich, Germany

G. BOMMELAER
Professor of Medicine, Service d'Hépato-Gastro-Enterologie, Hôtel Dieu, Clermont-Ferrand, France

K.G. BOTROS
Deparment of Anatomy, Faculty of Medicine, Mansoura University, Mansoura, Egypt

P. BOUTELIER
Professor of Surgery, Hôpital Jean Verdier, Bondy, France

H.W. BOYCE Jr., MD
Professor of Medicine, Centre for Swallowing Disorders, USF Medical Center, Tampa, Florida, USA

C.G. BREMNER, MB, ChB (Wits), ChM (Wits), FRCS (Eng), FRCS (Edin)
Professor of Surgery, Department of Surgery, USC Healthcare Consultation Center, Los Angeles, California, USA

R.M. BREMNER
Department of Surgery, USC Healthcare Consultation Center, Los Angeles, California, USA

E. BROSSARD
Otolaryngology Department, CHU Vaudois, Lausanne, Switzerland

S. BRULEY DES VARANNES
Service d'Hépato-Gastroentérologie, Hôpital Guillaume et René Laënnec, Nantes, France

R. BUMM
Department of Surgery, Klinikum Rechts der Isar, Technical University of Munich, Munich, Germany

G. CADIOT
Department of Gastroenterology, Hôpital Bichat-Claude Bernard, Paris, France

A.J. CAMERON, MD
Gastroenterology and Internal Medicine, Mayo Clinic, Rochester, Minnesota, USA

N. CAMPIONI
Surgical-Oncological Division, Istituto Regina Elena, Rome, Italy

D.O. CASTELL, MD
Professor of Medicine and Chairman, Department of Medicine, The Graduate Hospital, Philadelphia, Pennsylvania, USA

I. CECCONELLO
Digestive Surgery Division, São Paulo University School of Medicine, São Paulo, Brazil

M. CELERIER
Professor of Surgery, Hôpital Saint Louis, Paris, France

G. CHAMPAULT
Professor of Surgery, Hôpital Jean Verdier, Bondy, France

T.K. CHAUDHURI, MD, FACG
Professor and Chief, Nuclear Medicine, Eastern Virginia Medical School, Hampton, Virginia, USA

M.Y.M. CHEN, MD
Research Assistant Professor, Department of Radiology, The Bowman Gray School of Medicine, Winston-Salem, North Carolina, USA

S. COHEN, MD
Professor of Medicine, Chairman, Department of Medicine, Temple University Health Sciences Center, Philadelphia, Pennsylvania, USA

J.-M. COLLARD, MD
Department of Surgery, St. Luc University Clinics, Brussels, Belgium

S. CORRENTI, MD
Department of Surgery, R. Silvestrini Hospital, Perugia, Italy

D. COUTURIER
Professor Gastroenterology, Hôpital Cochin, Paris, France

P. CUBERTAFOND
Professor of Surgery, Hôpital Universitaire Dupuytren, Limoges, France

P.-H. CUGNENC
Professor of Surgery, Hôpital Laënnec, Paris, France

K.M. DAS, MD, PhD, FRCP, FACP
Professor of Medicine, Molecular Genetics, UMDNJ, Robert Wood Johnson Medical School, New Brunswick, New Jersey, USA

J.S. DE CAESTECKER, MD, MRCP
Consultant Physician, The Glenfield Hospital, Leicester, United Kingdom

J.M. DEBONNE
Hepatology-Gastroenterology, Hôpital d'Instruction des Armées A. Laveran, Marseilles, France

M. DEI POLI
Professor of Surgery, General Surgery Division, University of Turin, Turin, Italy

A. DEL GENIO
Professor of Surgery, Division of Esophageal Surgery, Naples University, Naples, Italy

G. DELPRE
Institute of Gastroenterology, Beilinson Medical Center, Petah-Tikva, Israel

T.R. DeMEESTER, MD, FACS
Professor of Surgery, Department of Surgery, USC Healthcare Consultation Center, Los Angeles, California, USA

N.J. DEMOS, MD
Clinical Associate, Professor of Surgery, 142 Palisada Avenue, Jersey City, Jersey, USA

M.D. DIEBOLD
Professor of Pathology, Hôpital Robert Debré, Reims, France

M.F. DIXON
Reader in Gastrointestinal Pathology, Academic Unit of Pathology, School of Medicine, Leeds, United Kingdom

E.D. DORVAL
Professor of Gastroenterology, Hôpital Trousseau, Tours, France

F. DUBOIS, MD
Professor of Surgery, Chirurgie Digestive, Centre Medico-Chirurgical de la Porte de Choisy, Paris, France

C. DUPONT
Professor of Pediatrics, Hôpital Saint-Vincent-de-Paul, Paris, France

A. DURANCEAU, MD
Professor of Surgery, Hôtel-Dieu de Montréal, Montréal, Québec, Canada

O. EKBERG, MD
Department of Diagnostic Radiology, Malmö General Hospital, Malmö, Sweden

M. ENDO, MD
Professor of Surgery, 1st Department of Surgery, School of Medicine, Tokyo Medical and Dental University, Tokyo, Japan

M.K. FERGUSON, MD
Associate Professor of Surgery, Section of Thoracic Surgery, Department of Surgery, University of Chicago Medical Center, Chicago, Illinois, USA

H. FEUSSNER, MD
Department of Surgery, Poliklinik Rechts der Isar, Technical University of Munich, Munich, Germany

R.S. FISHER, MD
Professor of Medicine, Chief of Gastroenterology Section, Temple University, Philadelphia, Pennsylvania, USA

J.-B. FLAMENT
Professor of Surgery, CHRU Reims - Hôpital Robert Debré, Reims, France

J.-F. FLEJOU
Anatomy-Cytology-Pathology, Hôpital Beaujon, Clichy, Paris, France

P. FOUCAUD
Departement of Pediatrics, Hôpital André Mignot, Versailles, France

B. FRAITAG
Jouveinal Research Institute, Fresnes, France

J.W. FRESTON, MD, PhD
Department of Medicine, University of Connecticut Health Center, Farmington, Connecticut, USA

P. FUENTES
Professor of Surgery, Department of Thoracic Surgery, Hôpital St. Marguerite, Marseilles, France

J.-P. GALMICHE
Professor of Gastroenterology, Hepato-gastroenterology, CHRU, Hôpital G. et R. Laënnec, Nantes, France

H.S. GAREWAL, MD, PhD
Associate Professor of Medicine, Cancer Prevention and Control Program, Hematology-Oncology and Gastroenterology Division, Arizona Cancer Center, Tucson, Arizona, USA

C. GAUTIER-BENOIT
Professor of Surgery, Centre Hospitalier Dr. Schaffner, Lens, France

K. GEBOES
Professor of Pathology, University Ziekenhuis St. Rafael, Leuven, Belgium

K.R. GEISINGER, MD
Professor and Director, Department of Pathology, The Bowman Gray School of Medicine, Winston-Salem, North Carolina, USA

R.J. GINSBERG, MD
Chief Thoracic Surgery, Memorial Sloan-Kettering Cancer Center, New York, USA

R. GIULI, MD, FACS, FCCP
Professor of Surgery, Department of Digestive Surgery, Hôpital Beaujon, Paris VII, University Clichy, Paris, France

S.N. GLICK, MD
Professor of Radiology and Chairman, Department of Diagnostic Radiology, Hahnemann University Hospital, Philadelphia, Pennsylvania, USA

H.G. GOOSZEN, MD, PhD
Professor of Surgery, University Hospital, Leiden, The Netherlands

J.C. GRIMAUD
Professor of Gastroenterology, Hepato-Gastroenterology, Hôpital Nord, Marseilles, France

V. GUARNER
Professor of Surgery, Department of Surgery, Hospital Angeles del Pedregal, Mexico City, Mexico

Y. HAMANAKA, MD
2nd Department of Surgery, Yamaguchi University, School of Medicine, Ube, Yamaguchi, Japan

S.R. HAMILTON, MD
Professor of Pathology and Oncology, Johns Hopkins University, Ross Research Building, Baltimore, Maryland, USA

J.W. HARMON, MD
Professor of Surgery, Chief Surgical Division, Department of Veterans Affairs, Medical Center, Washington DC, USA

E. HASSALL, MB ChB, FRCP (C)
Head, Division of Pediatric Gastroenterology, University of British Columbia and BC Children's Hospital, Vancouver, British Columbia, Canada

R.C. HEADING
Professor of Medicine, Department of Medicine (RIE), University of Edinburgh, Edinburgh, United Kingdom

T.P.J. HENNESSY, MCh, FRCS, FRCSI
Regius Professor of Surgery, Department of Clinical Surgery, St James's Hospital, Dublin, Ireland

C.A. HIEBERT, MD, FACS
Professor of Surgery, Maine Medical Center, Potland, Maine, USA

L.D. HILL, MD
Department of Vascular Thoracic Surgery, Health Resources Building, Seattle, Washington, USA

R.A. HINDER, MD, FACS
Professor of Surgery, Creighton University, School of Medicine, Omaha, Nebraska, USA

A.H. HÖLSCHER, MD
Assistant Professor, Department of Surgery, Technical University of Munich, Munich, Germany

D. HOPWOOD, MD, PhD
Department of Pathology, Ninewells Hospital and Medical School, Dundee, United Kingdom

C.W. HOWDEN , MD, FRCP, FACG, FCP
Professor of Medicine, Division of Digestive Diseases and Nutrition, University of South Carolina, Columbia, South Carolina, USA

R.H. HUNT, FRCP, FRCP (Edin), FRCPC, FACG
Professor of Medicine, Head of Gastroenterology Division, McMaster University Medical Center, Hamilton, Ontario, Canada

C. IASCONE
Professor of Surgery, General Clinical Surgery, Università degli Studi la Sapienza, Rome, Italy

W. INAUEN
Department of Gastroenterology, University Hospital, Inespital, Berne, Switzerland

J. ISOLAURI, MD
Department of Surgery, Tampere University Hospital, Tampere, Finland

G.G. JAMIESON, MB, MS, FRACS, FACS
Professor of Surgery, Department of Surgery, Royal Adelaide Hospital, Adelaide, Australia

J. JANSSENS, MD
Professor of Gastroenterology, University Ziekenhuizen, Leuven, Belgium

K. JEYASINGHAM, ChM, FACSE, FRCS
Department of Thoracic Surgery, Frenchay Hospital, Bristol, United Kingdom

L.F. JOHNSON, MD, FACP
Professor of Medicine, Director, Digestive Disease Division, F. Edward Hebert School of Medicine, Bethesda, Maryland, USA

S.G. JOLLEY, MD, Chtd
Surgery of Newborn Infants, Children and Adolescents, Las Vegas, Nevada, USA

P.J. KAHRILAS, MD
Associate Professor of Medicine, Gastroenterology Section, Northwestern University Medical School, Chicago, Illinois, USA

P. KEELING
Department of Clinical Surgery, St. James's Hospital, Dublin, Ireland

A. KESHAVARSIAN, MD, FACP
Gastroenterology Division, Loyola University Medical Center, Maywood, Illinois, USA

E. KLINKENBERG-KNOL
Department of Gastroenterology, Free University Hospital, Amsterdam, The Netherlands

F. KLOTZ
Professor of Surgery, Hepatology-Gastroenterology, Hôpital d'Instruction des Armées A. Laveran, Marseilles, France

S.J.M. KRAEMER, MD
Department of Surgery, Technical University of Munich, Munich, Germany

R. LAMBERT
Professor of Gastroenterology, Hepato-Gastroenterology, Hôpital Edouard Herriot, Lyons, France

B. LAUNOIS, MD, FACS
Professor of Surgery, Hôpital de Pontchaillou, Rennes, France

L. LE BODIC
Professor of Gastroenterology, Hepato-Gastroenterology, CHRU, Hôpital Guillaume et René Laënnec, Nantes, France

T. LERUT, MD, FACS
Professor of Surgery, University Ziekenhuizen Leuven, Leuven, Belgium

M.S. LEVINE, MD
Professor of Radiology, Department of Radiology, Hospital of the University of Pennsylvania, Philadelphia, Pennsylvania, USA

K.J. LEWIN, MD, FRCPath
Professor of Pathology and Medicine, Department of Pathology, UCLA Health
Sciences Center, Los Angeles, California, USA

D. LIEBERMANN-MEFFERT, MD
Professor of Surgery, Department of Surgery, Klinikum rechts der Isar, Technical
University of Munich, Munich, Germany

A.G. LITTLE, MD
Professor of Surgery, Chairman, Department of Surgery, University of Nevada,
School of Medicine, Las Vegas, Nevada, USA

L. LUNDELL, MD, PhD
Department of Surgery, Laboratory of Gastroenterology, Sahigren's Hospital,
Gothenburg, Sweden

C. MAURAGE
Professor of Pediatrics, Hôpital de Clocheville, Tours, France

R.W. McCALLUM, MD, FACP, FRACP (Australia), FACG
Professor of Medicine, Division of Gastroenterology, University of Virginia,
Charlottesville, Virginia, USA

N. MEADOWS
Consultant Pediatrician, Queen Elizabeth Hospital for Children, London, United
Kingdom

E.H. METMAN
Professor of Internal Medicine, Hôpital Trousseau, Tours, France

M. MIGNON, MD
Professor of Gastroenterology, University of Paris VII, Hôpital Bichat-Claude
Bernard, Paris, France

J. MILLS
International Medical Affairs Department, Glaxo Group Research Ltd., Uxbridge,
United Kingdom

R.K. MITTAL, MD
Division of Gastroenterology, Health Sciences Center, University of Virginia,
Charlottesville, Virginia, USA

K. MOGHISSI, BSc, MD, FRCS (Ed), FRCS (Eng)
Consultant Thoracic Surgeon, BUPA Hospital Hull and East Riding, Hull, United
Kingdom

A. MORALDI
Professor of Surgery, Ospedale S. Eugenio, University of Rome 'Tor Vergata', Rome,
Italy

G.C. O'SULLIVAN, Mch., FRCSI
Department of Surgery, Mercy Hospital, Cork, Ireland

H. OBERTOP
Professor of Surgery, Academic Medical Center, Amsterdam, The Netherlands

L.C. OLBE
Department of Surgery II, Sahlgren's Hospital, Gothenburg, Sweden

J.-B. OLLYO
Maladies des Voies Digestives, rue des Terreaux 20, 1003 Lausanne, Switzerland

S.R. ORENSTEIN, MD
Associate Professor of Pediatrics, University Pediatric Gastroenterology, Children's Hospital, Pittsburgh, Pennsylvania, USA

R.C. ORLANDO, MD
Professor of Medicine and Physiology, Gastroenterology Section, Tulane University Medical Center, New Orleans, Louisiana, USA

W.C. ORR, PhD
Sleep and GI Physiology Laboratories, Baptist Medical Center, Oklahoma City, Oklahoma, USA

M.B. ORRINGER, MD
Professor of Surgery, Head of Thoracic Surgery Section, Taubman Health Care Center, Ann Arbor, Michigan, USA

D.J. OTT, MD
Department of Radiology, Bowman Gray School of Medicine, Wake Forest University, Winston-Salem, North Carolina, USA

D. PAREKH, MD
Department of Surgery, USC Healthcare Consultation Center, Los Angeles, California, USA

C.A. PELLEGRINI, MD, FACS
Professor of Surgery, University of Washington Medical Center, Seattle, Washington, USA

A. PERACCHIA, MD, FACS
Professor of Surgery, Department of General Surgery and Clinical Oncology, Hospital Policlinico Monteggia, Milan, Italy

J.H. PETERS, MD
Department of Surgery, USC Healthcare Consultation Center, Los Angeles, California, USA

H.W. PINOTTI, MD, FACS
Professor of Surgery, Head of Digestive Surgery Division, São Paulo University, São Paulo, Brazil

C.E. POPE II, MD
Professor of Medicine, Division of Gastroenterology, Department of Medicine, University of Washington School of Medicine, Seattle, Washington, USA

F. POTET
Professor of Pathology, University of Paris VII, Hôpital Bichat-Claude Bernard Paris, France

S. RAMEL, MD
Department of Surgery, Ersta Hospital, Stockholm, Sweden

J.E. RICHTER, MD
Professor of Medicine, Director of Clinical Research, University of Alabama, Birmingham, Alabama, USA

R.H. RIDDELL, MD, FRCPath, FRCP (C)
Professor of Pathology, Department of Pathology, McMaster University, Hamilton, Ontario, Canada

M. ROBASZKIEWICZ
Professor of Gastroenterology, Hepatology-Gastroenterology, CHU Brest, Hôpital Augustin Morvan, Brest, France

J.A. ROTH, MD
Professor of Surgery and Chairman, Department of Thoracic Surgery, University of Texas, M.D. Anderson Cancer Center, Houston, Texas, USA

C.O.H. RUSSELL, MB, ChB, MS, FRACS
GI Surgery, Mornington Peninsula Hospital, Frankston, Victoria, Australia

F. SAIDI
Department of Surgery, Modarress Hospital, Saadatabad, Tehran, Iran

J.A. SALO, MD
Department of Thoracic and Cardiovascular Surgery, Helsinki University Central Hospital, Helsinki, Finland

R.E. SAMPLINER, MD
Professor of Medicine, Chief of Gastroenterology Section, Department of Internal Medicine, Arizona Health Sciences Center, Tucson, Arizona, USA

J. SAROSIEK, MD, PhD
Research Associate Professor, Division of Gastroenterology, Virginia Health Sciences Center, Charlottesville, Virginia, USA

R.T. SATALOFF, MD, DMA
Professor of Otolaryngology, Thomas Jefferson University, Philadelphia, Pennsylvania, USA

C. SCARPIGNATO, FCP, FACG
Professor of Pharmacology, Institute of Pharmacology, Maggiore Hospital, University of Parma, Parma, Italy

M. SCHAPIRO, MD, FACP, FACG
Clinical Professor of Medicine, Center for the Health Sciences, University of California, Los Angeles, California, USA

M.N. SCHOEMAN, MBBS, FRACP
Gastroenterology Department, Academic Medical Center, Amsterdam, The Netherlands

A. SICULAR, MD, FACS
800 A 5th Avenue, New York, NY 10021, USA

J.R. SIEWERT
Professor of Surgery, Head of Surgery Clinic, Poliklinik Rechts der Isar, Technical University of Munich, Munich, Germany

D.B. SKINNER, MD, DsC (Hon), FACS
Professor of Surgery, President of The New York Hospital, Cornell Medical Center, New York, USA

S. SLOAN, MD
Section of Digestive Diseases, Rush-Presbyterian-St. Luke's Medical Center, Chicago, Illinois, USA

A. SMOUT, MD
Department of Gastroenterology, Academisch Ziekenhuis Utrecht, Utrecht, The Netherlands

T.C. SMYRK, MD
Anatomic and Clinical Pathology, Clarkson Hospital, Omaha, Nebraska, USA

S.J. SONTAG, MD, FACG, FACP
Director of Endoscopy Clinics, Veterans Affairs Hospital, Ambulatory Care, Hines, Illinois, USA

S.J. SPECHLER, MD
Gastroenterology Division, Beth Israel Hospital, Boston, Massachusetts, USA

H.J. STEIN, MD
Department of Surgery, Technical University of Munich, Munich, Germany

J. TESTART
Professor of Surgery, Surgery Clinic, Hôpital Charles Nicolle, Rouen, France

R.J.S. THOMAS
Professor of Surgery, Department of Surgery, Western Hospital, Footscray, Victoria, Australia

L. TIBBLING, MD, PhD
Associate Professor, Department of Otorhinolaryngology, University Hospital, Linköping, Sweden

E. TISSOT
Professor of Surgery, Department of Digestive Surgery, Hôpital Edouard Herriot, Lyons, France

N.A. TOBEY, PhD
Gastroenterology Research, Tulane University Medical Center, New Orleans, Louisiana, USA

H. TONNESEN, MD
Department of Surgery, University of Copenhagen, Herlev County Hospital, Herlev, Denmark

G. TOUGAS, MD
Division of Gastroenterology, McMaster University Medical Center, Hamilton, Ontario, Canada

F.V. TRASTEK, MD
Thoracic Surgery, Mayo Clinic, Rochester, Minnesota, USA

G. TRIADAFILOPOULOS, MD, FACP
Associate Professor of Medicine, Chief of Section of Gastroenterology, Stanford University School of Medicine, Palo Alto, California, USA

G.N.J. TYTGAT
Professor of Gastroenterology, Department of Gastroenterology-Hepatology, Academic Medical Center, Amsterdam, The Netherlands

H.C. URSCHEL Jr., MD
Department of Thoracic-Cardiac and Vascular Surgery, 3600 Gaston, Suite 1201, Dallas, Texas, USA

P. VINCENT
Department of Bacteriology and Virologie A, Faculty of Medicine, Lille, France

T.N. WALSH, MCh, FRCSI
Department of Clinical Surgery, St. James's Hospital, Dublin, Ireland

A. WATSON, MD, FRCS (Ed), FRCS (Eng), FRACS
Professor of Surgery, The Wellington Hospital, London, United Kingdom

M. WIENBECK, MD
Professor of Medicine, Department of Internal Medicine 3, Zentralklinikum Augsburg, Augsburg, Germany

W.A. WILLIAMSON, MD
Department of Thoracic and Cardiovascular Surgery, Lahey Clinic Medical Center, Burlington, Massachusetts, USA

G.H. WILLITAL
Professor of Surgery, Pediatric and Surgical University Clinic, Münster, Germany

A. YASUI, MD
Department of Surgery, Saiseikai General Hospital, Shizuoka, Japan

G.P. YOUNG, MD, FRACP
Department of Medicine, The Royal Melbourne Hospital, Melbourne, Victoria, Australia

G. ZANINOTTO, MD
Department of Surgery, Istituto di Chirurgia Generale II, University of Padova, Padova, Italy

B. ZILBERSTEIN
Digestive Surgery Division, São Paulo University Medical School, São Paulo, Brazil

Squamous mucosa and reflux

Anatomy-Physiology

What is the relationship between anatomic variants of the hiatus and the efficiency of the antireflux barrier?

K.G. Botros (Mansoura)

Introduction

Many anatomical studies of human diaphragms have provided considerable information about the formation of the esophageal hiatus (EH) [1—11]. These studies have described multiple anatomical variations in the formation of the EH and have given inconsistent results. The variations described include the formation of the hiatus by: a) the right crus only; b) equal portions of the two crura; and c) the two crura, mainly the right crus. However, the previous authors make no mention of any role played by the median arcuate ligament of the diaphragm in the formation of the EH.

This study describes the anatomical arrangement of the crural muscle fibers of the human diaphragm and the different anatomical variations in the formation of the human EH. A new anatomical description of the human EH is given in this investigation.

Materials and Methods

Fifty human diaphragms (31 male and 19 female) were used in this study. Their ages varied from 10 to 60 years. The autopsies were carried out between 6 and 10 h after death. Each specimen was removed as one mass and mounted on a wooden frame, 40 × 60 cm. The margins of the specimens were evenly pulled from all directions to the frame using strong silk threads. Each specimen was then fixed in the stretched position in 5% formalin for about 24 h. Fixation of the specimens in the stretched position was beneficial in avoiding shrinkage and distortion of the fleshy fibers. After fixation, the peritoneum, pleura, pericardium, fat and fascia were carefully removed from both surfaces of the diaphragm and an accurate anatomical dissection of the different muscle fibers of each crus was performed.

For each diaphragm an accurate sketch for the arrangement of the crural muscle fibers around the EH was made on drafting paper in such a way that the resulting illustration of the EH would be identical to the specimen.

Results

Arrangement of the crural muscle fibers

In 98% of the cases (49 diaphragms), the fleshy fibers of the right crus (RC) were divided into three bundles of fibers:
— lateral (LR);
— medial (MR);
— middle (Mid-R).
The LR bundle was derived from the lateral surface of the tendon of origin of the RC, passed forward and to the right of the central tendon and took no part in the formation of the EH. Mid-R bundle was derived also from the lateral surface of the tendon of origin of the RC. In 36 out of 50 cases (72%) this bundle was the sole constituent of the right border of the hiatus and shared in the formation of the anterior border. MR bundle took origin from the medial surface of the tendon of the RC. In 82% (41 cases) MR bundle was the sole constituent of the left border and contributed to the formation of the anterior. In 10% it was the sole constituent of the posterior margin and in 88% there was supplementation from the medial bundle of the left crus.

In the remaining 2% of the cases (one diaphragm), the RC remained undivided and took no part in the formation of the EH.

In 45 out of 50 diaphragms (90%) the fleshy fibers of the left crus (LC) were divided into two bundles:
— lateral bundle (LL); and
— medial bundle (ML).
In one case, LL bundle was the sole constituent of the left margin and shared with the ML bundle in the formation of the anterior margin. In six cases (12%) ML bundle was the sole constituent of the right margin and contributed to the formation of the anterior border.

In the remaining 10% (five cases) the LC remained undivided and took no role in the formation of the EH.

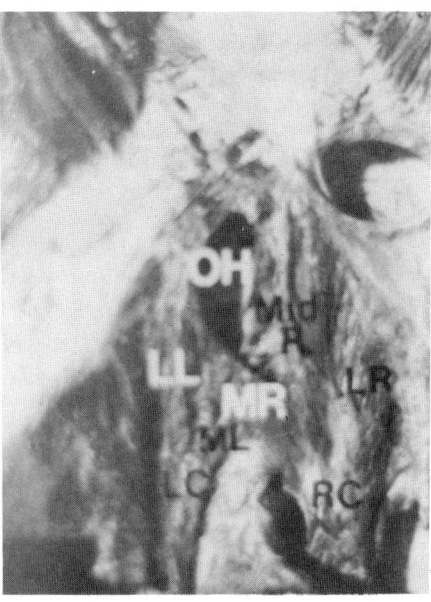

Fig. 1. Superior surface of a human diaphragm (62% of the cases). Note the arrangement of the crural muscle fibers (MR, Mid-R, LR bands of RC and ML and LL bands of LC) around the EH (please note that EH is indicated by OH in this figure).

Patterns of variation in the formation of the EH

In 62% (31 cases), the EH was bounded mainly by muscle fibers of the RC. In these cases (Figs. 1 and 2): Mid-R bundle formed the right border; MR bundle formed the posterior and left margins; the two bundles crossed each other anterior to the EH, forming the anterior margin. ML bundle was seen to be directed forward and to the right either superior (25 cases) or inferior (six cases) to the MR bundle and shared in the formation of the posterior margin.

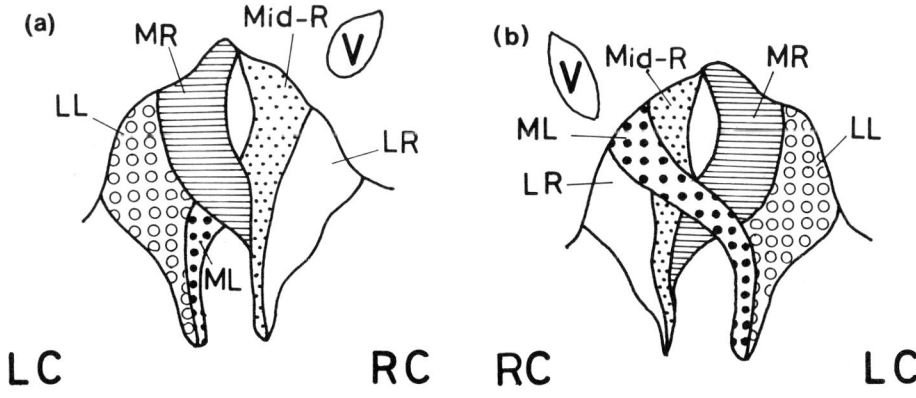

Fig. 2. The formation of the EH, as seen on the superior (a) and inferior (b) surfaces of the diaphragm.

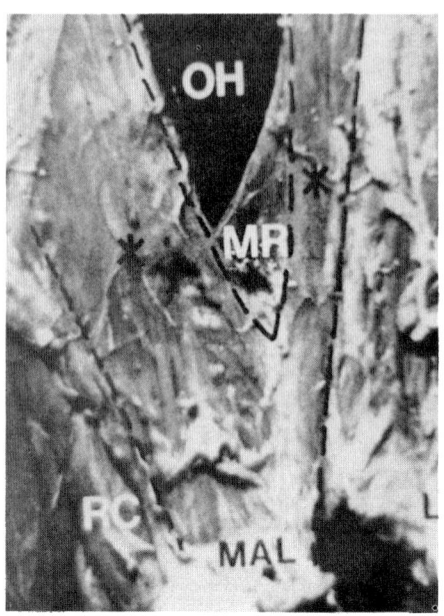

Fig. 3. Inferior surface of a human diaphragm (16% of the cases) showing a band of fibers (*) originating from the median arcuate ligament (MAL) and bounding the right, left and anterior margins of the hiatus. MR band of RC bounds the posterior margin (please note that EH is indicated by OH in this figure).

In 16% of the cases, a band of fleshy fibers were seen to originate from the median arcuate ligament (MAL) and bounded the anterior, right and left margins of the EH (Figs. 3 and 4). In these cases, MR and ML bundles crossed each other posterior to the hiatus, forming its posterior margin (ML bundle on the thoracic surface and MR bundle on the abdominal surface).

In 10% of the cases, the EH was bounded exclusively by fibers of the PC. MR fibers formed the left and posterior margins, while Mid-R fibers formed the right margin. The two bundles crossed each other anterior to the EH, forming its anterior

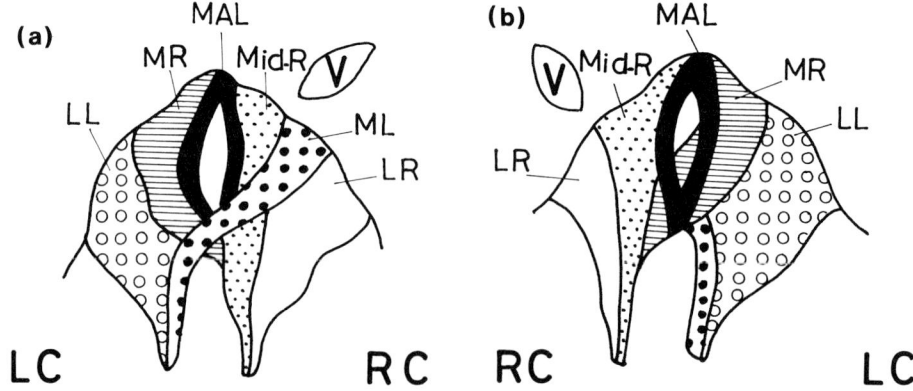

Fig. 4. Diagram illustrating the formation of the EH. (a) superior surface; (b) inferior surface.

6

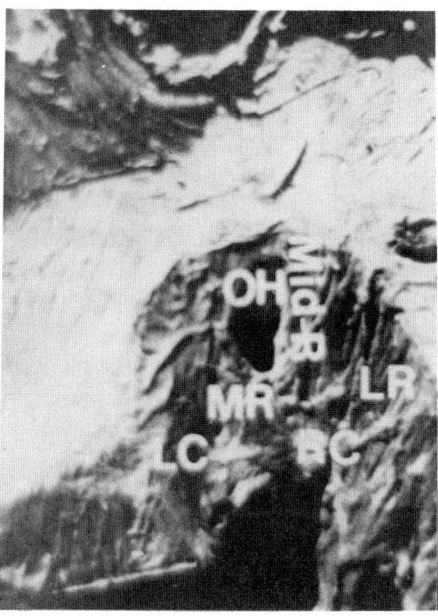

Fig. 5. Superior surface of a human diaphragm (10% of the cases). The hiatus is bounded by MR and Mid-R bands. LR band and LC have no relation to the hiatus (please note that EH is indicated by OH in this figure).

margin (Figs. 5 and 6).

In another 10% of the cases (Figs. 7 and 8), the two crura contributed equally to the formation of the EH. The medial bundles of the two crura (MR and ML) crossed the midline to form the contralateral margin of the EH. The anterior and posterior margins were formed by the crossing MR bundle on the abdominal surface and ML bundle on the thoracic surface.

In the remaining 2% (one diaphragm), the EH was bounded only by the LC (Figs. 9 and 10). The right and posterior margins were formed by the ML bundle, while the left margin was formed by the LL bundle. The anterior border was formed by the

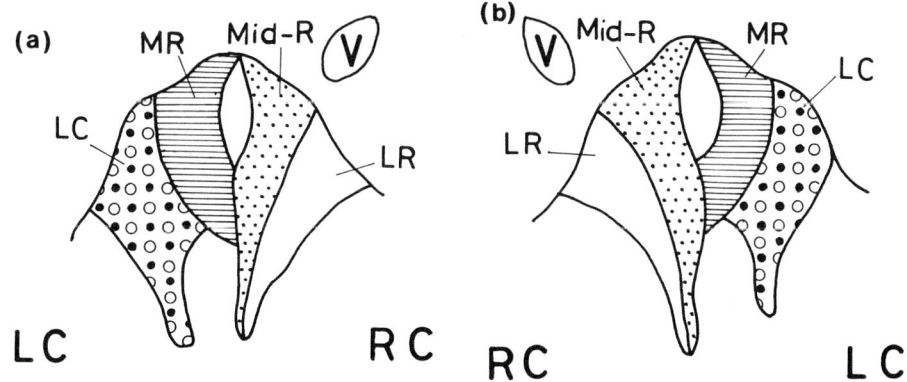

Fig. 6. Diagrammatic illustration of the superior (a) and inferior (b) surfaces of the diaphragm.

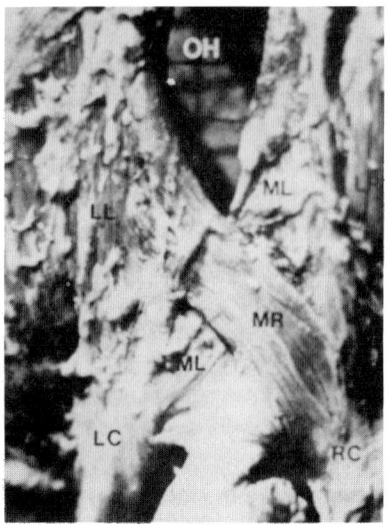

Fig. 7. Superior surface of the human diaphragm (10% of the cases). Note the arrangement of MR, Mid-R, LR, ML and LL bundles around the EH (please note that EH is indicated by OH in this figure).

crossing ML and LL bundles. The RC remained undivided and passed directly to the central tendon.

Table 1 shows a summary of the different anatomical variations in the formation of the EH.

Discussion

There has been controversy as to whether the EH is bounded only by the fleshy fibers of the RC of the diaphragm or by the fleshy fibers of the two crura. It has been reported that the EH is bounded exclusively by the RC in 100% of the cases

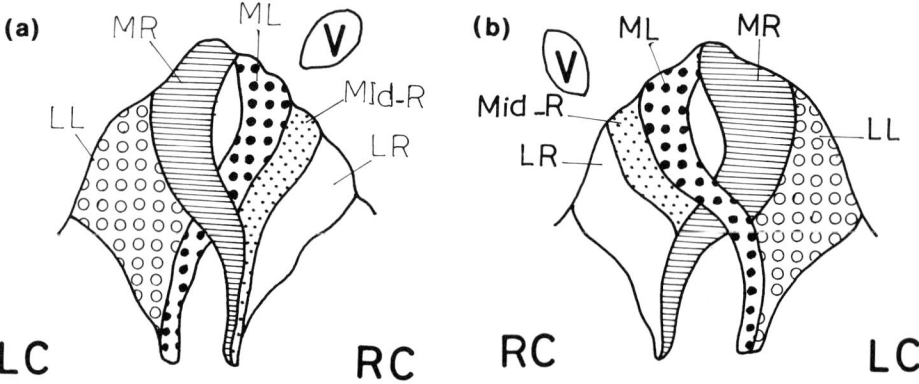

Fig. 8. Diagrammatic illustration of the superior (a) and inferior (b) surfaces of the diaphragm.

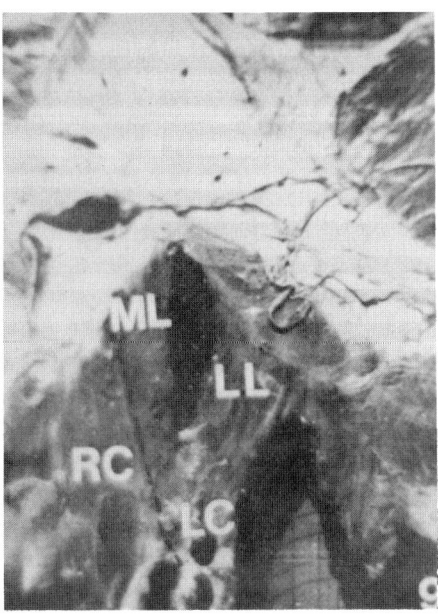

Fig. 9. Inferior surface of the human diaphragm (2% of the cases). Note that the hiatus is bounded by ML and LL bands of the LC. The RC is undivided.

[1,3,6,8,9], in 46% of the cases [4], in 58% of the cases [7], in 64% of the cases [12], in 36% of the cases [10] and in 75% of the cases [11]. In contrast to the previous studies, the results of this investigation showed that the EH was formed exclusively by the RC in only 10% of the cases. In these cases the EH appeared as a tunnel throughout the fleshy fibers of the RC between the medial and middle bundles. On the other hand, in one case (2%) the hiatus was formed exclusively by the LC. No such finding was found either by Low [1] or by Bowden and El-Ramli [10].

The formation of the EH by equal portions from the two crura, which was found in five out of 50 specimens (10%), has been previously reported by numerous authors who gave different incidences. Testut and Latarjet [2], Carey and Hollinshead [5]

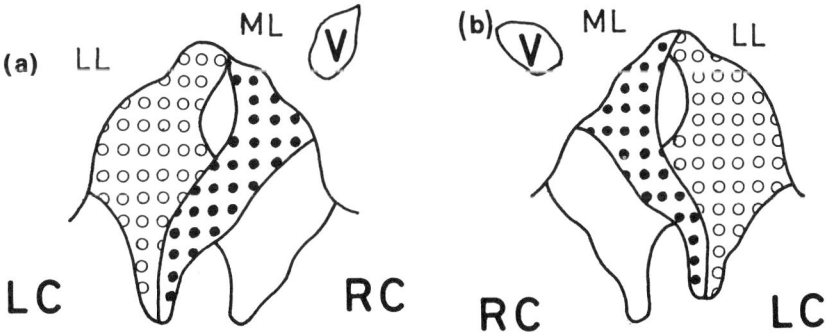

Fig. 10. Diagram illustrating the formation of the EH, (a) superior surface and (b) inferior surface.

Table 1. Summary of the mode of formation of the EH

% of cases	Right margin	Left margin	Anterior margin		Posterior margin	
62	Mid-R	MR	Mid-R,	MR	MR,	ML
16	MAL	MAL	MAL		MR,	ML
10	Mid-R	MR	Mid-R,	MR	M,	R
10	ML	MR	ML,	MR	ML,	MR
2	ML	LL	ML,	LL	M,	L

Note: Mid-R = middle bundle of RC; MR = medial bundle of RC; MAL = median arcuate ligament; ML = medial bundle of LC; LL = lateral bundle of LC.

recorded the highest incidence (100% of their cases). Bataro et al. [12] reported the lowest incidence (18%). Bowden, El-Ramli [10] and Juraniec [11] recorded a higher incidence (32% and 25%, respectively).

In the majority of the cases in this study (62%), the EH was formed by the two crura, mainly the RC. In these cases the right, the left and anterior margins were formed exclusively by the RC. The posterior margin was formed by the medial bundles of the crura (MR and ML). ML bundle crossed the midline forming a band of fleshy fibers which passed either superiorly (25 cases) or inferiorly (six cases) to the MR bundle posterior to the hiatus. Although several authors [1,3,9] described this medial band of the LC, they reported that it took no part in bounding the hiatus. Bowden and El-Ramli [10] found a similar slip which invariably made some contribution to the hiatal boundary.

Interestingly, in eight cases (16%) the two crura had no direct relation to the EH, except posteriorly where the posterior margin was formed by the crossing medial bundles of the two crura. The right, the left and anterior margins were formed by a band of fleshy fibers originating from the MAL of the diaphragm. This observation is a contribution which has not been reported before, although Figs. 2, 4, 5 and 6 of Bowden and El-Ramli [10] illustrated, to some degree, such a condition (without comment).

In all cases the anterior margin of the EH was formed by the fleshy fibers of the right and left margins which crossed each other in front of the hiatus before reaching their insertion into the central tendon. A similar observation has been reported by Marchand [8] and Bataro et al. [12].

Bowden and El-Ramli [10] reported that the anterior margin is more tendinous. Others found no fleshy fibers in front of the hiatus and reported that in all cases the anterior margin was tendinous and formed by the central tendon [6,13].

Although the functional significance of the EH was not the prime goal of this investigation, the fibers of the diaphragmatic crura are arranged around the esophagus in such a way as to be able to pinch the lower esophageal sphincter during active diaphragmatic contraction. This active diaphragmatic pinch may be an important factor in the antireflux barrier, since weak diaphragmatic performance, in cases of chronic pulmonary disease, is usually associated with a high incidence of gastro-esophageal reflux. Moreover, the anatomical variations in the formation of the EH might be of functional significance in causation of hiatal hernia and reflux esophagitis. More recently, it has been reported that active diaphragmatic contraction is an important factor in the generation of a high-pressure zone at the gastroesophageal junction, which might act as an extrinsic antireflux barrier [14,15] which complements the intrinsic barrier [16].

References

1. Low A. A note of the crura of the diaphragm and the muscle of treitz. J Anat Physiol 1907;42:93—96.
2. Testut L, Latarjet A. Traité d'Anatomie Humaine, vol 1, Barcelona: Salvat 1921;1:1027—1039.
3. Allison PR. Reflux oesophagitis, sliding hiatal hernia, repair and the anatomy of repair. Surg Gynecol Obstet 1951;92: 419—431.
4. Collis JL, Kelly JD, Wiley AM. The anatomy of the pillars of the diaphragm and surgery of the hiatus hernia. Thorax 1954;9:175—189.
5. Carey JM, Hollinshead WH. An anatomy of the oesophageal hiatus. Surg Gynecol Obstet 1955;100:196—200.
6. Madden JL. Anatomie et considerations techniques dans le traitement de la hernie hiatale. Surg Gynecol Obstet 1956;102:187—195.
7. Botha GSM. Radiological localization of the diaphragmatic hiatus. Lancet 1958;1:662—675.
8. Marchand P. The anatomy of oesophageal hiatus of the diaphragm and the pathogenesis of hiatus herniation. J Thoracic Cardiovasc Surg 1959;37:81—92.
9. Shehata R. The crura of the diaphragm and their nerve supply. Acta Anat 1966;63:49—54.
10. Bowden REM, El-Ramli HA. The anatomy of the oesophageal hiatus. Br J Surg 1967;54:983—989.
11. Juraniec J. The aortic and esophageral hiatus in the diaphragm of primates. Folia Morphol 1972;31:197—207.
12. Bataro VA, Piompo HS, Suarez DZ. Anatomical aspects of the oesophageal hiatus: distribution of the crura in its formation. J Int Coll Surg 1961;35:154—167.
13. Whillis J. A study on the lower end of oesophagus. J Anat 1930;54:132—133.
14. Welch RW, Gray JE. Influence of respiration on recordings of lower esophageal sphincter pressure in humans. Gastroenterology 1982;83:509—594.
15. Boyle JT, Altschuler SM, Nixon TE, Tuchman DN, Pack AI, Cohen S. Role of the diaphragm in the genesis of lower esophageal sphincter pressure in the cat. Gastroenterology 1985;88: 723—730.
16. Biancani P, Zabinski M, Kerstein M, Behar J. Lower esophageal sphincter mechanical, anatomical and physiologic relationship of the esophagogastic junction of the cat. Gastroenterology 1982;82:468—475.

How can one determine the function of the valve of the diaphragm
– in the normal individual?
– in cases of hiatus hernia?

S. Sloan (Chicago)

The answer to these questions assumes that the position and function of the diaphragm is vital in protecting the esophagus from gastric contents. Inherent in this assumption is that when there is an alteration of the esophagus and position of the diaphragmatic crura, there is an increased propensity for reflux. The clinical scenario would be the presence of a hiatus hernia and that under certain conditions, a patient with a hernia is more likely to reflux. A brief history of the relationship between gastroesophageal reflux disease (GERD) and the hiatus hernia is needed. The acceptance of hiatus hernia as an important factor in the pathogenesis of GERD has had a roller coaster history for the past half century. Symptoms ascribed to the hiatus hernia including epigastric pain, heartburn, and dysphagia were reported by Ritvo in 1930 [1]. The association between refluxed gastric acid and esophagitis was described by Winklestein soon thereafter [2]. It was approximately a decade later when reflux esophagitis and hiatus hernia became intertwined [3]. The type of hiatus hernia, described as associated with reflux esophagitis, was a sliding hiatal hernia (axial hiatal hernia) and treatment was directed toward the surgical repair of the anatomic defect [4]. For the next two decades, reflux esophagitis and hiatus hernia were viewed as almost synonymous. To this day, patients are influenced by the medical dogma of this period insisting that their reflux symptoms are caused by a hiatal hernia because there is a family history of such. Unfortunately, although the clinical observation was strong, epidemiologic evidence was not entirely supportive of the hernia/GERD association. Palmer found only 8% of 577 patients with hiatus hernia had typical symptoms of gastroesophageal reflux [5]. With this and other studies showing coincidental association of hiatus hernia and reflux disease, as well as the development in esophageal manometric technique, the focus of attention shifted away from the hiatus hernia and toward the lower esophageal sphincter (LES). Supporting this notion of LES pre-eminence was a study by Cohen and Harris demonstrating that the LES pressure was the main determinant for symptomatic reflux disease regardless of the presence or absence of a hiatal hernia [6]. The pendulum is swinging back with recent physiologic evidence now emerging that brings the hiatal hernia back into the gastroesophageal reflux fold, albeit, not to quite the same prominence as with the first go around. The weight of clinical evidence supports an association between the presence of a hiatal hernia and esophagitis. Animal and human physiologic studies have shown that the antireflux mechanism is comprised of both the smooth muscle lower esophageal sphincter and the striated muscle crural diaphragm component. The separation of these two components, such as might occur with a hiatal hernia, has significant pathophysiologic consequences with respect to GERD.

The antireflux barrier is comprised of the smooth muscle LES and the striated muscle right crus of the diaphragm which together form a sphincter. The resting LES pressure is measured during end-expiration with the tone primarily generated from the circular smooth muscle layer. What does the diaphragm have to do with the high pressure zone at the gastroesophageal junction (GEJ)? The contribution of the diaphragm to the antireflux barrier has been recently elucidated. In animal models, it has been shown that an augmentation of the GEJ pressure during inspiration in cats was caused primarily by diaphragmatic contraction [7]. With a pressure recording assembly anchored to the LES, in order to prevent axial movement during respirations, oscillations were recorded that corresponded to the respiratory rate. Peak high pressure zone measurements were correlated to the diaphragmatic electromyography (EMG) signal. In additional studies, the crural diaphragm in cats relaxed in response to swallows and was electrically dissociated from the costal diaphragm [8]. In these experiments balloon distension, as well as pharyngeal stimulation inducing a swallow, relaxed the smooth muscle LES and the crural diaphragm. These studies support the notion that the crural diaphragm works in concert with the smooth muscle LES. In humans, measurement and characteristics of the crural diaphragm have also been studied. In a series of elegant experiments, a modified esophageal manometric catheter with EMG electrodes attached opposite a Dent sleeve has been used to measure crural diaphragm activity. What has been demonstrated is that the increased pressure during inspiration at the GEJ is directly proportional to the force of diaphragmatic contractions [9]. With the smooth muscle LES in a relaxed state by distending the distal esophagus, contraction of the diaphragm was demonstrated to augment the GEJ pressure during maneuvers to increase intra-abdominal pressure [10]. In the setting of a hiatus hernia, the anatomic relationship between the diaphragm and the LES is altered, thus potentially weakening the response of the antireflux barrier, especially in response to transient increases in intra-abdominal pressure.

How does this translate into practical terms? Transient lower esophageal sphincter relaxations (tLESRs) have been written about as the most common LES profile in GERD patients and volunteers [11,12]. Another LES profile characterized in the same experiments identified a group of subjects with a baseline hypotensive sphincter that simply could not prevent gastroesophageal reflux with an abrupt rise in intra-abdominal pressure. Those reflux episodes during an increase in intra-abdominal pressure are termed stress reflux and can occur with coughing, straining for a bowel movement, bending over in the garden, wearing tight clothes, etc. Increased abdominal pressure occurs quite often on a daily basis and although tLESRs are proposed to be the most common sphincter profile during gastroesophageal reflux, it has been noted that during periods of cigarette smoking both controls and patients with esophagitis refluxed acid most often during coughing or deep inspiration when there was an abrupt increase in the intra-abdominal pressure [13]. This suggests stress reflux may be under represented as a mechanism for GERD. If the antireflux barrier is compromised or is simply overwhelmed during periods of abrupt increases in intra-abdominal pressure, then the potential for gastroesophageal reflux exists. Ideally ambulatory 24-h motility and pH monitoring could document these episodes of stress reflux. We recently studied this in a laboratory setting, mimicking those maneuvers that might occur in daily living. The effect of hiatus hernia and LES pressure on the competence of the GEJ was examined under conditions of increased abdominal pressure with resultant gastroesophageal reflux quantified [14]. During maneuvers including leg lifts, abdominal compression, coughing, Valsalva and Müller, both the presence and size of a hiatus hernia as well as a low LES pressure were found to be important and that these factors interact with each other to determine susceptibility to reflux. In these studies using simultaneous manometry and videofluoroscopy at the GEJ, subjects with larger hiatal hernias refluxed significantly more often than those subjects without a hiatal hernia and a similar resting LES pressure when undergoing these abdominal stress maneuvers. Part of the confusion with regards to the importance of the hiatus hernia in GERD, lies within the definition of the hiatal hernia itself. During the above mentioned stress reflux study, a hiatal hernia was qualified only if there was a persistence of barium between swallows within a hernia sac (nonreducing hiatal hernia). In GERD patients without a definable hiatal hernia and in asymptomatic volunteers, the diaphragmatic hiatus measured during mid-swallow was significantly smaller than the group of patients with a hiatal hernia. This suggests that not only are patients more susceptible to stress reflux when the crura and smooth muscle LES are separated, but the diaphragmatic hiatus is radiographically more lax in patients with a hiatal hernia. The nature of the reducibility of a hiatal hernia not only affects the propensity for stress reflux but also affects acid and volume clearance characteristics. In an earlier study, patients and volunteers without a nonreducing hiatal hernia had significantly shorter acid clearance times and better volume clearance of barium than those patients who had the presence of a nonreducing hiatal hernia [15].

In summary, the diaphragm has been demonstrated to be an essential component of the high pressure zone in animal models as well as humans. In the clinical setting of a hiatus hernia where there is separation of the smooth muscle LES and the diaphragm crus, there is impairment of the antireflux mechanism. When there is good apposition such as in individuals without a hernia, stress reflux is difficult to elicit in an experimental setting. The larger a hiatus hernia is, the less protection there is to stress reflux, which may ultimately lead to more severe disease from increased acid exposure.

References

1. Ritvo M. Hernia of the stomach through the esophageal orifice of the diaphragm. JAMA 1930;94:15–21.
2. Winlestein A. Peptic esophagitis. A new clinical entity. JAMA 1935;104:906–909.
3. Allison PR. Peptic ulcer of the esophagus. J Thoracic Surg 1946;15:308–317.
4. Allison PR. Reflux esophagitis, sliding hiatal hernia repair, and the anatomy of repair. Surg Gynecol Obstet 1951;92: 419–431.
5. Palmer ED. The hiatus hernia-esophagitis-esophageal stricture complex. Twenty-year prospective study. Am J Med 1968; 44:566–579.
6. Cohen S, Harris LD. Does hiatus hernia affect competence of gastroesophageal sphincter? N Engl J Med 1971;284:1053–1056.
7. Boyle JT, Altschuler SM, Nixon TE, Tuchman DN, Pack AI, Cohen S. Role of the diaphragm in the genesis of lower esophageal sphincter pressure in the cat. Gastroenterology 1985;88:723–730.
8. Altschuler SM et al. Simultaneous reflex inhibition of lower esophageal and crural diaphragm in cats. Am J Physiol 1985;249:G586–G591.
9. Mittal RK, Rochester DF, McCallum RW. Electrical and mechanical activity in the human lower esophageal sphincter during diaphragmatic contraction. J Clin Invest 1988;81:1182–1189.
10. Mittal RK, Rochester DF, McCallum RW. Sphincteric action of the diaphragm during a relaxed lower esophageal sphincter in humans. Am J Physiol 1989;256:G139–G144.
11. Dent J, Dodds WJ, Friedman RH, Sekiguchi T, Hogan WJ, Arndorfer RC, Petrie DJ. Mechanism of gastroesophageal reflux in recumbent asymptomatic subjects. J Clin Invest 1980;65:245–247.
12. Dodds WJ, Dent J, Hogan WJ, Helm JF, Hauser R, Patel GK, Egide MS. Mechanisms of gastroesophageal reflux in patients with reflux esophagitis. N Engl J Med 1982;307: 1547–1552.
13. Kahrilas PJ, Gupta RR. Mechanisms of acid reflux associated with cigarette smoking. Gut 1990;31:4–10.
14. Sloan S, Rademaker AW, Kahrilas PJ. Determinants of gastroesophageal junction incompetence: hiatus hernia, lower esophageal sphincter, or both? Ann Int Med 1992;117:977–982.
15. Sloan S, Kahrilas PJ. Impairment of esophageal emptying with hiatal hernia. Gastroenterology 1991;100:596–605.

What are the characteristics of the normal blood supply of the esophagus?

D. Liebermann-Meffert, M. Allgöwer, JR. Siewert (Munich)

The increasing range of operative procedures for diverticula, stenosis and malignancy of the esophagus, problems arising with leaking esophageal anastomoses and the supposition that the integrity of the anastomosis and the viability of the organ depends on an intact circulation required an accurate consideration of the related vascular anatomy. One might be concerned about fatal mediastinal bleeding from esophageal vessels, however, "blunt stripping" of the esophagus without thoracotomy for carcinoma has been shown to be relatively safe [1—3]. The remarkably low blood loss during the procedure and the frequency of postoperative anastomotic leaks suggested a primarily poor esophageal vascularization. Nevertheless, the surgically mobilized esophagus retained viability over a long distance when carefully handled [4—7].

Evaluations of previous workers were largely based on dissection specimens using a more or less coarse injection material. Neglecting the striking species differences in the vascular anatomy [3,8], results from experiments using animals were included which also produced apparent confusion in the various descriptions. More recently the smaller vessels, and in particular those entering the esophageal wall, could be clearly demonstrated by means of vascular corrosion casts [3]. The casts display the multidimensional arrangement of the extramural and intramural esophageal blood vessels [3,8]. They reproduce the macroscopic features of the esophagus by presenting vessels within the submucosa and down to microscopic dimensions [3]. The contours provided by the vascular network reflect the esophageal shape. The absence of tissues around the vascular casts and the ability to examine stereo pairs exclude potential misinterpretation of closely overlaying vessels [3,9].

Esophageal dimensions

The esophagus measured from the cricoid cartilage and cardiac notch, ranged from 21 to 34 cm (average of 27 cm) in 52 corpses in accordance with the height of the body (153 to 187 cm). It was 23 cm ± 2 SD in the female and 28 cm ± 3 SD in the male. The cervical portion was 3—4 cm, the thoracic 20—26 cm and the abdominal 3—6 cm in length.

Extramural arteries

The cervical esophagus is supplied via the paired superior and inferior thyroid arteries (Figs. 1 and 2) which derive from the right and left exterior carotid artery and the thyreocervical trunk of subclavian artery, respectively. The blood of both the cranial trachea and cervical esophagus is mainly provided by the inferior thyroid arteries [3,10–13] each giving off a 2 to 3 cm long branch called the tracheoesophageal artery, that travels on each side towards caudal and medial to approach the tracheoesophageal grove. The vessels of both sides are "joined by anastomotic twigs along the trachea [10]" and divide into three to four tracheal branches with two to three tributaries to the esophagus, which in turn subdivide within the periesophageal tissue into vessels of less than 500 μm luminal diameter, before entering the esophageal wall. Variants such as, direct esophageal branches from the subclavian artery, the superior thyroid artery, the thyroidea ima and the common carotid artery are infrequent and rather insignificant [3,8,10,11,13,14].

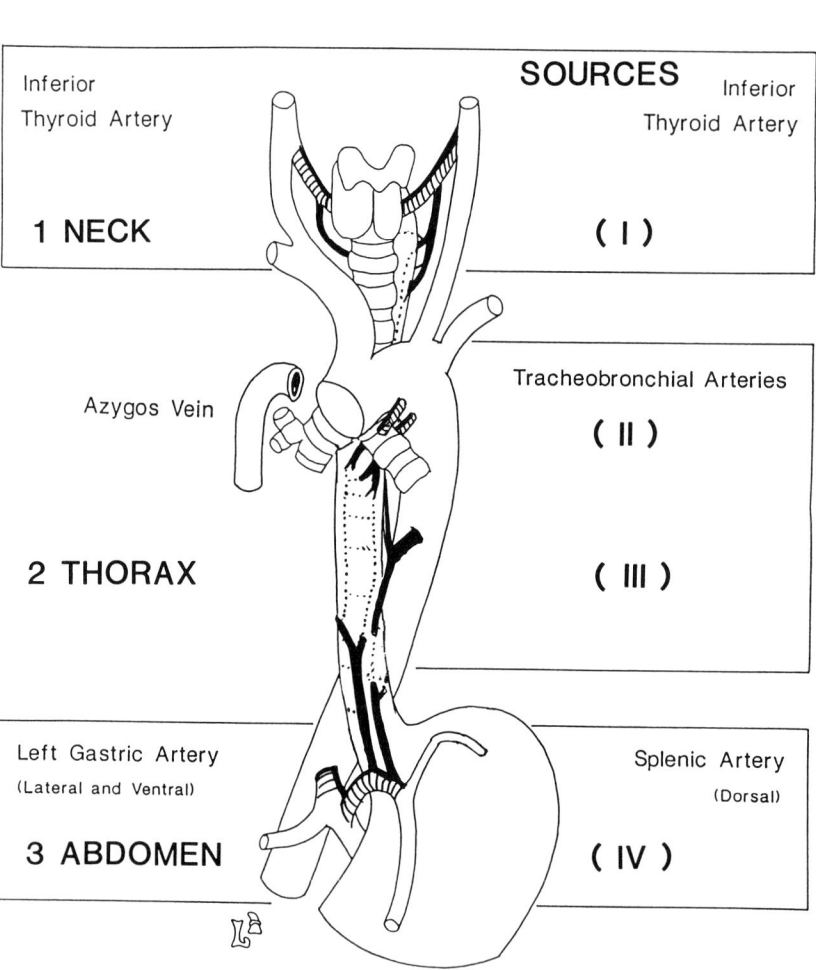

Fig. 1. Standard pattern of the angio-architecture of the esophagus. Size out of scale. Stem vessels are striped, esophageal branches black and the larger intramural vessels dotted.

COMMON EXTRINSIC BLOOD SOURCES OF THE ESOPHAGUS

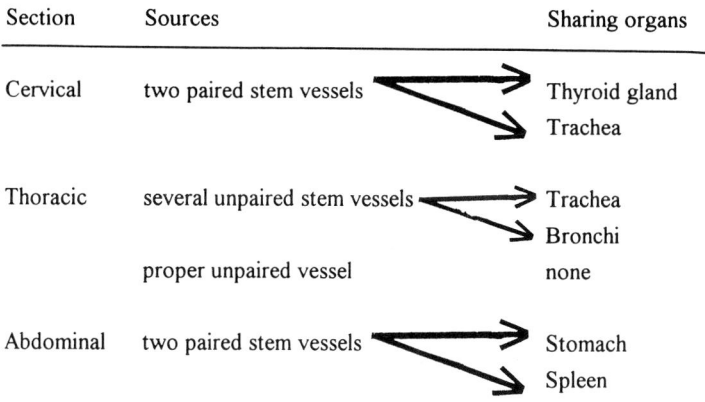

Section	Sources	Sharing organs
Cervical	two paired stem vessels	Thyroid gland Trachea
Thoracic	several unpaired stem vessels	Trachea Bronchi
	proper unpaired vessel	none
Abdominal	two paired stem vessels	Stomach Spleen

Fig. 2. Vessels of organs with which the esophagus shares its characteristic extramural pattern.

The intrathoracic esophagus receives blood from two origins (Figs. 1 and 2), which are described below:

— Up to four unpaired tracheobronchial arteries [3,8,11,12,14,15] which derive as a bundle from the inflexion of the aortic arch [3]. These give off several small branches to the esophagus which subdivide within the periesophageal tissue to vessels of 350—500 µm in diameter. Frequently one bronchoesophageal artery originates 1—3 cm caudal to the vascular bundle from the anterolateral aspect of the descending aorta [3]. In this area, which relates to the tracheal bifurcation, all the vessels are straight and short (less than 1.5 cm) and form a firm connection between the aorta, trachea and esophagus [3,8,14,15]. Variants, such as branches from intercostal arteries (if there are any) [3,8,11], seem to be insignificant for the blood supply of the human esophagus.

— One (or seldom two) unpaired proper esophageal artery with luminal diameter between 1—2 mm may arise more caudally from the anterior aspect of the descending aorta as an exclusive source (Fig. 2) for the esophagus [3,8,12,14—16]. If present, this vessel travels obliquely down towards the esophagus within the mediastinum, to divide into a recurrent ascending and a descending branch [12,14]. Both subdivide into several periesophageal vessels of less than 500 µm in diameter.

The abdominal esophagus and gastric cardia are supplied by the unpaired left gastric artery [3,8,12,14,15] and the splenic artery [3], which derive from the celiac axis (Figs. 1 and 2). With up to 11 arterial branches the left gastric artery supplies mainly the anterior and right lateral aspect of the esophageal wall, while the splenic artery is the source of blood for mainly the posterior and left lateral aspect (cardiac notch) by either one or two direct branches or via vessels of the gastric fundus including connections with the short gastrics. The branches from both stem vessels that supply the esophagus (Fig. 1) run straight up for 4—6 cm, within the periesophageal tissue across the diaphragmatic hiatus. At variable distances they give off small tributaries of less than 500 μm internal diameter before they penetrate the esophageal wall [3,15].

The dense continuous network of intramural vessels: structural appearance

Having reduced their diameter by approaching the periesophageal tissue, the extramural vessels pass perpendicularly through the layers of the tunica muscularis, give off a few small tributaries to the muscle bundles en route before they divide at the muscular side of the submucosa into one or two vessels of approximately 400 μm in diameter to follow the longitudinal axis of the esophagus. They give off vessels of 200–300 μm in diameter at right angles that pass around the circumference, in a circular manner, to anastomose with the vessels of the opposite site. During their course the transverse vessels subdivide into multiple fine branches throughout the submucosa. This pattern of supply is characteristic of the entire esophagus [3,10,16]. All these vessels form an uninterrupted, minute and dense network in the submucosa (Fig. 3) to supply the musculature and mucosa. The submucosal vasculature connects the extramural vessels with the intramural vessels in the esophagus without any visible segmental demarcation.

The microvascular connections are evident in detail after injection of low particle size resin and at a higher magnification. Scanning electron microscopy of the complete cast revealed a submucosal network of small arteries and arterioles down to capillary diameter. The venous system (venules and veins) is filled by retrograde infusion and is also displayed. The arteries may or may not be accompanied by veins. Their respective characteristically different endothelial (nuclear) impressions allow a ready distinction. In principle, the submucous network arteries are approximately 50 μm in diameter and the veins 60–80 μm. The arteries give off short arterioles which display a variety of vessel size (40–20 μm) and break up into capillaries of 5–20 μm in diameter. The capillary part revealed a complex polygonal meshwork of vessels that were connected to others, principally of similar diameter.

All together, this vascular intramural network provides a subtle but luxurious vascular supply to the esophagus.

Conclusion

The esophageal vascular casts provide the morphological basis for circulation. Sources of blood supply to the esophagus concern mainly three areas: from the neck by the paired inferior thyroid arteries; in the chest by the unpaired aortic arch arteries; from the abdomen by the unpaired left gastric and splenic artery. According to the dominant size of the extramural vessels, however, it is evident that the cervical and abdominal sources provide the major blood supply to the esophagus, while the small stem vessels at the level of the carina seem to be of minor importance.

The vascular pattern is developed in such a manner that with the exception of one

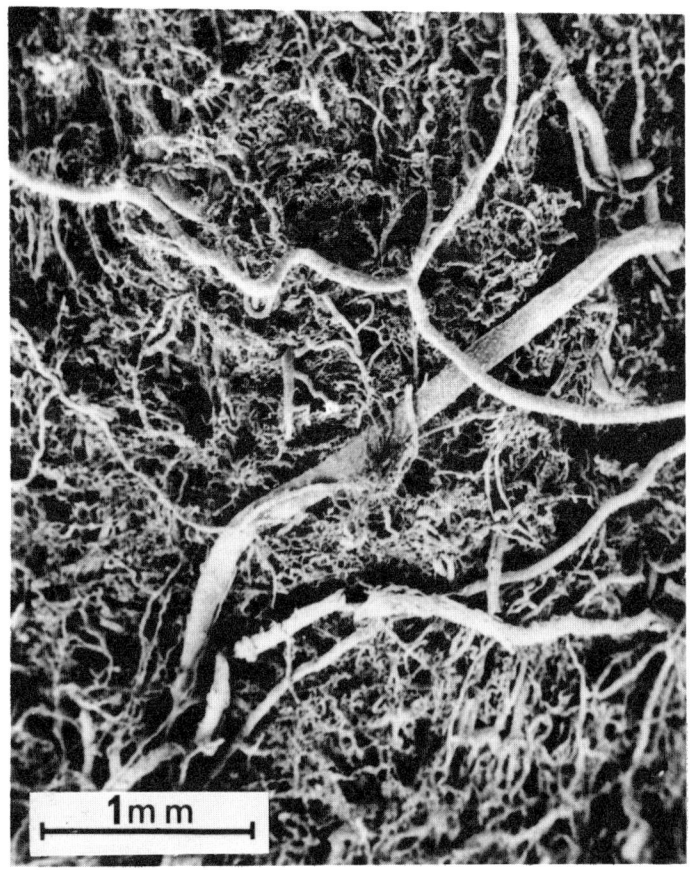

Fig. 3. Scanning electron microscopy of a vascular cast of the human intramural, submucosal blood supply. Vascular network in healthy human tissue. Sagittal section from the external to the luminal surface aspect showing the whole range of microvessels.

vessel of direct aortic origin, all others derive from the larger stem vessels of different organs (Fig. 2) which signifies that the esophagus depends on "a shared vasculature".

Branching subdivides the already primarily small esophageal vessels to be minute in the periesophageal tissue, before entering the wall of the esophagus. They, therefore, may undergo contractile hemostasis when torn.

A continuous regular network located in the submucosa connects all the extramural vessels. There is no short supplied or avascular zone. Besides, surgical experience has clearly shown that problems due to circulatory disturbances are by far, overestimated. Anastomotic failures practically always arise from the visceral substitute.

It is crucial that the esophagus itself is provided with an excellent blood supply through longitudinally oriented intramural vessels that permit the anastomosis being placed at which ever level. The intramural network thus provides a luxurious, although fine vascularity for the esophagus, by a system of small arteries, arterioles and capillaries which nevertheless needs careful surgical handling.

Acknowledgement

The International Foundation for Postgraduate Surgery, Basel, Switzerland lent its support in writing this article.

References

1. Akiyama H. Surgery for carcinoma of the esophagus. Curr Probl Surg 1980;17:53—120.
2. Orringer MB, Orringer JS. Esophagectomy without thoracotomy: a dangerous operation? J Thorac Cardiovasc Surg 1983;85:72—80.
3. Liebermann-Meffert D, Lüscher U, Neff U, Rüedi ThP, Allgöwer M. Esophagectomy without thoracotomy: is there a risk of intramediastinal bleeding? A study on blood supply of the esophagus. Ann Surg 1987;206:184—192.
4. MacManus JE, Dameron JT, Paine JR. The extent to which one may interfere with the blood supply of the esophagus and obtain healing on anastomosis. Surgery 1950;28:11—23.
5. Shek JL, Prietto CH, Tuttle WM, O'Brien EJ. An experimental study of the blood supply of the esophagus and its relation to esophageal anastomoses. J Thorac Cardiovasc Surg 1950;19:523—533.
6. Swenson O, Merrill K, Pierce EC, Rheinlander HF. Blood and nerve supply to the esophagus: an experimental study. J Thoracic Surg 1950;19:462—476.
7. Williams DB, Payne WS. Observations on esophageal blood supply. Mayo Clin Proc 1982;57:448—453.
8. Liebermann-Meffert D, Siewert JR. Arterial anatomy of the esophagus. A review of the literature with brief comments on clinical aspects. Gullet 1992;2:3—10.
9. Gannon B, Browning J, O'Brien P, Rogers P. Mucosal microvascular architecture of the fundus and of human stomach. Gastroenterology 1984;86:866—875.
10. Miura T, Grillo HC. The contribution of the inferior thyroid artery to the blood supply of the human trachea. Surg Gynecol Obstet 1966;123:99—102.
11. Shapiro AL, Robillard GL. The esophageal arteries. Their configurational anatomy and variations in relation to surgery. Ann Surg 1950;131:171—185.
12. Swigart LVL, Siekert RG, Hambley WC, Anson BJ. The esophageal arteries. An anatomic study of 150 specimens. Surg Gynecol Obstet 1950;90:234—243.
13. Vallee B, Hong R, Renelier B, Person H, Huu N. Les artères oesophagiennes d'origine cervicale. Etude anatomique de 23 dissections. Ann Otolaryngol 1982;99:29—34.
14. Gloor F. Die Gefäßversorgung der Speiseröhre. Thoraxchirurgie 1953/54;1:146—167.
15. Demel R. Die Gefäßversorgung der Speiseröhre. Ein Beitrag zur Oesophaguschirurgie. Arch Klin Chir 1924;128:453—504.
16. Colas M, Carret JP, Picq P, Le Pivert P, Cuilleret J. Etude de la vascularisation artérielle de l'oesophage par microangiographie. Bull Ass Anat 1976;60:489—496.

When is the esophageal mucosa normal?

K. Geboes (Leuven)

General organization of the esophageal mucosa

The luminal side of the normal esophagus is lined by mucosa composed of epithelium, lamina propria and a muscularis mucosae. Except for a short segment of columnar epithelium in the distal esophagus at the gastroesophageal junction, the normal esophageal epithelium is a tough, nonkeratinizing, stratified, squamous epithelium. The lower border of the squamous epithelium is irregular due to the presence of transitory folds of the lamina propria and more particularly, due to the presence of high conical papillae of connective tissue. These papillae are highly vascularized. On routine microscopy the squamous epithelium can be divided into basal, intermediate or prickle cell layers and superficial layers. In the superficial layers, functional and surface layers can be distinguished. The latter lay adjacent to the lumen. In many articles authors refer also to a basal zone. This is the area composed of the basal cell layer and several layers of cuboidal basophilic cells immediately above (the suprabasal cell layers). The upper extent of the basal zone has been arbitrarily defined as the level where the nuclei are separated by a distance equal to their diameter [1—3]. The parabasal cell layer or compartment, is roughly similar to the area classically described as intermediate or prickle cell layer.

Several parameters have been introduced to assess this organization. These include total epithelial thickness, papillary height and basal zone thickness. In morphometric studies, the values of these parameters have been determined in comparison with the total thickness of the epithelium. The basal zone normally comprises no more than 15—20% of the total epithelial thickness, while the normal value for papillary height ranges from 50%—75% [4—7] (Fig. 1). There is some variability in the criteria used in different studies. The organization and relative size of the different compartments of the squamous epithelium is generally the same throughout the whole length of the esophagus. Only small regional differences have been noted. From studies in normal control individuals it appears that the relative height of the papillae and of the basal zone may be greater in the distal (2—5 cm) esophagus. Weinstein [8] showed that the basal zone and papillary height can even be increased in an area between 2.5 and 10 cm of the distal esophagus in asymptomatic subjects. Yet, abnormal reflux was not excluded in these asymptomatic controls by objective methods. A low false positive rate of basal zone widening and increase of papillary height was found in a study on 18 asymptomatic volunteers in whom pH reflux tests were performed to exclude pathologic reflux [9].

In the early morphometric studies the histologic data have been determined on routinely hematoxylin and eosin (HE) or periodic acid schiff (PAS) stained, well oriented (suction) biopsies. The PAS stain was used to show the presence or absence

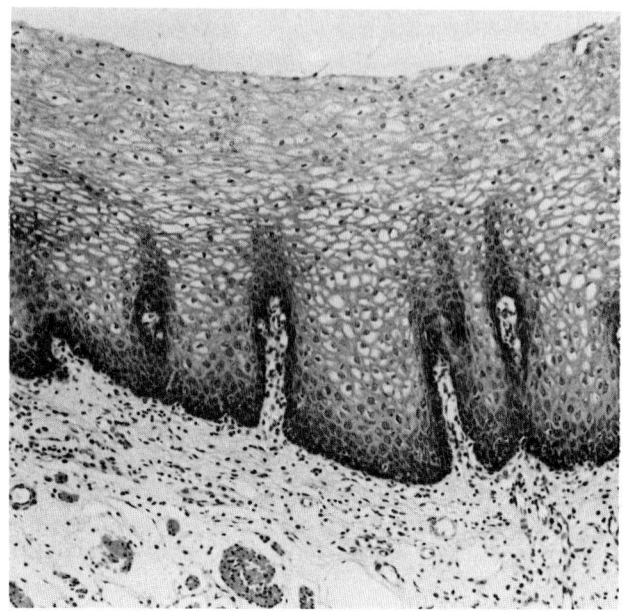

Fig. 1. Normal histology of the human esophagus showing the squamous surface epithelium with lower irregular border due to the presence of high conical lamina propria papillae. Papillary length and total epithelial thickness can be used for the evaluation of the histologic picture (HE ×40).

of glycogen. Cells of the basal cell layer lack glycogen. Accumulation of cytoplasmic glycogen starts above the basal zone and is considered a marker of maturation.

Routine histology and cell renewal

The squamous esophageal epithelium is a dynamic cell population which is renewed continuously. In health and in benign inflammatory conditions the proliferative indices remain in a steady state so that the cells produced are equivalent to those lost.

The different cell layers described in the squamous epithelium are the morphological expression of processes of proliferation, differentiation or maturation and dying cells. This was already realized when the basal zone was identified and its existence was explained by the presence of immature cells.

The proliferative compartment of the squamous epithelium resides in the basal cell layer. The basal or germinative layer is made up of one layer of cylindrical, basophilic cells resting on a basement membrane. The longitudinal axis of the cylindrical basal cells is oriented perpendicular to the basement membrane. Random mitotic figures can be observed by routine microscopy in this layer. Immunohistochemistry using antibodies directed against bromodeoxyuridine (BRDU), a compound which is incorporated in the nucleus during DNA synthesis, demonstrates the presence of S-phase cells in the same layer (Fig. 2). These cells are randomly

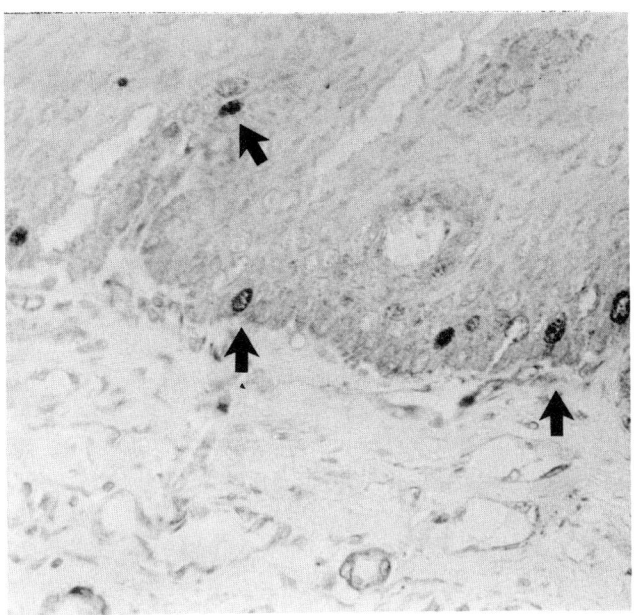

Fig. 2. Normal esophageal mucosa: immunohistochemistry using antibodies directed against BRDU, showing the presence of cells with positively staining nuclei in the basal cell layer (immunoperoxidase ×200).

distributed. For the normal esophagus, the labeling index of the basal cell layer indicating the ratio between the number of cells showing a positive nuclear staining for antibodies directed against BRDU and the sum of the labeled and unlabeled cells is 8.7%. For the entire mucosa the labeling index is 0.95% (pulse labeling). This indicates a slow rate of cell renewal [10]. The tissue turnover time (time taken for an entire epithelium to be regenerated) has been estimated to be approximately 2 weeks. The exact quantification of esophageal epithelial cell renewal and the most sensitive method to do so have, however, not yet been established. Various other in vitro and in vivo methods are available and have been used in different clinical conditions such as normal squamous mucosa and Barrett's esophagus. Cell proliferation studies with markers such as Ki67 (a nuclear antigen which is expressed in all phases of the cell cycle except Go) in squamous mucosa from patients with Barrett's esophagus show a mean percent of positive cells of 14.14 (± SD 12.70) [11]. Studies have also been performed with proliferating nuclear antigen (an auxiliary protein for DNA synthetase) and this topic is still in evolution [12]. Some basic concepts have already been established in animal studies. It appears that in rats virtually every cell of the basal layer becomes labeled after repeated injections with tritiated thymidine which indicates that all basal cells are capable of desoxyribonucleic acid synthesis and presumably of cell proliferation. One, both or neither of the two daughter cells of any mitosis can be transferred to the upper differentiating layers.

Cell proliferation and maturation is influenced by epidermal growth factor (EGF), a mitogenic polypeptide which in man is immunohistochemically demonstrable in the subepithelial capillaries [13]. Certain molecules, such as tumor necrosis factor and transforming growth factor β, can inhibit growth in the esophageal epithelium under normal circumstances. Both these factors are constitutively expressed in the human basal normal esophageal epithelium [14].

Epithelial cell layers

The basal cell layer can be divided in two topographically different but contiguous compartments, both forming the junction with the lamina propria connective tissue. One compartment is the flat layer laying parallel with the longitudinal axis of the esophagus. The second is lining the stromal lamina propria papillae and lying perpendicular to the luminal axis of the esophagus. These two compartments show some differences in cell properties as indicated by immunohistochemical studies on the presence of cytokeratins. Cytokeratin 14 is expressed diffusely in the cells of both compartments of the basal layer, whereas cytokeratin 19 is mainly expressed in the basal cells lining the stromal papillae [10].

As the cells leave the germinal layer, they disconnect from the basal lamina and become larger, polyhedral and subsequently more flattened and constitute the multilayered prickle cells. The deeply situated cells are the more immature cells (suprabasal layers). The cells mature as they migrate towards the surface. As indicated earlier, immaturity can be demonstrated by PAS but more recently immunohistochemical studies have been developed using other markers. In the esophagus the pairs of cytokeratins vary in the different compartments with the degree of differentiation of the epithelial cells. Keratin types 14 and 19 have been demonstrated in the cells of the basal compartment (basal cell layer and suprabasal cell layers) and types 1 and 10 have been found in the parabasal cells. A decreased expression of Lewis blood group antigens (markers of squamous maturity) has been shown in the parabasal cell compartment. Epidermal growth factor receptor (EGFR) is expressed in the basal and immediately suprabasal epithelial cell layers where it appears as a peripheral membranous staining and is absent from the more superficial layers. EGFR is an integral plasma membrane glycoprotein for which EGF is the ligand. In normal esophageal mucosa the proportion of epithelium staining positively for EGFR has been estimated to be 29% of the total (which is almost double the value normally accepted for the basal zone area using routine HE staining or PAS staining) (Fig. 3). The staining distribution for EGFR is the same at all levels of the esophagus. The immunohistochemical studies thus confirm the existence of a basal zone composed of immature cells but the normal quantitative values obtained with these techniques are not exactly the same as those assessed with more routine stainings [14]. Depending on the markers used, there may be transition zones between the basal cell layer, the suprabasal layers, the parabasal or intermediate layers and the superficial layers.

Above the basal zone the postmitotic epithelial cells mature. This process is characterized by nuclear pyknosis, loss of glycogen, loss of maturation markers and

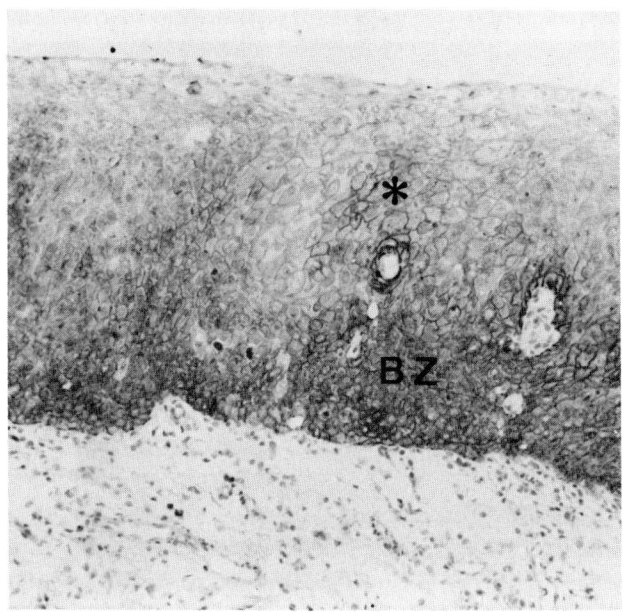

Fig. 3. Normal esophageal mucosa: immunohistochemistry using antibodies directed against Epidermal Growth Factor Receptor showing positive membranous staining of the lower cell layers in the basal zone (BZ) and along the stromal papillae * (×40; cryostat section).

a change in cell polarity from vertical to horizontal. The cells become more elliptical and increasing amounts of tonofilaments (keratins) and desmosomes can be observed with transmission electron microscopy (TEM) [15]. In situ hybridization allows identification of cytokeratin 4 mRNA expression starting in this (parabasal) area (Fig. 4).

As epithelial cells mature they move further away from the capillaries and oxygen. Cells in the outermost 4–6 layers accumulate lipid droplets with subsequent damage to cell organelles and intercellular junctions begin to loosen. Cell degeneration occurs in the surface layers. Superficial esophageal epithelial cells occasionally show features of programmed cell death characterized by the occurrence of apoptotic bodies but most cells seem to be lost by desquamation or exfoliation. This may be the result of lysis of desmosomes by endogenous proteinases.

Immunohistochemical studies can be used to identify markers associated with cell maturation but they can also identify other markers associated with cell activation or metabolism. Major histocompatibility class (MHC) antigens can be considered to some extent as activation markers. MHC class I antigens are normally expressed on the membrane of all nucleated cells and they appear also on esophageal epithelial cells. MHC class II antigens are mainly expressed on immunocompetent cells. Their presence has been associated with antigen processing and presentation and with cellular interactions. Increased or aberrant expression can be observed in inflammatory conditions and depends upon the release of cytokines. In the normal esophageal epithelium MHC class II antigens are expressed on a minority of epithelial cells.

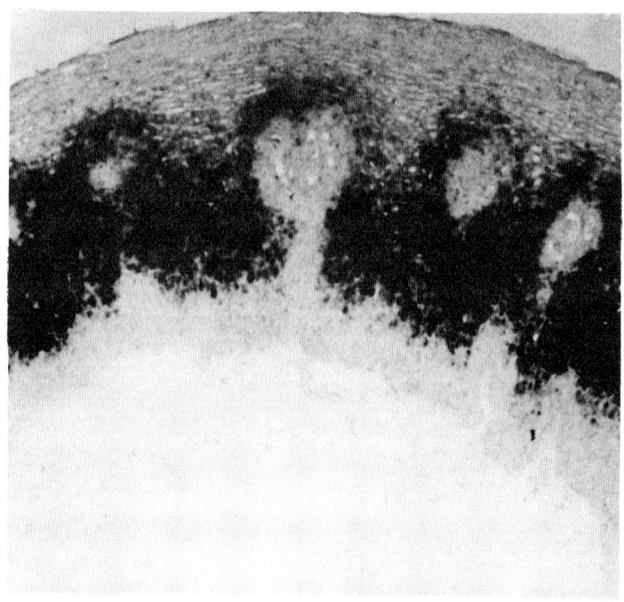

Fig. 4. Normal esophageal mucosa: localization of cytokeratin 4 mRNA in esophageal epithelium by nonradioactive in situ hybridization. Positivity starts in the parabasal compartment and extends into the lower superficial layers (provided by A. Viaene and J. Baert, IRC, KUL-Kortrijk; original magnification ×20).

Detailed analysis of biopsies shows that these are cells overlying lamina propria lymphoid follicles [15,16].

Specialized cells in the epithelium

A variety of cell types such as neuroendocrine cells (Merkel cells), rare melanocytes, lymphocytes and Langerhans cells are normally present within the squamous epithelium of the esophagus. Lymphocytes and Langerhans cells play a major role in the immunologic defense system of the esophagus. The Langerhans cells act as antigen-presenting cells. The interepithelial lymphocytes mainly belong to the suppressor/cytotoxic phenotype (CD8). On morphology they appear as small round cells with hyperchromatic nuclei. They show an uneven distribution within the epithelium with a higher number in certain areas which appear to be these overlying lamina propria lymphoid follicles [16,17]. The presence of small round lymphocytes and Langerhans cells within the esophageal epithelium can therefore not be considered as a sign of pathology. The appearance of wiggly cells or lymphocytes with squiggly nuclei is probably abnormal [18]. Occasionally mast cells and single eosinophils can be found in the epithelium. The meaning of this finding is not clear. According to some authors this would not be a sign of pathology in adults, but in children the presence of even single eosinophils would correlate with abnormal reflux.

Neutrophils are normally not present in biopsies from adults but might occur in small numbers in children. In fact this means that the upper limits of what is normal, or the lower limits of abnormality have not yet been determined, certainly not for the number of inflammatory cells infiltrating the squamous epithelium.

Lamina propria and muscularis mucosae

The lamina propria rests on a two-layered muscularis mucosae. The lamina propria contains lymphatics, blood vessels, nerve fibers and occasional inflammatory cells. Eosinophils can be observed in 10—33% of asymptomatic control patients. Lymphocytes can occur as scattered solitary cells or be organized in lymphoid follicles. The follicles may be associated with the excretory ducts of esophageal glands.

Conclusion

The value of the criteria that can be used to determine whether the esophageal mucosa is normal or abnormal depends upon the methods of investigation. The criteria established with routine microscopy may not be exact quantitatively, and routine staining may not be the most sensitive method to assess them, but in general they correlate rather well with the findings on cell maturation and cell renewal obtained by more sophisticated methods and hence with the physiology of the esophageal mucosa.

References

1. Ismail-Beigi F, Horton PF, Pope CE. Histological consequences of gastroesophageal reflux in man. Gastroenterology 1970;58:163—174.
2. Pope CE. Mucosal response to esophageal motor disorders. Arch Int Med 1976;136:549—554.
3. Geboes K, Desmet V. Histology of the esophagus. Front Gastrointest Res 1978;3:1—17.
4. Denardi FG, Riddell RH. The normal esophagus. Am J Surg Pathol 1991;15:296—309.
5. Eastwood GL. Histologic changes in gastroesophageal reflux. J Clin Gastroenterol 1986;8:45—51.
6. Hamilton SR. Reflux esophagitis and Barrett esophagus. In: Goldman H, Appelman H, Kaufman N (eds) Gastrointestinal Pathology. Baltimore: Williams & Wilkins, 1990:11—68.
7. Jarvis LR, Dent J, Whitehead R. Morphometric assessment of reflux esophagitis in fibreoptic biopsy specimens. J Clin Pathol 1985;38:44—48.
8. Weinstein WM, Bogoch ER, Bowes KL. The normal human esophageal mucosa. A histological reappraisal. Gastroenterology 1975;68:40—44.
9. Fink SM, Barwick KW, Winchenbach CL, DeLuca V, McCallum RW. Reassessment of esophageal histology in normal subjects: a comparison of suction and endoscopic techniques. J Clin Gastroenterol 1983; 5:177—183.
10. Geboes K, Haustermans K, Mebis J, Ectors N, Lerut T, Van der Schueren M. Cytokeratin 14; 18; 19 expression in squamous cancer of the esophagus. Fifth World Congress of the International Society for Diseases of the Esophagus, Kyoto, 1992.
11. Iftikhar SY, Steele RJC, Watson S, James PD, Dilks K, Hardcastle JD. Assessment of proliferation of squamous, Barrett's and gastric mucosa in patients with columnar lined Barrett's oesophagus. Gut 1992;33:733—737.
12. Jankowski J, McMenemin R, Yu C, Hopwood D, Wormsley KG. Proliferating cell nuclear antigen in oesophageal diseases: correlation with transforming growth factor alpha expression. Gut 1992;33:587—591.
13. Jankowski J, Coghill G, Tregaskis B, Hopwood D, Wormsley KG. Epidermal growth factor in the oesophagus. Gut 1992;33:1448—1453.

14. Jankowski J, Murphy S, Coghill G, Grant A, Wormsley KG, Sanders DSA, Kerr M, Hopwood D. Epidermal growth factor receptors in the oesophagus. Gut 1992;33:439—443.
15. Geboes K, Mebis J, Desmet V. The esophagus: normal ultrastructure and pathological patterns. In: Motta PM, Fujita H (eds) Ultrastructure of the Digestive Tract. Boston: Martinus Nijhoff Publishers, 1988:17—34.
16. Geboes K, Janssens J, Vantrappen G. Basic lesions in inflammatory disorders of the esophagus. In: Watanabe S, Sobrinho-Simoes M, Wolff M (eds) Digestive Disease Pathology. Philadelphia: Field & Wood Inc., 1992:1—34.
17. Geboes K, De Wolf-Peeters C, Rutgeerts P, Janssens J, Vantrappen G, Desmet V. Lymphocytes and Langerhans cells in the human oesophageal epithelium. Virch Arch 1983; 401:45—55.
18. Mangano M, Wang H, Schnitt S, Antonioli DO. Nature and significance of cells with irregular nuclear contours (CINC) in esophageal mucosa. Lab Invest 1991;64:38A.

What is basically wrong with the LES in reflux disease?

P.J. Kahrilas (Chicago)

Although gastroesophageal reflux disease (GERD) is multifactorial in etiology with potentially important modifying roles played by mucosal defensive factors, the effectiveness of esophageal acid clearance, and differences in the causticity of refluxate, the key event in the pathogenesis of GERD is reflux of noxious substances from the stomach into the esophagus. The modifiers alluded to above may change the threshold that distinguishes asymptomatic reflux from symptomatic reflux in terms of the number of reflux events required, but, regardless, reflux events are a prerequisite for the development of GERD. Under normal circumstances, gastroesophageal reflux is prevented by an antireflux barrier located at the gastroesophageal junction.

The antireflux barrier is an anatomically complex zone whose integrity has been attributed to lower esophageal sphincter (LES) pressure, extrinsic compression of the LES by the crural diaphragm, the intra-abdominal location of the LES, the phrenoesophageal ligament and maintenance of an acute angle of His. Although there is probably some merit to each of these possibilities, supporting evidence is more compelling in some cases than in others. Quite possibly, competence of the antireflux barrier is attributable to multiple factors and progressive incompetence occurs as more antireflux mechanisms are disabled. The antireflux barrier needs to be dynamic because it must guard against reflux in a variety of circumstances. For example, the intra-abdominal segment of the LES may be important in preventing reflux during swallowing, the diaphragmatic crus may be of cardinal importance during abdominal straining and resting LES pressure may be of primary importance during restful recumbency. The rate at which reflux events are incurred would then increase progressively as each of these protective mechanisms is compromised.

The complexity of the antireflux barrier has led investigators to a variety of conclusions regarding which is the most important mechanism of reflux. The three different prevailing opinions are that the dominant mechanism of reflux is by transient lower esophageal sphincter relaxations, a result of anatomic disruption of the diaphragmatic sphincter probably associated with a hiatal hernia, or simply a result of a hypotensive LES. Individuals can be found exemplifying each of these mechanisms; however, what proportion of the entire GERD population can be attributed to each mechanism remains a hotly debated issue. Rather than argue their relative importance, the aim of this discussion is to relay the evidence for these impairments of the antireflux barrier.

Transient lower esophageal sphincter relaxations

Studies in normal volunteers [1] and in GERD patients [2–4] have demonstrated the phenomenon of transient lower esophageal sphincter relaxation (tLESR). The descriptor "transient" distinguishes a tLESR from a swallow-induced LES relaxation. Transient LESRs appear without an antecedent pharyngeal contraction, persist for longer periods (5–30 s) than do swallow-induced LES relaxations, and are generally unaccompanied by esophageal peristalsis. There is compelling evidence that tLESRs account for the majority of reflux events in normal individuals or in patients with normal LES pressure at the time of reflux. However, the likelihood of reflux during a particular tLESR is influenced by both the circumstances of the recording and the temporal proximity to a meal, with different investigators reporting reflux during as many as 93% [1] or as few as 9–15% [5,6] of tLESRs. What has become increasingly clear is the role of tLESRs as a component of the belch reflex [7,8]. The frequency of tLESRs is greatly increased in humans [7,8] or dogs [9] by distension of the stomach by gas as it is in the upright as opposed to the supine posture [8]. Some investigators have suggested that tLESRs are "subthreshold swallows" in response to pharyngeal stimulation in the opossum [10] or humans. However, other investigators find no more than a chance co-occurrence of minor submental EMG activity and tLESRs [11]. In view of the circumstances in which they appear, it seems most likely that tLESRs are a physiologic response to gastric distension by food or gas and are the mechanism responsible for gas venting of the stomach.

Hypotensive lower esophageal sphincter

The LES is a 3–4 cm long segment of tonically contracted smooth muscle at the distal end of the esophagus. Resting tone of the LES normally varies from 10 to 30 mmHg relative to intragastric pressure. Lower esophageal sphincter pressure is lowest in the postprandial period and highest at night [1]. Intra-abdominal pressure, gastric distension, peptides, hormones, various foods, and many drugs affect the LES pressure. The mechanism of LES tonic contraction seems to be a property of the muscle itself rather than of nerves affecting the sphincter. Pressure within the sphincter is minimally affected following the elimination of neural activity by close intra-arterial injection of tetrodotoxin [12]. Furthermore, biochemical evidence suggests that the properties of the sphincter are defined by properties of the circular muscle. Nonetheless, 50–70% of LES tone of humans can be inhibited by atropine [13]. Such influences may be especially important in modification of closure force in response to stimuli such as feeding and fasting.

Diminished LES pressure can be associated with gastroesophageal reflux by two mechanisms, stress reflux and free reflux. Stress reflux results when a relatively hypotensive LES is overcome and "blown open" by an abrupt increase of intra-abdominal pressure. Substantial data have accumulated suggesting that stress reflux is unlikely when the LES pressure is greater than 10 mmHg [2,4,6]. However, it should be noted that these studies were not controlled for the potential effect of a hiatal hernia and a recent investigation suggests that for a given LES pressure, the susceptibility to stress reflux is directly related to the presence and size of hiatal hernia [14]. The other mechanism by which diminished LES pressure is associated with gastroesophageal reflux is free reflux. Free reflux is characterized by a fall in intraesophageal pH, without an identifiable change in either intragastric or LES pressure observed when the resting LES pressure is within 0–4 mmHg of intragastric pressure [2,4].

A puzzling clinical observation supporting the importance of tLESRs is that only a minority of individuals with GERD have a hypotensive LES when determined by isolated fasting measurements [15,16]. This observation can be somewhat reconciled when one considers the dynamic nature of LES pressure. The isolated fasting measurement is probably useful only in identifying patients with a grossly hypotensive LES who are constantly susceptible to stress reflux. However, there is probably a larger group of patients with mild or moderate GERD susceptible to stress reflux when their LES pressure has been temporarily diminished as a result of specific foods, drugs, or habits [2,6].

Hiatal hernia and the diaphragmatic sphincter

Manometric recordings of LES pressure are often characterized by inspiratory augmentation previously attributed to catheter movement. However, more recent evidence in both cats and humans suggests that these inspiratory increases result from contraction of the diaphragmatic crus that encircles the LES [17]. Despite pinning the manometric catheter in place, the inspiratory augmentation of LES pressure persists. The amplitude of respiratory oscillations increases with increased respiratory effort and are eliminated by manual hyperventilation. The augmentation of LES pressure observed during sustained inspiration, corresponds both temporally and quantitatively with the augmentation of crural EMG activity and this augmented LES pressure is observed to obscure the intrinsic LES relaxation induced by esophageal distension [18]. Intrinsic LES tone is equivalent to manometrically recorded end expiratory tone, suggesting that in normal circumstances the diaphragm contributes only to the inspiratory augmentation of LES pressure.

The physiologic relevance of the augmentation of gastroesophageal junction pressure attributable to the crural diaphragm pertains to the condition of hiatal hernia, a condition that may be associated with its anatomic disruption. Observations of the antireflux mechanism during stress maneuvers such as leg raising and abdominal compression suggest a "pinchcock effect" of crural contraction that effectively augments the antireflux barrier [18]. Patients with a substantial hiatal hernia, regardless of whether or not they had a hypotensive LES, have been shown to incur an increased number of acid reflux episodes in response to these same stress maneuvers [19].

References

1. Dent J, Dodds WJ, Friedman RH, Sekiguchi T, Hogan WJ, Arndorfer RC, Petrie DJ. Mechanism of gastroesophageal reflux in recumbent asymptomatic human subjects. J Clin Invest 1980;65:245–247.
2. Dodds WJ, Dent J, Hogan WJ, Helm JF, Hauser R, Pate GK, Egide MS. Mechanisms of gastroesophageal reflux in patients with reflux esophagitis. N Engl J Med 1982;307:1547–1552.
3. Dodds WJ, Kahrilas PJ, Dent J, Hogan WJ, Kern MK, Arndorfer RC. Analysis of spontaneous gastroesophageal reflux and esophageal acid clearance in patients with reflux esophagitis. J Gastroint Motil 1989;2:79.
4. Dent J, Holloway RH, Toouli J, Dodds WJ. Mechanisms of lower oesophageal sphincter incompetence in patients with symptomatic gastro-oesophageal reflux. Gut 1988;29:1020–1028.
5. Mittal RK, McCallum RW. Characteristics of transient lower esophageal sphincter relaxations in humans. Am J Physiol 1987;252:G636.
6. Kahrilas PJ, Gupta RR. Mechanisms of acid reflux associated with cigarette smoking. Gut 1990;31:4–10.
7. Kahrilas PJ, Dodds WJ. Dent J, Wyman JB, Hogan WJ, Arndorfer RC. Upper esophageal sphincter function during belching. Gastroenterology 1986;91:133.
8. Wyman JB, Dent J, Heddle R, Dodds WJ, Toouli J, Downton J. Control of belching by the lower esophageal sphincter. Gut 1990;31:639.
9. Patrikios J, Martin CJ, Dent J. Relationship of transient lower esophageal sphincter relaxation to postprandial gastro-esophageal reflux and belching in dogs. Gastroenterology 1986;90:545.
10. Paterson WG, Rattan S, Goyal RK. Experimental induction of isolated lower esophageal sphincter relaxation in anesthetized opossums. J Clin Invest 1986;77:1187.
11. Kahrilas PJ, Gupta RR, Jacob P, McLaughlin B, Rana F. Isolated transient LES relaxations are not "subthreshold swallows"? Gastroenterology 1988;95:873 (abstract).
12. Goyal RK, Rattan S. Genesis of basal sphincter pressure: effect of tetrodotoxin on lower esophageal sphincter pressure in opossum in vivo. Gastroenterology 1976;71:62.
13. Dodds WJ, Dent J, Hogan WJ, Arndorfer RC. Effect of atropine on esophageal motor function in humans. Am J Physiol 1981;240:G290.
14. Sloan S, Rademaker AW, Kahrilas PJ. Determinants of gastroesophageal junction competence: hiatal hernia, lower esophageal sphincter or both. Ann Int Med 1992;117:977–982.
15. Behar J, Biancani P, Sheahan DG. Evaluation of esophageal tests in the diagnosis of reflux esophagitis. Gastroenterology 1976;71:9.
16. Kahrilas PJ, Dodds WJ, Hogan WJ, Kern M, Arndorfer RC, Reece A. Esophageal peristaltic dysfunction in peptic esophagitis. Gastroenterology 1986;91:897.
17. Boyle JT, Altschuler SM, Nixon TE, Tuchman DN, Pack AI, Cohen S. Role of the diaphragm in the genesis of lower esophageal sphincter pressure in the cat. Gastroenterology 1985;88:723–733.
18. Mittal RK, Rochester DF, McCallum RW. Sphincteric action of the diaphragm during a relaxed lower esophageal sphincter in humans. Am J Physiol 1989;256:G139–G144.
19. Dent J, Dodds WJ, Hogan WJ, Toouli J. Factors that influence induction of gastroesophageal reflux in normal human subjects. Dig Dis Sci 1988;33:270.

Is there a disorder of esophageal clearance in cases of hiatus hernia?

R.K. Mittal (Charlottesville)

The existence of the hiatal hernia has been acknowledged for over 400 years. In this century, it has been the subject of much controversy, largely due to its unmistakable association with gastroesophageal reflux disease (GERD). In the 1950s and 60s, the presence of hiatal hernia was considered synonymous with GERD. The popularity of the role of hiatal hernia in reflux disease waned in the 1970s and 80s, as the focus of attention in literature shifted to the lower esophageal sphincter (LES) [1]. One observation that blurred the role of hiatal hernia in GERD was the finding that a significant number of patients with hiatal hernia do not have reflux symptoms. However, recent studies indicate that up to 90% of patients with significant reflux disease or endoscopic esophagitis, do indeed have hiatal hernias [2] There is a renewed interest in the relationship of hiatal hernia to GERD, partly due to the understanding of the role of the crural diaphragm as a sphincter mechanism at the lower end of the esophagus.

In order to understand the impact of hiatal hernia in GERD, it is important to review the anatomy of this region. The LES is 2.5–4.5 cm in length, 2 cm of which

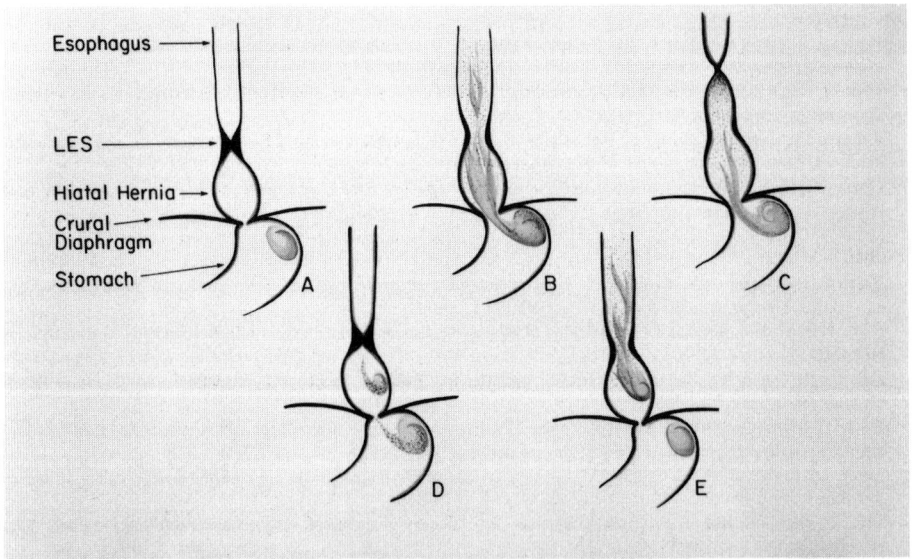

Fig. 1. Mechanism of delayed acid clearance in hiatal hernia. Acid reflux from the stomach (B) is cleared by a peristaltic contraction (C). At the end of the peristaltic contraction, a part of the bolus is retained in the hernial sac and the remainder returns back into the stomach (D). Re-reflux of acid during a swallow-induced LES relaxation from the hernial sac into the esophagus is seen in (E). This process of clearance and re-reflux from the hernial sac can occur swallow after swallow and markedly impair the acid clearance in the esophagus.

are located within the abdomen. The diaphragmatic hiatus is 1.5—2.0 cm in length, and surrounds the proximal half of the LES. The phrenoesophageal ligament, a loose condensation of areola tissue and subperitoneal facia originating from the undersurface of the diaphragm, connects the LES and crural diaphragm. In a normal situation, the crural diaphragm moves along with the rest of the diaphragm in a cranio caudal direction with inspiration and expiration. The LES, because of its attachment through the phrenoesophageal ligament, moves with the crural diaphragm. During swallowing, there is an axial shortening of the esophagus, resulting in movement of the LES in the orad direction of up to 2 cm. This orad movement results in herniation of most of the LES (and maybe even a part of the stomach), into the chest above the crural diaphragm. In some individuals, it appears that this movement may be excessive, resulting in a reducible type of hernia. A nonreducible hiatal hernia is usually defined as a protrusion of 2 cm, or more, of the stomach, above the crural diaphragm that does not return into the normal position in between the swallow. Obviously, the herniation could increase during swallowing in these individuals. The hiatal hernia predisposes to a unique problem of the esophageal acid clearance.

Acid clearance in the normal subjects is a two-step process: 1) bolus clearance; and 2) acid neutralization. Following a reflux episode, either a swallow-induced primary peristalsis or esophageal distention-induced secondary peristalsis clears 90% or more of the bolus from the esophagus into the stomach without affecting the esophageal pH. This step is called the bolus clearance. Following initial bolus clearance, it takes seven to ten swallows to restore the esophageal pH back to normal. This restoration of the esophageal pH is called acid-neutralization. It is due to the bicarbonate and other buffering proteins present in the saliva that travel into the esophagus along with swallow-induced peristalsis.

Longhi et al., using simultaneous barium and manometric studies, described a unique phenomenon in patients with hiatal hernia [3]. They observed that after a swallow of barium, a small amount of barium was trapped in the hiatal hernia sac. This trapped barium can reflux back into the esophagus during a swallow-induced LES relaxation. They described this phenomenon in one patient. We conducted systematic studies to confirm this phenomenon in a larger population [4]. Studies were conducted using simultaneous radionuclide esophageal emptying and esophageal pH monitoring. Following installation into the esophagus of a 15 ml bolus of 0.1 N HCl acid (labeled with 200 µc of 99 m technetium sulfur colloid), radionuclide transit and esophageal pH was monitored. We confirmed that, in the normal individual, a single esophageal contraction cleared the majority of the radionuclide activity from the esophagus back into the stomach without altering the esophageal pH. Esophageal pH increased in a step-wise fashion only with swallows, and it took seven to ten swallows to restore the esophageal pH to above 4. In patients with hiatal hernia, following initial bolus clearance, each swallow resulted in a biphasic pH response. This response consisted of an initial fall in the esophageal pH followed by a rise. This biphasic pH response was in contrast to the uniphasic (only the pH increase with the swallow) response in normal subjects without hiatal hernia. Radionuclide studies indicated that a part of the acid bolus during the initial bolus clearance phase was trapped in the hernial sac. During a swallow, there was initially a reflux of this trapped acid back into the esophagus followed by clearance. This initial reflux followed by clearance, corresponds with LES relaxation and peristaltic phase of the swallow respectively.

Recent studies by Sloan and Kahrilas confirm and extend these observations. They used techniques of simultaneous manometry and barium video fluoroscopy [5]. They observed the entrapment of barium bolus in the hiatal hernia sac following an initial bolus clearance phase. This trapped barium refluxed back into the esophagus during a subsequent swallow-induced LES relaxation. These investigators, furthermore, showed that this phenomenon of re-reflux from the hiatal hernia during a swallow was only present in those patients that demonstrated a nonreducing hiatal hernia. Therefore, based on all of these studies, it appears that hiatal hernia can interfere with the acid clearance mechanism mainly because of lack of swallow-induced peristalsis in the hiatal hernia sac, this then results in retention of a part of the bolus in between the LES and crural diaphragm.

DeMeester et al. demonstrated that acid clearance time markedly improved following Nissen's fundoplication [6]. Reduction of hiatal hernia is part of surgery in Nissen's fundoplication. Therefore, it may be that the improvement in acid clearance as observed by DeMeester et al. was indeed due to the reduction of hiatal hernia. It is tempting to speculate that acid secreted from the herniated stomach gets retained in the hernial sac, and can easily reflux into the esophagus either during a transient or swallow-induced LES relaxation, and can contribute to the pathogenesis of esophagitis in more than one fashion.

References

1. Cohen S, Harris LD. Does hiatus hernia affect competence of the gastroesophagal sphincter? N Engl J Med 1972;284:1053.
2. Sloan S, Kahrilas PJ, Smith CS, Richards CS. Does a nonreducing hiatal hernia predispose to the development of erosive esophagitis? Gastroenterology 1993;104:A193.
3. Longhi EH, Jordon PH. Pressure relationship responsible for reflux in patients with hiatal hernia. Surg Gynecol Obstet 1969;129:734–738.
4. Mittal RK, Lange RC, McCallum RW. Identification and mechanism of delayed esophageal acid clearance in subjects with hiatus hernia. Gastroenterology 1987;92:132–135.
5. Sloan S, Kahrilas PJ. Impairment of esophageal emptying with hiatal hernia. Gastroenterology 1991;100:596–605.
6. DeMeester TR, Lafontaine E, Joelsson BE et al. Relationship of hiatal hernia to the function of the body of the esophagus and the gastroesophageal junction. J Thorac Cardiovasc Surg 1981;82:547–558.

What information can be given by recording of evoked potentials of the esophagus?

G. Tougas, A.R.M. Upton, R.H. Hunt (Hamilton)

Altered esophageal function frequently manifests itself through a variety of symptoms such as dysphagia, heartburn and pain. However, esophageal function can also often be markedly abnormal without any significant symptoms being experienced by the patient, suggesting that under certain conditions the patient does not "perceive" or "sense" these abnormalities. Alternatively, a number of patients are very symptomatic, but do not demonstrate any significant abnormalities on standard esophageal investigations such as endoscopy, biopsies, pH metry and esophageal motility testing.

In recent years, it has been recognized increasingly that esophageal symptoms do not only result from abnormal esophageal motor function or mucosal injury, but can also be due to perceptual or sensory abnormalities. A number of patients are known to experience severe heartburn and to have strong reproduction of their symptoms during esophageal acid instillation (Bernstein's test), without any evidence of significant or pathological acid reflux on 24-h pH-metry or mucosal injury on biopsies. Similarly, it is possible in some patients to reproduce angina-like chest pains of esophageal origin with provocative tests such as balloon distension or edrophonium challenge [1]. However, although in a substantial proportion of patients this positive response was obtained without any discernible abnormalities of motility, in a number of patients the symptoms were reproduced at volumes below the perceptive threshold of control subjects [2].

If it is the perceptual threshold or the sensory perception that is altered in these patients, how can we study this alteration? While symptoms and dose–response relationships can be used, they are far from ideal. Symptoms are notoriously subjective end-points to study. Their perception depends on a large number of variables that include personality, previous experiences, and culture, as well as experimental variables [3]. The response to pain is also known to vary substantially between subjects and even within the same subject on different days [4].

Perception of a peripheral stimulus is a complex process involving peripheral sensors and sensory afferent pathways, but ultimately requiring the afferent signal to produce a response from the brain. In recent years, cortical-evoked responses (also known as cerebral-evoked potentials) have been proposed as a practical approach to the study of visceral sensory pathways. The following presentation will summarize the potential of this technique in the study of sensory pathways in humans.

Cerebral-evoked potentials

Cortical-evoked potentials represent the electrical brain activity produced in response to an external physical stimulus. They have been extensively used to study sensory response in a number of clinical settings in the past 15 years. They are recorded from the scalp of awake patients and volunteers using standard EEG electrodes, and can be precisely correlated with the subjective response produced by the external stimulus. A number of different methods have been used to produce the external stimulus, including electrical, mechanical, thermal, or even chemical stimulation. Evoked potentials have a number of significant advantages over other methods of study of sensory function. Firstly, they are noninvasive, objective, and reproducible. Secondly, they can provide an extremely precise analysis of the time course of the CNS response with resolution at the level of the millisecond. Thirdly, they can be used to examine the type of fibers involved. Finally, certain components of the evoked response have been found to correlate well with the intensity of the stimulus and with the subjective response reported by the subject to this same stimulus [5]. Therefore, evoked potentials provide a tool enabling the objective study of sensory pathways as well as the brain response observed, following peripheral sensory stimuli.

In recent years, brain-evoked potentials have been generally accepted as an objective and quantitative test for the evaluation of sensory function. Visual- and auditory-evoked potentials now have a well-defined clinical role. Somatosensory-evoked potentials have also been used to examine peripheral and spinothalamic afferent function. More recently, the cerebral-evoked potential produced by visceral stimulation has been examined, and the applicability of these methods to the study of visceral sensation demonstrated. Evoked responses produced by stimulation of the urinary bladder, urethra, and rectum have been published, and in some instances are used clinically [6].

Esophageal-evoked potentials

In a number of studies the cerebral-evoked responses to esophageal stimulation were examined [7–12]. Two types of stimulation have been used so far: balloon distension and electrical stimulation. While the evoked responses obtained by the two methods differ, these studies show that this approach can be used to study esophageal sensory pathways.

1. The stimulus used to evoke a cortical response must be of rapid onset, short duration and trigger the recording of evoked activity in a time-locked fashion. It must be of sufficient intensity as to be perceived by the subject. In our laboratory, balloon distension is done with volumes of 10–15 ml, produced through a pump capable of inflation at a rate of 170 ml/s, for 0.5 s. Electrical stimulation is done using a square pulse of 10–16 mA and of 0.2 ms duration. Our experience so far indicates that the number of stimuli should be kept under 25 because of rapid attenuation of the response when more repetitions are used.

2. The typical evoked response obtained is shown on Fig. 1. For both electrical and balloon stimulation a triphasic response is obtained, consisting of three negative (N1,N2,N3) and three positive peaks (P1,P2,P3). Two main end-points have been studied so far. The amplitude of each peak can be measured, as well as the respective latencies of each peaks. If stimulation is done at two different locations

36

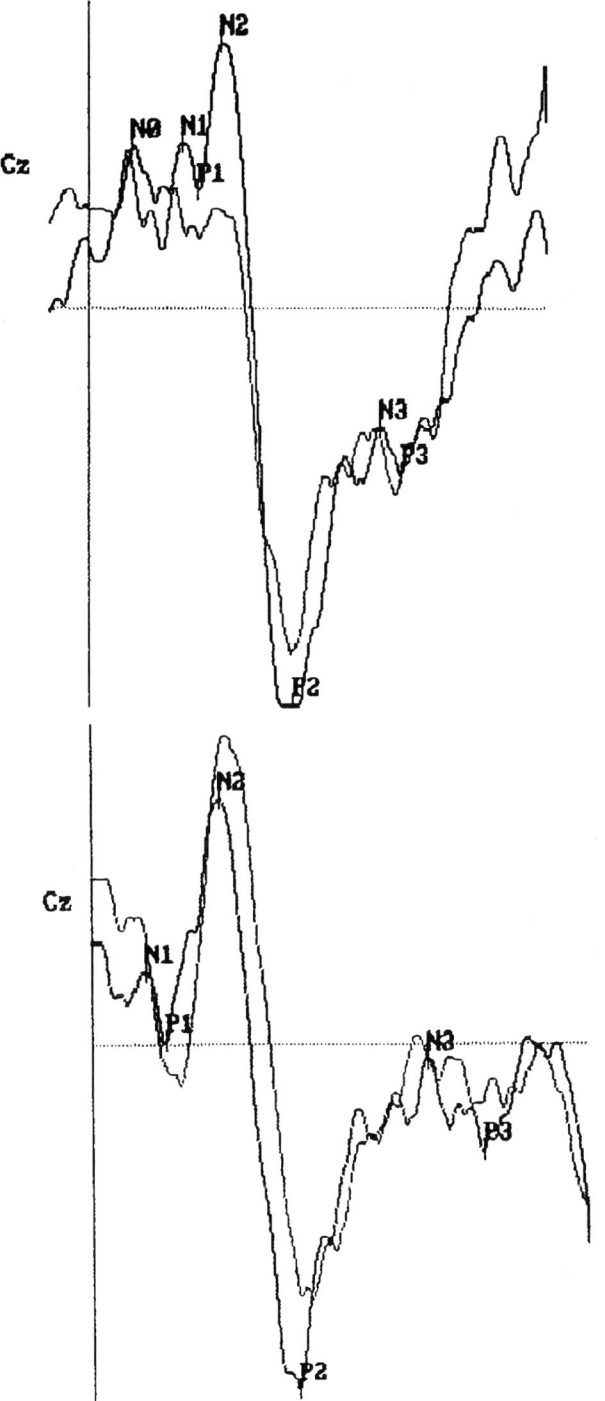

Fig. 1. Cortical-evoked responses obtained following proximal esophageal stimulation using electrical (top) and balloon (bottom) stimulation in a male subject; as can be seen, the responses are reproducible using both methodologies.

along the esophagus, the conduction velocity of the afferent impulse can be measured as the dividend of the distance between the two sites over the difference in latencies of each peak at both sites.

3. While the number of studies using both modalities of stimulation is small, there appear to be significant differences between the two. Firstly, it is much more difficult to obtain consistent and reproducible responses using balloon distension. This is probably due to the fact that the stimulus is much shorter in duration with electrical stimulation than with balloon distension. Balloon distension also tends to produce more swallowing and esophageal activity than electrical stimulation, causing variability of the response. Secondly, we have shown that the conduction velocities obtained by the two modalities differ: the conduction velocity measured with electrical stimulation has been reported by ourselves and by Frieling et al. [8,12] to be between 5 and 10 m/s, while conductions of less than 2 m/s have been reported by our group, as well as by Smout et al. [7,13]. This suggests that different afferent fibers are involved.

4. Using further signal-processing and brain-mapping techniques we have also shown that it is possible to produce topographic maps of the brain response to stimulation [10]. Recent advances in "dipole localization" modelling, used in conjunction with a large number (20) of scalp recording electrodes, now allow a much more precise localization of the site involved in the response [14].

Perspectives

The exact role of sensory afferent pathways in esophageal physiological and pathological processes can now be objectively defined using approaches such as those described here. A limited number of studies have already demonstrated changes in the response obtained in patients with diabetes mellitus [15,16], as well as in patients with noncardiac chest pain [17]. The exact place of these techniques in the diagnosis of esophageal disorders remains to be studied.

References

1. Richter JE, Bradley LA, Castell DO. Esophageal chest pain: current controversies in pathogenesis, diagnosis, and therapy. Ann Int Med 1989;110:66–78.
2. Richter JE, Barish CF, Castell DO. Abnormal esophageal perception in patients with esophageal pain. Gastroenterology 1986;91:845–852.
3. Wolff BB. Behavioral measurements of human pain. In: Steinbach RA (ed) The Psychology of Pain. New York: Raven Press, 1978:128–168.
4. DeVault KR, Castell DO. Esophageal balloon distention and cerebral evoked potential recording in the evaluation of unexplained chest pain. Am J Med 1992;92(suppl 5A):20S–26S.
5. Chen ACN, Chapman CR, Harkins SW. Brain evoked potentials are functional correlates of induced pain in man. Pain 1979;6:305–314.
6. Loening-Baucke V, Read NW, Yamada T. Further evaluation of the afferent nervous pathways from the rectum. Am J Physiol Gastrointest Liver Physiol 1992;262:G927–G933.
7. Smout AJPM, DeVore MS, Castell DO. Cerebral potentials evoked by esophageal distension in humans. Am J Physiol Gastrointest Liver Physiol 1990;259:G955–G959.
8. Frieling T, Enck P, Wienbeck M. Cerebral responses evoked by electrical stimulation of the esophagus in normal subjects. Gastroenterology 1989;97:475–478.

9. Castell DO, Wood JD, Frieling T, Wright FS, Vieth RF. Cerebral electrical potentials evoked by balloon distention of the human esophagus. Gastroenterology 1990;98:662–666.
10. Tougas G, Fitzpatrick D, Hunt RH, Clarke B, Upton ARM. Vagal and esophageal-evoked potentials in normal, epileptic and diabetic patients. Ann Neurol 1992;(abstract).
11. Upton ARM, Tougas G, Tallalla A, White AM, Hudoba P, Fitzpatrick D, Clarke B, Hunt RH. Neurophysiological effects of left vagal stimulation in man. Pacing Clin Electrophysiol 1991;14:70–76.
12. Tougas G, Hudoba P, Fitzpatrick D, Hunt RH, Upton ARM. Cerebral-evoked potential responses following direct vagal and esophageal electrical stimulation in humans. Am J Physiol Gastrointest Liver Physiol 1993;264:G486–G491.
13. Tougas G, Fitzpatrick D, Upton ARM, Hunt RH. The cortical evoked responses produced by balloon distention and electrical stimulation of the esophagus involve different afferent vagal fibres. Gastroenterology 1993;104(abstract):A592.
14. Chen ACN. Human brain measures of clinical pain: a review. I. Topographic mappings. Pain 1993;54:115–132.
15. Rathmann W, Enck P, Frieling T, Gries FA. Visceral afferent neuropathy in diabetic gastroparesis. Diabet Care 1991;14:1086–1089.
16. Tougas G, Hunt RH, Fitzpatrick D, Upton AR. Evidence of impaired afferent vagal function in patients with diabetes gastroparesis. Pacing Clin Electrophysiol 1992;15:1597–1602.
17. Smout AJPM, DeVore MS, Dalton CB, Castell DO. Cerebral potentials evoked by oesophogeal distention in patients with noncardiac chest pain. Gut 1992;33:298–302.

Epidemiology

What is physiological gastroesophageal reflux?

J.R. Bennett (Hull)

This paper will discuss the phenomenon of gastroesophageal reflux disease (GERD) which is not accompanied by symptoms nor endoscopic abnormalities and does not lead to complications. It is at present detectable only by intraesophageal pH monitoring. There are many technical aspects of pH monitoring which affect the results of such tests but they will not be dealt with except where variations of methodology cause registrable acid reflux which would not be revealed by other techniques.

pH recordings in "normal" individuals

Although esophageal pH had been measured over short periods since the 1950s, it was not until the 1960s that prolonged recordings were made. It was immediately seen [1—3] that "normal" subjects had short episodes of acid reflux mainly after meals but uncommonly at night.

This has since been repeatedly observed [4] but it poses a question about the selection of "normal" subjects. Careful epidemiological studies show that only one-third of British subjects *never* experience heartburn [5]. Few studies have been as careful as that of Johnsson et al. (1987) [6] whose normal subjects had "no *past* or present symptoms of gastrointestinal disease... " and all had normal endoscopic examination (9% of their asymptomatic subjects had an endoscopic abnormality and were rejected). They also pointed out that the resulting pH data was skewed, and so used the 95th percentile as the upper reference limit. Having obtained clear discrimination between 20 normal and 20 symptomatic patients the study was enlarged. Overlap then resulted, four patients having results within the normal range and one normal subject being above it. All other studies have also shown an overlap between their symptomatic patients and normal controls, however, the latter were selected [7–12].

Moreover, Smout found a correlation between age and duration of acid reflux, so that in subjects over 45 the 95th percentile figure for % time below 4 was 12, which was much higher than generally recognised "normal values". However, Kruse-Andersen et al. [13] did not find any increase in reflux values when 10 healthy subjects were studied 8 years apart. Alternative analysis using receiver operator characteristics (ROC) to identify the best discriminatory values [9] indicate pH 4 as the best cut-off point and demonstrate threshold values similar to those derived by standard statistical methods. Nevertheless, overlap between values for normal and symptomatic subjects remains.

It is therefore apparent that in prolonged recording of the lower esophageal pH, falls below pH 4, presumptively indicating acid gastresophageal reflux, can be detected in almost every asymptomatic, endoscopically normal person. Furthermore, in some of these apparently normal individuals the frequency and duration of such episodes can be greater than in some patients with symptoms attributable to reflux or with endoscopic changes of reflux esophagitis, even when matched for age. Some subjects (especially older ones) may have values for pH exposure well into the "pathological" range.

pH recording related to symptoms

A study of 86 patients with "symptoms typical of gastroesophageal reflux" graded by severity showed the usual correlation between severity of symptoms and mean pH reflux time, but 18 were within the normal range including four with the most severe symptoms [10].

Twelve patients with endoscopic esophagitis also fell into the normal range of pH recording, three of them with confluent erosions, ulcer/stenosis or Barrett's.

When 304 patients had pH monitoring for suspected GERD, heartburn occurred in 48% of the 138 with normal pH results compared to 68% of them with abnormal reflux.

Schlesinger and colleagues [14] found that of 30 patients with "reflux symptoms" and a normal endoscopy, only 21% had pH reflux outside normal values (although the group as a whole were significantly greater than normal). Ninety-three percent of those with normal studies responded to antireflux therapy.

Correlation between pH studies and endoscopy show a limited concordance of only 60% [15].

Reflux episodes related to symptoms

The studies above relate the sum of reflux episodes in a given period (usually 24 h) to symptoms extending over longer periods (days, months). There have been attempts to relate specific symptomatic episodes to single reflux events. The symptom usually investigated has been chest pain rather than more characteristic heartburn. The frequency of a close correlation of reflux with pain has varied from 24 to 62% [16–18] but it is not stated how many pH recorded reflux events were painless. Ghillebert et al. (1990) [19], used a binomial formula to indicate a probability of pain associated with reflux being due to chance, while Armstrong and colleagues (1992) [20] developed a computer program which compared the frequency distributions of pH events associated with pain, with the frequency distribution of symptom-unrelated pH events.

Acid sensitivity of the esophagus has traditionally been determined by standardised acid perfusion of the lower esophagus ("Bernstein test"). Correlation between the results of this test and scores for pain related to acid reflux during ambulatory monitoring, are poor.

In Hewson and colleagues (1989) [21] study, only 48% of Bernstein-positive patients had acid-related pain by pH monitoring; Kruse-Andersen (personal communication) found no difference in the frequency of pain episodes related to reflux between patients who were acid perfusion positive or negative.

Conclusion

Intraesophageal pH is a continuous variable in the community, with a distribution skewed to the right. The greater the acid exposure of the esophagus, the more likely the subject is to have reflux symptoms or esophagitis, but other factors must be important in determining these consequences. The corollary of this is that it is simplistic to define results of pH recording as being "normal" or "abnormal". The quantitative result of such recordings must be considered as one piece of evidence to be analysed in combination with symptoms and endoscopic changes; where possible, a score relating reflux episodes to symptoms is desirable.

References

1. Miller FA, Dovale J, Gunther T. Utilization of underlying pH probe for evaluation of acid-peptic diathesis. Arch Surg 1964;89:199–203.
2. Miller FA, Doberneck RC. Diagnosis of the acid-peptic diathesis by continuous pH analysis. Surg Clin North Am 1967; 47:1325–1334.
3. Spencer J. Prolonged pH recording in the study of gastro-oesophageal reflux. Br J Surg 1969;56:912.
4. Wallin L, Madsen T. Twelve hour simultaneous registration of acid reflux and peristaltic activity in the oesophagus: a study in normal subjects. Scand J Gastroenterol 1979;14:561–566.
5. Jones R, Lydeard S. Prevalence of symptoms of dyspepsia in the community. Br J Med 1989;298:30–32.
6. Johnsson F, Joelsson B, Isberg PE. Ambulatory 24-hour intra-esophageal pH-monitoring in the diagnosis of gastro-esophageal reflux disease. Gut 1987;28:1145–1150.
7. Branicki FJ, Evans DF, Ogilvie AL, Atkinson M, Hardcastle JD. Ambulatory monitoring of oesophageal pH in reflux oeso-phagitis using a portable radiotelemetry system. Gut 1982;23:992–998.

8. Vitale GC, Cheadle WG, Gadek S, Michel ME, Cuschieri A. Computerized 24-hour ambulatory esophageal pH-monitoring and esophageal gastro-duodenoscopy in the reflux patient. Ann Surg 1984;200:724−729.
9. Schindlbeck NE, Heinrich C, Konig A, Dendorfer A, Pace F, Muller-Lissner A. Optimal thresholds, sensitivity and specificity of long term pH monitoring for the detection of gastroesophageal reflux disease. Gastroenterology 1987;93: 85−90.
10. Mattioli V, Pilotti V, Zannoli R, Carvui N, Loria P, Felice V, Conci A, Castellini A, Gozzetti G. Twenty-four Hour Home Esophago-gastro pH Monitoring: Standardisation of the Method. Third European Symposium on Gastrointestinal Motility, Bruges, 1986:91.
11. Wiener GJ, Morgan TM, Copper JB, Wu WC, Castell DO, Sinclair JW, Richter JE. Ambulatory 24-hour esophageal pH monitoring. Dig Dis Sci 1988;33:1127−1133.
12. Smout AJPM, Breedijk M, van der Zouw C, Akkermans LMA. Physiological gastroesophageal reflux and esophageal motor activity studied with a new system for 24-hour recording and automated analysis. Dig Dis Sci 1989;34:372−378.
13. Kruse-Andersen S, Wallin L, Madsen T. The influence of age on esophageal acid defense mechanism and spontaneous acid gastroesophageal reflux. Am J Gastroenterol 1988;83:637−639.
14. Schlesinger PK, Donahue PE, Schmid B, Layden TJ. Limitations of 24-hour intraesophageal pH monitoring in the hospital setting. Gastroenterology 1985;89:797−804.
15. Armstrong D, Fraser R. Diagnosis and assessment of gastro-oesophageal reflux disease. Gullet 1993;3(suppl):31−41.
16. Peters L, Maas L, Petty D, Dalton C, Penner D, Wu WC, Castell DO, Richter JE. Spontaneous noncardiac chest pain. Gastroenterology 1988;94:878−886.
17. DeMeester TR, O'Sullivan GC, Bermudez GA, Midell A, Cimochowski GE, O'Drobinak J. Esophageal function in patients with angina-type chest pain and normal coronary angiogram. Ann Surg 1982;4:488−498.
18. Janssens J, Vantrappen G, Ghillebert G. 24-hour recording of esophageal pressure and pH in patients with noncardiac chest pain. Gastroenterology 1986;90:1978−1984.
19. Ghillebert G, Janssens J, Vantrappen G, Nevens F, Piessens J. Ambulatory 24-hour intraoesophageal pH and pressure recordings vs. provocation tests in the diagnosis of chest pain of oesophageal origin. Gut 1990;31:738−744.
20. Armstrong D, Emde C, Inauen W, Blum AL. Diagnostic assessment of gastroesophageal reflux disease: what is possible vs. what is practical. Hepato Gastroenterol 1992;39(suppl):3−13.
21. Hewson EG, Sinclair JW, Dalton CB, Wu WC, Castell DO, Richter JE. Acid perfusion test: does it have a role in the assessment of noncardiac chest pain? Gut 1989;33:305−310.

J. Janssens (Leuven)

Brief episodes of acid reflux occur in healthy subjects, especially in the postprandial period. During the day the intraesophageal pH is less than 4, for about 2% of the recording time; nocturnal episodes of reflux are normally very rare. These short-lived episodes of reflux remain asymptomatic and do not result in esophagitis; they correspond to what is called physiological reflux.

Symptoms and lesions of esophagitis appear when the episodes of reflux become more frequent and more prolonged; the reflux is then considered to be pathological. In normal subjects, as in patients with pathological reflux, nearly all the episodes of reflux obey one of the following three mechanisms:

− total transient relaxation of the gastroesophageal sphincter;

− a transient increase in intra-abdominal pressure;

− spontaneous reflux through a very hypotonic sphincter.

Physiological reflux nearly always follows transient relaxation of the lower esophageal sphincter (LES) (94% of cases); while in patients with esophagitis this mechanism is responsible for only 65% of the episodes of reflux. A transient increase in intra-abdominal pressure and spontaneous reflux are responsible for 17 and 18% of episodes of reflux respectively in patients with esophagitis [1].

The mechanism responsible for the induction of transient lower esophageal sphincter (tLES) relaxations is unclear. Some authors believe that transient LES relaxations are triggered by partial or incomplete swallowing [2,3]. Others feel that gastric distension is the major factor that induces the transient LES relaxations via vagovagal reflexes initiated by stimulation of mechanoreceptors in the gastric wall [4]. This mechanism could also explain the increased rate of transient LES relaxations and reflux during the postprandial period [5]. Transient LES relaxations may also occur at night, but almost exclusively during periods of being awake.

Relatively little is known about the occurrence and control of transient LES relaxations in patients with reflux disease. Dodds and Dent found a higher rate of transient LES relaxations in reflux patients [1,6], while Mittal and McCallum found that normals and patients had the same rate of tLES relaxations, but that the tLES relaxations were more frequently accompanied by reflux in the patient group [2,7]. When an episode of reflux has occurred, it is important that the refluxed material be evacuated from the esophagus as fast as possible. Besides the more or less irritant nature of the refluxed material, it is the duration of contact with the mucosa which determines whether or not esophagitis develops. Esophagitis seems to be more particularly related to long-lasting episodes of reflux.

In the upright position, gravity plays an important role in the elimination of this refluxed material. This is why patients with orthostatic reflux develop esophagitis less frequently than those with decubitus reflux or mixed reflux. In the prone position, (primary or secondary) esophageal peristalsis is mainly responsible for the clearance of acid. Although gravity and peristalsis are capable of returning nearly all the reflux material to the stomach, that in itself does not alter the pH of the tiny amount which still remains in contact with the esophageal mucosa. This residue must be neutralized chemically by saliva [8]. Physiological reflux is rapidly cleared from the lumen: it almost exclusively occurs in the upright position when gravity clears the lumen; if reflux occurs in the prone position normal peristalsis guarantees a fast clearance.

Twenty-four hour intraesophageal pH recording has become a routine procedure in clinical practice. Automatic analysis calculates various reflux parameters (i.e., the number of reflux episodes, the percentage of time of the recording when the pH is below 4, which is an expression of the total exposure of the esophageal mucosa to acid), the mean duration of the reflux episodes and the number of long lasting (> 5 min) reflux episodes (which reflect the efficiency of the acid clearing function). When these variables are determined in a group of healthy controls, they define in another way what is called "physiological reflux" [9]. If one uses the numerical parameters of a 24-h pH recording to distinguish normal subjects from patients with gastrocsophageal reflux disease (GERD), the technique is excellent to distinguish normals from patients with erosive esophagitis; however, when patients with symptoms without lesions are included, the distinction is less clear [10,11]. Patients with symptomatic GERD, as a group have on intraesophageal pH measurements an increased exposure to acid as compared to control subjects [12]. Patients with almost continuous symptoms have a much greater acid exposure than patients with daily symptoms or with occasional symptoms only [13]. However, symptomatic reflux and/or a positive acid perfusion test may be found in patients with normal esophageal acid exposure time during pH monitoring [14].

Although heartburn is the regular symptom induced by acid reflux, in some patients reflux may be responsible for pseudoanginal chest pain rather than heartburn. Prolonged measurements of esophageal pH has shown that, in subjects with angina-like chest pain of esophageal origin, most of the painful episodes appear to be caused by reflux, with or without a disorder of esophageal motor function [15]. In a recent overview it was shown that of all chest pain episodes that were of proven esophageal origin, as many as 71% of them appeared to be acid related [16]. In some patients with esophageal angina-like chest pain, an identical painful episode may be provoked either by isolated reflux (without motor disorder) or by severe alterations in motor function (without reflux) or again, at other times, by the association of reflux and motor disorders. Esophageal acid perfusion (Bernstein's test) may sometimes provoke this typical painful episode in patients in whom spontaneous episodes of pain seem to be connected solely with motor disorders without reflux. There therefore seems to be a group of patients in whom the esophagus is sensitive to numerous stimuli which are different from each other; it is this entity that has been called "irritable esophagus" [17].

Numerical analysis of the 24-h pH recording in these patients frequently appears to fall into normal limits.

Conclusions

Physiological reflux should be defined as the amount of reflux which occurs in a normal subject, who does not complain of reflux symptoms and has no endoscopic esophagitis. This physiological reflux can be quantified by numerical analysis of a 24-h pH recording. However, some patients with typical reflux symptoms and especially patients with atypical reflux symptoms (i.e., chest pain) have a numerical analysis of a 24-h pH recording which is in the normal range, although their reflux clearly is not physiological.

References

1. Dodds WJ, Dent J, Hogan WJ et al. Mechanism of gastroesophageal reflux in patients with reflux esophagitis. N Engl J Med 1982;307:1547—1552.
2. Mittal RK, McCallum RW. Characteristics and frequency of transient relaxations of the lower esophageal sphincter in patients with reflux esophagitis. Gastroenterology 1988;95:593.
3. Paterson WG, Rattan S, Goyal RK. Experimental induction of isolated lower esophageal sphincter relaxation in anesthetized opossums. J Clin Invest 1986;77:1187—1193.
4. Holloway RH, Hongo M, Berger K et al. Gastric distension: A mechanism for postprandial gastroesophageal reflux. Gastroenterology 1985;89:770.
5. Holloway RH, Kocyan P, Dent J. Provocation of transient lower esophageal sphincter relaxations by meals in patients with symptomatic gastroesophageal reflux. Dig Dis Sci 1991;8:1034—1039.
6. Dent J, Holloway RH, Toouli J, Dodds WJ. Mechanisms of lower oesophageal sphincter incompetence in patients with symptomatic gastroesophageal reflux. Gut 1988;29:1020.

7. Freidin N, Fisher MJ, Taylor W, Boyd D, Surratt P, McCallum RW, Mittal RK. Sleep and nocturnal acid reflux in normal subjects and patients with reflux oesophagitis. Gut 1991;32:1275—1279.
8. Helm JF, Dodds WJ, Pele LR et al. Effect of esophageal emptying and saliva on clearance of acid from the esophagus. N Engl J Med 1984;310:284—288.
9. Johnson LF. New concepts and methods in the study and treatment of gastroesophageal reflux disease. Med Clin North Am 1981;65:1195—1222.
10. Euler AR, Byrne WJ. Twenty-four hour esophageal intraluminal pH probe testing: a comparative analysis. Gastroenterology 1981;80:957—961.
11. Janssens J, Vantrappen G, Peeters T, Ghillebert G. How do 24-hour pH measurements distinguish the disease spectrum of reflux patients. Gastroenterology 1985;88:1431(abstract).
12. DeMeester TR, Johnson LF, Joseph GJ, Toscano MS, Hall AW, Skinner DB. Patterns of gastroesophageal reflux in health and disease. Ann Surg 1976;1984:459—470.
13. Joelsson B, Johnsson F. Heartburn — the acid test. Gut 1989;30:1523—1525.
14. Howard PJ, Maher L, Pryde A, Heading RC. Symptomatic gastro-oesophageal reflux, abnormal oesophageal acid exposure, and mucosal acid sensitivity are three separate, though related, aspects of gastro-oesophageal reflux disease. Gut 1991; 32:128—132.
15. Janssens J, Vantrappen G, Ghillebert G. 24-hour recording of esphageal pressure and pH in patients with noncardiac chest pain. Gastroenterology 1986;90:1978—1984.
16. Janssens J, Vantrappen G. Irritable esophagus. Am J Med 1992;92(suppl 5A):27S—32S.
17. Vantrappen G, Janssens J, Ghillebert G. The irritable esophagus — a frequent cause of angina-like pain. Lancet 1987;I:1232—1234.

R.S. Fisher (Philadelphia)

Gastroesophageal reflux is defined as the retrograde movement of the stomach contents across the gastroesophageal junction into the esophagus. Reflux can be regarded as physiological as long as it does not cause symptoms or damage the esophageal mucosa. In this monograph the composition, measurement and regulation of physiological gastroesophageal reflux will be discussed.

Composition of the refluxate

Over time the composition of the gastroesophageal refluxate reflects the stomach contents. During a 24-h period the stomach contains variable quantities of hydrochloric acid, pepsinogen/pepsin (proteolytic enzyme), mucus, and digestive products derived from food. The stomach contents change continuously depending upon the quantity of acid secreted, the ratio between the inactive pepsinogens and active pepsins, the amount of mucus and bicarbonate secreted by the gastric mucosa, and the composition of ingested meals. In some situations enterogastric reflux may occur introducing bile salts and, perhaps, pancreatic enzymes into the stomach and making them available to regurgitate into the esophagus. Bacterial overgrowth in the stomach or proximal small intestine can alter the digestive products and/or the structure of bile salts within the stomach. These changes may be important because they could alter the potency of the refluxate.

Gastric acid secretion has been studied basally and in response to meals and secretagogues such as pentagastrin. In addition, 24-h intragastric pH profiles have characterized the effects of different meals, gastric emptying, and sleep. It is important to recognize that there are times during the day when the normal stomach contains little acid. Therefore, gastroesophageal reflux would not be detected by intraesophageal pH monitoring. Of interest, these periods of physiologic gastric alkalinity may occur postprandially when the lower esophageal sphincter (LES) pressure may be reduced by transient lower esophageal sphincter relaxations.

Measurement of gastroesophageal reflux

Much of our knowledge about gastroesophageal reflux is based upon detection of acid within the esophagus using glass or antimony, hydrogen-detecting electrodes placed at varying distances, usually 5 cm, above the LES. Using 24-h intraesophageal pH monitoring, esophageal pH has been reported to be less than 4 for approximately 6% of the total time, 8% of the upright (postprandial) time and 2% of the recumbent (sleeping) time [4,5,25]. These "normal values" are approximations based on numerous reports. Although esophageal pH monitoring may be useful to correlate symptoms with acid reflux episodes into the esophagus and to establish guidelines for acid exposure, this technique has a number of limitations. First, 24-h intraesophageal pH monitoring does not record the volume of reflux, but only measures acid concentrations in the microenvironment of the pH electrode. Secondly, pH monitoring detects acid reflux, but not reflux of bile salts (primary or secondary), pancreatic enzymes, or abnormal digestive products. Also, it is well established that the intragastric pH is not below 4 continuously throughout the day. Therefore, reflux episodes which occur during nonacid periods would not be detected by pH monitoring. Thirdly, esophageal pH monitoring could be affected by salivary volume and composition and by bicarbonate secretion from the esophageal, stomach and duodenal mucosa and from the pancreas.

Gastroesophageal scintigraphy has been employed in some centers to evaluate gastroesophageal reflux [9]. This technique utilizes γ emitting radionuclides mixed with the stomach contents, not only to detect, but also to quantitate reflux. If the radionuclide mixes homogeneously with the gastric contents, counting γ scintillations over the esophagus will reflect gastroesophageal reflux of both the acid and nonacid gastric contents. Unfortunately, gastroesophageal scintigraphy is limited by gastric emptying. Once the γ labeled gastric contents have emptied from the stomach, this technique will not demonstrate gastroesophageal reflux. Therefore, it cannot be used for prolonged studies beyond 1 or 2 h. Roentgenographic techniques utilizing radiopaque barium have also been used to detect reflux, but are insensitive and non-quantitative.

Whether bile salts, pancreatic enzymes, or high pH (alkaline) liquid regurgitate normally from the duodenum into the stomach and then, perhaps, into the esophagus remains unresolved [16–18,22–24,28]. Several techniques have been introduced to detect "enterogastroesophageal" reflux. The most direct technique employs an indwelling esophageal tube to aspirate the esophageal contents and measure bile salts, bilirubin or pancreatic enzymes. Scintigraphic methods have been introduced employing γ labeled hepatocystic agents, usually derivatives of iminodiacetic acid (IDA), to mark bile salts so that their regurgitation into both the stomach and the esophagus can be identified. To date, this technique has been used mostly to detect and quantify enterogastric (bile) reflux in patients who have undergone peptic ulcer surgery. Recently, bilirubin and bile acid-sensing probes have been introduced to detect and quantitate enterogastric and enterogastroesophageal reflux. To date, little published data are available from studies using these new probes.

Determinants of physiological gastroesophageal reflux

The gastroesophageal pressure gradient is between 5 and 10 mmHg throughout much of the day. Therefore, if it were not for the antireflux barrier at the gastroesophageal junction, reflux would be continuous. Exceptions occur after swallowing or esophageal distension when primary or secondary peristaltic contractions, respectively, migrate aborally through the esophagus. Reflux could occur at times of increased intra-abdominal pressure during exercise, bending or straining to move the bowels. Intragastric pressures increase during the fed or postprandial period when antral contractions become more pronounced and regular. However, despite a pressure gradient conducive to reflux for most of the day, esophageal pH is below 4 for only one twentieth of the total time. Of course, this does not include nonacid reflux which would not be detected by intraesophageal pH monitoring.

The major antireflux factors are the gastroesophageal junction high pressure zone, constituted by the lower esophageal sphincter and the crural diaphragm, and the distal paraesophageal pressure. It is generally accepted that the lower esophageal sphincter contributes a tonic junction pressure of 12 to 26 mmHg above the intragastric pressure [1,2,4,26–28]; the crural diaphragm is mostly responsible for phasic changes in the high pressure zone but also, perhaps, for a component of the tonic pressure [3,19,20]. The high pressure zone pressure may be affected by a number of external factors. The most obvious are certain foods such as fat, xanthines (chocolate, cola), onions, peppermint and smoking which may decrease the resting LES pressure by a variety of mechanisms. When food-induced physiologic decreases in resting LES pressure are accompanied by increased postprandial antral contractility, this may theoretically predispose to physiologic reflux events. However, the most important factor in the production of physiological reflux is spontaneous (inappropriate or transient) LES relaxation which occurs independently of swallowing, mostly during the postprandial or fed period [7,8,21,29]. Dent and his colleagues have attributed more than 60% of physiological reflux episodes to these spontaneous LES relaxations. The mechanism for spontaneous LES relaxation may be an aberrant swallowing mechanism, which does not stimulate esophageal peristalsis, as evidenced by submental EMG recording. Another mechanism for physiologic reflux episodes may be swallows associated with abnormal or incomplete esophageal peristalsis which may account for up to 10%. A minority of reflux episodes are due to repetitive swallows over a short time period leading to prolonged LES relaxation. It is of interest that physiologic increases in intra-abdominal pressure alone, which occur during exercise, do not usually cause gastroesophageal reflux because of adaptive pressure increases at the high pressure zone which more than compensate for the elevated intra-abdominal pressure [1,2]. These adaptive high pressure zone responses are mediated by cholinergic mechanisms.

Coordination between esophageal contractions, LES relaxation and increased postprandial gastric motility may be important in determining physiologic gastro-esophageal reflux. However, to date, gastric contractions have not been measured in most studies of this phenomenon.

Esophageal motility is undoubtedly an important determinant of physiological esophageal acid exposure [6,10]. After some reflux episodes, a secondary esophageal contraction strips the refluxate from the body of the esophagus [13,15]. In addition, abnormal primary esophageal contractions have been reported during some physiologic reflux episodes. Equally important in limiting esophageal acid exposure is the saliva and its bicarbonate content which neutralizes the acid refluxate in a stepwise fashion [14]. Fortunately, in normal subjects little reflux occurs in the recumbent position during sleep when swallowing and primary peristaltic contractions are reduced to one to three per hour and salivation is diminished.

To summarize, the factors which separate physiological from nonphysiological (pathogenic) gastroesophageal reflux are not clear. Most likely, the composition and volume of the refluxate, the contact time between the refluxate and the esophageal mucosa, and the defenses of the esophageal mucosa determine whether gastroesopha-geal reflux will be physiological or whether it will produce symptoms and complications.

References

1. Cohen S, Harris DL. Lower esophageal sphincter pressure as an index of lower esophageal sphincter strength. Gastro-enterology 1970;58:157—163.
2. Cohen S, Harris DL. Does hiatal hernia affect competence of the lower esophageal sphincter. N Engl J Med 1971;284: 1053—1056.
3. Csendes A, Miranda M, Espinoza M et al. Parameter and location of the muscular gastroesophageal position or cardia in control subjects and in patients with reflux esophagitis or achalasia. Scand J Gastroenterol 1981;16:951—956.
4. De Caestecker JS, Heading RC. Esophageal pH monitoring. Gastroenterol Clin North Am 1990;19(3):645—669.
5. DeMeester TR, Johnson LF, Joseph GJ et al. Patterns of gastroesophageal reflux in health and disease. Am Surg 1976; 184:459—465.
6. Dent J, Dodds WJ, Friedman RH et al. Mechanism of gastroesophageal reflux in recumbent asymptomatic human subjects. J Clin Invest 1980;65:256—262.
7. Dent J, Holloway RH, Toouli J et al. Mechanisms of lower esophageal sphincter incompetence in patients with symp-tomatic gastroesophageal reflux. Gut 1988;29:1020—1025.
8. Dent J, Dodds WJ, Hogan WJ, Toouli J. Factors that influence induction of gastroesophageal reflux in normal human subjects. Dig Dis Sci 1988;33:270—277.
9. Fisher RS, Malmud LS, Roberts GS et al. Gastroesophageal (GE) scintiscanning to detect and quantitate GE reflux. Gastroenterology 1976;70:301—308.
10. Dodds WJ, Hogan WJ, Helm JF et al. Pathogenesis of reflux esophagitis. Gastroenterology 1981;81:376—384.
11. Giacosa A, Bocchini R, Molinari F. Reflux esophagitis and duodenogastric reflux. Scand J Gastroenterol 1981;16(suppl 67): 115—122.

12. Goyal RK, Rattan S. Neurohormonal, hormonal and drug receptors for the lower esophageal sphincter. Gastroenterology 1979;74:598—617.
13. Helm JF, Dodds WJ, Pelc LR et al. Effect of esophageal emptying and saliva on clearance of acid from the esophagus. N Engl J Med 1984;310:284—288.
14. Helm JF, Dodds WJ, Hogan WJ et al. Acid neutralizing capacity of human saliva. Gastroenterology 1982;83:69—74.
15. Helm JF, Dodds WJ, Riedel DR et al. Determinants of esophageal acid clearance in normal subjects. Gastroenterology 1983;85:607—612.
16. Liebermann-Meffert D, Allgöwer M, Schmid P et al. Muscular equivalent of the lower esophageal sphincter. Gastro-enterology 1979;76:31—38.
17. Lillemoe KD, Johnson LF, Harmon JW. Alkaline esophagitis: A comparison of the ability of components of gastroduodenal contents to improve the rabbit esophagus. Gastroenterology 1983;85:621—628.
18. Matikamen M, Lactikainer T, Kalima T et al. Bile acid composition and esophagitis after total gastrectomy. Am J Surg 1982;143:196—201.
19. Mittal RK, Fisher M, McCallum RW et al. Human lower esophageal sphincter pressure response to increased intra-abdominal pressure. Am J Physiol 1990;21:G624—G630.
20. Mittal RK, Rochester DF, McCallum RW. Electrical and mechanical activity in the human lower esophageal sphincter during diaphragmatic contraction. J Clin Invest 1988;81:1182—1189.
21. Mittal RK, McCallum RW. Characteristics of transient lower esophageal sphincter relaxation in humans. Am J Physiol 1987;252:G636—G641.
22. Orlando RC, Bozymski EM. Heartburn in pernicious anemia — a consequence of bile reflux. N Eng J Med 1973;289:522—525.
23. Paterson WG, Rattan S, Goyal RK. Experimental induction of isolated lower esophageal sphincter relaxation in anesthetized opossums. J Clin Invest 1986;77:1187—1189.
24. Safaie-Shirazi S, DenBesten L, Zike WL. Effect of bile salts on the ionic permeability of the esophageal mucosa and their role in the production of esophagitis. Gastroenterology 1975;68:728—734.
25. Spencer J. Prolonged pH recording in the study of gastroesophageal reflux. Br J Surg 1967;56:912—917.
26. Tottrup A, Forman A, Uldbjez N et al. Mechanical properties of isolated human esophageal smooth muscle. Am J Physiol 1990;21:G329—G337.
27. Tottrup A, Forman A, Funch-Jensen P et al. Effects of transmural field stimulation in isolated muscle strips from the human esophagus. Am J Physiol 1990;21:G344—G351.
28. Wickrenesinghe PC, Dayrit PP, Manfredi OL et al. Quantitative evaluation of bile diversion surgery using Tc-99m HIDA scintigraphy. Gastroenterology 1983;84:354—363.

What is the role of alcoholism in GER and esophagitis?

H. Tønnesen (Copenhagen)

In clinical practice, about one-third of chronic alcohol abusers suffers from upper abdominal dyspepsia, predominantly esophagitis [1]. So far, the underlying mechanism is not clear. It is probably multifactorial, and differs with different drinking habits, but is independent of administration form, i.e intravenous or peroral.

Acute consumption

Acute alcohol intake in healthy volunteers decreases the lower esophagus sphincter pressure and allows more reflux episodes to occur [2]. The mechanism is direct both on nerves and smooth muscles as well as indirect by stimulation of, for instance, the gastrin production, which will lower the sphincter pressure. Simultaneously, alcohol stimulates the gastric acid output, which may result in a lower pH in the reflux material [3], but also may decrease the gastrin production by feedback, see Table 1.

Acute drinking impairs acid clearance by a delay in the restoration of pH, which may be aggravated by changes in the salivary flow and composition [4]. Even a very moderate alcohol intake in the evening is associated with measurable nocturnal reflux episodes, but without clinical symptoms [5].

Acute intoxication may exert direct toxic damage on the mucosa together with a near abolition of mucosal blood flow [6]. The effects of acute alcohol consumption are transient only, but they may, in combination with other risk factors, precipitate or participate in maintaining an esophagitis.

Chronic alcohol abuse

Most investigations on chronic alcohol abusers are actually performed during the withdrawal period. However, two small studies suggest that active drinkers have abnormal motility, especially nutcracker esophagus. Contrary to the results with healthy volunteers, alcohol administration to active drinkers increases the lower esophageal sphincter pressure. It inhibits the relaxation of the sphincter to a lesser degree, indicating development of some compensatory resistance to the influence of ethanol. However, at the same time, the esophageal contraction amplitude is elevated, suggesting that chronic alcoholism affects all segments of the esophagus, but differentially (Table 1) [7—8].

An animal model supports the findings of gastrointestinal tolerance to chronic alcohol intake by the finding of normal pressure of the lower sphincter during long-term ethanol administration [9].

Composition changes of the cell membranes from several parts of the body are seen in alcohol abusers [10]. Corresponding changes of the esophageal cells may be part of the explanation for the above mentioned gastrointestinal resistance. Furthermore, the generalized alcoholic neuropathy could be responsible for some of the esophageal motility disturbances. [11], and theoretically, an alcohol-induced myopathy may add to the dysfunction.

Development of esophagitis in chronic abusers is probably a result of the combination of the constant dysmotility and a long-term irritant effect on the mucosa.

Table 1. Influence of different alcohol administration on esophageal manometry.

	Acute intake	Chronic intake	Withdrawal from alcohol
LES-P	decrease	small increase	increase
Relaxation of LES-P	inhibition	less inhibition	—
GER	decrease	small increase	increase

Abstinence from alcohol

At alcohol withdrawal the esophageal contraction amplitude increases more than during chronic alcohol intake, and the duration prolongs without effect on velocity of the contractions (Table 1) [7].

The potentiation of the high pressure peristaltic waves develops during decline of the ethanol concentration of the blood, which does not necessarily need to be zero before the symptoms are present.

Alcohol infusion to withdrawing abusers normalizes the esophageal contraction amplitude and decreases the high pressure of the lower sphincter [7].

Withdrawal from alcohol is characterized by an overactivity of the sympathetic nervous system [12] resulting in an imbalance between the sympathetic and the parasympathetic reaction. This imbalance may be responsible for the esophageal dysmotility, most pronounced in abstinent alcohol abusers.

One month after abstinence from alcohol the lower esophagus sphincter pressure and esophageal contraction amplitude return to normal [13].

Therapy of gastroesophageal reflux disease and esophagitis in patients drinking alcohol should start with recommendation of changing their lifestyle. Complaints from esophagitis disappear in half of the alcoholic patients after 2 weeks of abstinence without medical treatment [1]. Abstinence from alcohol (and tobacco) is necessary for the effectiveness of the medical therapy [14], which besides should follow the common outlines for treatment.

Future investigations should focus on the multifactorial pathogenesis and therefore include a more holistic view of the alcoholic patients or volunteers studied. For instance, smoking habits and intake of food products should be described together with information on concomitant hiatus hernia [15], esophageal varices or strictures, as well as chronic obstructive pulmonary disease [16] and other conditions that may influence the gastroesophageal reflux.

References

1. Tønnesen H, Andersen JR, Christoffersen P, Kaas-Claesson N. Reflux oesophagitis in heavy drinkers. Digestion 1987;38: 69–73.
2. Hogan WJ, Viegas de Andrade SR, Winship DH. Ethanol-induced acute esophageal motor dysfunction. J Appl Physiol 1971;32:755–760.
3. Jurgen LH, Ferrari-Taylor J, Isenberg JI. Wine and 5% ethanol are potent stimulants of gastric acid secretion in humans. Gastroenterology 1983;85:1082–1087.
4. Kjellen G, Tibbling L. Influence of body position, dry and water swallows, smoking and alcohol on esophageal acid clearing. Scand J Gastroenterol 1978;13:283–288.
5. Vitale GC, Cheadle WG, Patel B, Sadek SA, Mitchel ME, Cuschieri A. The effect of alcohol on nocturnal gastroesophageal reflux. JAMA 1987;258:2077–2079.
6. Bass BL, Trad KS, Harmon JW, Hakki FZ. Capsaicin-sensitive nerve mediate esophageal mucosal protection. Surgery 1991;110.419–426.
7. Keshavarzian A, Polepalle C, Iber FL, Durkin M. Esophageal motor disorder in alcoholics: result of alcoholism or withdrawal? Alcohol Clin Exp Res 1990;14:561–567.
8. Keshavarzian A, Polepalle C, Iber FL, Durkin M. Secondary esophageal contractions are abnormal in chronic alcoholics. Dig Dis Sci 1992;37:517–522.
9. Keshavarzian A, Rizk G, Urban G, Willson C. Ethanol-induced esophageal motor disorder: development of an animal model. Alcohol Clin Exp Res 1990;14:76–81.
10. Sun GY, Sun YA. Ethanol and membrane lipids. Alcohol Clin Exp Res 1985;9:164–180.

11. Winship DH, Caflisch CR, Zbolske FF, Hogan WJ. Deterioration of esophageal peristalsis in patients with alcoholic neuropathy. Gastroenterology 1968;55:173—178.
12. Linnoila M. Alcohol withdrawal and noradrenergic function. Ann Int Med 1987;107:875—889.
13. Keshavarzian A, Iber FL, Ferguson Y. Esophageal manometry and radionuclide emptying in chronic alcoholics. Gastroenterology 1987;92:651—657.
14. Harvey RF, Gordon PC, Hadley N et al. Effects of sleeping with the bed-head raised and of ranitidine in patients with severe peptic oesophagitis. Lancet 1987;II:1200—1203.
15. Berstad A, Weberg R, Larsen IF, Hoel B, Jensen MH. Relationship of hiatus hernia to reflux oesophagitis. Scand J Gastroenterol 1986;21:55—58.
16. Andersen LI, Jensen G. Risk factors for benign oesophageal disease in a random population sample. J Intern Med 1991; 230:5—10.

What factors are predictive of esophageal ulceration in GER?

G. Cadiot, J. Vatier, M. Mignon (Paris)

There are many differences between gastroesophageal reflux (GER) patients with esophagitis and those without esophagitis, when considering the patients as a group. However, to our knowledge, none of these differences can predict the occurrence of esophageal erosions, when considering a given individual with GER disease (GERD).

Those differences are the characteristics of the patients (sex, age) [1], the existence of exogenous factors (tobacco, alcohol, NSAID) [2], the clinical characteristics of GERD (quantitative extent of reflux [3], nycterohemeral periods of reflux [3–5], duration of disease [2]) and finally, the pathophysiological factors of GERD. Among the latter, the abnormalities of esophageal clearance, which determines the duration of the contact between refluxate and esophageal mucosa, the composition of the gastroesophageal refluxate and the esophageal mucosal resistance are probably the most significant factors of esophagitis.

Esophageal clearance of the refluxate is determined by secondary esophageal peristalsis and salivary secretion (neutralization of acid by salivary bicarbonates) [6]. The association of esophageal clearance abnormalities to lower esophageal sphincter (LES) incompetence and to gastric emptying delay, suggests that GERD is a primary motor disorder of the esophagus [7], whose origin might be vagal for some authors [8]. The fact that esophageal peristalsis and clearance abnormalities are not modified after esophagitis healing, is in favor of the existence of a primary motor disorder [9]. Our group showed, using a multifactorial approach with a logistic regression, that esophageal clearance abnormalities, reflected by the number of refluxes lasting more than 5 min, was one among the three significant factors differentiating GER patients without esophagitis from those with esophagitis [10]. However, when considering a given individual, measuring esophageal clearance (by scintigraphy [11] or pH-metry) did not predict the occurrence of esophageal erosions since there was a big overlap of the individual values between the two groups of patients. Esophageal motor perturbances (aperistalsis, low amplitude contraction waves) and LES hypotonia are correlated with esophagitis grade [12]. However, when considering a given individual, they also do not allow prediction of the occurrence of esophagitis [12].

Esophagitis is more frequent when hiatal hernia is present; in our experience hiatal hernia was present in 73% of patients with esophagitis, as compared to 39% in the patients without esophagitis [10]. Hiatal hernia favors esophageal clearance abnormalities, especially when it is irreducible [13]. However, its presence cannot allow prediction of the occurrence of esophageal erosions.

It is reasonable to anticipate that the composition of the refluxate, which in turn depends upon that of the gastric juice, is a factor of esophagitis. However, this remains a matter of debate in spite of evidence obtained in animals and humans [14–16]. We have shown that 25% of GER patients without esophagitis and 31% of those with esophagitis had gastric acid hypersecretion [15]. These percentages did not differ significantly. However, pentagastrin-stimulated peptic outputs were significantly higher in the patients with esophagitis than in the others [15]. Nevertheless, secretory parameters were not significant after multifactorial analysis [10]. The importance of a high concentration of pepsin in the refluxate has been recently emphasized by Gotley et al., but only in high grade esophagitis [17]. The relevance of duodenogastric reflux remains debatable.

The other major pathophysiological factor of esophagitis is probably the esophageal mucosal resistance. Modifications of mucosal resistance might explain why esophagitis develops in some patients when it does not in others who do not have significantly different GERD, both from quantitative and qualitative points of view. Esophageal mucosal resistance includes pre-epithelial, epithelial and postepithelial defense mechanisms and also mucosal regenerative factors [18]. However, to our knowledge, none have studied modifications of these different mechanisms in patients with esophagitis as compared to patients without esophagitis.

It is theoretically possible to determine, after multifactorial analysis, a mathematical equation which allows prediction of the risk of esophagitis in a given patient. However, taking into account the high number of potential factors to study and the high number of patients necessary to obtain a good statistical analysis, such a study is difficult to realize. Our multifactorial analysis, imperfect since some pathophysiological factors of esophagitis were not studied (especially mucosal resistance), aimed to determine the factors significantly associated to esophagitis [10]. The number of refluxes lasting more than 5 min, the amplitude of the esophageal contraction waves and male sex were the three factors which were significant after logistic regression [10].

In conclusion, if numerous factors or parameters are most often present or abnormal in cases of esophagitis, when considering the patients as a group, it is difficult to predict the occurrence of esophageal erosions when deliberating a given individual.

References

1. Wienbeck M, Barnert J. Epidemiology of reflux disease and reflux esophagitis. Scand J Gastroenterol 1989;24(suppl 156): 7–13.
2. Dedieu P, Gaillard F, Lavignolle A et al. Oesophagite par reflux: aspects épidémiologiques, anatomopathologiques et évolutifs (123 cas). Gastroenterol Clin Biol 1981;5:266–274.
3. DeMeester TR, Wang CI, Wernly JA, Pellegrini CA, Little AG, Klementschitsch P, Bermudez G, Johnson LF, Skinner DB. Technique, indications, and clinical use of 24 hour esophageal pH monitoring. J Thorac Cardiovasc Surg 1980;79: 656–670.
4. DeCaestecker JS, Blackwell JN, Pryde A, Heading RC. Daytime gastro-oesophageal reflux is important in oesophagitis. Gut 1987;28:519–526.
5. Freidin N, Fisher MJ, Taylor W, Boyd D, Surratt P, McCallum RW, Mittal RK. Sleep and nocturnal acid reflux in normal subjects and patients with reflux oesophagitis. Gut 1991;32:1275–1279.
6. Katzka DA, DiMarino AJ. Pathophysiology of gastroesophageal reflux disease: LES incompetence and esophageal clearance. In: Castell DO (ed) The Esophagus. Boston: Little, Brown and Company, 1992:449–461.
7. Castell DO. Gastroesophageal reflux disease is a motility disorder. In: Scarpignato C (ed) Advances in drug therapy of gastroesophageal reflux disease. Front Gastrointest Res, Basel: Krager 1992;20:11–16.
8. Cunningham KM, Horowitz M, Riddell PS et al. Relations among autonomic nerve dysfunction, oesophageal motility and gastric emptying in gastro-oesophageal reflux disease. Gut 1991;32:1436–1440.
9. Singh P, Adamopoulos A, Taylor RH, Colin-Jones DG. Oesophageal motor function before and after healing of oesophagitis. Gut 1992;33:1590–1596.
10. Cadiot G, Bruhat A, Hetzel D et al. Multivariate analysis of pathophysiological factors of gastroesophageal reflux and peptic esophagitis in 74 patients. Gastroenterology 1992;102:A46(abstract).
11. Stanciu C, Bennett JR. Oesophageal acid clearing: one factor in the production of reflux oesophagitis. Gut 1974;15:852–857.
12. Kahrilas PJ, Dodds WJ, Hogan WJ, Kern M, Arndorfer RC, Reece A. Esophageal peristaltic dysfunction in peptic esophagitis. Gastroenterology 1986;91:897–904.
13. Sloan S, Kahrilas PJ. Impairment of esophageal emptying with hiatal hernia. Gastroenterology 1991;100:596–605.
14. Goldberg HI, Doods WJ, Gee S, Montgomery C, Zboralske FF. Role of acid and pepsin in acute experimental esophagitis. Gastroenterology 1969;56:223–230.
15. Sekera E, Cadiot G, Poitevin C, Vallot T, Vatier J, Mignon M. Gastric proteolytic content in gastroesophageal reflux and esophagitis. Gastroenterol Clin Biol 1992;16:141–147.
16. Hirschowitz BI. A critical analysis, with appropriate controls, of gastric acid and pepsin secretion in clinical esophagitis. Gastroenterology 1991;101:1149–1158.
17. Gotley DC, Morgan AP, Ball D, Owen RW, Cooper MJ. Composition of gastro-oesophageal refluxate. Gut 1991;32:1093–1099.
18. Orlando RC. Pathophysiology of gastroesophageal reflux disease: Esophageal epithelial resistance. In: Castell DO (ed) The Esophagus. Boston: Little, Brown and Company, 1992;463–478.

What is the frequency of gastroesophageal reflux in young subjects?

J.M. Debonne, P. Berthezene, F. Klotz, J.C. Grimaud, J.P. Durbec (Marseilles)

Gastroesophageal reflux disease (GERD) represents a major health problem in the industrialized countries due to its frequency and economic cost. Even though modern digestive functional exploration methods have brought improvements in the understanding of its physiopathology and symptomatology, there are still some technical difficulties in the study of its epidemiology, such as the choice of diagnostic criteria, of the methods of data collection and of the samples to be studied [1]. Moreover, the complexity and multifactorial nature of its pathogenesis also limits the possibilities of using epidemiological studies to look for extrinsic and intrinsic factors. For all these reasons, we felt it would be interesting to study the main features of heartburn in the young adult using simple standardized criteria on a perfectly defined large homogeneous sample. The aims of the study were to study the prevalence of heartburn in a changing population of young men embarking on military service, to describe its main characteristics and to look for determinant factors through descriptive and analytic statistical analysis.

Population and Methods

Population

During the Army medical examinations in February, April and June 1990, 6,397 young French men conscripted for military service were questioned about any functional digestive symptoms they may have. The interview was performed on an individual basis by a team of physicians and nurses and included around 100 multiple choice and closed questions. The main question used to identify and quantify heartburn was: "Have you ever felt burning going up into the chest from the stomach sometimes with an acid taste in the mouth?". A further question specifying the daily, weekly or monthly frequency was asked for any positive replies to the first question. Those with occasional heartburn (less than once a month) were considered negative. All those taking part in the study had to reply to all the questions relating to their socioeconomic (geographic origin, social status, profession and family details) and physiological details (age and body mass index (BMI) = weight in kg/height in m^2), the state of their physical and mental health, family and personal history, any digestive or nondigestive symptoms they may have, their alcohol and tobacco consumption, a rough outline of their usual diet and the number of times they had sought medical advice.

Analysis of the results

The relationship between heartburn and the various items studied was analyzed using frequency tables and the distributions compared by the Chi^2 test together with calculation of the coefficient Phi (VChi^2/N, varying ± 1). Phi enabled a comparison to be made of the extent to which heartburn was related to the variables being studied. Here we only describe the analysis of the results of this bivariate analysis. The results of the multivariate study with an analysis of any associations between the various factors and stepwise conditional logistic regression, which is described in detail in the reference article [2], are not presented here. This noninvasive study was performed with the consent of the participants and of the Army Health Department.

Table 1. Frequency of the features of heartburn

	H1[a]	H2[b]	H3[c]	Total	χ^2
N	75 (100)	217 (100)	447 (100)	739 (100)	
Continuous	45 (61.6)	139 (64.4)	148 (45.2)	382 (52.6)	S
Occurring at night	22 (29.3)	66 (30.4)	94 (21)	182 (24.6)	NS
Bending down	27 (36)	62 (28.6)	130 (29)	219 (29.6)	NS
Effort	40 (53.3)	99 (45.6)	178 (39.8)	317 (42.9)	NS
Meals	55 (73.3)	124 (59.4)	275 (61.5)	459 (62.1)	NS

Numbers in parentheses represent percentage; [a]H1: daily heartburn; [b]H2: weekly heartburn; [c]H3: monthly heartburn.

Results

A total of 6,385 completed questionnaires were suitable for analysis. The mean age of the participants was 19.6 ± 2.9 years, and they were from all over France, especially from the Southeast region.

The number of participants who admitted having heartburn was 11.57% (739/6,385). In 75 of them (P1 = 1.17%) heartburn occurred daily, in 217 (P2 = 3.4%) weekly and in 447 (P3 = 7%) monthly. In addition, 1,148 (18%) said that they had occasionally experienced heartburn, whereas 4498 (70.45%) had never had it. Of 6,385 participants, 1,133 (17.74%) stated that they had acid regurgitation, but 810 (12.68%) did not have heartburn. Therefore 24.24% of the people questioned had symptoms suggestive of GERD (heartburn and/or acid regurgitation). Fifty-three percent of these suffered the symptoms continually throughout the year (Table 1), especially in more severe cases. The rest only had heartburn from time to time. The symptoms occurred at night (25%) or after meals (62%), were brought on by certain postures (30%) or by effort (43%) irrespective of the frequency of the symptom. Twenty-nine percent had also consulted for this condition, of whom 41% had already been investigated, 28% had followed a diet and 69% had been prescribed medical treatment. Another 26% had already treated themselves with medicines (Table 2). Overall 4.8% of all those interviewed stated that they were troubled by this symptom

Table 2. Heartburn and treatment

	[a]H1	[b]H2	[c]H3	Total
N	75 (100)	217 (100)	447 (100)	739 (100)
Consultation	36 (49)	67 (31)	111 (25)	216 (29)
Investigations	25 (33)	23 (11)	41 (9)	89 (12)
Dict	17 (23)	24 (11)	20 (4.5)	61 (8)
Medication	32 (43)	45 (21)	72 (16)	149 (20)
Self medication	17 (23)	66 (30)	111 (25)	194 (26)
Significant discomfort	50 (66.7)	105 (48.4)	152 (34)	307 (41.5)

Numbers in parentheses represent percentage; [a]H1: daily heartburn; [b]H2 weekly heartburn; [c]H3 monthly heartburn.

and 3.4% had already sought treatment.

Bivariate analysis did not show any link between heartburn and socioeconomic factors, age or body mass index. There was, however, a significant association between heartburn and respiratory and otorhinolaryngological disorders, thoracic pain and digestive symptoms. Also, those who complained of having heartburn had the highest frequency of other psychological problems and had the greatest tendency to mention various other problems that they had (Fig. 1). With respect to diet, bivariate analysis revealed a weak but significant association between heartburn and the consumption of alcohol, fizzy and/or sweet drinks, coffee, fat and spices. There was a slightly stronger association for tobacco or a sedentary lifestyle (Fig. 2).

Discussion

The results of studies looking into the epidemiology of GERD [3–9] should be interpreted in the light of the population studied and the methods employed. This makes any direct comparison of results difficult. We studied young men embarking on military service. This created an important bias because anyone who was exempted form military service was not included in the study. Because of this, a similar questionnaire was performed at the Army Selection Center to which almost the entire young male French population is called up, to see if they are fit for military service. Amongst the 500 people questioned, the prevalence of heartburn was 11%, not very different from that which was obtained with the questionnaire at the time of incorporation. Our results can therefore be taken as representative of the 18 to 22 year-old age group, rarely studied in the literature.

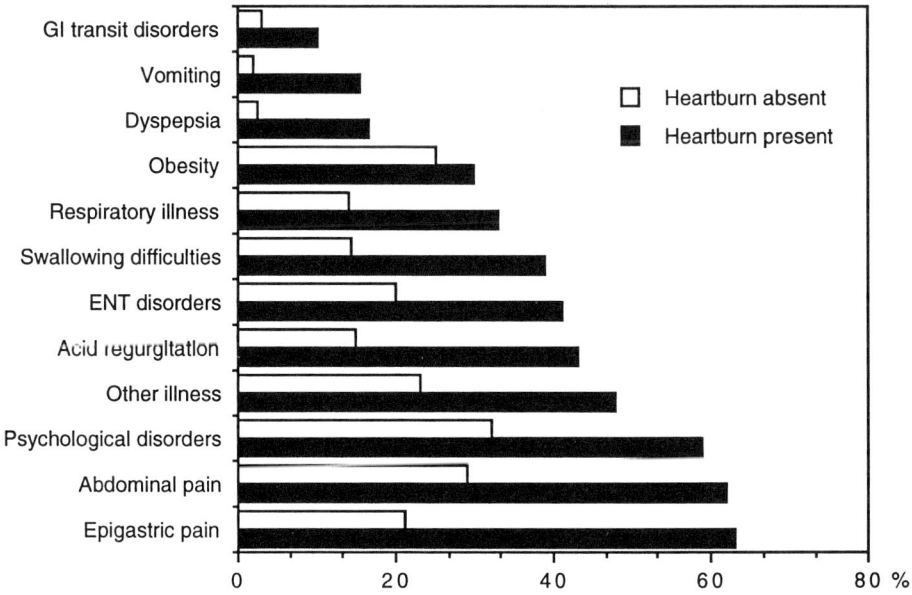

Fig. 1. Frequency of associated disorders in the presence or absence of heartburn.

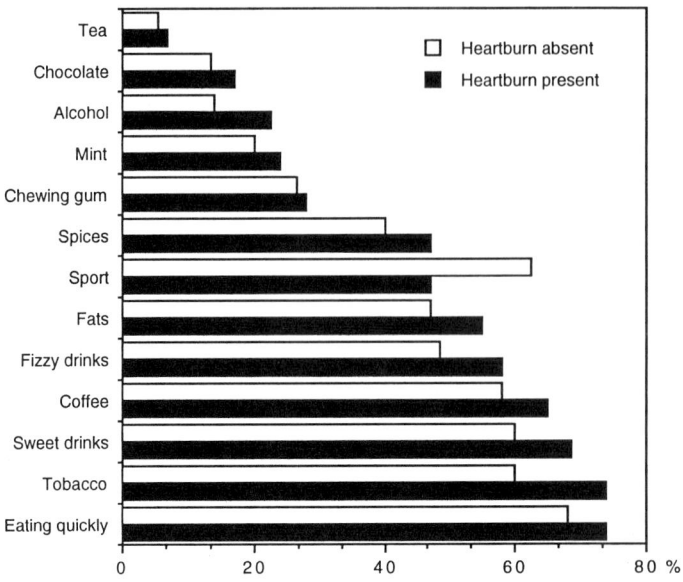

Fig. 2. Frequency of dietary factors in the absence and presence of heartburn.

The considerable homogeneity and large size of this group are two features which make this study a useful and original contribution to research into heartburn. The percentage of the sample who reported having heartburn at least monthly was 11.6% which is lower than the rates described in the literature (Table 3). Apart from the sampling methods, these differences could be explained by the diversity of symptoms studied and the way the data was collected. Our main criterion was heartburn, a symptom which is simple to describe, specific to GERD and very often causes people to seek medical help. Using the same criteria, Nebel [6] obtained a larger prevalence of heartburn (36%) in his controls who had not consulted for this symptom. Nebel [6], Smart [8], Welch [9], Ruth [7] and Thompson [10] also quantified heartburn according to its frequency. The first three of these authors found 7, 7 and 8.5%,

Table 3. Prevalence of heartburn in the literature

Year	Author	N	[a]Rep	[b]DS	[c]Method	Rate	Ref
1976	Nebel	335	NR	H	Q	36%	(6)
1981	Kjellen	2095	NR	H/A	SQ	16%	(5)
1986	Bommelaer	1200	NR	H	SQ	38.5%	(3)
1986	Smart	150	NR	H/A	Q	26%	(8)
1988	Bruley	1798	R	A	Q	27.1%	(4)
1990	Welch	285	NR	H/A	Q	20%	(9)
1991	Ruth	337	NR	H/A	SQ	26%	(7)

[a] REP : NR = non representative, R = representative; [b] DS: digestive symptoms, H = heartburn, A = acid regurgitation; [c] Method: Q= direct questionnaire, SQ= self questionnaire.

respectively, of their patients to be suffering from heartburn daily compared with 3% for Ruth, 4% for Thompson and 1.2% in this study. If acid regurgitation is included in heartburn, the prevalence of symptoms suggestive of GERD reaches 25%, this being similar to data found in the literature. Heartburn is a frequent reason, even amongst young men, to seek medical advice. This is confirmed by the literature where GERD is considered as one of the main reasons for gastrointestinal endoscopy [2], for a gastroenterological opinion [11–13] or for self-medication [14]. In our sample, as a result of the consultation, four out of 10 cases needed further investigation and seven out of 10 began medical treatment. The economic consequences are even more important because it is a chronic illness often treated by self-medication.

We did not find a clear association between heartburn and the socioeconomic factors studied. The strong link between heartburn and gastrointestinal and non-gastrointestinal, respiratory and otorhinolaryngological symptoms does not have any bearing on the pathophysiology of this condition because as our study showed, these patients have a tendency to somatize and to complain of a large number of symptoms. We did not find that excess weight had an influence, although the body weights in our sample were very evenly distributed around the normal value for age and sex (BMI = 22). Heartburn does, however, tend to be more frequent towards the extreme limits (BMI >23 or < 21). We noted a strong link between heartburn and certain psychological disorders, mostly severe anxiety, adaptation difficulties and immaturity. These people also had a marked tendency to somatize their symptoms as for example in irritable bowel syndrome. The relationship between GERD and psychological disorders has been emphasized recently by other authors [15,16].

The relationship between heartburn and dietary factors was studied using a preliminary bivariate analysis. This type of analysis, which has already been employed in the literature, often shows multiple significant associations, although these are usually of limited clinical interest [4,6,7,12,13,17–23]. The influence of alcohol and tobacco consumption remains unclear, whereas dietary factors, which have not been studied much, would appear to have an influence, for example fats as well as sugar, coffee, spices and tea, although these have not yet been sufficiently documented in the literature. Our results confirm most of these findings although they emphasize that the associations are weak, except for tobacco consumption and a sedentary lifestyle which are more strongly linked. The extent to which these factors are linked to heartburn is specified by descriptive and analytical multivariate analysis [2].

In conclusion, gastroesophageal reflux disease is, in its usual symptomatic form, a frequent finding in young men. The prevalence that we found was lower than in previous studies of the general population, but this may well be due to the different methods used and to the age of those studied. Even in this age group, many seek medical help for heartburn, which is often associated with dietary factors and a certain psychological pattern, something that would doubtless be worth clarifying by further studies.

References

1. Howard PJ, Heading RC. Epidemiology of gastroesophageal reflux disease. World J Surg 1992;16:288–293.
2. Debonne JM. Le pyrosis et l'homme jeune. Etude épidémiologique et analyse statistique multivariée de 6385 sujets. Mémoire de DEA, Marseille, 1991.
3. Bommelaer G, Rouch M, Dapoigny M et al. Epidémiologie des troubles fonctionnels intestinaux dans une population apparemment saine. Gastroenterol Clin Biol 1986;10:7–12.
4. Bruley des Varannes S, Galmiche JP, Bernades P, Bader JP. Douleurs épigastriques et régurgitations: épidémiologie descriptive dans un échantillon représentatif de la population française adulte. Gastroenterol Clin Biol 1988;12:721–728.
5. Kjellen G, Tibbling L. Manometric oesophageal function, acid perfusion test and symptomatology in a 55 year old general population. Clin Physiol 1981;1:405–415.
6. Nebel OT, Fornes MF, Castell DO. Symptomatic gastroesophageal reflux: incidence and precipitating factors. Am J Dig Dis 1976;11:953–956.
7. Ruth M, Mansson I, Sandberg M. The prevalence of symptoms suggestive of esophageal disorders. Scand J Gastroenterol 1991;26:73–81.
8. Smart HL, Nicholson DA, Atkinson M. Gastro-oesophageal reflux in the irritable syndrome. Gut 1986;27:1127–1131.
9. Welch WG, Pomare EW. Functional gastrointestinal symptoms in a Wellington community sample. N Zealand J Med 1990; 418–420.
10. Thompson WG, Heaton KW. Heartburn and globus in apparently healthy people. J Can Med Assoc 1982;126:46–48.
11. Carteret E, Renard P, Aucouturier JP et al. Hernie hiatale et oesophagite: hasard ou nécessité? Gastroenterol Clin Biol 1990;14(suppl 2B):A111.
12. Glaxo Laboratoires. Douleurs épigastriques. Etude prospective endoscopique. Conc Med 1989;111:1425.
13. Poynard T, Galmiche JP, Bernades P et al. Prévalence et facteurs de risque des maladies oeso-gastro-duodénales bénignes chez des patients consultants en gastroentérologie pour symptomatologie douloureuse haute. Gastroenterol Clin Biol 1989; 13(suppl 2B):A165.
14. Graham DY, Smith JL, Patterson DJ. Why do apparently healthy people use antacid tablets? Am J Gastroenterol 1983; 78:257–260.
15. Johnston BT, Lewis SA, Love AHG. Patients with heartburn have a specific personality profile. Gut 1992;33:S36.
16. Scarinci IC, Schan CA, Halle JM. Psychological distress and health care seeking behavior among persons with symptoms of gastroesophageal reflux disease. Gastroenterology 1992;102:A509.
17. Carteret E, Pasqual JC, Renard P, Zeitoun P. Fréquence et facteurs prognostiques de l'oesophagite par reflux. Gastroenterol Clin Biol 1988;12(suppl 2B):A44.
18. Dedieu P, Gaillard F, Lavignolle A et al. Oesophagite de reflux: aspects épidémiologiques, anatomo-pathologiques et évolutifs (123 cas). Gastroenterol Clin Biol 1981;5:266–274.
19. Micaleff A, Richard-Berthe C, Huyghe JL. Oesophagite de reflux: résultats d'une enquête épidémiologique et endoscopique chez 679 patients, réalisée par 146 gastroentérologues de ville. Med Chir Dig 1985;(special issue):8–14.
20. Stene-Larsen G, Weberg R, Froyshov Larsen I et al. Relationship of overweight to hiatus hernia and reflux oesophagitis. Scand J Gastroenterol 1988;23:427–432.
21. Stocker DL, Williams JG, Leicester RG, Colin-Jones DG. Oesophagitis: a five year review. Gut 1988;29:A1450.
22. Wienbeck M, Barnert J. Epidemiology of reflux disease and reflux esophagitis. Scand J Gastroenterol 1989;24(suppl 156): 7–13.
23. Carteret E, Renard P, Zeitoun P. Epidémiologie hospitalière de l'oesophagite érosive établie à partir d'une série consécutive de 20598 patients. Gastroenterol Clin Biol 1989;13(suppl 2B):A69.

What is the prevalence of gastroesophageal reflux disease and of reflux esophagitis?

R.C. Heading (Edinburgh)

To determine prevalence values for reflux disease and for reflux esophagitis in the population it is necessary to: 1) define the two conditions; and 2) undertake studies in the community to identify the occurrence of the conditions so defined. There are formidable difficulties in meeting these two requirements and in consequence no truly satisfactory prevalence data are yet available which compare directly the occurrence of reflux disease and esophagitis. Nevertheless, some inferences may be drawn from the data which do exist.

Prevalence of symptomatic reflux disease

Reflux disease may be defined as the occurrence of symptoms, tissue damage or both, attributable to gastroesophageal reflux. Although this definition is broadly satisfactory for patients coming under the care of physicians, the label "reflux disease" seems inappropriate for individuals who suffer only very mild or infrequent symptoms. This in turn implies that some threshold of symptom frequency or severity, or of patient distress, should be set to justify application of the term "reflux disease", but because any such threshold is necessarily arbitrary, the definition of "reflux disease" is thereby rendered less robust. Prevalence data based on the definition are then correspondingly less certain.

Simple enquiry about dyspeptic symptoms has produced broadly similar data in the United Kingdom and the United States. The 6 month prevalence in the United Kingdom is reported to be 41%, with just over half of symptomatic individuals experiencing both upper abdominal symptoms and heartburn, and heartburn alone in about one fifth [1]. Only one quarter of the sufferers had sought medical advice for their symptoms. In a Gallup poll conducted in the United States, 44% of respondents described suffering heartburn at least once a month and approximately one third of symptomatic individuals had never discussed their complaint with a doctor. In a well known study of hospital staff [2], Nebel and colleagues found 7% of individuals suffering heartburn on a daily basis, 14% weekly and 15% approximately monthly [3]. Thomson and Heaton reported figures of 4 and 10% for the proportion of the population suffering daily and weekly heartburn respectively [4].

The principal difficulty in interpreting these data to estimate the prevalence of reflux disease centres on the inadequacy of heartburn as an indicator of symptomatic reflux. Klauser and colleagues have shown that when heartburn is a dominant symptom, it serves as a relatively specific (though insensitive) predictor of reflux disease. In contrast, simple enquiry about the presence or absence of heartburn is not reliable as an indicator of the presence or absence of reflux disease [5]. Among individuals with proven reflux disease, the most common symptom pattern seems to be a complex dyspepsia which is not a basis for specific clinical diagnosis. These data therefore indicate that it is not possible to identify reflux disease reliably on the basis of symptom questionnaires alone. The published literature concerning the occurrence and frequency of so called reflux symptoms in the population must be interpreted in this context.

Prevalence of esophagitis

In comparison with symptomatic reflux, more accurate information about the prevalence of esophagitis might reasonably be expected but difficulties of definition arise here also, especially with mild forms of the disease. There is much observer variation in the endoscopic recognition of mild esophagitis and because mild disease is more common than severe disease, estimates of the incidence of abnormality among any population may be more variable than endoscopists would wish. Nevertheless, there is a measure of agreement around a figure of 20% for the presence of esophagitis in patients undergoing endoscopy for upper gastrointestinal symptoms [6,7]. An interesting study from Norway suggests that among individuals in the community who admit to dyspeptic symptoms on enquiry, approximately 12% have esophagitis at endoscopy whereas in a matched group of controls, who deny dyspeptic symptoms, approximately 8% have esophagitis [8].

Conclusion

For the reasons given above, figures which claim to represent the prevalence of reflux disease and esophagitis must be accepted with caution. Nevertheless, numbers can be useful as broad indicators of the occurrence of the condition in the population. Reflux symptoms are reported by approximately 10% of the adult population with a frequency or severity which would seem to justify the term "reflux disease". It seems likely, however, that an additional group of individuals, perhaps almost as numerous, suffers dyspeptic symptoms which are not obviously of reflux type but are in fact caused by gastroesophageal reflux. Esophagitis is found in approximately 20% of patients with upper gastrointestinal symptoms coming to gastroenterologists. For every two patients with such symptoms found to have esophagitis, a further one patient with similar symptoms but without esophagitis, can be shown to have abnormal 24-h esophageal pH monitoring [9]. The prevalence of reflux disease among symptomatic individuals is thus approximately 1.5 times the prevalence of esophagitis.

References

1. Jones RH, Lydeard SE, Hobbs FDR et al. Dyspepsia in England and Scotland. Gut 1990;31:401—405.
2. A Gallup survey on heartburn across America. Princeton, NJ Gallup Organization Inc., March 1988.
3. Nebel OT, Fornes MF, Castell DO. Symptomatic gastroesophageal reflux: Incidence and precipitating factors. Dig Dis Sci 1976;21:953—956.
4. Thompson WG, Heaton KW. Heartburn and globus in apparently healthy people. J Can Med Assoc 1982;126:46—48.
5. Klauser AG, Schindlbeck NE, Muller-Lissner SA. Symptoms in gastro-oesophageal reflux disease. Lancet 1990;335:205—208.
6. Ainley CC, Forgacs AC, Keeling PWN, Thompson RPH. Outpatient endoscopic survey of smoking and peptic ulcer. Gut 1986;27:648—651.
7. Stoker DL, Williams JG, Leicester RG, Colin-Jones DG. Oesophagitis: A five year review. Gut 1988;29:A1450.
8. Bernersen B, Johnsen R, Bostad L et al. Is Helicobacter pylori the cause of dyspepsia? Br Med J 1992;304:1276—1279.
9. Klauser AG, Voderholzer WA, Knesewitsch PA, Schindlbeck NE, Muller-Lissner SA. What is behind dyspepsia? Dig Dis Sci 1993;38:147—154.

Is there a relationship between esophagitis and duodenal ulcer?

G. Champault, J.C. Kikassa (Paris)

Although duodenal ulcer disease (DUD) and acid reflux esophagitis occur concurrently relatively frequently (10–15%) [1,2], the reasons for this are not fully understood [3]. A retrospective study of the mutual incidence of these two disorders, which are both caused by damaging acid action, was carried out in order to assess the therapeutic consequences.

Patients and Methods

Patients

All subjects who underwent esogastroduodenal endoscopy during 1992 in the Gastrointestinal Endoscopy department (Prof J.P. Ferrier) of the Jean Verdier Hospital in Bondy.

Selection criteria: symptomatic patients with:
— isolated duodenal lesions;
— isolated esophageal lesions;
— both these types of lesions;
— neither of these types of lesions.
Exclusion criteria:
— patients under 18 years of age;
— hemorrhage of the upper or lower gastrointestinal tract;
— patients known to have cirrhosis of the liver;
— esophageal-gastric varices;
— patients surgically treated for duodenal ulcer or gastroesophageal reflux (GER);
— endoscopic examination after medical treatment for duodenal ulcer or esophagitis;
— endoscopic gastric lesions: ulceration, inflammation, tumor.

Methods

The study involved retrospective analysis of endoscopy reports. The following lesions were taken into account:
— duodenal lesions:
    — acute inflammation of the duodenum;
    — superficial ulcerations;
    — newly formed ulcers;
    — chronic ulcers;

— esophageal lesions (Savary's classification):
  — erythematous lesions;
  — hemorrhagic lesions;
  — ulceration;
  — stenosing lesion or ulcer.

Results

A total of 1,600 patients satisfied the selection criteria. Their mean age was 39 ± 17 years and the sex ratio was 3:1.

Lesions: distribution

Duodenal lesions
— 274 patients (17%) had duodenal lesions comprising:
  — 164 cases of duodenal inflammation (59%);
  — 110 ulcers (6.8% of the study population) of which 92 were newly formed and 18 were chronic (18.8% of duodenal lesions).

Esophageal lesions
— 253 patients (15.8%) had esophageal lesions:
  — 170 cases of stage I esophagitis;
  — 38 cases of stage II esophagitis (2% of the study population);
  — 45 cases of stage III and IV esophagitis (3% of the study population);
    89 patients (5.6%) had both esophageal and duodenal lesions.

Lesions: combination

Table 1. Incidence of esophagitis in patients with duodenal lesions

Duodenal lesions	N	Esophagitis	%
Inflammation	164	22	13.4
Ulceration	110	67	60.9
· Newly formed	92	51	55.4
· Chronic	18	16	88.8

Table 2. Incidence of duodenal lesions in patients with esophagitis

Esophagitis	N	Duodenal lesion	%
Stage I	170	26	15.2
Stages II and III	38	21	55.2
Stage IV	45	32	71.1
· Stenosis	4	3	75
· Barrett's esophagus	17	12	70
· Ulcers	24	17	70

Discussion

This study confirmed the results published in the literature [3,4], especially with regard to the reciprocal incidence of the most severe effects of these two disorders. Although the incidence of esophagitis was only 13.4%, among subjects with superficial acute duodenal lesions, it was significantly greater among patients with proven ulcer disease (55%, p = 0.001) and especially among those with chronic ulcers (88.8%, p = 0.0001). The same was true for esophagitis: while (mostly superficial) duodenal lesions were found in 15.2% of patients with mild esophagitis, the incidence of duodenal lesions increased to 55 and 77% in those patients in which the disease was at a more advanced stage. This increase was statistically significant (p = 0.001). In contrast, however, there was no significant difference between the patients exhibiting different forms of advanced esophageal lesions (stenosis or ulceration; 75 vs. 70%), including Barrett's esophagus (70%).

In this study only 89 patients, 5.5% of the global study population, were suffering from both a severe form of esophagitis and chronic duodenal ulcer indicating that such cases are rare. It would appear that the risk of having both types of lesions together increases with increasing severity of one or other of the lesions. This raises interesting therapeutic problems, at both medical and surgical levels.

It appears that therapeutic measures must be taken whose effects are of immediate onset and long-lived. Despite the success of drug therapy, and especially that based on the proton pump inhibitors (PPI) [4], this combination of disorders requires an initial treatment of at least 8 weeks to heal the lesions (90% of esophageal lesions). Subsequently, maintenance treatment with H_2 receptor antagonists [5] should be given to consolidate the response and to reduce the likelihood of complications in these patients at risk. Surgical treatment also presents a problem, especially whether or not to combine antireflux surgery with vagotomy [6]. This procedure, which can now be carried out by laparoscopic route, would seem to be the best solution in men under 50 and women under 65 years of age, in view of its effectiveness and an estimated annual recurrence rate of 1.5%.

Conclusions

If there is a relation between esophagitis and duodenal ulcer, it only really concerns the severe forms of the disease. Patients with this pathological combination (5.6%) present an interesting therapeutic problem, although surgical treatment, especially by laparoscopy, would seem a good alternative to medical treatment.

References

1. Lahoti D, Misra SP, Malhotra V, Vij JC. Relationship of heartburn with histopathological changes in esophagus and stomach in patients with duodenal ulcer. J Gastroenterol 1991;10(2):54–55.
2. Stol DW, Murphy GM, Collis JL. Duodenogastric reflux acid and secretion in patients with symptomatic hiatal hernia. Scand J Gastroenterol 1974;9:97–101.

3. Hirschowitz BI. A critical analysis with appropriate controls of gastric acid and pepsin secretion in clinical oesophagitis. Gastroenterology 1991;101:1149–1158.
4. Walan A. The clinical utility and safety of omeprazole. Scand J Gastroenterol 1989;(suppl 166):140–144.
5. Bender SW. Therapie mit H₂ rezeptor antagonisten im kindersalter. Einsatz von ranitidin über ulcers duodeni, ventriculi und refluxoesophagitis. Fortsc d Medizin 1992;110(33):629–632.
6. Chernousov AF, Rishko VV, Bopołskii PM, Efendiev VM. Combined surgical treatment of duodenal ulcer and reflux esophagitis. Vest Khirurg Imen 1989;142(3):34–38.

What data do the prospective epidemiologic studies of esophagitis provide?

F. Klotz, J.M. Debonne, J.C. Grimaud (Marseilles)

The epidemiology of reflux esophagitis (RE) is known retrospectively with its major and minor clinical features being manifested in different ways in each individual. Only a prospective study of a cohort of patients presenting gastroesophageal reflux (GER) and followed up clinically, endoscopically and histologically until esophagitis occurs, then throughout its progression, would allow a greater knowledge of the determinant epidemiological factors in this condition. Although it would seem that there are some trials of this sort in progress, none has so far appeared in the literature. For a knowledge of the epidemiology of RE, the secrets of its natural history need to be understood. There have been many retrospective studies on the epidemiological features of patients presenting RE and a few partially isolated prospective studies which already provide some answers to these questions.

Historical background

If only RE is looked at, without taking into account the studies of the prevalence of GER and its features, the first prospective study began in 1946 and was published in 1968 by Palmer [1], and involved the follow-up of patients presenting RE. It was, however, really a progressive follow-up study using old classification criteria without specifically looking at epidemiological factors. In Nantes in 1981, Dedieu published an epidemiological study of a series of 123 cases of esophagitis [2]. Apart from that, in the 1980s, many retrospective studies including personal studies and literature reviews were published, the most important being those by Savary [3] and Zeitoun [4]. Also, the results of Micaleff's study of the epidemiological factors seen by private gastroenterologists in 679 cases of RE, published in 1986, appear to be of interest [5].

Frequency of RE

The incidence of RE in the general population is difficult to quantify, in the USA it has been estimated at 2% [6]. However, in a study of 1,000 autopsies, it was found to be present in 27% of cases, although this high incidence is, of course, not applicable to the general population [7]. In studies of patients who have had an endoscopy, the incidence of RE varies from 10 to 20% depending on the region and on the author [4,8–10]. Amongst the patients consulting for symptoms of GER, the incidence of RE varies from 50 to 65% [11,12]. In Micaleff's multicentric study [5], it was 86%.

Age and sex

More men than women are affected by RE, the sex ratio being more than two [9,13]. This moderate male predominance becomes much more pronounced in severe RE (71% men and 29% women) [5]. The incidence of esophagitis increases markedly with age, the mean age of patients who present RE being around 55 years old [3,14]. Fifty percent of Pantin's patients were over 70 years old, the women being affected at a significantly older age than the men [15]. This correlates well with the GER annual incidence curve [16] (Fig. 1). Tibbling [17] found RE to affect 5% of the population over 55 years old.

What are the determinant factors of RE?

Alcohol. Alcoholism is certainly an important factor. Many studies have found that the higher the alcohol consumption, the more severe is the esophagitis, with an overall rate of confirmed alcoholism in 55% of cases [2,5]. In Lausanne [18], the incidence was found to be the same, with a large majority of cases being in men. Alcohol may act in potentiating the toxic action of the reflux fluids by stimulation of the gastric acid secretion and by modification of esophageal clearance and saliva secretion [19].

Tobacco. Tobacco consumption is also found to be increasing with frequency, which is proportional to the severity of the RE and greater than the incidence in the general population [2,5]. The role of tobacco in the functioning of the lower esophageal sphincter (LES), on the resistance of the esophageal mucosa and on acid secretion has already been clearly demonstrated. Other general or dietetic factors have not proved to be important in the etiology of RE, nevertheless they are significant determinant factors in reflux.

The role of nonsteroidal anti-inflammatory drugs (NSAIDS). In Savary's study, it was found that severe or complicated RE occurred more frequently in patients taking NSAIDS, with 24% of them presenting Barrett's esophagus (BE), 27% with peptic

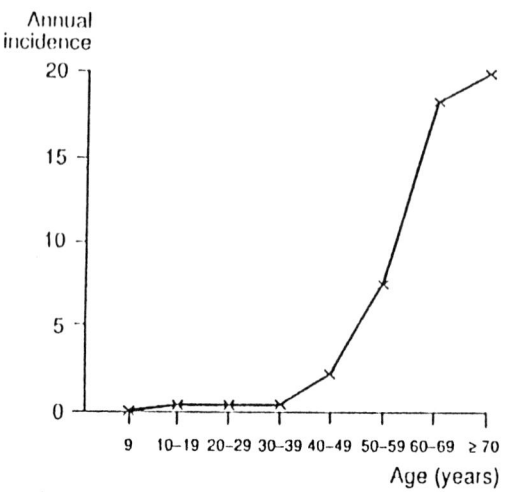

Fig. 1. Annual occurrence of the disease related to GER [16].

stenosis and 40% with esophageal ulceration taking medication known to cause esophagitis [18]. Wilkins found that 49% of patients with esophageal stenosis were taking NSAIDS [20].

Associated gastrointestinal pathology. Hiatus hernia has been viewed for a long time as an important factor in RE. In the studies reviewed by Stadelmann [21], hiatus hernia was found in 46–96% of patients presenting RE. Amongst the more recent important studies, Savary found hiatus hernias in 37% of cases [3], Zeitoun in 42.1% [4], whereas in the general population, it is only 10%. Hiatus hernia would therefore appear to have a definite role in promoting the occurrence of RE. The link with gastroduodenal ulcers is more controversial. Zeitoun noted 11.7% of patients with RE to have a duodenal ulcer, compared with 6.2% in a total of 20,598 patients studied [4]. Gastric ulcers were found in 5.9 and 4.4% of cases, respectively. In Savary's study of complicated RE, no clear link was found with ulcer disease [18].

Is there a link between the severity of the symptoms and the grade of the RE?

Dedieu found that there were symptoms of GER overall in 61% of cases of RE, without any noticeable difference between the different stages of RE [2]. In his study of 679 cases of RE, Micaleff observed symptomatology suggestive of GER in 88% of cases, with atypical ENT, respiratory and pseudocoronary symptoms occurring in 23% of cases [5]. There would not seem to be any link between the severity of the symptoms and the grade of RE except in cases where stenosis is present, in which dysphagia predominates the picture.

70

Frequency of the various grades of RE

This is difficult to assess from the studies in the literature, because the classifications used are not the same. With reference to the studies using Savary and Miller's classification:

— Schindlbeck [22] studied a group of 160 patients with characteristic GER and found 32% to have RE of which 11% was grade I, 9% grade II, 7% grade III and 5% grade IV.

— Savary's study of 2,673 cases of RE [3] found a predominance of grades I and IV with 50.7% being grade I, 13.6% grade II, 5.1% grade III and 30.6% grade IV.

According to Spechler [6], the incidence of RE with associated complications lies between 10 and 15% for BE, is 2–7% in esophageal ulcers, less than 0.2% in perforation and from 4–20% for peptic stenosis. Among 1,047 cases of esophagitis with complications studied by the Lausanne team, in 64% there was BE, in 34% stenosis, in 20% ulcer, and in 27% brachy-esophagus. The incidence of BE in the literature varies from 9–12.4% in those who are endoscoped [23]. In their study of 2,448 cases of RE, the Reims team [13] found fewer complicated cases including only 2.4% with peptic stenosis. This would seem to be closer to what is currently seen in most gastroenterological endoscopic centers.

Evaluation of the risk of progression of RE

No prospective study has so far been published on the progression of RE, although a retrospective study by the Lausanne team showed that 32.5% of their cases of RE progressed to stenosis, an ulcer or to BE in the end [24]. In patients with BE, there is a genuine risk of malignant transformation, they being 300–1,200 times more likely than the general population to develop an adenocarcinoma [25]. In a group of 360 cases of BE, the Lausanne team discovered that in 12% there was an adenocarcinoma [18]. This justifies an annual endoscopic surveillance of all patients with Barrett's esophagus. The occurrence of peptic stenosis appears to be encouraged directly by NSAID consumption in 31 and 49% of cases, respectively [20,26] compared with 14 and 12%, respectively, in the controls.

These drugs are therefore an aggravating factor for RE, by reducing the tissue concentration of prostaglandins, whose protective role on the esophageal mucosa is well known.

Can it be a complication of surgery?

About 15 to 20% of cases of peptic stenoses are thought to occur as a result of surgery with nasogastric intubation [27], this occurs within 6 months of the operation in 50% of cases. Included amongst the determinant factors are prolonged peri- or postoperative GER and the use of a nasogastric tube. All these epidemiological data about RE highlight the complexity of the etiological factors and the lack of knowledge of the long-term effects of the condition, there being notable differences between the various groups of patients studied. The numerous retrospective studies and the few incomplete prospective studies suggest that a large multicenter prospective trial of GER with a long-term follow-up is necessary.

References

1. Palmer ED. The hiatus hernia esophagitis, esophageal structure complex: twenty year prospective study. Am J Med 1968; 44:566—579.
2. Dedieu P, Gaillard F, Lavignolle A et al. Oesophagites par reflux: aspects épidémiologiques, anatomo-pathologiques et évolutifs (123 cas). Gastroenterol Clin Biol 1981;5:266—274.
3. Savary M, Ollyo J-B. L'oesophagite par reflux et ses complications: ulcère, sténose, endobrachy-oesophage. Encycl Med Chir Paris, ORL 1986;20822 A[10](16p).
4. Zeitoun P, Carteret E, Thiefin G, Renard P, Le Louargant M. Histoire naturelle des oesophagites par reflux. Med Hyg 1989;47:2641—2643.
5. Micaleff A, Richard-Berthe C, Huyghe J-L. Oesophagite de reflux. Résultats d'une enquête épidémiologique et endo-scopique chez 679 patients, réalisée par 146 gastroentérologues de ville. Med Chir Dig 1986;15:8—14.
6. Spechler SJ. Epidemiology and natural history of gastroesophageal reflux disease. Digestion 1992;51(suppl 1):24—29.
7. Postlethwait RW, Musser AW. Changes in the esophagus in 1000 autopsy specimens. J Thorac Cardiovasc Surg 1974;68: 953—956.
8. Heading RC. Epidemiology of esophageal reflux disease. Scand J Gastroenterol 1989;24(suppl 168):33—37.
9. Savary M, Monnier P, Miller G. L'oesophagite par reflux. Cham, Switzerland: Clyancourt Corporation S.A., 1983.
10. Klotz F, Debonne J-M. Ya-t-il une pathologie du reflux gastro-oesophagien en Afrique noire? Med Afr Noire 1991;38(1): 41—47.
11. Behar J. Gastroesophageal reflux disease and its complications with a critical analysis of treatment. In: Cohen S and Soloway RD (eds) Diseases of the Esophagus. New York: Churchill Livingstone, 1982;195—213.
12. Johansson KE, Ask P, Boeryd B, Fransson SG, Tibbling L. Esophagitis, signs of reflux and gastric acid secretion in patients with symptoms of gastroesophageal reflux disease. Scand J Gastroenterol 1986;21:837—847.
13. Carteret E, Renard P, Zeitoun P. Epidémiologie hospitalière de l'oesophagite érosive établie à partir d'une série consécutive de 20598 patients. Gastroenterol Clin Biol 1989;13(suppl 2B):A69.
14. Carteret E, Pasqual J-C, Renard P, Zeitoun P. Fréquence et facteurs pronostiques de l'oesophagite par reflux. Gastroenterol Clin Biol 1988;12(suppl 2B):A44.
15. Pantin B, Bacq Y, Metman EH, Bertrand J. Particularités cliniques des hemies hiatales du sujet âgé. Rev Méd 1983;6: 251—255.
16. Brunnen PL, Karnody AM, Needham C-D. Severe peptic esophagitis. Gut 1969;10:831—837.
17. Tibbling L. Epidemiology of gastroesophageal reflux disease. Scand J Gastroenterol 1984;19(suppl 109):14—18.
18. Ollyo J-B, Wellinger J, Monnier P, Levi F, Savary M. Etiopathogénie et dégénérescence des oesophagites par reflux com-pliquées. Rev Fr Gastroenterol 1988;244(24):1083—1086.
19. Debongnie J-C. Rôle de l'alcool éthylique dans l'étiopathogénie de l'oesophagite par reflux. Revue de la littérature. Acta Gastroenterol Belg 1985;48:493—500.
20. Wilkins WE, Ridley MG, Pozniak AL. Benign structure of the esophagus role of nonsteroidal anti-inflammatory drugs. Gut 1984;25:478—480.
21. Stadelmann O, Elster K, Ottenian R. Esophagitis. Pathology and clinical findings inflammation. Gut 1970;2:45.
22. Schindlbeck NE, Klauser AG, Berghammer G, Londong W, Muller Lissner SA. Three year follow-up of patients with gastroesophageal reflux disease. Gut 1992;33:1016—1019.
23. Jutel P, Galmiche J-P. Endobrachy-oesophage. In: Galmiche J-P, Colin R (eds) Troubles de la motricite de l'oesophage, Reflux Gastro-oesophagien. Paris: Doin Edit, 1987;177:186.
24. Brossard E, Monnier P, Ollyo J-B, Fontolliet C, Levi F, Krayenbuhl M, Savary M. Serious complications stenosis, ulcer and Barrett's epithelium develop in 21.6% of adults with erosive reflux esophagitis. Gastroenterology 1991;100(5,part 2): A36.
25. Bell RCW. Barrett's esophagus. N Engl J Med 1987;316:277.
26. Heller SR, Fellows IW, Ogilvie AL, Atkinson M. Nonsteroidal anti-inflammatory drugs and benign esophageal stricture. Br J Med 1982;285:167—168.
27. Savary M, Ollyo J-B, Monnier P. L'oesophagite sténosante par reflux. In: Galmiche J-P, Colin R (eds) Troubles de la motricite de l'oesophage, Reflux Gastro-oesophagien. Paris: Doin Edit 1987:193—229.

Mucosa and symptoms

How can epithelial resistance be assessed? Is there a relationship between defects in epithelial resistance and symptoms?

R.C. Orlando (New Orleans)

What is esophageal epithelial resistance? Esophageal epithelial resistance can be defined in two ways.

One, a structure-function definition, refers to the third-tier in the esophageal defense against injury by gastroesophageal reflux. In this respect, esophageal epithelial resistance is a group of mucosal structures and functions that protect the esophageal epithelium from injury upon exposure to noxious substances within the lumen [1,2]. These structures and functions and their individual roles in protection of the esophageal epithelium against acid injury have been described elsewhere in this book.

The other, an electrophysiological definition, is a measure of the ability of the epithelium to resist the flow of ions across it. In this sense, the resistance of the epithelium is a reflection of the tissue's permeability to ions, and this parameter can be given in specific measurable units, usually $\Omega \cdot cm^2$

How can esophageal epithelial resistance be assessed? Based on the structure-function definition above, esophageal epithelial resistance can be assessed in a variety of ways, either morphologically (i.e., as an effect on tissue structure), and/or functionally (i.e., as an effect on tissue functions, such as passive permeability and active transport). For example, the esophageal epithelial resistance to damage by any given noxious luminal agent can be determined at appropriate time intervals by examining the tissues structures in one or more of the following ways:

— by inspection for gross defects [3];
— by examination with light microscopy [3];
— by examination with scanning or transmission electron microscopy [4]; and
— by examination of the junctions with freeze fracture techniques [4].

Alternatively the esophageal epithelial resistance can be determined by examining the effects of a potentially noxious agent on tissue functions, the most prominent being its ability to transport Na^+ ions and its ability to act as a permeability barrier [5]. These can be assessed in one or more of the following ways:

— by monitoring the change in esophageal potential difference [5,6];
— by monitoring the change in esophageal electrical resistance [5,7] (see below);
— by measuring the change in the bidirectional net flux of radio-labeled Na^+ ions [5];
— by measuring the change in flux of a radio-labeled nontransported molecule such as mannitol [5]; or
— by visualizing with the electron microscope an increase in tissue permeation of an electron dense tracer such as horseradish peroxidase [4].

Based on the electrophysiological definition, esophageal epithelial resistance can be measured in vitro by mounting sections of esophageal epithelium as flat sheets within an Ussing chamber [5,7]. The chamber is designed in such a way as to permit two sets of electrodes (calomel and Ag-AgCl) to be placed in the bathing solutions contacting each side of the tissue. These electrodes permit the direct measurement of potential difference and by passage of a current, to negate the spontaneous potential difference, the measurement of a short-circuit current. Based on the potential difference and short circuit current and, using Ohm's Law (potential difference = current × resistance), an electrical resistance for the tissue can be calculated. The electrical resistance of esophageal epithelium predominantly reflects the permeability across the paracellular (as opposed to transcellular pathway and correlates over a wide range of values with lumen-to-serosal or serosal-to-lumen mannitol flux (flux measured by monitoring the appearance of ^{14}C-labeled mannitol in the serosal bath with luminally placed marker or vice versa) [5]. The values for esophageal epithelial resistance are usually 1,000–2,000 $\Omega \cdot cm^2$, which places the tissue in a category of being electrically "tight". Since the resistance of the cell membranes so greatly exceeds these values, electrical tightness implies limited diffusion of ions and molecules through the paracellular pathway. Thus, mannitol permeability across the healthy esophageal epithelium is in the range of 0.005 $\mu mol/h/cm^2$. If one studies an agent such as HCl (which damages the esophageal epithelium), a common pattern for injury to evolve is by altering the intercellular junctions such that paracellular permeability increases, and the latter will be reflected by both a decline in electrical resistance and increase in mannitol permeability [5].

Is there a relationship between defects in epithelial resistance and symptoms? The answer to this question can be developed in two ways, depending on the definition chosen for epithelial resistance. Based on the structure-function definition, the answer to this is in part *no* and in part *possibly*. The reason for the *no* is, that it is well known that the severity of esophagitis, as assessed by endoscopic mucosal appearance, fails to correlate with the degree of patient complaints (primarily heartburn) in that patients with severe disease may present little symptoms and those with mild (microscopic) disease may have severe symptoms [1]. The reason for any disagreement with this conclusion such that resistance may possibly correlate with symptoms has to do with the stage at which the disease is studied. Thus, for instance, the lack of significant symptoms in patients with gross disease may reflect chronic injury to sensory neurons within the mucosa. In contrast, those with mild disease may have more symptoms despite less disease because the sensory neurons remain intact and therefore are still capable of responding to noxious stimuli.

If the answer is to be based on the electrophysiologic definition of electrical resistance, the answer is a qualified *yes*. However there are not, nor are there likely to be, any in vivo data on the measurement of esophageal electrical resistance in humans. The reason for this is that, unlike the measurement of potential difference, the measurement of electrical resistance is potentially unsafe in as much as current would have to be passed across the epithelium to make the appropriate measurements for calculation of resistance (see above) [5]. As an alternative the potential difference can be measured and from its change, a change in electrical resistance can be inferred by reference to data from the Ussing chamber (the latter a technique in which both the potential difference and electrical resistance can be measured). Therefore, the data in humans showing that acid perfusion of the esophagus can elicit symptoms at a time when the esophageal potential difference falls to very low levels are consistent with the concept that a fall in electrical resistance may correlate with the presence of symptoms, at least for patients with early or mild disease [8]. It is clear, however, that in those with severe disease, the potential difference is already very low and this is true whether or not they are exhibiting symptoms at the time [6].

References

1. Orlando RC. Reflux esophagitis. In: Yamada T, Alpers DH, Owyang C, Powell DW, Silverstein FE (eds) Textbook of Gastroenterology. Philadelphia: JB Lippincott Company, 1991;1123–1147.
2. Orlando RC. Esophageal epithelial resistance. In: Castell DO (ed) The Esophagus. Boston: Little Brown Inc, 1992;463–478.
3. Orlando RC. Pathology of reflux oesophagitis and its complications. In: Jamieson GG (ed) Surgery of the Oesophagus. London: Churchill Livingstone, 1988;189–200.
4. Orlando RC, Lacy ER, Tobey NA, Cowart K. Barriers to paracellular permeability in rabbit esophageal epithelium. Gastroenterology 1992;102:910–923.
5. Orlando RC, Powell DW, Carney CN. Pathophysiology of acute acid injury in rabbit esophageal epithelium. J Clin Invest 1981;68:286–293.
6. Orlando RC, Powell DW, Bryson JC et al. Esophageal potential difference measurements in esophageal disease. Gastroenterology 1982;83:1026–1032.
7. Tobey NA, Powell DW, Schreiner VJ, Orlando RC. Serosal bicarbonate protects against acid injury to rabbit esophagus. Gastroenterology 1989;96:1466–1477.
8. Orlando RC, Powell DW. Studies of esophageal epithelial electrolyte transport and potential difference in man. In: Allen A, Flemstrom G, Garner A, Silen W, Turnberg LA (eds) Mechanisms of Mucosal Protection in the Upper Gastrointestinal Tract. New York: Raven Press, 1984:75.

Which factors lead to esophageal inflammation in GERD?

J. Janssens (Leuven)

Twenty-four hour pH recordings have clearly shown that patients with reflux eso-phagitis have a significantly greater exposure to acid reflux (% time, pH < 4) than control subjects and patients with reflux symptoms only. This is due to an increased number of reflux episodes which last longer due to an impaired acid clearing function. These factors are discussed in detail elsewhere.

The composition of the reflux fluid is a deciding factor in determining whether or not it harms the esophageal mucosa. The concentration of H^+ ions and, to a certain extent, the concentration of pepsin are generally considered to be the most important factors. Reflux of alkaline fluid containing bile salts, pancreatic enzymes, and lysolecithin, due to an increase in duodeno-gastric reflux, may play an important role in some patients. In some cases, it is the sole factor responsible for esophagitis, particularly after total gastrectomy [1]. The frequency of alkaline reflux is not well known, because this type of reflux is difficult to measure. Some studies suggest that this frequency might be higher than is generally thought [2]. However, other authors have concluded that alkaline reflux is rare. In a recent study by Gotley et al., in 52 patients with pathological reflux only one patient was found to have conjugated bile acids in the esophageal aspiration in concentrations likely to be cytotoxic [3]. The observation that reflux esophagitis heals in more than 95% of the cases if acid secretion is almost completely abolished, indicates that alkaline reflux cannot be the single most important factor in the pathogenesis of reflux esophagitis. Chung et al., have shown that the harmful effect of the H^+ ions depends both on their concentration and on the duration of exposure of the esophageal mucosa to these aggressive agents. The damaging effect of 80 mmol of HCl for 1 h is comparable to that of 20 mmol for 3 h [4]. There is no evidence that, as a group, patients with reflux have greater acid secretion than subjects without reflux [5]. Even in patients with refractory esophagitis, basal and maximal acid (and pepsin) secretion are not higher than in patients who heal after standard therapy [6]. It is only when the pH of the reflux fluid is sufficiently acidic that its damaging effect depends on the concentration of pepsin present. Maximal esophageal damage coincides with peptic solutions at pH 1.5–2.5 [7]. The reflux of pancreatic enzymes such as trypsin and amylase is probably not significant except after total gastrectomy or in patients with a reduced or absent hydrochloric acid content because an acid gastric pH irreversibly denatures these enzymes. It is generally accepted that bile salts reduce the resistance of the mucosal barrier. In themselves (i.e., in the absence of H^+ ions), they are not very toxic, but during acid reflux they potentiate the deleterious effect of the H^+ ions [8].

The resistance of the esophageal epithelium is another important and decisive factor in whether or not esophagitis develops. Although the mechanism of this mucosal resistance is less well investigated in the esophagus than in the stomach, the studies available show that the underlying mechanisms are roughly comparable.

The layer of mucus which carpets the mucosa of the esophagus is an important line of defense. The mucus probably comes both from the saliva and from the submucosal glands located in the proximal and distal parts of the esophagus. It is then drawn along by esophageal peristalsis and carpets the median part of the esophagus.

The aggressive elements which manage to cross this protective layer are stopped in their turn by the second line of defense, situated at the level of the mucosal cells. This epithelial permeability barrier consists of both the cell membranes and the intercellular junctional complexes. In the human esophagus, these junctional complexes are intercellular lamellar corpuscles, rich in lipids, rather than true tight junctions. The intercellular lamellar corpuscles act as cement plugs preventing the H^+ ions from spreading inside the cells. The paracellular pathway is the major route by which mucosal HCl enters and then damages the esophageal epithelium [9]. The permeability barrier consisting of the cell membrane itself rests on a phenomenon of active sodium transport from the lumen towards the blood. This transport of ions is reflected by a negative potential difference between the mucosa and the serosal membrane [10], the lumen being electrically negative in relation to the serosa. It is primarily via the basolateral membrane that hydrogen ions may enter the cell [11,12].

It is possible that in the esophagus, as in the stomach, bicarbonate brought by the blood may allow some elimination of H^+ ions which have crossed the epithelial barrier and may thus act as a postepithelial protection factor. Studies by Geboes et al., have shown that capillaries develop very early in the epithelium in patients suffering from reflux [13]. Also Zijlstra et al., have provided evidence that microvascular permeability increases early in the course of acid induced esophageal injury [14]. These observations seem to confirm that this defense mechanism might also play an important role in the esophagus.

When cell necrosis has occurred, the rate of cell regeneration is a major determinant of the severity of the lesions.

References

1. Stoker SL, Williams JG. Alkaline reflux oesophagitis. Gut 1991;32:1090–1092.
2. Pellegrini CA, DeMeester TR, Wernly JA et al. Alkaline gastroesophageal reflux. Am J Surg 1978;135:177–183.
3. Gotley DC, Morgan AP, Ball D, Owen RW, Cooper MJ. Composition of gastro-oesophageal refluxate. Gut 1991;32: 1093–1099.
4. Chung RSK, Magri J, DenBesten L. Hydrogen ion transport in the rabbit esophagus. Am J Physiol 1975;229:496–500.
5. Hirschowitz DI. A critical analysis, with appropriate controls of gastric acid and pepsin secretion in clinical esophagitis. Gastroenterology 1991;101:1149–1158.
6. Hirschowitz BI. Acid and pepsin secretion in patients with esophagitis refractory to treatment with H_2 antagonists. Scand J Gastroenterol 1992;27:449–452.
7. Zaninotto G, DiMario F, Costantini M, Baffa R, Germana B, Dalsanto PL, Rugge M, Bolzan M, Naccarato R, Ancona E. Oesophagitis and pH of refluxate: an experimental and clinical study. Br J Surg 1992;79:161–164.
8. Harmon JW, Johnson LF, Maydonovitch CH. Effects of acid and bile salt on the rabbit esophageal mucosa. Dig Dis Sci 1981;26:280–285.
9. Tobey NA, Powell DW, Schreiner VJ, Orlando RC. Serosal bicarbonate protects against acid injury to rabbit esophagus. Gastroenterology 1989;96:1466–1477.
10. Orlando RC, Powell DW, Bryson JC et al. Esophageal potential difference measurements in esophageal disease. Gastroenterology 1982;83:1026–1032.
11. Orlando RC, Powell DW, Carney CN. Pathophysiology of acute acid injury in rabbit esophageal epithelium. J Clin Invest 1981;68:286–293.

12. Tobey NA, Orlando RC. Mechanisms of acid injury to rabbit esophageal epithelium. Gastroenterology 1991;101:1220–1228.
13. Geboes K, Desmet V, Vantrappen G, Mebis J. Vascular changes in the esophageal mucosa: an early histologic sign of esophagitis. Gastrointest Endosc 1980;26:29–32.
14. Zijlstra FG, Hynna-Liepert TT, Dinda PK, Beck IT, Paterson WG. Microvascular permeability increases early in the course of acid-induced esophageal injury. Gastroenterology 1991;101:295–302.

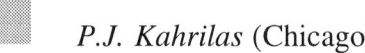

P.J. Kahrilas (Chicago)

Concomitant with the refinement in our knowledge of the mechanisms which underlie reflux events, the hypothesis which has emerged is that the extent of esophageal mucosal injury is determined by the duration of time that the mucosa is exposed to refluxate and by the caustic potency of refluxed fluid [1–3]. Symptomatic gastro-esophageal reflux disease (GERD) results when the balance between aggressive forces (reflux, potency of refluxate) and defensive forces (esophageal acid clearance, mucosal resistance) tilts in favor of the aggressive forces. The intermittent nature of symptoms in some individuals with GERD suggests that the aggressive and defensive forces are part of a rather delicately balanced system. Significant aberration in any one of these pathophysiologic influences can result in tipping the balance of forces acting on the esophageal mucosa from a compensated condition to a decompensated condition (heartburn, esophagitis).

Reflux esophagitis is a condition in which the esophageal epithelium is damaged by gastroesophageal reflux of predominant acid and pepsin. High grade changes in gastroesophageal reflux are characterized by severe epithelial injury or destruction, usually accompanied by neutrophil and/or eosinophilic infiltration of the mucosa. Low grade reflux esophagitis is detected histopathologically by reactive epithelial changes, rather than by the presence of inflammatory cells. The presence of more than very rare intraepithelial polymorphonuclear neutrophils or eosinophils is more consistent with high grade changes. The histopathologic criteria for low grade esophagitis, developed from a study of well-oriented capsule biopsies taken 2 cm above the manometrically defined lower esophageal sphincter (LES), are:

— the basal zone comprises more than 15% of the total thickness of the epithelium; and
— the papillae extend more than two thirds of the distance to the surface [4,5].

These criteria have been modified by other authors who pointed out additional features including, increased mitotic figures and an increased proportion of basal cells incorporating tritiated thymidine [6], vascularization of the epithelium with dilated vessels or "lakes" at the tops of the papillae [7], increased numbers of papillae [8], loss of the longitudinal orientation of the surface epithelial cells due to the presence of ovoid immature cells at the surface and balloon cells [9]. Except for vascular lakes and balloon cells, these additional features are morphologic consequences of the increased epithelial proliferation resulting from mild reflux injury [10]. Balloon cells probably result from increased cellular permeability due to reflux injury.

Mediators of tissue injury and mucosal defense

The development of esophagitis on a cellular level is the result of hydrogen ion diffusion into the mucosa leading to cellular acidification and necrosis. The esophageal mucosa possesses several morphologic and physiologic defenses against cellular acidification.

The esophageal mucosa is a 25–30 cell thick layer, nonkeratinized squamous epithelium functionally divided into a proliferating basal cell layer (stratum basalis), a midzone layer of metabolically active squamous cells (stratum spinosum), and a 5–10 cell thick layer of dead cells (stratum corneum) [11]. The epithelium also contains a few submucosal glands that may secrete bicarbonate into the submucosa, mucosa and lumen [12]. There is high inherent resistance to ionic movements in the esophageal mucosa at the intercellular as well as the cellular level, making it a relatively "tight" epithelium [13]. High intercellular resistance is a result of the complexity of the zona occludens (tight junctions) reflected both by the number of strands between cells and by the matrix of lipid rich material in the intercellular space [14]. The importance of tight junctions in retarding diffusion of noxious substances has been demonstrated experimentally with horseradish peroxidase and ionic lanthanum, as indicators of paracellular permeability. When the markers were applied luminally, their paracellular movement was restricted in the first few layers of the stratum corneum by tight junctions. In contrast, when applied serosally, they permeated freely through the basal cell and stratum spinosum layers and were retarded only within the intracellular space of the stratum corneum, seven to nine cell layers from the lumen [15]. These observations regarding the function of the stratum corneum highlight the vulnerability of the esophageal mucosa to injury once the superficial cell layers have been lost.

The effectiveness of the esophageal mucosal barrier is highlighted by the observation that this mucosa can effectively retard H^+ ion penetration when contacted by ion gradients of greater than 1:100,000 (5 pH units) [16]. The barrier function of epithelium can be demonstrated physiologically by its ability to maintain an electrochemical gradient across the mucosa, measured experimentally by the potential difference (PD) [14]. Luminal perfusion of rabbit esophageal mucosa (which closely resembles human esophageal mucosa) with a low concentration of HCl, results in a sustained increase in PD which would defend cellular integrity [17,18]. Available evidence suggests that the increased PD results from H^+ ion back diffusion that is at least partly attributable to a newly described Na^+/H^+ antiport of mucosal cell membrane, activated by cytoplasmic acidification [19]. Perfusion of esophageal mucosa with a higher concentration of HCl results in an initial increase in the PD followed by a reduction [17,18]. The initial increase presumably is by the same mechanism as in perfusion with a lower concentration hydrogen ion and the subsequent decrease probably reflects increased paracellular conductance resulting from disruption of the fine structure of epithelium. Increased paracellular conductivity was confirmed in studies showing increased mucosal to serosal flux of the inert nonionic marker mannitol [20]. Finally, when the mucosa is no longer able to maintain a significant PD, cells in the stratum spinosum appear ballooned and necrotic suggesting that acidification causes regulation of cell volume to fail. Balloon cells are a histopathologic marker of reflux esophagitis.

Although the eventual mediator of cellular injury is probably the hydrogen ion, several investigations have demonstrated that pepsin, bile acids, trypsin [21] and food hyperosmolarity facilitate susceptibility of the esophageal mucosa to acid injury. Since gastroesophageal refluxate is a heterogeneous mixture, containing all of these substances to varying degrees, it is reasonable to implicate them as facilitators of tissue injury.

The facilitative roles of pepsin and bile acids have been subjected to the most scrutiny. Pepsin is a proteolytic enzyme secreted in the stomach and, activated by gastric acid, is implicated as a coparticipant in acid-induced esophageal injury (i.e., peptic esophagitis) [2,21—23]. In vivo rabbit perfusion studies have demonstrated that at pH 2, pepsin, in concentration dependent fashion, significantly disrupts the histologic integrity of the mucosal barrier, increases hydrogen ion permeability and causes hemorrhage [21,24]. On the other hand, an esophagus exposed to a pepsin perfusate at pH 7.5 followed by a solution at pH 2, shows minimal mucosal disruption or changes in permeability. Thus, pepsin's ability to cause mucosal injury is pH dependent, reflecting the optimal pH activity range of its major isoenzymes (below pH 4).

Bile acids have also been implicated in the development of esophagitis, especially in instances of increased duodenogastric reflux [25]. Although bile acid concentration is notoriously difficult to quantify, concentrations of 0.5 mmol/l have been detected in the gastric aspirates of control subjects and up to 10.6 mmol/l in gastric aspirates from patients with gastric ulcer or gastrectomies. It stands to reason that the esophageal mucosa would be exposed to these same concentrations in the event of gastroesophageal reflux. Experimentally administered bile salts increase hydrogen ion absorption in the esophagus and accelerate tissue injury. For example, in rabbit esophageal mucosa, bile salts cause significant ion back diffusion and mucosal damage at intraluminal pH values of only 4.0, which is two pH units higher than what is needed for tissue penetration when the hydrogen ion is present alone [26]. Furthermore, there is evidence that bile acids can cause mucosal injury independent of acid, presumably by acting as detergents capable of solubilizing membranes [19,27].

References

1. DeMeester TR, Johnson LF, Joseph GJ, Toscano MS, Hall AW, Skinner DB. Patterns of gastroesophageal reflux in health and disease. Ann Surg 1976;184:459.
2. Goldberg HI, Dodds WJ, Gee S, Montgomery C, Zboralske FF. Role of acid and pepsin in acute experimental esophagitis. Gastroenterology 1969;56:223.
3. Johnson LF. 24-hour pH monitoring in the study of gastroesophageal reflux. J Clin Gastroenterol 1980;2:387.

4. Ismail-Beigi F, Horton PF, Pope CE II. Histological consequences of gastroesophageal reflux in man. Gastroenterology 1970;58:163–174.
5. Ismail-Beigi F, Pope CE II. Distribution of the histological changes of gastroesophageal reflux in the distal esophagus of man. Gastroenterology 1974;66:1109.
6. Livstone EM, Sheahan DG, Behar J. Studies of esophageal epithelial cell proliferation in patients with reflux esophagitis. Gastroenterology 1977;73:1315–1319.
7. Geboes K, Desmet VJ, Vantrappen G, Mebis J. Vascular changes in the esophageal mucosa: an early histologic sign of esophagitis. Gastrointest Endosc 1980;26:29.
8. Kobayashi S, Kasugai T. Endoscopic and biopsy criteria for the diagnosis of esophagitis with a fiberoptic endoscope. Am J Dig Dis 1974;19:345.
9. Jessurun J, Yardley JH, Giardello FM, Hamilton SR. Intracytoplasmic plasma proteins in distended esophageal squamous cells (balloon cells). Modern Pathol 1988;1:175.
10. Hamilton SR. Reflux esophagitis and Barrett esophagus. Monographs In Pathology 1990;31:11.
11. Yassin TM, Toner PG. Fine structure of squamous epithelium and submucosal glands of human esophagus. J Anat 1977; 123:705.
12. Hamilton BH, Orlando RC. In vivo alkaline secretion by mammalian esophagus. Gastroenterology 1989;97:640.
13. Powell DW. Barrier function of epithelia. Am J Physiol 1981;241:G275.
14. Elias PM, McNutt NS, Friend DS. Membrane alterations during cornification of mammalian squamous epithelia: a freeze-fracture, tracer, and thin-section study. Anat Rec 1977;189:577.
15. Lacy ER, Tobey NA, Cowart K. The esophageal mucosal barrier: structural correlates. Orlando RC. Gastroenterology 1989; 96:A281.
16. Chung RSK, Magri J, DenBesten L. Hydrogen ion transport in the rabbit esophagus. Am J Physiol 1975;229:496.
17. Orlando RC, Bryson JC, Powell DW. Mechanism of H^+ injury in rabbit esophageal epithelium. Am J Physiol 1984;246: G718.
18. Orlando RC, Powell DW, Carney CN. Pathophysiology of acute acid injury in rabbit esophageal epithelium. J Clin Invest 1981;68:286.
19. Layden TJ, Agnone LM, Schmidt LN, Hakim B. Rabbit esophageal cells possess an Na^+, H^+ antiport. Goldstein JL. Gastro-enterology 1990;99:909.
20. Goldstein JL, Schlesinger PK, Mozwecz HL, Layden TJ. Esophageal mucosal resistance A factor in esophagitis. Gastro-enterol Clin North Am 1990;19(3):565.
21. Lillemoe KD, Johnson LF, Harmon JW. Alkaline esophagitis: a comparison of the ability of components of the gastro-duodenal contents to injure the rabbit esophagus. Gastroenterology 1983;85:621–628.
22. Safaie-Shirazi S. Effect of pepsin on ionic permeability of canine esophageal mucosa. J Surg Res 1977;22:5.
23. Goldberg HI, Dodds WJ, Montgomery C et al. Controlled production of acute esophagitis. Invest Radiol 1970;5:254.
24. Lillemoe KD, Johnson LF, Harmon JW. Taurodeoxycholate modulates the effects of pepsin and trypsin in experimental esophagitis. Surgery 1985;97:662.
25. Safaie-Shirazi S, DenBesten L, Zike WL. Effect of bile salts on the ionic permeability of the esophageal mucosa and their role in the production of esophagitis. Gastroenterology 1975;68:728–734.
26. Lalyre Y, Subach C, Schmidt L, Barrett T, Layden T. Mechanism of combined bile salt and acid induced esophageal injury. Gastroenterology 1984;86:1149A.
27. Palmer ED. Subacute erosive ("peptic") esophagitis associated with achlorhydria. N Engl J Med 1960;262:927.

What features are evidence of reflux-related esophageal lesions?

A. Duranceau (Montreal)

Symptoms by themselves are known to be unreliable to diagnose gastroesophageal reflux disease [1,2]. Symptoms may suggest an esophageal investigation to rule out esophageal disease but cannot be used to establish the diagnosis of pathological reflux. Similarly radiological demonstration of gastroesophageal reflux cannot imply reflux disease. This observation shows a low sensitivity when compared to more specific diagnostic techniques [3,4]. Jamieson et al. [5] suggested the use of a staging process to classify reflux disease. This staging concept is based on what is considered at present the most objective evidence of mucosal and functional damage from reflux disease.

Histologic evidence

The normal esophagus has a mucosa made up of an epithelial layer of squamous cells supported by a lamina propria and a muscularis mucosa. The squamous epithelium itself is not keratinized in its outer layer. Its middle layer shows plumper cells while the basal layer shows cylindrical cells. The cells of the basal layer usually form less than 15% of the epithelium. The surface epithelium is supported by the lamina propria and the underlying muscularis mucosa. The lamina propria pushes papillae toward the surface of the epithelium but these papillae usually do not extend over more than two-thirds of the thickness of the epithelium.

The initial events leading to early mucosal damage were documented initially in the early 1970s. Ismail-Beigi and Pope [6], studying suction biopsies, suggested that when an increase in the basal layer thickness resulted in this part of the mucosa taking more than 15% of the total epithelium this indicated reflux disease. In parallel, when the papillae of the lamina propria were seen to penetrate over more than 66% of the epithelium thickness to come in close proximity to the esophageal lumen this was also considered as evidence of reflux disease. They observed, however, that these changes were distributed at random over the distal 8 cm of the esophagus and that 20% of their normal controls showed similar changes. Weinstein [7], looking at a different normal control population, found that over 50% of them actually showed these histological changes in the distal 2.5 cm of their esophagus.

The explanation for these changes is that the esophageal mucosa is usually impermeable to hydrogen ion. When stimulated by acid or even more by acid mixed with bile salts, pepsin and trypsin, the mucosa loses this impermeability and allows diffusion of hydrogen ions. Damage results in the subepithelial and basal layers of the epithelium [8]. This may stimulate a repair mechanism by causing direct damage to the basal layer of the epithelium. It has been shown that irritative stimulation of the esophageal mucosa leads to increased turnover of the basal layer and eventually to basal hyperplasia. This increased cellular activity leads to an increased blood supply, resulting in more prominent papillae pushing toward the surface of the epithelium. The initial changes in the lamina propria considered to be the best indicator of reflux damage are the presence of neutrophils and eosinophils: they increase in proportion with the mucosal damage. Progression in this damage leads to destruction of the epithelium with erosions and ulcerations. These acute changes then allow chronic inflammatory changes to occur in the lamina propria and in the submucosa. This inflammation rarely penetrates deeper than the submucosa and the muscularis is rarely affected. Despite the circular and longitudinal layers being spared, periesophageal inflammation and fibrosis are frequent when a stricture affects the esophagus. Thus periesophagitis does not imply panmural esophagitis.

If the ulceration, inflammation, granulation, fibrosis and the repair process continue overtime, stricture and re-epithelialization may occur [9]. The ulcerated part of the squamous mucosa will become progressively covered by a columnar mucosa which may grow slowly in a cephalad direction. This abnormal epithelium leads to the formation of a columnar lined esophagus with the columnar cells being gastric junctional or specialized in appearance. With persistent reflux the mucosal junction between the squamous epithelium and the columnar epithelium tends to be damaged with the same repetition of early and progressive changes of mucosal insult [10,11]. When damage occurs in the columnar lined esophagus, away from the mucosal junction, these ulcerations behave like gastric ulcers with a potential for penetration bleeding, perforation and fistulization.

When considering documented changes in the esophageal wall in reflux disease, the normal epithelium[H-0] and the epithelium showing only basal cell hyperplasia[H-1] are considered at present only equivocal in suggesting esophageal reflux mucosal damage. And this is mostly due to the fact that between 20% and 50% of a normal population (depending on the area of mucosal biopsies) may present these minimal changes of reflux disease.

If, however, esophageal mucosal biopsies show acute inflammation with erosions or ulcerations[H-2], or if they reveal the fibrosis of a stricture or the columnar lined epithelium of a Barrett's mucosa this can be considered unequivocal evidence of mucosal damage by reflux (Table 1).

Table 1. Histology

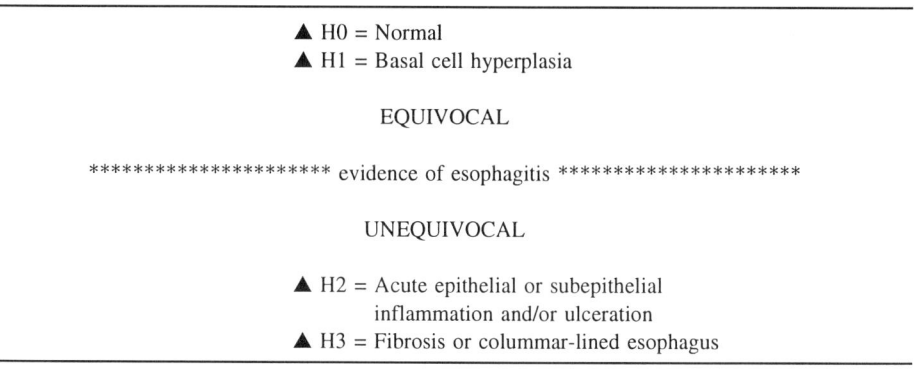

▲ H0 = Normal
▲ H1 = Basal cell hyperplasia

EQUIVOCAL

******************** evidence of esophagitis ********************

UNEQUIVOCAL

▲ H2 = Acute epithelial or subepithelial
       inflammation and/or ulceration
▲ H3 = Fibrosis or columnar-lined esophagus

Endoscopic evidence

Endoscopic assessment of esophageal mucosa damage remained limited when only rigid instruments were available. Attempts at classifying the mucosal disease have multiplied with the use of flexible instruments. Even early in these efforts, it became evident that the minimal damage situation, the minor degrees of inflammation, were the stage of the mucosal disease producing more difficulties with the classification [12,13]. When esophagitis was diagnosed endoscopically it did not always correlate with the histologic diagnosis. Siegel and Hendrix [14] found a correlation in 72% of their patients, Ward in 62.5% of his group. Schuman confirmed the endoscopic esophagitis in 32%. The explanation given for this discrepancy between observation and histology was mostly sampling errors due to the patchy nature of refluxed induced mucosal inflammation. Another reason for these differences might be related to the method of biopsy. Suction biopsies seem to show better the minimal histologic changes than the daily used pinch biopsies. When minimal damage exists different endoscopists will view the damage with different interpretations. Overinterpretation of mucosal alterations is easily done. Endoscopy for these reasons does not reliably detect lesser degrees of damage and chronic changes.

Whenever severe esophagitis exists the objectivity of observers is improved with an expected better correlation between observers and the existing damage.

One of the most recent classification has been proposed by Armstrong et al. [15]. Four categories of mucosal damage are reported: Metaplasia, Ulcers, Stricture and Erosions (MUSE). Each has an objective damage level quantified on its own and no place is given to minimal damage situations as viewed endoscopically. This classification seems to provide better visual information for easier and more precise reporting.

To provide the most objective information on endoscopic damage at present a normal mucosa[E-0] or a mucosa presenting only erythema[E-1] should be seen as presenting very unreliable evidence of esophagitis.

On the other hand, endoscopic documentation of erosions and ulcerations[E-2] is unequivocal proof of mucosal damage. Just as the presence of stricture and columnar lined mucosa[E-3] will also be taken as evidence of severe reflux disease (Table 2).

Motor function of the esophagus

Motor function studies of the esophagus provide evidence for the physiologic abnormalities which are most commonly seen with reflux disease. Those abnormalities may be present in the esophageal body and at the lower esophageal sphincter (LES) level.

Lower esophageal sphincter

The lower esophageal sphincter was described as hypotensive in nine of 10 patients first described by Atkinson [16]. However, Winans [17] and Pope [18] suggested that motility systems could not offer reliable enough recordings of the LES. Haddad [19] reported that patients with pH documented free reflux had the lowest basal pressures in the LES. High lower esophageal sphincter pressures (LESP) are usually not associated with reflux, whereas low LESP in the range of 0–10 mmHg above gastric baseline pressure are usually associated with reflux. Behar et al. [20] observed in their study that the presence of endoscopic esophagitis was usually associated with poor

Table 2. Endoscopy

▲ E0 = Normal	
▲ E1 = Erythema	

EQUIVOCAL

********************* evidence of esophagitis *********************

UNEQUIVOCAL

▲ E2 = Erosions and ulceration
▲ E3 = Stricture or columnar-lined esophagus

LES tone. They also observed that when a very low tone existed in the lower sphincter that the chances of altering sphincter function by medical management were nonexistent overtime. Kahrilas [21] showed that patients with increased reflux damage have significantly weaker LES resting pressures. Patients with a documented columnar lined esophagus show the worst changes with a virtually nonexistent lower sphincter accompanied by higher exposure to acid reflux [22–25].

When the LES is below 10, although suggestive of poor tone at the G-E junction, much variation exists at this level and it is too imprecise for identifying a potential for reflux. If the pressure in the LES is less than 6 mmHg, this shows a reasonably high specificity for the presence of abnormal reflux as documented by pH testing. When LES sphincter pressures are extremely low or nonexistent this suggests a more severe degree of reflux and a poorer prognosis for long-term medical therapy [24].

Esophageal body

Quantifying measurement of peristaltic activity and pressure amplitude are also of importance. Active esophagitis results in significantly altered function. There is an increase in failed peristalsis and significantly weaker contractions in the esophageal body [22]. Here again it is in patients with a columnar lined esophagus that the

Table 3. Manometry

▲ M0 = Normal esophageal motilityLES >10 mmHg
▲ M1 = Normal esophageal motilityLES 6–10 mmHg

EQUIVOCAL

***************evidence of functional abnormality*****************
associated with reflux

UNEQUIVOCAL

▲ M2 = Normal esophageal motilityLES <5 mmHg
▲ M3 = Aperistaltic esophagusLES <5 mmHg

functional abnormalities are worst [22–25].

With these studies in perspective motility studies offer objective and prognostic information on the physiologic damage present with reflux disease (Table 3). When motor function is normal in the esophageal body with LES pressure values above 10 mmHg[M-0], this is very equivocal evidence of functional damage. If esophageal contractions are propulsive with a LES between 6 and 10 mmHg[M-1], this is interpreted as being at the lower limits of normal and too imprecise to conclude a functional damage leading to reflux. When the LES is virtually absent (below 5 mmHg) this is considered as strong evidence of the physiologic abnormality necessary to cause significant reflux disease. In this situation normal motility[M-2] implies adequate defense mechanisms while the aperistaltic and powerless esophagus[M-3] suggests deficient function and a high probability of damage.

Twenty-four hour pH monitoring

The amount, frequency and time of acid exposure in the esophagus can be measured objectively by placing an electrode 5 cm above the manometric LES. Multiple pH probes can measure the esophageal exposure to acid reflux at different levels in the esophagus and correlate the observations with oropharyngeal, pulmonary or atypical chest pain symptoms.

Twenty-four hour pH monitoring has become the gold standard in establishing the presence of acid in the esophageal body [26]. When Johnson [27] and DeMeester [28] looked at their normal population, the total time of acid exposure in the control was always less than 4.2%. When Hölscher and Weiser [29] looked at their normal group, they suggested 7% of total acid exposure as being the normal acceptable level seen. Kraus [30] et al. suggested that the mean acid contact time measured during 24-h pH monitoring better indicates possible reflux injury. The mucosal injury level correlated to the period of acid exposure when Parilla et al. [23,24] reported their patients and compared them to a normal group. The esophagitis group showed exposure to an acid environment during 15% of the recording time. Columnar lined esophagus patients showed a mean acid exposure of 26%. Stein et al. [25] also reported a higher acid exposure in their esophagitis group with an even more significant increase if the patients had a columnar lined esophagus. They suggested that alkaline exposure could play a major role in the extent of mucosal damage.

With the notion that there is good correlation between endoscopic esophagitis and pH parameter of acid reflux, objective documentation of reflux disease could be reported (Table 4), where mean acid contact time and percentage of acid exposure when less than 7% represent equivocal proof of reflux disease[R-1]. Exposure to acid between 8 and 12%[R-2] or above 12%[R-3] usually correlates with more damage to the esophageal mucosa and represents unequivocal evidence of reflux.

The acid perfusion or Bernstein test is used to reproduce and assess symptoms. It is qualitative and by itself does not provide information on the severity of reflux. The acid emptying test as employed by Booth [31] measures the emptying capacity of the esophagus when it is exposed to an acid bolus. It is a measure of one of the

Table 4. pH monitoring

▲ R0 = No reflux
▲ R1 = < 3 reflux episodes — SART or 4–7% — 24-h pH

EQUIVOCAL

*************************** evidence of reflux ***************************

UNEQUIVOCAL

▲ R2 = >3 reflux episodes — SART or > 7% — 24-h pH
▲ R3 = >12% — 24-h pH

---

esophagus defense mechanism and may be abnormal in up to 50% of reflux esophagitis patients. Both the acid perfusion test and the acid clearance test are recorded in some way by the 24-h pH recording which measures acid exposure overtime as well as symptoms.

Conclusion

The pathology of established complications from reflux disease is at present the most objective evidence of damage in this condition. None of the existing diagnostic techniques are perfect by themselves. Their association, however, may prove useful to classify gastroesophageal reflux disease by grouping patients in categories of damage.

References

1. Gibson MA, Varghese A, Clarke KE, Irwin WG, Love AG. Heartburn for the patient — heartache for the doctor? Br Med J 1983;287:465–466.
2. Costantini M, Crookes PF, Bremner RM, Hoeft SF, Ehsan A, Peters JH, Bremner CG, DeMeester TR. Value of physiologic assessment of foregut symptoms in a surgical practice. Surgery 1993;114:780–787.
3. Morgan FH. Studies of intraluminal pressure and pH at the gastroesophageal junction. Q Bull NorthWest Univ Med Sch 1962;36:258–267.
4. Ott DJ, Gelfand DW, Wu WC. Reflux esophagitis: Radiographic and endoscopic evaluation. Diag Radiol 1979;130:583–588.
5. Jamieson CG, Duranceau A. Gastroesophageal Reflux. Staging of severity of GER. Philadelphia: WB Saunders, 1988; 105–111.
6. Ismail-Beigi F, Horton PF, Pope CE. Histological consequences of gastroesophageal reflux in man. Gastroenterology 1970;58:163–174.
7. Weinstein WM, Bogoch ER, Bowes KL. The normal human esophageal mucosa: A histological reappraisal. Gastroenterology 1975;68:40–44.
8. Kiroff GK, Mukerjhee K, Dixon B, Devitt PG, Jamieson GG. Morphological changes caused by the exposure of rabbit esophageal mucosa to hydrochloric acid and sodium taurocholate. Aust NZ J Surg 1987;57:119–126.
9. Sandry RJ. The pathology of chronic esophagitis. Gut 1962;3:189–200.
10. Bremner CG, Lynch VP, Ellis FH. Barrett's esophagus: congenital or acquired? An experimental study of esophageal mucosal regeneration in the dog. Surgery 1970;68:209–216.
11. Pollara WM, Zilberstein B, Cecconello I, Filho UL, Pinotti WH. Regeneration of esophageal epithelium in the presence of gastroesophageal reflux. In: DeMeester TR, Skinner DB (eds) Esophageal Disorders Pathophysiology and Therapy. New York: Raven Press, 1985.

12. Schuman BM, Rinaldo JA. Relative frequency of esophagitis and gastritis in patients with symptomatic hiatus hernia. Gastrointest Endo 1966;12:14—16.
13. Ward AS, Wright DH, Collis JL. The assessment of esophagitis in hiatus hernia patients. Thorax 1970;25:568—572.
14. Siegel CI, Hendrix TR. Esophageal motor abnormalities induced by acid perfusion in patients with heartburn. J Clin Invest 1963;42:686—695.
15. Armstrong D, Monnier Ph, Nicolet M, Blum AL, Savary M. Endoscopic assessment of oesophagitis. Gullet 1991;1:63—67.
16. Atkinson M, Edwards DAW, Honour AJ, Rowlands FN. The oesophagogastric sphincter in hiatus hernia. Lancet 1957;2:1138—1142.
17. Winans CS, Harris LD. Quantitation of lower esophageal sphincter competence. Gastroenterology 1967;52:773—778.
18. Pope CE. A dynamic test of sphincter strength: Its application to the lower esophageal sphincter. Gastroenterology 1967;52:779—786.
19. Haddad JK. Relation of gastroesophageal reflux to yield sphincter pressures. Gastroenterology 1970;58:175—184.
20. Behar J, Sheahan DG, Biancani P, Spiro HM, Storer EH. Medical and surgical management of reflux esophagitis. A 38 month report on a prospective clinical trial. N Engl J Med 1975;293:263—268.
21. Kahrilas PJ, Dodds WJ, Hogan WJ, Kern M, Arndorfer RC, Reece A. Esophageal peristaltic dysfunction in peptic esophagitis. Gastroenterology 1986;91:897—904.
22. Iascone C, DeMeester TR, Little AG, Skinner DB. Barrett's esophagus: Functional assessment proposed pathogenesis and surgical therapy. Arch Surg 1983;118:543—549.
23. Parilla P, Ortiz MA, Martinez De Haro LF, Aguayo JL, Ramirez P. Evaluation of the magnitude of gastroesophageal reflux in Barrett's esophagus. Gut 1990;31:964—967.
24. Parilla P, Martinez De Haro LF, Ortiz MA, Ruiz G, Aguayo JL, Morales G, Garcia Marcilla JA. Correlation between endoscopic and pH-metric findings and motor oesophageal alterations in reflux oesophagitis. Dig Surg 1991;8:210—214.
25. Stein HJ, Hoeft SM, DeMeester TR. Reflux and motility pattern in Barrett's esophagus. Dis Esophagus 1992;5:21—28.
26. Castell DO. pH monitoring versus other tests for gastroesophageal reflux disease: Is this the gold standard? In: Richter JE (ed) Ambulatory Esophageal pH Monitoring. New York: Igaku-Shoin, 1991;101—113.
27. Johnson LF, DeMeester TR. Twenty-four hour pH monitoring in the distal esophagus. Am J Gastroenterol 1974;62:325—332.
28. DeMeester TR, Johnson LF, Joseph GJ, Toscano MS, Hall AW, Skinner DB. Patterns of gastroesophageal reflux in health and disease. Ann Surg 1976;184:459—470.
29. Hölscher AH, Weiser HF. Reflux characteristics in health and disease. Gastrointestinal Motility, Lancaster: MTP Press Ltd, 1984;63—72.
30. Kraus BB, Wu WC, Castell DO. Comparison of lower esophageal sphincter manometrics and gastroesophageal reflux measured by 24-hour pH recording. Am J Gastroenterol 1990;85:692—696.
31. Booth DJ, Kemmerer WT, Skinner DB. Acid clearing from distal esophagus. Arch Surg 1968;96:731—740.

What are the particular features of purely diurnal reflux?

J.S. de Caestecker (London)

What is diurnal reflux?

Patterns of acid gastroesophageal reflux (GER) can be defined by prolonged esophageal pH monitoring. Diurnal reflux is that occurring during the daytime or "upright" period, as opposed to the night-time or "supine" period. The main features of waking hours (for these purposes) compared to sleep, are upright posture, physical activity and meals. Since lower esophageal sphincter pressure is lower after meals [1,2] and in the erect compared to the supine position [1,2], it is not surprising that even healthy individuals are more likely to reflux during the day than at night [3]. Furthermore, more reflux can be recorded in ambulant outpatients than hospital inpatients with restricted activities [4]. Graded physical activity itself has been shown to provoke reflux [5]. Thus, diurnal reflux is particularly evident in the 3 h period during and following meals [1,2], particularly the evening meal [6], and is enhanced by physical exertion.

How common is diurnal reflux?

It is well established that healthy asymptomatic control subjects characteristically reflux by day [1,3]. The majority of such individuals do not reflux at night, though a small number may have marked nocturnal reflux [7,8]. Abnormal diurnal reflux is defined quantitatively when the amount of acid reflux exceeds statistically defined upper limits established in healthy controls. These upper limits are now most commonly defined in terms of percentage of time that esophageal pH is less than 4, using a method (such as 95th centile of the range) [9] which does not assume a normal distribution of values. Reported upper limits for percentage of daytime pH 4 have varied widely, between 1.55% [10] and 10.5% [7]. A recent large multicentre series of 110 patients found a value of 8.15% [11]. It is clear therefore, that the distinction of normal from abnormal diurnal reflux on these grounds is far from clear cut. It is often more clinically helpful to separate normal from abnormal diurnal reflux on the basis of "symptom-reflux correlation" [12].

In patients presenting reflux symptoms, 9–31% have purely diurnal reflux (Table 1). However, it should be appreciated that these are selected groups of reflux patients referred for specialist care and as such they represent the "tip of the GERD iceberg". The patterns of reflux may not accurately represent that in the majority of patients in the community with reflux symptoms. A larger proportion could have purely diurnal reflux, but no data exists to address this issue.

Table 1. Patterns of reflux related to proportions with esophagitis in some hospital-based series

Reference	No.	Comments	Pattern of reflux		
			Upright	Supine	Combined
DeMeester et al. [17]	217		10%	26%	64%
	217	proportion with esophagitis	33%	46%	75%
Vitale et al. [28]	11	no esophagitis	18%	18%	27%
	40	esophagitis	20%	18%	43%
Schindlbeck et al. [7]	29	no esophagitis	21%	24%	45%
	16	esophagitis	31%	13%	56%

Notes: All patients had typical reflux symptomatology. Where percentages do not add up to 100%, the remainder did not have "abnormal" quantities of reflux.

What are the clinical features of diurnal reflux?

Typical symptoms are of postprandial and sometimes postural (on bending) or exertional heartburn. A definite positive relationship has been shown between the amount of acid reflux, particularly during the day, with frequency and severity of heartburn [13]. However, it is curious that a minority of acid reflux episodes are associated with symptoms [14]. Painful reflux episodes tend to be longer than painless episodes and also tend to have been preceded by other painful reflux episodes [14]. This implies that esophageal mucosal sensitivity is an important factor in determining whether symptoms occur. In this respect, an important minority of patients with purely diurnal reflux have "normal" amounts of acid reflux during prolonged pH monitoring, but frequent association of symptoms with reflux episodes [15]. These individuals, who have an abnormally acid sensitive esophagus, can be identified by calculating the "symptom index" [12,15].

DeMeester's group have characterized patients with pure diurnal reflux as "air swallowers" who reflux because they belch a great deal [3]. Consequently, if such individuals undergo antireflux surgery, they are more likely to suffer postoperative complications such as "gas bloat". Support for this clinical observation comes from the recent demonstration using ambulatory monitoring of esophageal pH, motility and sphincter pressure that the majority of daytime reflux episodes are associated with belching [16]. Furthermore, a relatively small number of patients with purely diurnal reflux have esophagitis, and of those that do, most have mild mucosal damage only (Table 1) [17].

What is the relationship of diurnal to nocturnal reflux?

DeMeester identified three patterns of reflux: "upright" or daytime reflux, "supine" or nocturnal reflux and "combined" daytime and night-time reflux [3]. All are defined in relation to "normal" reflux, observed in healthy controls. It appears that, with worsening degrees of reflux disease, not only does diurnal reflux increase but nocturnal reflux appears and contributes a progressively larger proportion to the total [18,19]. The concept is consistent with current research, indicating that in patients with severe esophagitis a large proportion of reflux episodes occur across an atonic lower esophageal sphincter, whereas in normal subjects and those with mild reflux disease most reflux occurs during transient lower esophageal sphincter relaxations [1,20]. Indeed, the classic manometric hallmark of lower esophageal dysfunction, a very low pressure sphincter (< 10 mmHg), occurs predominantly in those with severe esophagitis [21]. It is not difficult to understand why such individuals reflux during the night as well as during the day. On the other hand, it is unclear why some patients should only reflux abnormally at night; there is no evidence at present that these individuals have a different mechanism of reflux. It would be of interest to perform duplicate studies in patients with pure "supine" reflux to determine whether this pattern remains consistent.

Is nocturnal or diurnal reflux more damaging to the esophagus?

There has been considerable recent controversy surrounding this issue. Table 1 shows that the largest proportion of patients with esophagitis reflux both during the day and at night, and these individuals include a high proportion with severe esophagitis [17]. Patients with pure diurnal reflux also develop esophagitis which tends to be mild [17]. Significant correlations exist between increasing diurnal or nocturnal acid exposure and grade of esophagitis, the best correlation being obtained with diurnal and postprandial reflux [18]. As observed above, with worsening reflux disease, both diurnal and nocturnal reflux increase. Quantitatively, there is more diurnal than nocturnal acid exposure, but it has been pointed out that the relative increase (compared to healthy controls) is far greater at night [19,22]. Additionally, reflux at night is more slowly cleared, both because of sleep [23] — since swallow-initiated peristalsis and saliva delivery to the esophagus are inhibited — and the recumbent posture [24]. Reflux patients are in "double jeopardy" at night since they also commonly have impaired distal esophageal motor function [25]. For these reasons, some authors feel that nocturnal reflux is the more damaging to the esophagus.

Undoubtedly, grade of esophagitis is most closely correlated with the total 24 h acid exposure (usually expressed as % time pH < 4) [18,19,26]. Therefore, it is total acid contact, whether during the day or at night, which results in esophageal mucosal damage. Studies examining correlations between grade of esophagitis and reflux during different periods cannot differentiate between cause and effect. What of the argument that reflux episodes during the night are longer lasting than those during the day? There is now evidence to suggest that the most damaging form of reflux is intermittent and repeated [27]; this would support a damaging potential for diurnal reflux. Despite differing interpretations of the available data, there is a clear and practical message which emerges; all acid reflux, in whatever portion of the 24-h period, is potentially damaging to the esophagus. Therapy is most likely to succeed when 24 h reduction in esophageal acid exposure is achieved.

References

1. Dent J, Dodds WJ, Friedman RH et al. Mechanism of gastroesophageal reflux in recumbent asymptomatic human subjects. J Clin Invest 1980;65:256–267.
2. Dodds WJ, Dent J, Hogan WJ et al. Mechanisms of gastroesophageal reflux in patients with reflux esophagitis. N Engl J Med 1982;307:1547–1552.
3. DeMeester TR, Johnson LF, Joseph GJ et al. Patterns of gastroesophageal reflux in health and disease. Ann Surg 1976; 184:459–470.
4. Branicki FJ, Evans DF, Ogilvie AL, Atkinson M, Hardcastle JD. Ambulatory monitoring of oesophageal pH in reflux oesophagitis using a portable radiotelemetry system. Gut 1982;23:992–998.
5. Schofield PM, Bennett DH, Whorwell PJ et al. Exertional gastro-oesophageal reflux: a mechanism for symptoms in patients with angina pectoris and normal coronary angiograms. Br J Med 1987;294:1459–1461.
6. Gudmundsson K, Johnsson F, Joelsson B. The time pattern of gastroesophageal reflux. Scand J Gastroenterol 1988;23: 75–79.
7. Schindlbeck NE, Heinrich C, Konig A et al. Optimal thresholds, sensitivity and specificity of long-term pH-metry for the detection of gastroesophageal reflux disease. Gastroenterology 1987;93:85–90.
8. Cheadle WG, Vitale GC, Sadek SA, Cuschieri A. Computerised ambulatory esophageal pH monitoring in 50 asymptomatic volunteer subjects: results and clinical implications. Am J Surg 1988;155:503–508.

9. Johnsson F, Joelsson B, Isberg PE. Ambulatory 24 hour intraesophageal pH-monitoring in the diagnosis of gastroesophageal reflux disease. Gut 1987;28:1145—1150.
10. Johansson KE, Boeryd B, Fransson SG, Tibbling L. Oesophageal reflux tests, manometry, endoscopy, biopsy and radiology in healthy subjects. Scand J Gastroenterol 1986;21:399—406.
11. Richter JE, Bradley LA, DeMeester TR, Wu WC. Normal 24-h ambulatory esophageal pH values: influence of study center, pH electrode, age and gender. Dig Dis Sci 1992;37:849—856.
12. Wiener GJ, Richter JE, Coopper JB, Wu WC, Castell DO. The symptom index: a clinically important parameter of 24-h esophageal pH monitoring. Am J Gastroenterol 1988;83:358—361.
13. Joelsson B, Johnsson F. Heartburn — the acid test. Gut 1989;30:1523—1525.
14. Lacey Smith J, Opekun AR, Larkai E, Graham DY. Sensitivity of the esophageal mucosa to pH in gastroesophageal reflux disease. Gastroenterology 1989;96:683—689.
15. Howard PJ, Maher L, Pryde A, Heading RC. Symptomatic gastro-oesophageal reflux, abnormal oesophageal acid exposures and mucosal acid sensitivity are three separate, though related, aspects of gastro-oesophageal reflux disease. Gut 1991;32: 128—132.
16. Barham CP, Gotley DC, Miller R, Mills A, Alderson D. Ambulatory measurement of oesophageal function: clinical use of a new pH and motility recording system. Br J Surg 1992;79:1056—1060.
17. DeMeester TR, Wang CI, Wernly JA et al. Technique, indications and clinical use of 24 hour esophageal pH monitoring. J Thorac Cardiovasc Surg 1980;79:656—667.
18. de Caestecker JS, Blackwell JN, Pryde A, Heading RC. Daytime gastro-oesophageal reflux is important in oesophagitis. Gut 1987;28:519—526.
19. Jenkinson LR, Norris TL, Barlow AP, Watson A. Acid reflux and oesophagitis — day or night? Gullet 1990;1:36—44.
20. Dent J, Holloway RH, Toouli J, Dodds WJ. Mechanisms of lower oesophageal sphincter incompetence in patients with symptomatic gastro-oesophageal reflux. Gut 1988;29:1020—1028.
21. Kahrilas PJ, Dodds WJ, Hogan WJ et al. Esophageal peristaltic dysfunction in peptic esophagitis. Gastroenterology 1986; 91:897—904.
22. Kruse-Andersen S, Wallin L, Madsen T. Reflux patterns and related oesophageal motor activity in gastro-oesophageal reflux disease. Gut 1990;31:633—638.
23. Orr WC, Johnson LF, Robinson MG. Effect of sleep on swallowing, esophageal peristalsis and acid clearance. Gastroenterology 1984;86:814—819.
24. Kjellen G, Tibbling L. Influence of body position, dry and water swallows, smoking and alcohol on oesophageal acid clearing. Scand J Gastroenterol 1978;13:283—288.
25. Johnson LF. Methods of testing esophageal clearance. In: Dubois A, Castell DO (eds) Esophageal and Gastric Emptying. Florida: CRC Press, 12—27.
26. Rokkas T, Sladen GE. Ambulatory esophageal pH recording in gastroesophageal reflux: relevance to the development of esophagitis. Am J Gastroenterol 1988;83:629—632.
27. Cassidy HT, Geisinger KR, Kraus BB, Castell DO. Continuous versus intermittent acid exposure in production of esophagitis in a feline model. Dig Dis Sci 1992;37:1206—1211.
28. Vitale GC, Cheadle WG, Sadek S, Michel ME, Cuschieri A. Computerised 24-hour ambulatory esophageal pH monitoring and esophagogastroduodenoscopy in the reflux patient: a comparative study. Ann Surg 1984;200:724—728.

Can the rumination syndrome be differentiated from physiologic reflux?

A.J.P.M. Smout, R. Breumelhof (Utrecht)

Definition

Rumination is usually defined as the repetitive regurgitation of small amounts of gastric contents into the mouth, in the absence of organic disease. The term rumination is derived from the latin word rumen, one of the stomachs of herbivores who, as part of their normal eating behavior, bring up undigested food into the mouth. In humans rumination is considered abnormal.

Mechanisms of rumination

In ruminant herbivores, regurgitation of gastric contents into the mouth is accomplished by cyclic, sequential contractions of the reticulum and rumen. This is followed by forceful inspiration which sucks food into the distal esophagus, whereafter a high velocity antiperistaltic wave is believed to carry the contents to the pharynx and the oral cavity [1]. In man, elevation of the intra-abdominal pressure caused by contraction of the abdominal wall is the most important driving force in the retropulsion of the material. In this process, the antireflux barrier, constituted by the lower esophageal sphincter, must be overcome. Some studies indicate that transient lower esophageal sphincter (LES) relaxations, induced by intra-abdominal pressure rises, play a role [2,3].

Differential diagnosis

Clinically the rumination syndrome may mimic gastroesophageal reflux disease (GERD) and idiopathic vomiting. Careful history taking may, however, distinguish the rumination syndrome from these disorders in the majority of cases. Most patients with a rumination syndrome have been ruminating since infancy. Rumination always occurs in the early postprandial period which may help to differentiate it from reflux disease. The aliquots of food that reach the pharynx and mouth are small, in contrast to the situation in vomiting. In rumination there is no nausea and no retching. The act of rumination is not preceded by, or associated with, vasomotor symptoms, such as palpitation, sweating and light-headedness. In fact, most patients with the rumination syndrome may admit that the symptom itself is not really unpleasant. Usually the retropelled food is reswallowed, which is seldom the case in vomiting. Patients with the rumination syndrome seldom complain of heartburn. They may, however, have macroscopic esophagitis and the enamel of the teeth may be affected by prolonged acid exposure.

The above described characteristics usually allow the differentiation between rumination, reflux disease and vomiting on the basis of the history itself. If not, careful observation of the patient during a postprandial period may provide the necessary information.

Manometric differentiation

An objective diagnosis of the rumination syndrome requires esophago-gastrointestinal manometry, preferably combined with esophageal pH monitoring. Several authors

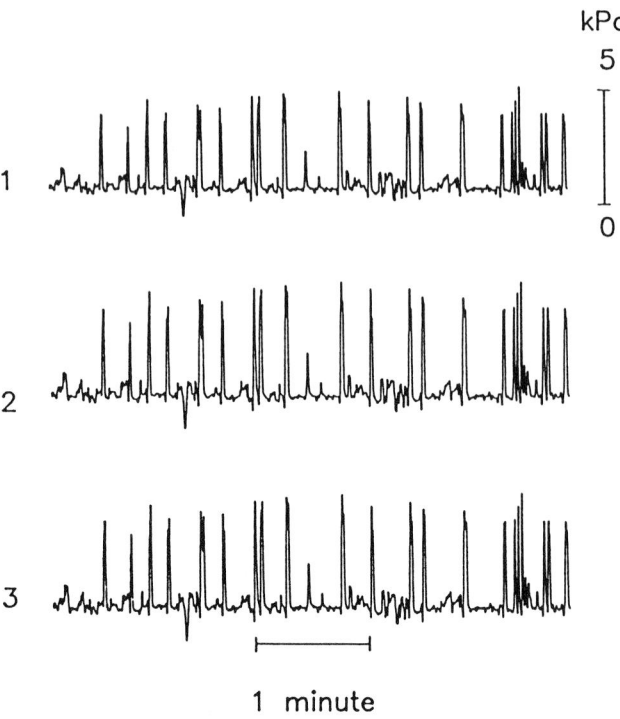

Fig. 1. Antral manometry in a patient with the rumination syndrome. In the postprandial period simultaneous pressure spikes at all pressure sites can be seen. These are not caused by antral contractions but by voluntary contractions of the abdominal wall, giving rise to increased intra-abdominal pressure. Sensors 1, 2 and 3 were located 3 cm apart in the antrum.

have reported a characteristic pressure spike pattern, recorded simultaneously at all manometric sites in the abdomen [2–6]. These simultaneous pressure spikes (Fig. 1) are brought about by contraction of the abdominal wall. In typical cases these pressure spikes occur at a rate of up to 4/min. The amplitude of these spikes may be as high as 60 mmHg. When simultaneous esophageal pH monitoring is carried out, one sees a precipitous fall in esophageal pH immediately after all, or most of these pressure spikes (Fig. 2). When this is observed, one has proven that the reflux is not spontaneous but induced voluntarily by abdominal contractions.

Treatment

Some anecdotal reports about biofeedback training as a successful treatment modality for the rumination syndrome were reported. Controlled studies in large groups of patients are still lacking, however, in a substantial proportion of cases, supportive therapy (explanation and gastric acid secretion inhibitors) is sufficient treatment.

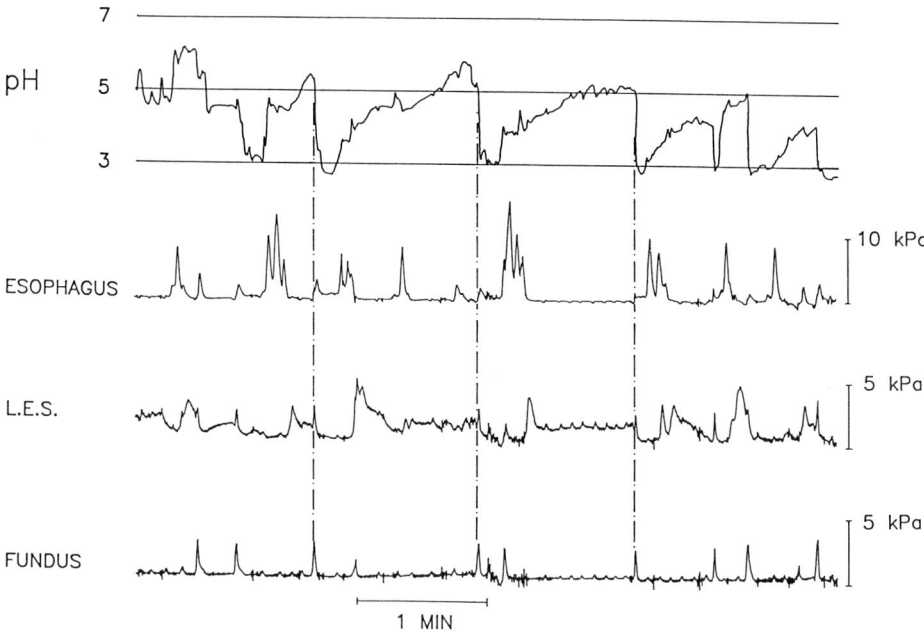

Fig. 2. Simultaneous esophageal pH monitoring and manometry of the esophagogastric junction in a patient with the rumination syndrome. The LES pressure was monitored with a Dent sleeve. Several intra-abdominal pressure peaks can be seen which are followed by a reflux episode. In the episodes indicated by the dashed lines, transient LES relaxations appear to be involved.

Experience with antireflux surgery in the rumination syndrome appears to be nonexistent.

Summary

Usually the differentiation between rumination syndrome and other disorders in which gastric contents are retropelled (such as reflux disease or idiopathic vomiting), can be made on the basis of the clinical history. If doubt persists, esophagogastric manometry combined with esophageal pH-metry will enable the differentiation. The treatment of the rumination syndrome has not been well established.

References

1. Winship DH, Zboralske FF, Weber WN et al. Esophagus in rumination. Am J Physiol 1964;207:1189−1194.
2. Smout AJPM, Breumelhof R. Voluntary induction of transient lower esophageal sphincter relaxations in an adult patient with the rumination syndrome. Am J Gastroenterol 1990;85:1621−1625.
3. Breumelhof R, Smout AJPM, Depla ACTM. The rumination syndrome in an adult patient. J Clin Gastroenterol 1990;12:232−234.
4. Amarnath RP, Abell TL, Malagelada JR. The rumination syndrome in adults. A characteristic manometric pattern. Ann Int Med 1986;105:513−518.
5. Reynolds RPE, Lloyd DA. Manometric study of a ruminator. J Clin Gastroenterol 1986;82:127−130.
6. Levine DF, Wingate DL, Pfeffer JM et al. Habitual rumination: a benign disorder. Br J Med 1983;287:255−256.

What is the correlation between mucosal damage and symptoms?
Are symptoms adequate for the classification of esophagitis?

W.C. Orr (Oklahoma City)

Establishing a correlation between symptoms, gastroesophageal reflux (GER) events, and the presence or absence of mucosal pathology has proven to be complicated and difficult. The complicated interactions can be viewed at several different levels. For example, one can simply consider the relationship between the presence or absence of erosive lesions and the presence or absence of classic symptoms such as heartburn or regurgitation, or more specifically, at the relationship between a specific GER event and the presence or absence of a subsequent symptom. The latter entails dealing with a very complicated epistemological question of cause and effect and assessment of various contingencies of symptoms and reflux events, in order to establish the presence or absence of a true predictive relationship. It is simply not enough to assume that if every symptom is associated with a reflux event, there is a true cause-effect relationship. This ignores the basal frequency of both reflux events and symptoms, and the fact that these two events could easily be associated by chance alone. Thus, the utilization of the classic symptom index described by Wiener et al., is not adequate [1]. This measure relies solely on the occurrence of symptoms and reflux events, while ignoring the basal rate of GER. The establishment of any cause-effect relationship must be done via a contingency table analysis which takes into account the basal frequency of reflux events, symptoms, and the various combinations of the occurrence of these events. This then creates a four-way contingency table for proper analysis [2].

Adding to the complexity of this issue is the well-established fact that the majority of recorded reflux events are not accompanied by a report of a symptom, by the patient [3,4]. However, it does appear that a symptom could be associated with reflux events (i.e., the presence of esophagitis increases the likelihood that a reflux event will produce a symptom) [3]. Reproducing a specific typical symptom in a patient with acid perfusion also fails to be sufficiently discriminating to be clinically useful [5]. The problem with the acid perfusion test is the high rate of false-negatives. That is, the test is quite likely to reproduce symptoms in patients who actually have esophagitis, but a negative test in no way excludes individuals with esophagitis [5,6]. Another variable which further complicates the relationship between reflux and symptomatology is the finding that, as might be expected, the lower the pH of the refluxant, the greater the probability of symptoms occurring [3].

Symptoms alone appear to be a rather poor predictor of the presence or absence of esophagitis [4,7]. Utilizing pH monitoring alone as the criterion for the presence or absence of GER disease, it was shown that the frequency of heartburn and acid regurgitation differed significantly between groups with normal and abnormal pH monitoring. However, the specificity and sensitivity, as well as results from a multivariate discriminant analysis, did not produce particularly convincing results in terms of the ability of these physiological measures to predict the clinical status of the patient [4]. Another study found that a confident clinical diagnosis could be obtained in less than half of the patients with esophagitis [8]. In addition, a recent study confirmed the relative inadequacy of symptoms in distinguishing patients with erosive and nonerosive esophagitis [7]. These investigators noted that the mean severity of reflux symptoms and the number of symptomatic reflux events per week did not distinguish patients with erosive and nonerosive esophagitis. They concluded that assessment of symptoms is an inadequate substitute for endoscopy in predicting the presence or absence of esophagitis. Also, it would appear that other tests, such as the acid perfusion test and even the 24-h pH test, are relatively poor predictors of the presence or absence of esophagitis.

References

1. Wiener GJ, Richter JE, Cooper JB, Wu WC, Castell DO. The symptom index: A clinically important parameter of ambulatory 24-hour esophageal pH monitoring. Am J Gastroenterol 1988;83(4):358−361.
2. Orr WC. Noncardiac chest pain: Conundrum of cause and effect (Editorial). Am J Gastroenterol 1991;86(10):1548−1550.
3. Baldi F, Ferrarini F, Longanesi A, Ragazzini M, Barbara L. Acid gastroesophageal reflux and symptom occurrence. Analysis of some factors influencing their association. Dig Dis Sci 1989;34(12):1890−1893.
4. Klauser AG, Schindlbeck NE, Muller-Lissner SA. Symptoms in gastro-oesophageal reflux disease. Lancet 1990;335:205−208.
5. Kaul B, Petersen H, Grette K, Myrvold HE, Halvorsen T. The acid perfusion test in gastroesophageal reflux disease. Scand J Gastroenterol 1986;21:93−96.
6. Winnan GR, Meyer CT, McCallum RW. Interpretation of the Bernstein test: A reappraisal of criteria. Ann Int Med 1982;96:320−322.
7. Sloan S, Kahrilas PJ, Richards CS, Rubinstein AM. Symptom assessment does not predict severity of disease in GERD patients. Gastroenterology 1993;104:A23.
8. Wienbeck M, Berges W. Esophageal disorders in the etiology and pathophysiology of dyspepsia. Scand J Gastroenterol 1985; 20(suppl 109):133−137.

Can severe reflux symptoms without endoscopic evidence of esophagitis be due to irritation of the nerve of the submucosa?

Y. Hamanaka, Y. Hirose, H. Hayashi, T. Murakami
(Yamaguchi)

There have been many studies regarding the effects of reflux content, such as hydrochloric acid, pepsin, bile and pancreatic juice, on the esophageal mucosa. Each has been shown to play an important role in causing reflux esophagitis [1]. However, clinically and potentially, the relative contributions of each factor of the refluxate to the reflux esophagitis have not been elucidated. Although the pH of the refluxate in the esophagus and/or the stomach have been recently elucidated using 24-h pH monitoring, the clinical relationship between the above mentioned barrier breakers and pH remains unclear. There are many questions to be answered, such as:

— Why can we not find early esophagitis by endoscopy in patients with severe reflux symptoms?
— Microscopically, where are the initial foci of the esophagitis?

Experimental study using canine esophagus [2]

Under general anesthesia, right thoracotomy was performed and a double lumen tube was inserted orally into the esophagus, the esophagogastric junction was then occluded with rubber tape. The perfusion system incorporated a reservoir, a water bath and a microtube pump. Esophageal perfusion was performed for 2 h with 200 ml of perfusate. Perfusate solutions consisted of 100 mM HCl and various concentrations of pepsin (0, 1, 2 g/l) and sodium taurocholate (Na-Tc) (0, 10, 20 mM) in different combinations.

Histochemical examination

After 2-h perfusion, the esophageal segment was removed and opened longitudinally. Macroscopic findings were then assessed. The full thickness of the mucosa was fixed in 10% phosphate buffered formalin, embedded in paraffin and sectioned. The sections were stained with hematoxylineosin, alcian blue (pH 2.5) and high iron diamine [3] to detect mucins and submucosal glands.

On gross inspection, pepsin-perfused segments of the esophagus showed fine unevenness compared to marked mucosal edema in Na-Tc perfused segments of the esophagus. Pepsin injury was characterized by substantial mucosal erosion and inflammatory cell infiltrations in the lamina propria, while the esophageal glands in the submucosal layer were not involved (Fig. 1). Submucosal edema, destruction of esophageal glands and leakage of mucins were pathognomonic in the Na-Tc perfused esophageal mucosa (Fig. 2). These characteristic findings (i.e., mucosal erosion and destruction of esophageal glands) were graded according to the following scale: 0 = none; 1 = slight; 2 = moderate; 3 = severe (Table 1). Also, it is conceivable that bile induced reflux esophagitis initially develops not only in the mucosa but also in the submucosal layer. This hypothesis, if correct, might explain pathogenesis of reflux esophagitis in patients with severe reflux symptom but without endoscopic findings of esophagitis.

Selection of experimental animals

Human esophagi have a few but obvious esophageal glands [2,4] which may serve as protection against several injurious substances. Although many investigators have

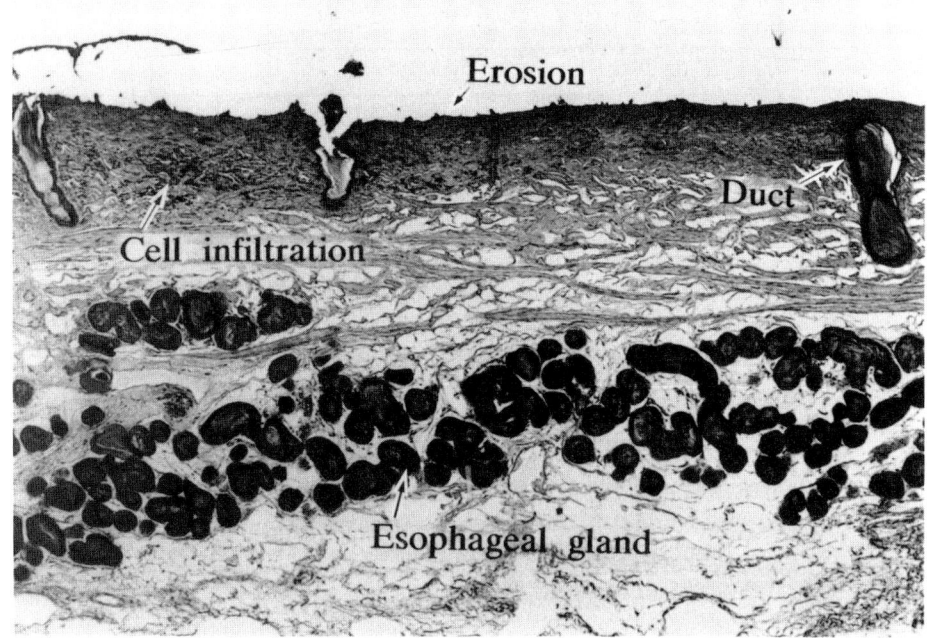

Fig. 1.

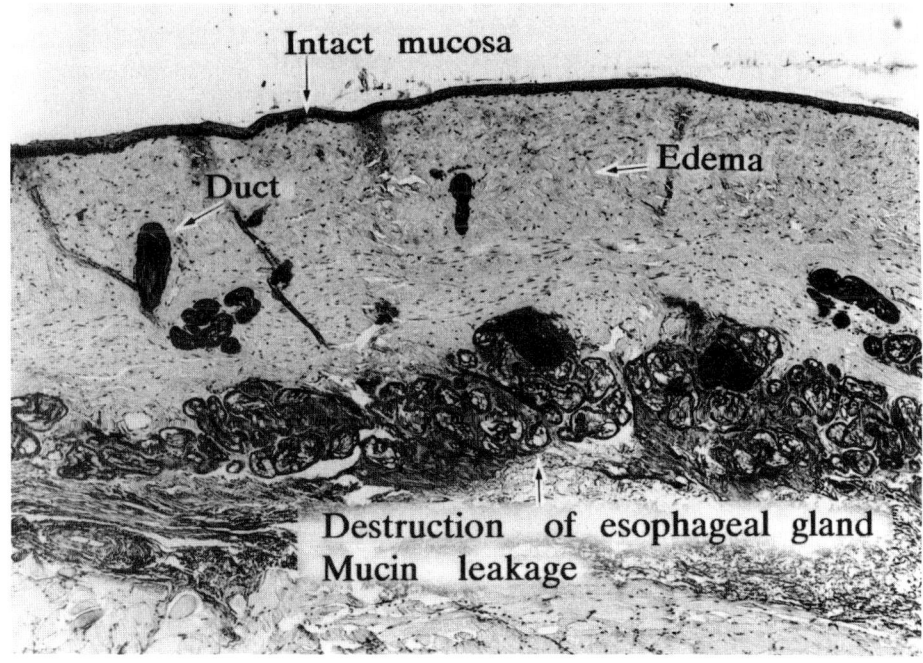

Fig. 2.

Table 1. Histochemical findings in pepsin (P) and/or sodium taurocholate (Na-Tc) perfused canine esophagus (n = 18)

	Na-Tc 0 mM		Na-Tc 10 mM		Na-Tc 20 mM	
	erosion	destruction	erosion	destruction	erosion	destruction
P 0 g/l	0.1	0.0	0.0	1.3	0.0	2.3
P 1 g/l	2.2	0.1	0.1	0.0	1.1	1.1
P 2 g/l	3.3	0.1	0.0	2.2	0.2	0.3

Note: 0 = none; 1 = slight; 2 = moderate; 3 = severe.

used rabbit esophagi for a model of esophagitis, there are no esophageal glands in this animal. In contrast, an opossum or a dog have many esophageal glands in the submucosal layer [5]. It is important and of interest to clarify whether the submucosal gland and its duct or orifice are relevant to the development of reflux esophagitis as a site of origin.

Detailed examination of each barrier breaker

Under general anesthesia, a canine esophagus was opened longitudinally and fixed horizontally by stay sutures. Several chambers (made of Teflon, content volume 2 ml, weight 5 g) were placed on the esophageal mucosa. Saline used as a control and several combinations of barrier breakers (i.e., HCl, pepsin, Na-Tc, bile, pancreatic juice) were added to the chamber for 30 min.

Figure 3 shows that 100 mM HCl plus pepsin 2 g and 100 mM HCl plus Na-Tc 20 mM was added to the chamber. After 30 min, the resected esophagus revealed fine unevenness in the case of pepsin and mucosal edema in Na-Tc (Fig. 4). The specimen was fixed in formalin for microscopic analyses and 2% glutaraldehyde for scanning electron microscopy (SEM). Figure 5 shows SEM findings of normal canine eso-phageal mucosa after being treated with saline. A fine microridge was seen on the surface of the mucosa. After being treated with canine bile, the microridge had disappeared and squamous cell exfoliation was seen (Fig. 6). Na-Tc caused more severe exfoliation of the superficial squamous cell layer (Fig. 7). Pepsin induced complete desquamation, exposing collagen fibers and fibrine (Fig. 8). This procedure has the following advantages:
— It is easy to change the combination of barrier breakers.
— It is easy to change the contact time.
— Several breakers can be applied at the same time in various parts of the same esophagus in vivo.
— Both the surface and deeper layers of the esophagus can be examined using light and electron microscope.

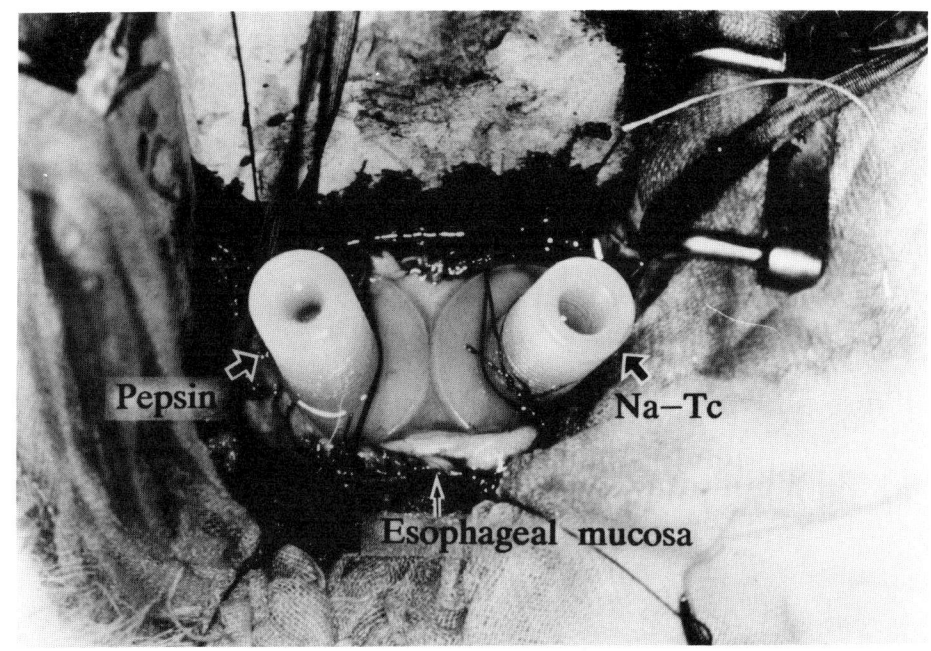

Fig. 3.

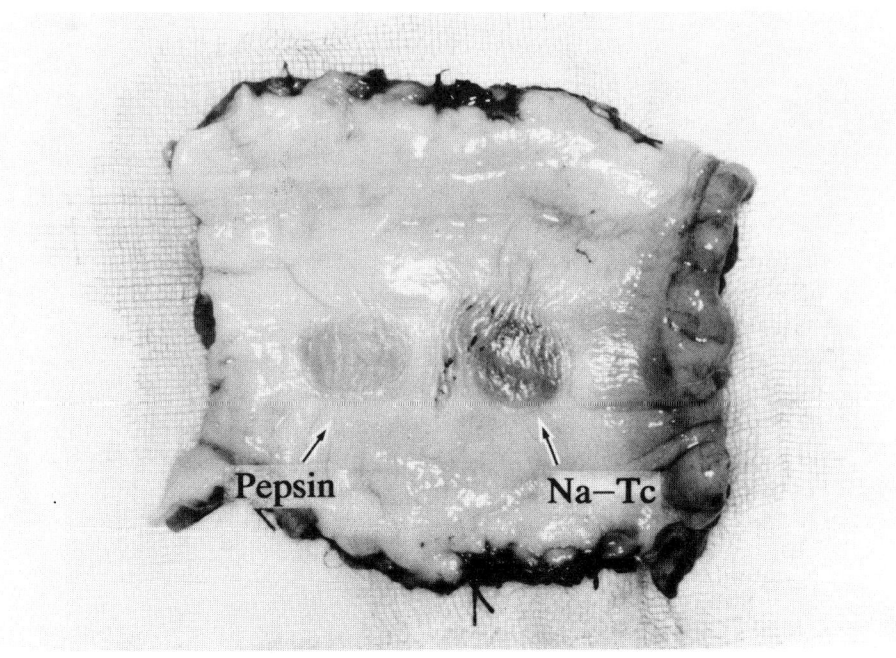

Fig. 4.

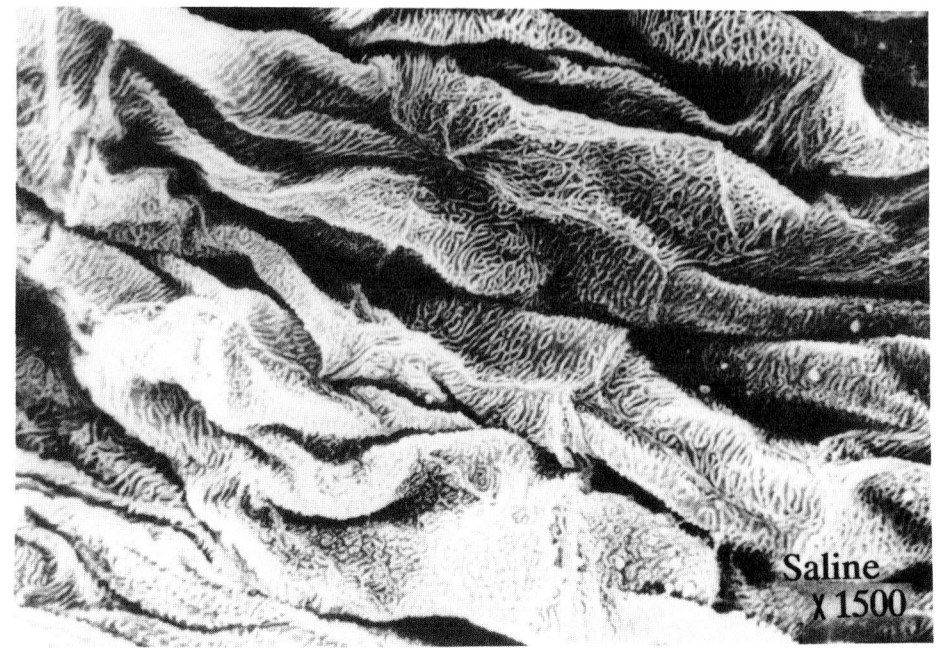

Fig. 5.

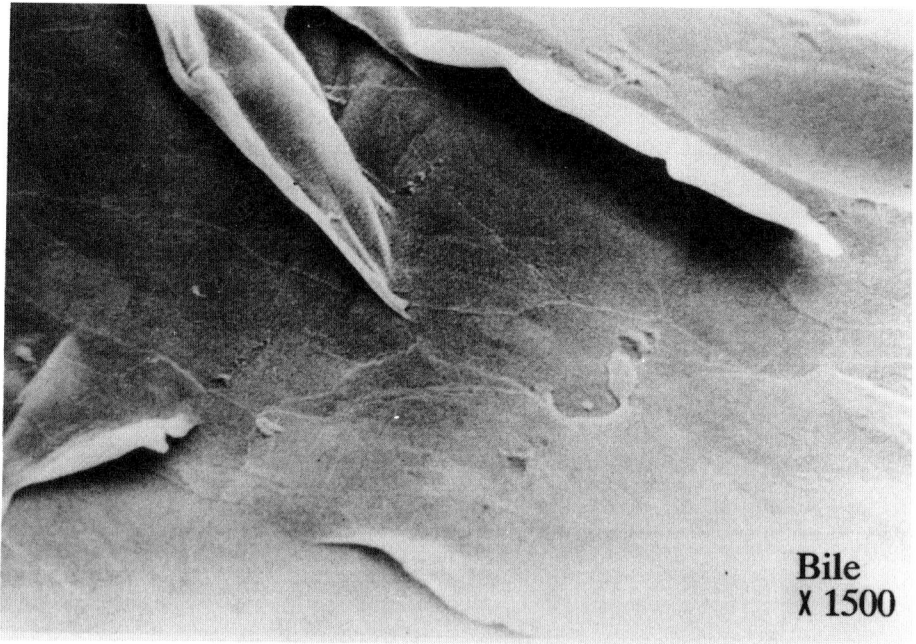

Fig. 6.

102

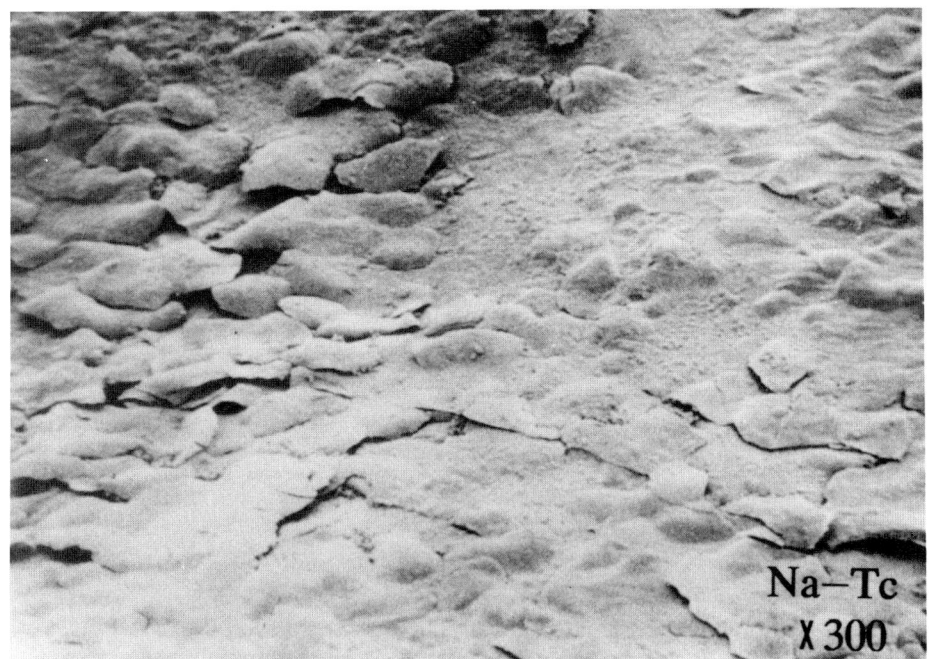

Fig. 7.

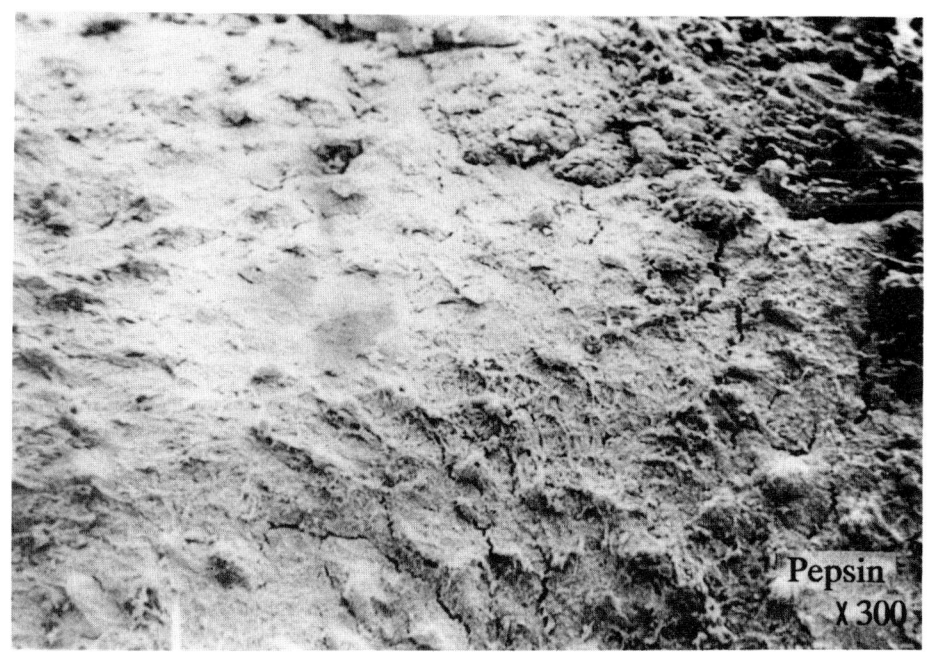

Fig. 8.

Summary

Based on our experimental findings, Na-Tc acted on deeper layers of the canine esophagus while pepsin acted superficially. Therefore, we hypothesized that the early stage of bile reflux esophagitis may develop in the orifices of the esophageal gland and submucosal glands.

References

1. Goldstein JL, Schledinger PL, Mozwecz HL et al. Esophageal mucosa resistance. A factor in esophagitis. Gastroenterol Clin North Am 1990;19:565–586.
2. Hamanaka Y, Ishigami K, Murakami T et al. Pathogenesis of reflux esophagitis in relation to the characteristic difference between acid-pepsin and bile as an aggressive factor. Dis Eso 1988;1:119–127.
3. Gad A, Sylven B. On the nature of the high-iron diamin method for sulfomucins. J Histochem Cytochem 1969;17:156–160.
4. Hamilton BH, Orlando RC. In vivo alkaline secretion by mammalian esophagus. Gastroenterology 1989;97:640–648.
5. Harmon JW, Johnson LF, Maydonovitch CL. Effects of acid and bile salts on the rabbit esophageal mucosa. Dig Dis Sci 1981;26:65–72.

The otorhinolaryngologic manifestations of esophagitis: peptic laryngitis

R.T. Sataloff, D.O. Castell, M.J. Hawkshaw, J.R. Spiegel
(Philadelphia)

Occult chronic gastroesophageal reflux (GER) is an etiologic factor in a high percentage of patients with laryngological complaints. Patients with reflux laryngitis (RL) frequently have characteristic histories and physical findings which lead to the diagnosis. Although it is seen in general otolaryngologic practice in patients of all ages, the problem is particularly common in professional singers. In 1991, Sataloff et al. reported reflux in 265 of the 583 consecutive professional voice users (45%) who sought medical care during a 12-month period, although RL was often diagnosed incidentally and was not always responsible for the patient's primary voice complaint [1]. The incidence may be lower in patients with other vocations. However, it is interesting to note that Koufman, et al. found increased GER in 78% of patients with hoarseness [2]. Nevertheless, convincing studies of the prevalence of RL are not available.

Professional voice users: a special case

Acid reflux is especially common in singers for several reasons. First, the technique of singing involves "support," forceful compression of the abdominal muscles designed to push the abdominal contents superiorly and pull the sternum down. This compresses the air in the thorax and generates force for the stream of expired air. However, it also compresses the stomach and works against the lower esophageal sphincter (LES). Singing is an athletic endeavor, and the mechanism responsible for reflux in voice users is similar to that associated with reflux following other athletic activities, lifting, and pregnancy (in addition to hormonal factors). Secondly, many singers do not eat before performing because a full stomach interferes with abdominal support and promotes reflux. Performances usually take place at night. Consequently, the singer returns home hungry and eats a large meal before bed. Thirdly, performance careers are particularly stressful, and this factor may be associated with increased acid production. Fourthly, many singers pay little attention to good nutrition, frequently consuming caffeine, fatty foods, spicy foods, citrus products (especially lemons), tomatoes (including pizza and spaghetti), and fatty "fast foods."

Symptoms

Common symptoms of RL include morning hoarseness, prolonged warm up time (greater than 20–30 min), halitosis, excessive phlegm, frequent throat clearing, dry mouth, coated tongue, sensation of a lump in the throat, throat tickle, dysphagia, chronic sore throat, nocturnal cough, chronic or recurrent cough, difficulty breathing (especially at night), closing off of the airway ("laryngospasm"), regurgitation of food, poorly controlled asthma (which causes dysphonia by interfering with the support mechanism), pneumonia, and occasionally dyspepsia. However, dyspepsia is frequently absent. Interestingly, if patients stop reflux treatment after a period of a couple of months or more, classic dyspepsia is frequently present when symptoms recur. In addition to prolonged vocal warm up time, professional singers and actors may also complain of voice practice intolerance. This involves frequent throat clearing and excessive phlegm especially during the first 10 to 20 min of vocal exercises or songs. Although the majority of otolaryngologists have only begun to acknowledge the importance of reflux in causing otolaryngologic disease recently, many authors have recognized the association over a period of more than 2 decades [3–27].

Signs

Laryngoscopic examination typically reveals erythema and edema of the mucosa overlying the arytenoid cartilages, the posterior aspect of the larynx, and often the posterior portion of the true vocal folds. In severe cases, the erythema and edema may be more extensive. Mild, nonspecific laryngitis and halitosis are also commonly present. In some patients with laryngitis severe enough to involve the oral cavity, there is also loss of dental enamel. Transparency of the lower portion of the central incisors may be seen occasionally in reflux patients, although it is more common in patients with bulimia.

In addition to erythema and edema, more significant vocal fold pathology may be caused by reflux laryngitis. In 1968, Cherry and Margulies [28] recognized that reflux laryngitis might be a causative factor in contact ulcers and granulomas of the posterior portion of the vocal folds. They also observed that treatment of peptic esophagitis resulted in resolution of vocal process granulomas. Delahunty and Cherry [29] followed up on this observation by applying gastric juice to the vocal processes of two dogs, and applying saliva in a similar fashion to the vocal processes of a third dog who was used as a control. The control dogs' vocal folds remained normal, the other dogs developed granulomas at the sites of repeated acid application. Since then, numerous authors have recognized the importance of reflux laryngitis as a causative factor in laryngeal ulcers and granulomas, including intubation granuloma [2,4,7,8, 30–36]. In addition to its etiological involvement in intubation granuloma, reflux laryngitis has long been recognized as contributing to posterior glottic stenosis, especially following intubation [37]. Olson has suggested that it may also be involved in causing cricoarytenoid joint arthritis through chronic inflammation and ulceration, beginning on the mucosa and involving the synovial cricoarytenoid joint [32]. In addition to posterior glottic and supraglottic stenosis, subglottic stenosis has also been reported as a complication of reflux [3,38].

Vocal fold pathology may also occur secondary to aspiration of gastric juice. Severe coughing may cause vocal fold hemorrhage or mucosal tears, sometimes leading to permanent dysphonia. Aspiration also makes reactive airway disease difficult to control. Even mild pulmonary obstruction impairs voice support. Consequently, afflicted patients subconsciously strain to compensate with muscles in the neck and throat, designed for delicate control, not for power source functions [39]. This behavior is typically responsible for vocal nodules and other voice abuse lesions.

It appears likely that RL is also causally related to laryngeal carcinoma. The association of GERD with Barrett's esophagus and esophageal carcinoma has been well established. Delahunty biopsied the posterior laryngeal mucosa in a RL patient and reported epithelial hyperplasia with parakeratosis and papillary downgrowth [25]. Olson reported five patients with posterior laryngeal carcinoma, in whom he believed reflux to be a cofactor [32]. This issue was also addressed by Morrison [40]. Although the causal relationship between reflux and laryngeal cancer has not been established with absolute certainty, it appears likely.

In addition to its possible carcinogenic potential, the chronic irritation of reflux laryngitis may be responsible for failure of wound healing, another sign of reflux. Reflux appears to delay the resolution not only of vocal process ulcers and granulomas, but also of surgical vocal fold disruptions. For this reason, otolaryngologists are becoming increasingly aggressive about diagnosing and treating reflux before subjecting patients to vocal fold surgery, even for conditions unrelated to the reflux.

Tests

Tests to confirm the presence of reflux laryngitis are discussed elsewhere in this book, and will not be reviewed in this chapter. However, a couple of points are worth special consideration. At present, 24-h pH monitoring is considered the most definitive study and should be used to confirm abnormal reflux in many of these patients. Studies in our laboratory have shown that dual electrode pH recording can document abnormal distal and proximal esophageal reflux induced by singing (Fig. 1). However, occasionally patients will show abnormalities on barium swallow with water siphonage, but normal 24-h pH monitor studies. Although this is usually regarded as a "false-positive" barium study, this assumption may require further investigation. In professional singers and actors especially, barium swallow with water siphonage provides a good clinical approximation of daily activities. In order to optimize mucosal function, it is essential for singers and actors to remain well hydrated. Consequently they drink large quantities of water, routinely carry water bottles with them, and drink substantial quantities shortly before they sing. This routine behavior is similar to the water siphon portion of the barium swallow, and this raises the question of whether positive water siphonage tests may provide useful information

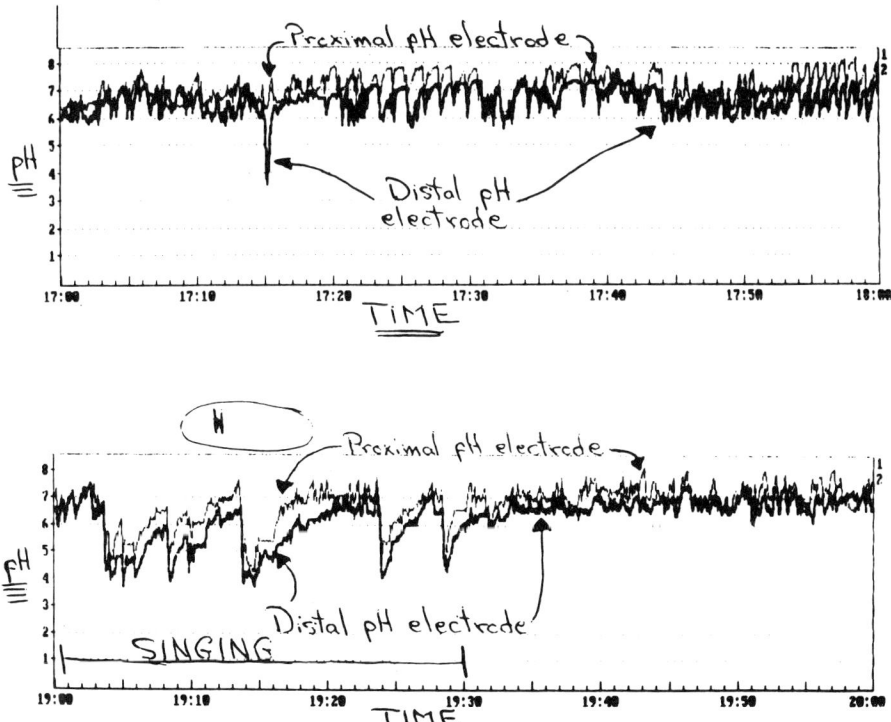

Fig. 1. Dual electrode pH probe monitoring while singing for a 30 min period of the 1 h shown. The patient experienced typical heartburn, and increased proximal and distal acid exposure was prominent during singing.

at least in professional voice users, even when 24-h pH monitor studies are normal, much like the singing challenge (Fig. 1).

Other otolaryngologic manifestations of GERD

Other otolaryngologic manifestations of GERD are beyond the scope of this chapter. However, chronic recurrent sore throat, "globus hystericus," chronic aspiration, recurrent airway problems in infants, Zenker's diverticulum, oropharyngeal dysphagia, halitosis, possibly geographical tongue, and other problems encountered commonly by laryngologists may all be caused by, or associated with, reflux. Otolaryngologists are becoming increasingly diligent about recognizing GERD as the underlying problem, and beginning to treat it as the primary approach to these conditions, as well as to the many laryngeal abnormalities discussed above.

Treatment

Treatment considerations in reflux patients are discussed elsewhere in this book. However, it should be noted that patients with reflux laryngitis frequently require more intensive therapy with higher doses of H2 blockers than patients with dyspepsia in the absence of laryngeal symptoms and signs. In addition to monitoring symptoms and signs of RL, response to treatment is best judged by combined intraesophageal and intragastric pH monitoring of patients while they are receiving treatment. Research into appropriate treatment regimens is ongoing, and extensive additional investigation is needed on the consequences of reflux upon the larynx, and upon all of the other mucosal surfaces above the cricopharyngeus muscle.

References

1. Sataloff RT, Spiegel JR, Hawkshaw MJ. Strobovideolaryngoscopy: Results and clinical value. Ann Otol Rhinol Laryngol 1991;100(9):725—727.
2. Koufman JA, Wiener GJ, Wu WC, Castell DO. Reflux laryngitis and it's sequelae: The diagnostic role of ambulatory 24-hour pH monitoring. J Voice 1988;2(1):78—89.
3. Bain WM, Harrington JR, Thomas LE et al. Head and neck manifestations of gastroesophageal reflux. Laryngoscope 1983; 93:175—179.
4. Cherry J, Siegal C, Margulies S et al. Pharyngeal localization of symptoms of gastroesophageal reflux. Ann Otol Rhinol Laryngol 1970;79:912—915.
5. Chodosh P. Gastro-esophago-pharyngeal reflux. Laryngosocope 1977;87:1418—1427.
6. Hallewell JD, Cole TB. Isolated head and neck symptoms due to hiatus hernia. Arch Otolaryngol 1970;92:499—501.
7. Johnson LF. New concepts and methods in the study and treatment of gastroesophageal reflux disease. Med Clin N Am 1981;65:1195—1222.
8. Ward PH, Zwitman D, Hanson D, et al. Contact ulcers and granulomas of the larynx: New insights into their etiology as a basis for more rational treatment. Otolaryngol Head Neck Surg 1980;88:262—269.
9. Olsen NR. The problem of gastroesophageal reflux. Otolaryngologic Clin North Am 1986;19(1):119—133.
10. Sataloff RT. Professional singers: The science and art of clinical care. Am J Otolaryngol 1981;8(3):251—266.
11. Ward PH, Berci G. Observations on the pathogenesis of chronic nonspecific pharyngitis and laryngitis. Laryngoscope 1982; 92:1377—1382.
12. Ossakow SJ, Elta G, Colturi T, Bogdassarian R, Nostrant TT. Esophageal reflux and dysmotility as the basis for persistent cervical symptoms. Ann Otol Rhinol Laryngol 1987;96(4):387—392.

13. Kuriloff DB, Chodosh P, Goldfarb R, Ongseng F. Detection of gastroesophageal reflux in the head and neck: The role of scintigraphy. Ann Otol Rhinol Laryngol 1989;98:74–80.
14. Lumpkin SMM, Bishop SG, Katz PO. Chronic dysphonia secondary to gastroesophageal reflux disease (GERD): Diagnosis using simultaneous dual probe prolonged pH monitoring. J Voice 1989;3(4):351–355.
15. McNally PR, Maydonovitch CL, Prosek RA, Collette RP, Wong RKH. Evaluation of gastroesophageal reflux as a cause of idiopathic hoarseness. Dig Dis Sci 1989;34(12):1900–1904.
16. Wiener GJ, Koufman JA, Wu WC, Cooper JB, Richter JE, Castell DO. Chronic hoarseness secondary to gastroesophageal reflux disease: Documentation with 24-h ambulatory pH monitoring. Am J Gastroenterol 1989;84(12):1503–1507.
17. Katz PO. Ambulatory esophageal and hypopharyngeal pH monitoring in patients with hoarseness. Am J Gastroenterol 1990; 85(1):38–40.
18. Sataloff RT. Reflux and other gastroenterologic conditions that may affect the voice. Professional Voice: The Science and Art of Clinical Care. New York: Raven Press Ltd, 1991;179–183.
19. Freeland AP, Ardran GM, Emrys-Roberts E. Globus hystericus and reflux oesophagitis. J Laryngol Otol 1974;88(10): 1025–1031.
20. Koufman JA. Otolaryngologic manifestations of gastroesophageal reflux disease (GERD): A clinical investigation of 225 patients using ambulatory 24 hr pH monitoring and an experimental investigation of the role of acid and pepsin in the development of laryngeal injury. Laryngoscope 1991;101(4)(suppl 53):2.
21. Pesce G, Caligaris F. Posterior laryngitis in the pathology of the digestive system (Le laringiti posteriori nella pathologia dell'apparato digerente). Arch Ital Laringol 1966;74(2):77–92 (in Italian).
22. Vaughan CW, Strong MS. Medical management of organic laryngeal disorders. Otolaryngol Clin North Am 1984;17(4): 705–712.
23. Barkin RL, Stein ZL. GE reflux and vocal pitch [letter; comment] Hospital Pract, 1989;Oct. 30 24(10A):20.
24. Kambic V, Radsel Z. Acid posterior laryngitis. Aetiology, histology, diagnosis and treatment. J Laryngol Otol 1984;98(12): 1237–1240.
25. Delahunty JE. Acid laryngitis. J Laryngol Otol 1972;86(4):335–342.
26. Jacob P, Kahrilas PJ, Herzon G. Proximal esophageal pH-metry in patients with reflux laryngitis. Gastroenterology 1991; 100(2):305–310.
27. Wilson JA, White A, von Haacke NP, Maran AG, Heading RC, Pryde A, Piris J. Gastroesophageal reflux and posterior laryngitis. Ann Otol Rhinol Laryngol 1989;98(6):405–410.
28. Cherry J, Margulies S. Contact ulcer of the larynx. Laryngoscope 1968;78:1937–1940.
29. Delahunty JE, Cherry J. Experimentally produced vocal cord granulomas. Laryngoscope 1968;78:1941–1947.
30. Goldberg M, Noyek A, Pritzker KPH. Laryngeal granuloma secondary to gastroesophageal reflux. J Otolaryngol 1978;7: 196–202.
31. Ohman L, Tibbling L, Olafsson J et al. Esophageal dysfunction in patients with contact ulcer of the larynx. Ann Otol Rhinol Laryngol 1983;92:228–230.
32. Olson NR. Effects of stomach acid on the larynx. Proc Am Laryngol Assoc 1983;104:108–112.
33. Sataloff RT. Professional Voice: The Science and Art of Clinical Care. New York: Raven Press, 1991.
34. Gould WJ, Sataloff RT, Spiegel JR. Voice Surgery. St. Louis, Missouri: C.V. Mosby Co, 1993.
35. Teisanu E, Hecioia D, Dimitriu T, Calarasu R, Marinescu A. Tulburari faringolaringiene la bolnavii cu reflux gastro-esofagian. Otorinolaringologia 1978;23(4):279–286.
36. Miko TL. Peptic (contact ulcer) granuloma of the larynx. J Clin Pathol 1989;42:800–804.
37. Bogdassarian RS, Olson NR. Posterior glottic laryngeal stenosis. Otolaryngol Head Neck Surg 1980;88:765–772.
38. Fligny I, François M, Algrain Y, Polonovski JM, Contencin P, Narcy P. Subglottic stenosis and gastroesophageal reflux (Sténoses sous-glottiques et reflux gastro-oesophagien). Ann Otolaryngol Chir Cervicofac 1989;106(3):193–196.
39. Sataloff RT. The human voice. Scientific American 1993;267(6):108–115.
40. Morrison M. Is chronic gastroesophageal reflux a causative factor in glottic carcinoma? Otolaryngol Head Neck Surg 1988; 99(4):370–373.

Are GER and asthma related?

S.J. Sontag (Hines)

Historians are not certain whether Adam first had heartburn or wheezing when he finally realized that God knew about the apple [1]. Ancient philosophers and Talmudic scholars, realizing the importance of Adam's symptoms, openly discussed the possible relationship of heartburn to wheezing. In the last millennium, numerous theologians have suggested a link between many types of pulmonary abnormalities and gut symptoms such as gastroesophageal reflux (GER) [2–7]. In modern times, the focus of attention has centered on two specific entities: GER and asthma. Does GER cause asthma? Does asthma cause GER? Are GER and asthma even related? Indeed, some skeptics have dared to imply that GER and asthma may not be related [8,9]. Such skepticism must be stopped, lest it spread to the scientific community. There is simply too much evidence suggesting that in certain patients an exacerbating or even causative relationship exists between GER and asthma.

By the late 1970s, at least 16 articles on the relationship between GER and pulmonary disease already had been published [2–7,10–18]. No less than six of these studies showed improvement in pulmonary status with antireflux surgery. Since 1977, numerous investigators have reported on the epidemiology, studied the mechanisms and conducted clinical trials in an effort to piece together the GER/asthma puzzle.

Epidemiological evidence for the GER/asthma association suggests that about three-fourths of asthmatics, independent of the use of bronchodilators [19–22], have acid GER [19], increased frequency of reflux episodes [19], or heartburn [20]; and 40% have reflux esophagitis [21].

Three factors reported to promote GER in asthmatics are the use of bronchodilators [23–25], assuming the supine position [26,27] and overeating [15,28]. The exact mechanism by which the GER promotes the bronchospasm, however, still remains unknown. The results of previous work [29] and of other published studies on mechanisms [26,30–34] have failed to provide a diagnostic test with a degree of certainty high enough to identify patients with GER-induced asthma. It has been suggested, however, that the occurrence of a GER-induced exacerbation of asthma is dependent on a number of factors. These factors include reflux of gastric acid into the esophagus, an acid sensitive esophagus (positive Bernstein), and a low nocturnal threshold to bronchoconstrictive stimuli [26], which may result from the normal circadian variations in bronchial reactivity and/or a waning of the effect of bronchodilator medications [35].

Bronchodilators

Asthmatics who require bronchodilators might be expected to be at risk for nocturnal asthma because of increased drug-induced GER followed by decreased bronchodilating activity as the drug is eliminated throughout the night. Indeed, asthma drug therapy, by relaxing the lower esophageal sphincter (LES), has been reported to adversely influence GER [24,36–40] and potentially contribute to or worsen asthma [41,52].

Recent studies, however, demonstrated similar reflux patterns both in the group receiving and in the group not receiving bronchodilators [19]. There appeared to be no adverse effects of bronchodilators on any of the GER parameters during the upright, supine, postprandial or nonpostprandial periods. Although GER parameters in each subject were not studied before and after, it was demonstrated that asthmatics receiving bronchodilators had no worse reflux than those not receiving bronchodilators, suggesting that bronchodilators do not promote postprandial or nocturnal reflux. Indeed, two placebo controlled studies also could not demonstrate an adverse effect of asthma medications on acid reflux or frequency of reflux episodes [25,42].

Supine position

The prevalence of night cough and nocturnal wheezing is significantly greater in asthmatics with GER than in asthmatics without GER [27], and GER has been implicated as an etiologic factor in nocturnal wheezing [43]. In a clinical trial of 18 patients with asthma and symptomatic GER, night-time asthma scores improved significantly in the group receiving cimetidine [44], suggesting that acid reflux has a role in nocturnal wheezing. Although nocturnal reflux is similar in bronchodilator-requiring and bronchodilator-nonrequiring asthmatics, when compared to controls they had more than 4 times the acid reflux and 19 times the frequency of prolonged reflux episodes. Thus, with or without bronchodilator therapy, asthmatics have significantly more acid reflux when asleep than do nonasthmatics.

Postprandial reflux

Since esophageal acid clearance time is increased in the supine position 3 h after eating [45], lying down immediately after a meal might be expected to result in even greater GER. Indeed, even during the upright period, the greatest acid reflux occurs after eating [46] in both refluxers and controls. Thus, a large meal at supper time in an individual with delayed emptying might be expected to remain in the stomach after bedtime, promote nocturnal GER, and contribute to night-time bronchoconstriction. It still is unknown whether the bronchoconstriction is due to a vagal reflex or direct aspiration.

More than 50 years ago, Bray [15] observed in some of his patients that dietary indiscretion could lead to asthmatic attacks. He believed that gastric distention from late evening overeating could cause a vagally mediated reflex bronchoconstriction. More recently, Mansfield et al. [47] demonstrated in dogs a significant fall in respiratory conductance and functional residual capacity after distention of the esophagus and intraesophageal hydrochloric acid infusion.

Evidence also suggests that two separate mechanisms are involved in the GER/asthma relationship. The presence of a vagally mediated reflex arc is supported by the findings that acid infusion of the esophagus in asthmatics leads to increased airway flow resistance that rapidly reverses with antacids [48] and infusion of acid into the distal esophagus of asthmatic children during sleep induces bronchoconstriction [26]. Microaspiration as a cause of asthma is supported by the findings of: a) a large vagally-mediated increase in airway flow resistance when minute quantities of hydrochloric acid are infused into the trachea of cats [49]; b) a high prevalence rate of hiatus hernias and GER in patients with idiopathic pulmonary fibrosis [11] or severe asthma [7]; c) GER in 60% of children with recurrent bronchitis [50]; d) and GER in 63% of children with chronic asthma or recurrent pneumonia [51].

The evidence of a GER/asthma relationship also has gained support by the results of certain clinical trials. The effect on asthma of medical therapy of GER has been previously reported. An open trial of antacids and postural therapy reported improvement in pulmonary symptoms but not function [52]. Four studies using cimetidine or ranitidine for up to 8 weeks produced results ranging from no benefit to modest improvement of only nocturnal asthma symptoms [44,52–55]. Unfortunately, such short-term studies using low dosages of H_2 blockers are unreliable in assessing improvement. One patient with disabling asthma, however, reportedly obtained dramatic improvement in pulmonary symptoms and function when gastric acid was suppressed with omeprazole [56].

The effect on asthma of surgical correction of GER has also been reported. In earlier, uncontrolled studies, surgical repair of GER resulted in partial or complete remission of asthma in 17 of 18 patients [6], 24 of 27 patients [12], all of 16 patients [57], and 70% of adolescent asthmatic patients [58]. Pulmonary function tests, unfortunately, were not performed before and after surgical repair. Despite the lack of objective data, many patients had dramatic subjective improvement in asthma from antireflux surgery.

Three uncontrolled, but more recent, surgical studies do provide objective data both before and after treatment:
- 12 of 13 asthmatics improved after antireflux surgery, and most were able to reduce or discontinue completely the pulmonary medications [29];
- seven of 10 asthmatics had at least temporary improvement in pulmonary function [59];
- of 44 asthmatics who received surgical correction of GER at least 5 years earlier, marked improvement or cure occurred in 41% and moderate improvement was achieved in 27% [60].

Unfortunately, there is no acceptable diagnostic method available to confirm the presence of GER-induced asthma. Scintigraphic monitoring under controlled conditions has been largely unsuccessful. Therefore, it appears that clinical trials are the only available means to assess whether medical or surgical treatment of GER in patients with both GER and asthma improves the symptoms of asthma and decreases the need for pulmonary medications.

Finally, in the only study of its kind, Larrain et al. [61] conducted an initial 6 month study as well a 5-year follow-up. Of the 142 patients screened, 94 had GER and asthma and 90 consented to randomization. Nine patients dropped out or refused their assigned treatment, leaving 28 patients in the placebo group, 27 patients in the cimetidine 300 mg q.i.d. group, and 26 patients in the surgical group.

By the end of 6 months, the mean symptom score and medicine score was significantly better in the surgical group and cimetidine group than in the placebo group. The cimetidine group required less medication, the surgical group required substantially less medication, but the placebo group required the same or needed even more. By 5 years, only the surgical group had maintained its symptom free status; the placebo and cimetidine groups were unchanged.

Improvement in asthma occurred at 6 months in 80% of 26 patients randomized to the surgical group, 80% of 27 patients randomized to the cimetidine group and 33% of 28 patients randomized to the placebo group. Eight of 11 surgical patients, two of 13 cimetidine patients and none of 14 placebo patients could stop steroids. Eleven cimetidine patients, nine surgical patients and one placebo patient were free of wheezing for 6 months. Thus, treatment of the reflux substantially altered the course of the asthma. The authors, using their clinical acumen, came up with certain markers that, they suggest, might help identify patients who could benefit from antireflux treatment. These predictors include:
— onset of reflux symptoms before the onset of pulmonary symptoms;
— the presence of nocturnal asthma;
— signs of laryngeal irritation;
— an initial pulmonary response to medical reflux management.
No longer can the coexistence of both wheezing and indigestion be ignored. However, how and in whom these two common afflictions coexist needs further study.

References

1. God. The Hebrew Scriptures (The Bible) Genesis 3:12.
2. Friedland GW, Yamare M, Marinkovich VA. Hiatal hernia and chronic unremitting asthma. Pediatr Radiol 1973;1:156—160.
3. Babb RR, Notrangelo J, Smith VM. Wheezing: a clue to gastroesophageal reflux. Am J Gastroenterol 1970;53:230—233.
4. Kennedy JH. "Silent" gastroesophageal reflux: an important but little known cause of pulmonary complications. Dis Chest 1962;42:42—45.
5. Klotz SD, Moeller RK. Hiatal hernia and intractable bronchial asthma. Ann Allergy 1971;29:325—328.
6. Overholt RH, Ashraf MM. Esophageal reflux as a trigger in asthma. NY State J Med 1966;66:3030—3032.
7. Mays EE. Intrinsic asthma in adults, association with gastroesophageal reflux. JAMA 1976;236:2626—2628.
8. Tan WC, Martin RJ, Pandey R, Ballard R. Effects of spontaneous and simulated gastroesophageal reflux on sleeping asthmatics. Am Rev Respir Dis 1990,141.1394—1399.
9. Ekstrom T, Tibbling L. Gastro-oesophageal reflux and triggering of bronchial asthma: a negative report. Eur J Respir Dis 1987;71:177—180.
10. Clemencon GH, Osterman PO. Hiatal hernia in bronchial asthma: The importance of concomitant pulmonary emphysema. Gastroenterologia (Basel) 1961;95:110—120.
11. Mays EE, Dubois JJ, Hamilton GB. Pulmonary fibrosis associated with tracheobronchial aspiration: A study of the frequency of hiatal hernia and gastroesophageal reflux in interstitial pulmonary fibrosis of obscure etiology. Chest 1976;69:512—515.
12. Urschel HC, Paulson DL. Gastroesophageal reflux and hiatal hernia: Complications and therapy. J Thorac Cardiovasc Surg 1967;53:21—32.
13. Meadows CT. Clinical observations regarding sliding hiatal hernia. Dis Chest 1965;47:629—631.
14. Davis MV. Evolving concepts regarding hiatus hernia and gastroesophageal reflux. Ann Thorac Surg 1969;7:120—133.
15. Bray GW. Recent advances in the treatment of asthma and hay fever. Practitioner 1934;34:368—371.
16. Belsey R. The pulmonary complications of oesophageal disease. Br J Dis Chest 1960;54:342—348.

17. Overholt RH, Voorhees RJ. Esophageal reflux as a trigger in asthma. Dis Chest 1966;49:464−466.
18. Lichter I. Measurement of gastro-oesophageal acid reflux: its significance in hiatus hernia. Br J Surg 1974;61:253−258.
19. Sontag S, O'Connell S, Khandelwal S, Miller T, Nemchausky B, Serlovsky R, Schnell T. Most asthmatics have gastroesophageal reflux with or without bronchodilator therapy. Gastroenterology 1990;99:613−620.
20. O'Connell S, Sontag SJ, Miller T, Kurucar C, Brand L, Reid S. Asthmatics have a high prevalence of reflux symptoms regardless of the use of bronchodilators. Gastroenterology 1990;98(2):A97.
21. Sontag S, Schnell T, Khandelwal S, O'Connell S, Chejfec G. Asthmatics have endoscopic esophagitis regardless of bronchodilator therapy. Am J Gastroenterol 1989;84:A1153.
22. Sontag S, O'Connell S, Khandelwal S, Miller T, Nemchausky B, Schnell T, Serlovsky R. Effect of positions, eating and bronchodilators on gastroesophageal reflux in asthmatics. Dig Dis Sci 1990;35:849−856.
23. Berquist WE, Rachelefsky GS, Kadden M et al. Gastroesophageal reflux-associated recurrent pneumonia and chronic asthma in children. Pediatrics 1981;68:29−35.
24. Stein MR, Towner TG, Weber RW et al. The effect of theophylline on the lower esophageal sphincter pressure. Ann Allergy 1980;45:238−239.
25. Berquist WE, Rachelefsky GS, Rowshan N, Siegel S, Katz R, Welch M. Quantitative gastroesophageal reflux and pulmonary function in asthmatic children and normal adults receiving placebo, theophylline, and metaproterenol sulfate therapy. J Allergy Clin Immunol 1984;73:253−258.
26. Davis RS, Larsen GL, Grunstein MM. Respiratory response to intraesophageal acid infusion in asthmatic children during sleep. J Allergy Clin Immunol 1983;72:393−398.
27. Perrin-Fayolle M, Bel A, Kofman J et al. Asthma and gastroesophageal reflux. Results of a survey of over 150 cases. Poumon Coeur 1980;36:225−230.
28. Mitsuhashi M, Tomomasa T, Tokuyama K, Morikawa A, Kuroume T. The evaluation of gastroesophageal reflux symptoms in patients with bronchial asthma. Ann Allergy 1985;54:317−320.
29. Sontag SJ, O'Connell SA, Greenlee HB, Schnell TG et al. Is gastroesophageal reflux a factor in some asthmatics? Am J Gastroenterol 1987;82:119−126.
30. Herbst JJ, Minton SD, Book LS. Gastroesophageal reflux causing respiratory distress and apnea in newborn infants. J Pediatr 1979;95:763−768.
31. Pellegrini CA, DeMeester TR, Johnson LF, Skinner DB. Gastroesophageal reflux and pulmonary aspiration: incidence, functional abnormality, and results of surgical therapy. Surgery 1979;86:110−119.
32. Reich SB, Earley WC, Rawin TH, Goodman M et al. Evaluation of gastropulmonary aspiration by a radioactive technique. J Nucl Med 1977;18:1079−1081.
33. Ghaed N, Stein M. Assessment of a technique for scintigraphic monitoring of pulmonary aspiration of gastric contents in asthmatics with gastroesophageal reflux. Ann Allergy 1979;42:306−308.
34. Chernow B, Johnson LF, Janowitz WR, Castell DO. Pulmonary aspiration as a consequence of gastroesophageal reflux. Dig Dis Sci 1979;24:839−844.
35. Nelson HS. Gastroesophageal reflux and pulmonary disease. J Allergy Clin Immunol 1984;73:547−556.
36. Berquist WE, Rachelefsky GS, Kadden M et al. Effect of theophylline on gastroesophageal reflux in normal adults. J Allergy Clin Immunol 1981;67:407−411.
37. Johannesson N, Andersson KE, Joelsson B, Persson CG. Relaxation of lower esophageal sphincter and stimulation of gastric secretion and diuresis by antiasthmatic xanthines. Role of adenosine antagonism. Am Rev Respir Dis 1985;131:26−30.
38. Goyal RK, Rattan S. Mechanism of the lower esophageal sphincter relaxation. Action of prostaglandin E1 and theophylline. J Clin Invest 1973;52:337−341.
39. DiMarino AJ, Cohen S. Effect of an oral beta 2-adrenergic agonist on lower esophageal sphincter pressure in normals and in patients with achalasia. Dig Dis Sci 1982;27:1063−1066.
40. Zwass AM, Prince R, Allen FN, Farrar T. Inhibitory beta adrenergic receptors in the human distal esophagus. Dig Dis Sci 1970;15:303−310.
41. Barish CF, Wu WC, Castell DO. Respiratory complications of gastroesophageal reflux. Arch Int Med 1985;145:1882−1888.
42. Hubert D, Gaudric M, Guerre J, Lockhart A, Marsac J. Effect of theophylline on gastroesophageal reflux in patients with asthma. J Allergy Clin Immunol 1988;81:1168−1174.
43. Martin ME, Grunstein MM, Larsen GL. The relationship of gastroesophageal reflux to nocturnal wheezing in children with asthma. Ann Allergy 1982;49:318−322.
44. Goodall RJR, Earis JE, Cooper DN, Bernstein A, Temple JG. Relationship between asthma and gastroesophageal reflux. Thorax 1981;36:116−121.
45. Johnson LF, DeMeester TR. Evaluation of elevation of the head of the bed, bethanechol, and antacid foam tablets on gastroesophageal reflux. Dig Dis Sci 1981;26:673−680.
46. Fink SM, McCallum RW. The role of prolonged esophageal pH monitoring in the diagnosis of gastroesophageal reflux. JAMA 1984;252:1160−1164.
47. Mansfield LE, Hameister HH, Spaulding HS, Smith NJ, Glab N. The role of the vagus nerve in airway narrowing caused by intraesophageal hydrochloric acid provocation and esophageal distention. Ann Allergy 1981;47:431−434.
48. Mansfield LE, Stein MR. Gastroesophageal reflux and asthma: a possible reflex mechanism. Ann Allergy 1978;41:224−226.
49. Tuchman DN, Boyle JT, Pack AI. Comparison of airway responses following tracheal or oesophageal acidification in the cat. Gastroenterology 1984;87:872−881.

50. Danus O, Casar C, Larrain A, Pope CE II. Esophageal reflux — an unrecognized cause of recurrent obstructive bronchitis in children. J Pediatr 1976;89:220—224.
51. Euler AR, Byrne WJ, Ament ME et al. Recurrent pulmonary disease in children: A complication of gastroesophageal reflux. Pediatrics 1979;63:47—51.
52. Kjellen G, Tibbling L, Wranne B. Effect of conservative treatment of oesophageal dysfunction on bronchial asthma. Eur J Respir Dis 1981;62:190—197.
53. Harper PC, Bergner A, Kaye MD. Antireflux treatment for asthma. Improvement in patients with associated gastroesophageal reflux. Arch Int Med 1987;147:56—60.
54. Ekstrom T, Lindgren BR, Tibbling L. Effects of ranitidine treatment on patients with asthma and a history of gastro-oesophageal reflux: a double-blind crossover study. Thorax 1989;44:19—23.
55. Nagel RA, Brown P, Perks WH, Wilson RSE, Kerr GD. Ambulatory pH monitoring of gastro-oesophageal reflux in "morning dipper" asthmatics. Br Med J 1988;297:1371—1373.
56. Depla AC, Bartelsman JF, Roos CM, Tytgat GN, Jansen HM. Beneficial effect of omeprazole in a patient with severe bronchial asthma and gastro-oesophageal reflux. Eur J Respir Dis 1988;1:966—968.
57. Lomasney TL. Hiatus hernia and the respiratory tract. Ann Thorac Surg 1977;24:448—450.
58. Johnson DG, Syme WC, Matlak ME, Black RE, Herbst SJ. Gastro-oesophageal reflux and respiratory disease: the place of the surgeon. Aust NZ J Surg 1984;54:405—415.
59. Tardiff C, Nouvet G, Denis P, Tombelaine R, Pasquis P. Surgical treatment of gastroesophageal reflux in ten patients with severe asthma. Respiration 1989;56:110—115.
60. Perrin-Fayolle M, Gormand F, Braillon G et al. Long-term results of surgical treatment for gastroesophageal reflux in asthmatic patients. Chest 1989;96:40—45.
61. Larrain A, Carrasco E, Galleguillos F, Sepulveda R, Pope CE II. Medical and surgical treatment of nonallergic asthma associated with gastroesophageal reflux. Chest 1991;99:1330—1336.

Strategy of investigations

 ## What are the radiologic signs of reflux esophagitis?

M.S. Levine (Philadelphia)

Gastroesophageal reflux disease is by far the most common inflammatory disease involving the esophagus. Barium studies have been advocated for patients with reflux symptoms, primarily to document the presence of a hiatal hernia or gastroesophageal reflux, to detect complications such as deep ulcers or strictures and to rule out other organic or motor abnormalities in the esophagus that can mimic reflux disease. By permitting a more detailed assessment of the esophageal mucosa, double contrast radiographic techniques have made it possible to detect superficial ulceration and other changes of mild or moderate esophagitis before the development of deep ulcers or strictures. Thus, esophagography has become a valuable technique for evaluating patients with suspected gastroesophageal reflux disease.

Reflux esophagitis may be manifested radiographically by a spectrum of findings, including abnormal motility, mucosal nodularity, thickened folds, ulceration, and scarring or strictures. These findings are discussed separately in the following sections.

Abnormal motility

Between 25 and 50% of patients with reflux esophagitis have abnormal esophageal motility, manifested by weakened or absent primary peristalsis which is associated with an increased frequency of nonperistaltic contractions [1]. This abnormal motility may be secondary to neuronal damage in Auerbach's plexus, caused by direct extension of the inflammatory process into the esophageal wall. Conversely, pre-existing esophageal motor disorders may predispose to the development of reflux esophagitis by impairing clearance of refluxed peptic acid from the esophagus. In any case, the combination of abnormal motility and gastroesophageal reflux may lead to progressively severe esophagitis and stricture formation.

Mucosal nodularity

In early reflux esophagitis, mucosal edema and inflammation may be manifested on double contrast radiographs by a granular or finely nodular appearance in the distal third or half of the thoracic esophagus (Fig. 1) [2,3]. Although mucosal granularity is best seen with maximal esophageal distention, it can also be recognized in the collapsed esophagus by lobulation or nodularity of the longitudinal folds. Less frequently, these patients may have coarse nodularity of the mucosa. However, the nodules tend to have poorly defined borders that fade peripherally into the adjacent mucosa, so that discrete nodules are rarely detected in patients with reflux esophagitis.

Thickened folds

In other patients with reflux esophagitis, submucosal edema and inflammation may lead to the development of thickened longitudinal folds (Fig. 2). Thickened folds are best seen on mucosal relief views of the collapsed esophagus, where folds wider than 3 mm are thought to be abnormal. These thickened folds may have a smooth, nodular, or scalloped appearance. Occasionally, they may be quite tortuous or serpiginous, mimicking the appearance of esophageal varices.

Ulceration

Shallow ulcers and erosions associated with reflux esophagitis may appear on double contrast radiographs as one or more tiny collections of barium in the distal esophagus at or adjacent to the gastroesophageal junction (Fig. 3) [4,5]. The ulcers are often associated with surrounding mounds of edema, radiating folds, or puckering and sacculation of the adjacent esophageal wall. Other patients may have long, flowing ulcers that are oriented longitudinally in the distal esophagus (Fig. 4).

When superficial ulceration is detected in patients with reflux esophagitis, the

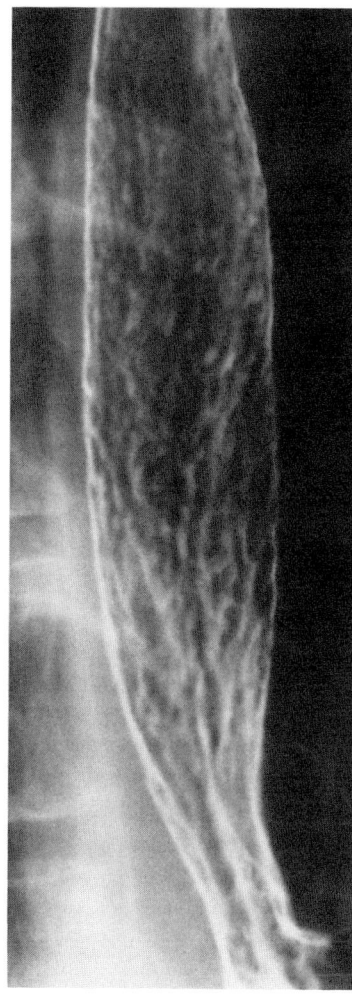

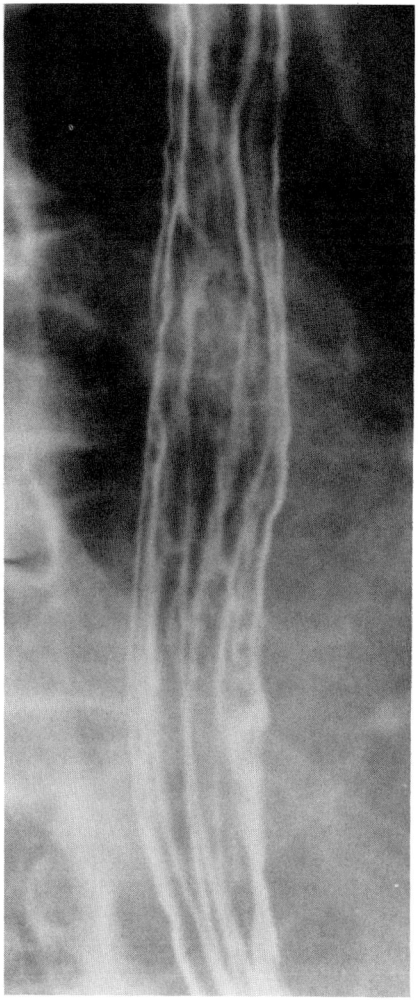

Fig. 1. Reflux esophagitis with a finely nodular or granular mucosa in the distal half of the eso- phagus. This appearance is caused by mucosal edema and inflammation.

Fig. 2. Reflux esophagitis with thickened, irregu- lar folds in the esophagus due to submucosal edema and inflammation.

correct diagnosis is almost always suggested by the distal location of the ulcers, the presence of a hiatal hernia or gastroesophageal reflux, and the clinical presentation of the patient. Some individuals may have relatively diffuse ulceration in the distal half or even two-thirds of the thoracic esophagus. However, ulceration in reflux esophagitis tends to occur as a continuous area of mucosal disease extending proximally from the gastroesophageal junction, so that the presence of superficial ulcers in the midesophagus with distal esophageal sparing should suggest another cause of the patient's esophagitis.

In advanced reflux esophagitis, the esophagus may have a grossly irregular contour

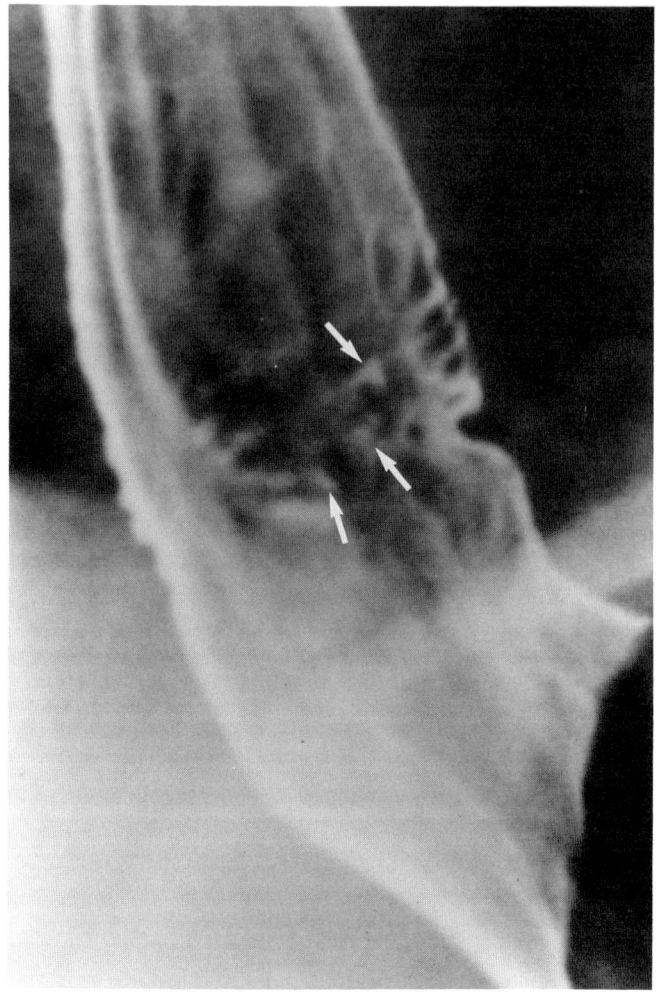

Fig. 3. Reflux esophagitis with superficial ulceration. Tiny ulcers (arrows) are seen en face in the distal esophagus near the gastroesophageal junction. The ulcers are associated with radiating folds and puckering of the adjacent esophageal wall.

with serrated or spiculated margins, wall thickening, and decreased distensibility due to extensive ulceration, edema, and spasm. Without a clinical history, such cases may be difficult to distinguish from other types of severe esophagitis. However, predominant involvement of the distal esophagus and the presence of an associated hernia and gastroesophageal reflux should suggest the correct diagnosis.

Scarring and strictures

Depending on the degree of scarring, reflux esophagitis eventually may lead to

120

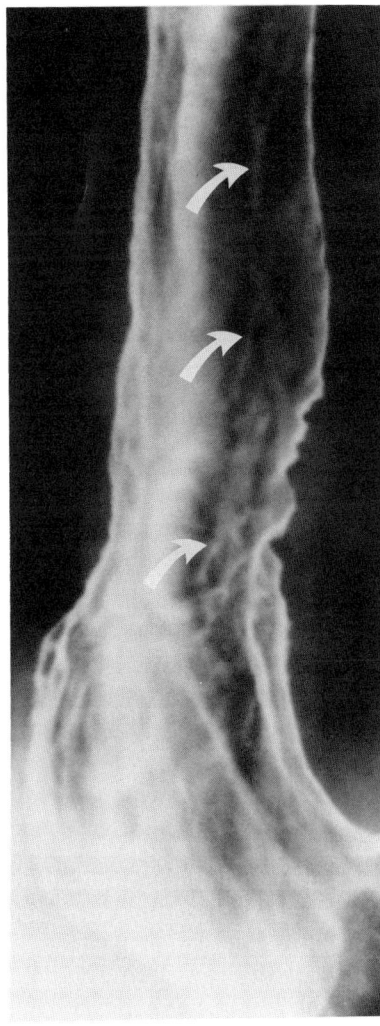

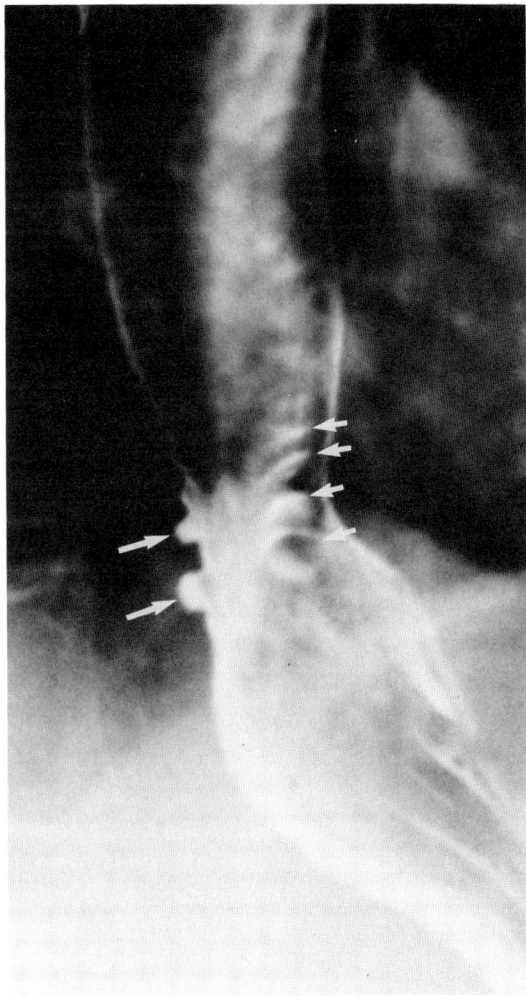

Fig. 4. Reflux esophagitis with long, flowing ulcers (arrows) in the distal esophagus. There also is puckering and deformity of the anterolateral wall of the distal esophagus.

Fig. 5. Peptic scarring with multiple sacculations seen both in profile (long arrows) and en face (short arrows) in the distal esophagus.

stricture formation. However, esophageal scarring may occur without the development of a circumferential stricture. It is often possible to detect slight flattening or puckering of the esophageal wall and/or radiating folds at the site of previous ulceration. Scarring caused by reflux esophagitis may also lead to focal outpouching or sacculation of the distal esophagus with outward ballooning of the esophageal wall between areas of fibrosis (Fig. 5). Sacculations are particularly common in patients with scleroderma as a result of the severe esophagitis which occurs in these

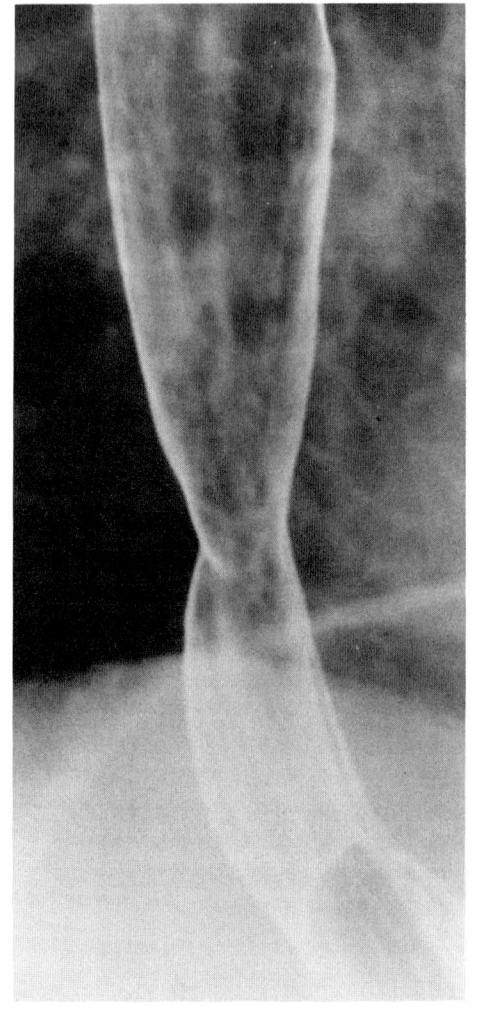

Fig. 6. Peptic stricture with a smooth, tapered area of concentric narrowing in the distal esophagus. This is the classic appearance of a benign reflux-induced stricture.

individuals. Sacculations may resemble active ulcer craters but usually can be differentiated from ulcers by their changing shape and appearance at fluoroscopy.

Scarring from reflux esophagitis may also be manifested by fixed transverse folds in the distal esophagus, producing a characteristic "stepladder" appearance [6]. These transverse folds are usually 2–5 mm wide and do not extend more than halfway across the esophagus. The folds tend to be relatively few in number, and they cannot be obliterated with esophageal distention. In most cases, there is other evidence of scarring from reflux esophagitis, and these transverse folds extend proximally a variable distance from the site of a distal stricture or scar. The folds probably represent areas of heaped-up or crinkled mucosa, due to simultaneous longitudinal scarring from reflux esophagitis.

Between 10 to 20% of patients with reflux esophagitis develop peptic strictures as a result of circumferential scarring of the distal esophagus. Accurate radiologic diagnosis of peptic strictures requires continuous drinking of low-density barium in the prone position for optimal esophageal distention to demonstrate mild or even moderate strictures that are not visible on the double contrast phase of the examination. The routine esophagram should therefore be performed as a biphasic study that includes upright double contrast and prone single contrast views of the esophagus. With careful technique, esophagography has a sensitivity of almost 95% in diagnosing peptic strictures and occasionally may demonstrate strictures which are missed at endoscopy.

The classic appearance of a smooth, tapered area of concentric narrowing in the distal esophagus above a hiatal hernia should be virtually pathognomonic of a benign peptic stricture (Fig. 6). However, many peptic strictures have an asymmetric appearance with puckering, deformity, or sacculation of one wall of the stricture, due to asymmetric scarring from reflux esophagitis. Other strictures may involve a longer segment of the distal esophagus and may have irregular margins due to associated reflux esophagitis. As a result, a benign peptic stricture cannot always be distinguished from an infiltrating carcinoma, particularly an adenocarcinoma arising in Barrett's esophagus. Endoscopy should therefore be performed to rule out a malignant lesion when the radiographic findings are equivocal.

References

1. Kahrilas PJ, Dodds WJ, Hogan WJ et al. Esophageal peristaltic dysfunction in peptic esophagitis. Gastroenterology 1986; 91:897–904.
2. Graziani L, Bearzi I, Romagnoli A et al. Significance of diffuse granularity and nodularity of the esophageal mucosa at double-contrast radiography. Gastrointest Radiol 1985;10:1–6.
3. Kressel HY, Glick SN, Laufer I et al. Radiologic features of esophagitis. Gastrointest Radiol 1981;6:103–108.
4. Laufer I. Radiology of esophagitis. Radiol Clin North Am 1982;20:687–699.
5. McDermott P, Wallers KJ, Holden R et al. Double-contrast examination of the oesophagus: the radiological changes of peptic oesophagitis. Clin Radiol 1982;33:259–264.
6. Levine MS, Goldstein HM. Fixed transverse folds in the esophagus: a sign of reflux esophagitis. Am J Radiol 1984;143: 275–278.
7. Ott DJ, Wu WC, Gelfand DW. Reflux esophagitis revisited: prospective analysis of radiologic accuracy. Gastrointest Radiol 1981;6:1–7.
8. Ott DJ, Gelfand DW, Lane TG et al. Radiologic detection and spectrum of appearances of esophageal strictures. J Clin Gastroenterol 1982;4:11–15.

Should endoscopy be routine before the treatment of GERD?

P. Renkes, M.A. Bigard (Nancy)

Despite the difficulty in evaluating the prevalence of gastroesophageal reflux disease (GERD), this complaint can be considered as the most frequent esophageal disease, leading frequently to consultation. According to epidemiologic studies done on the French population, the number of adult subjects who periodically present symptoms classically suggestive of GERD is about 10% [1]. The more and more frequent use of endoscopy on this population allowed a better understanding of GERD and its consequences. However, should this examination be systematic before treatment of GERD?

In order to answer this question, the present indications of endoscopy when GERD occurs shall be considered. One of these indications could be the detection of esophagitis. In this case, the imbalance between the importance of the clinical symptoms of GERD and the reality of macroscopic esophagitis can be pointed out [2]. In a multicentric study [3], a gastroscopy was performed on patients with a persistent reflux after 2 weeks treatment with alginate and antacid (7.2% of all cases). An esophagitis was discovered in only 40% of cases. Minor forms of esophagitis were described in healthy subjects [4], nevertheless erosive esophagitis remains exceptional in this case. On the other hand, 50% of the patients with GERD symptoms have no esophagitis lesions, as shown by endoscopy [5]. This difference could be partially due to the criteria chosen for the diagnosis of esophagitis and to the lack of sensibility and specificity of the histologic diagnosis. This can explain the bad diagnostic efficiency of endoscopy in GERD. Moreover, in cases of grade I and II esophagitis lesions, complete healing is not absolutely necessary because severe complications such as stenosis will not develop [6]. Thus, endoscopy will be prescribed straightaway for patients with a high risk of hemorrhage, particularly in cases of anticoagulant therapy and for elderly subjects who are more likely to suffer from more severe forms of esophagitis. The second reason for prescribing esophago-gastroscopy in case of reflux, is the possibility of a neoplastic lesion. The probability of detecting a cancer is the same with patients with typical symptoms of GERD as with asymptomatic subjects, therefore, endoscopy will not be used straightaway in this case. On the contrary, endoscopy will be performed in case of GERD with atypical or alarming revealing symptoms (dysphagia, anaemia, hematemesis) in order to detect a neoplastic lesion or possible complications such as severe peptic csophagitis, stenosis and Barrett's esophagus. Endoscopy will also be performed straightaway in the case of cancerophobia as a routine test that will reassure the patient.

The prescription of treatment depends on the clinical symptomatology revealing the GERD. If pyrosis and regurgitation, which are specific of GERD, are the main symptoms, an anti-H_2 receptor therapy can be started without any complementary investigation and particularly without endoscopy. Even if dietetical measures seem to be justified, their efficiency is not well established. These measures are often restricting and more often uncomfortable than beneficial for the patient. Among them, the elevation of the head of the bed leads to a moderate decrease of the exposure time to a pH inferior to 4 [7]. Moreover, one knows that acid reflux occurs more often in the daytime [8,9]. In the same way, because antacids and alginates have an efficiency that is limited in time, they require multiple administrations in the course of a day. The evolution under H_2-blockers is evaluated in 4 to 6 weeks. In the case of lack of improvement, worsening of the symptoms and/or occurrence of complications, endoscopy is then essential. The majority of subjects who have clinical symptoms of reflux do not consult because their symptoms are intermittent and not very severe. A great number of them will resort to self-medication during the painful period, particularly with antacids and will consult only in case of the inefficiency of the treatment or worsening of the symptoms. The simple modification of the treatment will often entail the disappearance of the symptoms and endoscopy will not be necessary.

Resorting to first intent endoscopy in the case of typical reflux symptoms does not only raise the question of a precise diagnosis based on macroscopy, possibly supplemented by esophageal biopsy, but also the question of the validity of a negative examination in a symptomatic patient. The increase in number and the efficiency of GERD therapies has very often made it possible, in cases of typical reflux and when there were no alarm symptoms, not to resort to the systematic prescription of endoscopy before treatment.

References

1. Bruley des Varannes, Galmiche JP, Bernades P, Bader JP. Douleurs épigastriques et régurgitations: Epidémiologie descriptive dans un échantillon représentatif de la population française adulte. Gastroenterol Clin Biol 1988;12:721−728.
2. Galmiche JP, Denis P, Desechalliers JP. Valeur diagnostique des examens complémentaires au cours du reflux gastro-oesophagien de l'adulte. Gastroenterol Clin Biol 1981;5:1024−1025.
3. Bigard MA, Colin JP, Galmiche JP, Rampal P, De Meynard C. Evolution des symptômes de reflux gastro-oesophagien (RGO) après 2 semaines de traitement par alginate-anti-acide. Facteurs prédictifs et données endoscopiques chez les non-répondeurs. Gastroenterol Clin Biol 1990;14(2 bis):A110.
4. Johansson KE, Boeryd B, Fransson SG, Tibbling L. Oesophageal reflux tests, manometry, endoscopy, biopsy and radiology in healthy subjects. Scand J Gastroenterol 1986;21:399−406.
5. Johansson KE, Ask P, Boeryd B et al. Oesophagitis, signs of reflux and gastric acid secretion in patients with symptoms of gastro-oesophageal reflux disease. Scand J Gastroenterol 1986;21:837−847.
6. Schindlbeck NE, Klauser AG, Berghammer G, Londong W, Muller-Lissner SA. Three year follow-up of patients with gastroesophageal reflux disease. Gut 1992;33:1016−1019.
7. Hamilton JW, Boisen RJ, Yamamoto DT, Wagner JL, Reichelderfer M. Sleeping on a wedge diminishes exposure of the esophagus to refluxed acid. Dig Dis Sci 1988;33:518−522.
8. Robertson D, Aldersley M, Shepherd H, Smith CL. Patterns of acid reflux in complicated oesophagitis. Gut 1987;28:1484−1488.
9. De Caestecker JS, Blackwell JN, Pryde A, Heading RC. Daytime gastro-oesophageal reflux is important in oesophagitis. Gut 1987;28:519−526.

Does retroflexed endoscopic examination of the cardia allow prediction of reflux status?

*S.J.M. Kraemer, L.D. Hill, R.B. Kozarek, R.W. Aye,
C.E. Pope II* (Seattle)

Thirty years ago, there were many explanations for the absence of gastroesophageal reflux (GER) in normal individuals. Most papers of that era stated that there was no anatomic evidence for a sphincter at the lower end of the esophagus; therefore other explanations for continence must be sought. Several structures which might prevent reflux (many of which were difficult to verify experimentally) were suggested — a mucosal rosette, a flap valve, or the angle of His.

When manometric evidence for a lower esophageal sphincter was offered by Code and associates [1], all attention was focussed on this newcomer to the collection. As time has gone on it seems unlikely that the lower esophageal sphincter is the only barrier to reflux. The contribution of the diaphragmatic crural fibers has been recognized especially during times of exertion or sudden rises in intra-abdominal pressure [2]. Whether or not there is a flap valve mechanism in addition remains an open question.

In experiments done in cadavers with the stomach left in situ, a barrier to the flow of water from the stomach to the esophagus has been demonstrated [3]. This barrier can be disrupted by manual pressure on the gastric fundus or by freeing the attachments of the lower esophageal area. This suggests that passive mechanisms such as a mechanical valve might play a role in the prevention of GER in life.

It was decided to see if there was a grossly recognizable difference in the appearance of the cardia when viewed from below between control subjects and those with reflux. In a preliminary study to seek such a difference, 12 control subjects without a history of heartburn, regurgitation or other esophageal symptoms were examined endoscopically, and the appearance of the gastric fundus distended with air was recorded on videotape. Eleven patients who were being endoscoped for reflux symptoms were also videotaped and the appearance of the cardia in the two groups was compared.

The majority of control subjects revealed a ridge of tissue which tightly closed around the endoscope. This was scored as grade I (Fig. 1). Occasionally, the orifice seemed to open but closed promptly again. This was termed grade II. The patients with reflux tended to have very minimal ridges, and the lumen to the esophagus often gaped open (grade III, Fig. 2). Especially in the patients with erosive esophagitis, there was often a large hiatal hernia and no ridge surrounding the scope. The esophageal mucosa could occasionally be seen through this open orifice (grade IV, Figs. 3A and 3B).

The videotapes were coded and presented to a panel of five gastroenterologists and surgeons who independently graded each tape. There was an interobserver agreement of 80%. There was never more than a one-grade disparity between different

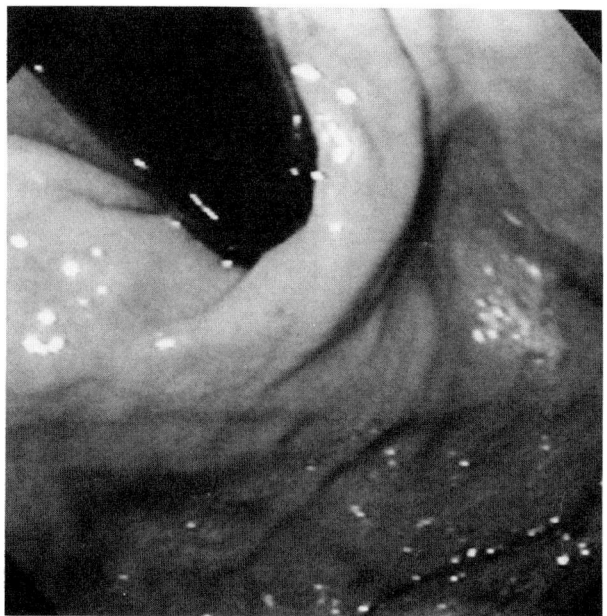

Fig. 1. Grade I valve. The ridge of tissue seems to grip the endoscope, and there is no space around the scope.

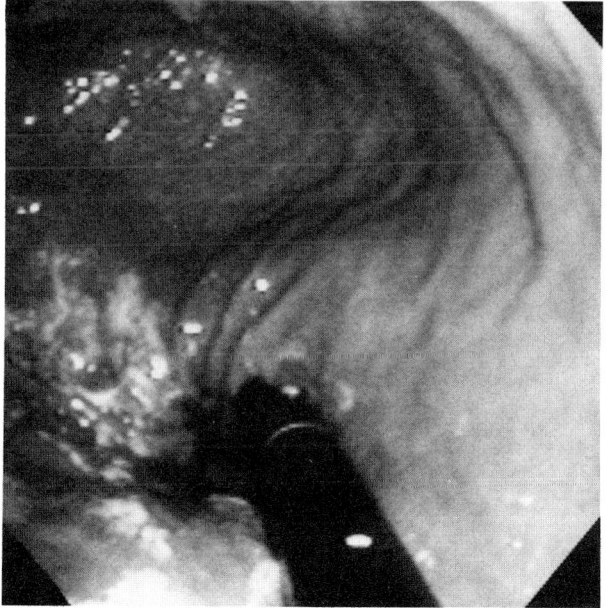

Fig. 2. Grade III valve. The normal ridge of tissue is absent and the esophageal lumen is intermittently visible.

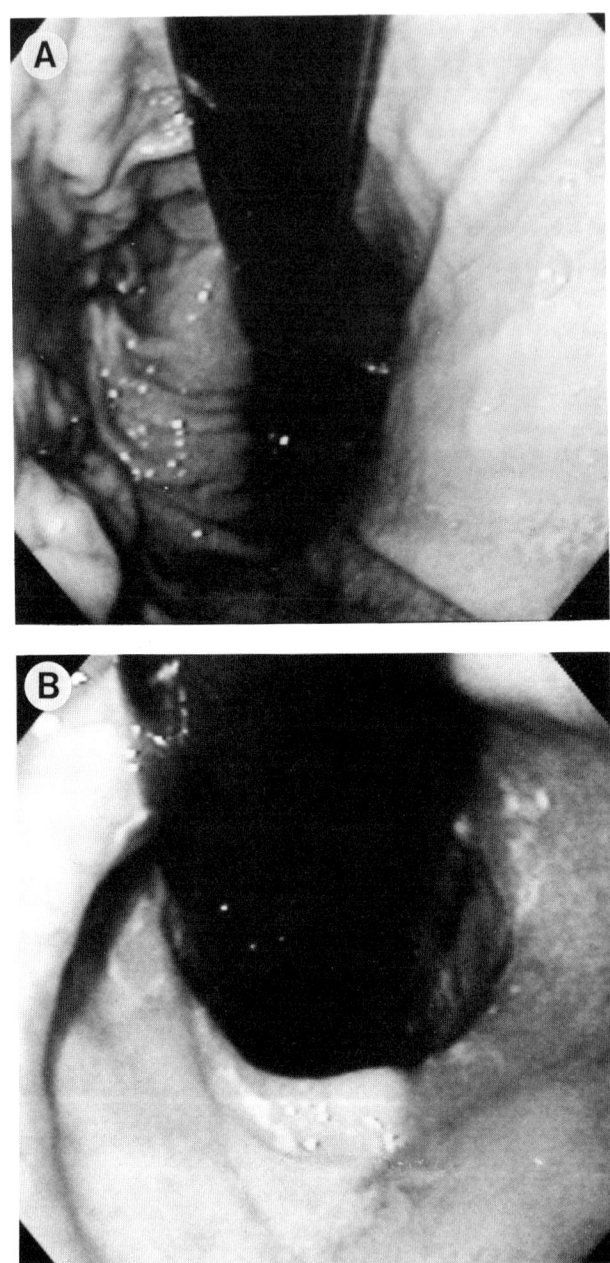

Fig. 3A. Grade IV valve. The crural impression defining a hiatal hernia is easily seen, and the endoscope seems to disappear into the fundal sac.

Fig. 3B. Grade IV valve. This is the same patient, only the endoscope has been pulled up so that the entrance into the esophageal lumen can be seen. Note that there is a wide gap between the endoscope and the wall which allows the esophageal mucosa to be seen from below.

observers. The greatest difficulty was experienced in separating grade I from grade II. In the initial group of control subjects, seven had grade I and five had grade II appearances. It was decided to consider either a grade I or a grade II appearance as

Table 1.

Patient no.	Clinical diagnosis	Esophagitis	pH reflux	LESP	Valve grade
1.	GERD	+	+	32	IV
2.	GERD	+	+	17	III
3.	GERD	+	+	18	IV
4.	GERD	−	+	12	IV
5.	Dysphagia	+			III
6.	Bleeding	+			IV
7.	GERD	+	+	12	IV
8.	UGI Bleed	+	+		IV
9.	GERD	−	+		II
10.	GERD	+	+	18	IV
11.	Dysphagia	+			IV
12.	Barrett's	+			II
13.	Scleroderma	+			III
14.	Stricture	+	+	11	IV
15.	GERD	+			IV
16.	GERD	+	+	10	IV
17.	Barrett's	+			IV
18.	GERD	+			III
19.	Barrett's	+	+	0	IV
20.	Barrett's	+			IV
21.	GERD	+			III
22.	Barrett's	+	+		IV
23.	Barrett's	+	+	10	IV
24.	Dysphagia	+			IV
25.	Pain	+			III
26.	GERD	+			IV
27.	Barrett's	+			III
28.	GERD	+			IV
29.	GERD	+			IV
30.	GERD	+			III
31.	GERD	−	+	0	IV
32.	GERD	+	+	0	IV
33.	GERD	+	+	0	IV
34.	GERD	+	+	0	IV
35.	GERD	+	+	50	IV
36.	GERD	+	−		IV
37.	GERD	+	+	8	IV
38.	GERD	+	−		IV
39.	GERD	+	−		IV
40.	GERD	+	+	20	IV
41.	GERD	+	+	22	IV
42.	GERD	+	+	22	IV
43.	GERD	+	+	13	IV
44.	GERD	+	+	17	IV

129

a "nonreflux" appearance and a grade III or IV was considered to suggest reflux.

Next a prospective study was designed and executed. The definition of a control subject for this study required no esophageal symptoms and a normal 24-h pH monitor value. The reflux group consisted of 44 patients with symptoms of esophageal reflux and either endoscopic appearance of reflux changes or short-term (SART) pH values in the abnormal range. The retroflexed appearance of the gastroesophageal junction was graded by one of three experienced endoscopists who had viewed the original tapes. A summary of the reflux patients is given in Table 1.

If grades I and II are considered normal and grades III and IV considered to suggest reflux, a 2 × 2 table shown in Table 2 can be constructed. The sensitivity and specificity of an abnormal cardia in predicting reflux was 91%. The positive predictive value was 95% and the negative predictive value was 87%.

How did the lower esophageal sphincter pressure fare as a predictor of reflux? Figure 4 shows lower esophageal sphincter pressure (LESP) as a function of both endoscopic grade and reflux status. It can be seen that in the population studied, LESP is a relatively poor predictor of reflux status unless the value is below 10 mmHg. High values of LESP do not mean that reflux is not present.

Table 2.

	Grades III–IV	Grades I–II
Reflux +	42	2
Reflux −	2	20

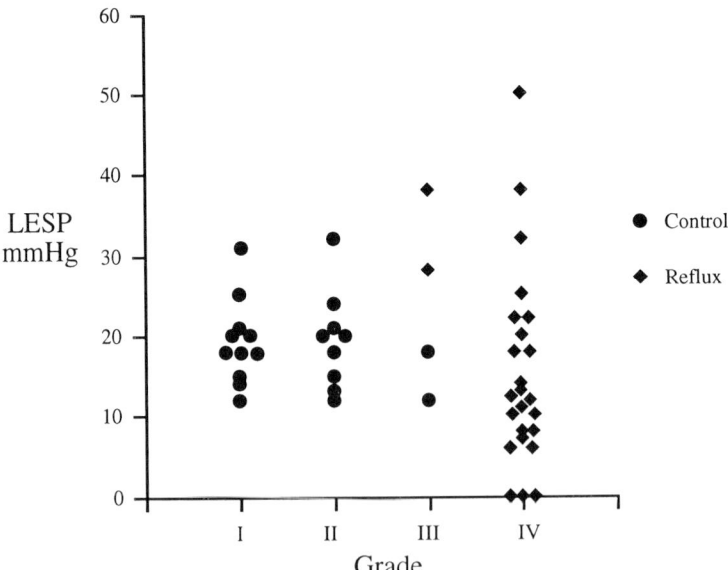

Fig. 4. Endoscopic grade and lower esophageal sphincter pressure (LESP) in controls and patients with reflux. Note that the endoscopic grade separates control subjects and reflux patients almost completely. LESP does not separate the two groups.

130

Discussion

The advent of flexible endoscopes has allowed inspection of the esophagogastric junction from the gastric side. The appearance of the normal gastroesophageal junction has been well-described by Boyce [4]. His description tallies very well with our observations. He also describes the appearance of a hiatal hernia as seen from the gastric side and comments on how tightly or loosely the tissues were applied to the endoscope.

The observations we have made by first examining some control subjects and some patients with esophageal reflux, developing criteria for normality and abnormality, and then prospectively applying these criteria to more control subjects and patients with reflux suggest that such observations may serve a useful clinical purpose. The sensitivity and specificity in this group of subjects and patients is very high, and of a great deal more value in the prediction of reflux status than was the measurement of lower esophageal sphincter pressure in the same individuals. Subsequent experience of several of the investigators in their endoscopic suites has led us to believe that similar studies would produce the same good correlation between endoscopic appearance and the presence or absence of reflux.

The actual physical structures which go into the creation of the gastric fold which surrounds the endoscope are not certain. Direct observation of the gastroesophageal junction through a previously created PEG tract shows that the cardia appears like a closed slit which is very difficult to find until water issues forth from it. In one sense the tissue ridge seen in the retroflexed position is a creation of the endoscope. Yet this appearance is very useful in the prediction of reflux. It is of interest that in 32 patients who were studied after antireflux surgery, the ridge was present whereas it had been absent preoperatively.

We hope that these simple observations, which can be easily made during any endoscopy without unduly prolonging the period of observation, will be of benefit in the evaluation of our patients both preoperatively and postoperatively.

References

1. Fyke FE, Code CF, Schlegel JF. The gastroesophageal sphincter in healthy human beings. Gastroenterologia 1956;86: 135—150.
2. Mittal RK, Fisher M, McCallum RW, Rochester DF, Dent J, Sluss J. Human lower esophageal sphincter pressure response to increased intra-abdominal pressure. Am J Physiol 1990;258:G624—G630.
3. Thor KB, Hill LD, Mercer CD, Kozarek RD. Reappraisal of the flap valve mechanism in the gastroesophageal junction. A study of a new valvuloplasty procedure in cadavers. Acta Chir Scand 1987;153:25—28.
4. Boyce HW. Hiatal hernia and peptic disease of the esophagus. In: Sivak MV Jr (ed) Gastroenterologic Endoscopy. Philadelphia: WB Saunders, 1987:401—418.

Do the motor disorders of esophagitis precede the development of a stricture or a Barrett's esophagus?

M. Wienbeck, A. Moll, J. Barnert (Augsburg)

Heartburn is a widespread phenomenon; about 15% of the population suffer from heartburn at least once a month [1]. Even in asymptomatic persons pathological reflux is said to occur at a rate of 15% [2]. Thus, reflux disease is a widespread gastrointestinal disturbance and therefore deserves appropriate consideration. The prevalence of esophagitis induced by reflux is approximately 3—5% [3], which is about one third of the prevalence of heartburn. About 50% of this group finally develop complications, such as esophageal strictures or Barrett's esophagus. The question, therefore, is which factors cause simple heartburn to develop into esophagitis or its complications, such as esophageal strictures. This article will look more closely at the influence of esophageal motility disturbances in the pathogenesis of esophageal strictures and Barrett's esophagus.

Due to ethical reasons, prospective studies on esophageal motility leaving patients with esophagitis and without therapy are not feasible. Therefore the following questions will be further discussed in order to clarify the situation in an indirect way.

*

Which motility disturbances appear in esophagitis and do they differ from disorders appearing in simple heartburn (i.e., without esophageal inflammation)?

The effects of different pH of swallowing samples on esophageal motility were examined in healthy test persons [4]. They showed that the lower the pH was [5—7], the smaller the volumes were which induced secondary peristalsis. With respect to the occurrence and frequency of simultaneous contractions, no significant difference between the various pH values was detected. Depending on the severity of esophagitis, the pressure in the lower esophageal sphincter (LES) drops [8]; in patients with severe esophagitis, esophageal motility dissipated and stopped more frequently than in mild esophagitis [8]. With respect to contractions in the tubular esophagus, severity of esophagitis, in general, increases as the amplitudes of contractions become smaller [9]. In a further study 16 patients were examined after gastrectomy with regard to the appearance of esophagitis and disturbances of esophageal motility [10]: 13 out of 16 patients suffered from esophagitis; a resting pressure too low at the esophageal exit may be an important pathogenetic factor. There was no significant difference in the duration of contractions and their propulsion between patients and controls, but the amplitudes of contractions were significantly decreased in the gastrectomy patients (Fig. 1). Kruse-Andersen et al. were able to prove that pathological reflux time (pH < 4) was longer in patients

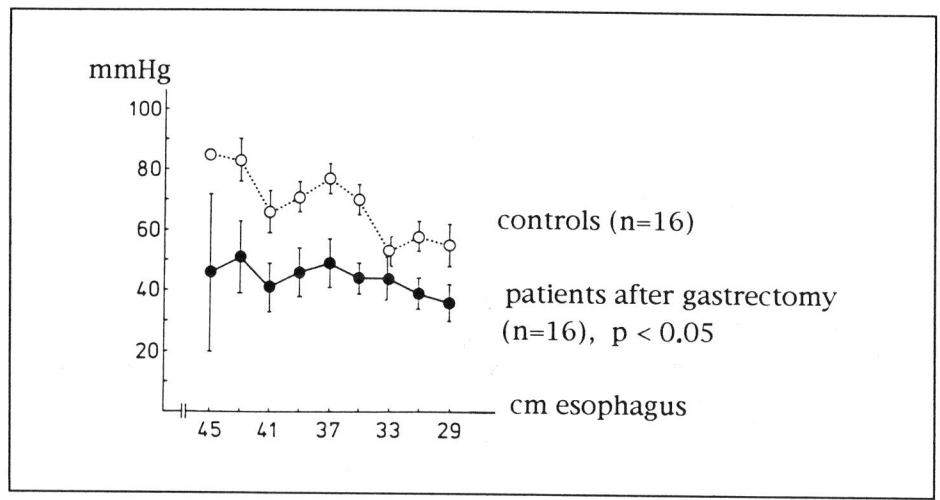

modified according to [10].

Fig. 1. Median amplitudes of contractions in the esophageal body of 16 patients after gastrectomy and 16 healthy volunteers.

suffering from reflux esophagitis than in patients with reflux disease and no inflammation, which in turn was longer than in normal controls [11]. In this study simultaneous, retrograde and segmentary contractions appeared significantly more frequently during reflux phases in patients with esophagitis than in reflux patients without inflammation (in these patients it was about 20 times more frequent than in normal controls).

Scleroderma deserves special consideration in the pathogenesis of the reflux esophagitis; about 50% of patients with scleroderma develop esophagitis [12,13]. Disturbed esophageal motility is thought to be the reason; in these patients motility gradually deteriorates from distal to proximal esophagus and in the final stage peristaltic activity is found only in the proximal esophagus. In the late stages of the disease the resting pressure of the lower esophageal sphincter (LES) also drops [14,15].

Another possible mechanism for the development of reflux needs attention: Disturbances of gastric emptying. Cunningham et al. provided evidence for a disturbance of the enteric nervous system in 44% of reflux patients (n = 48) [16]. Esophageal transit was delayed in patients with autonomic dysfunction. Furthermore, simultaneous contractions occurred more frequently. In 46% of the 48 patients, delayed gastric emptying was also stated. McCallum et al. [17] detected delayed gastric emptying in 41% of 20 symptomatic reflux patients. It is possible that delayed gastric emptying weakens the antireflux function of the LES.

No correlation was found between LES pressure and disturbed esophageal peristalsis [9].

Acid reflux alters esophageal motility even in healthy persons, and this can be looked upon as a physiological protective mechanism. Low LES pressures and a deterioration of esophageal peristalsis occur, corresponding to the severity of the reflux disease.

∗

Which specific motility disturbances are found in esophageal strictures and in Barrett's esophagus?

Zaninotto et al. examined motility disturbances in healthy volunteers, reflux patients, patients with esophagitis, patients with esophageal strictures and Barrett's esophagus [18]. LES pressure decreased continuously in this order; it was significantly lower in Barrett's esophagus than in volunteers and patients with simple reflux disease. All patients with reflux disease, with or without complications, had significantly lower LES pressures than healthy volunteers. Also, patients with esophageal strictures and Barrett's esophagus had significantly lower contraction amplitudes in the lower two thirds of the esophagus than controls. This tendency also appeared in patients with esophagitis or simple reflux disease without reaching statistical significance. Furthermore, patients with esophageal strictures had significantly more nonpropagated contractions than normal subjects; this trend was not significant in Barrett's esophagus.

Murphy et al. got the same results with respect to amplitudes and duration of esophageal contractions, but propulsive activity and acid clearance was not disturbed in reflux patients [19].

In eight patients with esophageal stenosis predominantly simultaneous contractions were observed distal to the stenosis [20]. The other results are listed in Table 1 (mean ± SD).

There were no differences found with regard to motility in patients with Barrett's esophagus, with and without complications [5], although the time of exposure to alkaline reflux (pH > 7) in the esophagus of patients with complications of Barrett's esophagus was significantly longer than in patients with an uncomplicated Barrett's esophagus.

The motility disturbances in esophageal strictures or Barrett's esophagus, respectively, are of the same kind as in uncomplicated esophagitis, but they are more severe.

Table 1. Esophageal motility in patients (n = 8) with esophageal stenosis (modified according to [20])

	Prestenotic	Poststenotic	Controls
Mean ampl. (mmHg)	36.4 ± 10.4	19.1 ± 8.3	39.9 ± 9.6
Mean duration (s)	4.5 ± 1.2	5.7 ± 1.1	3.3 ± 0.8
Mean velocity of propagation (cm/s)	4.9 ± 0.7	1.8 ± 0.7[a]	5.0 ± 0.8
Nonpropulsive contractions	40%	>90%	

[a]pre- vs. poststenotic, p < 0.001.

*

Can esophageal motility disorders be reversed by reversing the morphological alterations?

Eastwood and his colleagues showed in cats that LES pressure decreased after induction of esophagitis by exposure of the esophagus to hydrochloric acid [21]. LES pressures returned to their initial levels after healing of esophagitis. Thus motility disturbances seem to be first of all a consequence of acid reflux; secondly pathological reflux may increase due to a weakening of the antireflux barrier which then sets off a vicious cycle. However, other observations contradict this hypothesis. They were unable to find a rise in LES pressure after healing of a reflux esophagitis in man [22]. Singh et al. measured not only LES pressures but also esophageal transit time, duration of contractions, amplitude of contractions and the propulsive activity in esophagitis and after its healing, by omeprazole [23]; none of these variables changed significantly after healing. The authors therefore conclude that a primary motility disturbance is present, which then favors the development of reflux esophagitis. On the other hand, in a single patient suffering from esophagitis, motility disturbances and esophageal diverticuli were successfully treated with antacids and raising of the head-part of the bed [6]. Both the diverticuli and the motility disturbances disappeared.

Brand et al. showed in 10 patients suffering from Barrett's esophagus, that four of them lost their Barrett's epithelium after successful antireflux surgery; one patient developed an esophageal carcinoma, five kept their Barrett's syndrome [7]. Interestingly, LES pressures increased slightly in mean value only in some patients, but in other healed patients LES pressures did not rise. On the other hand, in four out of five patients, who were not healed, LES pressures rose. Changes in LES pressure, therefore, do not appear to be a prognostic indicator with respect to healing in Barrett's esophagus.

Healing of reflux esophagitis in man did not affect esophageal motility in some studies, but in others, further investigations were necessary to clarify the situation.

Conclusions

Motility disorders consisting of decreased propulsive force in the esophageal body and basal pressure in the LES, can be demonstrated in esophagitis. Their quantity is increased in Barrett's syndrome and esophageal strictures, but no new quality of motor disorders appears in these conditions. LES pressure alone does not appear to be a major determinant in healing of Barrett's esophagus, which makes it unlikely that LES pressure is decisive in the development of Barrett's esophagus. Also, in congenital Barrett's syndrome, the hypothesis of motility disturbances as the initial event fails.

There is a strong argument that esophageal motility disturbances precede the development of esophagitis and are not solely secondary to esophagitis. Disturbed motility could therefore be an indicating factor in the development of esophagitis.

Once reflux disease is present, the acid reflux is likely to intensify esophageal motility disturbances and could trigger a vicious cycle.

Since interventional studies with the aim of inducing stricture and Barrett's esophagus are not feasible in man, further evidence has to come from animal experiments and from long-term observations in man. Until then, the initial question has to be answered: it is very likely that motor disorders of esophagitis precede the development of a stricture or a Barrett's esophagus, but final proof is still missing.

References

1. Nebel O, Fornes M, Castell D. Symptomatic gastroesophageal reflux: incidence and precipitating factors. Dig Dis Sci 1976;21:953–956
2. Venkatachakam B, DaCosta L, Beck I. What is a normal esophagogastric junction? Gastroenterology 1972;62:521–528
3. Wienbeck M, Barnert J. Epidemiology of reflux disease and reflux esophagitis. Scand J Gastroenterol 1989;24(suppl156): 7–13.
4. Corazziari E, Pozzessere C, Dani S et al. Intraluminal pH and esophageal motility. Gastroenterology 1978;75:275–271.
5. Attwood SEA, DeMeester TR, Bremner CG et al. Alkaline gastroesophageal reflux: implications in the development of complications in Barrett's columnar-lined lower esophagus. Surgery 1989;106:764–770.
6. Bender M, Haddad J. Disappearance of multiple esophageal diverticula following treatment of esophagitis. Gastrointest Endosc 1973;20:19–22.
7. Brand DL, Ylvisaker J, Gelfand M et al. Regression of columnar esophageal (Barrett's) epithelium after antireflux surgery. N Engl J Med 1980;302:844–848.
8. Olsen A, Schlegel J. Motility disturbances caused by esophagitis. J Thorac Cardiovasc Surg 1965;50:607–612.
9. Kahrilas PJ, Dodds WJ, Hogan WJ et al. Esophageal peristaltic dysfunction in peptic esophagitis. Gastroenterology 1986; 91:897–904.
10. Nier H, Wienbeck M, Berges W et al. Syndrome nach gastrektomie unter besonderer berücksichtigung der refluxösophagitis. Langenbecks Arch Chirurg 1983;360:71–80.
11. Kruse-Andersen S, Wallin L, Madsen T. Reflux patterns and related oesophageal motor activity in gastro-oesophageal reflux disease. Gut 1990;31:633–638.
12. D'Angelo WA, Fries JF, Masi AT et al. Pathologic observation in systemic sclerosis (Scleroderma). Am J Med 1964;46: 428–440.
13. Treacy WL, Baggenstoss AH, Slocumb CH et al. Scleroderma of the esophagus. Ann Int Med 1963;59:351–356.
14. Creamer B, Andersen HA, Code CF. Esophageal motility in patients with sleroderma and related diseases. Gastroenterologia 1956;86:763–775.
15. Heitmann P, Espinoza J. Funktionelle störungen des ösophagus bei patienten mit sklerodermie. Dtsch Med Wschr 1964;93: 1960–1966.
16. Cunningham KM, Horowitz M, Riddell PS et al. Relations among autonomic nerve dysfunction, oesophageal motility, and gastric emptying in gastro-oesophageal reflux disease. Gut 1991;32:1436–1440.
17. McCallum RW, Berkowitz DM, Lerner E. Gastric emptying in patients with gastroesophageal reflux. Gastroenterology 1981;80:825–291.
18. Zaninotto G, DeMeester TR, Bremner CG et al. Esophageal function in patients with reflux-induced strictures and its relevance to surgical treatment. Ann Thorac Surg 1989;47:362–370.
19. Murphy PP, Johnson BT, Collins JSA. Esophageal manometry and acid clearance: a comparison between patients with columnar-lined esophagus and those with erosive reflux. Gastroenterology 1993;104:A153.
20. Wienbeck M, Heitmann P, Dombrowski H et al. Das Barrett syndrom. Leber Magen Darm 1973;3:81–90.
21. Eastwood G, Castell DO, Higgs R. Experimental esophagitis in cats impairs lower esophageal sphincter pressure. Gastroenterology 1975;69:146–153.
22. Allen M, McIntosh D, Robinson MG. Healing or amelioration of esophagitis does not result in increased lower esophageal sphincter or esophageal contractile pressure. Am J Gastroenterol 1990;85:1331–1334.
23. Singh P, Adamopoulos A, Taylor RH et al. Oesophageal motor function before and after healing of oesophagitis. Gut 1992; 33:1590–1596.

Are barium studies useful in detecting abnormal esophageal motility as a manifestation of reflux esophagitis?

D.J. Ott (Winston-Salem)

Reflux esophagitis is part of the spectrum of gastroesophageal reflux disease (GERD) in which histologic or gross findings of esophageal inflammation are present [1,2]. Abnormal esophageal motility is often associated with reflux esophagitis, and radiologic evaluation of the esophagus can assess both the functional and structural abnormalities that may occur in this disorder [1—4]. In response to this question, the pathogenesis of GERD with emphasis on the potential role of abnormal esophageal function in this disease is reviewed briefly. Secondly, radiologic evaluation of the esophageal motility, particularly in reflux esophagitis, is discussed.

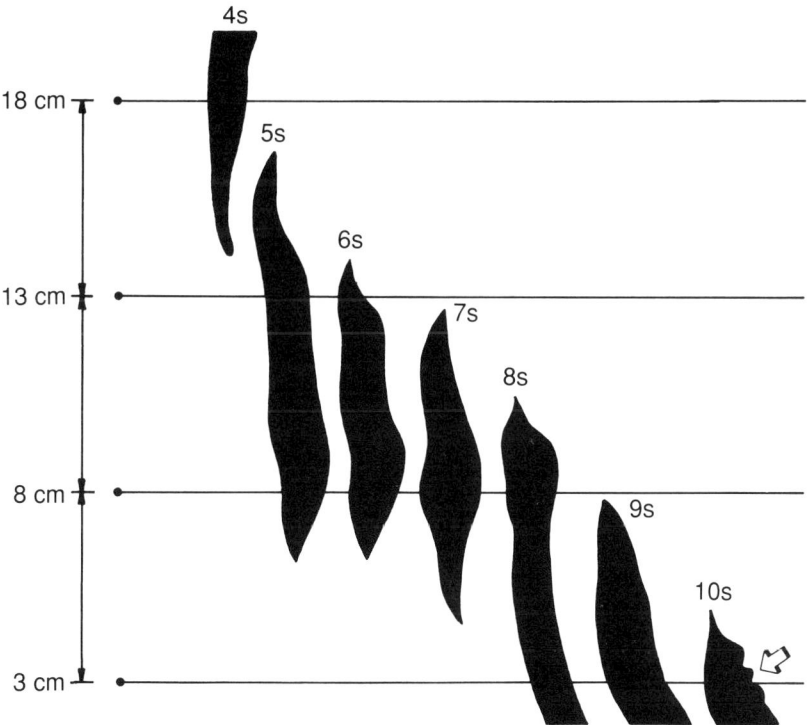

Fig. 1. Temporal tracings of a 5 ml barium bolus at 1-s intervals show normal primary peristalsis at fluoroscopy. The tapered tops of the barium column correspond to the peristaltic contraction wave seen at manometry. Mild tertiary activity (arrow) affects tracing at 10 s. Numbers on vertical axis represent positions of the catheter ports (with permission [16]).

Pathogenesis of GERD

Pathogenesis of GERD is multifactorial, and the following factors are thought to be contributory: 1) inadequacy of the antireflux mechanism; 2) volume and potency of the reflux material; 3) esophageal mucosal resistance; and 4) efficacy of esophageal clearance and gastric emptying [2]. Specific factors, or their combination, may predominate in different individuals as a cause of symptomatic reflux disease.

Inadequacy of the antireflux barrier manifested by lower esophageal sphincter (LES) dysfunction is generally accepted as the main cause of GERD. However, prolonged LES hypotension is uncommon in patients with reflux disease. Transient LES relaxations are more often associated with symptomatic reflux, and abnormal gastroesophageal reflux may also relate to patient position and temporally to meals and sleep [5–8]. Thus, other factors such as esophageal clearance must be considered in the pathogenesis of GERD.

Esophageal motility in reflux esophagitis

Although the frequency and duration of gastroesophageal reflux determines the

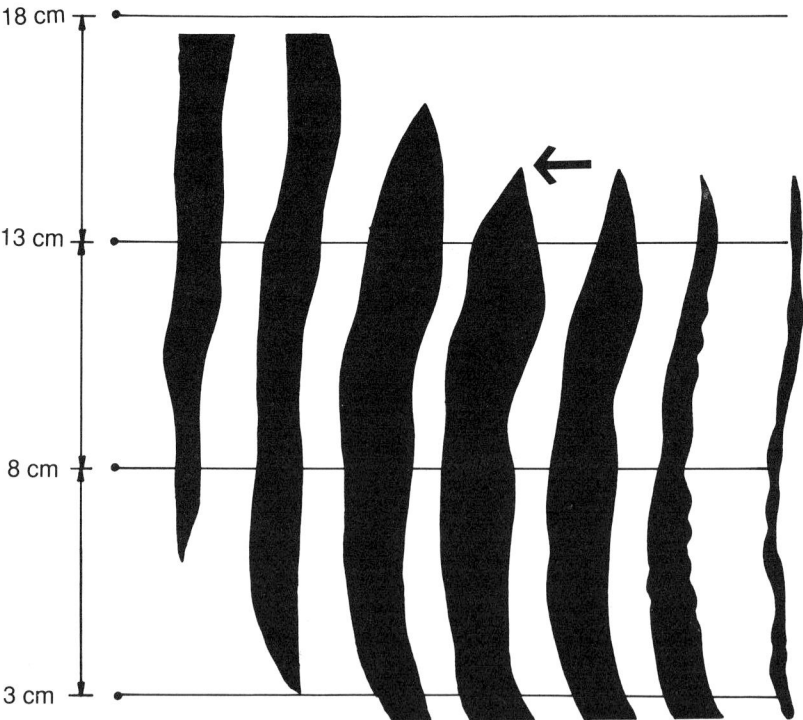

Fig. 2. Disruption of primary peristalsis (arrow) just above the 13 cm level with gradual and generalized clearance of barium from the esophagus over a 4-s interval. Simultaneous contractions were present at manometry. Tracings are at 1 s intervals (with permission [16]).

potential injury of the esophagus to gastric contents, esophageal clearance governs the temporal exposure to refluxed material [2]. Volume clearance and acid clearance, or neutralization by saliva, are interrelated processes. Primary esophageal peristalsis is most effective in clearing fluid from the esophagus and is important in counteracting the injurious effects of gastroesophageal reflux (Fig. 1) [2,5,9–11]. Secondary peristalsis and nonperistaltic contractions may also promote some esophageal volume clearance but are less important than the presence of normal primary peristalsis (Figs. 2 and 3).

Volume clearance is impaired when esophageal function is abnormal, especially with the patient recumbent which eliminates esophageal drainage by gravity. About half of patients with reflux esophagitis show some impairment of primary peristalsis on manometric examination [2,9]. Whether the peristaltic disturbances found in patients with reflux esophagitis precede and contribute to its development or are related secondarily to esophageal inflammation remains debated. Recent investigations have shown that abnormal esophageal function may persist after effective medical treatment of reflux disease [12–15]. Thus, in some patients, GERD may be considered a primary esophageal motility disorder.

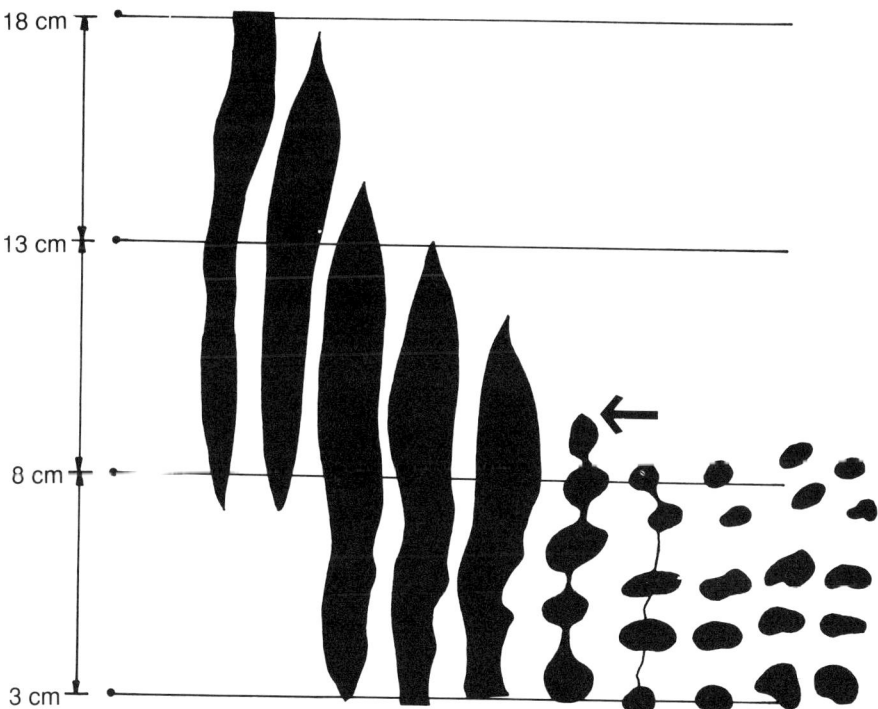

Fig. 3. Tracings at 1-s intervals with disruption of primary peristalsis (arrow) associated with segmental tertiary contractions that clear the barium bolus from the lower esophagus (with permission [16]).

139

Radiologic evaluation of esophageal motility

The barium esophagram and radionuclide transit and emptying studies are useful in detecting esophageal motility disturbances and abnormal clearance that may accompany reflux esophagitis [1,3,4]. Fluoroscopic observation or videotape recording during the barium esophagram using multiple barium swallows reliably evaluates primary esophageal peristalsis [16,17]. In an investigation of synchronous videotape fluoroscopy and esophageal manometry, a 92% agreement between the examinations was found using a total of five single barium swallows for radiologic evaluation [16].

Esophageal functional disturbances that may be seen radiographically in patients with reflux esophagitis include nonperistaltic contractions, incomplete or intermittently absent primary peristalsis, and rarely aperistalsis (Figs. 4 and 5) [1,3,4,18]. Secondary motility disorders, such as scleroderma, should be considered if aperistalsis accompanies reflux esophagitis. The lower half of the esophagus is typically affected in areas of active inflammation and peristaltic disturbances are more common in that location.

The barium esophagram also provides a good estimate of esophageal clearance. In normal recumbent individuals, a single peristaltic sequence usually strips most or

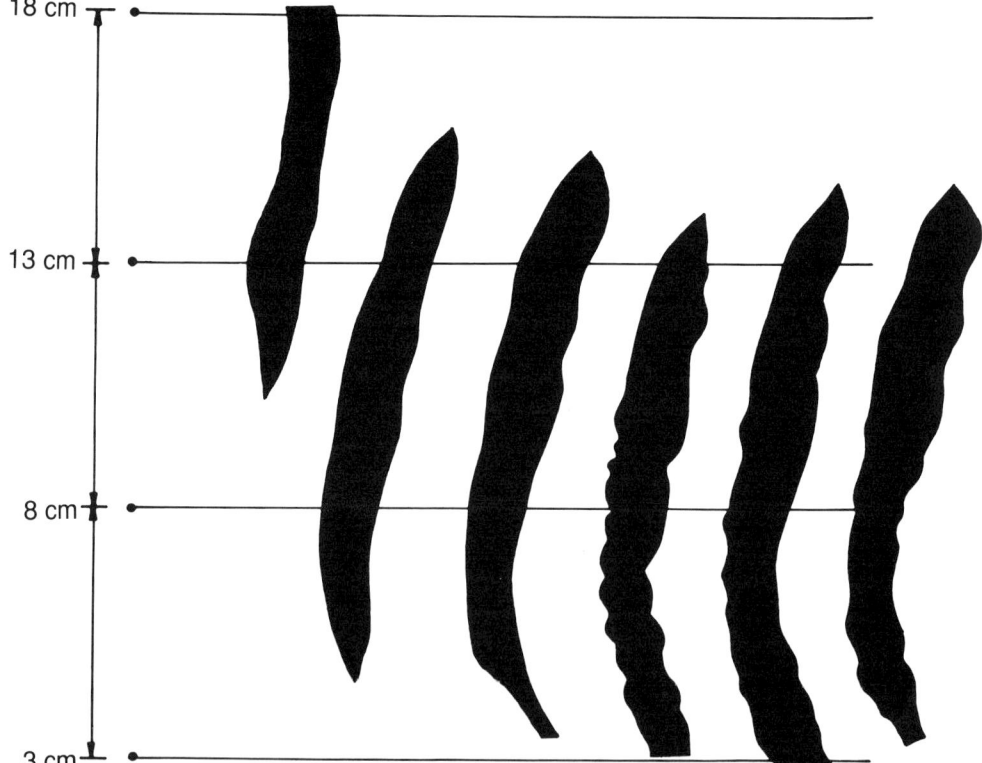

Fig. 4. Tracings of a 10 ml barium bolus at 2-s intervals show disrupted primary peristalsis between the 13 cm and 18 cm levels. Prolonged stasis of barium and nonsegmental tertiary activity are seen (with permission [16]).

140

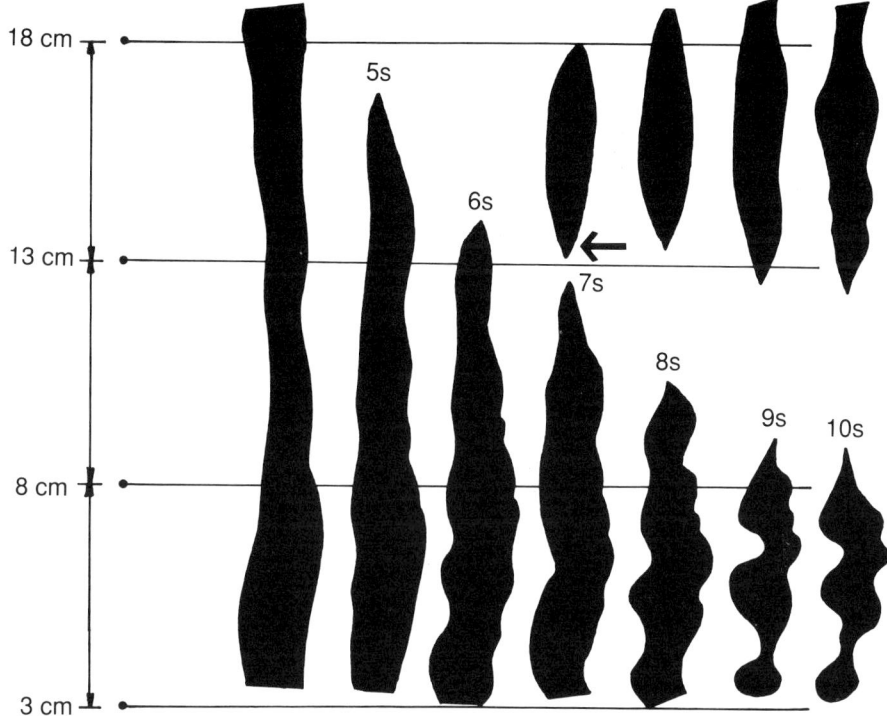

Fig. 5. Tracings of a 5 ml bolus at 1-s intervals show proximal escape (arrow) and disruption of primary peristalsis just above the 8 cm level. Nonsegmental tertiary activity is also present (with permission [16]).

all of the swallowed barium bolus from the esophagus (Fig. 1) [1–5]. Occasionally, proximal escape of some barium occurs at the level of the aortic arch, especially in older patients, and several swallows may be needed to empty the esophagus completely (Fig. 6). Nonperistaltic esophageal contractions may also contribute, but less effectively, to clearance of the barium bolus from the esophagus (Figs. 2 and 3) [16].

The efficacy of the radiologic evaluation of esophageal functional impairment in patients with reflux esophagitis will depend largely on the technique used and the experience of the examiner. Careful fluoroscopic observation or videotape recording of multiple, single swallows of barium are necessary to accurately assess esophageal function. Fluoroscopic observation of five barium swallows by an experienced radiologist will correlate well with manometric findings.

Summary

In summary, abnormalities of esophageal function are common in patients with reflux esophagitis. The barium esophagram can detect the structural changes seen in moderate to severe reflux esophagitis and also demonstrate the functional disturbances that may accompany reflux disease. If properly performed, the radiologic evaluation

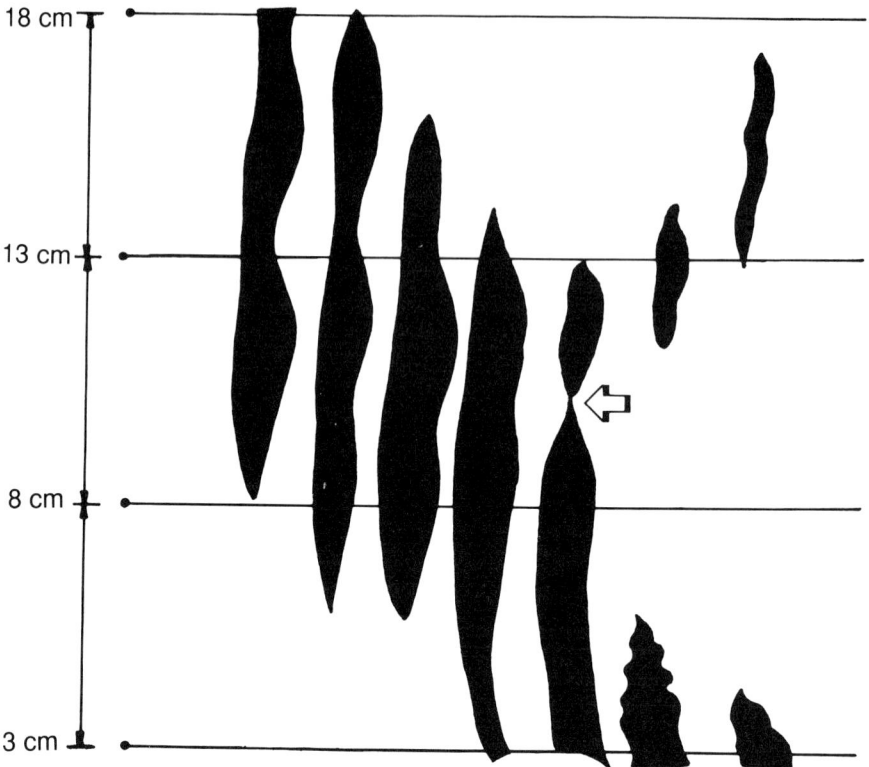

Fig. 6. Similar 1-s tracings of a 5 ml bolus of normal primary peristalsis associated with proximal escape of barium (arrow). The lower esophagus is normally stripped of barium below the arrow. Nonsegmental tertiary activity affects the lower barium columns of the last two tracings (with permission [16]).

of esophageal motility and its impairment compares favorably to manometric examination.

References

1. Ott DJ, Dodds WJ, Wu WC, Gelfand DW, Hogan WJ, Stewart ET. Current status of radiology in evaluating for gastro-esophageal reflux disease. J Clin Gastroenterol 1982;4:365–375.
2. Dodds WJ. The pathogenesis of gastroesophageal reflux disease. AJR 1988;151:49–56.
3. Ott DJ, Cowan RJ, Gelfand DW, Wu WC, Chen YM, Munitz HA. The role of diagnostic imaging in evaluating gastro-esophageal reflux disease. Postgrad Radiol 1986;6:3–14.
4. Ott DJ. Barium esophagram. In: Castell DO, Wu WC, Ott DJ (eds) Gastroesophageal Reflux Disease. New York: Futura Publ. Co., 1985:109–128.
5. Dodds WJ. Current concepts of esophageal motor function: clinical implications for radiology. AJR 1977;128:549–561.
6. DeMeester TR, Johnson LF, Guy JJ, Toscano MS, Hall AW, Skinner DB. Patterns of gastroesophageal reflux in health and disease. Ann Surg 1976;184:459–470.
7. Dent J, Dodds WJ, Friedman RH, Sekiguchi T, Hogan WJ, Arndorfer RC, Petrie DJ. Mechanism of gastroesophageal reflux in recumbent asymptomatic human subjects. J Clin Invest 1980;65:256–267.
8. Dodds WJ, Dent J, Hogan WJ, Helm JF, Hauser R, Patel GK, Egide MS. Mechanisms of gastroesophageal reflux in patients with reflux esophagitis. N Engl J Med 1982;307:1547–1552.
9. Kahrilas PJ, Dodds WJ, Hogan WJ, Kern MK, Arndorfer RC, Reece A. Esophageal peristaltic dysfunction in peptic esophagitis. Gastroenterology 1986;91:897–904.

142

10. Kahrilas PJ, Dodds WJ, Hogan WJ. Effect of peristaltic dysfunction on esophageal volume clearance. Gastroenterology 1988;94:73—80.
11. Dodds WJ, Kahrilas PJ, Dent J, Hogan WJ, Kern MK, Arndorfer RC. Analysis of spontaneous gastroesophageal reflux and esophageal acid clearance in patients with reflux esophagitis. J Gastrointest Motility 1990;2:79—89.
12. Burns TW, Venturatos SG. Esophageal motor function and response to acid perfusion in patients with symptomatic reflux esophagitis. Dig Dis Sci 1985;30:529—535.
13. Eckardt VF. Does healing of esophagitis improve esophageal motor function? Dig Dis Sci 1988;33:161—165.
14. Baldi F, Ferrarini F, Longanesi A, Angeloni M, Ragazzini M, Miglioli M, Barbara L. Oesophageal function before, during, and after healing of erosive oesophagitis. Gut 1988;29:157—160.
15. Singh P, Adamopoulos A, Taylor RH, Colin-Jones DG. Oesophageal motor function before and after healing of oesophagitis. Gut 1992;33:1590—1596.
16. Ott DJ, Chen YM, Hewson EG, Richter JE, Dalton CB, Gelfand DW, Wu WC. Esophageal motility: assessment with synchronous video tape fluoroscopy and manometry. Radiology 1989;173:419—422.
17. Massey BT, Dodds WJ, Hogan WJ, Brasseur JG, Helm JF. Abnormal esophageal motility — an analysis of concurrent radiographic and manometric findings. Gastroenterology 1991;101:344—354.
18. Simeone JF, Burrell M, Toffler R, Walker Smith GJ. Aperistalsis and esophagitis. Radiology 1977;123:9—14.

What is the proportion of cases of pathological reflux with a normal sphincter pressure?

G.C. O'Sullivan (Cork)

The introduction of esophageal manometry and the flexible gastrointestinal pH probe established that the distal esophageal segment of humans functions as a sphincter and provides a barrier to the reflux of gastrointestinal contents into the esophagus [1]. Sphincter dysfunction and/or its destruction by myotomy leads to incompetence of the antireflux barrier and a risk of esophagitis and stricture. In contrast, restoration of sphincter function by surgery restores competence and permanently eliminates reflux and its long-term sequelae [2].

The contact time between the esophageal mucosa and the destructive elements of gastroesophageal reflux (GER) is important in the genesis of esophagitis. The contact time is thought to be increased by a more severe degree of incompetence and/or by impairment of the esophageal clearance mechanisms. Studies with 24-h pH monitoring have shown that the acid mucosal exposure time is more prolonged in patients with reflux symptoms, in contrast with control subjects. This difference is more marked when patients are recumbent. An important finding was that radiographic or endoscopic evidence of esophagitis did not exist in many patients with symptoms and with evidence of pathological GER on pH monitoring [3—5]. Thus, neither symptoms, nor the absence of endoscopic evidence of mucosal injury are a reliable guide to the presence or absence of GER.

The measurement of a hypotensive distal esophageal sphincter is used by many as an indicator of reflux. Initial studies of highly selected populations suggested that distal esophageal sphincter measurements could distinguish control subjects from patients with severe symptoms [6]. Subsequent larger studies showed extensive overlap of the sphincter pressure measurements between control subjects and reflux patients [5]. This suggests that pressure measurements have limited diagnostic usefulness. In this study we examine the diagnostic accuracy of sphincter pressure measurements in symptomatic patients assessed by 24-h pH monitoring.

Methods

One hundred and seventy-five patients with symptoms suggestive of GER were studied by esophageal manometry, 24-h pH monitoring of the distal esophagus, the standard acid reflux test (SART), and by upper intestinal barium and endoscopic studies. Esophageal manometry was performed according to the technique of Winans and Harris [6]. Using a single catheter assembly of three fluid-filled polyethilene tubes perfused with distilled water from a pneumohydrolic pump system (Arndorfer). The amplitude of pressure in the distal esophageal sphincter was measured as the difference (in mmHg) between the resting gastric pressure and the maximum DES pressure at the respiratory inversion point. The length of sphincter above and below the respiratory inversion point was assessed. The mean of three measurements were used for analysis.

Twenty-four hour pH monitoring was performed according to the technique of Johnson and DeMeester [3]. Patients with a DeMeester score of ≥18 were classified as refluxers [5].

The SART was performed as described by Skinner and Booth [7]. A SART score of ≥4 indicated a positive test.

On endoscopy esophagitis was scored as grade 0: normal mucosa; grade I: erythema; grade II or greater: erosions, ulceration or stricture.

Test criteria

Patients were classified as refluxers if there was a positive 24-h pH test or grade II esophagitis. Reflux patients with a positive SART were considered to have a mechanical and functional abnormality of the gastroesophageal junction (common cavity syndrome). Reflux patients with negative SART were considered to have a functional abnormality of the lower esophageal sphincter, that is GER in the presence of a mechanically adequate barrier.

Statistical evaluation of data

Results were evaluated by an analysis of variance-incorporating techniques for unequal numbers after a two-way classification of the data.

Results

Of 175 patients studied, 118 were found to have a positive 24-h pH test. The SART was positive in 57 of 118 reflux patients and 11 of 57 patients with a negative 24-h pH test. Out of 118 with reflux on pH testing, 38 were found to have endoscopic esophagitis of grade II or more. Three patients had grade II esophagitis in the presence of a negative SART and 24-h pH test.

The relationship between sphincter measurements and prevalence of GER is outlined in Table 1. These data indicate that competence of the cardia is determined by the level of pressure in the sphincter, the length of sphincter below the respiratory inversion point, and an interaction between both. The relationship between sphincter measurements and the degree of esophagitis and the SART test in reflux patients is outlined in Table 2. The sphincter pressures were reduced in the presence of esophagitis irrespective of the SART status of the patients. Similarly the pressure was lower in SART-positive patients irrespective of the severity of esophagitis. Patients with severe esophagitis and a positive SART had the lowest sphincter pressures.

Out of 71 patients with the pressure <10 mmHg, 12 did not have GER. Out of 118 patients with reflux, 58 (approximately 50%) had sphincter pressures >10 mmHg. Thus a sphincter pressure index of 10 mmHg has a low sensitivity and specificity.

Discussion

Measurements of distal esophageal sphincter pressures are not a reliable guide to the presence or absence of GER. This study also confirms previous findings that competence of the gastroesophageal junction requires both a minimal sphincter pressure and a minimal length of sphincter exposed to the positive pressure environment of the abdomen [8]. In determining competence, the pressure and length effects are not strictly additive, but have an interactive relationship. This has

Table 1. The percentage of incidence of abnormal GER stratified for length and pressure of DES

Pressure of DES in mmHg	Length of DES below respiratory inversion point		
	0–1 cm	1–2 cm	>2 cm
0–<5	100% (n = 12/12)	100% (n = 8/8)	100% (n = 1/1)
5–<10	100% (n = 10/10)	70.8% (n = 16/23)	70.6% (n = 12/17)
10–<15	83% (n = 5/6)	70.4% (n = 19/27)	61.9% (n = 13/21)
15–<20	100% (n = 1/1)	62.5% (n = 4/8)	61.5% (n = 1/16)
20+	100% (n = 1/1)	50% (n = 4/8)	6.25% (n = 1/16)

n = number of patients in each cell (total: 175); total number of refluxers: 118; DES: distal esophageal sphincter.

Determinants of competence: Pressure $P_{(4,7)}$ 8.8 P 0.025
Length $P_{(2,7)}$ 18.49 P 0.01
Interaction $P_{(1,7)}$ 20.5 P 0.01

Table 2. The sphincter pressure, length of sphincter and abdominal esophagus in reflux patients

	24-h pH positive (n = 118)					
	Grade 0 (n = 56)		Grade I (n = 24)		Grade II (n = 38)	
	SART + (n = 22)	SART − (n = 34)	SART + (n = 14)	SART − (n = 10)	SART + (n = 22)	SART − (n = 16)
P	10.54 ± 4.52	11.85 ± 6.34	8.37 ± 3.54	15.12 ± 9.11	7.72 ± 5.13	8.86 ± 5.22
LS	3.60 ± 0.82	3.49 ± 1.19	3.76 ± 1.11	3.67 ± 1.11	4.05 ± 1.34	2.99 ± 1.11
LA	1.41 ± 0.73	1.55 ± 0.91	1.24 ± 0.1	1.65 ± 1.0	1.25 ± 0.97	1.40 ± 0.69

Results are stratified for the grade of esophagitis and the results of the SART; they are expressed in mean ± SD.

Analysis of variance − Pressure Grade $F_{(2,112)}$ 3.849 P 0.05
SART $F_{(1,112)}$ 6.390 P 0.025
Interaction $F_{(2,112)}$ 5.427 P 0.025

important implications for manometric diagnosis and therapy. Strict manometric criteria for diagnosis of sphincter incompetence are difficult to determine because the interaction of pressure and length measurements must be considered. Similarly, because of this interactive effect competence may not be restored to the gastro-esophageal junction by correcting just the pressure deficit alone.

In the presence of reflux, low sphincter pressures are found in patients with esophagitis and/or a positive SART. The question is whether esophagitis is important in the cause of sphincter hypotension − perusal of the data suggests that at most it can only be one of many factors. The wide standard deviation of the groups show that many patients with low sphincter pressures do not have esophagitis and some patients with esophagitis have pressures in the region of the nonreflux patients with a normal mucosa. It has been suggested that esophagitis is not related to the lowering of the distal esophageal sphincter pressure as sphincter tone did not improve in patients where esophagitis healed on medication. However, the results of those studies may not be conclusive as it is not known whether the changes to the neuro- or myogenic control mechanisms are reparable. On balance the findings in this study support the experiments of Higgs [9], that inflammation in the sphincter region may be one factor in the genesis of hypotension and could be a late event in the evolution of reflux disease.

Many patients with GER have sphincter pressures >15 mmHg and abdominal segments >2 cm, suggesting that factors other than sphincter competence may be important in the genesis of reflux disease. These factors may be diurnal variations of sphincter pressure in relation to the different phases of the migratory motor complexes [10], transient lower esophageal sphincter relaxations [11,12], and failure of the esophageal acid clearance mechanisms [4].

In conclusion, GER is a multifactorial disease. Lower esophageal sphincter competence is determined by many factors, including sphincter pressure. Measurements of sphincter pressure are not a reliable guide to the presence or absence of GER.

References

1. Tuttle SG, Grossman MI. Detection of gastroesophageal reflux by simultaneous measurements of interluminal pressure and pH. Proc Soc Exp Biol Med 1958;98:225.
2. DeMeester TR, Bonavina L, Albertucci M. Nissen fundoplication for gastroesophageal reflux disease. Ann Surg 1986; 204:9.
3. Johnson LF, DeMeester TR. Twenty-four hour pH monitoring of the distal esophagus. Am J Gastroenterol 1974;62:325.
4. Johnson LF, DeMeester TR, Haggitt RG. Esophageal epithelial response and gastroesophageal reflux: a quantitative study. Am J Dig Dis 1978;23:498.
5. DeMeester TR, Wang CI, Wernly JA et al. Technique indications and clinical use of 24-hour esophageal pH monitoring. J Thorac Cardiovasc Surg 1980;79:636.
6. Winans CS, Harris LD. Quantitation of lower esophageal sphincter competence. Gastroenterology 1967;52:773.
7. Skinner DB, Booth DG. Assessment of distal esophageal function in patients with hiatal hernia and/or gastroesophageal reflux. Ann Surg 1970;172:627.
8. O'Sullivan GC, DeMeester TR, Joelsson BE et al. The interaction of lower esophageal sphincter pressure and length of sphincter in the abdomen as determinants of gastroesophageal competence. Am J Surg 1982;143:40.
9. Higgs RH, Castell DO, Eastwood GC. Studies of the mechanism of esophagitis-induced lower esophageal sphincter hypotension in cats. Gastroenterology 1976;71:51.
10. Gill RC, Kellow JE, Wingate DL. Gastroesophageal reflux and the migrating motor complex. Gut 1987;28:929.
11. Dodds WJ, Dent J, Hogan WJ. Mechanisms of gastroesophageal reflux in patients with reflux esophagitis. N Engl J Med 1982;307:1547.
12. Mittal RK, McCallum RW. Characteristics and frequency of transient relaxation of the lower esophageal sphincter in patients with esophagitis. Gastroenterology 1988;95:593.

Is it important to distinguish between voluntary motor activity and involuntary contractions?

M.N. Schoeman, R.H. Holloway (Adelaide)

Meltzer first made the distinction between voluntary and involuntary esophageal contractions in 1906 and defined esophageal contractions induced by the voluntary act of deglutition as primary peristalsis, while secondary peristalsis referred to the involuntary response to esophageal distension [1].

Since this time, considerable data have been published about the luminal pressure patterns of primary peristalsis with regard to their reproducibility, manometric characteristics and abnormalities in various disease states [2,3]. Conversely, secondary peristalsis has received minimal attention in health and disease.

Secondary peristalsis occurs in response to esophageal distension [4–10]. Under normal circumstances, this usually occurs if food, fluid or air are retained in the esophagus after a failed primary peristaltic sequence or after reflux of gastric contents into the esophagus. Secondary peristalsis results in the mechanical volume clearance of the distending esophageal bolus and is considered to be of protective importance, as it is the major mechanism which maintains an empty esophagus [11]. This is

147

particularly important after gastroesophageal reflux where secondary peristalsis assists in the initial volume clearance of the refluxate and so contributes to esophageal acid clearance [12]. In patients with gastroesophageal reflux disease (GERD), secondary peristalsis is seen less often after spontaneous reflux episodes [13] than in normal subjects [14], which suggests that there may be a defect of secondary peristalsis in this condition. Consistent with these findings, motor responses to prolonged balloon distension have also been reported to be abnormal in patients with gastroesophageal reflux disease. This defect appears to correlate with delayed esophageal acid clearance [15]. It is doubtful, however, that balloon distension is the most appropriate method of evaluating reflux-induced esophageal motor responses, as the balloon results in a fixed, focal esophageal distension, more analogous to acute esophageal obstruction, compared to the less focal distension of the esophagus by refluxed fluids.

In addition to delayed esophageal acid clearance, defective secondary peristalsis may lead to prolonged bolus retention within the esophagus and so cause dysphagia. This may be particularly important in the pathogenesis of symptoms in patients with nonobstructive dysphagia who, by definition, have no structural lesion to account for their symptoms. In these patients it is widely believed that the dysphagia is due to an esophageal motor disorder [16]. In a significant number of these patients there are clear abnormalities of primary peristalsis. In the remainder of the patients, standard manometric assessment of primary peristalsis fails to reveal any abnormality and the aetiology of the dysphagia remains unclear in this group [16–20]. There is indirect evidence for an abnormality of secondary peristalsis, as a possible explanation for the dysphagia in patients with nonobstructive dysphagia from the studies of Deschner et al. and Williams et al. which showed abnormal esophageal motor responses to prolonged balloon distension [21,22]. In these patients it was postulated that this abnormality contributed to the pathogenesis of nonobstructive dysphagia.

Secondary peristalsis in gastroesophageal reflux disease and nonobstructive dysphagia

Debate persists about the nature of the secondary esophageal motor response and its similarity to primary peristalsis [7,23]. In our studies [8], primary peristalsis, using 5 ml water swallows, was compared to secondary peristalsis induced by three stimuli. Secondary responses were triggered by both inflation of an intraesophageal balloon to a diameter of 1, 2 and 3 cm and intraesophageal injection of boluses of 5, 10, and 20 ml of air and 2, 5 and 10 ml boluses of water. Each distension volume was tested in triplicate in the upper, middle and lower esophagus.

Primary peristalsis was normal in all subjects, with a propagated contraction that progressed down the esophageal body. Secondary peristaltic responses, on the other hand, varied with the type of esophageal distension used. Both air and water boluses produced complete secondary peristaltic responses that, regardless of the level of injection, started at the most proximal esophageal recording site and traversed the entire length of the esophageal body. For both air and water boluses, the response rate of complete peristalsis increased significantly as the injected volume increased

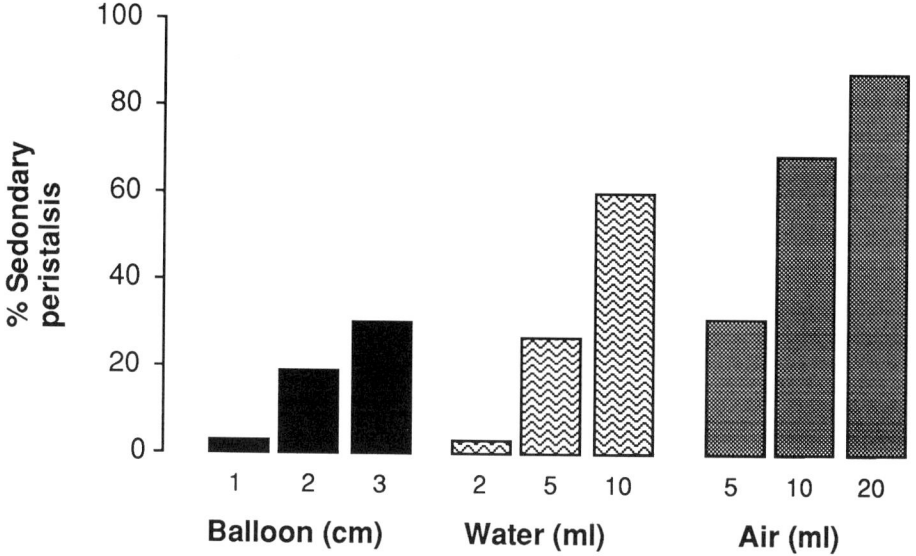

Fig. 1. Effect of bolus volume on the secondary peristaltic responses to air, water and balloon in normal subjects. Data for the three esophageal sites are combined and data are expressed as mean response rates for each volume. The frequency of secondary peristaltic responses increased significantly with bolus volume (p < 0.0001). There was no difference in the frequency of secondary peristalsis, however, when equal bolus volumes of air and water were compared.

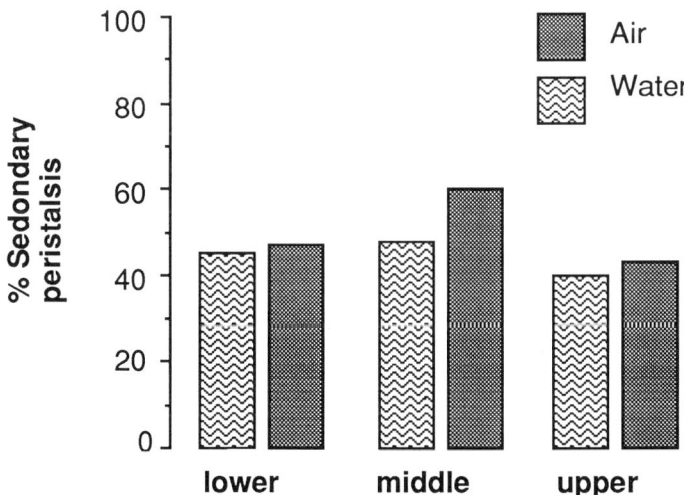

Fig. 2. Effect of the site of injection on the proportion of secondary peristaltic responses to air and water boluses in the normal subjects. Combined data for the 5 and 10 ml boluses are shown. The columns represent the mean response rates for each stimulus at each site. The frequency of secondary peristalsis in response to air and water boluses are not influenced by the site of injection.

(p < 0.0001) and were similar for air and water boluses of equal volume (Fig. 1). In addition, when equal bolus volumes of air and water were compared, the level of injection did not influence the number of complete peristaltic responses (Fig. 2).

In contrast to the responses induced by the air and water boluses, balloon distension produced a different esophageal motor pattern. Characteristically, during distension there was a high amplitude synchronous contraction above the balloon, while below there was motor quiescence. After distension, the synchronous contraction above the balloon subsided and a peristaltic contraction wave progressed distally from the level of the balloon. The ability to trigger secondary peristalsis below the balloon was also volume dependent with a 3 cm distension and was more likely to elicit a response than a 1 cm distension. In addition, the middle balloon was more likely to stimulate a peristaltic response than the upper or lower balloons (data not shown).

In subsequent studies, secondary peristalsis was evaluated with the same stimulus in patients with GERD [24] and nonobstructive dysphagia [25]. In these subjects, a simplified approach was used. Esophageal distension was tested with a single esophageal balloon, located in the mid-esophagus, and a single infusion port located immediately above the balloon for the rapid injection of boluses of air or water. In addition, the distensions used were limited to the 3 cm diameter balloon and 10 ml boluses of air or water. Each distension was tested 5 times in each subject.

In the reflux patients, seven of the 11 subjects exhibited normal primary peristalsis with a mean response rate of 76% which was comparable to the normal subjects (Table 1). In the nonobstructive dysphagia patients only six of the 16 patients had normal primary peristalsis with a mean response rate of successful primary peristalsis in this group of 55%, which was less than that seen in the normal subjects. The frequencies of successful secondary peristalsis, in response to esophageal distension with air and water injections, were significantly higher in the normal subjects than in the reflux or nonobstructive dysphagia patients (Table 1). The mean response rate with air injection was 80% in the normal subjects, 24% in the reflux patients and 18% in the patients with nonobstructive dysphagia (p < 0.05). Similarly, the mean success rate with water injections was 60% in the normal subjects, 16% in the reflux patients, and 20% in the nonobstructive dysphagia patients (p < 0.05). Within each

Table 1. Frequency of secondary peristalsis in patients with GERD and patients with nonobstructive dysphagia

Stimulus	Response (%)		
	Normal subjects	Reflux patients	NOD patients
Primary peristalsis			
Water swallows	98	76	55[a]
Secondary peristalsis			
Air bolus	80	24[a]	18[a]
Water bolus	60	16[a]	20[a]
Balloon distension	53	31	47

[a]p < 0.05 compared to normal subjects.

group, however, the frequency of secondary peristalsis in response to air bolus injection did not differ from that in response to water bolus injection.

The major pattern of failure, in response to the air and water bolus injections, in the two patient groups compared to the normal subjects was a complete absence of secondary peristalsis in response to esophageal distension. The proportion of failed and synchronous responses, however, was similar in the two groups. In contrast, the frequency of secondary peristalsis after balloon distension in the patients with reflux disease (31%) and nonobstructive dysphagia (47%) was similar to that in the normal subjects (53%). This difference probably relates to the different physical characteristics of the distending stimuli or to the greater degree of local distension induced by the balloon, which often resulted in chest discomfort.

Commentary

From our studies it is clear that most patients with reflux disease and nonobstructive dysphagia have grossly defective triggering of secondary peristalsis in response to esophageal distension with boluses of air and water. The implication of this finding is that these patients will also manifest defective secondary peristaltic responses to the esophageal distension induced by gastroesophageal reflux or by a retained bolus within the esophagus. We believe that this defect may contribute to the delayed esophageal acid clearance seen in reflux disease or to the prolonged esophageal transit often documented in patients with nonobstructive dysphagia.

The nature of the distending stimulus determined the manometric pattern of the secondary peristaltic responses recorded. The air and water boluses were distributed rapidly along the length of the esophagus and triggered an integrated response that swept the length of the esophagus. Distension with air or water produces a pattern of distension analogous to the esophageal distension induced by reflux; the 10 ml bolus producing a common cavity pressure rise which is similar to that seen after reflux events. Air and water boluses were also more effective stimuli than balloon distension in discriminating normal subjects from patients with reflux disease and nonobstructive dysphagia. These observations would suggest therefore, that air and water boluses are the most appropriate method of examining secondary peristalsis.

Fixed balloon distension produces a manometric response more analogous to acute esophageal obstruction [10], with the propagated response only occurring below the site of distension after balloon deflation. Balloon inflation produces a focal and often uncomfortable feeling retrosternally, whereas, the distending air and water are distributed immediately along the esophageal body and produce no symptoms. The fact that the balloon caused symptoms suggests that it produces a greater degree of local distension and perhaps exceeded the threshold required to trigger a motor response. This may also explain why the balloon responses failed to discriminate between normal subjects and the patients. Certainly, the balloon diameter of 3 cm used in the study exceeded the threshold volume used by Deschner et al. [21]. In addition, technical factors such as balloon rupture and patient discomfort, limit its usefulness in clinical manometry.

In summary, it is clear that the evaluation of both voluntary and involuntary motor patterns is both physiologically relevant and clinically important. The particular motor response being evaluated depends on the type of stimulus used. Testing of secondary peristalsis by esophageal distension with boluses of air or water is technically easier to perform than balloon distension, better tolerated and appears to be the most sensitive test for assessing secondary peristaltic dysfunction in both reflux disease and nonobstructive dysphagia. The evaluation of involuntary esophageal motor responses is readily incorporated into standard clinical manometry where traditionally only voluntary motor activity is examined in any detail.

References

1. Meltzer SJ. Secondary peristalsis of the esophagus − a demonstration on a dog with a permanent esophageal fistula. Proc Soc Exp Biol Med 1906;3:35−37.
2. Dodds WJ, Hogan WJ, Reid DP, Stewart ET, Arndorfer RC. A comparison between primary esophageal peristalsis following wet and dry swallows. J Appl Physiol 1973;35:851−857.
3. Richter JE, Wu WC, Johns DN, Blackwell JN, Nelson JL, Castell JA et al. Esophageal manometry in 95 healthy adult volunteers. Dig Dis Sci 1987;32:583−592.
4. Creamer B, Schlegel J. Motor responses of the esophagus to distension. J Appl Physiol 1957;10:498−504.
5. Dornhurst AC, Harrison K, Pierce JW. Observations on the normal oesophagus and cardia. Lancet 1954;1:695−698.
6. Fleschler B, Hendrix TR, Kramer P, Ingelfinger FJ. The characteristics and similarity of primary and secondary peristalsis in the esophagus. J Clin Invest 1959;38:110−116.
7. Paterson WG, Rattan S, Goyal RK. Esophageal responses to transient and sustained esophageal distension. Am J Phyiol 1988;255:G587−G595.
8. Schoeman MN, Tippett M, Ireland A, Dent J, Holloway RH. Stimulation and characteristics of secondary peristalsis in normal subjects. Gastroenterology 1991;100:A491.
9. Siegel Cl, Hendrix TR. Evidence for the central mediation of secondary peristalsis in the esophagus. Bull Johns Hopkins Hosp 1961;108:297−307.
10. Winship DH, Zboralske FF. The esophageal propulsive force: Esophageal response to acute obstruction. J Clin Invest 1967; 46:1391−1401.
11. Helm JF, Dodds WJ, Pelc LR, Palmer DW, Hogan WJ, Teeter BC. Effect of esophageal emptying and saliva on clearance of acid from the esophagus. N Engl J Med 1984;310:284−288.
12. Helm JF. Esophageal acid clearance. J Clin Gastroenterol 1986;8(suppl 1):5−11.
13. Dodds WJ, Kahrilas PJ, Dent J, Hogan WJ, Kern MK, Arndorfer RC. Analysis of spontaneous gastroesophageal reflux and esophageal acid clearance in patients with reflux esophagitis. J Gastrointest Motility 1989;1:105−114.
14. Dent J, Dodds WJ, Friedman RH, Sekiguchi T, Hogan WJ, Arndorfer RC et al. Mechanism of gastroesophageal reflux in recumbent asymptomatic human subjects. J Clin Invest 1980;65:256−267.
15. Williams D, Thompson DG, Marples M, Heggie L, O'Hanrahan T, Mani V et al. Identification of an abnormal esophageal clearance response to intraluminal distension in patients with esophagitis. Gastroenterology 1992;103:943−953.
16. Jacob P, Kahrilas PJ, Vanagunas A. Peristaltic dysfunction associated with nonobstructive dysphagia in reflux disease. Dig Dis Sci 1990;35:939−942.
17. Barish CF, Castell DO, Richter JE. Graded esophageal balloon distension: A new provocative test for noncardiac chest pain. Dig Dis Sci 1986;31:1292−1298.
18. Katz PO, Dalton CB, Richter JE, Wu WC, Castell DO. Esophageal testing of patients with noncardiac chest pain or dysphagia − Results of three years experience with 1161 patients. Ann Int Med 1987;106:593−597.
19. Ott DJ, Richter JE, Chen YM, Wu WC, Gelfand DW, Castell DO. Esophageal radiography and manometry: correlation in 172 patients with dysphagia. Am J Roentgenol 1987;149:307−311.
20. Triadafilopoulos G. Nonobstructive dysphagia in reflux esophagitis. Am J Gastroenterol 1989;84:614−618.
21. Deschner WK, Maher KA, Cattau EL, Benjamin SB. Manometric responses to balloon distension in patients with nonobstructive dysphagia. Gastroenterology 1989;97:1181−1185.
22. Williams D, Thompson DG, Marples M, O'Hanrahan T, Bancewicz J. Motor responses to mechanoreceptor stimulation in the normal oesophagus and in patients with oesophageal symptoms. J Gastrointest Motility 1990;2:163.
23. Paterson W, Hynna-Liepert T, Selucky M. Comparison of primary and secondary esophageal peristalsis in humans: effect of atropine. Am J Physiol 1991;260:G52−G57.
24. Schoeman MN, Tippett M, Dent J, Holloway RH. Integrity and characteristics of secondary peristalsis in patients with gastroesophageal reflux disease. Gastroenterology 1991;100:A157.
25. Schoeman MN, Tippett M, Dent J, Holloway RH. Integrity and characteristics of secondary peristalsis in patients with nonobstructive dysphagia. Gastroenterology 1991;100:A157.

Which manometric criteria should be observed in the assessment of an esophagitis?

A. Watson (London)

The principal manometric criteria in the assessment of patients with esophagitis relate to lower esophageal sphincter (LES) characteristics and those of the esophageal body. Abnormalities of the upper esophageal sphincter may occur in a small proportion of patients with gastroesophageal reflux disease (GERD), but these are neither related to the presence or degree of esophagitis, nor of therapeutic relevance.

The characteristics of the LES which are believed to be of relevance are the resting pressure, intra-abdominal length and total length. It is well recognized that resting LES pressure may be entirely normal in a significant proportion of patients with GERD, and particularly those with mild disease. The mechanism of reflux in these patients is believed to be transient LES relaxations as described by Dent et al. [1]. However, in patients with more severe GERD, as assessed by grade of esophagitis or level of acid exposure, several workers have reported a greater association with low values of resting lower esophageal sphincter pressure (LESP). Kahrilas et al. reported a progressive decrease in mean resting LESP with increasing grade of esophagitis [2] and Dent et al. reported absent basal LESP being a progressively more important mechanism in the genesis of reflux episodes as the grade of esophagitis increased [1]. Zaninotto et al. showed that 60% of patients with pathological acid exposure had a mechanically incompetent sphincter, and when resting LESP fell below 6 mmHg, being the 2.5 percentile in control subjects, 79% had increased acid exposure [3]. A similar level of 6 mmHg was found by Jenkinson et al. in our laboratory to be the threshold which predisposed to severe degrees of acid exposure fell below the fifth percentile in control subjects, and probably represents the minimum pressure to maintain competence at the cardia [4]. We found an inverse relationship between resting sphincter pressure and degree of acid exposure, 45% of patients with a resting LESP below 6 mmHg exhibiting a total time, the pH was <4 of >20%. A similar inverse relationship between resting LESP and degree of acid exposure was found by Johnsson et al [5]. These findings probably explain the high incidence of LES hypotension in patients with complications of GERD, such as stricture and Barrett's columnar-lined esophagus [6,7].

Other manometric characteristics of the LES which have been studied and related to the likelihood and severity of reflux include the intra-abdominal length and overall length of the LES. In the study by Zaninotto et al., 80% of patients with an intra-abdominal length of < 1 cm had pathological acid exposure. Thirty-eight per cent of their patients with pathological acid exposure and resting LESP below 6 mmHg also had an intra-abdominal length of < 1 cm. In our laboratory, a similar proportion (39%) of patients with resting LESP below 6 mmHg had an intra-abdominal length of < 1 cm, and in both of the studies and that of Johnsson et al., there was an inverse correlation between the degree of acid exposure and intra-abdominal length. A short overall sphincter length (< 2 cm) was found by the Zaninotto group to be associated with pathological acid exposure in 79% of cases, although present in only 25% of their reflux population. Our studies and those of Johnsson et al. found a sphincter length of < 2 cm to be a very unusual occurrence, the combination of resting pressure below 6 mmHg and intra-abdominal length of <1 cm having a specificity of 97% in the prediction of GERD [4,5].

While the LES characteristics which imply sphincter failure or a mechanically incompetent cardia correlate accurately with the presence of reflux, lesser degrees of LES dysfunction and particularly isolated recordings of resting LES pressure correlate poorly with the presence of reflux and indeed with successful surgical correction of reflux. In order to try to take into account the radial asymmetry of the LES, Castell et al. [8] investigated a computer-aided analysis of the LES, and Bombeck et al. developed this further, finding that computer generated three dimensional LES vector volume correlated very accurately with the presence or absence of reflux and with the effects of antireflux surgery [9].

In the esophageal body, the manometric features which have received most attention in GERD are peristaltic amplitude and the incidence of nonpropagated peristalsis, both of which impact upon the ability of the esophageal "pump" mechanism to clear refluxed material, demonstrated in the elegant simultaneous manometric and fluoroscopic studies of Kahrilas et al. [10]. This group found an inverse relationship between peristaltic amplitude in the distal esophagus and severity of esophagitis [2], and the studies of Johnsson et al. [5] and Jenkinson et al. in our laboratory [4] found an inverse relationship between peristaltic amplitude and level of acid exposure. The threshold for significant increase in acid exposure and grade of esophagitis in all these studies was around 30 mmHg, a level below which had a 90% specificity for the presence of reflux in our laboratory. Fifty per cent of patients with a peristaltic amplitude below this level exhibited a total time that the pH was <4 in excess of 20%, compared with only 8% of patients with normal peristaltic amplitude who had acid exposure of this magnitude. It seems likely that the level of 30 mmHg represents the minimum value to allow luminal occlusion in order to enable peristalsis to occur.

Another important factor in esophageal body function is propagation of the primary peristaltic wave, which has also been studied extensively in control subjects and those with GERD and esophagitis. Kahrilas et al. observed a correlation between percentage of failed primary peristalsis and severity of esophagitis, >50% of failed primary peristalsis representing the 95th percentile in control subjects [2]. They have postulated that both propagated primary peristalsis and an adequate peristaltic amplitude are necessary for esophageal volume clearance, such that the esophageal lumen is occluded and the occluded segment passes progressively down the esophagus, resulting in rcturn of the refluxed bolus to the stomach and delivery of saliva to neutralize the residual acid [10]. In Kahrilas' series, peristaltic dysfunction assessed by a combination of these phenomena was present in 25% of patients with mild and 48% with severe esophagitis. As with LES dysfunction, the increasing incidence of peristaltic dysfunction with increasing severity of esophagitis is reflected in the increased incidence in patients with complications of esophagitis, particularly

Barrett's CLE [6,7] In our laboratory, 65% of patients with Barrett's CLE had low amplitude contractions and 31% had >50% nonpropagated peristalsis, compared to 35 and 5% respectively in patients with uncomplicated erosive esophagitis.

Overall in our series, 45% of reflux patients had an incompetent cardia and 59% had peristaltic failure. In most patients, however, these manometric abnormalities were combined, with 67% of patients with an incompetent cardia also exhibiting peristaltic failure, and 50% of patients with peristaltic failure also having an incompetent cardia [4]. The importance of a detailed manometric evaluation involving esophageal body measurements at six levels was illustrated in our study. When the distal half of the esophagus was subdivided into three levels, it was found that low amplitude peristalsis was present at all three levels in only 23%, and was present at a single level in 49%.

The mechanism of the various manometric abnormalities in GERD has been the subject of considerable debate as to whether they are primary or the consequence of esophagitis by damage to the enteric nervous system. Healing of esophagitis on medical therapy does not generally influence resting LESP or peristaltic dysfunction [11,12], which presumably accounts for the almost universal relapse of reflux symptoms after cessation of medication, even when treated with omeprazole [13]. While antireflux surgery generally results in an increase in the resting high pressure zone, opinion is divided as to the reversibility of peristaltic dysfunction. Russell et al. found an incidence of impaired radionuclide transit in 52% of patients with GERD requiring antireflux surgery, but no improvement following surgery [14]. However, two studies have shown improvement in peristaltic dysfunction when studied a year, or longer, after antireflux surgery [15,16]. It therefore remains controversial whether GERD is part of a diffuse upper gastrointestinal motility disturbance, the cause of which persists after treatment of the reflux, or whether components of upper gastrointestinal dysmotility may be secondary phenomena which may resolve in time after successful reflux correction.

While many of the manometric features described are pathophysiological observations in the genesis of GERD, there are some practical applications to be drawn from these measurements. Many workers believe that patients with a mechanically defective LES are unlikely to respond to medical treatment and a prospective study of a group of unselected reflux patients, referred to our laboratory, showed that among the factors which differed between those patients responding to medical treatment and those requiring antireflux surgery were LES failure, peristaltic dysfunction and grade of esophagitis [17]. These factors are, as discussed, all interrelated and it has been shown that patients with the more severe grades of esophagitis are less responsive to medical treatment [13]. The manometric profile may, therefore, make a contribution to the selection process for antireflux surgery and the duration of medical treatment, particularly in the presence of a mechanically defective sphincter in younger patients. The degree of peristaltic dysfunction may also be relevant to the type of antireflux procedure performed in surgically treated patients, as obstructive complications are more likely to occur after total fundoplication in patients with severe degrees of peristaltic dysfunction, particularly in patients with scleroderma, reflux induced stricture and achalasia. In these circumstances, it is generally considered that one of the partial fundoplication procedures is preferable [18,19].

Finally, the ability of the LES to relax on swallowing is an important manometric measurement, although not in the evaluation of esophagitis once a diagnosis of GERD has been made. Impairment of the ability of the LES to relax on swallowing has been cited as one of the mechanisms responsible for obstructive complications following Nissen fundoplication [15,20], It is an important measurement in the postoperative evaluation of the success of antireflux surgery, particularly in the context of evaluation of newer procedures [21] or the laparoscopic adaptation of existing procedures [22].

References

1. Dent J, Holloway RH, Toouli J, Dodds WJ. Mechanisms of lower oesophageal sphincter incompetence in patients with symptomatic gastro-oesophageal reflux. Gut 1988;29:1020−1028.
2. Kahrilas PJ, Dodds WJ, Hogan WJ et al. Esophageal peristaltic dysfunction in peptic esophagitis. Gastroenterology 1986; 91:897−904.
3. Zaninotto G, DeMeester TR, Schwizer W et al. The lower esophageal sphincter in health and disease. Am J Surg 1988; 155:104−110.
4. Jenkinson LR, Ball CS, Barlow AP, Watson A. A re-evaluation of the manometric assessment of oesophageal function in reflux oesophagitis. Gullet 1991;1:135−142.
5. Johnsson F, Joelsson B, Gudmundsson K. Determinants of gastro-oesophageal reflux and their inter-relationships. Br J Surg 1989;76:241−244.
6. Attwood SEA, Barlow AP, Watson A, Norris TL. Barrett's oesophagus: Effect of antireflux surgery on symptom control and development of complications. Br J Surg 1992;79:1050−1053.
7. Bremner CG. Barrett's oesophagus. Br J Surg 1989;76:995−996.
8. Castell DO, Dubois A, Davis CR et al. Computer-aided analysis of human esophageal peristalsis. Technical description in comparison with manual analysis. Dig Dis Sci 1984;29:65−72.
9. Bombeck CT, Vaz O, Desalvo J et al. Computerised axial manometry of the esophagus. Ann Surg 1987;206:465−472.
10. Kahrilas PJ, Dodds WJ, Hogan WJ. Effect of peristaltic dysfunction on esophageal volume clearance. Gastroenterology 1988;94:73−80.
11. Katz PO, Knuff TE, Benjamin SB, Castell DO. Abnormal esophageal pressures in reflux esophagitis: Cause or effect? Am J Gastroenterol 1986;81:744−747.
12. Baldi F, Ferrarini F, Longanesi A et al. Oesophageal function before, during and after healing of erosive oesophagitis. Gut 1988;29:157−160.
13. Hetzel DJ, Dent J, Reed WB et al. Healing and relapse of severe peptic oesophagitis after treatment with omeprazole. Gastroenterology 1988;95:903−912.
14. Russell COH, Pope CE, Gannan RM et al. Does surgery correct esophageal motor dysfunction in gastroesophageal reflux? Ann Surg 1981;194:290−295.
15. Gill RC, Bones KL, Murphy PD, Chingman YJ. Esophageal motor abnormalities in gastroesophageal reflux and the effects of fundoplication. Gastroenterology 1986;91:364−369.
16. Escandell AO, DeHaro LFM, Paricio PP et al. Surgery improves defective oesophageal peristalsis in patients with gastro-oesophageal reflux. Br J Surg 1991;78:1095−1097.
17. Barlow AP, Jenkinson LR, Watson A et al. Can failure of medical treatment be predicted in gastro-oesophageal reflux? Gut 1989;30:730.
18. DeMeester TR. Management of benign esophageal strictures. In: Stipa S, Belsey RHR, Moraldi A (eds) Medical and Surgical Problems of the Oesophagus. London: Academic Press, 1981;173−176.
19. Crookes WG, Wilkinson AJ, Johnston GW. Heller's myotomy with partial fundoplication. Br J Surg 1989;76:99−100.
20. Dent J, Toouli J, Sidey P, Barnes B. Incomplete relaxation of the lower esophageal high pressure zone − possible mechanism of action of fundoplication. Gastroenterology 1982;82:1042−1044.
21. Watson A, Jenkinson LR, Ball CS et al. A more physiological alternative to total fundoplication for the surgical correction of resistant gastro-oesophageal reflux. Br J Surg 1991;78:1088−1094.
22. Watson A. Expectations of surgery for benign oesophageal disease. In: Paterson-Brown S, Garden OJ (eds) Principles and Practices of Surgical Laparoscopy. London: WB Saunders, 1994 (in press).

What may be expected from the new manometric techniques based on the three-dimensional sphincter pressure profile?

H.J. Stein (Munich)

P.F. Crookes, T.R. DeMeester (Los Angeles)

The lower esophageal sphincter (LES) represents a unique one way valve which provides a pressure barrier between the negative intrathoracic and positive intra-abdominal pressure environment and allows only a minimum amount of physiologic gastroesophageal reflux to occur. An inadequate barrier function of the LES inevitably leads to increased esophageal exposure to gastric contents, symptoms of heartburn, regurgitation and chest pain and eventually causes esophageal mucosal injury. Microdissection studies of the human gastroesophageal junction have shown that the manometric LES correlates to an asymmetric thickening of the muscle layer at the esophagogastric junction, which is highest at the greater curvature side and corresponds to the location of the gastric sling fibers. This radial asymmetry of muscle thickness at the gastroesophageal junction, mirrors the asymmetric distribution of sphincter pressures measured with radial pressure transducers [1].

Since the first description of a high pressure zone at the gastroesophageal junction by Fyke et al., manometry has been the classic test to examine LES function [2–4]. Today, manometry is usually performed by a stepwise manual or continuous motorized pullback of pressure sensitive transducers across the gastroesophageal junction (Fig. 1). The peak resting pressure or pressure at the respiratory inversion

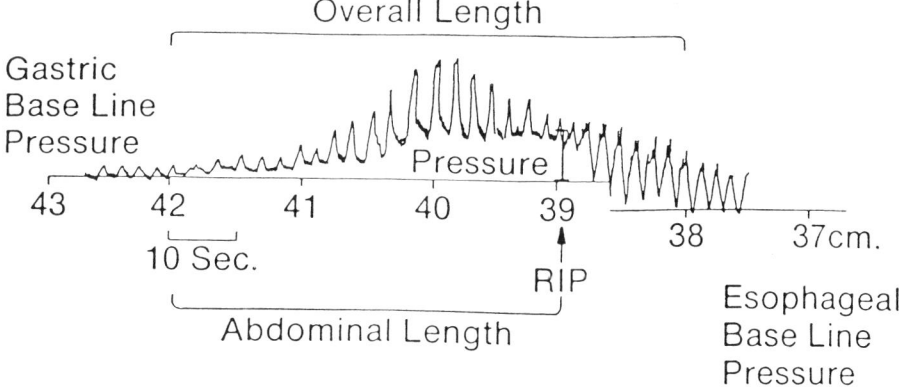

RIP = Respiratory Inversion Point

Fig. 1. A sample manometric record of a stepwise pullback of a pressure transducer across the gastroesophageal junction. From [6] with permission.

point are commonly used to assess sphincter resistance to reflux of gastric juice. Various studies have confirmed that this single pressure measurement is lower in patients with gastroesophageal reflux disease (GERD) as compared to controls and decreases with increasing severity of esophageal mucosal injury [5,6]. Due to a large overlap with normal subjects, measurement of sphincter pressure alone is, however, not adequate to identify individual patients with a mechanically defective sphincter. Subsequent investigations have shown that the position of the sphincter (i.e., how much of the sphincter is exposed to the positive intra-abdominal pressure environment) and the overall length of the sphincter, also contribute to sphincter resistance, in that a short overall or abdominal length can nullify a normal sphincter pressure [6]. Measurement of the sphincter resting pressure, overall length, and abdominal length is, however, still insufficient to identify subtle sphincter defects which may result in increased esophageal acid exposure.

From a mechanical standpoint, the pressures at each point along the sphincter and around its circumference must be taken into account as contributing to the overall resistance. Consequently the barrier function of the LES is determined by the integrated effects of radial pressures exerted over the entire length of the sphincter. This can be quantified by the volume circumscribed by the three-dimensional sphincter pressure image. With the recent introduction of personal computers and multichannel manometry catheters into the esophageal function laboratory, three-dimensional manometric imaging of the LES pressure profile has become available even for routine clinical use and offers several advantages over standard manometric techniques.

Technique of three-dimensional manometric LES imaging

Three-dimensional pressure images of the LES may be obtained with a continuous or stepwise pullback of a catheter with four to eight radially oriented electronic pressure transducers or water perfused tubes with radial openings connected to external transducers. The rapid pullback technique proposed by some investigators (i.e., a pullback speed of 3–5 mm/s) requires that the patient hold the breath in the end-expiratory situation until the pressure transducers have passed across the sphincter. This can be difficult for some patients and does not allow the determination of the respiratory inversion point and the position of the sphincter. We therefore prefer a slow motorized pullback (pullback speed of 1 mm/s or less) or a stepwise manual pullback technique.

The three-dimensional pressure image of the LES is constructed by plotting radial pressures measured in each channel at each station of the pullback, radially around a zero axis representing gastric baseline pressure. Alternatively, sphincter pressures may also be plotted as radial vectors directed to the center of a cylinder (Fig. 2). Commercially available computer programs can easily create three-dimensional sphincter images within fractions of a second and allow rotation of the sphincter image on the computer screen and inspection from various angles for asymmetry.

The volume circumscribed by the three-dimensional sphincter image integrates

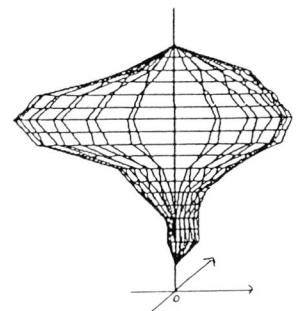

"POSITIVE PRESSURE IMAGE"

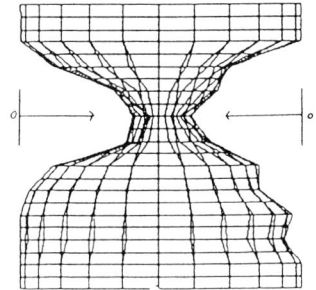

"NEGATIVE PRESSURE IMAGE"

Fig. 2. "Positive" and "negative" three-dimensional manometric LES pressure images. "Positive" images show radial sphincter pressures plotted around an axis representing gastric baseline. "Negative" images show radial sphincter pressures as indentations in a cylinder which represents gastric baseline.

pressures exerted over the entire length and around the circumference of the sphincter into one number representing sphincter resistance to reflux. This has been termed the sphincter pressure vector volume (SPVV) [7]. The SPVV can be calculated using standard trigonometric formulas and is expressed in units of mmHg*mmHg*mm. With a stepwise or slow motorized pullback technique the intrathoracic and intra-abdominal portions of the SPVV (i.e., the portions of the SPVV located above and below the respiratory inversion point), can be determined separately [8].

Validation studies have shown that calculation of the SPVV with four radially oriented transducers, is sufficient to reliably evaluate sphincter resistance. A stepwise pullback technique with a catheter, containing radial side holes located at the same level or placed sequentially in 5 cm intervals, was found to be superior to a rapid pullback in discriminating patients with GERD from control subjects [8]. The use of a catheter with radial transducers spaced in 5 cm intervals to each other has the additional advantage that sphincter relaxation and esophageal body function can be assessed in the same session without changing the catheter.

Three-dimensional LES imaging in GERD

A mechanically defective LES is the major cause of increased esophageal exposure to gastric juice and predisposes to the development of complications (i.e., esophagitis, strictures and Barrett's esophagus with its known premalignant potential) [9]. Medical therapy in patients with a mechanically defective sphincter is plagued by high failure and relapse rates. On the other hand, antireflux surgery is designed to correct a mechanically defective sphincter and can effectively prevent reflux of any gastric content. It is important to identify the patients with a mechanically defective LES prior to the development of complications, in order to avoid the loss of esophageal body function which is known to occur as mucosal injury progresses.

Using three-dimensional manometric sphincter imaging, Bombeck et al. were the first to show that the SPVV is superior to all individual sphincter parameters in identifying those patients with GERD who would not respond to medical therapy or those who recur as soon as medical therapy is discontinued [7]. In a recent study we confirmed these findings and showed that both the total and abdominal SPVV are markedly lower in patients with increased esophageal acid exposure compared to healthy volunteers, and decrease with the increasing severity of mucosal injury [8]. When the SPVV was compared with standard sphincter parameters (i.e., resting pressure, overall length and abdominal length) in a large population of patients with

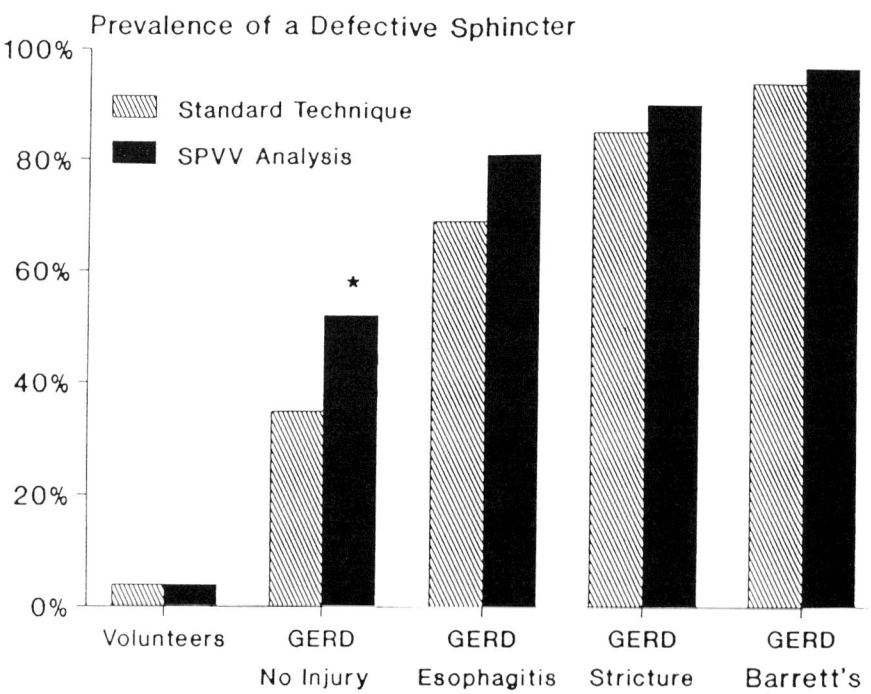

Fig. 3. Prevalence of a mechanically defective LES in patients with GERD and various degrees of esophageal mucosal injury: standard manometric techniques versus SPVV analysis. From [8] with permission. ★: p < 0.05 versus standard techniques.

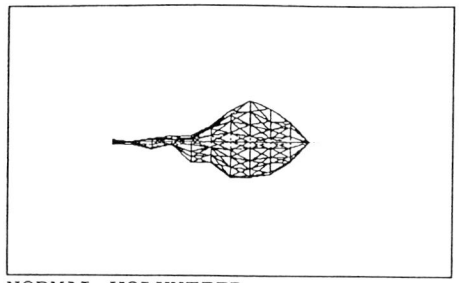

NORMAL VOLUNTEER

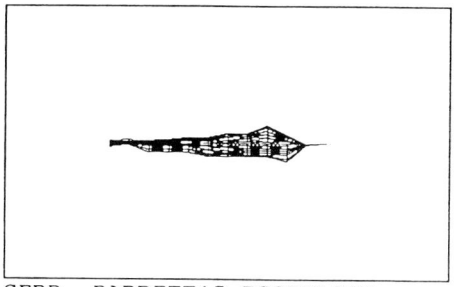

GERD, BARRETT'S ESOPHAGUS

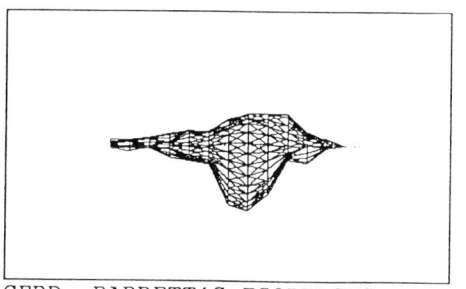

GERD, BARRETT'S ESOPHAGUS,
s/p NISSEN FUNDOPLICATION

Fig. 4. The three-dimensional LES pressure image in a normal volunteer (top), a patient with Barrett's esophagus (center), and the same patient after Nissen fundoplication (bottom) (stomach is to the left).

increased esophageal acid exposure, both techniques showed an increasing prevalence of a mechanically defective sphincter with increasing severity of mucosal injury [8]. Calculation of the SPVV had no significant advantage over the standard parameters in detecting a defective sphincter in patients with advanced complications of GERD. However, it did significantly increase the sensitivity of manometry in identifying a mechanically defective sphincter in patients with increased esophageal acid exposure but no mucosal damage (Fig. 3). This indicates that measurement of sphincter pressure, overall length and abdominal length, can reliably identify gross sphincter defects but is insufficient to detect subtle sphincter abnormalities.

Despite the advance of the SPVV in assessing sphincter resistance, there still remains a number of patients with increased esophageal acid exposure and an apparently normal LES. A marked asymmetry of the sphincter, which is not taken into account when assessing the SPVV, may be responsible for reflux in some of these patients [10]. Although, the exact role of a marked sphincter asymmetry in the

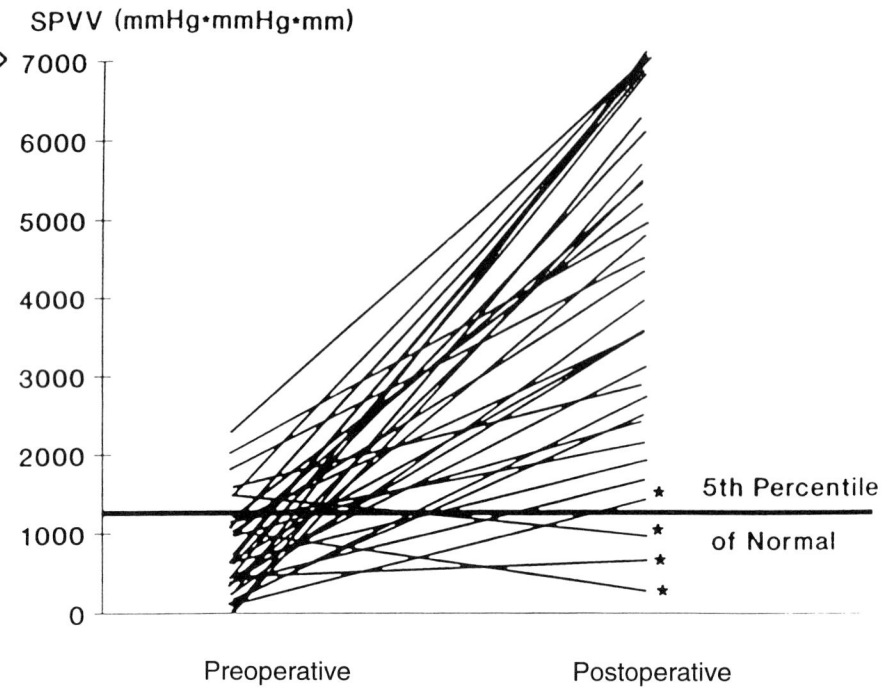

Fig. 5. Individual pre- and postoperative SPVVs in 32 patients undergoing antireflux surgery. From [8] with permission. *: patients with persistent or recurrent reflux.

pathogenesis of GERD is not clear at the present time, three-dimensional imaging of the sphincter pressure profile is the only means to detect and assess sphincter asymmetry. Calculation of the SPVV and assessment of the three-dimensional sphincter pressure profile for asymmetry should therefore become the standard technique to evaluate LES in patients with GERD.

Three-dimensional manometric LES imaging after antireflux surgery

In patients with increased esophageal acid exposure due to a mechanically defective LES, reconstruction of a functional sphincter by an antireflux procedure effectively abolishes reflux of any gastric contents in over 90% of patients. Gauging operative success only by the lack of postoperative symptoms is, however, inadequate. Rather, the success of an antireflux procedure depends on relief from symptoms, in combination with objective documentation on 24-h esophageal pH monitoring that reflux has been reduced to physiologic levels, and evidence on esophageal manometry that the mechanical defect of the LES has been corrected.

The effect of antireflux procedures on LES resistance has been difficult to quantify with standard manometric techniques. Although an increase in sphincter resting pressure and abdominal length after Nissen fundoplication have been reported by

162

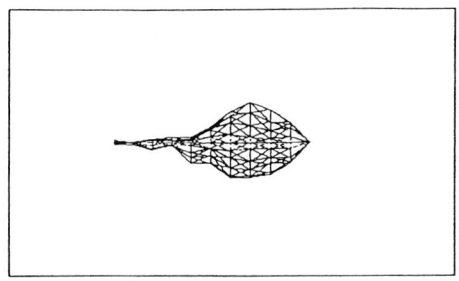

NORMAL VOLUNTEER

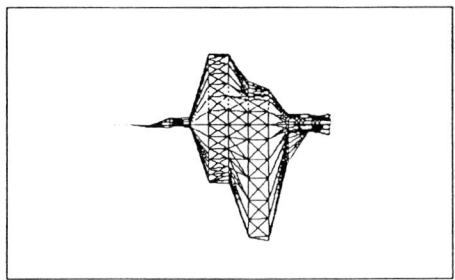

CLASSIC ACHALASIA

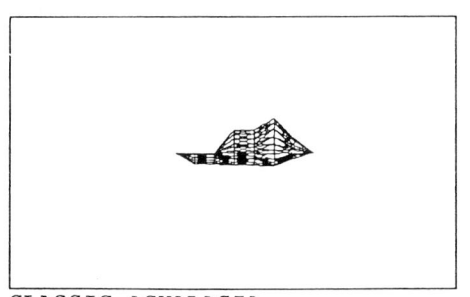

CLASSIC ACHALASIA,
s/p MYOTOMY AND DOR FUNDOPLASTY

Fig. 6. The three-dimensional LES pressure image in a normal volunteer (top), a patient with achalasia before therapy (center), and the same patient after myotomy and Dor-fundoplasty (bottom). Note the increased esophageal baseline pressure in the patient with classic achalasia which disappears after myotomy. (Stomach is to the left).

some investigators, this has not been consistently so with other antireflux procedures. In addition there is no clear relationship between postoperative sphincter pressure and success of the procedure [11,12]. When we compared the preoperative and postoperative findings of three-dimensional manometric sphincter imaging in patients who had a 360 degree Nissen fundoplication and patients who had a 270 degree Belsey type antireflux operation, the mean total and abdominal SPVV was markedly increased with both procedures [8]. Nissen fundoplication usually resulted in a 80–100-fold augmentation of the SPVV above preoperative values and a normalization of the three-dimensional sphincter pressure profile (Fig. 4).

Figure 5 shows the individual SPVVs in 32 patients before and after Nissen fundoplication. Subjective and objective control of reflux was associated with an increase of the SPVV to the normal range in 28 patients. Four patients had persistent or recurrent reflux on 24-h esophageal pH monitoring following the antireflux procedure. In three of these patients the postoperative SPVV was below the fifth percentile of normal. This indicates that reflux control by Nissen fundoplication is achieved by normalizing the total and abdominal SPVV. Failure to restore the three-dimensional sphincter pressure profile to normal, or a breakdown of the repair, are associated with persistent or recurrent reflux.

Three-dimensional manometric LES imaging in patients with achalasia

A hypertensive LES with incomplete or absent relaxation on swallowing is the primary defect causing dysphagia in patients with achalasia [4]. The dynamics of LES relaxation are best assessed on standard manometry with one pressure transducer positioned within the sphincter, a distal transducer located within the stomach and a proximal transducer within the esophageal body [4]. Three-dimensional manometric sphincter imaging can illustrate the hypertensive sphincter with its marked asymmetry and the effect of a surgical myotomy with and without a concomitant antireflux procedure in patients with achalasia (Fig. 6).

References

1. Liebermann-Meffert D, Stein HJ, DeMeester TR, Siewert JR. Three-dimensional pressure image and muscular structure of the human lower esophageal sphincter. Presented at the 35th World Congress of the International Society of Surgery. Hong Kong, August 1993.
2. Fyke FE, Code CF, Schlegel JF. The gastroesophageal sphincter in healthy human beings. Gastroenterologia 1956; 86:135–150.
3. Winans CS, Harris LD. Quantitation of lower esophageal sphincter competence. Gastroenterology 1967;52:773–778.
4. Castell DO, Richter JE, Dalton CB (eds) Esophageal Motility Testing. New York: Elsevier, 1987.
5. Haddad JE. Relation of gastroesophageal reflux to yield sphincter pressures. Gastroenterology 1970;58:175–184.
6. Zaninotto G, DeMeester TR, Schwizer W et al. The lower esophageal sphincter in health and disease. Am J Surg 1988; 155:104–111.
7. Bombeck CT, Vaz O, DeSalvo J et al. Computerized axial manometry of the esophagus. Ann Surg 1987;206:465–472.
8. Stein HJ, DeMeester TR, Naspetti R, Jamieson J, Perry RE. The three-dimensional lower esophageal sphincter pressure profile in gastroesophageal reflux disease. Ann Surg 1991;214:374–384.
9. Stein HJ, Barlow AP, DeMeester TR, Hinder RA. Complications of gastroesophageal reflux disease: Role of the lower esophageal sphincter, esophageal acid/alkaline exposure, and duodenogastric reflux. Ann Surg 1992;216:35–43.
10. Crookes PF, Kaul BK, DeMeester TR, Stein HJ, Oka M. Manometry of individual segments of the distal esophageal sphincter. Its relation to functional incompetence. Arch Surg 1993;128:411–415.
11. Mughal MM, Bancewicz J, Marples M. Oesophageal manometry and pH recording does not predict the bad results of Nissen fundoplication. Br J Surg 1990;77:43–45.
12. Lundell L, Abrahamsson H, Ruth M, Sandberg N, Olbe LC. Lower esophageal sphincter characteristics and esophageal acid exposure following partial or 360 degree fundoplication. World J Surg 1991;15:115–121.

Is there a criterion of pH measurement capable of distinguishing a population of patients at high risk of esophagitis, recurrence, or deterioration?

L.F. Johnson (Bethesda)

The answer to this question began with the development of the 24-h pH composite score described by Johnson and DeMeester [1]. This composite score, using 6 pH parameters from the 24-h period, differentiated symptomatic patients from asymptomatic controls so that other pH monitoring parameters could be used to make intragroup comparisons. Two obvious pH parameters that seemed to further characterize the patient population were acid exposure (% time pH < 4) during both the upright (daytime) and recumbent (night-time) segments of the 24-h record. Thus, when compared to asymptomatic controls, some symptomatic patients had excessive acid exposure during the day, but were normal at night (upright refluxers); others had excessive acid exposure at night, but were normal during the day (supine refluxers); and some had excessive acid exposure both day and night (combined refluxers, Fig. 1) [2]. These refluxer types have been corroborated by others [3], with the only difference being the percentage of patients that comprised each type.

These three refluxer groups, with respect to the assigned question, provided an

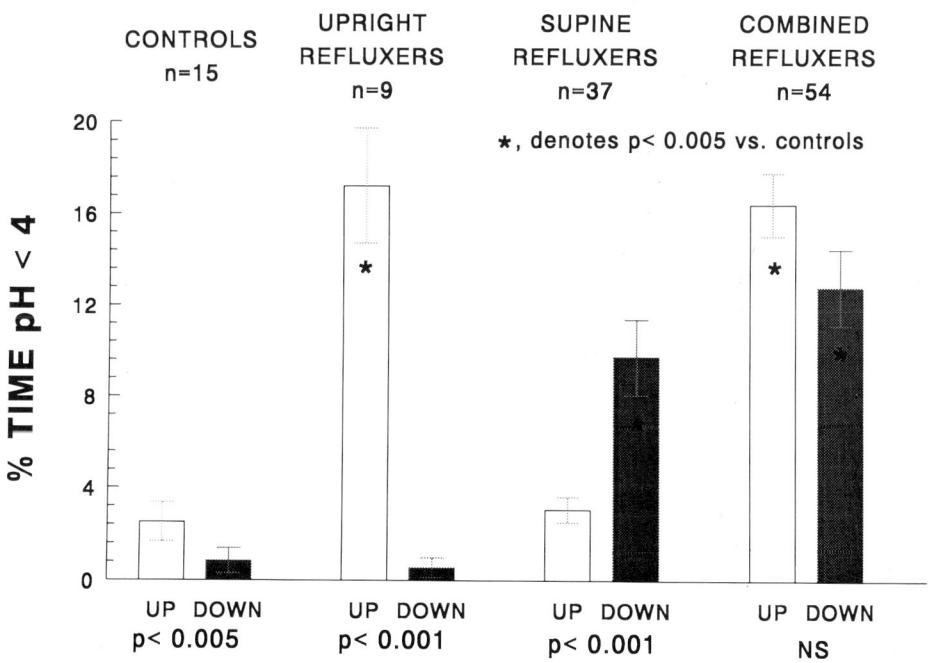

Fig. 1. Three refluxer types compared to asymptomatic controls [2]. UP, indicates upright acid exposure and DOWN, recumbent acid exposure (n denotes the number of individuals).

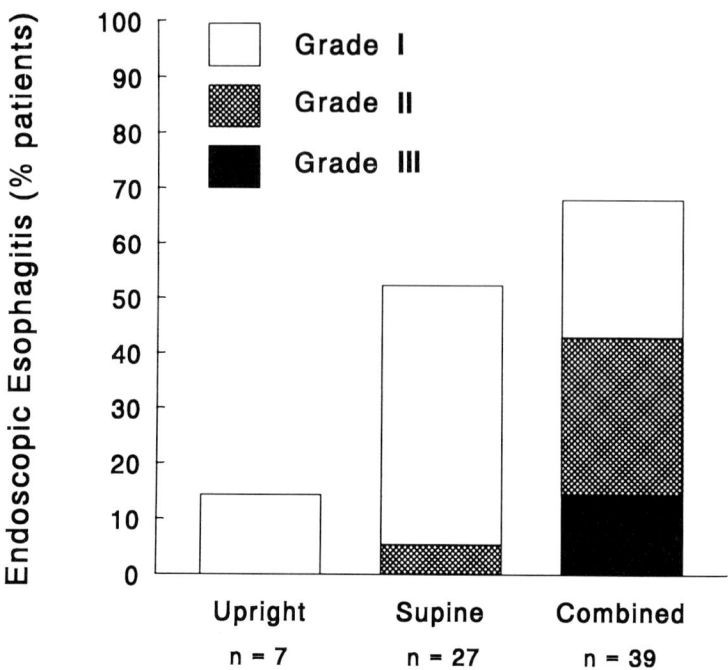

Fig. 2. The effect of refluxer type on the incidence (%) and severity of reflux esophagitis (grade I–III). Upright, Supine and Combined denote refluxer group.

opportunity to determine if a particular type(s) influenced the incidence and/or severity of esophagitis. Clearly, it did (Fig. 2) [2]! Notice that upright refluxers had the lowest incidence and mildest form of esophagitis characterized by friability and/or granularity (grade I) as opposed to the supine or combined refluxers who not only had an increased incidence of esophagitis, but more severe forms such as linear erosions and exudate (grade II) or strictures (grade III). While this publication [2] indicated subpopulations of symptomatic patients at added risk for esophagitis, it failed to show how or why they became at risk i.e., differences in reflux patterns.

Using the same three refluxer types, a subsequent publication in 1978 [4] utilized reactive epithelial change or the percentage papillary extension (% PE) [5] to examine the effect that reflux patterns had on the severity of esophagitis. This study also included additional pH parameters such as absolute acid exposure (minutes pH < 4) for the 24-h, the upright and recumbent periods. For the latter two periods, the mean number of reflux events per hour and the mean esophageal acid clearance time (minutes) were also determined. As in our previous study [2], upright refluxers had the lowest degree of reactive epithelial change (% PE, Fig. 3A) [4]. In contrast, the highest values for % PE were seen in those with the most recumbent acid exposure (i.e., the recumbent and bipositional refluxers, Fig. 3B). These two types received a large degree of recumbent acid exposure as a result of increased reflux frequency compared to the upright refluxers (Fig. 3C) and a significant increase in their

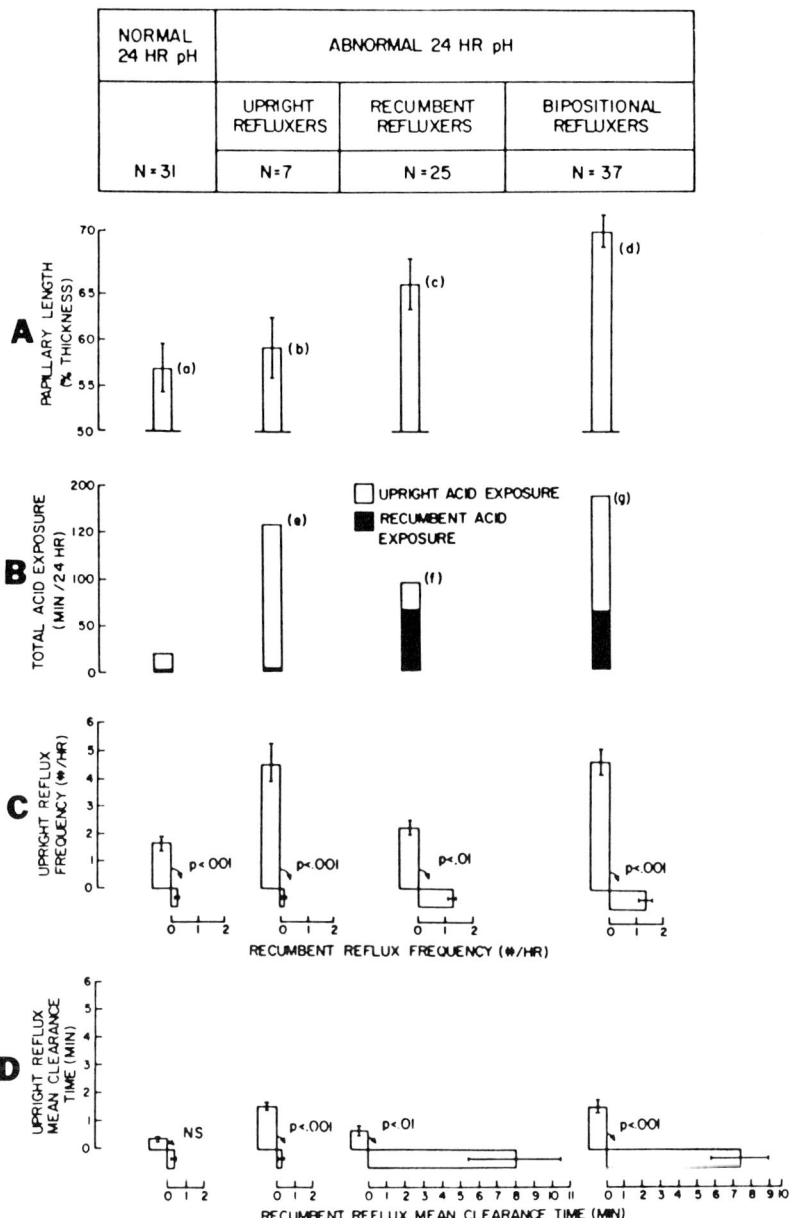

Fig. 3. Influence of reflux patterns on percent papillary extension. N = number of patients. All bars show mean and ± 1 SEM. Papillary length (d) and (c) both more than (a) with p < 0.001 and 0.05, respectively; (d) more than (b) with borderline significance (0.1 > p > 0.05). Minutes of total acid exposure shown by the entire bar; unshaded area equals minutes upright, and shaded area equals minutes recumbent. Total acid exposure (f) is less than both (g) (p < 0.001) and (e) (0.1 > p > 0.05). The sign (↘) and adjacent "p" denote significance of change in reflux measure in each group after upright-to-recumbent posture change. Upright reflux frequency and clearance measures on vertical bar and comparable recumbent measures on horizontal bar. "NS" means not statistically significant.

esophageal acid clearance time (Fig 3D). Thus, nocturnal reflux events which were poorly cleared provoked the greatest epithelial reactive change, given comparable total absolute acid exposure (Fig. 3B) [4].

In reflecting on the importance of this study since its publication in 1978 [4], I regretted that reactive epithelial change (i.e., % PE) was used for reflux esophagitis instead of endoscopic signs [6]. I feel that the latter criteria would have been more relevant and better portrayed the important clinical implications of this study. The O.E.S.O. meeting and my assigned question provided an opportunity to revisit unpublished data from the 1978 study [4], and use endoscopic signs [6] to depict the incidence and severity of reflux esophagitis. This change in diagnostic criteria for esophagitis also illustrates better how certain pH monitoring criteria can distinguish a population of patients at high risk of esophagitis.

Materials and Methods

The study population consisted of 69 patients with symptoms of gastroesophageal reflux (GER) and abnormal 24-h pH composite scores from the previous publication [4]. Based on values from asymptomatic controls (n = 15) [1], they were divided into upright, recumbent, and bipositional refluxers, as reported in 1978 [4].

Fortunately, the author still had the original flow sheets which contained their data. Endoscopic grading for evidence of reflux esophagitis was attained in these patients and duly recorded on the flow sheets; however, this information was not used in the 1978 manuscript [4], since it was a dissertation on epithelial response to GER. No alterations or reinterpretations of data on the original flow sheets was undertaken in preparing the current manuscript.

Criteria for endoscopic evidence of reflux esophagitis

In accordance with our previous publications [2,6], the esophagus was graded at endoscopy as follows:
— 0 = normal appearance;
— grade I esophagitis = granularity and/or friability;
— grade II esophagitis = linear erosion and exudate;
— grade III esophagitis = stricture.
All patients had fiberoptic endoscopy prior to 24-h esophageal pH monitoring. The chi-square test for heterogeneity or independence was used to determine if a statistically significant difference existed in the incidence and severity of esophagitis between the three refluxer groups. Statistical significance was considered p < 0.05.

Results

Notice the low incidence and mild degree of esophagitis in the upright refluxers, despite practically comparable total absolute acid exposure to that of the bipositional refluxers who had a significantly higher incidence and more severe degree of esophagitis (Fig. 4). In fact, total absolute acid exposure actually decreased in the recumbent refluxers compared to the upright refluxers, yet their incidence and severity of esophagitis increased. The same incongruous relationship exists when one relates absolute upright acid exposure to esophagitis.

In contrast, those refluxers with the highest incidence and most severe form of esophagitis (i.e., the recumbent and bipositional refluxers) have the most recumbent acid exposure (Fig. 4). Despite all groups diminishing significantly their reflux frequency after assuming the recumbent posture, those with the most recumbent acid exposure still had more frequent reflux events at night than the upright refluxers (Fig. 4). However, most importantly, while recumbent they experienced a significant increase in their mean esophageal acid clearance time as opposed to a significant

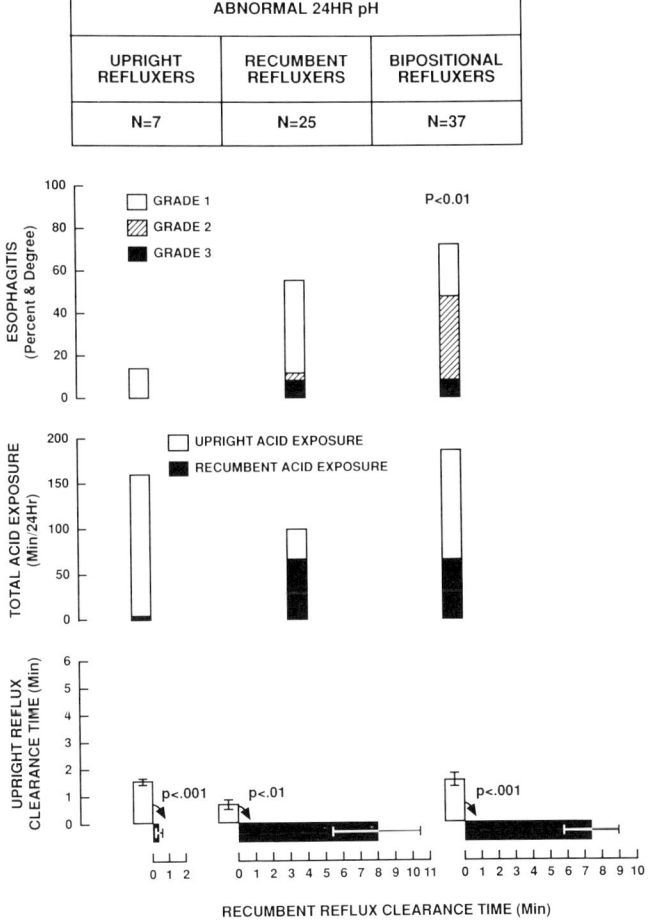

Fig. 4. Influence of reflux frequency (n/h) in three refluxer types on the incidence and severity of endoscopic esophagitis. Where appropriate, bar shows mean value ± 1 SEM. p < 0.01, denotes significant difference in incidence and severity of reflux esophagitis between the refluxer groups.

decrease in that of the upright refluxers (Fig. 5). Thus, patterns of reflux more than total absolute acid exposure, or even absolute upright acid exposure, determine the incidence and severity of reflux esophagitis. Clearly, nocturnal reflux events that are poorly cleared denote a subpopulation at risk for esophagitis.

Discussion

Whether reactive epithelial change (% PE) [4] or endoscopic signs of esophagitis as used in this paper and an earlier study [2], there are certain 24-h pH monitoring criteria that distinguish patients at increased risk for esophagitis. These criteria, upright and recumbent acid exposure (% time pH < 4), classify symptomatic patients into three types of refluxers with widely divergent propensities for esophagitis. The

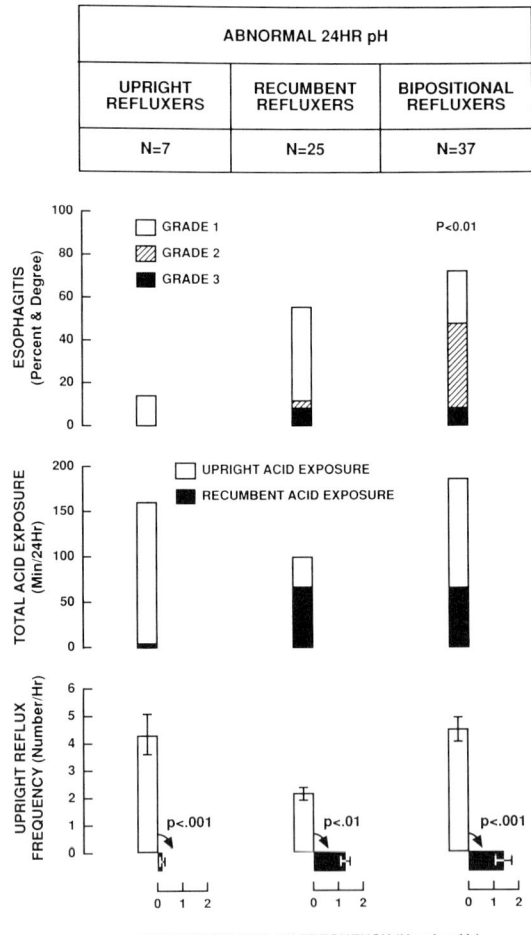

Fig. 5. Influence of mean esophageal acid clearance time (min) in three refluxer types on the incidence and severity of endoscopic esophagitis. Where appropriate, bar shows mean value ± 1 SEM.

unifying concept for the risk of esophagitis, the involved pH criteria and the subpopulations of patients, consist of when the reflux events occur. Night-time is detrimental, as is the duration of mucosal contact determined by the esophageal acid clearance time. That nocturnal reflux is deemed important in the development of reflux esophagitis and its complications have also been confirmed by others [7].

While the effects that posture and the awake-sleep cycle exerts on reflux patterns that influence esophagitis seemed mystical in the late 1970s, recent clinical investigation has now supported these findings. That reflux events occur more during the day than at night, would now be explained by the phenomenon of transient relaxations in lower esophageal sphincter pressure that predispose to reflux events. These relaxations occur predominantly during the day [8], especially with meals [9], cigarette smoking [10], and rarely at night while asleep [9]. In a similar manner, sudden increases in intra-abdominal pressure that provoke reflux events [8] occur more during the day than at night while asleep [11].

Most important, the effect that posture and the awake-sleep cycle exert on the esophageal acid clearance time, have also been clarified. For instance, the upright as opposed to the recumbent posture decreases the number of dry swallows to clear 15 ml of 0.1NHCl from the esophagus [12]. A more upright posture such as "head of bed" elevation even facilitates esophageal acid clearance during the sleeping period [13]. In terms of the awake-sleep cycle, patients with reflux esophagitis must content with the following triple jeopardy. First, they reflux more at night than asymptomatic controls [14] or upright refluxers [4]. Secondly, sleep impairs their esophageal acid clearance time [15]. Thirdly, some patients may have an esophageal peristaltic defect that can further impair their clearance [16]. The duration of acid-mucosal contact is important in predisposing to esophagitis is also supported by animal studies. For instance, a single exposure to an acid-bile salt solution or acid alone results in a significant direct relationship between the duration of contact and the magnitude of either hydrogen ion back diffusion or the degree of esophagitis [17,18]. Thus, recent clinical investigation has demystified the effect that different segments of the circadian cycle have on acid reflux and its clearance, as well as the way these phenomena influence the risk for esophagitis.

Conclusions

In summary, there are 24-h esophageal monitoring criteria that denote subpopulations of patients at greater risk for esophagitis.

Acknowledgements

The opinions or assertions contained herein, are those of the author and are not to be construed as reflecting the views of The Department of the Army or The Department of Defense.

References

1. Johnson LF, DeMeester TR. Twenty-four hour pH monitoring of the distal esophagus, a quantitative measure of gastro-esophageal reflux. Am J Gastroenterol 1974;62:325−332.
2. DeMeester TR, Johnson LF, Guy GJ, Toscano MS, Skinner DB. Pattern of gastroesophageal reflux in health and disease. Ann Surg 1976;184:459−470.
3. Vitale GC, Cheadle WG, Sadek S, Michel ME, Cuschieri A. Computerized 24-hour ambulatory esophageal pH monitoring and esophagogastroduodenoscopy in the reflux patient. A comparative study. Ann Surg 1984;200:724−728.
4. Johnson LF, DeMeester TR, Haggitt RC. Esophageal epithelial response to gastroesophageal reflux, a quantitative study. Am J Dig Dis 1978;23(6):498−509.
5. Ismail-Beigi F, Horton PF, Pope CE. Histological consequences of gastroesophageal reflux in man. Gastroenterology 1970; 58:163−174.
6. Johnson LF, DeMeester TR, Haggitt RC. Endoscopic signs for gastroesophageal reflux objectively evaluated. Gastrointest Endo 1976;22:151−155.
7. Robertson D, Aldersley M, Shepherd H, et al. Patterns of acid reflux in complicated oesophagitis. Gut 1987;28:1484−1488.
8. Dent J, Holloway RH, Toouli J, et al. Mechanisms of lower oesophageal sphincter incompetence in patients with symptomatic gastroesophageal reflux. Gut 1988;29:1020−1028.
9. Mittal RK, McCallum RW. Characteristics and frequency of transient relaxations of the lower esophageal sphincter in patients with reflux esophagitis. Gastroenterology 1988;95:593−599.
10. Kahrilas PJ, Gupta RR. Mechanisms of acid reflux associated with cigarette smoking. Gut 1990;31:4−10.
11. Shay SS, Johnson LF, Wong RKH, Curtis DJ, Rosenthal R, Lamott JR, Owensby LC. Rumination, heartburn and daytime gastroesophageal reflux: a case study with mechanisms defined and successfully treated with biofeedback therapy. J Clin Gastroenterol 1986;8:115−126.
12. Kjellen G, Tibbling L. Influence of body position, dry and water swallows, smoking and alcohol on esophageal acid clearing. Scand J Gastroenterol 1978;13:283−287.
13. Johnson LF, DeMeester TR. Evaluation of elevation of the head of the bed, bethanechol, and antacid foam tablets on gastroesophageal reflux. Dig Dis Sci 1981;26:673−680.
14. Dodds WJ, Dent J, Hogan WJ, Helm JF, et al. Mechanism of gastroesophageal reflux in patients with reflux esophagitis. N Engl J Med 1982;307:1547−1552.
15. Orr WC, Robinson MG, Johnson LF. Acid clearing during sleep in patients with esophagitis and controls. Dig Dis Sci 1981;26:423−427.
16. Kahrilas PJ, Dodds WJ, Hogan WJ. Effect of peristaltic dysfunction on esophageal volume clearance. Gastroenterology 1988;94:73−80.
17. Harmon JW, Johnson LF, Maydonovitch CL. Effects of acid and bile salts on the rabbit esophageal mucosa. Dig Dis Sci 1981;26:65−72.
18. Geisinger KR, Cassidy KT, Nardi R, Castell DO. The histologic development of acid-induced esophagitis in the cat. Mod Pathol 1990;3:619.

What are the indications for pH measurement, both conventional and combined with event markers, in evaluating the symptoms of GER?

S. Bruley des Varannes, J.P. Galmiche (Nantes)
C. Scarpignato (Parma)

Esophageal pH monitoring is considered as the method of choice for investigating patients with gastroesophageal reflux disease (GERD). Twenty-four-hour pH-monitoring is of high diagnostic value when used in patients with typical symptoms of

172

heartburn and regurgitation and/or esophagitis. In these patients, the sensitivity and specificity of esophageal pH monitoring usually run between 90 and 100% [1]. However, in clinical practice, esophageal pH-metry is primarily indicated in patients with atypical symptoms and no lesions at endoscopy.

Twenty-four-hour pH-monitoring measures esophageal acid exposure. With currently available automated system analysis, many variables can easily be determined during various periods (total, upright, supine). Among these variables, the percentage of time spent below pH 4 appears to be the best and most useful discriminator between normal subjects with physiological reflux and patients with abnormal esophageal acid exposure [1].

In fact, abnormal esophageal acid exposure is not sufficient proof that reflux episodes cause the symptoms. To establish the direct role of GER in symptoms, it is necessary to demonstrate a temporal relationship between reflux episodes and the occurrence of symptoms. Commercially available ambulatory pH recorders now make it possible to detect such temporal relationships. By pressing the event-marker button, the patient indicates the occurrence of a symptom or an event. When the pH recording is analyzed, it can be determined whether or not the symptom occurred simultaneously with a reflux episode.

Although analysis of pH recordings supplements interpretation of pH monitoring, several problems are involved.

First of all, no strict criteria have been defined to indicate that a symptom is associated with reflux episodes. A symptom is usually considered as reflux-related if it occurs within 2 min before or after the reflux episode.

Table 1. Main indices proposed to evaluate the strength of the relationship between reflux and symptoms

---

Symptom index [3]

$$\frac{\text{Number of symptom events associated with reflux episodes}}{\text{Number of marked events}} \times 100$$

Symptom sensitivity index [6]

$$\frac{\text{Number of refluxes perceived by the patient}}{\text{Total number of refluxes during recording}}$$

Probability of association by chance [7]

$$P = \sum \frac{n!}{r! \, (n-r)!} \cdot p^{r}(1 - p)^{n-r}$$

n: total number of pain episodes;
r: ranges from the actual number of pain episodes that occur during or within 2 min of a drop in pH < 4 to n;
p: probability that a pain episode occurs only by chance during or within 2 min of a drop in pH < 4.

Evaluation of the strength of such a relationship remains difficult. During a pH recording, patients frequently have both reflux-related symptoms and reflux-unrelated symptoms [2]. To establish a definite relationship, several indexes are used (Table 1). Castell's group first proposed the use of a symptom index [3] which, however, has major drawbacks. As the number of reflux episodes are not taken into account, this index does not allow for the probability that an association between reflux and symptoms might occur only by chance. Moreover, the cut-off values of the symptom index (i.e., the percentage considered to reflect a high likelihood of a causal relation between symptoms and reflux) are arbitrary and vary between groups [2,4,5]. Breumelhof and Smout [6] have suggested the inclusion of a symptom sensitivity index (the percentage of reflux perceived by the patient during recording). By taking into account the number of refluxes, the number of symptoms, the duration of the recording and total acid exposure, it is possible to calculate the probability that symptoms and reflux could occur simultaneously by chance [7]. Although none of these indexes has so far been universally accepted, it must be recognized that some patients, in spite of reflux symptoms during the pH-monitoring period, have a normal esophageal acid exposure (percentage of time with pH < 4). Some of these patients probably suffer from an "acid-hypersensitive esophagus", as suggested by the temporal relationship between symptoms (indicated by the event marker) and the reflux episodes.

In a recent work, we tried to determine the prevalence and characteristics of patients with normal esophageal acid exposure and a statistically significant association between symptoms and reflux episodes [8; unpublished personal results]. Among 417 consecutive patients referred to the laboratory for 24-h pH-metry, because of symptoms suggestive of gastroesophageal reflux, esophageal acid exposure was normal for 250 (63%), 175 of whom (70%) used the event marker at least once during pH monitoring (median 8, range 1—37). The probability of the association between events and reflux episodes occurring by chance was calculated [7], and the relationship was regarded as significant if $p < 0.05$. Acid-hypersensitive esophagus patients were defined as those with normal acid exposure (pH < 4 for < 4.2% of time) and a probability of under $p < 0.05$ of association by chance.

An acid-hypersensitive esophagus was present in 60 (33 women, 27 men) out of 175 patients (34%) with normal esophageal acid exposure. Age ranged from 13 to 73 years (mean 50 years). The predominant symptoms were distributed as follows: digestive complaints (67%), noncardiac chest pain (16%) and respiratory (15%) or cervical (2%) symptoms. The mean percentage of time spent below pH 4 was 2% in these patients. The symptom index was ≥75% in seven patients, < 25% in seven, and between 25% and 75% in 46. Endoscopy (n = 54) was normal in 43 cases and showed erosions in 11. Manometry (n = 37) showed hypotonic lower esophageal sphincter (LES) in 16 patients. The Bernstein test (n = 15) was positive in only six patients, whereas the esophageal balloon distension test was positive in 10 of these 15 patients.

These results show that, despite normal esophageal acid exposure, acid-hypersensitive esophagus may be the cause of symptoms in about one-third of patients who manifest their usual complaints during 24-h pH-monitoring. The discrepancy between sensitivity to endogenous and exogenous acid [9], as well as the frequent abnormal response to mechanical stimuli, suggests that factors other than acid are involved.

References

1. Galmiche JP, Scarpignato C. Esophageal pH monitoring. In: Functional Investigations in Esophageal Disease. Front Gastrointest Res. Basel: Karger Publications, 1993;71–108.
2. Barré P, Bruley des Varannes S, Masliah C, Cloarec D, Le Bodic L, Galmiche JP. Le marqueur d'événements: un progrès dans l'interprétation de la pH-métrie oesophagienne. Gastroenterol Clin Biol 1989;13:32–37.
3. Wiener GJ, Richter JE, Coopper JB, Wu WC, Castell DO. The symptom index: a clinically important parameter of ambulatory 24-hour esophageal pH-monitoring. Am J Gastroenterol 1988;83:358–361.
4. Johnston BT, McFarland RJ, Collins JSA, Love AHG. Symptom index as a marker of gastro-oesophageal reflux disease. Br J Surg 1992;79:1054–1055.
5. Howard PJ, Maher L, Pryde A, Heading RC. Symptomatic gastro-oesophageal reflux, abnormal oesophageal acid exposure, and mucosal acid sensitivity are three separate, though related, aspects of gastrooesophageal reflux disease. Gut 1991;32:128–132.
6. Breumelhof R, Smout AJPM. The symptom sensitivity index: a valuable additional parameter in 24-hour esophageal pH monitoring. Am J Gastroenterol 1991;86:160–164.
7. Ghillebert G, Janssens J, Vantrappen G, Nevens F, Piessens J. Ambulatory 24-hour intraoesophageal pH and pressure recordings vs. provocation tests in the diagnosis of chest pain of oesophageal origin. Gut 1990;31:738–744
8. Bruley des Varannes S, Le Rhun M, Simon J, Galmiche JP. The acid hypersensitive esophagus: a frequent cause of symptoms in patients with normal esophageal acid exposure. Gastroenterology 1992;102:A432.
9. Richter JE, Hewson EG, Sinclair JW, Dalton CB. Acid perfusion test and 24-hour esophageal pH monitoring with symptom index. Comparison of tests for esophageal acid sensitivity. Dig Dis Sci 1991;36:565–571.

What is the short-term reproducibility of the results of 24-h pH measurement in GER?

D.O. Castell (Philadelphia)

Over the past few years prolonged ambulatory esophageal pH monitoring has evolved as the preferred method for detecting the presence of abnormal reflux, because it measures the actual exposure time of the distal esophageal mucosa to acid gastric juice. This test records reflux during normal daily activities such as upright activity, eating and sleeping or lying recumbent. It does not stress the lower esophageal sphincter (LES) with unnatural respiratory maneuvers or unphysiologic abdominal compression.

Ambulatory pH monitoring is the most physiologic test currently available for studying reflux and additionally, frequent refinements in technique allow accurate recording over prolonged time intervals. It is generally accepted as the gold standard for identification of reflux. However, it is important to understand the limitations of this technique and to accept that the findings are not absolute. In the study by Schlesinger et al. a group of 64 hospitalized patients with typical reflux symptoms were compared with 20 age-matched controls [1]. The patients were divided into two groups, 30 with reflux symptoms and normal endoscopic examination (group 1) and 34 with similar symptoms and erosive esophagitis (group 2). As in prior studies, the patients with typical reflux symptoms had significantly more reflux than did the controls, but only 48% in group 1 had abnormal results. Furthermore, only 71% of patients with erosive esophagitis (group 2) had an abnormal 24-h pH monitoring result. These results suggest that esophageal pH monitoring lacks sensitivity or accuracy and that a negative test must be interpreted with caution.

A similar observation has recently been reported by Klauser et al. [2]. Their studies showed that 17% of patients with endoscopic esophagitis had normal pH testing. In addition, only 72% of patients characterized as having "definite" gastroesophageal reflux by symptoms assessment were found to have abnormal pH monitoring. In the latter situation, in which the presence of gastroesophageal reflux disease (GERD) is based on typical reflux symptoms, no true criterion is available to serve as a basis for comparative diagnosis. Much of the information in the literature comparing the sensitivity and specificity of the various tests for GERD has utilized such symptomatic assessment. In addition, since there is ample documentation that reflux can occur in the absence of esophagitis, the endoscopic assessment does not provide a reliable absolute diagnostic criterion. The assessment of whether false positive results of pH testing occur is very difficult to determine with the current state of knowledge in this field.

These observations underscore the difficulty in placing numerical values for true sensitivity and specificity for any test of GERD. In order to define these characteristics for any test, valid criteria discriminating between the presence and absence of the disease in question must be available. The presence of erosive esophagitis on endoscopic examination provides such strong evidence for the presence of GERD that one must accept the potential for pH monitoring to provide false negative results. Possible explanation for this finding are discussed below. The relatively low frequency of abnormal pH studies in patients with symptoms suggestive of reflux provides considerably weaker evidence. Due to the fact that symptoms suggestive of reflux may be produced by a variety of other causes, these findings do not provide a meaningful indictment against the status of pH monitoring as a gold standard.

As noted above, discrepancies between pH monitoring and documented endoscopic esophagitis support the conclusion that false negative pH monitoring studies do occur. An explanation for this phenomenon is supported by recent studies from our laboratory, in which two pH probes were placed at the same level (5 cm above the LES) in a group of patients with reflux [3]. Considerable discrepancies were noted between simultaneous readings from the two probes in the same patient. These differences would have resulted in a change in diagnosis (normal vs. abnormal) in 20% of the patients, using time below pH 4 as the critical factor. This effect was hypothesized to be due to the potential for the pH electrode at the tip of the probe to be buried within the esophageal mucosa and actually miss adjacent acid.

Other studies from our laboratory, involving two ambulatory pH tests performed within 10 days, yielded comparable results which are shown in Fig. 1 [4]. When patients and controls were compared, similar variability was noted in the same subjects between the 2 days of testing, with the pH monitoring results producing a change in diagnosis (normal or abnormal based on percentage of the time the pH was below 4) in 11% of cases. Evaluated from the opposite view, these data also indicate that the same diagnosis was obtained in 89% of the cases. This study was also dependent on the variability in the amount of reflux that occurs in any one individual from day to day. The observation that 7% of the patients with endoscopic esophagitis

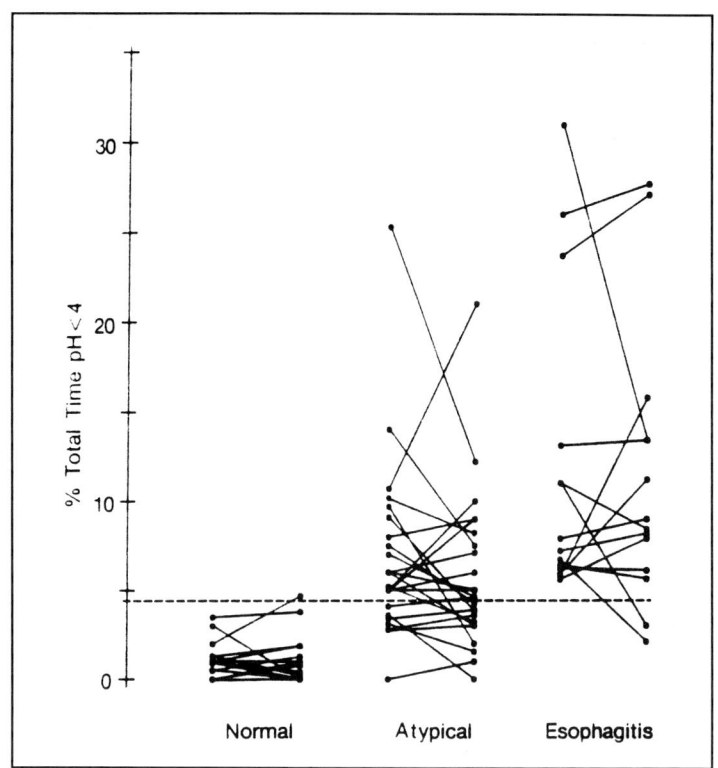

Fig. 1. Absolute values for total percentage of time with pH < 4 in 53 subjects studied by ambulatory 24-h esophageal pH monitoring performed on two separate days. The total group can be divided into three subgroups representing the clinical spectrum of GERD normal volunteers, patients with atypical reflux symptoms (e.g., chest pain, asthma), and patients with esophagitis. The dotted line represents the X + 2 standard deviations for total percentage of time with pH < 4 derived from 20 asymptomatic volunteers (i.e., the diagnostic discrimination value for abnormal gastroesophageal reflux). (Weiner GJ et al. Dig Dis Sci 1988;33:1127–1133.)

had at least one entirely normal pH study, underscores the fact that even pH monitoring is not an absolute discriminator for GERD.

It seems reasonable to conclude that the ambulatory pH monitor may not be a true gold standard, although it is a reasonably reliable diagnostic test once its limitations are understood. It is arguably the best test to document the presence of abnormal reflux. Ambulatory pH monitoring can also provide accurate information on the relationship of specific symptoms to reflux, if the symptoms index is calculated during the period of testing. This technique may be considered an endogenous Bernstein test.

References

1.   Schlesinger PK, Donahue PE, Schmid B et al. Limitations of 24-hour pH monitoring in the hospital setting. Gastroenterology 1985;89:797–804.

2. Klauser AG, Heinrich C, Schindlbeck NE et al. Is long-term esophageal pH monitoring of clinical value? Am J Gastro-enterol 1989;84:362—365.
3. Murphy D, Yuan YU, Castell DO. Does the intraesophageal pH probe accurately detect acid reflux? Simultaneous recording with two pH probes in humans. Dig Dis Sci 1989;34:649—656.
4. Wiener GJ, Morgan TM, Coopper JB, Wu WC, Castell DO, Sinclair JW, Richter JE. Ambulatory 24-hour esophageal pH monitoring: Reproducibility and variability of pH parameters. Dig Dis Sci 1988;33:1127—1134.

Is it possible to define the abnormal parameters of pH measurement in elderly subjects?

J.E. Richter (Birmingham, Alabama)

Schlesinger et al. [1] first raised the possibility that increasing age had an effect on esophageal pH parameters. They studied 20 control male subjects matched by age with their male patients (58.8 ± 6.9 (SD) and 55 ± 13.3 years, respectively). It was found that the controls' mean values for five of the six reflux variables were markedly higher than those previously reported by Johnson and DeMeester [2], among 15 younger healthy volunteers. However, these older controls were obtained from a hospitalized veterans population, with a high prevalence of coronary artery disease, liver disease, hypertension and diabetes mellitus. These diseases and their treatment may have influenced the pH parameters. Spence et al. [3] also examined the possible relationship between physiologic gastroesophageal reflux and age but could not find any reliable associations. However, their sample size was small (14 subjects) and only young and "middle aged" controls were studied (the middle aged controls ranged from 39—61 years, with a mean age of 49 years). Thus, the restricted age range of the sample may have precluded any positive findings. In an 8-year longitudinal study, Kruse-Andersen et al. [4] found that aging among healthy adults (n = 10, age range 30—53 years at end of study) did not alter the results of their overnight intraesophageal pH records. Nevertheless, this negative result may have been due to the use of a small study subset and a relatively small time period between baseline and final pH assessment.

The best evidence to date suggesting the amount of gastroesophageal reflux (GER) encountered in healthy adults is age dependent was reported by Smout et al. [5]. They compared 16 young healthy volunteers (mean age 31 years) and a similar number of healthy older volunteers (mean age 61 years, range 45—73 years), thereby eliminating the problem of restricted age ranges associated with the two previous early studies. The subject samples included 16 men and 16 women but the authors did not describe how the men and women were distributed within the two age groups. It was found that older subjects produced significantly higher values of total and upright % time pH < 4, as well as the total number of reflux episodes >5 min. However, no attempt was made to assess possible interactions of age and gender on these pH parameters. Moreover, these data were unusual, in that five of the 16 (31%) older subjects had total acid exposure times >10%. These latter patients may have represented occult refluxers, as routine endoscopy was not done on the healthy volunteers.

Our group has recently published a large study involving 110 healthy subjects, in order to better understand the influence of multiple factors on ambulatory 24-h esophageal values [6]. By using this large sample size, we hoped to overcome many of the limitations of these previous investigations. All of the subjects involved were healthy individuals without prior history of heartburn or regurgitation. About half of these individuals had undergone prior endoscopy and/or barium esophagram. The older subject group was relatively large in size (n = 24) and the groups were substantially different in age (younger controls' mean age 36 years, range 29–49; older controls' mean age 64 years, range 50–84 years). Unlike Smout et al., we did not find any independent effect of age on pH parameters, although men seemed to have more reflux than women (Fig. 1). However, age and gender showed strong interactive influences on the total number of episodes >5 min and the longest reflux episode in which the older males produced the highest values on these parameters. Our data also differed from those of Smout et al. in that both the younger and older subjects produced values substantially lower, on nearly all of the pH parameters, than those of their counterparts in Smout's study. It is possible that a type II error may be present in our data analysis. However, a power analysis suggests that approximately 100 older and 100 younger subjects would need to be studied, to detect an age effect with 80% power at $p < 0.05$. Thus, for clinical purposes we do not believe that age generally has an important effect on the physiologic parameters of acid reflux.

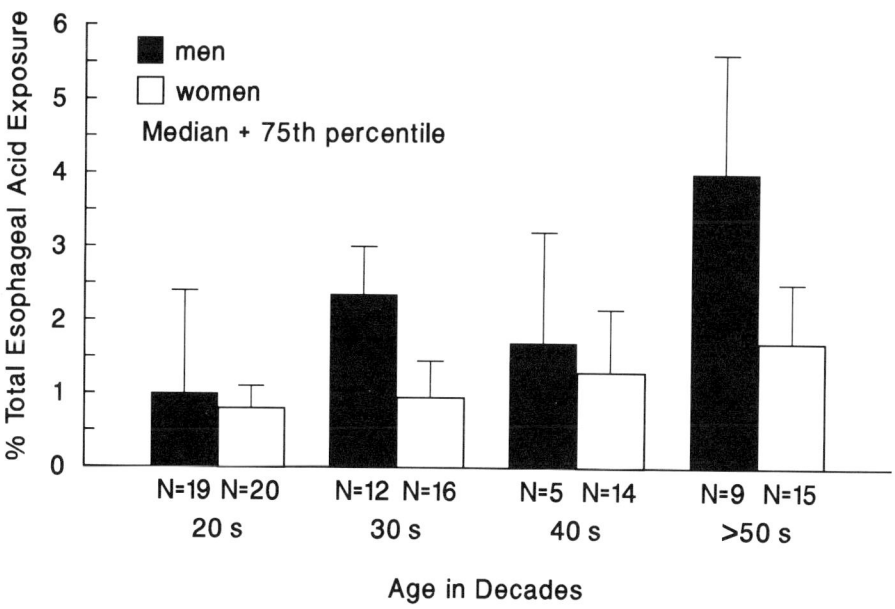

Fig. 1.

In support of our results, Johnston et al. [7] recently presented a preliminary report at the AGA, assessing the effects of age, gender, body mass and cigarette smoking in 103 consecutive heartburn sufferers who agreed to esophageal pH monitoring. Of all the variables assessed, they found that only age (r = 0.29, p = 0.004) correlated with esophageal acid exposure, defined by total percentage time pH < 4. For each decade increase in age, esophageal acid exposure increased by 23%. However, the clinical relevance of aging and acid reflux parameters was better defined by a multiply regression analysis. This model suggested that age predicted less than 13% of the variance in esophageal acid exposure.

Although not in total agreement, the studies to date suggest that aging alone does not have a marked effect on the normal physiological parameters of esophageal acid reflux. Age may be associated with some increase in acid exposure times, particularly total number of episodes >5 min, but the change appears to be of minimal clinical importance and does not warrant the establishment of separate standards for the elderly population.

References

1. Schlesinger PK, Donahue PE, Schmid B, Layden TJ. Limitations of 24-h intraesophageal pH monitoring in the hospital setting. Gastroenterology 1985;89:797–804.
2. Johnson LF, DeMeester TR. 24-hour pH monitoring of the distal esophagus. Am J Gastroenterol 1974;62:325–332.
3. Spence RAJ, Collins BJ, Parks TG, Love AHG. Does age influence normal gastroesophageal reflux. Gut 1985;26:799–801.
4. Kruse-Andersen S, Wallin L, Madsen T. The influence of age on esophageal acid defense mechanisms in spontaneous acid gastroesophageal reflux. Am J Gastroenterol 1988;83:637–639.
5. Smout AJPM, Breedijk M, Van der Zouw C, Akkermans LMA. Physiological gastroesophageal reflux and esophageal motor activity studied with a new system for 24-hour recording and automated analysis. Dig Dis Sci 1989;34:372–378.
6. Richter JE, Bradley LA, DeMeester TR, Wu WC. Normal 24-hour ambulatory esophageal pH values. Influence of study center, pH electrodes, age and gender. Dig Dis Sci 1992;37:849–856.
7. Johnston BT, Collins JSA, McFarland RJ, Love AHG. Esophageal acid exposure increases with age but does not correlate with other factors. Gastroenterology 1993;104:A111.

Do preoperative measurements of alkaline reflux and the concentration of biliary acids make it possible to avoid certain postoperative complications?

C.A. Pellegrini (Seattle)

Preoperative evaluation of esophageal function is important on at least three counts:
— it allows the surgeon to understand the problem in a given patient;

— it allows the surgeon to plan therapy appropriately; and
— it is essential to evaluate the results of operations.

The majority of patients with abnormal gastroesophageal reflux (GER) have a mechanically incompetent sphincter (i.e., a sphincter pressure less than 6 mmHg, length less than 2 cm or intra-abdominal length less than 1 cm). Other factors related to esophageal and gastric function (such as poor gastric motility, excessive acid secretion, inadequate esophageal clearance, etc.) may aggravate the effects of reflux. When the sphincter is incompetent, gastric contents regurgitate easily into the esophagus. The time the refluxate remains in contact with the esophageal mucosa (esophageal exposure) determines, to some extent, the damage to the lining of the esophagus.

Depending on the nature of gastric contents, patients may regurgitate primarily acid, a mixture of acid and alkaline juices, or primarily alkaline substances into the esophagus. A great deal of experimental and clinical work has shown that alkaline reflux particularly when it contains bile salts and is mixed with gastric acid, can produce serious damage to the esophageal mucosa [1–4]. Although not entirely agreed upon by all, it is believed that alkaline reflux into the esophagus plays an important role in the development of esophageal strictures [1] and Barrett's esophagus [2].

How does alkaline material get into the esophagus? It is now believed that the majority of patients with alkaline material in the esophagus have associated abnormal duodenogastric reflux. Lin et al. [1] have shown that epigastric pain is more common among these patients than it is among those with pure GER; strictures and a columnar-lined esophageal mucosa are also more commonly seen in this group of patients. Lin et al. also showed that alkaline reflux was more prevalent in the 30 min following an episode of duodenogastric reflux, suggesting that the latter caused the former. Similarly, Attwood et al. have shown that patients with greater degrees of alkaline reflux tend to develop strictures and Barrett's more often than those with lesser amounts of alkaline reflux [2]. Thus, the noxious effects of alkaline reflux appear to be well documented.

Can alkaline reflux be measured? Although the method of 24-h pH monitoring was initially developed to measure acid reflux, we found that it could also be used to identify alkaline reflux [5]. Logic indicates that the sensitivity of this method should be inferior, for example, alkaline reflux has a pH much closer to saliva and when mixed with gastric juice, alkaline substances may reflux to the esophagus with a pH in the 4–5 range, rather than in the expected 7–8 range. This may decrease the sensitivity of the method to identify abnormal alkaline reflux. Due to this, other methods have been devised to aid in the identification of abnormal alkaline GER. For example, the sensitivity of 24-h esophageal pH monitoring can be increased by simultaneous measurement of gastric pH [6], which identifies abnormal duodenogastric reflux. The presence of abnormal duodenogastric reflux in a patient with a mechanically incompetent gastroesophageal sphincter, should raise the serious possibility of abnormal alkaline exposure of the esophageal mucosa. Nevertheless, to be certain the esophagus is exposed to duodenal contents, direct measurement of bile acids [3,7] or other markers contained within the duodenal fluid (such as bilirubin, tripsin, etc.) may in the future provide a more reliable determination of alkaline reflux.

Does identification of abnormal alkaline reflux lead to a different form of surgical therapy? We believe that it does not, but others disagree. This controversy can be examined: Lin et al. showed that, for alkaline GER to occur, two elements must be present, a defective sphincter and abnormal duodenogastric reflux [1]. In the absence of one of these two conditions, alkaline reflux does not reach the esophagus. The implication of these findings is that correction of the sphincter by an antireflux procedure should abolish abnormal reflux. That is why we perform a standard Nissen fundoplication in these patients. Nevertheless, there are claims by Csendes and others, that restoration of gastroesophageal competency alone, without correction of associated abnormal duodenogastric reflux in patients with Barrett's esophagus, is followed by an unacceptably high rate of recurrence. These authors have proposed that when abnormal duodenogastric reflux and abnormal GER have been identified, both these conditions should be corrected to obtain good long-term results. They also propose the use of the "duodenal switch" operation [8], described by DeMeester et al., to address the duodenogastric reflux problem and the use of Nissen fundoplication to restore the competency of the cardia. They base their recommendation on the fact that, in their experience, up to 40% of patients with this condition, subjected only to a Nissen fundoplication, develop recurrence of GER within 5 years. Since abnormal duodenogastric reflux presumably continues unchecked, failure of the operation to prevent GER leads to further alkaline exposure of the esophageal mucosa. This in turn leads to stricture formation and may increase the risk of esophageal adenocarcinoma. Overall, then, we believe there is insufficient data, at this time, to support the position of these authors, and prefer to address the problem of abnormal gastroesophageal sphincter function only (within a Nissen fundoplication) as the initial treatment of choice for patients with abnormal alkaline reflux. For patients with recurrent reflux, we believe that functional evaluation of the esophagus should guide the reoperation. This may mean, in some instances, a duodenal switch and a redo Nissen, a redo Nissen alone, a subtotal gastrectomy with a Roux-Y procedure or even — in some situations — a total gastrectomy with a Roux-Y esophagojejunostomy.

In summary, preoperative evaluation should always include measurement of esophageal alkaline exposure, by 24-h pH monitoring, or more sensitive methods if available. This information provides meaningful data to understand the nature of the underlying disease, which then allows the surgeon to plan adequately the kind of operation most likely to succeed.

References

1. Lin KM, Ueda RK, Hinder RA, Stein HJ, DeMeester TR. Etiology and importance of alkaline esophageal reflux. Am J Surg 1991;162:553−557.
2. Attwood SEA, DeMeester TR, Bremner CG et al. Alkaline gastroesophageal reflux: implications in the development of complications in Barrett's columnar-lined lower esophagus. Surgery 1989;106:764−770.
3. Gotley DC, Morgan AP, Cooper MJ. Bile acid concentrations in the refluxate of patients with reflux oesophagitis. Br J Surg 1988;75:587−590.
4. Kivilaakso E, Fromm D, Silen W. Effects of bile salts and related compounds on esophageal mucosa. Scand J Gastroenterol 1981;16(supp 167);119−121.

5.   Pellegrini CA, DeMeester TR, Wernly JA, Johnson LF, Skinner DB. Alkaline gastroesophageal reflux. Am J Surg 1978; 134:177–184.
6.   Fuchs KH, DeMeester TR, Hinder RA, Stein HJ, Barlow AP. Computerized identification of pathologic duodenogastric reflux using 24-hour gastric pH monitoring. Ann Surg 1991;213:13–20.
7.   Mittal RK, Reuben A, Whitney JO, McCallum RW. Do bile acids reflux into the esophagus? A study in normal subjects and patients with gastroesophageal reflux disease. Gastroenterology 1987;92:371–375.
8.   DeMeester TR, Fuchs KH, Ball CS et al. Experimental and clinical results with proximal end-to-end duodenojejunostomy for pathologic duodenogastric reflux. Ann Surg 1987;206:414–426.

Can one specify unequivocal indications for pH measurement?

J.-P. Galmiche, S. Bruley des Varannes (Nantes)
C. Scarpignato (Parma)

Gastroesophageal reflux disease (GERD) is a disorder which is due to the reflux of gastric juice into the esophagus. At one end of the spectrum of the disease are subjects with mild, intermittent symptoms who do not seek medical help or who are seen by primary care physicians and managed with conservative measures. In contrast, at the other end are patients with chronic relapsing disease, persistent disabling symptoms and/or severe esophagitis [1,2]. Even if GERD is not a life threatening condition, severe complications such as strictures, columnar-lined (Barrett's) esophagus or respiratory manifestations may occur. Moreover, GERD may also be causally related to a variety of nondigestive symptoms (e.g., hoarseness, chronic nocturnal cough, asthma, recurrent pneumonitis and even angina like chest pain) [1]. Symptoms of GERD and lesions of esophagitis do not necessarily coexist in the same patient, therefore making the diagnosis more difficult for those patients who present with atypical symptoms and no lesions at endoscopy. In that clinical situation, monitoring esophageal pH has become an increasingly popular test [3–5]. Indeed, the development of portable data loggers not only allows objective measurement of the esophageal acid exposure but also, thanks to the event marker, it enables the investigation of the relationship between symptoms and reflux episodes.

In this paper, the diagnostic and nondiagnostic usefulness of esophageal pH monitoring will be discussed, in order to address the question: "What are the unequivocal indications for esophageal pH measurement?"

Diagnostic applications

Measure of acid exposure

In the majority of studies, the diagnostic accuracy of pH-metry to discriminate between patients and controls has been evaluated by reference to a clinical definition of GERD based on typical symptoms of heartburn and regurgitations and/or on the presence at endoscopy of various degrees of lesions of esophagitis. When these groups of patients are compared to healthy volunteers, the sensitivity and specificity of 24-h pH monitoring are very high and range usually between 90–100%. However, in clinical practice, the majority of reflux patients do not have lesions at endoscopy [7]. A recent study by Klauser et al. [8] addressed the important issue of the diagnostic value of symptoms and whether GERD can be reasonably diagnosed by means of a well-taken history or a discriminant analysis of symptoms. In this study the diagnosis of GERD was based on 24-h pH metry and a standard questionnaire was used for the search of typical and atypical symptoms. The only symptoms differing significantly between the groups of patients with normal and pathological pH metry were heartburn and regurgitations. However, those two symptoms were also reported by nearly half the patients with normal pH metry. Overall, the discriminant analysis of symptoms was inferior to the subjective impression of an experienced gastroenterologist. However, 34% of the 304 patients in this study could not be classified clinically by a thorough history. Moreover, when heartburn or regurgitation, and to a lesser extent epigastric burning, clearly dominated the patient's complaints the specificity of these symptoms were good (but the sensitivity was low). These authors concluded that only heartburn and regurgitations can be considered typical symptoms of reflux. On the other hand, GERD cannot be excluded in the absence of these symptoms.

Relationship between symptoms and reflux episodes

One of the most important aspects of ambulatory pH-metry is its ability to detect a temporal relationship between symptoms and reflux episodes. Although strict criteria have not yet been defined, a symptom or event is usually considered associated with GERD if it occurs during the reflux episodes or within the 2 min before or after the reflux episode. To measure the strength of such kinds of relationships, different indexes have been suggested. Castells' group [9] first proposed the use of a symptom index (number of symptom events associated with reflux episodes/ number of marked events ×100). With more experience it became obvious that this simple index had major drawbacks; for instance, it does not take into account the number of reflux episodes and therefore the probability that association between reflux and symptoms occurs merely by chance. Moreover, the cut-off values of the symptom index (i.e., the percentages considered to reflect a high likelihood of causal relation between symptoms and reflux) are arbitrary and vary from one study to another. Several remedies have been proposed, including the calculation of a symptom sensitivity index [10] (i.e., the percentage of reflux perceived by the patients during 24-h) or the determination of the probability that reflux and symptoms occur simultaneously by chance [11]. However, so far none of these indexes have been universally accepted. Finally, it must be recognized that some patients may present normal esophageal acid exposure, despite a highly significant correlation between symptoms and reflux at pH monitoring. The recently described concept of "acid burden" [12], sensitizing the mucosa to further reflux episodes, may be useful to explain these apparent discrepancies and also the fact that pH-monitoring and the Bernstein test led to different results in a substantial proportion of patients with symptoms suggestive of GERD. In fact, sensitivity to exogenous acid (Bernstein test) and pH monitoring explore different — though related — phenomena [13].

In summary, although there is no true "gold standard" for the diagnosis of GERD, 24-h esophageal pH-monitoring is the best available diagnostic test for discriminating between physiological reflux and pathological acid exposure (i.e., patients with GERD). The diagnostic accuracy in GERD is better than all other functional tests including the standard acid reflux test, the Bernstein test, histological criteria of esophagitis or the finding of an hypotonic lower esophageal sphincter (LES) at manometry. However, 24-h pH monitoring also has its own limitations. For example, pH monitoring does not provide any information about the volume of the material which actually refluxes from the stomach into the esophagus.

Nondiagnostic applications

Predictive value of acid exposure

There is a definite relation between the duration of esophageal acid exposure and the frequency and severity of heartburn [14]. Similarly, several studies [15] have established a statistically significant association between the severity of lesions seen at endoscopy and the duration of acid exposure. Nonetheless, all these studies show considerable overlap between individual values measured in the different groups (e.g., patients with and without esophagitis). The question is, therefore: "Can measurement of acid exposure predict the natural history of the disease in an individual patient?" In a study of 106 patients with moderate to severe symptoms of GERD and esophagitis, Olden and Triadafilopoulos [16] found no differences in the various pH parameters analyzed between 58 patients who responded to an 8-week H_2 antagonist therapy and the 48 patients who were refractory to medical therapy. Similarly, Boesby et al. [17] found 12 h overnight pH monitoring of no value in selecting candidates for surgery because there was a considerable overlap of pretreatment acid exposure values between patients who responded to medical therapy and those who needed antireflux surgery. In contrast, in a recent trial of omeprazole vs. ranitidine performed in patients with refractory esophagitis, Bianchi Porro ct al. [18] found by multivariate analysis that the pretreatment acid exposure was the only factor (apart from the type of treatment) related to healing. However, it must be underlined that only borderline significance was detected. Taken together, these results suggest that at least in the individual patient, the pretreatment acid exposure does not accurately predict the responsiveness of symptoms and esophagitis to medical therapy.

Presently there is very little information on long-term outcome and acid exposure. Schindlbeck et al. [19] suggested that supine reflux is an unfavorable prognostic factor. In contrast, in a small series of initially endoscopy negative patients, Pace et al. [20] found no difference in esophageal acid exposure between those patients who subsequently developed erosive esophagitis and those who did not. Our own experience in infants is similar [21], since we failed to identify any pH monitoring values which were predictive of the course of the disease in 141 consecutive infants, followed for a mean of 18 months. Irrespective of the definition of GERD (i.e., typical symptoms or abnormal acid exposure), univariate as well as multivariate analyses indicated that a bad prognosis was only associated with the presence of hiatal hernia and respiratory symptoms.

Evaluation of treatment

During the last decade, pH monitoring has been used increasingly to assess many new or old drugs potentially useful in the treatment of GERD. Obviously pH monitoring is very appealing because it offers an excellent opportunity to objectively and quantitatively compare different drugs at various dosages or dosing regimens. There is now considerable evidence showing that the degree of reduction of acid exposure is a good predictor of the therapeutic response to antisecretory drugs, at least in the short term. Indeed, it has been shown that nonresponders to standard treatment with H_2 antagonists have less reduction of acidity and more prolonged acid exposure than responders [22–24]. Similarly, several studies have shown that patients in whom surgery has failed have more reflux than those in whom it was successful [25]. Moreover, even asymptomatic patients with an abnormal reflux pattern a few months after surgery have shown to carry an increased risk of further deterioration in the long term.

However, even if the diagnosis of GERD by pH-monitoring is reproducible, it is now largely established that there is substantial variability of acid exposure from day to day [26]. Consequently, interpretation of data in an individual patient should remain very cautious. The only relevant criteria is whether medical or surgical therapy is able or not to bring acid exposure within the normal range. This variability also has important consequences with regard to the risk of type-II error in pharmacological studies. Indeed, the number of patients included must be sufficient to detect a significant reduction of acid with a moderately or slightly effective drug [27].

Conclusion

In clinical practice, esophageal pH-metry is primarily indicated in patients with atypical symptoms and no lesions at endoscopy (Fig. 1). In that context, esophageal pH monitoring not only detects pathological acid exposure but, provided that there is a good relationship between reflux episodes and symptoms, the test is also able to demonstrate the responsibility of reflux in the patient's complaints. In contrast, esophageal pH-monitoring is not necessary for the diagnosis of GERD in patients with typical symptoms and/or erosive or ulcerative esophagitis at endoscopy. In these patients the specificity of symptoms and/or lesions is sufficiently high to start with therapeutic trial. Finally, the test is also indicated in patients who previously failed to respond to medical treatment or in whom surgery seems indicated.

186

INDICATIONS OF OESOPHAGEAL pH-MONITORING
IN THE INDIVIDUAL PATIENT

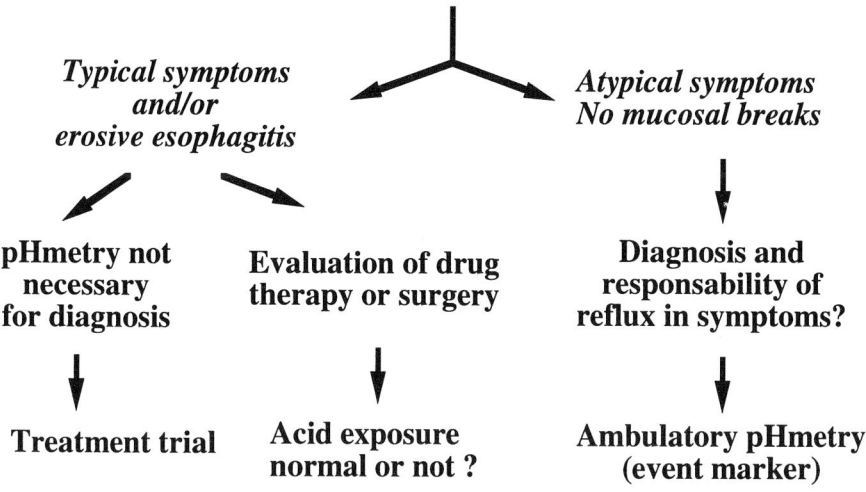

Fig. 1. Suggested flow-chart for the use of esophageal pH-monitoring.

References

1. Traube M. The spectrum of the symptoms and presentations of gastroesophageal reflux disease. Gastroenterol Clin North Am 1990;19:609–616.
2. Galmiche JP, Bruley des Varannes S. Symptoms and disease severity in gastro-oesophageal reflux disease (GORD). Scand J Gastroenterol (in press).
3. Galmiche JP, Scarpignato C. Esophageal pH-metry. Front Gastrointest Res (in press).
4. Mattox HE, Richter JE. Prolonged ambulatory esophageal pH monitoring in the evaluation of gastroesophageal reflux disease. Am J Med 1990;89:345–356.
5. Bianchi Porro G, Pace F. The role of continuous oesophageal pH monitoring in the diagnosis of gastroesophageal reflux. Eur J Gastroenterol Hepatol 1991;3:501–509.
6. Jamieson JR, Stein HJ, DeMeester TR, Bonavina L, Schwizer W, Hinder RA, Albertucci M. Ambulatory 24-h esophageal pH monitoring: normal values, optimal thresholds, specificity, sensitivity, and reproducibility. Am J Gastroenterol 1992; 87:1102–1110.
7. Johnsson F, Joelsson B, Gudmundsson K, Greiff L. Symptoms and endoscopic findings in the diagnosis of gastroesophageal reflux disease. Scand J Gastroenterol 1987;22:714–718.
8. Klauser AG, Schindlbeck NE, Müller-Lissner SA. Symptoms in gastro-oesophageal reflux disease. Lancet 1990;335:205–208.
9. Wiener GJ, Richter JE, Coopper JB, Wu WC, Castell DO. The symptom index: a clinically important parameter of ambulatory 24-hour esophageal pH monitoring. Am J Gastroenterol 1988;83:358–361.
10. Breumelhof R, Smout AJPM. The symptom sensitivity index: a valuable additional parameter in 24-hour esophageal pH recording. Am J Gastroenterol 1991;86:160–164.
11. Ghillebert G, Janssens J, Vantrappen G, Nevens F, Piessens J. Ambulatory 24-hour intraoesophageal pH and pressure recordings vs. provocation tests in the diagnosis of chest pain of oesophageal origin. Gut 1990;31:738–744.
12. Janssens J, Vantappen G, Vos R, Ghillebert G. The acid burden over an extended period preceding a reflux episode is a major determinant in the development of heartburn. Gastroenterology 1992;102:A90 (abstract).
13. Howard PJ, Maher L, Pryde A, Heading RC. Symptomatic gastro-oesophageal reflux, abnormal oesophageal acid exposure, and mucosal acid sensitivity are three separate, though related, aspects of gastro-oesophageal reflux disease. Gut 1991;32: 128–132.
14. Joelsson B, Johnsson F. Heartburn — the acid test. Gut 1989;30:1523–1525.
15. Stein HJ, Barlow AP, DeMeester TR, Hinder RA. Complications of gastroesophageal reflux disease. Ann Surg 1992;216:35–43.

16. Olden K, Triadafilopoulos G. Failure of initial 24-hour esophageal pH monitoring to predict refractoriness and intractability in reflux esophagitis. Am J Gastroenterol 1991;86:1142−1146.
17. Boesby S, Wallin L, Myrhoj T, Andersen LI. Twelve hour overnight oesophageal pH monitoring in patients with reflux symptoms. Gut 1991;32:10−11.
18. Bianchi Porro G, Pace F, Peracchia A, Bonavina L, Vigneri S, Scialabba A, Franceschi M. Short-term treatment of refractory reflux esophagitis with different doses of omeprazole or ranitidine. J Clin Gastroenterol 1992;15:192−198.
19. Schindlbeck NE, Klauser AG, Berghammer G, Londong W, Müller-Lissner S. Three year follow-up of patients with gastro-oesophageal reflux disease. Gut 1992;33:1016−1019.
20. Pace F, Santalucia F, Bianchi Porro G. Natural history of gastro-oesophageal reflux disease without oesophagitis. 1992;32:858−848.
21. Masliah C, Galmiche JP, Cloarec D, Gérard P, Czernichow P, Bruley des Varannes S. Twenty-four hour oesophageal pH monitoring in infants with suspected gastro-oesophageal reflux disease: relationships with symptoms, endoscopy and evolution. Eur J Gastroenterol Hepatol 1990;2:137−142.
22. Johansson KE, Tibbling L. Gastric secretion and reflux pattern in reflux oesophagitis before and during ranitidine treatment. Scand J Gastroenterol 1986;21:487−492.
23. Robertson DA, Aldersley MA, Shepherd H, Lloyd RS, Smith CL. H2 antagonists in the treatment of reflux esophagitis: can physiological studies predict the response? Gut 1987;28:946−949.
24. Collen J, Lewis JH, Benjamin SB. Gastric acid hypersecretion in refractory gastroesophageal reflux disease. Gastroenterology 1990;98:654−661.
25. Galmiche JP, Tenière P, Ducrotté P, Denis P, Colin R, Testart J. Traitement du reflux gastro-oesophagien acide par hémi-fundoplicature postérieure. Résultats cliniques et pH-métriques. Gastroenterol Clin Biol 1983;7:385−391.
26. Wiener GJ, Morgan TM, Coopper JB, Wu WC, Castell DO, Sinclair JW, Richter JE. Ambulatory 24-hour esophageal pH monitoring. Reproducibility and variability of pH parameters. Dig Dis Sci 1988;33:1127−1133.
27. Galmiche JP, Scarpignato C. Pharmacodynamic assessment of drugs in gastro-oesophageal reflux disease. In: Tytgat GNJ (ed) The Medical Management of Oesophageal Reflux Disease, Round Table Series 22. London: Royal Society of Medicine Services, 1990;12−32.

What is the comparative value of histologic study of the mucosa and 24-h pH measurement in the diagnosis of reflux esophagitis?

E. Bollschweiler, A.H. Hölscher, J.R. Siewert (Munich)

There is very little information about the correlation between damage of mucosa of the esophagus and the amount of acid. Most of the studies describe relations between histomorphology and endoscopy [1−3]. Other studies give information about the correlation between results of endoscopy and pH monitoring [4,5].

The esophageal mucosa has very little protection against the aggressive factors of gastroduodenal reflux. The tissue resistance is a function of the intact epithelium layer, which is maintained by sufficient cell regeneration originating in the basalis and by a sufficient blood supply, provided by the capillaries within the tips of the papillae.

The intense and prolonged contact of the esophageal mucosa with the contents of the reflux leads to damage of the uppermost epithelial cells, which can be visualized by necroses and desquamation of single cells. This is probably caused by a leukotactic effect of the degenerating cells or caused directly by the contents of the refluxate, single eosinophilic of neutrophilic leukocytes beginning to migrate into the epithelial layer. This phenomenon is thought to be a very sensitive sign of reflux disease. The increased cell loss is compensated for by an intensified cell regeneration as is visualized by a broadening of the basal layer. The higher demand for blood supply causes a dilatation of capillaries and an elongation of the papillae. These phenomena were first described by Ismail-Beigi et al. [6,7] and can be noted in 90% of patients with reflux, but also in 57% of normal patients in the distal 2.5 cm of the esophagus. These early changes probably have no endoscopic correlation and represent the histological stage A of reflux disease [1].

Histologic examinations are necessary to determine the exact depth of the lesions in the esophageal wall. Such histologically visible alterations of the esophageal mucosa in patients with symptoms of gastroesophageal reflux GER have been described as follows: increased thickness of the basal cell zone and proximity of the dermal papillae to the epithelial surface [6,8]. These alterations closely correlate with the severity of reflux symptoms and the endoscopic signs of esophagitis. Similar results were reported by other authors, however, the close correlation with the symptoms was not always confirmed [7,9,10]. Heilmann et al. [1] looked at patients with symptoms of reflux esophagitis and described a good correlation between the histological results of biopsy and the endoscopic classification of GER according to Savary and Miller [11]. However, remarkably in stages I and II, fibrin-coated erosions showed more severe alterations and damages up to the mucosa than those without fibrin. Heilmann described the histomorphology of erosions coated with fibrinous membranes as a "deep and clearly visible defect of the epithelium, coated by a fibrinous exudate and a dense leukocyte infiltrates in the epithelium as well as in the mucosa". The basal cell layer is increased in thickness and the papillae expand to more than 70% of the depth of the epithelium. In contrast, an erosion without visible fibrinous coating appears flat with a superficially damaged epithelium containing a small number of eosinophilic leukocytes with slightly extended papillae (Fig. 1).

According to these results, Siewert and Ottenjann [12] extended the endoscopic classification of reflux esophagitis by Savary and proposed two subgroups for stages I and II: one subgroup for lesions with, and the other for lesions without fibrinous coat. Other endoscopic classifications also showed that fibrin-coated erosions indicate a more severe form of esophagitis [2,13,14].

Another study done by Ottenjann and Steib [3] confirmed this classification. They studied 59 patients with reflux esophagitis and red lesions (n = 23) or white lesions (n = 36) who underwent endoscopically controlled biopsy of selected particles. Histologic analysis confirmed the hypothesis that white lesions are nearly always necroses involving all layers of the squamous epithelium with fibrin deposits (and rarely epithelial hyperplasia), while red lesions are caused by local granulocytic inflammation or granulation tissue with partial re-epithelialization. These results suggest that reflux esophagitis Savary stages I and II can be rationally subclassified into reflux esophagitis with red spots (Stage Ia), white spots (Stage Ib), red streaks (Stage IIa), and white streaks (Stage IIb).

Geisinger [15] studied the histologic development of acid-induced esophagitis in

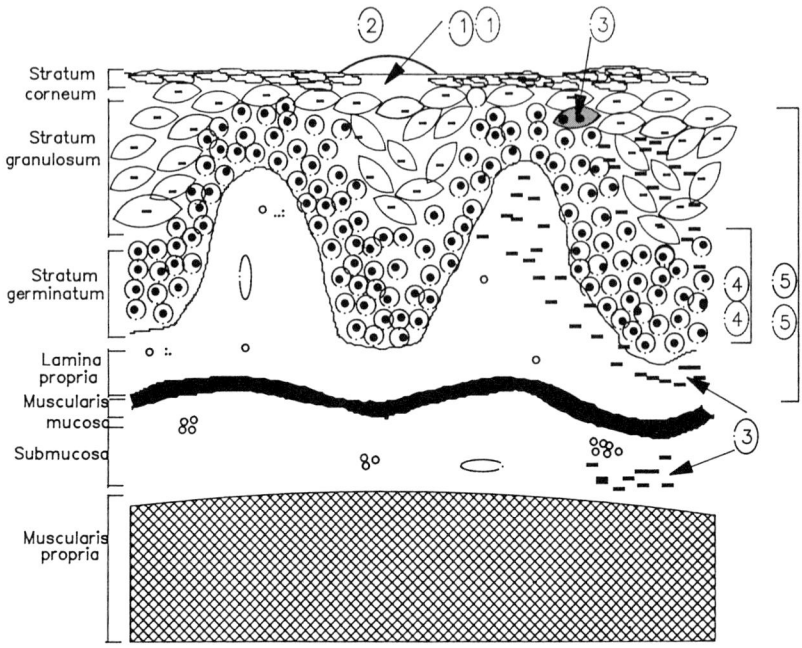

Fig. 1. Histomorphology of esophageal reflux disease (according to Heilmann [1]).

Stage A: 1) Damaging uppermost epithelial cells with flat erosions; 3) Eosinophilic of neutrophilic leukocytes migrate into the epithelial layer; 4) Basal cell layer < 20% of epithelial thickness; 5) Papillae extend no more than 70% of the way into the epithelium.

Stage B: 1) Severe and clearly visible epithelial damage with deep erosions; 2) Superficial defects in the form of erosions with a fibrinous exudate; 3) Dense leukocytic infiltrates in the epithelium and submucosa. 4) Basal cell layer >20% of epithelial thickness; 5) Papillae extend more than 70% of the way into the epithelium.

the cat. The feline model is produced by the infusion of 0.1 N HCl at the rate of 1 ml/min into the distal esophagus of adult cats for varying periods of time. Basal cell hyperplasia appeared to be the most sensitive marker of acid injury; ulcers denoted severe injury associated with longer exposure periods.

Black et al. [16] assessed the incidence of histological esophagitis in infants less than 2 years old with symptoms of GER. Thirty-five infants were studied with esophageal suction biopsy and pH probe monitoring. Ninety-three percent of the patients with histological esophagitis had significant reflux as determined by pH probe monitoring.

Johnson et al. [17] provided further evidence for the importance of basal cell thickness and lamina propria length, when they found a direct correlation between histologic changes and the degree of abnormal reflux determined by 24-h pH monitoring. In five patients they found that successful antireflux surgery reversed these changes.

We looked for a correlation between the sequence of these esophagitis stages according to Savary and the severity of GER measured by 24-h pH monitoring [18].

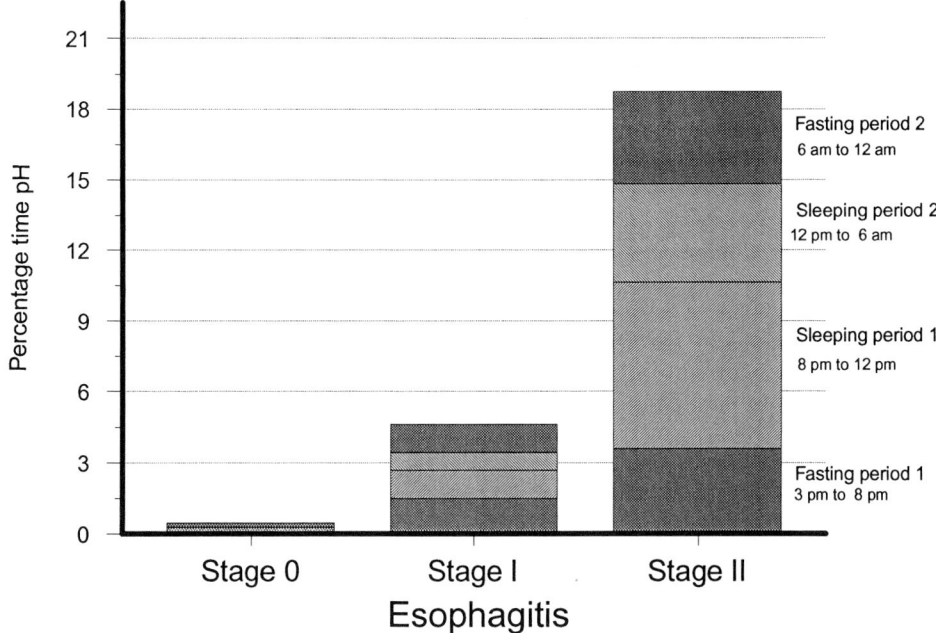

Fig. 2. Gastroesophageal reflux and esophagitis. Median time with pH < 4 during 24-h period of measurement.

The number of patients with symptoms of GER having endoscopy and 24-h pH monitoring was 153. The median time of reflux (% of measurement period) for pH < 4 and pH < 5 differed significantly among the stages 0, I and II for the total measurement time (p < 0.01) and for the different fasting and sleeping periods (p < 0.05) (Fig. 2). It was shown that patients with esophagitis, according to Savary, evidence different quantities of acid reflux. Published evidence indicates the same results [4,5,19].

These results suggest that the histological damage to the mucosa of the esophageal wall correlates to the amount of pathological acid reflux. In addition, correlation between the results of 24-h pH monitoring and the endoscopic classification, according to Siewert and Ottenjann, was looked at [3]. Our results showed a significant difference between the subgroups of the stages I and II: lesions with fibrinous coats had longer duration of acid reflux than those without fibrin (Fig. 3). The subgroups also differed significantly with regard to the intensity of acid reflux, shown on the graph as the area under the curve. The reflux episodes of long duration are especially important for these differences. Normally the esophagus reacts to acid exposure with an increased clearance activity [19,20]. The number of reflux episodes longer than 5 min differed significantly between the subgroups but they did not differ between the erosions with different sizes without fibrinous coats. Obviously the esophageal clearance function does not seem to work when patients have esophagitis with a fibrin-coated lesion. Therefore the mucosa is exposed to the injuring

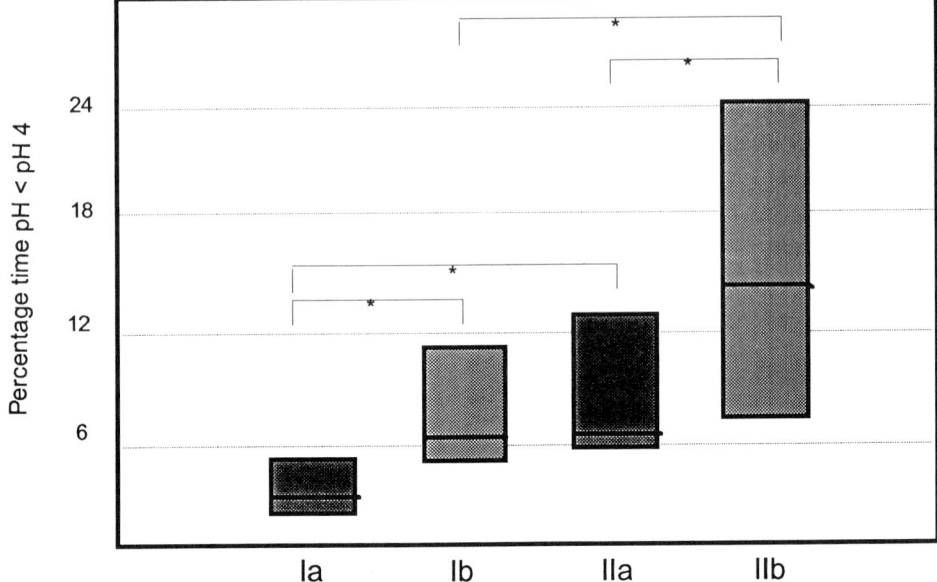

Fig. 3. Gastroesophageal reflux and subgroups of esophagitis according to Siewert and Ottenjann. Median time with pH < 4. (* = p < 0.05).

substances to a greater degree. Consequently they can cause more damage to the deeper layer of mucosa. Small and large erosions without fibrinous coats show an equal number of long reflux episodes. Other authors again say that reflux episodes of long duration do correlate closely with the severity of esophagitis [5,11].

In conclusion we can say that the amount of acid measured with 24-h pH monitoring correlates with histomorphological changes in epidermoid mucosa of the esophagus.

References

1. Heilmann KL, Siewert JR, Ottenjann R, Neiss A, Döpfer H. Histomorphology of esophageal reflux disease: Results of biopsy histology in a multicentre trial with cimetidine. In: Siewert JR, Hölscher AH (eds) Diseases of Esophagus. Berlin, Heidelberg, New York, London, Paris, Tokyo: Springer, 1986;1130−1136.
2. Kobayashi S, Kasugai T. Endoscopic and biopsy criteria for the esophagitis with a fiberoptic esophagoscope. Dig Dis 1974; 19:345−352.
3. Ottenjann R, Seib NJ. Endoskopisch-bioptische studie zur stadieneinteilung der refluxösophagitis. Z Gastroenterol 1991;29: 360−362.
4. Bollschweiler E, Feussner H, Hölscher AH, Siewert JR. Reflux-esophagitis: Correlation between endoscopic classification and gastroesophageal reflux pattern in 24-h pH-metry. Gastroenterology 1989,96.A50.
5. Jenkinson LR, Norris TR, Watson A. The role of acid exposure in the initiation and progression of reflux esophagitis. In: Fuchs KH, Hamelmann H (eds) Gastrointestinale Funktionsdiagnostik in der Chirurgie. Berlin: Blackwell Wissenschaft, 1991.
6. Ismail-Beigi F, Horton PF, Pope CE. Histological consequences of gastroesophageal reflux in man. Gastroenterology 1970; 58:163−174.
7. Ismail-Beigi F, Pope CE. Distribution of the histological changes of gastroesophageal reflux in the distal esophagus of man. Gastroenterology 1974;66:1109−1113.

8. Hopwood D, Milne G, Logan KR. Electron microscopic changes in human oesophageal epithelium in esophagitis. J Pathol 1979;129:161–166.
9. Knuff TE, Benjamin SB, Worsham GF, Hancock JE, Castell DO. Histologic evaluation of chronic gastroesophageal reflux. Dig Dis Sci 1984;29:194–201.
10. Seefeld U, Krejs GJ, Siebenmann RE, Blum AL. Esophageal histology in gastroesophageal reflux. Dig Dis 1977;22:956–964.
11. Savary M, Miller C. L'expression endoscopique de l'oesophagite par reflux. SIMEP, 1971.
12. Siewert JR, Ottenjann R, Heilmann K, Neiss A, Döpfer H. Therapie und prophylaxe der refluxoesophagitis. Ergebnisse einer multicenterstudie mit cimetidin. Teil I: Epidemiologie and ergebnisse der schubtherapie. Z Gastroenterol 1986; 24:381–395.
13. Bollschweiler E, Hölscher AH. Wertigkeit verschiedener diagnostischer verfahren bei refluxkrankheit – eine prospektive klinische untersuchung. In: KH Fuchs, H Hamelmann (eds) Gastrointestinale Funktionsdiagnostik in der Chirurgie. Berlin: Blackwell Wissenschaft, 1991;75–85.
14. Skinner DB, Belsey RHR. Surgical management of esophageal reflux and hiatus hernia. J Thorac Cardiovasc Surg 1967; 33:53.
15. Geisinger KR, Cassidy KT, Nardi R, Castell DO. The histologic development of acid induced esophagitis in the cat. Mod Pathol 1990;3(5):619–624.
16. Black DD, Haggitt RC, Orenstein SR, Whitington PF. Esophagitis in infants. Morphometric histologic diagnosis and correlation with measures of gastroesophageal reflux. Gastroenterology 1990;98(6):1408–1414.
17. Johnson LF, DeMeester TR, Haggitt RC. Esophageal epithelial response to gastroesophageal reflux: a quantitative study. Am J Dig Dis 1978;23:498–509.
18. Bollschweiler E, Hölscher AH, Feussner H, Dittler NJ, Siewert JR. Classification of reflux esophagitis according to the severity of gastroesophageal reflux pattern in 24-h pH metry. Dysphagia 1993 (in press).
19. Weiser HF, Bollschweiler E, Lange R, Siewert JR. Update on esophageal pH-monitoring. In: DeMeester TR, Matthews HR (eds) Benign Esophageal Disease, vol 3. St. Louis: C.V. Mosby Company, 1987;31–39.
20. Henderson RD. Reflux and primary motor disorders. In: The Esophagus. London, Baltimore: Williams & Wilkins, 1980;76.

Is there any effect of pH probes and pressure catheters on the function of the LES?

R.K. Mittal (Charlottesville)

The lower esophageal sphincter (LES) is a valvular mechanism at the lower end of the esophagus which prevents reflux of gastric contents into the esophagus. This valvular mechanism is due to the tonic contractions of the smooth muscles of the LES. The intraluminal LES pressure is a parameter of the strength of the valvular mechanism. The intraluminal LES pressure can only be measured by placing a tube inside the lumen of the LES. Therefore, the strength of the antireflux barrier can only be measured under nonphysiological situations, using a tube positioned in the lumen of the LES. Therefore, the key question is: does placement of a tube across the LES affect the intraluminal LES pressure? Since one cannot measure intraluminal LES pressures without placing a tube across the LES, this question can only be answered through an indirect approach. One approach is to answer the following question: does the increasing size of the manometric probe affect the LES pressure? Biancani et al. showed that there is a direct correlation between the size of the pressure probe and the LES pressure measured in a given individual over the probe diameters ranging from 0.25—1.0 cm [1]. There was minimal difference between the probe diameters of 0.25—0.5 cm but a significant increase as the diameter increased to 0.75 cm and 1 cm. This increase in pressure with the increasing size of the probe was seen in the normal individuals as well as in patients with incompetent LES (reflux esophagitis). The commonly used size of manometric pressure probe is 0.3—0.45 cm. One could safely say that the probe diameters commonly used in clinical practice (up to 0.5 cm), may not have a major influence on the LES pressure measurement.

The function of the LES is to prevent reflux of gastric contents. Another question which can be asked is: does a tube across the LES affect the frequency or acid exposure times in the esophagus? There are three possible ways by which a tube across the LES can affect movement of acid contents from the stomach into the esophagus:
- a tube placed across the LES can act as a wick (like a cotton swab) and suck acid from the gastric pool into the esophagus;
- through a weakening or reduction of the LES pressure; or
- induction of transient LES relaxations.

The data against the wick-like effect of the manometric catheter is quite convincing. Fisher et al., using simultaneous radionuclide studies and manometry, failed to find any such effect [2]. Indirect evidence against a wick-like effect is provided by the observations made during simultaneous manometry and pH recordings of the esophagus. The reflux event occurs as discreet drops in intraesophageal pH, in association with transient LES relaxation [3], rather than a continuous pH fall, as would be the case if the acid reflux were to be occurring due to the wick-like effect.

The third possibility, whether a manometry catheter can induce transient LES relaxation, has recently been explored. Transient LES relaxation is an eponym given to a unique event in the LES that is frequently associated with acid reflux [3]. Normally, the LES can relax in response to either swallowing, which is initiated through the pharyngeal receptors and is accompanied by a peristaltic contraction in the esophagus, or alternatively, through distention in the esophagus caused either by a bolus or a balloon. The swallow-induced LES relaxation is 6—9 s long and is almost never associated with reflux events. The third type of LES relaxation is transient LES relaxation. It is usually 5—45 s in duration, is not associated with a swallow event and is frequently seen in association with acid reflux. Transient LES relaxation occurs in the awake state and ceases during sleep.

Transient LES relaxation is not a local event but is mediated through the central nervous system and the efferent pathway is in the vagus nerve [4]. The afferent receptors which mediate transient LES relaxation may be either in the stomach or pharynx. The stomach receptors are most likely distention sensitive and are located in the fundus or the lesser curvature of the stomach close to the cardia. The receptors in the pharynx are sensitive to mechanical stimulation. One possibility that has recently been explored is whether the mechanical irritation of the pharynx by manometry catheter can induce transient LES relaxation. We recently conducted a study where LES pressure was recorded through a manometry catheter placed via a gastrostomy tube into the esophagus [5]. The rationale was that, by eliminating the manometry catheter from the pharynx, does the frequency of transient LES relaxation change? The LES monitoring was performed with the catheter placed via the

Table 1. The frequency of transient LES relaxation under two circumstances (without a manometry catheter in the pharynx and with a manometry catheter in the pharynx)

	Catheter in	Catheter out	t	p
Complete transient relaxations	5.4 ± 1.5	1.6 ± 1.4	3.60	0.015
Total transient LES relaxations	6.4 ± 2.2	2.0 ± 1.1	3.56	0.016

gastrostomy tube into the esophagus and LES. In the same subjects, the frequency of transient LES relaxation was determined by placing an additional catheter, that rested in the nose and pharynx (Table 1).

The data show that there is a marked increase in the frequency of complete as well as incomplete transient LES relaxation when there was a catheter in the pharynx. This lends support to the hypothesis that a catheter placed across the pharynx increases the frequency of transient LES relaxation. Since these transient LES relaxations are the mechanism of gastroesophageal reflux in normal subjects as well as patients with esophagitis, a tube in the pharynx may increase the frequency of acid reflux by increasing the frequency of transient LES relaxation. It is likely that increase in the frequency of acid reflux, observed after a nasogastric catheter [6], is not due to either the wick-like effect of the catheter or the effect of the tube across the LES on the basal sphincter tone, rather it is due to the effect of the manometry catheter in the pharynx on the transient LES relaxation.

The effect of the size of a catheter in the pharynx on the frequency of transient LES relaxation is not known. The manometry catheters are usually 3–5 mm in diameter. The pH probe is usually smaller, 1–2.5 mm in diameter. Whether the size of the pH probe is enough to induce mechanical irritation in the pharynx, and then, induce transient LES relaxation, is not known. However, I think it is not an unlikely possibility. If this indeed were to be the situation, it may explain the relative high frequency of acid reflux episodes recorded during prolonged pH monitoring in normal healthy subjects. This observation could also account for the large overlap in acid exposure times recorded during esophageal pH monitoring in control subjects and patients with reflux disease [7].

References

1. Biancani P, Zabinski MP, Behar J. Pressure, tension, and force of closure of the human lower esophageal sphincter and esophagus. J Clin Invest 1975;56.476–483.
2. Fisher RS, Malmud LS, Roberts GS et al. Gastroesophageal (GE) scintiscanning to detect and quantitate GE reflux. Gastroenterology 1976;70:301–308.
3. Holloway RH, Dent J. Pathophysiology of gastroesophageal reflux: lower esophageal sphincter dysfunction in gastroesophageal reflux disease. Gastroenterol Clin North Am 1990;517–531.
4. Martin CG, Patrikios J, Dent J. Abolition of gas reflux and transient lower esophageal sphincter relaxation by vagal blockade in the dog. Gastroenterology 1986;91:890–896.
5. Mittal RK, Stewart WR, Schirmer BD. Effect of catheter in the pharynx and the frequency of transient lower esophageal sphincter relaxation. Gastroenterology 1992;103:1236–1240.
6. Nagler R, Spiro HM. Persistent gastroesophageal reflux induced during prolonged gastric intubation. N Engl J Med 1963;269:495–500.
7. Schlesinger PK, Donahue PE, Schmid B, Layden T. Limitation of 24-hour intraesophageal pH monitoring in the hospital setting. Gastroenterology 1985;89:797–804.

In what cases is isotopic esophageal scintigraphy highly advisable?

M.K. Ferguson (Chicago)

Scintigraphic techniques for evaluating esophageal function were initially developed by Kazem in 1972 [1] and since that time have been applied to a variety of pathophysiologic states. Esophageal scintigraphy, which was introduced in 1976 [2] as a means to evaluate gastroesophageal reflux (GER), offered the promise of an accurate noninvasive means to diagnose and quantify reflux, but has not been enthusiastically adopted by the medical community. The reasons for this are numerous and include:
— the lack of a standard means for performing and interpreting the tests;
— substantial intrapatient variability in test results; and
— the failure of scintigraphy to achieve a sensitivity similar to that of other tests, particularly esophageal pH monitoring, in diagnosing reflux.
Nevertheless, there are compelling reasons to continue to consider scintigraphy for the evaluation of esophageal function. It provides quantitative data on esophageal transit, exposes patients to only a low dose of irradiation, enables study of the esophagus globally or in segments, and is noninvasive and therefore does not alter typical esophageal function.

Background

Scintigraphic evaluation of patients with suspected gastroesophageal reflux disease (GERD) is performed using two general techniques. The first technique, gastroesophageal scintigraphy, involves ingestion of ^{99m}technetium sulfur colloid in acidified orange juice. Patients are placed supine, followed by scintiscanning of the stomach and esophagus before and during provocation, such as the use of abdominal binders and Valsalva maneuvers. In infants and children, a modification of this technique includes scanning of the lungs to evaluate for pulmonary aspiration of the tracer. Data assessment is performed by eye or with the use of computer-generated time-activity curves. The initial description of this technique demonstrated a sensitivity of 90% [2], but data from subsequent publications have not always substantiated this. Reported sensitivities range from 14–98%, averaging 73% in all patients and 71% in the pediatric population (Table 1) [2–16].

With the second technique, esophageal transit is measured with patients in the supine position beginning with the swallowing of ^{99m}technetium sulfur colloid in 10–20 ml water. A region of interest (ROI) is identified over the distal esophagus or the whole esophagus, and the percentage of esophageal emptying after one or more swallows, and the time required for counts in the region of interest to drop below a specified level are determined. This technique does not measure frequency or quantity

Table 1. Sensitivity of radionuclide studies in diagnosing GER

Author	Year	Patients	Diagnostic reference	Sensitivity (%)
Fisher et al. [2]	1976	30	symptoms	90
Heyman et al. [3]	1979	39[a]	barium study	70
Rudd and Christie [4]	1979	25[a]	symptoms; acid reflux test	80
Arasu et al. [5]	1980	45[a]	acid reflux test	55
Blumhagen et al. [6]	1980	65[a]	acid reflux test	88
Jona et al. [7]	1981	125[a]	symptoms	77
Seibert et al. [8]	1983	47[a]	24-h pH probe	79
Velasco et al. [9]	1984	54	acid reflux test	84
Berger et al. [10]	1985	18[a]	symptoms	44
Fung et al. [11]	1985	51	symptoms; endoscopy	14
Kaul et al. [12]	1986	101	symptoms; endoscopy	98
Gonzalez Fernandez et al. [13]	1987	90[a]	symptoms	92
Babic et al [14]	1990	54	symptoms; endoscopy	85
Tolia et al. [15]	1990	69[a]	24-h pH probe	65
Vandenplas et al. [16]	1992	65[a]	pH probe	33

[a]Pediatric patients.

of GER but assesses the nonspecific disruption of normal motility which often accompanies acid reflux. Representative reports demonstrate that the prevalence of abnormal transit ranges from 17–92%, averaging 58% (Table 2) [17–24].

Given the large number of children and adults who develop symptoms of GERD and the relatively low diagnostic accuracy of gastroesophageal scintiscanning, the routine use of this radionuclide technique as an initial screening tool in symptomatic individuals is not cost effective. Similarly, the routine assessment of esophageal motility in patients with proven GERD is currently best performed using manometric techniques, despite the high percentage of patients who have abnormal transit as determined by esophageal scintigraphy.

Possible indications for scintigraphic studies

Although the overall accuracy of gastroesophageal scintiscanning is not good when

Table 2. Radionuclide measurement of abnormal esophageal transit in GERD

Author	Year	Patients	Diagnostic reference	Abnormal (%)
Russell et al. [17]	1981	29	acid reflux test; symptoms	52
Ferguson et al. [18]	1985	26	24-h pH probe	87
Van Heukelem et al. [19]	1985	23	24-h pH probe	17
Taillefer et al. [20]	1986	25	24-h pH probe	60
Bartlett et al. [21]	1987	20	endoscopy	55
O'Connor et al. [22]	1988	13	24-h pH probe	54
Taillefer et al. [23]	1990	48	24-h pH probe	92
Eriksen et al. [24]	1991	58	symptoms	46

compared to pH monitoring, radionuclide techniques sometimes may detect reflux episodes other than those recorded by pH probe. Shay et al. performed simultaneous comparisons of postprandial scintigraphy and pH monitoring in patients with endoscopic features of GER and abnormal 24-h pH monitoring. They found that reflux episodes were recorded by both techniques, but that each technique detected unique reflux events [25]. These findings were supported by Tolia et al. who demonstrated poor correlation between pH monitoring and scintigraphy in infants with reflux [15]. Vandenplas et al. also performed simultaneous pH monitoring and scintigraphy in children and found that among 123 separate reflux episodes detected, only six were recorded by both techniques [16].

The results suggest that these two methods of detecting reflux measure different pathophysiologic phenomena and record reflux events under different conditions. There has always been concern that the use of pH as a marker for reflux events is artificially limiting. These studies support the long-held contention that reflux of neutral gastric contents does occur and that acid reflux episodes may be masked when the intraesophageal pH is already low. The two techniques, therefore, are not interchangeable, but may be complimentary in the assessment of GER. Scintigraphy may be particularly useful in patients in whom reflux is suspected on the basis of clinical symptoms but is not detected by standard pH monitoring. Typical patients may include those who are achlorhydric or in whom alkaline duodenogastric reflux occurs, resulting in an intragastric pH that is not always acidic (Table 3).

In addition to gastroesophageal radionuclide studies, scintigraphic measurement of esophageal transit may provide unique information about GER problems, particularly following fundoplication operations. In one of the original reports assessing esophageal transit, Russell et al. demonstrated disordered transit in patients with GERD that persisted following antireflux surgery [17]. This lack of improvement in esophageal transit, even in the presence of normal postoperative manometric studies, has been confirmed by others [22,26]. These data suggest that underlying disorders of esophageal transit and clearance are present in a substantial number of patients with GER and persist despite successful surgical correction of reflux. Crisci et al. have shown that scintigraphic transit abnormalities correlate well with postoperative symptoms of dysphagia even in the presence of normal pH and manometric studies [27]. Esophageal scintigraphy is more sensitive than manometry in the assessment of esophageal motility postoperatively, and may be useful for evaluating patients who are symptomatic following fundoplication surgery (Table 3).

As the above data indicates, measurement of esophageal transit using scintigraphic

Table 3. Suggested indications for scintigraphy in assessing patients with symptoms of GERD

Gastroesophageal scintigraphy
    Gastric achlorhydria
    Duodenogastric reflux

Esophageal transit
    Postoperative dysphagia
    Normal endoscopy and pH monitoring

techniques detects esophageal motor abnormalities in reflux patients more often than do manometric studies. However, the reproducibility of scintigraphy using single swallow techniques has sometimes been questioned. Recent investigations demonstrate that analysis of multiple swallows (one radiolabeled swallow followed by several "dry" swallows) provides better accuracy and substantially reduces intrasubject variability [21,28,29]. Use of this improved methodology may yield even better diagnostic results in the future.

Finally, esophageal scintigraphy has been used to assess patients with typical reflux symptoms but without the expected clinical findings. Eriksen et al. investigated patients with severe reflux symptoms who had normal 24-h esophageal pH monitoring and no evidence of esophagitis at endoscopy [24]. They found that nearly half of the patients had prolonged esophageal transit due to segmental delays, intraesophageal shuttling or nonspecific causes. Possible explanations for these findings include the presence of nonacidic reflux (possibly including alkaline reflux), an increased sensitivity of the esophagus to refluxed material leading to symptoms in the absence of esophagitis, or the irritable esophagus syndrome. Esophageal scintigraphy may be a useful study in these patients, who present a true diagnostic dilemma (Table 3).

Conclusion

Current techniques of scintigraphic assessment of the esophagus are not indicated for routine use in patients with GER. However, these methods appear to provide unique information in select subgroups of patients, that is not available through standard tests such as radiography, manometry and pH studies. This overview summarizes patient subgroups in which scintigraphy may be of value. Additional study is necessary to define more clearly the indications for scintigraphy in the evaluation of GERD.

References

1. Kazem I. A new scintigraphic technique for the study of the esophagus. AJR 1972;115:682–688.
2. Fisher RE, Malmud LS, Roberts GS, Lobis IF. Gastroesophageal (GE) scintiscanning to detect and quantitate GE reflux. Gastroenterology 1976;70:301–308.
3. Heyman S, Kirkpatrick JA, Winter HS, Treves S. An improved method for the diagnosis of gastroesophageal reflux and aspiration in children (milk scan). Radiology 1979;131:479–482.
4. Rudd TG, Christie DL. Demonstration of gastroesophageal reflux in children by radionuclide gastroesophagography. Radiology 1979;131:483–486.
5. Arasu TS, Wyllie R, Fitzgerald JF, Franken EA, Siddiqui AR, Lehman GA, Eigen H, Grosfeld JL. Gastroesophageal reflux in infants and children — comparative accuracy of diagnostic methods. J Pediatr 1980;96:798–803.
6. Blumhagen JD, Rudd TG, Christie DL. Gastroesophageal reflux in children: radionuclide gastroesophagography. AJR 1980; 135:1001–1004.
7. Jona JZ, Sty JR, Glicklich M. Simplified radioisotope technique for assessing gastroesophageal reflux in children. J Pediatr Surg 1981;16:114–117.
8. Seibert JJ, Byrne WJ, Euler AR, Latture T, Leach M, Campbell M. Gastroesophageal reflux — the acid test: scintigraphy or the pH probe? AJR 1983;140:1087–1090.
9. Velasco N, Pope CE II, Gannan RM, Roberts P, Hill LD. Measurement of esophageal reflux by scintigraphy. Dig Dis Sci 1984;29:977–982.
10. Berger G, Bischof-Delaloye A, Reinberg O, Roulet M. Esophageal and pulmonary scintiscanning in gastroesophageal reflux in children. Prog Pediatr Surg 1985;18:68–77.

11. Fung WP, Van der Schaaf A, Grieve JC. Gastroesophageal scintigraphy and endoscopy in the diagnosis of esophageal reflux and esophagitis. Am J Gastroenterol 1985;80:245–247.

12. Kaul B, Halvorsen T, Petersen H, Grette K, Myrvold HE. Gastroesophageal reflux disease. Scintigraphic, endoscopic, and histologic considerations. Scand J Gastroenterol 1986;21:134–138.

13. Gonzalez Fernandez F, Arguelles Martin F, Rodriguez de Quesada B, Gonzalez Hachero J, Sanchez de Puerta AV, Gentles M. Gastroesophageal scintigraphy: a useful screening test for GE reflux. J Pediatr Gastroenterol Nutr 1987;6:217–219.

14. Babic Z, Ugarkovic B, Ivancevic D, Babic D. Dynamic scintigraphy of the oesophagus in the evaluation of reflux oesophagitis. Nucl Med Commun 1990;29:204–209.

15. Tolia V, Calhoun JA, Kuhns LR, Kauffman RE. Lack of correlation between extended pH monitoring and scintigraphy in the evaluation of infants with gastroesophageal reflux. J Lab Clin Med 1990;115:559–563.

16. Vandenplas Y, Derde MP, Piepsz A. Evaluation of reflux episodes during simultaneous esophageal pH monitoring and gastroesophageal reflux scintigraphy in children. J Pediatr Gastroenterol Nutr 1992;14:256–260.

17. Russell COH, Pope CE II, Gannan RM, Allen FD, Velasco N, Hill LD. Does surgery correct esophageal motor dysfunction in gastroesophageal reflux? Ann Surg 1981;194:290–296.

18. Ferguson MK, Ryan JW, Little AG, Skinner DB. Esophageal emptying and acid neutralization in patients with symptoms of esophageal reflux. Ann Surg 1985;201:728–735.

19. Van Heukelem HA, Blom H, Camps JAJ, Gooszen HG, Pauwels EKJ, Biemond I. Assessment of esophageal motility by radionuclide transit studies in patients with reflux esophagitis and a pathologic 24-hour pH study. In: DeMeester TR, Skinner DB (eds) Esophageal Disorders: Pathophysiology and Therapy. New York: Raven Press, 1985;83–86.

20. Taillefer R, Beauchamp G, Duranceau AC, Lafontaine E. Nuclear medicine and esophageal surgery. Clin Nucl Med 1986;11:445–460.

21. Bartlett RJV, Parkin A, Ware FW, Riley A, Robinson PJA. Reproducibility of oesophageal transit studies: several "single swallows" must be performed. Nucl Med Commun 1987;8:317–326.

22. O'Connor MK, Byrne PJ, Keeling P, Hennessy TP. Esophageal scintigraphy: applications and limitations in the study of esophageal disorders. Eur J Nucl Med 1988;14:131–136.

23. Taillefer R, Jadliwalla M, Pellerin E, Lafontaine E, Duranceau A. Radionuclide esophageal transit study in detection of esophageal motor dysfunction: comparison with motility studies (manometry). J Nucl Med 1990;31:1921–1926.

24. Eriksen CA, Cullen PT, Sutton D, Kennedy N, Cuschieri A. Abnormal esophageal transit in patients with typical reflux symptoms but normal endoscopic and pH profiles. Am J Surg 1991;161:657–661.

25. Shay S, Eggli D, Maydonovitch C, Johnson L. Postprandial gastroesophageal reflux event frequency and clearance: a simultaneous comparison of scintigraphy vs. pH monitoring. Gastroenterology 1986;90:1630 (abstract).

26. Maddern GJ, Jamieson GG. Oesophageal emptying in patients with gastro-oesophageal reflux. Br J Surg 1986;73:615–617.

27. Crisci R, De Vincentis N, Pona C, Lococo A, Lenti R, Coloni GF. Scintigraphy, radiology and pH-manometry in patients after antireflux surgery. J Nucl Med Allied Sci 1987;31:303–306.

28. Tatsch K, Schrottle W, Kirsch C-M. Parametric scintigrams of the oesophageal passage of multiple swallows: comparisons of a new method with a standard oesophageal transit test. Nucl Med 1990;29:195–203.

29. Klein HA. Improving esophageal transit scintigraphy (editorial). J Nucl Med 1991;32:1371–1374.

What is the overall planning of functional investigation of a patient with esophagitis?

S. Cohen (Philadelphia)

The investigation of patients with gastroesophageal reflux (GER) depends to a great extent upon the basic question that is to be answered. The investigation must be designed to resolve the specific question, not to address the general problem of GER or esophagitis.

The questions that occur most often are 5-fold:
— Are the symptoms experienced by this patient due to GER?
— Does this patient have esophagitis or any other sequelae of GER?
— Is this patient at high risk form developing a complication of reflux disease?
— Does this patient have an unusual laryngeal or respiratory complication of GER?
— Is this patient a candidate for prolonged medical or surgical therapy?

The five questions can be viewed in three major parts: first, symptom assessment; secondly, determination of disease complications; and thirdly, disease outcome and therapeutic guidelines.

Symptom assessment

The assessment of unusual symptoms beyond the classical symptom of heartburn requires a great number of tests. In this area, prolonged pH reflux testing with concomitant motility studies provides the best direct way of determining the temporal association of symptoms to a specific event (pH or motor). This approach is especially helpful in studying noncardiac chest pain, wheezing, apnea, or hoarseness. In patients with unexplained symptoms standard manometry, provocative tests (Tensilon or acid perfusion), and endoscopy are of value. It is most important to exclude coronary artery disease before seeking an esophageal cause of pain.

In recent years, many clinicians have discovered the inexpensive therapeutic trial of using omeprazole (20 mg b.i.d.) to determine if pain subsides. The follow-up evaluation of a positive or beneficial therapeutic trial has been more difficult to design.

Overall, symptom assessment with current testing has been of great value, leaving very few patients with an uncertain diagnosis of GER.

Evaluation of disease complications or sequelae of gastroesophageal reflux disease

The complications of GER are best evaluated by fiberoptic endoscopy with biopsy. Endoscopy allows one to assess the presence of esophagitis with appropriate grading, stricture, Barrett's metaplasia, and possibly adenocarcinoma. No other study provides the direct evidence of complications as does endoscopy. Barium swallow with air contrast is a reasonable study for stricture assessment or detection of cancer, but is much less sensitive in defining esophagitis and Barrett's metaplasia. In most clinical settings, barium swallow is being abandoned because of the overall superiority of fiberoptic endoscopy with biopsy.

Esophageal manometry is of value in assessing motor disorders that may be associated with esophagitis. This is especially helpful in patients with atypical chest pain or dysphagia.

Disease outcome and therapeutic guidelines

One of the major difficulties in evaluating GER is assessing disease progression and determining whether surgical therapy is indicated. Unfortunately, most diagnostic studies have not been done prospectively in order to determine the factors that lead to complicated disease. Many studies demonstrate the physiological abnormalities seen in each complication, suggesting that these factors contributed to the complication.

The factors that have been implicated as being predictive of complicated disease are:
— Esophagitis (high grade) or other sequelae of reflux at the time of presentation;
— Prolonged acid exposure with upright and supine reflux during 24-h pH monitoring;
— Lower esophageal sphincter (LES) pressure below 5 mmHg;
— Peristaltic abnormalities;
— Scleroderma or mixed connective tissue disease;
— Zollinger-Ellison syndrome.
These findings alone or in combination suggest complicated disease but prospective evaluation of large numbers of patients is not available.

Severity and duration of heartburn or sliding hiatus hernia are not good predictors of disease severity.

The requirement for surgery, based upon complications of disease or physiological measures, is not possible. Indication for surgery is based upon clinical judgement at this time. The overall assessment of the patient with endoscopy and physiological measurements determines this clinical decision.

Summary

The investigation of each patient must be considered on an individual basis. Assessment is based upon the specific question to be answered. Predictors of outcome and choice of therapy are the most difficult questions to resolve at this time.

Alkaline duodenogastric reflux

What factors contribute to alkaline reflux and why?

S.J.M. Kraemer, H.J. Stein, H. Feussner, J.R. Siewert
(Munich)

Reflux of "alkaline" duodenal juice into the stomach is a naturally occurring sporadic event. However, the explanations for this phenomenon are still not satisfactory. Nonetheless, excessive duodenogastric reflux (DGR) is accused of being associated with a variety of symptoms, such as:
— epigastric pain (89%); and
— bilious vomiting (94%) [1].
DGR with intragastric bile collections is heavily disputed as a cause for:
— gastric ulcerations;
— development of antral gastritis;
— atrophic gastritis;
— gastric carcinoma; and
— "alkaline" gastroesophageal reflux (GER) [1–3].
The main components of the alkaline duodenal juice are:
— bile salts;
— activated pancreatic; and
— other intestinal enzymes, which ultimately lead to gastric mucosal barrier damage.
Bile acids, for example, are capable of disrupting the gastric mucosa, allowing back diffusion of hydrogen ions into the stomach wall, initiating one of the pathways to gastritis and ulceration [4,5]. It has been demonstrated that most enzymes are highly

effective — and more harmful — in an almost neutral environment and that the pH does not correlate well with their cell toxicity or the patients pain.

Physiologically, the antropyloroduodenal segment (APD) is an antireflux barrier. This "biosphincter" nevertheless allows, as an intermittent sporadic natural event, "physiologic" DGR in fasting and fed states, primarily occurring postprandial and during the early morning hours (in the supine position). The physiologic process presumably turns pathologic when the exposure time of the duodenal juice to the gastric mucosa is extended as a result of dysmotility of the APD and an anatomically intact, but increasingly incompetent pylorus. As a result, the refluxed duodenal juice has a prolonged contact time with the gastric mucosa, caused by:
— frequent reflux episodes;
— insufficient gastric clearance; or
— diminished gastric secretion [6].

Secondary and probably more frequent factors for intractable symptoms of DGR due to inadequate biliary drainage, like pain and bilious vomiting, are postoperative situations after:
— vagotomies (?);
— pyloroplasties;
— distal gastric resections with Billroth I or II reconstructions; and
— total gastrectomies with the resection of the lower esophageal sphincter (LES) [7–13].

Excessive DGR may also occur in patients with previous biliary surgery or cholecystectomy [14,15], probably due to an increased and steady flow of bile into the duodenum. Yet the relation of cause and effect is still unclear. In the discussion are:
— the absence of a bile reservoir;
— pooling of bile in the duodenum;
— an incriminated duodenal motility;
— alteration of the normal anatomy;
— changes in neurohormonal reactions on gastrin, cholecystokinin (CCK) and others.

In patients with general systemic disorders and intestinal motility disorders, DGR is not an uncommon phenomenon (e.g., in scleroderma or diabetes) [16].

Finally, DGR may occur in patients with small or large bowel obstructions and in those patients suffering from intra-abdominal benign or, more commonly, malignant tumors or tumor recurrences. Tumor growth either leads to a mechanical obstruction of the gut, which ultimately results in DGR and finally GER, or the intra-abdominal pressure increases with the increasing volume of the tumor, thus leading to DGR or alkaline or mixed gastroesophageal reflux disease (GERD). A similar cause can be found in women with both forms of temporary reflux disease during pregnancy.

The discussion about the phenomenon of "alkaline DGR" after previous gastric or biliary surgery and also the dispute concerning "alkaline" esophagitis, which frequently seems to be one of the sequelae of prolonged excessive DGR, are still very controversial.

Acid or biliary GERD may lead to such complications as heartburn, esophagitis, ulceration, dysphagia, stricture, upper GI-bleeding, Barrett's esophagus and cancer.

GERD is the most common disorder of the upper gastrointestinal tract in humans. It accounts for significant morbidity, which may be as high as 50% in the affected patient population [17,18]. A large body of experimental and clinical evidence demonstrates that GERD results from a partial or complete loss of the gastroesophageal antireflux barrier (GEARB):

— loss of the gastroesophageal valve mechanism (GEV);
— a nonfunctioning lower esophageal sphincter (LES);
— a compromised esophageal clearance function; and the
— exposure of the esophageal mucosa to refluxed gastric contents;

have been identified as predisposing factors to the development of these complications [19–21].

As part of the standard acid reflux testing (SART), acid GER is measured routinely by pH-testing with an H^+ ion sensitive antimony or glass probe. However, refluxed gastric juice may contain alkaline duodenal contents, lipophilic bile salts, lysolecithin and activated pancreatic and other intestinal enzymes, of which all also promote esophageal mucosal injury in patients with GERD [20,22,23]. These combined forms of acidic and alkaline reflux are frequently found in patients with severe intractable GERD [24].

These cases of alkaline or mixed GER are extremely hard to assess so far, since pH-testing has its limitations in the alkaline environment [25]. It has often been discussed that the "alkaline" reading on the pH-probe is due to saliva coming down into the stomach. If bile salts and enzymes are actually identified, one can say that there is alkaline or mixed reflux present.

The problem of measuring alkaline reflux is not a problem of measuring (OH–) groups, but it is a problem of a direct analysis of the quality and quantity of the components of the refluxed alkaline or mixed alkaline/acid duodenogastric juice. With new methods like the ambulatory 24-h reflux aspiration test, in combination with the high performance liquid column chromatography (HPLC), new standards are being developed [7,16].

Conclusions

"Alkaline" reflux — per se — is not the villain. It is rather the excessive DGR and GERD with its bile salts, activated pancreatic and other intestinal enzymes, which can exist in an acid environment and are more harmful and which seem to be responsible for a number of symptoms and histological changes in the foregut.

Whereas a dysfunctional or destroyed antroduodenal segment is an absolute precondition for DGR, alkaline or mixed GER is due to a combination of the presence of excessive DGR and a partial or complete loss of the GEARB. If GER is stopped by creating an adequate GEARB with a good antireflux repair, then alkaline GER is corrected as well.

A prevention or reduction of postoperative DGR can best be achieved by an adequate biliary drainage operation, preferably — according to experience — a Roux en Y derivation procedure.

References

1. Ritchie WP. Alkaline reflux gastritis: late results on a controlled trial of diagnosis and treatment. Ann Surg 1986; 203:537—544.
2. Ritchie WP. Alkaline gastritis: a critical reappraisal. Gut 1984;25:975—987.
3. Lawson HH. Effect of duodenal contents on the gastric mucosa under experimental conditions. Lancet 1964;1:469—472.
4. Davenport HW. Destruction of the gastric mucosal barrier by detergents and urea. Gastroenterology 1968;54:175.
5. Pazzi P, Scalia S, Stabellini G, Trevisani L, Alvisi V, Guarneri M. Bile reflux gastritis in patients without prior gastric surgery: Therapeutic effects of ursodeoxycholic acid. Curr Ther Res 1989;45(3):476—487.
6. Welch NT. Diagnosis and treatment of duodenogastric reflux. In: Nyhus LM, Hinder RA (eds) Problems in General Surgery, vol 9, 1st edn. Philadelphia: J.B. Lippincott, 1992;1:184—194.
7. Feussner H, Weiser HF, Liebermann-Meffert D, Siewert JR. Intestino-ösophagealer reflux nach gastrektomie. Wirkungsmechanismus und effektivität der oesophagojejunoplicatio. Chirurg 1988;59:665—669.
8. Gillison EW, De Castro VAM, Nyhus LM, Kusakari K, Bombeck CT. The significance of bile in reflux esophagitis. Surg Gynecol Obstet 1972;134:419—424.
9. Morrow D, Passaro ER Jr. Alkaline reflux esophagitis after total gastrectomy. Am J Surg 1976;132:287—291.
10. Nier H, Wienbeck M, Berges W, Kremer K. Syndrome nach gastrektomie unter besonderer berücksichtigung der refluxösophagitis. Langenbecks Arch Chir 1983;360:71—80.
11. Matikainen M, Laatikainen T, Kalima T, Kivilaakso E. Bile acid composition and esophagitis after total gastrectomy. Am J Surg 1982;143:196—198.
12. Cabrol J, Navarro X, Sancho J, Simo-Deu J, Segura R. Bile reflux in postoperative alkaline reflux gastritis. Ann Surg 1989;211(2):239—243.
13. Spychal RT, Savalgi RS, Marrero JM, Saverymuttu SH, Kirkham JS, Northfield TC. Thermodynamic effects of bile acids in the stomach. Gastroenterology 1990;99:305—310.
14. Brown TH, Walton G, Cheadle WG, Larson GM. The alkaline shift in gastric pH after cholecystectomy. Am J Surg 1989; 157:58—65.
15. Warshaw AL. Bile gastritis without prior surgery: contributing role of cholecystectomy. Am J Surg 1979;137:527—531.
16. Feussner H. Öesophageale refluxkrankheit: Qualitative und quantitative refluatanalyse. Klinische Bedeutung des "Nicht-Sauren" Refluxes. Habilitationsschrift, Medizinische Fakultät, Technische Universität, München, 1992.
17. Hill LD, Aye RW, Ramel SO. Antireflux surgery. A surgeon's look. Gastroenterol Clin N Am 1990;19:745—775.
18. DeMeester TR, Stein HJ. Gastroesophageal reflux disease. In: Moody FG, Carey LC, Jones RC, Kelly KA, Nahrwold DL, Skinner DB (eds) Surgical Treatment of Digestive Disease, 2nd edn. Chicago: Year Book Medical Publishers, 1989; 65—108.
19. Thor KBA, Hill LD, Mercer CD, Kozarek RA. Reappraisal of the flap valve mechanism: a study of a new valvuloplasty procedure in cadavers. Acta Chir Scand 1987;153:25—28.
20. Stein HJ, Barlow AP, DeMeester TR, Hinder RA. Complications of gastroesophageal reflux disease: Role of the lower esophageal sphincter, esophageal acid/alkaline exposure and duodenogastric reflux. Ann Surg 1992;216:35—43.
21. Bremner RM, Crookes PF, DeMeester TR, Peters J, Stein HJ. Concentration of refluxed acid and mucosal injury. Am J Surg 1992;164:522—527.
22. Bateson MC, Hopwood D, Milno G. Oesophageal epithelial ultrastructure after incubation with gastrointestinal fluids and their components. J Pathol 1981;133:33—38.
23. Johnson LF, Harmon JW. Experimental esophagitis in a rabbit model. J Clin Gastroenterol 1986;8(suppl):26—44.
24. Lin KM, Ueda RK, Hinder RA, Stein HJ, DeMeester TR. Etiology and importance of alkaline esophageal reflux. Am J Surg 1991;162:553—557.
25. Mittal RK, Reuben A, Whitney JO, McCallum RW. Do bile acids reflux into the esophagus? A study in normal subjects and patients with gastroesophageal reflux disease. Gastroenterology 1987;92(2):371—375.

Can low oxygen tension levels mimic alkaline reflux?

L. Tibbling, U. Gustafsson, F. Sjöberg (Linköping)

The concentration of bile in the esophagus has been found to be 15–2,330 µmol/l in patients from whom bile-stained fluid had been aspirated at esophageal endoscopy [1]. The pH of this bile-stained fluid ranged from 1.5–7.8 units. In patients with acid gastroesophageal reflux (GER), the fasting total gastric bile content has been found to range from 0 to 940 µmol/l [2]. From these data, it would seem unlikely that a pH of more than 8 units exists in the esophagus, even if the gastric refluxate contains high levels of bile.

False pH values

Since the introduction of antimony electrodes for esophageal pH monitoring, pH values of 8.0, and more, have often been recorded and sometimes even claimed to be due to alkaline reflux. The difference in results between different laboratories with regard to normal 24-h pH patterns made us investigate if the antimony electrodes may give false high pH values [3]. So, for instance, the upper normal limit for the time that pH values are below 4.0 during a 24-h period in the esophagus was set at 1.0% in healthy adults by Johansson et al. [4], and at 1.2% in children and adolescents by Gustafsson and Tibbling [5], both groups using antimony electrodes. In the study by Johnson and DeMeester [6], glass electrodes were used and the normal value was set at 4.2% or below. A study by Sjöberg et al. [3] in 52 patients with suspected GER showed that the esophageal pH, as measured with antimony electrodes, was higher than 8.0 for 7% of the time (range 0–60%).

Glass and antimony electrodes

Several factors other than pH are known to affect the corrosion potential of antimony electrodes. Among these, the effect of oxygen is the most important, and it has even been shown that antimony electrodes can be used for the measurement of tissue oxygen tension [7]. By placing glass electrodes and antimony electrodes at the same esophageal level simultaneously, the oxygen influence on the antimony electrodes was calculated as the difference between pH values of glass and antimony electrodes. It was found that antimony electrodes gave higher pH values due to decreased oxygen tension levels during night-time esophageal inactivity as well as in older people [8]. An increase in oxygen tension was seen during eating and when acid reflux caused irritation of the esophageal mucosa. When comparing antimony and glass electrodes [3], the values recorded by antimony electrodes were found to be 2.1 ± 0.8 pH units higher than by glass electrodes (p < 0.001).

It is concluded that the diagnosis of alkaline reflux seems to be valid only when pH monitoring is performed with glass electrodes or when values obtained with antimony electrodes are adjusted for the influence of the oxygen tension in the esophagus. In addition, our biomedical engineering department is developing an antimony electrode capable of differentiating pH and oxygen tension.

References

1. Stoker DL, Williams JG, Dewar EP, Colin-Jones DG. The pH and concentration of bile in the oesophagus. Gut 1988;128: 728–729.
2. Smith MR, Buckton GK, Bennett JR. Bile acid levels in stomach and oesophagus of patients with acid gastro-oesophageal reflux. Gut 1984;26:A556.
3. Sjöberg F, Gustafsson U, Tibbling L. Alkaline oesophageal reflux — an artefact due to oxygen corrosion of antimony pH electrodes. Scand J Gastroenterol 1992;27:1084–1088.
4. Johansson KE, Boeryd B, Fransson SG, Tibbling L. Oesophageal reflux tests, manometry, endoscopy, biopsy and radiology in healthy subjects. Scand J Gastroenterol 1986;21:399–406.
5. Gustafsson PM, Tibbling L. 24-hour oesophageal two-level pH monitoring in healthy children and adolescents. Scand J Gastroenterol 1988;23:91–94.
6. Johnson LF, DeMeester TR. Twenty-four hour pH monitoring of the distal esophagus: a quantitative measure of gastro esophageal reflux. Am J Gastroenterol 1974;62:325–332.
7. Sjöberg F, Thorborg P, Wranne B, Lund N. Oxygen sensitivity of a multichannel antimony electrode for tissue surface oxygen pressure measurements. Microcirc Endothel Lymphatics 1990;6:127–148.
8. Tibbling L, Sjöberg F. Variations in esophageal oxygen tension measured with intraluminal antimony electrodes. Dysphagia (accepted for publication).

What would justify making a positive diagnosis of alkaline reflux?

R.K. Mittal (Charlottesville)

The duodenal secretions have an alkaline pH which is due to the bicarbonate secreted by the duodenal mucosa and secretions from the liver and pancreas. In an experimental situation, perfusion of the esophagus with pancreatico-biliary secretions can induce mucosal inflammation and esophagitis. Based on this observation and case reports of the presence of esophagitis in patients with pernicious anemia, who do not have acid in the stomach, investigators have been led to believe that alkaline pancreatico-duodenal contents can reflux back into the esophagus, and induce esophagitis. Several investigators have indicated that even those patients who have acid in their stomach may reflux pancreatico-biliary secretion along with or in between acid reflux episodes and exacerbate the noxious potential of the refluxate material. There are three important questions that are relevant to this area: 1) can the pancreatico-biliary secretion injure the esophagus; 2) do pancreatico-biliary secretions reflux all the way back into the esophagus in the human setting; and 3) is the concentration of bile salts and trypsin in the esophageal refluxate high enough to induce mucosal injury?

In the acute experimental animals, it appears that bile salts in concentrations of 3–5 mM range or larger in the presence or absence of HCl can induce significant esophagitis [1,2]. Taurine and glycine conjugate of bile salts potentiate the HCl in inducing esophagitis, because they can remain in the solution at low pH. However, most of the animal studies are acute studies and do not provide data on the minimal concentration needed to induce esophagitis, if the esophagus were to be exposed to it on a chronic basis.

Do pancreatico-biliary secretions indeed reflux all the way back into the esophagus in enough concentrations to induce mucosal damage? The investigators have attempted to answer this question with the following methodology: 1) measuring esophageal pH — it is suggested that an esophageal pH of >7 represents reflux of pancreatico-biliary material into the esophagus [3]; 2) nuclear imaging of the radio labeled bile acid in the stomach [4]; 3) aspiration of esophageal refluxate material and its analysis for the presence of bile acids; and 4) measurement of bilirubin in the esophagus using a bili-probe, the rationale being that if bilirubin was present in the esophagus, then other pancreatico-biliary secretions must be present as well.

Does an esophageal pH of >7 represent reflux of pancreatico-biliary secretions into the esophagus? The pH of the pancreatico-biliary and duodenal secretions is 7.5–8.0. Therefore, intuitively, it seems correct that if the pH in the esophagus was above 7, it could represent pancreatico-biliary secretions. However, the major problem with this supposition is that it assumes that there are no other secretions in the esophagus that may have a pH of >7. It is clear that the pH of saliva is 7.5–8.0. In addition, esophageal mucosal glands may secrete bicarbonate that could make esophageal pH close to 7.5–8.0. Therefore, an esophageal pH of >7 could represent one of three things: 1) saliva in the esophagus; 2) esophageal secretions; or 3) pancreatico-biliary secretions. It is impossible to differentiate between the three materials just based on the esophageal pH measurement alone [5]. The other argument that makes the pH > 7 as representative of pancreatico-biliary secretions less likely is that pancreatico secretions must pass through the stomach in order to reach the esophagus. Gastric pH is usually 1.0–2.0 and it is more than likely that the duodenal secretions are quickly acidified as they enter into the stomach.

Can radionuclide studies document biliary bile reflux into the esophagus? The bile salt pool can be labeled by ingestion of bile acid isotope, which can subsequently be aspirated from the gastric lumen and measured. Cholescintigraphy, employing intra-venous radio isotope that is secreted into the bile, can also demonstrate duodenogas-tric reflux. The isotope can be measured by γ-cameras positioned on the abdomen. Using these techniques, one can document duodenogastric reflux in the postsurgical stomachs. A newly developed technology involves a γ-detector which is small enough to be passed into the gastric lumen for detection of radiolabeled bile acids. These studies can qualitatively document gastroduodenal bile reflux in a variety of patho-logical states, and in about 10% of the normals. However, none of these techniques are sensitive enough to be able to demonstrate reflux of bile salts in the esophagus.

The direct demonstration of esophageal reflux of bile requires esophageal aspiration and quantification of bile salts through one of the bile acid assays [6,7]. The esophageal refluxate can be collected via a salem sump tube positioned proximal to the gastroesophageal junction. Since the reflux is an intermittent and unpredictable phenomenon, continuous aspiration over prolonged periods is required to capture the esophageal refluxate material. The esophageal refluxate can then be analyzed for the presence of bile acids through either the enzymatic assay (3 α-hydroxy steroid dehydrogenaze), or liquid chromatography, or mass spectrometry. The type of assay used is important because the enzymatic assay, even though sensitive, can produce false positive results. High performance liquid chromatography (HPLC), even though less commonly reported, is fairly sensitive (detection range of 10–20 µM) and a specific assay. Similarly, the liquid ion mass spectrometry, again, is fairly sensitive and specific for detection of bile acids.

There are a total of seven studies, including a total of 159 patients, in which the bile salts in the esophageal refluxate were analyzed. The majority of these studies were on patients with an intact stomach. Of the patients, 36% had no bile salts detected in the esophagus, and only 13% of the patients had bile salt concentrations of >200 µM. Of the control subjects, 93% had no bile salts detected, and the highest concentration recorded was 40 µM. One reason that the concentrations of bile in the esophageal refluxate are small may be because of an inherent problem in the aspiration methodology to collect the esophageal samples. Esophageal refluxate obtained by continuous esophageal aspiration is likely to contain swallowed saliva, which can cause dilution of the refluxed material. Some investigators have made an attempt to aspirate the saliva from the mouth in order to prevent mixing of the saliva with the esophageal refluxate. However, even with the most compulsive oral suctioning, some saliva is bound to trickle down the esophagus and dilute the esophageal samples significantly.

If we assume that the bile salt concentrations in the refluxate, reported in these studies, are true, then these concentrations are similar to plasma concentration of bile acid. These concentrations are generally 100–1,000 times lower than those used in experimental models of bile esophagitis. It is highly unlikely that these small concentrations of bile salts can induce damage, at least in an acute situation. Whether these small concentrations over prolonged periods of time can induce esophagitis or potentiate HCl acid remains to be seen.

Recently, Champion et al. [8] have used a bilitec 2000 probe (Synectics, Inc.) to identify the presence of bilirubin as a marker of pancreatico-biliary reflux in the esophagus. These authors found that when using bilirubin as a marker of alkaline reflux, esophageal pH of >7 correlated poorly with duodenogastric reflux. Bilirubin reflux correlated highly with the acid reflux. In other words, no bilirubin was detected in the esophagus when the esophageal pH was >7, suggesting that bile acid reflux occurs in the esophagus in the acidic and not in the alkaline environment. However, this technique cannot provide the quantitative data regarding the concentration of bile acids in the esophagus and cannot answer the questions whether significant concentrations of bile salts capable of inducing mucosal damage do indeed reflux into the esophagus.

I feel that a positive diagnosis of biliary reflux would require direct demonstration of bile acid and trypsin in the esophageal refluxate. Furthermore, these substances should be present in enough concentration to induce mucosal damage. Two things that can unequivocally establish the role of pancreatico-biliary reflux in reflux disease would be: 1) the development of a bile probe, very similar to a pH or bilirubin probe, that can sit in the esophagus and indicate not only the qualitative but quantitative aspects of the pancreatico-biliary reflux; or 2) I think inhibition of bile acids and trypsin in the esophagus with specific pharmaceutical agents, along the lines similar to inhibition of acid, may indirectly indicate the true role of the bile salts and pancreatic enzymes in the pathogenesis of reflux disease. Unfortunately, neither the bile acid probe nor the pharmaceutical substances for neutralization of the bile and trypsin in the esophagus are on the horizon in the immediate future. Therefore, determination of the true role of pancreatico-biliary reflux in reflux esophagitis will have to wait.

References

1. Harmon JW, Johnson LF, Maydonovitch CL. Effect of acid and bile salts on the rabbit esophageal mucosa. Dig Dis Sci 1981;26:65—72.
2. Salo J, Kivilaakso E. Role of bile acid salts and trypsin in the pathogenesis of experimental esophagitis. J Surg 1983;93:525—532.
3. Pellegrini CA, DeMeester TR, Wernly JA, Johnson LF, Skinner DB. Alkaline gastroesophageal reflux. Am J Surg 1978; 135:177—184.
4. Eriksson B, Emas S, Jacobsson H, Larsson SA, Samuelsson K. Comparison of gastric aspiration and HIDA scintigraphy in detecting fasting duodenogastric bile reflux. Scand J Gastroenterol 1988;23:607—610.
5. Singh S, Bradley LA, Richter JE. Determinants of esophageal alkaline "pH environment in a control and patients with gastroesophageal reflux disease". Gastroenterology 1992;102:A166.
6. Mittal RK, Reuben A, Whitney JO, McCallum RW. Do bile acids reflux into the esophagus?: A study in normal subjects and patients with reflux esophagitis. Gastroenterology 1987;92:371—375.
7. Gotley DC, Morgan AP, Ball D, Owen RW, Cooper MJ. Composition of gastro-oesophageal refluxate. Gut 1991;32:1093—1099.
8. Champion G, Singh S, Bechi P, Richter JE. Duodenal gastric reflux: relationship to esophageal pH in response to omeprazole. Gastroenterology 1993;104—A51.

Are there histologic changes in esophagus and stomach indicative of alkaline reflux?

T.C. Smyrk (Omaha)

Duodenal contents refluxed into the stomach produce chemical gastritis. Histologic markers of chemical gastritis include elongation and tortuosity of gastric pits (foveolar hyperplasia), mucosal congestion and edema, prominence of mucosal smooth muscle fibers, and paucity of inflammation. The histology is distinctive but not specific; similar changes result from mucosal injury by nonsteroidal anti-inflammatory drugs (NSAIDs), alcohol, and probably other agents as well.

Histological abnormalities of the gastric mucosa are common after gastric operations, and the best descriptions of reflux gastritis come from studies of postgastrectomy subjects. Chronic superficial gastritis, chronic atrophic gastritis and active gastritis have all been described in one or more studies, but foveolar hyperplasia is the most consistent finding. The surface epithelium is often slightly flattened and depleted of mucin, resulting in a "regenerative" appearance that may be mistaken for dysplasia by the unwary pathologist. At least three studies of post-gastrectomy gastritis have shown regression of foveolar hyperplasia after bile diversion, suggesting that the mucosal changes do in fact reflect bile reflux injury. [1–3].

Dixon studied the relationship between foveolar hyperplasia and postgastrectomy alkaline reflux in the 1986 paper "Reflux Gastritis: Marked Distinct Histopathologic Entity?" [4]. He made the important observation that inflammation need not accompany the other changes of reflux gastritis. Dixon warned that foveolar hyperplasia does not invariably accompany alkaline reflux and that foveolar hyperplasia is not specific for alkaline reflux, but concluded that the combination of foveolar hyperplasia and paucity of inflammation is highly suggestive of reflux gastritis in the postoperative stomach.

The nonspecificity of foveolar hyperplasia as a marker of reflux gastritis is particularly apparent when histologic criteria are applied outside the postgastrectomy setting. Dixon's group recently studied a series of biopsied patients with intact stomachs [5]. Ninety-one biopsies were histologically normal and 47 were classified as "reflux gastritis" on the basis of foveolar hyperplasia. (Patients with other diagnoses were excluded from further analysis.) The reflux gastritis group was significantly more likely to be using NSAIDs. Only one patient in the study had high bile acid concentrations in the stomach; that patient did have reflux gastritis on gastric biopsy. The authors concluded that the histologic features of "reflux gastritis" might better be termed "chemical gastritis", and that, in the intact stomach, such changes are much more likely to be related to NSAIDs than alkaline reflux.

Our own work in patients with intact stomachs and symptoms suggestive of alkaline reflux has given similar results [6]. We studied 73 patients with symptoms of alkaline reflux who underwent ^{99m}Tc HIDA scan, 24-h gastric pH monitoring, and endoscopy with gastric biopsy [6]. The sensitivity and specificity of foveolar hyperplasia for alkaline reflux were 45% and 74%, when reflux was defined as either a positive ^{99m}Tc HIDA scan or positive pH study. The false positive diagnoses were made in patients who were using NSAIDs.

Dixon clarified the histology of alkaline reflux gastritis (and chemical gastritis from any cause) by emphasizing the fact that inflammation need not accompany the process. He did, however, acknowledge that inflammation may be present. In my experience, the inflammation that sometimes accompanies chemical gastritis is distinctive. It consists of active inflammation in the form of neutrophils localized to the lamina propria. This is distinctly different from the active inflammation that accompanies *Helicobacter pylori* infection, in which the neutrophils are localized to the epithelial cells in gastric pits and the mucous neck region of gastric glands. In our study of alkaline reflux gastritis, the sensitivity of biopsy was 75% if a positive biopsy was considered to be foveolar hyperplasia or foveolar hyperplasia with active gastritis.

In summary, I prefer the term "chemical gastritis", as proposed by Dixon, to describe biopsies with foveolar hyperplasia, mucosal congestion and edema and prominence of smooth muscle fibers in the lamina propria. The presence of acute inflammation in the lamina propria does not prevent a diagnosis of chemical gastritis; instead, I use the diagnosis "foveolar hyperplasia with active gastritis". Whether the diagnosis is chemical gastritis or foveolar hyperplasia with active gastritis, I add a comment to the effect that the condition probably reflects mucosal injury due to NSAIDs, alcohol or bile reflux.

The esophagus has a limited repertoire of responses to injury, and I know of no histologic marker specific for alkaline reflux esophagitis. There is abundant animal evidence that duodenal juice is more injurious to esophageal mucosa than gastric juice [7]. Some human studies have suggested that duodenal gastric reflux with subsequent esophageal reflux is important to the development of reflux esophagitis [8]. Our own work with Barrett's esophagus has indicated that complicated Barrett's esophagus (stricture, ulcer, dysplasia) is more likely than uncomplicated Barrett's to be associated with duodenal gastroesophageal reflux [9]. We pursued the idea that the presence of Paneth cells in Barrett's esophagus might indicate alkaline reflux, but there was no correlation between that histologic feature and clinical markers of alkaline reflux (unpublished data).

In summary, no study has shown histologic features of esophageal injury that are suggestive of alkaline reflux.

References

1. Mosimann F, Sorgi M, Wolderson RL et al. Gastric histology and its relationship to enterogastric reflux after duodenal ulcer surgery. Scand J Gastroenterol 1984;19(suppl 92):142.
2. Bechi P, Amorosi A, Mazzanti R et al. Short-term effects of bile diversion on postgastrectomy gastric histology. Dig Dis Sci 1988;33:1288.
3. Hollands MJ, Filipe I, Edwards S et al. Clinical and histological sequelae of Roux-en-Y diversion. Br J Surg 1989;76:481.
4. Dixon MS, O'Connor HJ, Axon ATR, King RFG, Johnston D. Reflux gastritis: Distinct histopathological entity? J Clin Pathol 1986;39:524.
5. Sobala GM, King RFG, Axon ATR, Dixon MF. Reflux gastritis in the intact stomach. J Clin Pathol 1990;43:303.
6. Rouse J, Stein HJ, DeMeester TR, Hinder RA, Smyrk TC. Gastric biopsy in the diagnosis of alkaline reflux gastritis. Mod Pathol 1990;3:86A.
7. Lillemoe KD, Johnson LF, Harmon JW. Alkaline esophagitis: A comparison of the ability of components of gastroduodenal contents to injure a rabbit's esophagus. Gastroenterology 1983;85:621–628.
8. Giacosa A, Bocchini R, Molinari F. Reflux esophagitis and duodenal gastric reflux. Scand J Gastroenterol 1981;16(suppl 67):115.
9. Attwood SEA, DeMeester TR, Bremner CG, Barlow AP, Hinder RA. Alkaline gastroesophageal reflux: Implications in the development of complications in Barrett's columnar-lined lower esophagus. Surgery 1989;106:764–770.

Can the action of taurocholate be precised by means of histochemistry?

J.A. Salo (Helsinki)

Reflux esophagitis has also been observed in conditions where hydrochloride acid secreted by the stomach is lacking, or is quantitatively very slight. Such conditions ensue, for example, total gastrectomy, extensive gastric resection or pernicious anemia. In addition patients with acidic stomachs, who have severe reflux disease, often have periods of alkaline reflux diagnosed in esophageal pH-monitoring [1].

The pathogenesis of this alkaline reflux esophagitis is different from acid reflux and different secretions of the gastrointestinal track are responsible for its development. In the presence of gastric acid pepsin, conjugated bile salts and lysolecithin are the offending agents in the refluxed material that are responsible for the esophageal mucosal damage [2]. Under nonacidic or alkaline conditions bacterial colonization of the upper gastrointestinal tract occurs. The colonizing flora usually includes bacteria capable of deconjugating bile salts. Experimentally, it has been shown that deconjugated bile salts, such as deoxycholate and chenodeoxycholate, as well as the conjugated bile salt taurodeoxycholate, are the injurious agents under these conditions. In addition pancreatic enzymes, trypsin and lipase, can cause significant esophageal mucosal damage [3–6].

Quantitatively, the most important bile salts are cholate and chenodeoxycholate, which together comprise almost 80% of the whole bile salt pool. Conjugated bile salts, especially taurine conjugates, remain soluble even at relatively low pH. Taurocholate, having pKa = 1.8, is the most soluble bile salt in acid solution. In clinical reflux esophagitis conjugated bile salts, especially glycochenodeoxycholate and taurocholate, are detected in the esophagus of most patients, and may play a role in the pathogenesis of reflux esophagitis in patients with nocturnal gastroesophageal reflux [7]. Morphologically, in electron-microscopic studies, taurocholate affects primarily cell membranes and intracellular organelles and later causes the detachment of cells from esophageal mucosa, whereas pepsin digests intercellular substances, causing detachment of epithelial cells. The presence of acid in itself does not affect the quality of esophageal mucosal damage. The action of pepsin, taurocholate and deoxycholate can be examined by histochemistry. In an experimental situation, distinct uptake of antinuclear antibodies and trypan blue can be observed in esophagi perfused by deoxycholate [8]. The effect of taurocholate may be similar. In contrast, no uptake of trypan blue or antinuclear antibodies has been observed in esophagi perfused with pepsin and HCl.

In clinical reflux esophagitis the esophageal mucosal damage is caused by multifactorial pathogenetic mechanism. Therefore, the morphological damage caused by the individual agent, i.e., taurocholate, is very difficult to study. Under nonacidic or alkaline conditions the effect of taurocholate in esophageal mucosa is very weak [9], and the action of taurocholate is not very important in alkaline or nonacidic reflux esophagitis. On the contrary taurocholate, due to its pKa = 1.8, may play an important role in the pathogenesis of acid reflux esophagitis.

References

1. Little AG, DeMeester TR, Kirchner PT, O'Sullivan GC, Skinner DB. Pathogenesis of esophagitis in patients with gastro-esophageal reflux. Surgery 1980;88:101–105.
2. Salo JA, Kivilaakso E. Role of luminal H$^+$ in the pathogenesis of experimental esophagitis. Surgery 1982;92:61–67.
3. Lillemoe KD, Johnson LF, Harmon JW. Alkaline esophagitis: A comparison of the ability of components of gastroduodenal contents to injure the rabbit esophagus. Gastroenterology 1983;85:621–624.
4. Salo JA, Kivilaakso E. Role of bile salts and trypsin in the pathogenesis of experimental alkaline esophagitis. Surgery 1983;93:525–560.
5. Salo JA, Lehto V-P, Karonen S-L, Kivilaakso E. Role of lipase in the pathogenesis of experimental esophagitis in the rabbit. Arch Surg 1987;122:1160–1164.
6. Salo JA, Lehto V-P, Myllärniemi HS, Kivilaakso E. Morphological alterations in tryptic esophagitis: An experimental light microscopic and scanning, and transmission electron microscopic study in rabbits. J Surg Res 1990;49:14–17.
7. Gotley DC, Morgan AP, Cooper MJ. Bile acid concentrations in the refluxate of patients with reflux oesophagitis. Br J Surg 1988;75:587–590.
8. Salo JA, Lehto V-P, Kivilaakso E. Morphological alterations in experimental esophagitis. Light microscopic and scanning, and transmission electron microscopic study. Dig Dis Sci 1983;28:440–444.
9. Salo JA, Kivilaakso E. Contribution of trypsin and cholate to the pathogenesis of experimental alkaline reflux esophagitis. Scand J Gastroenterol 1984;19:875–878.

Does alkaline reflux produce mucolysis on the esophageal mucosa as it does on the gastric and duodenal mucosa?

K. Boumcheda, G. Cadiot, J. Vatier, M. Mignon (Paris)

The gastric and duodenal epithelia are lined with a surface layer of mucus, the composition and the properties of which are now well-known. The mucus mainly derives from the mucus cells localized at the epithelium surface and from the submucosal glands. Duodenogastric alkaline reflux induces duodenal and gastric mucolysis by mechanisms that are not yet well-known. Some of these mechanisms are the proteolytic action of pepsin, the pancreatic proteolytic activity and the detersion due to bile salts [1]. Measurement of sialic acid outputs represents an approach to evaluate duodenal and gastric mucolysis [1,2]. Very few studies have been made concerning esophageal mucus. Very recently, McCallum's team showed 1) that mucus is present at the surface of the esophageal epithelium; 2) that esophageal mucus is a heterogeneous mixture of mucin and nonmucin proteins; and 3) that esophageal mucosa contains its own pre-epithelial defense, similar to that observed within other parts of the digestive tract [3]. In man, esophageal mucus-secreting glands are only localized in the submucosa of the proximal and the distal esophagus. It is, therefore, very likely that the esophageal mucus production is not important enough to ensure a correct epithelial protection. Mucus secreted by salivary glands probably takes part in this protection, in association with other factors secreted by the salivary glands and the esophagus (bicarbonates, EGF).

In animals, the aggressivity of duodenogastric reflux for the esophageal mucosa through one or several of its constituents (bile salts, pancreatic enzymes) is well-known experimentally [4]. In man, the pathogenic action of duodenogastric reflux has also been demonstrated [5]. However, as far as is known, no study has been made concerning the esophageal mucolysis by duodenogastric reflux. In a work published by our group, comparing patients with esophagitis to patients with uncomplicated gastroesophageal reflux, gastric sialic acid outputs (presumed marker of mucolysis) and choline outputs (presumed marker of duodenogastric reflux) did not differ between the two groups [6]. No conclusion concerning esophageal mucolysis could be drawn from this study, however, since no distinction between the gastric mucolysis and a possible esophageal mucolysis could be made. Other studies are necessary to progress in that field.

References

1. Vatier J, Poitevin C, Vitré MT, Mignon M. Caractérisation et évaluation du caractère pathogène du reflux duodénogastrique par la mesure de la choline et de l'acide sialique intragastriques chez le sujet normal et l'ulcéreux duodénal. Gastroenterol Clin Biol 1988;12:207–213.
2. Vatier J, Poitevin C, Mignon M. Sialic acid content and proteolytic activity in gastric juice in man: an approach for appreciating glycoprotein erosion. Dig Dis Sci 1988;33:144–151.
3. Namiot Z, Rourk RM, Sarosiek J, Hetzel DP, McCallum RW. Evidence for the presence of esophageal mucin as a major mucus component among various nonmucin proteins in human esophageal secretion. Boston: American Gastroenterological Association Congress, 1993:A385 (abstract).
4. Orlando RC. Pathophysiology of gastroesophageal reflux disease: Esophageal epithelial resistance. In: Castell DO (ed) The Esophagus. Boston: Little, Brown & Co, 1992:463–478.
5. Stocker DL, Williams JG. Alkaline reflux oesophagitis. Gut 1991;32:1090–1092.
6. Sékéra E, Cadiot G, Poitevin C, Vallot T, Vatier J, Mignon M. Sécrétion gastrique de pepsine dans le reflux gastro-oesophagien compliqué ou non d'oesophagite peptique. Gastroenterol Clin Biol 1992;16:141–147.

How high are serum gastrin levels in case of esophageal alkaline reflux exposure?

T.N. Walsh (Dublin)

Only one study to date has addressed the question of serum gastrin levels in alkaline esophageal reflux. DeMeester's group measured fasting serum gastrin levels in 22

Barrett's patients and compared 11 patients who had increased esophageal alkaline exposure with 11 who had normal alkaline exposure [1]. The mean (SEM) gastrin level in the former group were 59 pg/ml compared with 35 (7.5) pg/ml in patients with normal alkaline exposure (p < 0.05). No comparable data were available from patients with reflux but without Barrett's esophagus, or from normal controls. Gastric hypersecretion was also identified in 10 of 23 Barrett's patients tested. It is not clear whether these had normal or elevated levels of gastrin or how many were represented in the alkaline reflux group.

There is no evidence that alkaline or acid reflux into the esophagus influences gastrin secretion. Gastrin, produced by the G cells of the lateral walls of the antral portion of the gastric mucosa, is secreted in response to stimuli from receptors in the microvilli which mediate the gastrin response to changes in the gastric lumen. Its release is also stimulated by increased vagal discharge and blood-borne factors such as calcium and epinephrine. It is inhibited by luminal acid, and by secretin, GIP, VIP, glucagon and calcitonin.

The effect of alkaline duodenogastric reflux on gastrin secretion was the subject of considerable debate as some workers could detect no increase in serum gastrin in response to an acute change in gastric antral alkalinisation [2–4]. Peters et al. [5] found, however, that when the antrum was exposed to alkaline perfusate for up to 5 h, serum gastrin levels rose significantly from 25 to 37 pg/ml (p < 0.05). In the clinical context of chronic duodenogastric alkaline reflux the findings have been less clear. Wilson et al [6] could find no difference between basal gastrin levels in bile reflux patients (18.8 pmol/l), bile diverted patients (20.6 pmol/l) and normal controls (16.0 pmol/l) while Niemela [7] has shown a positive correlation between the degree of duodenogastric reflux as measured by isotope studies and serum gastrin levels. In animal studies an amplified serum gastrin response to food was identified in animals with bile reflux, even where basal fasting levels were normal [8,9].

In our unit, the effect of cholecystectomy on alkaline duodenogastric reflux, serum gastrin levels and gastroesophageal reflux (GER) was examined in a series of studies. Nine patients were studied before and 3 months after cholecystectomy by dual channel gastric and esophageal pH monitoring, esophageal manometry and fasting blood sampling for gastrin, substance P and neurotensin [10]. Mean ± SEM gastrin levels increased significantly following cholecystectomy from 8.9 ± 1.8 ng/l to 17.9 ± 3.4 ng/l while substance P and neurotensin levels were unchanged. This was paralleled by a significant increase in gastric alkalinisation detected by the gastric pH probe and by an insignificant drop in the LES pressure from 15.4 ± 0.7 mmHg to 14.3 ± 0.9 mmHg. Further studies established that following cholecystectomy, alkaline duodenogastric reflux was associated with a significant increase in mixed GER [11]. While there was no change in the basal lower esophageal sphincter pressure, there was a significant reduction in the sphincter function index. This does not imply that the reduction was mediated through gastrin. McCallum demonstrated a rise in basal LES pressures in response to 0.4 M $NaHCO_3$ bolus ingestion which was not associated with alteration in serum gastrin levels [12].

The definition of esophageal alkaline reflux as pH > 7.0 reflects the lack of sophistication of the facilities hitherto available for monitoring duodenal contents, necessitating reliance on the pH of the refluxate to determine its presence. It does not reflect any belief in alkalinity per se as the source of esophageal pathology. While the term seems to imply that acid and alkaline reflux are mutually exclusive or that mixed alkaline and acid reflux is not as harmful as acid or alkaline reflux alone, there is obviously a continuum from pure acid reflux, to mixed reflux which is clinically significant, to alkaline reflux.

Serum gastrin levels in GERD are of interest because of the role of gastrin LES pressure modulation, in gastric acid secretion, and in the gastrin response to acid reduction. McCallum et al. found no difference between patients with GER and normal subjects with respect to serum gastrin levels, endogenous gastrin response, or antral gastrin concentration and concluded that gastrin played no role in the development of LES incompetence, or the pathophysiology of GER [13]. No correlation was observed between LES pressure and gastrin levels in patients with Zollinger-Ellison syndrome [14], or in patients with pernicious anaemia [15]. Despite elevated gastrin levels in Barrett's patients with alkaline GER LES pressures are invariably lower than normal [1]. These findings are in keeping with the observations that the dose of gastrin required to elevate LES pressure to the equivalent of that seen after a meal, would require serum gastrin levels 10 times greater than physiological values [16]. It is likely that while gastrin has a potential role in pharmacological doses, the complex interplay of other hormonal, neural and myogenic effects reduces this effect to insignificance.

In patients with GER, acid blockade with omeprazole therapy results in a significant elevation of serum gastrin levels from 8.6 to 16.9 pmol/l ($p < 0.05$) [17]. In another study cessation of long-term omeprazole therapy resulted in a rapid reduction in gastrin levels from 160 to 42 ng/l within 10 days and a parallel increase in gastric acid production with a rapid recurrence of esophagitis [18]. Robertson et al. described a predictive role for gastrin as patients who responded to ranitidine 300 mg had a mean (range) serum gastrin level of 4.52 (2.4—10) pmol/l, while patients with a level of 11.1 (3.5—21) pmol/l did not [19].

The introduction of monitoring equipment such as the Bilitec 2000 (Synectics Medical AB, Sweden) which can detect bile in the esophagus [20], the development of probes that can detect other duodenal constituents, and the availability of ambulatory manometry should shed further light on esophageal alkaline reflux and the effects of gastrin in a more physiological context.

References

1. DeMeester TR, Attwood SEA, Smyrk TC, Therkildsen DH, Hinder RA. Surgical therapy in Barrett's esophagus. Ann Surg 1990;212:528—542.
2. Levant JA, Walsh JH, Isenberg JI. Stimulation of gastric secretion and gastrin release by single oral doses of calcium carbonate in man. N Engl J Med 1973;289:555—558.
3. Higgs RH, Smyth RD, Castell DO. Gastric alkalinisation: effect on lower esophageal sphincter pressure and serum gastrin. N Engl J Med 1974;291:486—490.
4. Kline MM, McCallum RW, Curry N, Sturdevant RAL. Effect of gastric alkalinisation on lower esophageal sphincter pressure and serum gastrin. Gastroenterology 1975;68:1137—1139.
5. Peters MN, Feldman M, Walsh J, Richardson CT. Effect of gastric alkalinisation on serum gastrin concentrations in humans. Gastroenterology 1983;85:35—39.

6. Wilson P, Welch NT, Hinder RA et al. Abnormal plasma gut hormones in pathologic duodenogastric reflux and their response to surgery. Am J Surg 1993;165:169–177.
7. Niemela S. Duodenogastric reflux in patients with upper abdominal complaints or gastric ulcer with particular reference to reflux associated gastritis. Scand J Gastroenterol 1985;115(suppl):1–56.
8. Thomas WE, Lewin MR. The effect of duodenogastric reflux on serum gastrin levels in the dog. Eur Surg Res 1980;12:403–407.
9. Robbins FL, Broadie TA, Sosin H, Delaney JP. Reflux gastritis: the consequences of intestinal juice in the stomach. Am J Surg 1976;131:23–29.
10. Jazrawi S. Gallbladder disease and oesophageal function. MD Thesis, Trinity College Dublin 1992;155–174.
11. Jazrawi S, Walsh TN, Byrne PJ et al. Cholecystectomy and oesophageal reflux: a prospective evaluation. Br J Surg 1993;80:50–53.
12. McCallum RW. Studies on the mechanism of the lower esophageal sphincter pressure response to alkali ingestion in humans. Am J Gastroenterol 1985;80:513–517.
13. McCallum RW, Holloway RH, Callachan C, Avella J, Walsh JH. Endogenous gastrin release and antral gastrin concentration in gastroesophageal reflux patients and normal subjects. Am J Gastroenterol 1983;78:398–402.
14. McCallum RW, Walsh JH. Relationship between lower esophageal sphincter pressure and serum gastrin concentrations in Zollinger-Ellison syndrome and other clinical settings. Gastroenterology 1979;76:76–81.
15. Farrell RL, Nebel OT, McGuire AT, Castell DO. The abnormal lower oesophageal sphincter in pernicious anaemia. Gut 1973;14:767–772.
16. Freeland GR, Higgs RH, Castell DO, McGuigan JE. Lower esophageal sphincter and acid responses to intravenous infusions of synthetic human gastrin heptadecapeptide. Gastroenterology 1976;71:570–574.
17. Lundell L. Prevention of relapse of reflux oesophagitis after endoscopic healing. The efficacy and the safety of omeprazole compared with ranitidine. Digestion 1990;47(suppl 1):72–75.
18. Klinkenberg-Knol EC, Jansen JB, Lamers CB et al. Temporary cessation of long-term maintenance treatment with omeprazole in patients with H2-receptor antagonist resistant oesophagitis. Scand J Gastroenterol 1990;25:1144–1150.
19. Robertson DA, Aldersley MA, Shepherd H, Lloyd RS, Smith CL. H2 antagonists in the treatment of reflux oesophagitis: can physiological studies predict the response. Gut 1987;28:946–949.
20. Caldwell MTP, Evoy D, Byrne PJ et al. Ambulatory 24-hour bile reflux monitoring in Barrett's oesophagus. Br J Surg (in press).

What are the limitations of intragastric pH measurement in the diagnosis of duodenogastric reflux?

R.A. Hinder (Omaha)

The nonspecific symptoms of primary duodenogastric reflux (DGR) are easily confused with other upper gastrointestinal conditions, so objective tests are required to confirm the diagnosis (Table 1).

A number of techniques have been developed to diagnose and quantify the extent of DGR. These include the measurement of bile and pancreatic components in gastric aspirates, radiographic evidence of gastric reflux of barium instilled into the duodenum, radioisotopic evidence of reflux of radiolabeled bile or radiolabeled material introduced directly into the duodenum, electrolyte and pH changes in the gastric juice, endoscopic study, and specific histologic markers of reflux.

The endoscopic findings in primary DGR are relatively nonspecific. They include

Table 1. Tests used in the diagnosis of duodenogastric reflux

Test	Finding
Gastroscopy	Antral or global erythema and mucosal friability with or without gastric ulceration
Histology	Paucity of acute and chronic inflammatory cells; edema and smooth muscle fibers in the lamina propria; vasodilatation and congestion of superficial mucosal capillaries; elongation and tortuosity of the glands (foveolar hyperplasia)
Hepatobiliary scintigraphy [1,2]	DISIDA/HIDA scanning (± IV CCK to promote gallbladder emptying) positive ^{99m}Tc counts over the stomach region
24-h gastric pH monitoring [3]	Increased fasting % time pH > 3 (>10%) (Fig. 1); positive discriminant score
Gastric juice aspiration	Measurement of bile acids, bilirubin, pancreatic enzymes, or sodium concentration in gastric juice
Duodenal marker techniques	Duodenal instillation of barium, dyes, or radioisotopes and detection of their reflux into the stomach
Provocation techniques	Instillation of alkali or bile into the stomach to reproduce symptoms

DISIDA/HIDA: o-diisopropyl iminodiacetic acid/Sn-2,6-diethylacetanilidoiminodiacetate.

erythema and friability of the gastric mucosa, particularly in the prestomal area, and there may be associated gastric ulceration. Microscopic features in gastric biopsy specimens include a paucity of acute and chronic inflammatory cells, the presence of edema and smooth muscle fibers in the lamina propria, increased mucus content of the surface and pit cells, vasodilatation and congestion of superficial mucosal capillaries, and foveolar hyperplasia (elongation and tortuosity of the glands). The combination of these histologic features has been strongly correlated with excessive reflux of alkaline duodenal content into the stomach [1,2].

^{99m}Tc DISIDA (o-diisopropyl iminodiacetic acid) and ^{99m}Tc HIDA (Sn-2,6-diethylacetanilidoiminodiacetate) scanning can give an indication of the quantity of DGR, but overlap of the left lobe of the liver or small intestine into the gastric region of interest can complicate anatomic definition of the stomach on static imaging, and small volumes of transient reflux often remain undetected. The sensitivity and accuracy of measurement of DGR can be improved by techniques involving continuous infusion of ^{99m}Tc HIDA with counting of ^{99m}Tc activity in gastric aspirates.

Twenty-four-hour gastric pH monitoring can be useful in the diagnosis of DGR, because it accounts for diurnal variations in reflux. However, the interpretation of gastric pH recordings is difficult because the gastric pH environment is determined by a complex interplay of acid and mucus secretion, ingested food, swallowed saliva, regurgitated duodenal, pancreatic, and biliary secretions, and the effectiveness of the mixing and evacuation of chyme. The type of pH electrode and its positioning are important. Microglass electrodes with built-in reference electrodes are more accurate than antimony probes in the gastric environment. The tip of the electrode is placed 5 cm below the lower border of the lower esophageal sphincter, in the proximal stomach. For the quantitation of DGR, simple measurements of alkaline peaks have proved unreliable because of the effects of meals and nocturnal reduction in acid secretion, which results in sudden changes of gastric pH, mimicking alkaline reflux episodes. To overcome these problems, a scoring system for DGR was developed that uses a large number of computer-generated pH measurements. To quantitate alkaline reflux, the gastric pH record is divided into four periods: upright, supine, prandial pH plateau, and postprandial pH decline. For each of these periods the following parameters are calculated:

— The pH frequency distribution (i.e., the percentage time the gastric pH is at the pH interval 0–1, 1–2, 2–3, 3–4, 4–5, 5–6, 6–7, and >7).
— The frequency of pH changes (i.e., the incidence of pH movements from a lower into a higher pH interval).
— The duration of pH exposure expressed as the longest time the pH remains at a pH interval during the monitored period.
— The duration and frequency of pH exposure expressed as the number of times the pH remained at a pH interval longer than 5 min.

Using discriminant analysis, we have shown that a scoring system based on 16 of these parameters can differentiate the gastric pH profiles of healthy volunteers from those of patients with primary pathologic DGR [3]. When applied prospectively, this scoring system was superior to DISIDA scanning in the diagnosis of excessive DGR and detected the disease with a sensitivity of 90% and a specificity of 100%. Long-term gastric pH measurement is able not only to differentiate between normal and abnormal, but also has been shown to become more strongly positive with increasing

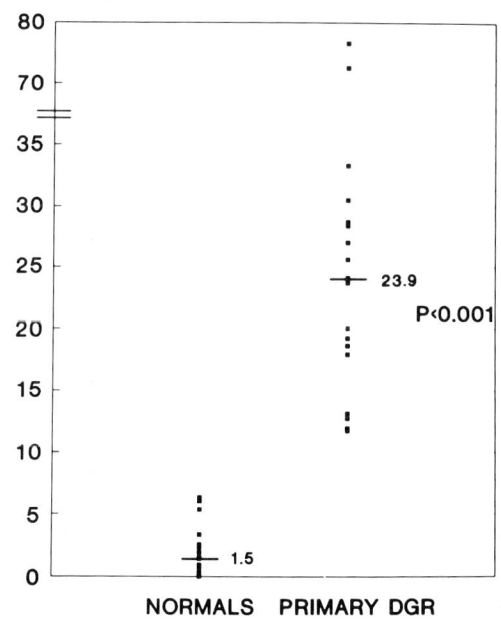

Fig. 1. Fasting % time gastric pH > 3 (excluding prandial plateau and postprandial decline phases) in 20 healthy people and 20 patients with primary duodenogastric reflux (DGR). Bars and figures show median values. This simple parameter completely discriminates between the two groups (p < 0.001, Mann-Whitney U-test).

221

severity of the disease.

The percentage of time the gastric pH was >3, excluding the prandial pH plateau and the postprandial pH decline phases, also can accurately reflect the degree of gastric alkaline exposure and discriminate between physiologic and pathologic DGR. When this simple parameter was compared in 20 healthy people and 20 patients with primary DGR, it discriminated between the two groups (Fig. 1).

References

1. DeMeester TR, Fuchs KH, Ball CS, Albertucci M, Smyrk TC, Marcus JN. Experimental and clinical results with end-to-end duodenojejunostomy for pathologic duodenogastric reflux. Ann Surg 1987;206:414–426.
2. Stein HJ, Hinder RA, DeMeester TR, Lloyd BA, Fuchs KH, Attwood SEA. Clinical use of 24-hour gastric pH monitoring versus DISIDA scanning in the diagnosis of pathologic duodenogastric reflux. Arch Surg 1990;125:966–971.
3. Fuchs KH, DeMeester TR, Hinder RA, Stein HJ, Barlow AP, Gupta NC. Computerized identification of pathologic duodenogastric reflux using 24-hour gastric pH monitoring. Ann Surg 1991;213:13–20.

Are there alternative methods for measuring "bile" reflux?

P. Bechi, F. Pucciani, F. Baldini, C. Cortesini (Florence)

Although enterogastric and nonacid gastroesophageal refluxes (GERs) are probably involved in relevant pathologic conditions (gastric ulcer, "chemical" gastritis, severe esophagitis, upper dyspeptic syndromes), none of the different techniques for their detection is completely effective. ^{99m}Tc HIDA cholescintigraphy and selenium-homocholic acid taurine scanning are stationary methods and require the consumption of radioactive reflux markers. Other methods involving the assessment of any of the components of enterogastric reflux (e.g., bile acid quantification in the gastric or esophageal aspirates) require what should simply be removed from the stomach or the esophagus, respectively. Monitoring of gastric and/or esophageal pH is almost universally recognized as being unsatisfactory for enterogastric and nonacid GER detection, since it is both an indirect technique and unable to evaluate postprandial periods [1]. Furthermore, all these techniques, with the exception of pH monitoring, are discontinuous and/or restrict data samplings to short periods.

Biases of each of these methods have spurred us to conceive and develop the present ambulatory technique based on the use of a completely new sensor named Bilitec 2000 [2]. The basic working principle of this fiberoptic system is that an absorption peak at $\cong 450$ nm (characteristic absorption peak of bilirubin) implies the presence of bilirubin in the sample under consideration [3–5]. Moreover, since the absorbance (intensity of light absorbed) at a particular wave-length is directly proportional to the concentration of the substance, with absorption at that particular wave-length, the fiberoptic system has the potential to assess bilirubin concentration in a given medium.

The bile reflux monitoring device consists of a probe, as well as a light emitting and signal-elaborating recording unit.

The miniaturized probe, which consists of a flexible fiberoptic bundle, carries the signal into the esophagus or the stomach and back to the optoelectronic unit. Its PVC tip is shaped (Fig. 1).

Two light-emitting diodes (at 470 and 565 nm) represent the sources for the measurement and the reference signals, respectively. The signals are processed by an integrated microcomputer which calculates the difference in the absorbencies at 470 and 565 nm. This value is directly proportional to the bilirubin concentration and, therefore, it is related to bile reflux. At the end of each 24-h monitoring period, the data stored in the buffer of the instrument are transferred to a personal computer for processing and filing.

In vitro studies have shown good precision, good stability, a sensitivity of 2.5 μmol/l bilirubin concentration, as well as a useful working range of 2.5—100 μmol/l bilirubin concentration (100 μmol/l bilirubin concentration corresponds to high reflux values).

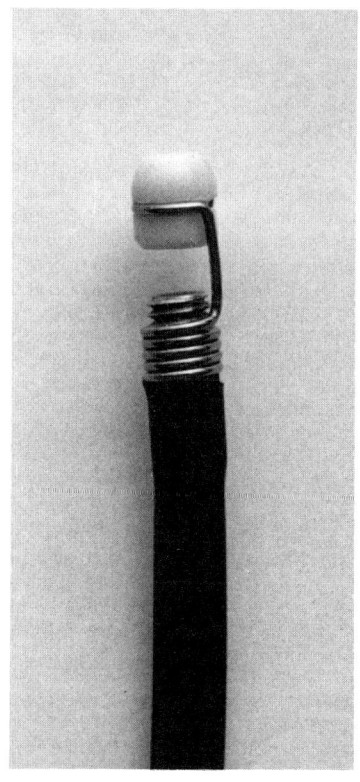

Fig. 1. The tip of the fiberoptic probe.

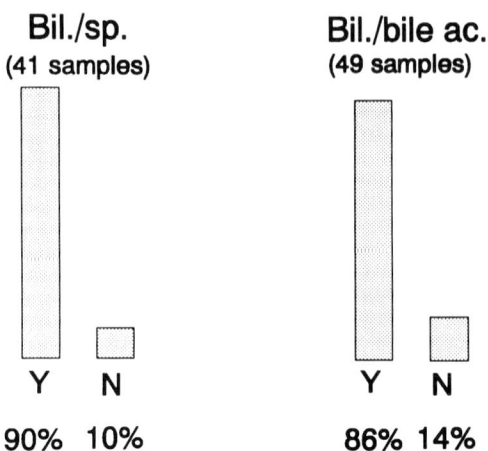

Fig. 2. Comparisons of in vivo fiberoptic system measurements (Bil.) with measurements in gastric aspirates of spectrophotometric absorbance (sp.) and bile acid concentration (bile ac.), respectively.

In vivo validation tests were performed on 29 dyspeptic subjects. Due to the lack of a "gold standard" for enterogastric reflux measurement, fiberoptic system absorbance values were compared with values obtained by means of the best methods presently available (i.e., gastric aspiration and ^{99m}Tc HIDA cholescintigraphy).

All the aspirated samples, when quantitatively sufficient, were homogenized and both analyzed spectrophotometrically and evaluated enzymatically for total bile acid concentration. Bilitec absorbance values, have shown a good correlation with the spectrophotometric (41 samples available) and bile acid concentration (49 samples available) assessment of gastric aspirates (r = 0.63, p < 0.01 and r = 0.71, p < 0.01, respectively; linear correlation). Moreover, fiberoptic system findings were considered to correspond to spectrophotometric and bile acid findings, when they agreed in being above or below conventionally established threshold values. Good concordance was shown (Fig. 2).

Fourteen subjects were studied using the fiberoptic system together with simultaneous ^{99m}Tc HIDA cholescintigraphy. In seven of these, both tests showed no reflux, while in six both methods of assessment detected reflux. In one case, bile reflux was detected by cholescintigraphy, but bilimetric assessment failed to detect it. Concordance, as regards the presence/absence of reflux, was significant (p <0.01; binomial test). Figure 3 shows the comparison of results of reflux detection by means of cholescintigraphy and the fiberoptic system. Concordance between the two methods, as far as mucosa/refluxate contact time is concerned, is impressive.

In view of these encouraging results, as a preliminary step for the establishment of normal limits for 24-h monitoring values of gastroesophageal and enterogastric bile reflux, control subjects were studied.

Five healthy volunteers (all males; mean age: 27.4 years, range: 21—36 years) were studied using 24-h esophageal monitoring. Results were compared with those obtained in a group of six subjects with symptoms suggestive of GER (three males, three

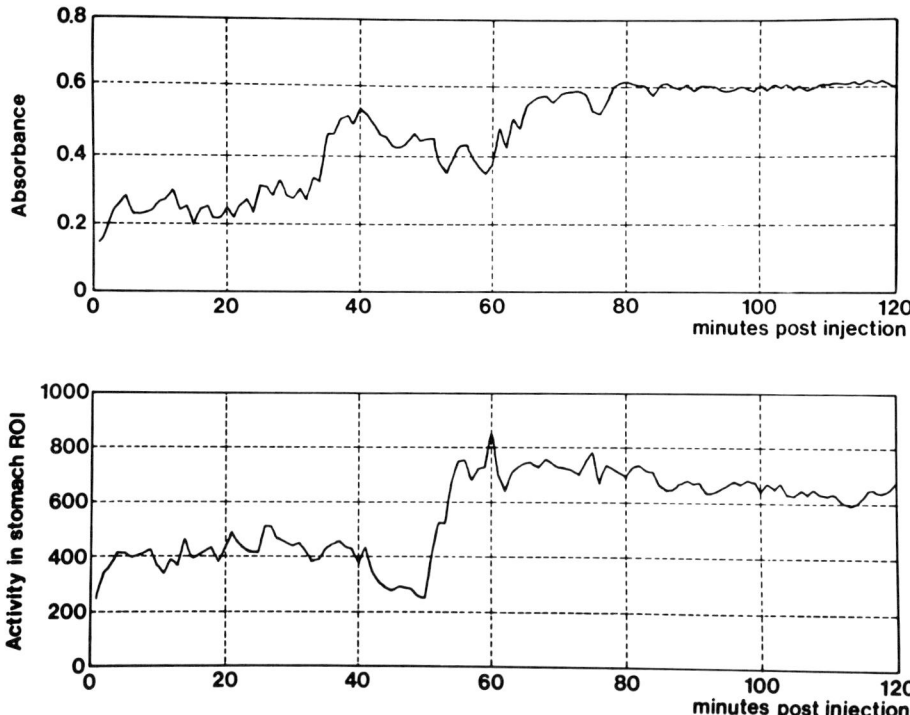

Fig. 3. An example of bilimetric (upper) and ^{99m}Tc-HIDA cholescintigraphic (lower) tracings. The contact time between refluxate and gastric mucosa agrees in the two methods of measurement.

females; mean age: 62.6 years, range: 43–80 years). The latter group included three subjects with Polya gastrectomy and one with Barrett's esophagus (Fig. 4). The fiberoptic probe was positioned 5 cm above the upper border of the LES (located by manometry) for esophageal monitoring in both volunteers and symptomatic subjects.

Moreover, 5 healthy volunteers (all males; mean age: 27.0 years, range: 26–28 years) were studied for enterogastric reflux (Fig. 5). In these subjects the tip of the probe was positioned fluoroscopically in the stomach between the vertical and the horizontal part of the corpus (Tables 1 and 2).

A greater number of controls will be needed in order to establish cut-off points for normal limits and this represents the next objective.

Conclusions

Bilitec 2000 is the only system at present, available for ambulatory enterogastric reflux and nonacid GER detection. In vitro tests and in vivo validation have demonstrated its reliability, precision and accuracy.

The experience with enterogastric reflux detection is quite satisfactory, and the utilization of the fiber optic system in the study of nonacid GER is even easier and

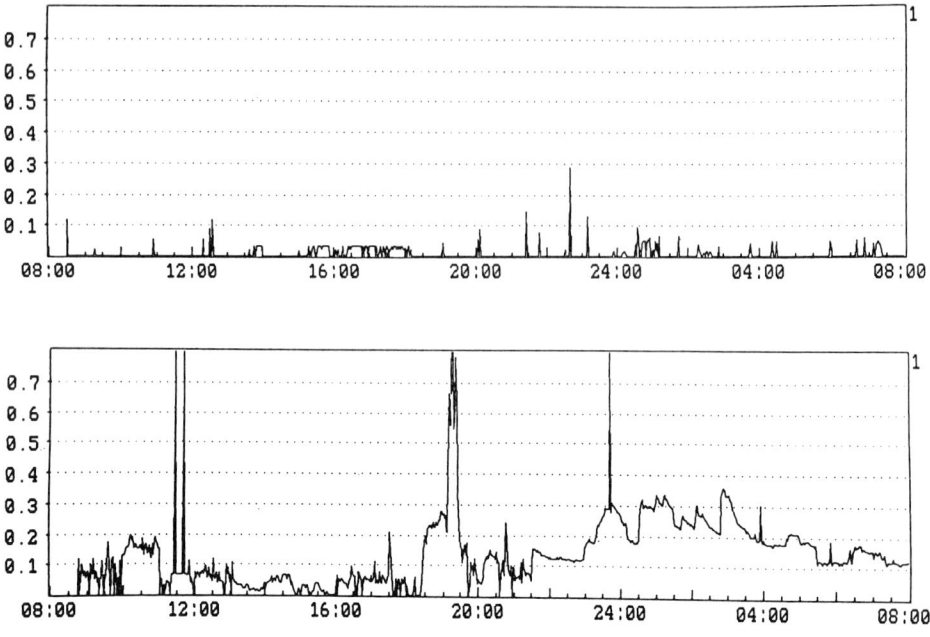

Fig. 4. Examples of 24-h esophageal tracings from a healthy volunteer (top) and from a symptomatic subject with Barrett's esophagus (bottom).

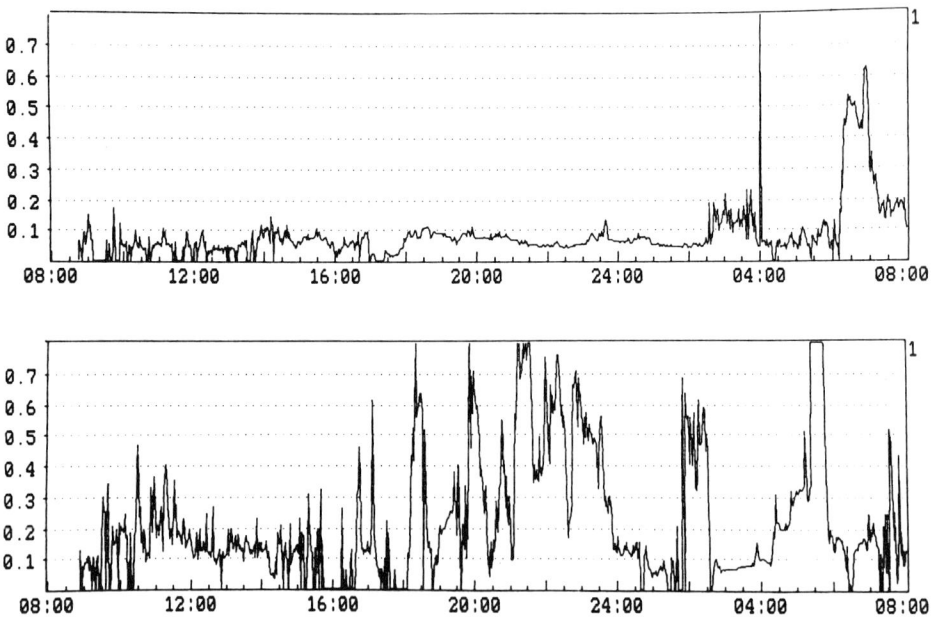

Fig. 5. Examples of 24-h gastric tracings from a healthy volunteer (top) and from a cholecystectomized subject (bottom).

Table 1. Values of nonacid GER obtained in control subjects and in symptomatic subjects. Reflux was considered to occur when absorbance detected by the esophageal probe exceeded 0.14 units

Component	Controls (n = 5)		Symptomatic subjects (n = 6)	
	Mean	SEM	Mean	SEM
Total time (%)	0.05	± 0.03	16.96	± 9.91
Upright time (%)	0.06	± 0.05	13.95	± 9.33
Supine time (%)	0.05	± 0.02	21.68	± 13.99
No. of episodes	1.20	± 0.73	22.83	± 9.48
No. of episodes >5 min	0	—	4.17	± 2.53
Longest episode (min)	0.43	± 0.12	124.47	± 74.89

Table 2. Values of enterogastric reflux obtained in control subjects. Reflux was considered to occur when absorbance detected by the gastric probe exceeded 0.14 absorbance

Component	Controls (n = 5)	
	Mean	SEM
Total time (%)	2.58	± 1.07
Upright time (%)	1.86	± 0.93
Supine time (%)	3.53	± 2.21
No. of episodes	13.00	± 5.67
No. of episodes >5 min	1.60	± 0.51
Longest episode (min)	15.80	± 7.74

results appear even more reliable (no need for fluoroscopic probe positioning, no displacement during 24-h monitoring). The combined use of the fiber optic probe and pH-monitoring in the esophagus, has shown that the presence of gastric content in the esophagus (i.e., GER can occur with a pH between 4–7) [6,7]. Therefore, it is restrictive to consider reflux as occurring only when esophageal pH drops below 4 (acid reflux with no or negligible enteric component) or — exceptionally — exceeds 7 (alkaline reflux with no or negligible gastric secretion component). Agreement must be reached on the term best fitted to define this reflux, which has been previously defined as "mixed reflux" [8] or "alkalacid" [9]. Probably the best solution is just to abandon the term "alkaline" and to define all GER with pH greater than 4 (upper limit for acid reflux) as nonacid [4,6].

A greater number of normal subjects must be studied in order to identify normal limits for enterogastric and nonacid GER. However, the results which have been obtained to date, give an idea of the entity of the physiological occurrence of these types of reflux.

The only relevant problem with the use of the fiberoptic system in the clinical setting, is that some foods (e.g., those with an absorption close to 450 nm) may affect measurements. A list of foods to be consumed at the three different meals is therefore

given to subjects prior to undergoing 24-h bilimetric monitoring [5], otherwise suitable commercial dietary products can be used. This minor drawback is overcome by the many positive aspects of Bilitec 2000:
— the straightforward basic working principle;
— the naturally occurring marker utilized (bilirubin); and
— the additional advantages linked to optical fibers (miniaturization, safety, low cost).
All these make this system an important device in the study of the functional disorders of the alimentary tract.

References

1. Hostein J, Bost R, Faure H, Lachet B, Fournet J. Valeur diagnostique de la pH-métrie gastrique au cours du reflux duodenogastrique. Gastroenterol Clin Biol 1987;11:206—211.
2. Falciai R, Scheggi AM, Baldini F, Bechi P. USA Patent 1990;4,976,265.
3. Bechi P, Falciai R, Baldini F, Cosi F, Pucciani F, Boscherini S. A new fiber-optic sensor for ambulatory enterogastric reflux detection. In: Katzir A (ed) Fiber Optic Medical and Fluorescent Sensors and Applications, Proc SPIE 1648. Bellingham: SPIE 1992;130—135.
4. Bechi P, Falciai R, Baldini F, Cosi F, Pucciani F, Travaglini F, Boscherini S. Ambulatory assessment of enterogastric and nonacid gastroesophageal reflux by means of a fiberoptic sensor. Gastroenterology 1992;102:A39.
5. Bechi P, Pucciani F, Baldini F, Cosi F, Falciai R, Mazzanti R, Castagnoli A, Passeri A, Boscherini S. Long-term ambulatory enterogastric reflux monitoring. Validation of a new fiberoptic technique. Dig Dis Sci 1993;38:1297—1306.
6. Bechi P, Falciai R, Baldini F, Pucciani F, Cortesini C. A new fiber-optic sensor for detection and measurement of duodenogastric and nonacid gastroesophageal reflux. Fourth World Cong ISDE, Chicago, 1989.
7. Champion G, Singh S, Bechi P, Richter JE. Duodenogastric reflux. Relationship to esophageal pH and response to omeprazole. Gastroenterology 1993;104:A51.
8. Cortesini C, Pucciani F. Usefulness of combined gastric and esophageal pH monitoring in detecting gastroesophageal alkaline and mixed reflux. Eur Surg Res 1984;16:378—382.
9. Mattioli S, Pilotti V, Felice V, Lazzari A, Zannoli R, Bacchi ML, Loria P, Tripodi A, Gozzetti G. Ambulatory 24-hr pH monitoring of esophagus, fundus and antrum. A new technique for simultaneous study of gastroesophageal and duodeno-gastric reflux. Dig Dis Sci 1990;35:929—938.

Reflux and mucosa

Does measurement of esophageal mucosal potential difference allow early recognition of injury?

R.C. Orlando (New Orleans)

What is an esophageal mucosal potential difference?

All gastrointestinal epithelia, including that of the esophagus, exhibit a mucosal (or transmural) electrical potential difference (PD) [1]. The PD, which is another name for voltage, is based on Ohm's law:

$$PD \text{ (mV)} = I \text{ (}\mu A\text{)} \times R \text{ (}\Omega \cdot cm^2\text{)},$$

where I is net current flow across the tissue and R is the electrical resistance of the tissue. Under steady state conditions, i.e., when the tissue is bathed on both sides by solutions of similar ion concentrations, the mucosal PD can be measured directly (see below) and represents a product of net active transcellular ion transport across the epithelium and the passive resistance to the flow of ions across the epithelium [1,2]. (While the resistance of an epithelium is comprised of the resistances of the apical and basolateral cell membranes and that of its junctional structures (primarily tight junctions and intercellular glycoconjugate), the very high values of the former result in the total resistance for the mucosa being dominated (and approximated) by junctional resistance.) In physicochemical terms, the PD can be viewed, therefore, as a force reflected by the separation of charges in space, that is created by the utilization of energy to place a relatively greater concentration of positively-charged ions on the serosal surface and leaving behind, as it were, a relatively greater concentration of negatively-charged ions on the luminal surface. For the esophageal epithelium, sodium ions are the actively transported positively-charged species and chloride the negatively-charged species remaining on the luminal side [2]. This separation results in a PD of −15 mV across the esophageal epithelium of humans and −30 mV across that of the rabbit [1].

How is the esophageal mucosal PD measured?

The technique for measuring the esophageal mucosal PD involves the positioning of the electrodes from a voltmeter in contact with opposing sides of the tissue, i.e., one contacts the luminal surface and the other contacts the serosal surface. The fact is, however, that contact with each of these surfaces does not require physical contact between electrode and tissue, since contact can be made via bathing solutions in contact with each surface. This means that for in vivo measurements a satisfactory luminal electrode can be achieved by perfusing the luminal surface with Ringer solution and a satisfactory serosal electrode can be achieved by placing a Ringer agar-bridge subcutaneously so that it is in contact with interstitial fluid [1]. (Note: interstitial fluid which serves as the reference electrode is of similar ion composition

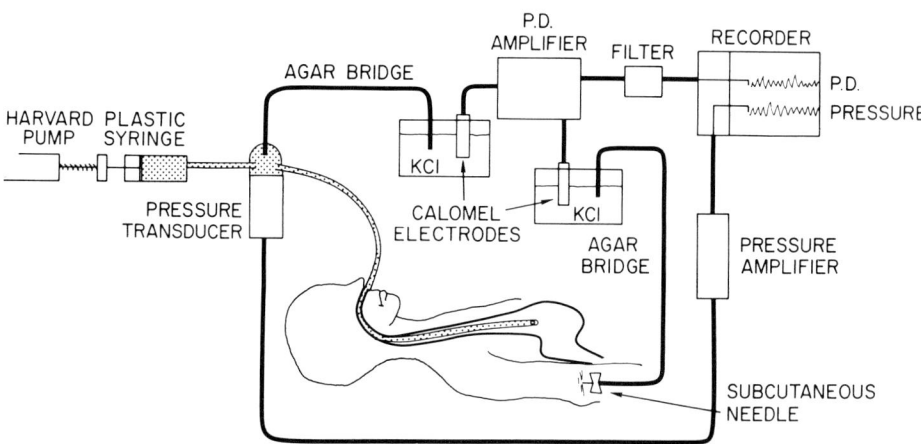

Fig. 1. Technique for in vivo measurement of the esophageal mucosal potential difference (PD) simultaneously with esophageal pressure. The traditional manometric catheter system is perfused with Ringer's solution via a Harvard pump utilizing a plastic syringe. The pressure transducer is modified so that a Ringer-agar-filled polyethylene bridge is inserted into the dome of the pressure transducer making contact with the perfusate. As a reference bridge, a similar Ringer-agar-filled scalp vein needle with tube is inserted subcutaneously. Both agar bridges are placed in beakers of KCl which contain calomel reference electrodes. These electrodes are connected to a low voltage, high impedance differential amplifier with a remote power source, and the signal is filtered of 60-cycle interference before being recorded simultaneously with pressures on a multichannel strip recorder. (Reprinted with permission from Turner et al. [1], p. 286.)

230

throughout the body, and so the subcutaneous fluid and interstitial fluid in esophagus are in continuity and reflect the same body compartment). Further, by modifying a standard manometric catheter system so that one perfusion port can measure the PD simultaneously with pressure, the PD of the human esophagus can be measured in vivo and localized by reference to the pressure profile (Fig. 1). For in vitro measurements of the esophageal mucosal PD, the esophageal mucosa can be sectioned, stripped of its muscle layers and mounted as flat sheets between two half-cells in an Ussing chamber [2–4]. The Ussing chamber set-up permits bathing each side of the tissue with Ringer solution, and these solutions have contact with electrodes that enable measurement of PD (by connection to a voltmeter) and passage of a current, known as the short circuit current (Isc) (by connection to a battery). The ability to pass a current through the tissue such that it negatives the spontaneously measured PD is of great value because it permits, using Ohm's law, the direct calculation of the esophageal mucosal electrical resistance (R) from the measured PD and Isc (see equation above).

Can the esophageal mucosal PD detect early injury?

Since the mucosal PD is a function of the ability of a tissue to both actively transport ions and to prevent passive diffusion (barrier function), any process that alters either or both of these functions will affect the PD. Indeed, a common means of altering the

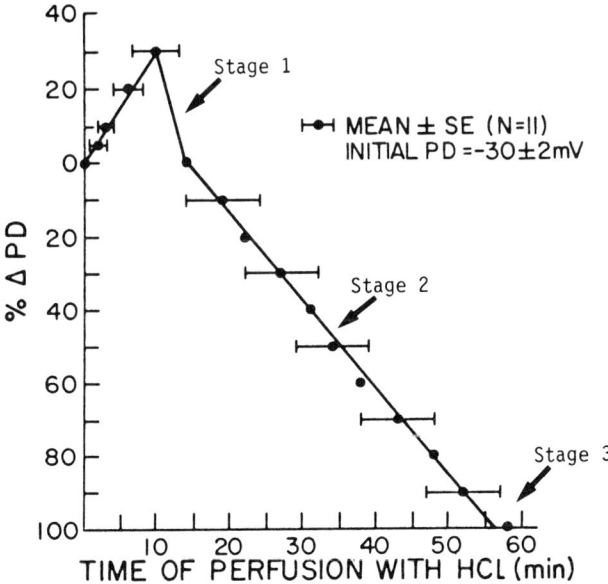

Fig. 2. The percent change in rabbit esophageal transmural potential difference (Δ PD) is shown plotted against the time of exposure to 80 mmol HCl-80 mmol NaCl. A transient increase in PD occurs during the first 10 min. This is followed by a progressive decline in PD to zero at 1 h. Values are the means ± SEM (n = 11); initial PD = –30 ± 2 mV. (Reprinted by copyright permission of The American Society for Clinical Investigation from Orlando et al. [3].)

PD experimentally is to damage the cells or junctions of the tissue in some way, and for esophageal epithelium this has been done using exposure to HCl [3,4]. In the acid-perfused esophagus, the PD can be observed to change with time, first rising above normal, then declining until it ultimately reaches zero (Fig. 2). Notably when acid perfusion has abolished the PD, the esophageal mucosa often exhibits gross evidence of epithelial necrosis [3]. This finding of an abnormally low or abolished PD is also seen in humans whose esophagi have been grossly damaged as a result of severe gastroesophageal reflux [5]. It is notable, however, that both experimentally in the acid-perfused rabbit esophagus and in some humans with reflux disease, a low PD is demonstrable in the absence of gross disease [3,5]. This implies that the PD can detect changes within the epithelium before gross change is apparent. In humans with reflux disease, the low PD could be correlated with the presence of histologic esophagitis [5]. However, even more intriguing is that in the rabbit model of esophagitis, a low PD developed *early* during the initiation of tissue damage to the extent that the only changes detected were an increase in mannitol permeability (measured by radiolabeled flux), and the presence of dilated intercellular spaces on electron microscopy (Fig. 3) [6]. From these observations, it is evident that the PD is capable of detecting early (or subtle) changes in esophageal epithelium, changes that would elude the currently used clinical techniques.

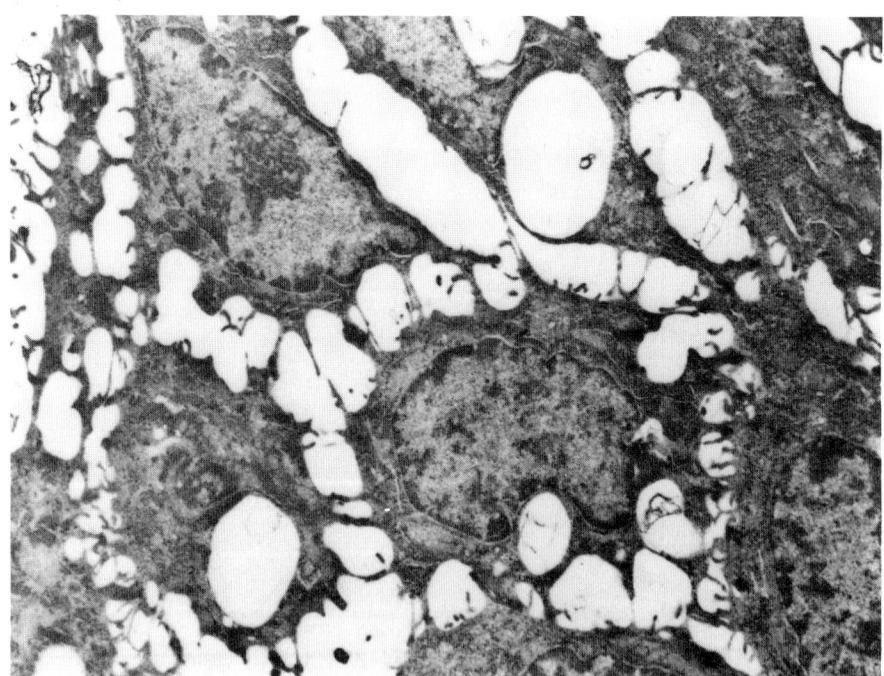

Fig. 3. Electron micrograph of lower stratum spinosum in rabbit esophagus after in vivo HCl exposure lowered potential difference by 50% (perfusion time approximately 30 min). There is prominent dilation of the intercellular spaces, but the cells themselves show no evidence of damage, ×6375. (Reprinted with permission from Carney et al. [6].)

Can measurement of the esophageal mucosal PD detect early injury due to alkaline duodenogastric reflux?

The general answer to this question is a qualified yes. The answer is qualified because it has never been demonstrated experimentally. The rationale for the affirmative statement is based on the known ability of duodenal contents to damage upon prolonged contact the esophageal epithelium. The most potentially noxious agents present in duodenum are the bile salts and pancreatic enzymes [7,8]. Notably what is not damaging to the esophageal mucosa is the pH of the duodenal fluid and this is true irrespective of whether pH is in the 7 or 8 range. The reason for this is that duodenal alkalinity is due to secreted bicarbonate and bicarbonate concentrations even up to aqueous solution saturability is not injurious to esophageal epithelium (unpublished observations). Nonetheless, alkaline (duodenal-gastric) esophageal reflux can damage the esophageal epithelium when there is prolonged contact with bile salts and/or pancreatic enzymes, and such damage would predictably lead to a decline in PD. While the decline in PD is likely to be a far more sensitive indicator of tissue damage than gross inspection or histology, independent verification of its sensitivity will be needed by the performance of permeability studies or electron microscopy.

References

1. Turner KS, Powell DW, Carney CN et al. Transmural electrical potential difference in the mammalian esophagus in vivo. Gastroenterology 1978;75:286–291.
2. Powell DW, Morris SM, Boyd DD. Water and electrolyte transport by rabbit esophagus. Am J Physiol 1975;229:438–443.
3. Orlando RC, Powell DW, Carney CN. Pathophysiology of acute acid injury in rabbit esophageal epithelium. J Clin Invest 1981;68:286–293.
4. Orlando RC, Bryson JC, Powell DW. Mechanisms of H^+ injury in rabbit esophageal epithelium. Am J Physiol 1984;246: G718–G724.
5. Orlando RC, Powell DW, Bryson JC et al. Esophageal potential difference measurements in esophageal disease. Gastroenterology 1982;83:1026–1032.
6. Carney CN, Orlando RC, Powell DW, Dotson MM. Morphologic alterations in early acid-induced epithelial injury of the rabbit esophagus. Lab Invest 1981;45:198–208.
7. Safaie-Shirazi S, DenBesten L, Zike WL. Effect of bile salts on the ionic permeability of the esophageal mucosa and their role in the production of esophagitis. Gastroenterology 1975;68:728–733.
8. Salo JA, Lehto V, Karonen S, Kivilaakso E. Role of lipase in the pathogenesis of experimental esophagitis in the rabbit. Arch Surg 1987;122:1160.

Is it necessary to perform a biopsy in erosive esophagitis?

C.E. Pope II (Seattle)

Endoscopic biopsy can provide added information to that obtained visually through the endoscope. Tissue removed serves as a permanent record of the state of the mucosa. Biopsy specimens may be examined at leisure, and by different observers. The risk to the patient of endoscopic biopsy with standard forceps is very small; bleeding post biopsy is very unusual unless the platelets or clotting factors are markedly depressed. Obtaining biopsies lengthens the procedure and the cost of disposable forceps (or processing of reusable forceps), and the cost of processing and interpreting the biopsies is not inconsiderable. This latter fact makes it essential to make certain that the information obtained by the endoscopic biopsy is needed.

When the issue of whether endoscopic biopsy is needed in erosive esophagitis is raised, many would answer in the affirmative. After all, is it not good medical practice to document observations (even those made through the endoscope) with objective proof of what was seen? The author would like to present the point of view that biopsy is only necessary in a few circumscribed circumstances; that biopsy in the usual case of erosive esophagitis is a waste of time and money.

A large portion of my opinion is based on the idea of discrimination in diagnosis [1,2]. That is, if one knows what the condition is with one form of test, then it is redundant to obtain other tests to confirm a diagnosis which has already been established. What will be the most common cause of erosive esophagitis? Clearly, reflux disease will be, by far and away, the most common cause. What are the endoscopic features of gastroesophageal reflux (GER) disease? Most authorities agree that erythema or friability are too nonspecific, and subject to too much observer variation [3]. More specific for reflux disease are longitudinal erosions which are usually located on the tops of the esophageal folds. Often the white erosions are surrounded by a rim of erythema. Biopsy of such a lesion will uniformly reveal polymorphonuclear leukocytes infiltrating the lamina propria, as well as an increase in the basal cell layer and elongation of the dermal papilla [4–6].

When the erosions became more confluent, as is found in more severe reflux disease, the endoscopic appearance becomes less diagnostic and the chance that biopsy may be useful rises. If the endoscopic appearance shows a confluent group of erosions and exudate in the lower tubular esophagus, often with an indistinct or absent Z line, reflux disease is still the best possibility, especially if this appearance is associated with a hiatus hernia as recognized endoscopically. A patulous G-E junction which gapes open increases the probability of reflux damage. If the gastroesophageal junction is viewed from below by retroflexing the instrument, absence of a valve-like structure is found in many patients with severe reflux. (See page 126).

If, however, the same endoscopic appearance is seen in the middle of the tubular esophagus, then biopsy is probably warranted. Samples should be taken not only of the eroded areas, but also distally from the intact mucosal zone below the area of inflammation, as this will usually be found to show columnar (Barrett's) epithelium. In this case, biopsy is to be used not only to document the presence of erosions and inflammation, but also to confirm the presence of columnar or metaplastic epithelium. Knowledge of the presence of this type of epithelium will set into motion other questions of evaluation and therapy covered elsewhere in this book.

The patient's clinical history can be of a great deal of help in deciding whether or not to biopsy an erosive lesion of the esophageal mucosa. If the patient has been taking certain pills (tetracyclines, quinidine, potassium chloride), and then develops sudden odynophagia, then endoscopy will usually show an eroded area in the mid-esophagus [7]. Yet again, it is necessary to ask whether biopsy is warranted, as it will show only nonspecific inflammation and will not add to the clinical diagnosis of pill esophagitis. In fact, the history is so specific that even endoscopy may not be necessary as the diagnosis can be firmly established on clinical grounds.

Are there other conditions which can mimic esophagitis from GER? An interesting paper suggested that candidal esophagitis (even in the nonimmunocompromised host) can present with a confluent eroded appearance, which can be difficult to distinguish from severe GER damage [8]. The presence of hyphae in the biopsy (best seen on silver or PAS stain) confirms the diagnosis and requires a change in therapeutic management. It seems likely that some such cases are missed even when biopsied, as the fungal organisms are difficult to recognize on ordinary hematoxylin and eosin (H and E) stains.

Erosive esophagitis in the immunocompromised host is one situation in which biopsy can be very helpful [9]. Involvement of the mucosa with herpes simplex virus (HSV) or cytomegalovirus (CMV) can produce not only vesicles and ulcers, but confluent esophagitis as well. With the use of suppressive mediums such as acyclovir and gancyclovir, such infections are becoming less common. However, in the untreated host, they are still encountered. In bone marrow patients, the presentation is often atypical with the patient complaining of nausea and vomiting instead of the more usual clinical manifestation of esophageal inflammation such as odynophagia or dysphagia [10]. Biopsies should be taken not only from the sides of the lesions (for herpes virus), but deep at the base of the erosions in order to sample CMV. Culture and immunostaining of the biopsies will show the viral lesions more often than standard histological changes, such as nuclear and cytoplasmic inclusions.

One situation in which endoscopic biopsy would be indicated in erosive esophagitis, is during investigations involving new drug therapy or the results of antireflux surgery. In this special situation, the need for biopsy is not to sort out the individual clinical situation, but rather to document the results of a clinical trial. The ability to pass around coded biopsies to several different investigators during such a trial allows a degree of objectivity which is difficult to reach with endoscopy alone.

There are other situations in which the role of biopsy of erosive lesions of the esophageal mucosa are less well defined. Damage to the mucosa by radiotherapy or chemotherapy may show characteristic changes on biopsy, but the clinical situation will still be the most useful diagnostic aid.

Does biopsy of erosive esophagitis, when treatment has not caused the lesions to regress, offer anything? Possibly, although even with biopsy results the usual clinical response will be to increase acid peptic therapy (switching to a proton-pump inhibitor if H2 blocking agents had been the prior form of therapy). Only in the failure of the latter type of therapy would it be worthwhile to check for an unexpected fungal or viral pathogen.

To summarize, it would appear that routine biopsy in erosive esophagitis would seem not to be a worthwhile strategy, as it increases time and cost of the procedure without increasing the diagnostic yield. Exceptions to this strategy would be in the immunocompromised host or when the erosive esophagitis is located in an atypical location. If biopsy is used in the patient suspected of viral or fungal invasion, then special stains and cultures should be performed.

References

1. Edwards DAW. Flow charts, diagnostic keys and algorithms in the diagnosis of dysphagia. Scot Med J 1970;15:378—385.
2. Edwards DAW. Discriminative information in diagnosis. Proc R Soc Med 1971;64:676—677.
3. Geisinger KR, Wu WC. Endoscopy and biopsy in gastroesophageal reflux disease. In: Castell DO, Wu WC, Ott DJ (eds) Pathogenesis, Diagnosis, Therapy. New York: Futura Publishing Co, 1985;149—166.
4. Ismail-Beigi F, Horton PF, Pope CE II. Histological consequences of gastroesophageal reflux in man. Gastroenterology 1970;58:163—174.
5. Behar J, Sheahan DC. Histologic abnormalities in reflux esophagitis. Arch Pathol Lab Med 1975;99:387—391.
6. Frierson HF. Histology in the diagnosis of reflux esophagitis. Gastroenterol Clin North Am 1990;19:631—644.
7. Eng J, Sabanathan S. Drug-induced esophagitis. Am J Gastroenterol 1991;86:1127—1133.
8. Kodsi BE, Wickremesinghe PC, Kozinn PJ, Iswara K, Goldberg PK. Candida esophagitis. Gastroenterology 1976;71:715—719.
9. McDonald GB. Esophageal diseases caused by infections, systemic illness, medications, and trauma in gastrointestinal disease. In: Sleisenger MH, Fordtran JS (eds) Pathophysiology/Diagnosis/Management. Philadelphia: W.B. Saunders, 1993; 427—477.
10. Spencer GD, Hackman RC, McDonald GB, Amos DE, Cunningham BA, Meyers JD, Thomas ED. A prospective study of unexplained nausea and vomiting after marrow transplantation. Transplantation 1986;42:602—606.

What are the histologic changes in reflux esophagitis?

P. Bechi, A. Amorosi, P. Romagnoli (Florence)

The critical question, "What is reflux esophagitis?" must first be answered. We know what acid gastroesophageal reflux (GER) is and what its range of "normality" is. We know that, when excessive, reflux causes reflux disease which includes typical and/or atypical symptoms and/or esophageal mucosal lesions (i.e., esophagitis). We know that eventually reflux may result in symptoms without any endoscopically detectable esophageal change, minor endoscopic abnormalities of the mucosa without erosive changes, and finally erosions or more severe mucosal lesions.

The presence of erosions is at present requested in order to diagnose esophagitis endoscopically, whereas nonerosive endoscopic abnormalities such as erythema, friability and granularity of the mucosa are subjective and aspecific features and are not sufficient for a diagnosis. Therefore, the answer to the question, "What are the histologic changes in reflux esophagitis?", would imply the description of the histologic changes which occur in erosive esophagitis. However, in this phase the clinical usefulness of obtaining tissue biopsies is questionable, since the presence of mucosal damage is testified by endoscopic changes and histology adds no new information regarding the etiology of esophagitis (acid and/or nonacid reflux, drug ingestion).

On the other hand, histology may have a more important role in the study of reflux disease without endoscopic esophagitis since it is able to provide evidence of nonendoscopically evident mucosal damage.

Although histology with its aspecific signs of mucosal injury has only a purely confirmatory value in true esophagitis, whilst when it is supposedly more helpful for the diagnosis of reflux disease true esophagitis is not present, both these conditions will be briefly illustrated.

Histologic changes in reflux disease without macroscopic esophagitis (low grade histologic changes)

Morphologic changes

Histologic abnormalities associated with reflux in the absence of macroscopic esophagitis were first described by Ismail-Beigi, Horton and Pope II [1]. Basal cell hyperplasia of the squamous epithelium and elongation of the lamina propria papillae (defined as a basal cell layer exceeding 15% of the total epithelial thickness, and papillae extending into the upper third of the epithelium) have been considered by these authors as indicative of low grade mucosal damage caused by GER. Since these changes are usually found in the lowermost 2 cm of the esophagus in control subjects, they are indicative of abnormal reflux when found above this level.

Additional histologic criteria of low grade damage have been proposed, namely the presence of intraepithelial eosinophils (their abnormal minimal number is debatable) [2] and dilated vascular channels at the tips of the papillae [3]. The diagnostic importance of squamous cells with abundant pale cytoplasm and shrunken nuclei (balloon cells) as well as of intraepithelial T-lymphocytes with irregular nuclear contours as isolated findings is questionable.

The histopathologic assessment of all these findings may be affected by several factors, including type, number and topography of biopsies, technique of tissue processing and sectioning; furthermore, it is subject to inter- and intraobserver variations.

It is worth underlining that histology sensitivity and specificity are 0.75 and 0.90 respectively when only the above-described changes can be found (i.e., in the absence of endoscopic esophagitis) [4].

Morphometric changes

In order to improve the unsatisfactory sensitivity of esophageal biopsies morphometric methods have been described [5–7]. Some of them have the additional advantage of circumventing the problem of poorly oriented biopsies obtained from grasp forceps. Morphometric methods based upon measurements of the number or size of nuclei at different depths of the epithelium [6,7], percent papillary length and basal zone hyperplasia measured in adequately-oriented biopsies [5], and the ratio between the surface area of the epithelium-lamina propria junction and the volume of the epithelium (P. Bechi et al., unpublished data) have been used.

Neither Jarvis et al. [6], nor Collins et al. [7], recommend their method as a diagnostic tool in the diagnosis of esophagitis, in spite of its usefulness in the assessment of individual therapeutic response. Johnson et al. [5] were able to demonstrate in well-orientated biopsies that papillary length and basal zone hyperplasia correlate directly with exposure of the esophagus to acid. However, data on the possible increase in sensitivity compared to the purely histologic assessment are not available, since this aspect is not considered in this paper.

Moreover, it was impossible to demonstrate an increase in sensitivity due to morphometry when compared with conventional histologic evaluation in discriminating subjects with and without pathologic reflux (unpublished data).

Histologic changes in reflux disease with erosive esophagitis (high grade histologic changes)

Endoscopic (i.e., erosive) esophagitis is characterized by epithelial injury and active inflammation. Epithelial injury is represented by edema, which appears as a widening of the intercellular spaces, loss of cell cohesion, necrosis and sloughing [3]. Regenerative changes may occur in the epithelium adjacent to the eroded area. The presence of neutrophil polymorphs in both the epithelium and lamina propria is the hallmark of active inflammation. Occasionally eosinophils may predominate. The intensity of cellular infiltrate usually correlates with the degree of epithelial injury. The recognition of these findings is not a diagnostic problem, provided the mucosal sampling is adequate.

Conclusions

From a diagnostic point of view, the role of histology appears to be that of merely confirming endoscopic esophagitis, since the presence of reflux injury is obvious from the macroscopic appearance. At most, in this stage of the disease, biopsies may be obtained to rule out an infectious process (i.e., subtle cases of Candida or Herpes esophagitis) and/or an esophageal neoplasm.

Histology seems more helpful in the diagnosis of reflux disease which is not associated with endoscopic esophagitis. At this stage of the disease it may reveal inflammatory and/or reactive epithelial changes indicative of mild reflux mucosal damage (low grade changes). However, in the latter, its sensitivity and specificity are not greater than 0.75 and 0.90, respectively [4]. The overall sensitivity and specificity of histology is 0.77 and 0.91, compared with a sensitivity and specificity of 24-h pH-monitoring claimed to be as high as 0.88 and 0.98, respectively [4].

Therefore, in spite of its low cost, simplicity and safety, collection and histologic evaluation of esophageal biopsies are of little help from a purely diagnostic point of view. Moreover, although histology may reveal signs of epithelial injury and active inflammation which are hypothetically relevant for the understanding of the evolution of the disease, it has not been shown to be helpful either for the indication of different therapeutic treatments or the follow-up [4]. Morphometric evaluation does not seem to add much to the purely histologic assessment.

Undoubtedly the most useful application of histology appears to be the surveillance of Barrett's esophagus for a correct timing and selection of type of treatment, but these aspects will be considered in different chapters.

References

1. Ismail-Beigi F, Horton PF, Pope CE II. Histological consequences of gastroesophageal reflux in man. Gastroenterology 1970;58:163−174.
2. Winter HS, Madara JL, Stafford RJ, Grand RJ, Quinlan J-E, Goldman H. Intraepithelial eosinophils: a new diagnostic criterion for reflux esophagitis. Gastroenterology 1982;83:816−821.
3. Hamilton SR. Esophagitis. In: Ming S-C, Goldman H (eds) Pathology of the Gastrointestinal Tract. Philadelphia: WB Saunders, 1992;383−438.
4. Klingman RR, Stein HJ, DeMeester TR. The current management of gastroesophageal reflux. In: Cameron JL, Balch CM, Langer B, Manick JA, Sheldon GF, Shires GT, Tomkins RK, Welch CE (eds) Advances in Surgery, vol 24. Mosby-Year Book, 1991;259−291.
5. Johnson LF, DeMeester TR, Haggitt RC. Esophageal epithelial response to gastroesophageal reflux. A quantitative study. Dig Dis 1978;23:498−509.
6. Jarvis LR, Dent J, Whitehead R. Morphometric assessment of reflux oesophagitis in fibreoptic biopsy specimens. J Clin Pathol 1985;38:44−48.
7. Collins JSA, Watt PCH, Hamilton PW, Collins BJ, Sloan JM, Elliott H, Love AHG. Assessment of oesophagitis by histology and morphometry. Histopathology 1989;14:381−389.

Does histochemistry offer better experimental definition of the effects of reflux on the mucosa than light microscopy alone?

D. Hopwood (Dundee)

The immediate consequence of gastroduodenal reflux (GDR) to the esophagus is the destruction of the most superficial of the esophageal squames [1]. This is due to pepsin-hydrochloric acid, the detergent bile acids/salts and trypsin [2,3]. The result of this damage is an increase in the rate of cell turnover of the squamous epithelium [4]. If the damage is continued, there is an increase in the length of the papillae and in the height of the basal cell compartment, the morphological counterparts [5]. The proportion of cells in the different compartments is also altered and more maturing/differentiating prickle cells and less functional cells are seen. The metabolic requirements of the maturing cells are greater than those of the mature functional cells and new longer capillaries are induced, extending higher into the epithelium, possibly also attracted by cell damage. These changes form the basis for the histopathological diagnosis of reflux esophagitis (discussed elsewhere in this volume, see page 271). The general basophilia of the basal/prickle cells can be seen in the standard haematoxylin and eosin (H and E) preparation. H and E sections will also show up basophilic dots in the cytoplasm of mature cells [1]. The latter are due to a gathering together of organelle debris, including rough endoplasmic reticulum. The presence of these dots argues for normal complete maturation of the squamous cells and against damage. H and E preparations will also demonstrate the presence of inflammatory cells. Amongst these, eosinophils have been described as markers of reflux [6]. However, from a practical viewpoint they are difficult to demonstrate in standard paraffin wax H and E sections. Nevertheless, they are easily shown in resin sections, but this is not a routine procedure.

Gastroesophageal reflux (GER) may damage the esophageal mucosa, allowing various pathogens entry or attachment. Some of these may be demonstrated in H and E preparations. Partly digested squames are sometimes associated with the numbers of bacteria attached to them. In esophageal cells, around peptic esophageal ulcers, herpes virus and their effects may be seen in 25% of cases. Also, candidal hyphae may sometimes be seen. Endoscopic white patches may also be due to large amounts of glycogen stored in squames (glycogenic acanthosis) [5].

Histochemical techniques can potentially offer a more sensitive and accurate picture of the effects of reflux of the esophageal mucosa. Some of the techniques involved are well known. For example, glycogen is not present in significant amounts in the basal cells. When this compartment increases in size, the glycogen demonstrated by the PAS reaction is much reduced in sections, being found in suprabasal cells only [7]. This forms a useful method for the histometric assessment of damage and regeneration in esophageal biopsies.

Other approaches have been made to apply histochemical findings to define or express changes in esophageal mucosa due to reflux. Alkaline phosphatase, for example, has been documented in the vascular loops of esophageal papillae, but not to any significant amount in the squames. This allowed a subsequent quantitative biochemical approach, where the amount of alkaline phosphatase correlated well with the length of the papillae and the histological degree of inflammation [8]. More recent reports have shown that capillary loops in inflamed skin are associated with the exhibition of ELAM-1 an adhesion molecule on the endothelium, directed toward inflammatory cells [9].

Cell damage has been associated with lysosomal activity. Lysosomal enzymes have been detected histochemically in esophageal mucosa. Acid phosphatase decreases with inflammation. This may be due to most of the large lysosomes being in the most superficial cells, which are decreased in inflammation [8]. Secondly, membrane coating granules also contain acid phosphatase. They are known to secrete their contents into the intercellular space in response to acid (as also happens in skin) [10]. β-Glucuronidase, on the other hand, increases with inflammation. This may be related to its synthetic activity [8].

Lipids have been demonstrated in the esophageal mucosa using Oil Red O on frozen sections which shows neutral lipids [11]. Droplets, nonmembrane limited, are most abundant in the superficial cells. Similar appearances have been noted with Nile Red (a probe for neutral lipids and cholesterol esters). Using disaggregated esophageal biopsies and flow cytometry [12], there was significantly less lipid in basal and prickle cells and in mature large squames from inflamed esophageal biopsies, compared with normal control biopsies [13]. The function of the neutral lipid is uncertain, it may simply reflect the anaerobic metabolism of mature squames at an increasing distance from the capillaries. Some of the lipid may be involved with a barrier function which appears to be the mechanism in keratinising epithelia. Biochemically, we have shown that there were significantly more neutral lipids (fatty acids, triglycerides and cholesterol esters) in normal biopsies than inflamed ones. Similarly, there was significantly more sphingomyelin than other phospholipids in normal biopsies.

ATP-ase has been briefly examined histochemically. Basal and prickle cells showed a small activity on the cell membrane. This may be related to sodium and potassium transport recently described in relation to maintenance of cell volume in rabbit esophagus. Higher activity was noted on Langerhans' cells in a study of esophageal striped muscle [14]. Changes in these cells have been noted in cervix and skin, in inflammatory and premalignant conditions [15]. It would seem that equivalent changes should be identifiable in the esophagus.

There has been no systematic histochemical study of the esophageal mucosa. Therefore, the question posed can be answered quite clearly. Although the standard H and E techniques can give much information, the histochemical approach can give much more refined information on the effects of reflux on the esophageal mucosa. The addition of immunoperoxidase methods extends and refines the information greatly.

References

1. Hopwood D. The oesophageal lining. In: Whitehead R (ed) Gastrointestinal and oesophageal pathology. Edinburgh: Churchill Livingstone, 1989;3−12.
2. Bateson MC, Hopwood D, Milne G, Bouchier IAD. Oesophageal epithelial ultrastructure after incubation with gastro-intestinal fluids and their components. J Pathol 1980;133:35−51.
3. Hopwood D, Bateson MC, Milne G, Bouchier IAD. Effects of bile acids and hydrogen ions on the fine structure of oesophageal epithelium. Gut 1981;22:306−311.
4. Livstone EM, Sheahan DG, Behar J. Studies of esophageal epithelial cell proliferation in patients with reflux esophagitis. Gastroenterol 1977;73:1315−1319.
5. Whitehead R. The Oesophageal Lining. Edinburgh: Churchill Livingstone, 1989;3:850−854.
6. Brown LF, Goldman H, Antonioli DA. Intraepithelial eosinophils in endoscopic biopsies of adults with reflux esophagitis. Am J Surg Pathol 1984;8:899−905.
7. Sanders DSA, Kerr MA, Hopwood D, Coghill G, Milne G. Expression of the 3-fucosyl N-acetyllactosamine (CD15) antigen in normal, metaplastic, dysplastic and neoplastic squamous epithelia. J Pathol 1988;154:255−262.
8. Hopwood D, Ross PE, Bouchier IAD. Reflux oesophagitis. Clin Gastroenterol 1981;10:505−520.
9. Norton J, Sloane JP, Al-Saffar N, Haskard DO. Vessel associated adhesion molecules in normal skin and acute graft-versus-host disease. J Clin Pathol 1991;44:586−591.
10. Hopwood D, Logan KR, Milne G. The light and electron microscopic distribution of acid phosphatase activity in normal human oesophageal epithelium. Histochem J 1978;10:159−170.
11. Hopwood D, Logan KR, Coghill G, Bouchier IAD. Histochemical studies of mucosubstances and lipids in normal human oesophageal epithelium. J Histochem Cytochem 1977;9:153−161.

12. Hopwood D, Jankowski J, Milne G, Wormsley KG. Flow cytometry of oesophageal mucosal biopsies; epidermal growth factor receptor and CD15. J Pathol 1992;167:321–326.
13. Hopwood D, Spiers E, Potts R, Ross PE, Callaghan C, Anderson J, Murray FE. Lipid in the esophageal mucosa. Gullet 1993 (submitted).
14. Leese G, Hopwood D. Muscle fibre typing in the human pharyngeal constrictors and oesophagus. Acta Anat 1986;127: 77–80.
15. Morris HHB, Gatter KC, Sykes C, Casemore V, Mason DY. Langerhans' cells in human cervical epithelium: effects of wart virus infection and intraepithelial neoplasia. Br J Obstet Gynecol 1983;90:412–420.

Does electron microscopy of the esophageal mucosa add useful information?

C.E. Pope II (Seattle)

If the total number of papers employing electron microscopy to evaluate the esophageal mucosa is used to determine the answer to this question, then one would have to conclude that the answer is negative. In spite of the numbers of electron microscopes available and the ease of endoscopic or suction biopsy of the esophageal mucosa, not much work using electron microscopy has been done on the esophageal epithelium. However, there have been some useful ultrastructural findings about the stratified squamous epithelium, and the opportunity for using this tool in future investigations would seem to offer a great deal of promise.

Table 1 lists some of the subjects of investigation by means of electron microscopy, both scanning (SEM) and transmission electron microscopy (TEM). A fair amount of effort has gone into the description of the normal esophageal epithelium [1–7]. It should be noted that most specimens used for "normal" studies were obtained from patients undergoing endoscopy for suspected or known upper gastrointestinal pathology. There were no endoscopic esophageal changes, but the reflux status of most of these "normal" patients is not known.

The appearance of the normal epithelium can be synthesized from these studies in normal patients. By SEM, the esophageal mucosa consists of an interlocking arrangement of polygonal cells with prominent raised intercellular ridges. On the surface of the cells are raised microridges in a whorled pattern. Some of the cells are

Table 1.

1.	Description of normal ultrastructural anatomy
2.	Study of damage by reflux
3.	Description of epithelial interfaces
4.	Studies of esophageal mucosal dysplasia
5.	Alterations of epithelial cells in carcinoma
6.	Effects of chemotherapy and radiotherapy

partially detached in the process of exfoliation, and occasionally the cell will be totally folded back on itself prior to exfoliation. On TEM, the luminal edge is coated with a 1000 A thick acidic glycocalyx [4]. The subsurface cells are tightly connected to each other by desmosomes. In the prickle cell layer, the number of desmosomes and membrane folds are increased. The basal cell layer is attached to the basement membrane by prominent hemidesmosomes. The intracellular spaces are narrow (Fig. 1). The capillaries in the dermal pegs are fenestrated, resembling the capillaries in the renal glomeruli and endocrine glands. Free-ending nerve fibers have been demonstrated within the epithelial layer [8]. These probably serve a sensory function.

In the few patients with esophageal reflux who have been studied, there is increased desquamation of cells and exudate is present over the surface as shown by SEM [7]. The intercellular ridges were usually preserved unless there was marked

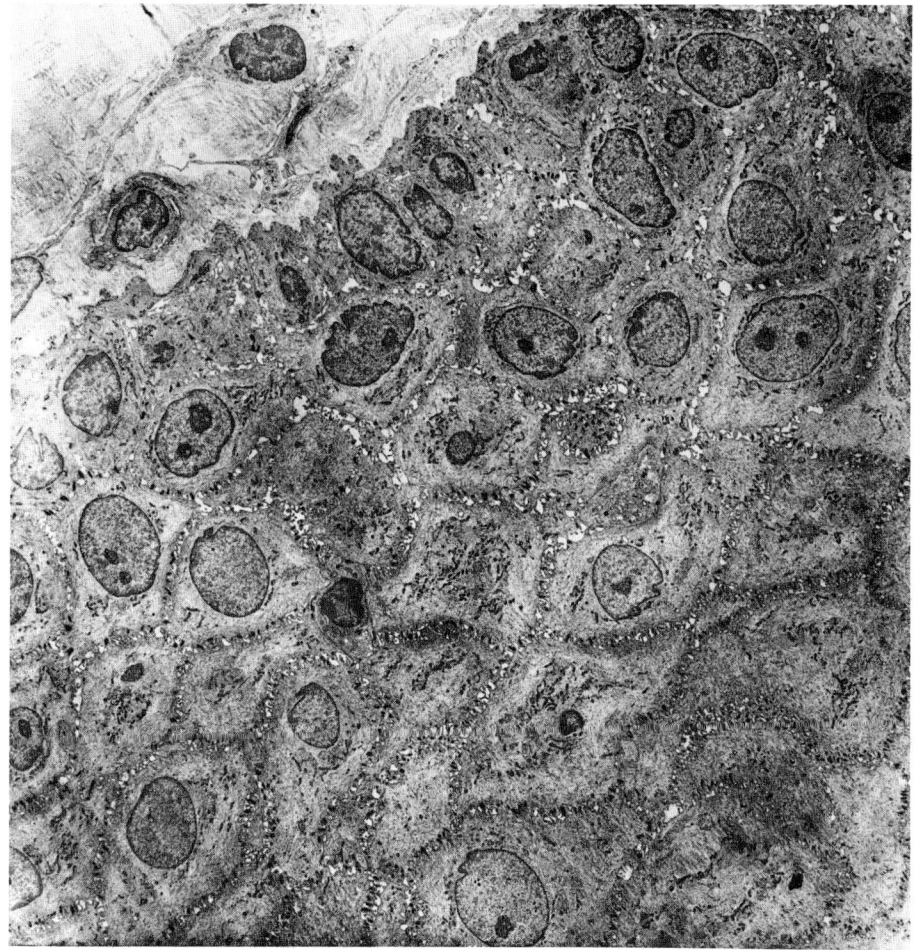

Fig. 1. Ultrastructural appearance of normal esophageal mucosa. The lamina propria is at the bottom right hand corner. A row of the basal cells is tightly connected to the basement membrane. Several rows of prickle cells are seen above the single row of basal cells. Note close apposition of the cells to one another.

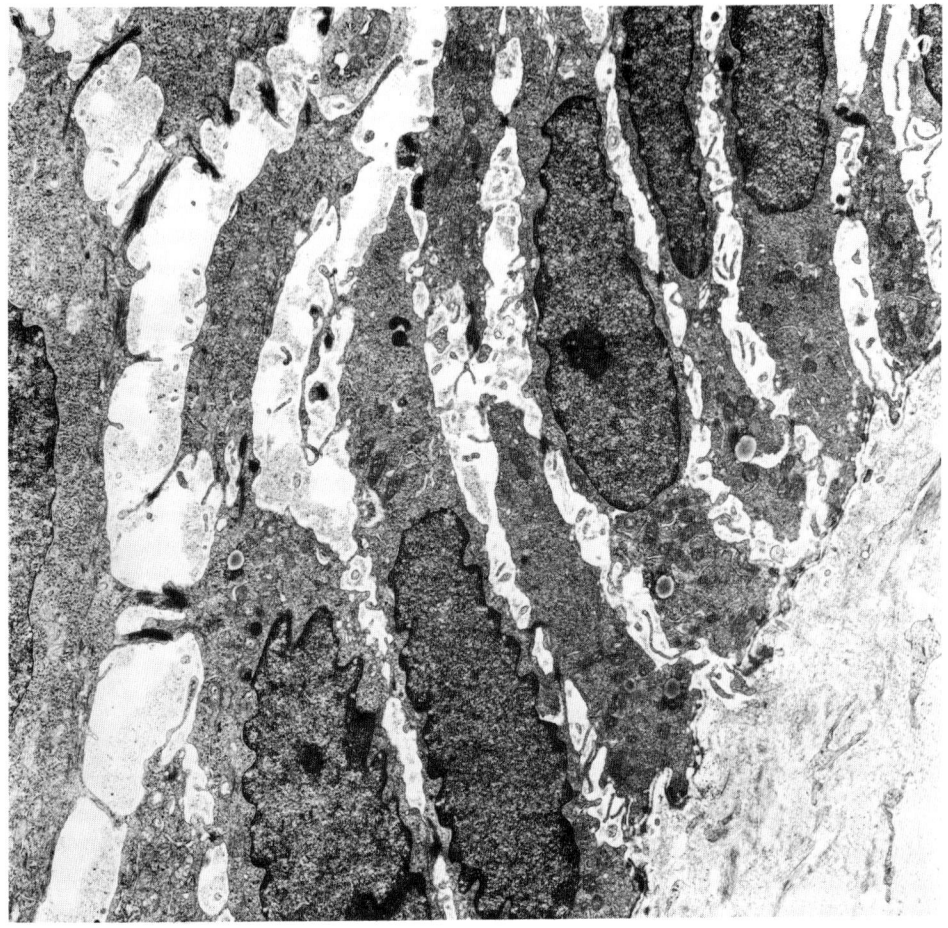

Fig. 2. Ultrastructural appearance of a biopsy from a patient with reflux esophagitis. The lamina propria is in the bottom right hand corner. The single row of basal cells shows elongation of nucleus and cytoplasm. The intercellular space is increased as is the space between the prickle cells above the basal cell row. Note increased debris in the intercellular spaces.

damage, but the microridges on each cell were reduced [9]. By TEM, there was increased space between the prickle cell layer (Fig. 2) [10]. The epithelium can be infiltrated by lymphocytes and polymorphonuclear leukocytes. When this occurs, the desmosomes which normally hold the cells together vanish in the area in which the infiltrating cell is located. The midzonal cells are relatively undisturbed.

Experimentally, production of such changes has been studied in biopsies cultured for short periods of time in solutions containing various concentrations of bile, gastric juice and acid [11–13]. Gastric juice at pH = 7 and 0.1 N HCl produces little damage. Bile salts at physiological concentrations (0.2 mM) also do not produce much damage, unless they are placed in an acid medium. Gastric juice at pH 1–3 (pepsin would be activated) causes a great deal of surface damage. These changes have been confirmed by in vivo studies using EM in rabbits [14]. In the rabbit experiments it was felt that the bile salts in an acid solution affected mostly the cell membranes and intracellular organelles, whereas the infusion of acid-pepsin solutions caused mainly damage to the intercellular connections with increased shedding of surface cells.

Electron microscopy has also been useful in studying aspects of metaplastic and neoplastic change in the squamous epithelium. A recent paper studied the interface between squamous epithelium and columnar (Barrett's) epithelium. In contradistinction to the normal situation where typical squamous cells abut gastric cells, a transitional cell interposed between squamous and gastric cells has been described in patients with Barrett's epithelium [15]. This cell has features of both squamous cells (surface microridges and well-formed intercellular ridges) and gastric surface cells (microvilli). In a few cells, both microridges (squamous) and microvilli (gastric) were present on the same cell. The microvilli were seen on top of the intercellular ridges, a situation never present in gastric cells — gastric cells are not connected by intercellular ridges.

Dysplasia of the squamous epithelium has also been investigated from biopsies obtained from areas surrounding frank squamous cell carcinoma [9]. In dysplasia, the intercellular ridges disappear and the microridges on each cell become more densely packed together. This is in contradistinction to the appearance seen in biopsies from patients with reflux esophagitis in which the intercellular ridges are preserved, but the microridges are more sparse than in control biopsies. These visual impressions of the relative densities of microridges between control, dysplastic and reflux esophagitis cells were confirmed by quantitative morphometric measurements.

Study of esophageal carcinomas by TEM reveals some very interesting findings. In 11 of 43 cases of esophageal cancer studied, multidirectional differentiation was demonstrated [16]. Five squamous cell carcinomas contained cells with glandular features; four adenocarcinomas showed cells with squamous cell characteristics. Of two small cell carcinomas of the esophagus, one had cells with squamous, the other cells with glandular characteristics. This suggests the possibility that esophageal cancers may arise from a stem cell precursor and only later differentiate into a predominantly squamous cell carcinoma or predominantly adenocarcinoma.

Electron microscopy has another potential use — to evaluate damage from chemotherapy and radiotherapy [17] or laser therapy [18]. In animal studies, graded doses of X-ray produce loss of microridges on the squamous cell [17]. Similar studies are possible in humans, and might offer an extremely sensitive index to cell damage by therapeutic agents, and a method whereby protection from such damage could be evaluated.

Electron microscopy does offer a unique method of evaluation of the esophageal mucosa. It is a tool which has only begun to be utilized, although the techniques of obtaining tissue and studying it are well advanced. It is expected that new and interesting information will be obtained by using SEM and TEM to study the esophageal mucosa in health and disease.

References

1. Dilly PN, Mallison CN. Ultrastructural characteristics of the oesophageal mucosa in man. Gut 1975;16:841−842.
2. Ackerman L, Piros J, deCarle D, Christensen J. A scanning electron microscopic study of esophageal mucosa. Scanning Electron Microscopy 1976;5:247−252.
3. Al Yassin TM, Toner PG. Fine structure of squamous epithelium and submucosal glands of human oesophagus. J Anat 1977;123:705−721.
4. Logan KR, Hopwood D, Milne G. Ultrastructural demonstration of cell coat on the cell surfaces of normal human oesophageal epithelium. Histochem J 1977;9:495−504.
5. Hopwood D, Logan KR, Bouchier IAD. The electron microscopy of normal human oesophageal epithelium. Virchows Arch B Cell Path 1978;26:345−358.
6. Logan KR, Hopwood D, Milne G. Cellular junctions in human oesophageal epithelium. J Pathol 1978;126:157−163.
7. Siew S, Goldstein ML. Scanning electron microscopy of mucosal biopsies of the human upper gastrointestinal tract. Scanning Electron Microscopy 1981;4:173−181.
8. Robles-Chillida EM, Rodrigo J, Mayo I, Arnedo A, Gomez A. Ultrastructure of free-ending nerve fibres in oesophageal epithelium. J Anat 1981;133:227−233.
9. Goran DA, Shields HM, Bates ML, Zuckerman GR, DeSchryver-Kecskemeti K. Esophageal dysplasia. Assessment by light microscopy and scanning electron microscopy. Gastroenterology 1984;86:39−50.
10. Hopwood D, Milne G, Logan KR. Electron microscopic changes in human oesophageal epithelium in oesophagitis. J Pathol 1979;129:161−167.
11. Bateson MC, Hopwood D, Milne G, Bouchier IAD. Oesophageal epithelial ultrastructure after incubation with gastrointestinal fluids and their components. J Pathol 1980;133:35−51.
12. Hopwood D, Bateson MC, Milne G, Bouchier IAD. Effects of bile acids and hydrogen ion on the fine structure of oesophageal epithelium. Gut 1981;22:306−311.
13. Gotley DC, Flaks B, Cooper MJ. Bile acids do not modify the effects of pepsin on the fine structure of human oesophageal epithelium. Austr NZ J Surg 1992;62:569−575.
14. Salo JA, Lehto V-P, Kivilaakso E. Morphological alterations in experimental esophagitis. Dig Dis Sci 1983;28:440−448.
15. Shields HM, Zwas F, Antonioli DA, Doos WG, Kim S, Spechler SJ. Detection by scanning electron microscopy of a distinctive esophageal surface cell at the junction of squamous and Barrett's epithelium. Dig Dis Sci 1993;38:97−108.
16. Newman J, Antonakopoulos GN, Darnton SJ, Matthews HR. The ultrastructure of oesophageal carcinomas: Multidirectional differentiation. A transmission electron microscopic study of 43 cases. J Pathol 1992;167:193−198.
17. Albertsson M, Cwikiel M, Hakansson CH, Palmegren M. Response of the esophageal epithelium to concomitant cis-dichlorodiamineplatinum (II) and radiation treatment. An electron microscopic study in rabbits. Scanning Microscopy 1992;6:1023−1033.
18. Schaarschmidt K, Stratmann U, Lehmann RR, Heinze H, Willital GH. The rat esophagus: ultrastructure and radiological aspects of tissue response after 1320 nm Nd:YAG laser irradiation. Exp Toxicol Path 1992;44:239−244.

What is the correlation between severity of mucosal damage and motor disorders of the esophagus?

R. Bumm (Munich)

The concept of an esophageal motor disorder in patients with gastroesophageal reflux (GER) was initiated by Siegel and Hendrix in 1963 when they observed "non-progressive, spastic as well as high amplitude" esophageal body contractions during esophageal acid perfusion in patients with reflux esophagitis [1]. Until now, subsequent workers have aimed to identify specific defects in esophageal peristalsis or sphincter function and tried to correlate observed changes with severity of mucosal damage in patients with GER. This article will review the relevant studies according to the specific defects of esophageal motility described and supply a preliminary conclusion.

GER and the lower esophageal sphincter

The lower esophageal sphincter (LES) is considered to be the major device for the prevention of reflux. The function of the LES was first monitored by balloon compression, unperfused catheters, and then determined by perfused catheter systems. Dent introduced the era of sleeve measurements of the LES [2] which enabled accurate continuous LES-pressure recordings. In subsequent studies it was demonstrated that GER requires episodes of low LES-pressure, i.e., transient relaxations or persistent hypotension [3]. The frequency of transient LES-relaxations is similar in normals and GER patients [4], although it can not represent the primary GER-mechanism. In the state of deterioration of esophageal mucosa (Barrett's esophagus [5], peptic strictures [6], scleroderma [7]) extremely low LES-pressure profiles have been demonstrated. Clinical studies have shown that LES-pressures are usually decreased in patients with GERD [3,8–10]; however, considerable overlap of LES-pressures of normals and GER patients exists.

More recently, 3-D imaging of LES-pressure recordings [11] was used in a trial incorporating patients with all stages of GERD and showed that LES-pressure (expressed as a vector volume) gradually decreased with increasing severity of mucosal injury [12].

Low LES-pressures can not usually be normalized by clinically successful medical therapy [8], although one author reported a significant improvement [3]. Surgical repair such as Nissen fundoplication reliably elevates LESP [12,13].

GER and esophageal body motility

GER and alterations of esophageal pressure waves

Conventional stationary manometry by means of perfused catheter systems and chart recording was engaged by a variety of investigators to study the effect of GERD on esophageal body motility. It is now generally accepted that patients with GERD develop a general hypotension of esophageal contractions with progressing disease [10], and frequently exhibit a peristaltic dysfunction [14] which impairs bolus transport [15,16] and often generates dysphagia symptoms. In a recent paper the presence of esophagitis did not impair the radionucleid transport compared to GER patients without esophagitis [17], but the incidence of peristaltic dysfunction is clearly related to the degree of esophagitis [18]. One paper describes an aperistalsis as a consequence of long-existing GERD which responded to medical treatment [19]. However, it is still controversial whether the "hypomotility" of advanced GERD can be reversed after medical or surgical treatment [8].

GER and "induced" pressure events

Siegel and Hendrix first described irregular esophageal contractions when they perfused the esophagus of GER patients with acid solutions [1]. Corazziari found in normal men that the bolus volume for eliciting secondary peristalsis was directly related to intraesophageal pH [20] and speculated about a possible mechanism of reflux defense. A similar experiment showed that this mechanism may be lost in GER patients [21]. Secondary and tertiary esophageal contractions linked to GER are frequently observed [22], but it remains a "hen and egg" question whether deterioration of esophageal mucosa effects esophageal motility or vice versa.

GER and circadian esophageal motility pattern

Recent technical advances have enabled the circadian analysis of esophageal motility and pH (MP24) by 24-h measurements with lightweight, high-capacity data loggers and computed data analysis [23,24]. The circadian motor pattern of the normal esophagus has been described [23]. Nowadays, digital recording is the preferred monitoring method and systems using intermittent data sampling are inadequate because they do not permit access to the full manometric data set and, therefore, do not allow for uninterrupted intercorrelation of esophageal motility and pH. Until now, only three trials engaging MP24 were published [14,25,26]; in one, which used intermittent recording but incorporated a large number of patients, an abnormal overall circadian motor pattern in GER patients [25] with an increased frequency of low amplitude and nonperistaltic contractions was found. These impairments depended on the degree of mucosal damage.

GER-inducing motor events and clearance motility

A different way to quantify GER-induced esophageal motor abnormalities is to analyze separately every incidence of GER and distinguish motility preceding, accompanying or following GER. In a recent paper [14], time periods were defined (induction period: 30 s before until start of GER; response period: time during GER and 240 s after end of GER). GER patients exhibited an increased percentage of abnormal, mostly segmental motor events during the induction period and a reduced peristalsis during the response period, if compared to controls. A second study engaging a similar study design [26] did not confirm these results; however, the authors used a monitoring system with intermittent data recording and data reduction during data sampling.

The contact time of refluxed material is strongly affected by the number of peristaltic contractions recorded during GER-episodes [14,27]. In patients, the clearance motility is reduced and the median time interval between onset of GER and the first esophageal contraction is prolonged. This is especially true for patients with esophagitis [28]. The mechanism for clearance of physiological GER is secondary peristalsis. In contrast to Corazziari's findings mentioned above, a more recent paper [29] does not support the hypothesis of a pH-sensitive esophagus; identical volumes of NaCl, HCl and balloon distension elicited similar secondary motor events in normal subjects.

Conclusion

The common motor defect in patients with GERD is hypotension of the LES, hypo-peristalsis of the esophagus and peristaltic dysfunction, and this defect is clearly linked to the degree of mucosal damage expressed as the stadium of esophagitis or presence of stricture and Barrett's esophagus. There is evidence that abnormal motility shortly before and hypoperistalsis during GER is a major pathogenetic mechanism in reflux patients. We believe that the circadian rhythm of esophageal motility in GERD patients is also affected, but it will require dedicated studies with long-term monitoring of esophageal body peristalsis, lower esophageal sphincter pressure and swallowing in large patient cohorts to determine these abnormalities. The therapeutic relevance of GER-related motor disorders is accepted for the lower esophageal sphincter and for hypomotility and hypoperistalsis, but less defined for the abnormalities in GER clearance. Future studies on circadian interaction of GER and motility may help to understand the pathogenesis of GERD better and find distinctive diagnostic tools for therapeutic decisions.

References

1. Siegel CI, Hendrix TR. Esophageal motor abnormalities induced by acid perfusion in patients with heartburn. J Clin Invest 1963;42:686–695.
2. Dent J. A new technique for continuous sphincter pressure measurement. Gastroenterology 1976;71:263–267.
3. Dodds WJ, Dent J, Hogan WJ, Helm JF, Hauser R, Patel G, Egide MS. Mechanisms of gastroesophageal reflux in patients with reflux esophagitis. N Engl J Med 1982;307:1547–1552.
4. Mittal RK, McCallum RW. Characteristics and frequency of transient relaxations of the lower esophageal sphincter in patients with reflux esophagitis. Gastroenterology 1988;95:593–599.
5. Knuff TE, Benjamin SB, Worsham F. Histologic evaluation of chronic gastroesophageal reflux: an evaluation of biopsy methods and diagnostic criteria. Dig Dis Sci 1984;29:194–201.
6. Ahtaridis G, Snape WJ, Cohen S. Clinical and manometric findings in benign peptic strictures of the esophagus. Dig Dis Sci 1979;24:858–860.
7. Chobanian SJ, Castell DO. Esophageal abnormalities in systemic disease. In: Castell DO, Johnson LF (eds) Esophageal Function in Health and Disease. New York: Elsevier Biomedical, 1983:273–294.
8. Katz PO, Knuff TE, Benjamin SB, Castell DO. Abnormal esophageal pressures in reflux esophagitis: Cause or effect? Am J Gastroenterol 1986;81:744–746.
9. Dent J, Holloway RH, Toouli J, Dodds WJ. Mechanisms of lower esophageal sphincter incompetence in patients with symptomatic gastroesophageal reflux. Gut 1988;29:1020–1028.
10. Burns TW, Venturatos SG. Esophageal motor function and response to acid perfusion in patients with symptomatic reflux esophagitis. Dig Dis Sci 1985;30:529–535.
11. Bombeck CT, Vaz O, DeSalvo J. Computerized axial manometry of the esophagus. Ann Surg 1987;206:465–472.
12. Stein HJ, DeMeester TR, Naspetti R, Jamieson J, Perry RE. Three-dimensional imaging of the lower esophageal sphincter in gastroesophageal reflux disease. Ann Surg 1991;214:374–384.
13. Eckardt VF. Does healing of esophagitis improve esophageal motor function. Dig Dis Sci 1988;33:161–165.
14. Bumm R, Feussner H, Hölscher AH, Jörg K, Dittler HJ, Siewert JR. Interaction of gastroesophageal reflux and esophageal

motility: evaluation by ambulatory 24-hour manometry and pH-metry. Dig Dis Sci 1992;37:1192−1199.

15. Eriksen CA, Sadek SA, Cranford C, Sutton D, Kennedy N, Cuschieri A. Reflux esophagitis and oesophageal transit: evidence for a primary motor disorder. Gut 1988;29:448−452.

16. Kahrilas PJ, Dodds WJ, Hogan WJ. Effect of peristaltic dysfunction on esophageal volume clearance. Gastroenterology 1988;94:73−80.

17. Maddern GJ, Jamieson GG. Oesophageal emptying in patients with gastroesophageal reflux. Br J Surg 1986;73:615−617.

18. Kahrilas PJ, Dodds WJ, Hogan WJ, Kern MK, Arndorfer RC, Reece A. Esophageal peristaltic dysfunction in peptic esophagitis. Gastroenterology 1986;91:897−904.

19. Moses FM. Reversible aperistalsis as a complication of gastroesophageal reflux disease. Am J Gastroenterol 1987;82: 272−275.

20. Corazziari E, Materia E, Pozzessere C, Anzini F, Torsoli A. Intraluminal pH and oesophageal motility in patients with gastroesophageal reflux. Digestion 1986;35:151−157.

21. Corazziari E, Pozzessere C, Dani S, Anzini F, Torsoli A. Intraluminal pH and esophageal motility. Gastroenterology 1978;75:275−277.

22. Triadafilopoulos G, Castillo T. Nonpropulsive esophageal contractions and gastroesophageal reflux. Am J Gastroenterol 1991;86:153−159.

23. Armstrong D, Emde C, Bumm R, Blum AL. Twenty-four hour pattern of esophageal motility in asymptomatic volunteers. Dig Dis Sci 1990;35:1190−1197.

24. Bumm R, Feussner H, Emde C, Hölscher AH, Siewert JR. Interaction of gastroesophageal reflux and esophageal motility in healthy men undergoing combined 24-hour mano/pH-metry. In: Little AG, Ferguson MK, Skinner DB (eds) Diseases of the Esophagus, vol 2. Mount Kisco, New York: Futura Publishing, 1990:102−112.

25. Stein HJ, Eypasch EP, DeMeester TR, Smyrk TC, Attwood SEA. Circadian esophageal motor function in patients with gastroesophageal reflux. Surgery 1990;108:769−778.

26. Timmer R, Breumelhof R, Nadorp JHSM, Smout AJPM. Oesophageal motor response to reflux is not impaired in reflux esophagitis. Gut 1993;34:317−320.

27. Kruse-Andersen S, Wallin L, Madsen T. Relationship between spontaneous nonpropagating pressure activity in the oesophagus and acid gastroesophageal reflux in pathological and nonpathological refluxers. Gut 1987;28:1478−1483.

28. Kruse-Andersen S. Extended recordings of intraesophageal pressures and pH. Booklet available through Dr. Kruse-Andersen.

29. Thompson DG, Andreollo NA, McIntyre AS, Earlam RJ. Studies of the esophageal clearance responses to intraluminal acid. Gut 1988;29:881−885.

30. Baldi F, Ferrari F, Longanesi A, Angeloni M, Raggazini M, Miglioli M, Barbara L. Oesophageal function before, during, and after healing of erosive oesophagitis. Gut 1988;29:157−160.

31. Jacob P, Kahrilas PJ, Vanagunas A. Peristaltic dysfunction associated with nonobstructive dysphagia in reflux disease. Dig Dis Sci 1990;35:939−942.

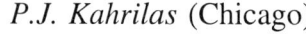 *P.J. Kahrilas* (Chicago)

Normal esophageal acid clearance

Following gastroesophageal reflux (GER), the period that the esophageal mucosa remains acidified is the esophageal acid clearance time. Acid clearance time can be determined by instilling 15 ml of 0.1 N HCl (pH 1.2) into the esophagus and monitoring the intraesophageal pH with an electrode positioned 5 cm above the LES, as the esophageal mucosal pH is restored to a value of 4. An elegant demonstration of the normal mechanism of acid clearance simultaneously assessed volume clearance (elimination of detectable fluid volume from the esophagus) and acid clearance (restoration of esophageal mucosal pH to a value of 4) using 0.1 N HCl radiolabeled with technetium sulfur colloid [1]. Esophageal volume clearance almost immediately follows acid instillation but volume clearance does not equate with acid clearance. Rather, the restoration of esophageal pH is achieved in increments with each subsequent swallow. Aspirating saliva from the mouth prolongs acid clearance suggesting that it is the swallowed saliva rather than the subsequent peristaltic contractions themselves that restore intraesophageal pH. Thus, the normal process of esophageal acid clearance is a two-step process; virtually all acid volume is cleared by esophageal peristalsis, leaving a minimal residue that sustains an acidic pH in the esophageal mucosa until neutralized by swallowed saliva.

Intraesophageal pH following esophageal volume clearance is restored in stepwise fashion with an incremental increase with each swallow. However, the swallow rate itself has minimal influence on the subsequent acid clearance time, because swallow rate is mainly determined by the rate of saliva secretion and it is the saliva that titrates the esophageal pH [2]. Thus, in individuals with normal esophageal volume clearance, the acid clearance time is solely dependent upon the rate of salivation and maneuvers that increased salivation, such as oral lozenges or bethanechol which hasten acid clearance, while aspiration of saliva or replacement of saliva by equal volumes of water prolongs acid clearance.

Esophageal acid clearance in GERD

Prolongation of esophageal acid clearance among patients with esophagitis was demonstrated along with the initial description of the acid clearance test [3]. The acid clearance time values of patients with hiatal hernias and symptomatic GER were found to be greater than the values of controls. Similarly, in 24-h distal esophageal pH recordings of 100 patients with reflux disease, the mean acid clearance time of "supine refluxers" was markedly prolonged, compared to the values of 15 control subjects [4]. Subsequent investigations have demonstrated heterogeneity within the patient population such that, although the mean acid clearance time value among patients with symptomatic reflux was greater than that of controls, about half of GERD patients had normal values and the other half had prolonged values [5]. That proportion of about half normal, half abnormal was also found by analysis of spontaneous reflux events in recumbent patients being monitored with both a manometric catheter and an intraesophageal pH electrode [6]. Finally, a review of a large data set on 24-h esophageal pH monitoring also suggested heterogeneity within the population of patients with symptomatic reflux disease such that individuals with known hiatal hernias tended to have the most prolonged recumbent acid clearance times [7].

Thus, in either the controlled setting of the acid clearance time test or in the setting of spontaneous reflux, GERD patients have acid clearance times that are, on average, 2–3 times longer than those of normal controls. It is, however, important to note that the GERD population is heterogeneous with respect to this measure such that some individuals have normal clearance values and other individuals have markedly abnormal values. From what we know regarding the mechanisms of acid clearance, the two major potential causes of prolonged esophageal acid clearance are impaired volume clearance and impaired salivary function. This discussion will focus exclusively on impaired volume clearance.

Esophageal volume clearance in GERD

As mentioned above, the role of volume clearance in the normal process of acid clearance is to empty the lion's share of fluid from the esophagus, leaving behind a small amount that is then neutralized in stepwise fashion by swallowed saliva. Impaired volume clearance in reflux disease was inferred by the observation that patients with abnormal acid clearance times were improved by an upright posture or by head-of-bed elevation, suggesting that gravity could improve abnormal clearing [5]. Subsequently, two mechanisms of impaired volume clearance have been identified: peristaltic dysfunction and "re-reflux" associated with some hiatal hernias.

Impaired esophageal motor function in esophagitis has been described by a number of investigators [8–10]. A recent analysis compared motor activity of subgroups of patients with reflux disease of varying severity, to groups of control subjects [8]. Peristaltic dysfunction was defined as either failed peristalsis or peristaltic sequences with contractions in the distal esophagus sufficiently feeble to impair esophageal volume clearance. The prevalence of peristaltic dysfunction increases dramatically with increasing severity of esophagitis, rising from 25% in individuals with mild esophagitis to 50% in patients with severe esophagitis. Whether peristaltic dysfunction associated with peptic esophagitis is reversible is disputed [5,11]. Current opinion suggests that the impaired motor function (both decreased LES pressure and diminished peristaltic amplitude) does not revert following effective medical or surgical therapy [12,13]. Further analysis of the relationship between peristaltic activity and volume clearance reveals that both patterns of peristaltic dysfunction (failed peristalsis and feeble peristaltic contractions) impair volume clearance [14]. Failed peristalsis results in very poor volume clearance while foci of feeble contractions clear most, but not all, barium from the esophagus. Further, the vigor of peristalsis required to effect complete volume clearance varies with location; i.e., very weak contractions proximally are effective, but contractions on the order of 30 mmHg are required distally, a finding supported also by other investigations [15].

Hiatal hernias also play a pathophysiologic role in impaired esophageal volume clearance [16,17]. Concurrent pH recording and scintiscanning demonstrate "re-reflux" from the hernia sac during swallowing in 15 of the 20 hiatal hernia patients studied. A more recent analysis suggests the importance of reduction of the hernia between swallows. Thus, early retrograde flow or "re-reflux" is seen only in patients with nonreducing hernias, and these patients have the greatest impairment of both esophageal volume clearance and acid clearance [17].

References

1. Helm JF, Dodds WJ, Pelc LR, Palmer DW, Hogan WJ, Teeter BC. Effect of esophageal emptying and saliva on clearance of acid from the esophagus. N Engl J Med 1984;310:284.
2. Helm JF, Dodds WJ, Hogan WJ, Soergel KH, Egide MS, Wood CM. Acid neutralizing capacity of human saliva. Gastroenterology 1982;83:69.
3. Booth DJ, Kemmerer WT, Skinner DB. Acid clearing from the distal esophagus. Arch Surg 1968;96:731.
4. DeMeester TR, Johnson LF, Joseph GJ, Toscano MS, Hall AW, Skinner DB. Patterns of gastroesophageal reflux in health and disease. Ann Surg 1976;184:459.
5. Stanciu C, Bennett JR. Oesophageal acid clearing: one factor in production of reflux esophagitis. Gut 1974;15:852—857.
6. Dodds WJ, Kahrilas PJ, Dent J, Hogan WJ, Kern MK, Arndorfer RC. Analysis of spontaneous gastroesophageal reflux and esophageal acid clearance in patients with reflux esophagitis. J Gastrointest Motil 1989;2:79.
7. Johnson LF. 24-hour pH monitoring in the study of gastroesophageal reflux. J Clin Gastroenterol 1980;2:387.
8. Kahrilas PJ, Dodds WJ, Hogan WJ, Kern MK, Arndorfer RC, Reece A. Esophageal peristaltic dysfunction in peptic esophagitis. Gastroenterology 1986;91:897—904.
9. Olsen AM, Schlegel JF. Motility disturbances caused by esophagitis. J Thorac Cardiovasc Surg 1965;50:607.
10. Ahtaridis G, Snape WJ, Cohen S. Clinical and manometric findings in benign peptic stricture of the esophagus. Dig Dis Sci 1979;24:858—860.
11. Gill RC, Bowes KL, Murphy PD, Kingma YJ. Esophageal motor abnormalities in gastroesophageal reflux and the effects of fundoplication. Gastroenterology 1986;91:364.
12. Behar J, Sheahan DG, Biancani P, Spiro M, Storer EH. Medical and surgical management of reflux esophagitis. A 38-month report on a prospective clinical trial. N Engl J Med 1975;293:263.
13. Eckardt VF. Does healing of esophagitis improve esophageal motor function? Dig Dis Sci 1988;33:161.
14. Kahrilas PJ, Dodds WJ, Hogan WJ. Effect of peristaltic dysfunction on esophageal volume clearance. Gastroenterology 1988;94:73.
15. Richter JE, Blackwell JN, Wu WC, Johns DN, Cowan RJ, Castell DO. Relationship of radionuclide liquid bolus transport and esophageal manometry. J Lab Clin Med 1987;109:217.
16. Mittal RK, Lange RC, McCallum RW. Identification and mechanism of delayed esophageal acid clearance in subjects with hiatus hernia. Gastroenterology 1987;92:130.
17. Sloan S, Kahrilas PJ. Impairment of esophageal emptying with hiatal hernia. Gastroenterology 1991;100:596.

May loss of sphincter function occur without mucosal injury?

C. Iascone, A. Moraldi, D. Castiglia, M. Barreca (Rome)

The development of mucosal injury in patients with gastroesophageal reflux disease (GERD) is the result of several factors such as the mechanical competency of the cardia, the amount and quality of refluxed material and the resistance of esophageal mucosa. Differences of opinion exist, however, in regard to the relative importance of each of these factors [1—4]. Therefore, "the loss of sphincter function" may be explained as:

— a mechanically defective cardia on manometry, regardless of the presence of abnormal reflux;
— a cardia that allows reflux to occur, as documented by 24-h pH monitoring of the esophagus, regardless the characteristics of its mechanical components; or
— a mechanically defective cardia that allows reflux to occur.

DeMeester and coworkers [5–7] defined a defective sphincter as having one or more of the following characteristics:
— an average resting pressure equal to or less than 6 mmHg;
— an average overall length equal to or less than 2 cm; or
— an average abdominal length of the sphincter equal to or less than 1 cm.
Furthermore, some reports focused on transient lower esophageal sphincter (LES) relaxations as one of the major mechanisms of reflux in normal subjects [8,9] and in patients with GERD [10,11]. According to personal findings and other authors' reports [5,12], the incidence of defective LES components, detected on manometry in patients with symptoms of GER, ranges from 11–49%, with a 42.6 to 75.3% overall frequency of mechanically defective cardia as shown in Table 1.

In the study of Pustorino et al. [12], endoscopic esophagitis was not present in 29 out of 88 patients (33%) with defective cardia. The prevalence of normal endoscopic findings decreased according to the number of defective LES components detected on manometry, as it was 43.2%, 25.8%, 18% and 0%, respectively, in the patients with one, two, three or four altered mechanical components. In our own series, 95 out of 184 patients (51.6%) with defective cardia did not show any mucosal injury on endoscopy. However, when esophagitis was assessed with multiple esophageal biopsies in a consecutive series of 115 patients, only eight patients (13%) out of 62 with mechanically defective LES had normal histologic findings. It must be underlined that no gross esophagitis was detected in 30 out of 62 patients (48%), indicating that histologic patterns of reflux were present in about 70% of patients (22/30) with normal endoscopy. In our study, 169 patients had abnormal reflux documented by 24-h pH monitoring of the distal esophagus. Sixty patients (35.5%) had normal esophageal mucosa on endoscopy. Similarly, when patients with abnormal reflux and defective cardia were selected, absent esophagitis was documented in 37 out of 94 patients (39.4%). Recently, Stein and DeMeester [13] reported that normal endoscopic findings were present in 23.2% of 112 patients with mechanically defective LES and positive 24-h pH monitoring of the esophagus, in addition to a 26.6% rate in patients with acid reflux and 5.6% in subjects with mixed acid/alkaline reflux (Table 2).

Table 1.

Author	Year	Overall with GER symptoms	LESP ≤6 mmHg (%Pts)	LES length ≤2 cm (%Pts)	Abdom LES ≤1 cm (%Pts)	Overall with one or more defective components (%Pts)
Bonavina	1986 [5]	448	24%	15%	25%	42.6%
Pustorino	1990 [12]	117	49%	34%	16%	75.3%
Personal Series	1992	323	29%	11%	42%	57%

Table 2.

	Absent mucosal injury	
	Personal series	Stein/DeMeester
Positive 24-h pH monitoring	60/169 (35.5%)	–
Positive 24-h pH monitoring and mechanically defective cardia	37/49 (34.4%)	26/112 (23.2%)
Acid reflux and mechanically defective cardia	–	25/94 (26.6%)
Acid/alkaline reflux and mechanically defective cardia	–	1/18 (5.6%)

Conclusion

Esophagitis is the multifactorial result of loss of protective barriers and activity of aggressive components of reflux material. As these factors are variously combined, it is not surprising that mucosal damages are not detected in all patients with reflux symptoms. It may be expected that about one third to one quarter of patients will not develop esophagitis, even though the cardia is defective in one or more of its components, reflux has been documented by 24-h pH monitoring or both abnormalities are present. However, the number of altered mechanical components, the quality of reflux and methods of scoring the esophagitis can greatly affect the detection of mucosal damages, as only 6% of patients with alkaline reflux do not develop esophagitis and histologic patterns of reflux are present in 87% of endoscopically obtained biopsy specimens.

References

1. Johnson LF, Harmon JW. Experimental esophagitis in a rabbit model. J Clin Gastroenterol 1986;8(suppl):26–44.
2. Lillemoe KL, Johnson LF, Harmon JW. Alkaline esophagitis: a comparison of the ability of components of gastroduodenal contents to injure the rabbit esophagus. Gastroenterology 1983;85:621–628.
3. Little AG, DeMeester TR, Kirchner PT. Pathogenesis of esophagitis in patients with gastroesophageal reflux. Surgery 1980;88:101–107.
4. Zaninotto G, DeMeester TR, Schwizer W. The lower esophageal sphincter in health and disease. Am J Surg 1988;155:104–111.
5. Bonavina L, Evander A, DeMeester TR, Walther B, Cheng SC, Palazzo L, Concannon JL. Length of the distal esophageal sphincter and competency of the cardia. Am J Surg 1986;151;25–33.
6. DeMeester TR, Wernly JA, Bryant GH, Little AG, Skinner DB. Clinical and in vitro analysis of determinants of gastroesophageal competence. A study of the principles of antireflux surgery. Am J Surg 1979;137:39–46.
7. O'Sullivan GC, DeMeester TR, Joelsson BE. Interaction of lower esophageal sphincter pressure and length of sphincter in the abdomen as determinants of gastroesophageal competence. Am J Surg 1982;143:40–47.
8. Dodds WJ, Dent J, Hogan WJ. Mechanism of gastroesophageal reflux in patterns with reflux esophagitis. N Engl J Med 1982;307:1547–1552.
9. Mittal RK, McCallum RW. Characteristics of transient lower esophageal sphincter relaxation in humans. Am J Physiol 1987;252:636–641.
10. Dodds DJ, Friedman RH. Mechanism of gastroesophageal reflux in recumbent asymptomatic human subject. J Clin Invest 1980;65:256–267.
11. Mittal RK, McCallum RW. Characteristics and frequency of transient relaxation of the lower esophageal sphincter in patients with reflux esophagitis. Gastroenterology 1988;95:593–599.
12. Pustorino S, Migliorato D, Ianni G, Martinez P, Guerrisi O, Federico G, Luzza G. Alterazione dei dispositivi meccanici e funzionali dello sfintere esofageo inferiore in pazienti con esofagite da reflusso. Recenti Progressi in Medicina 1990;81:6–11.
13. Stein HJ, Barlow AP, DeMeester TR, Hinder RA. Complication of gastroesophageal reflux disease. Ann Surg 1992;(July):35–43.

What is the relationship between esophageal exposure to gastric acidity and the severity of mucosal injury?

G. Zaninotto, M. Costantini, M. Anselmino, E. Ancona
(Padua)

Symptoms and complications of gastroesophageal reflux (GER) are commonly attributed to the effect of gastric secretions (HCl and pepsin) on the esophageal mucosa. In fact "peptic esophagitis" has often been used as a synonym for the expression "reflux esophagitis" since the disease was first described by Winkelstein in 1935 [1]. With the introduction nearly 20 years ago of a new diagnostic method (24-h pH monitoring of the distal esophagus), the disease was more correctly defined as "gastroesophageal reflux disease" (GERD), described as an "abnormal exposure of the distal esophagus to the refluxed acid contents of the stomach, as assessed by 24-h pH monitoring, and assuming a pH < 4 as a threshold for a reflux condition" [2]. This definition nonetheless fails to embrace the broad spectrum of the disease or explain differences in the severity of mucosal damage in patients with the same esophageal exposure at pH < 4 and no mathematical model has yet been constructed to describe differences in the severity of esophagitis based on the pH < 4 threshold [3]. This may be due to variability in the gullet's defensive capacity (e.g., mucosal resistance, saliva flow, motility) or differences in the composition of the refluxed gastrointestinal juice. Two mechanisms have been suggested to contribute to mucosal damage (both based on the action of proteolytic enzymes), i.e., the acid pepsin system and the alkaline, pancreatic enzymes and bile system. The ability of the acid pepsin system to cause mucosal injury in the esophagus has been demonstrated experimentally [4,5].

Pepsin is a powerful digestive enzyme, secreted as pepsinogen by gastric fundus chief cells and then activated to pepsin by gastric acid. The optimum pH for its maximum proteolytic activity is 0.6 to 2.5, depending on the substrate: in general, a lower concentration of hydrogen ions is needed when the substrates have been suitably denatured [6]. It is essential for hydrogen ions to be present for pepsin to take effect, as they activate the enzyme (from pepsinogen to pepsin), modifying the electric charges of the substrate and directly influencing the process of enzyme catalysis [7].

The acid directly affects the esophageal mucosa and a mucosal barrier to H^+ ion back diffusion, similar to the one observed in the stomach, has also been observed in the esophagus. Prolonged acid exposure at moderate concentrations of H^+ (80 mM HCl) or brief exposure at higher concentrations (120 mM HCl) produce a progressively lower potential difference in the esophageal mucosa, due to inhibition of Na-K-ATPase activity [8]. This leads to cell swelling and eventually to necrosis. Despite such observations, however, no correlation has been found between H^+ ion back diffusion and esophagitis [9]. This was confirmed in an experimental model using a rabbit esophagus perfused with solutions containing HCl and/or pepsin at different pH and concentrations: little or no esophageal damage was observed when the esophagus was perfused with HCl alone, and the presence of pepsin was required for mucosal injury to occur. In general, damage increased with higher concentrations of pepsin and was significantly more evident with solutions at pH 1.5 to 2.5 than with solutions at a higher pH [10]. These observations support the old theory that the gastric proteolytic enzyme, pepsin, is the main cause of esophagitis, but pepsin needs an acid environment at a pH between 1.5 and 2.5 to explicate its digestive power on the esophageal mucosa. In an environment with a slightly higher pH (pH 3), the harmful effect of pepsin is dramatically reduced.

These experimental findings were applied to the clinical field with a view to identifying GERD patients with different degrees of esophagitis. Various pH level intervals (< 4, 0—1, 1—2, 1.5—2.5, 2—3, 3—4, 4—5) of exposure to the distal esophagus during 24-h pH monitoring and lower esophageal sphincter (LES) characteristics (pressure, overall length and abdominal length) were considered as variables in a group of 58 patients with proven GER. A discriminating model of statistical analysis (stepwise regression test and linear regression) was applied to all variables. Eight patient-discriminating variables were identified, obtaining an accuracy of 76%. However, a combination of two of these variables (percentage of exposure in supine position at pH 1.5—2.5 and overall sphincter length) could correctly classify 75% of patients, which means that they alone account for 98% of the total discriminating ability of all eight variables. After exposure at pH 1.5—2.5, the second discriminating parameter emerging from the analysis was the overall length of the LES. A progressive shortening of the sphincter with increasingly severe esophagitis has also been reported elsewhere [11]. Whether this is a cause of the disease or a consequence of peptic damage is controversial. However, patients with a short sphincter and raised acid exposure at pH 2.5—1.5 should be considered as prone to developing esophagitis and suitable for treatment with aggressive medical or surgical therapy.

In conclusion, there is experimental and clinical evidence that, in a suitably acid environment (at a pH between 1.5 and 2.5), pepsin is the main cause of mucosal injury in the esophagus. A mathematical model based on this variable explains 75% of mucosal injury in patients with GERD.

Whether esophagitis in the 25% of patients unexplained by this model is due to a different defensive capability, refluxed pancreatic and/or biliary juice or a combination of the two, is still under debate.

References

1. Winkelstein A. Peptic esophagitis: a new clinical entity. JAMA 1935;104:906—909.
2. Johnson LF, DeMeester TR. Twenty-four hour pH monitoring of distal esophagus: a quantitative measure of gastro-esophageal reflux. Am J Gastroenterol 1974;62:325—332.
3. Schindlbeck NE, Heinrich C, Konig A et al. Optimal thresholds, sensitivity and specificity of long-term pH-metry for the detection of gastroesophageal reflux disease. Gastroenterology 1987;93:85—90.
4. Goldberg HJ, Dodds WJ, Sheldon G et al. Role of acid and pepsin in acute experimental esophagitis. Gastroenterology 1969;56:223—230.
5. Lillemoe KD, Johnson LF, Harmon JW. Role of the components of the gastroduodenal contents in experimental acid esophagitis. Surgery 1982;92:276—284.

6. Shlamowitz M, Peterson LU. Studies on the optimum pH for the action of pepsin on native and denatured bovine serum albumin and bovine hemoglobin. J Biol Chem 1959;34:3137−3145.
7. Cornish-Bowden AJ, Knowles JR. The pH dependance of pepsin catalysed reactions. Biochemistry 1969;113:353−362.
8. Orlando R, Bryson J, Powell DW. Mechanism of H⁺ injury in rabbit esophageal epithelium. Am J Physiol 1984;246(Gastro-intest Liver Physiol. 9):G718−G724.
9. Salo J, Kivilaasko E. Role of luminal H+ in the pathogenesis of experimental esophagitis. Surgery 1982;92:61−68.
10. Zaninotto G, Di Mario F, Costantini M et al. Oesophagitis and pH of refluxate: an experimental and clinical study. Br J Surg 1992;79:161−164.
11. Zaninotto G, DeMeester TR, Bremner CG et al. Esophageal function in patients with reflux-induced stricture and its relevance to clinical treatment. Ann Thorac Surg 1989;47:362−370.

Are the bile acids themselves toxic to the esophageal mucosa or mainly in the presence of acid?

J.W. Harmon, B.L. Bass, S. Batzri (Washington)

The recent clinical experience with omeprazole teaches a great deal about the pathophysiology of reflux esophagitis. Reducing gastroesophageal acidity with earlier forms of therapy, such as antacids and H_2-blockers, had only relatively small benefit for patients suffering from gastroesophageal reflux (GER). On the other hand, the hydrogen-potassium ATPase inhibitor omeprazole abolishes gastroesophageal acidity and dramatically benefits patients suffering from GER. This clinical experience strongly suggests an important role for acid in the pathophysiology of GER. As the bile acids remain constant in the gastroesophageal contents despite the presence of omeprazole treatment, this clinical experience suggests that bile acids alone are not particularly damaging to the esophageal mucosa.

Our experience with a laboratory rabbit model of gastroesophageal reflux disease (GERD), has shown two important ways in which the presence of gastroesophageal acidity is critical in amplifying the damaging effects of bile acids. The role of acid in bile induced injury in the rabbit model was so significant, that we are not surprised by the recent clinical experience with omeprazole in which the elimination of acidity eliminated bile induced injury.

Mechanism one: driving accumulation of intracellular bile acid

Our experiments with the rabbit model showed that luminal acidity drives a physiochemical mechanism, which results in the accumulation of bile within the cells at an intracellular concentration greater than 10-fold the luminal concentration. Without luminal acidity, this intracellular accumulation of bile does not occur. In this

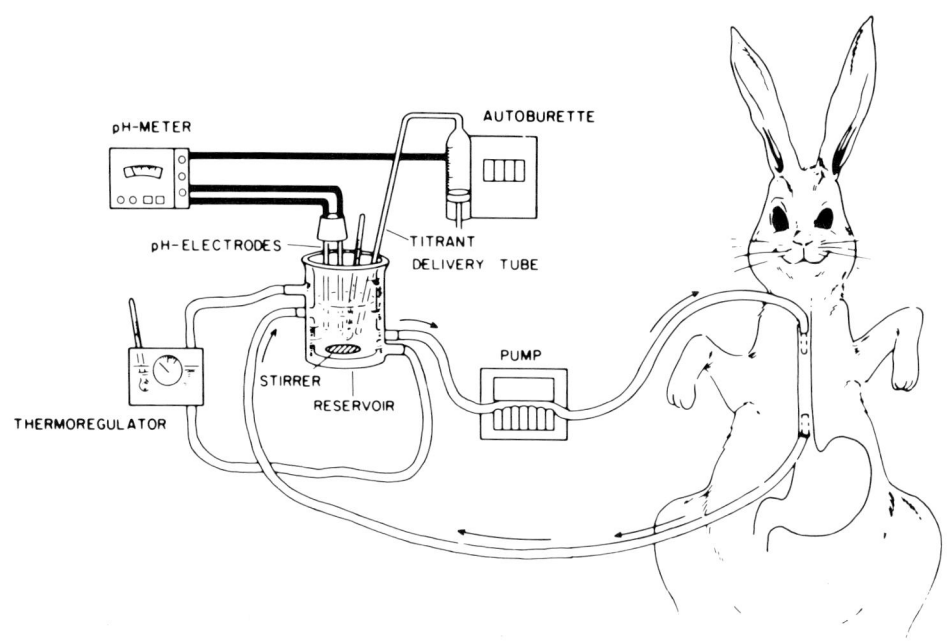

Fig. 1. Experimental setup.

study, experiments were carried out on New Zealand white rabbits, where the esophagus was perfused with a recirculating system (Fig. 1). The proximal and distal esophagus was ligated around the cannulas, in order that the components of the perfusate can be specifically controlled. Using this system, GER can be mimicked by matching the timing of exposure and the concentrations of the various luminal components to those found in patients with GER [1–3]. In our early experience, we were impressed to discover that the bile salts cholate and deoxycholate were rapidly absorbed into the esophageal mucosa in an acidic environment, but much more slowly absorbed at neutrality (Fig. 2) [4]. Thereafter we searched for an explanation of this observation. We concluded that, at neutrality, the bile acids were ionized and not lipid soluble and therefore, could not pass through the cell membrane. On the other hand, in an acidic environment, the bile salts were protonated in the acid form. They did not have a charge and could more readily pass through the cell membranes. This would explain the greater absorption of bile acids from the lumen into the cells in the presence of acid. We further show that the absorption of bile acids into the mucosa enhanced their injurious effect. The luminal fluid utilized contained labeled glucose as a permeability marker. Increased fluxes of glucose out of the lumen occur during mucosal injury, as the mucosa becomes more permeable. We correlated glucose flux out of the lumen with bile flux, and found a significant direct linear correlation (Fig. 3) [4,5].

At this point, we had shown that acid is important in facilitating the absorption of bile from the esophageal lumen, and that bile absorption from the lumen was

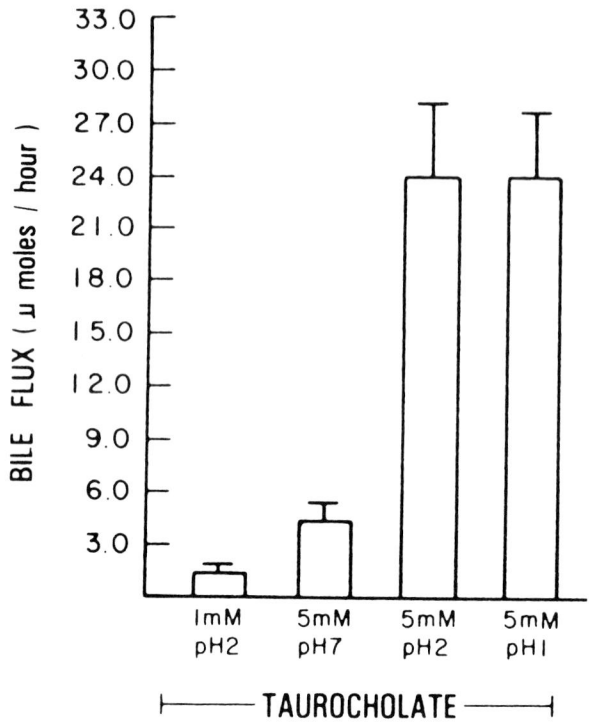

Fig. 2. Absorption of radioactively labeled bile acid at various concentrations and pHs. Notice that at 5 mm concentration the absorption of bile acid is greater at the acidic pH of 2 than at the neutral pH of 7 [4].

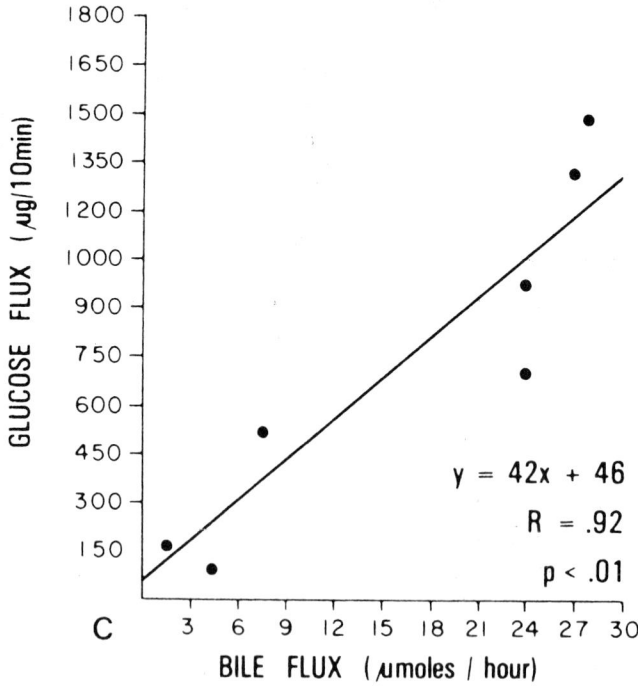

$$y = 42x + 46$$

$$R = .92$$

$$p < .01$$

Fig. 3. Glucose flux correlated with bile absorption. Notice that injury to the mucosa increases with increasing bile absorption. Increasing glucose flux is a sign of mucosal injury in this model [4].

associated with increased injury. Next, we developed experiments to measure the concentration of bile within the esophageal wall during luminal perfusion. We expected that luminal concentration of bile would greatly exceed the concentration of bile in the esophageal wall, and also that the blood flow to the esophageal wall would clear away bile as it was absorbed into the wall. Surprisingly, bile concentrations within the mucosa exceeded the luminal concentrations by more than 10-fold [6,7]. This accumulation was only seen in the presence of acid. This dramatic accumulation of bile within the esophageal wall required an explanation. Again, we turned to our physiochemical explanation, based on the interrelationship between acidity and bile (the explanation is shown schematically in Fig. 4). At an acid pH, the bile is protonated, it is electronically neutral and easily enters through the lipid cell membrane. Once in the cell, it encounters a pH of 7 where it loses its hydrogen ion and becomes ionized. In the negative ionized form, it is trapped within the cell (Fig. 4). Figure 4 shows how this would work: it is assumed that we are dealing with a glycolated bile acid with a pka of 5 and that gastric cells are involved. When the pH in the lumen equals the pka of the bile acid, half will be ionized and half will be protonated. At pH 7, on the other hand, the ionized will exceed the un-ionized by a ratio of 100:1. Thus, with a hypothetical 100 molecules of bile acid in the lumen, there is essentially no gradient for absorption of R-COOH at pH 7, while at pH 5 there is a significant gradient for absorption of R-COOH. Regardless of the luminal pH, within the cell, the pH 7 condition exists. The R-COOH which is absorbed into the cell is returned to the R-COOH form. This allows continued absorption of the protonated form and results in accumulation of bile within the cell.

This phenomenon can explain how relatively low luminal concentrations of bile salt can produce significant mucosal injury in the presence of acid. Without acid intracellular accumulation and damage would be minimal, whereas with acid the bile salts are absorbed into the cell and can produce significant damage.

SCHEMATIC REPRESENTATION OF GLYCOCHOLIC ACID UPTAKE

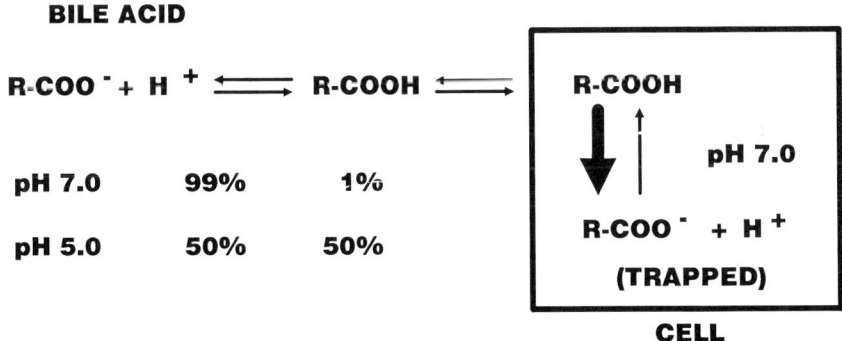

Fig. 4. Physiochemical mechanism accounting for bile acid accumulation within mucosal cells.

Mechanism two: acid acidity controls esophageal mucosal blood flow during bile injury

Our rabbit model of esophageal reflux injury allows the measurement of blood flow to the esophagus. Therefore we utilized radioactively-labeled microspheres to make these measurements; the same esophageal perfusion system can be utilized (Fig. 1). We have shown in a number of experiments that preserving or enhancing esophageal blood flow tends to protect the esophageal mucosa from luminal injury [8—10]. In fact, increasing esophageal mucosal blood flow may be a future strategy for protection and treatment of esophageal reflux disease. Increasing blood flow is also a natural response to injury (e.g., when bile salts are applied to the esophageal mucosa, the esophageal blood flow rises dramatically) [11]. This appears to be a natural protective response of the esophageal mucosa. This is another point at which acid interacts significantly and dramatically with bile acids on the esophageal mucosa.

Without luminal acidity, bile salts dramatically increase esophageal blood flow. However, in the presence of acid this effect is eliminated. Figure 5 shows that esophageal mucosal blood flow at baseline was approximately 25 ml/min × 100 grams of tissue. With exposure to 5 mM deoxycholate the blood flow increased to 125 ml per × 100 grams of tissue. This increase in blood flow was eliminated when hydrochloric acid was added to the luminal perfusate to reduce the pH from 7 to 2 [11]. Thus, the presence of acid eliminated the ability of bile salt to increase mucosal blood flow. This may represent the loss of a very serious protective mechanism for the esophageal mucosa. Again, we see how the presence of luminal acid dramatically changes the interaction between bile and the esophageal mucosa.

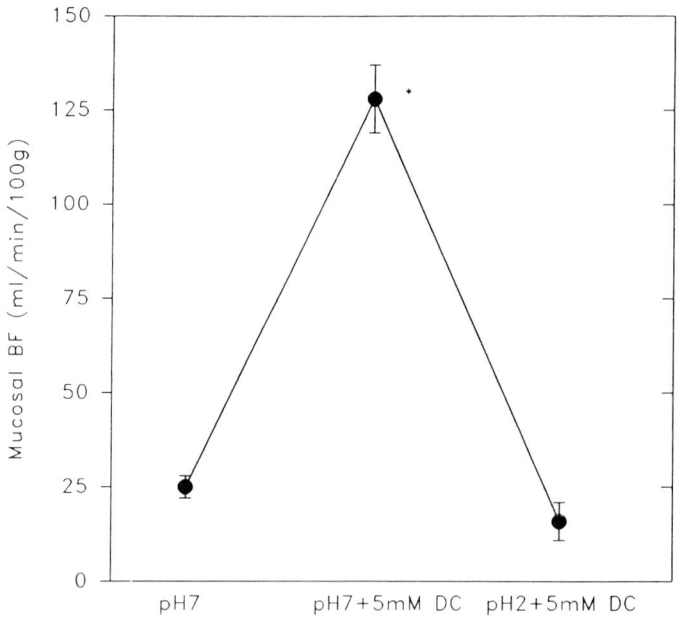

Fig. 5. Esophageal blood flow (ml/min × 100). The blood flow is baseline at pH 7, increases with the addition of the bile salt deoxycholate, and then diminishes when the lumen is acidified [11].

Conclusion

These experiments in a rabbit model of GER, show two important ways in which luminal acidity modulates the injurious effects of luminal bile. Acid can drive the accumulation of bile within the cells through physiochemical mechanisms and thereby enhance injury. Additionally, luminal acid can eliminate bile salt induced increases in esophageal mucosal blood flow, and thereby deprive the esophageal mucosa of one of its important defenses. In view of these observations it is not surprising that eliminating gastroesophageal acidity is beneficial for patients with bile associated esophageal reflux disease.

References

1. Harmon JW, Johnson LF, Maydonovitch CL. Effects of acid bile and bile acid salts on the rabbit esophageal mucosa. Dig Dis Sci 1981;26(10):65−72.
2. Lillemoe KD, Johnson LF, Harmon JW. Role of the components of gastroduodenal contents in experimental acid esophagitis. Surgery 1982;92:276−284.
3. Lillemoe KD, Johnson LF, Harmon JW. Alkaline esophagitis: A comparison of the ability of components of gastroduodenal contents to injure the rabbit esophagus. Gastroenterology 1983;85:621−628.
4. Lillemoe KD, Gadacz TR, Harmon JW. Bile absorption occurs during disruption of the esophageal mucosal barrier. J Surg Res 1983;35:57−62.
5. Schweitzer EJ, Harmon JW, Bass BL, Batzri S. Bile acid reflux precedes mucosal barrier disruption in the rabbit esophagus. Am J Physiol 1984;247(10):G480−G485.
6. Schweitzer EJ, Bass BL, Batzri S, Harmon JW. Esophageal mucosa: A bile acid sink in the rabbit. Surg Form 1983;34: 152−154.
7. Schweitzer EJ, Bass BL, Batzri S, Harmon JW. Bile acid accumulation by rabbit esophageal mucosa. Dig Dis Sci 1986; 31:1105−1113.
8. Trad KS, Fernicola MT, Hakki FZ, Dziki AJ, Harmon JW, Bass BL. Modulation of esophageal blood flow: A local effector function of sensory nerves. Surg Form 1990;41:122−124.
9. Petersen BM, Curcio LD, Trad KS, Harmon JW, Bass BL. Visceral afferent nerves mediate protection against acid-pepsin injury of the esophagus. Gastroenterology 1992;102:147.
10. Petersen BM, Curcio LD, Trad KS, Harmon JW, Bass BL. Visceral afferent nerves mediate protection against acid-bile injury of the esophagus. Surg Form 1992;43:143.
11. Bass BL, Schweitzer EJ, Harmon JW, Kraimer J. H⁺ back diffusion interferes with intrinsic reactive regulation of esophageal mucosal blood flow. Surgery 1984;96:404−413.

How can the sensitivity of the esophageal mucosa to acid be assessed quantitatively?

R.M. Bremner, T.R. DeMeester (Los Angeles)

Although the esophagus may be the origin of incapacitating symptoms, such as heartburn, dysphagia or chest pain, it is an organ of unreliable sensitivity. The receptors and mechanisms responsible at the cellular and neuronal level for initiating the pathways which culminate in a specific symptom are still unclear. Nociceptors of various forms have been described in the mucosa and submucosa, and irritation of these receptors by acid or alkaline reflux presumably results in a conscious subjective feeling but there is a great variability between patients in symptoms experienced [1]. For example, some patients with severe symptoms may be found on endoscopy to have minimal mucosal damage and on pH monitoring to have mild acid exposure, while others with severe mucosal damage and excessive acid exposure may be relatively asymptomatic. Attempts at correlating reflux episodes with symptoms has shown that up to 85% of reflux episodes, defined as a drop in esophageal pH to less than 4, are asymptomatic [2]. Consequently, symptom indexes have been devised in an effort to attribute a particular patient's symptoms to reflux disease [3–5]. They have suggested that more than 75% of the patients symptoms should be related to reflux episodes before reflux and symptoms can be causally related. Even on this basis, up to 25% of symptoms are unrelated to a reflux episode. Further, several investigators have shown, not surprisingly, that symptoms at night are far less frequent than during the day. Attempting to correlate symptoms at night with either motility abnormalities or changes in pH is almost useless, as patients are extremely unreliable at recording their symptoms during the night or symptoms readily experienced during the day may not be sufficiently severe to wake the patient from sleep during the night [6].

The subjective recognition of a symptom is probably multifactorial and understandably it is difficult to quantitate the sensitivity of the esophagus to naturally occurring reflux episodes. Smith et al., however, have provided valuable information relating symptoms to esophageal pH exposure [7]. They infused the esophagus with different concentrations of hydrochloric acid and recorded the pain experienced and the time to the onset of the experience in 25 patients with symptomatic GERD. There was a greater prevalence of pain and a more rapid onset of pain with infusions of increasing concentrations of acid (Fig. 1). They also noted on 24-h pH monitoring that reflux episodes resulting in pain were more often preceded with a recently painful episode, suggesting that pain episodes sensitize the patient for subsequent pain.

The results of Smith's infusion study are in keeping with our findings on pH monitoring studies that also showed mucosal damage to be more related to exposure of the esophagus to concentrated acid [8]. In this study we attempted to quantitate the sensitivity of the mucosa to injury by correlating mucosal damage with exposure to reflux of different concentrations of acid. We studied 154 patients with reflux disease and compared their patterns of pH exposure at different intervals to those of 50 normal subjects (Fig. 2). The percent time spent within the intervals pH 0–2, 2–3, 3–4 and 7–8 in patients with normal and injured mucosa are illustrated in Fig. 3. We found that 89% of the patients with abnormal exposure (defined as exposure greater than the 95 percentile of 50 normal subjects) to the pH interval 0–2, had mucosal injury. Logistic regression performed for specific pH intervals showed that the risk of mucosal damage was significant for total time that the esophagus was exposed to a pH of 0–2, 2–3, and 7–8 ($p < 0.0001$). Time spent at the interval 3–4 was not significant. Patients with mucosal injury had a higher exposure at all intervals with

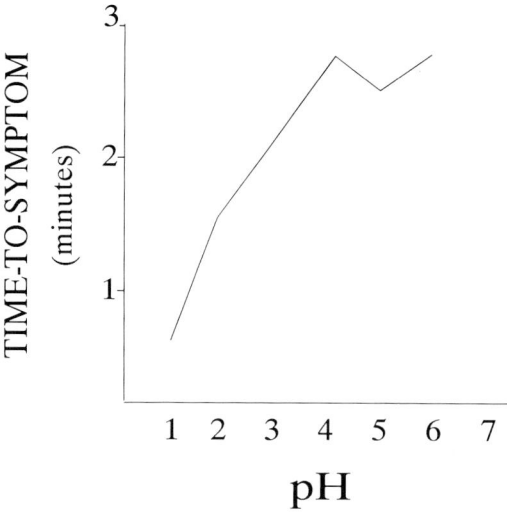

Fig. 1. Relationship between symptoms and duration of esophageal exposure to pH of different concentrations. Adapted from [7] (with permission).

the greatest difference in exposure occurring at the pH interval 0–2. It would be interesting to see if the daytime symptom index using a pH threshold of pH < 2 has a higher correlation with reflux episodes in symptomatic patients.

We are currently addressing the question of mucosal sensitivity using the new technology of simultaneous pH and motility monitoring in an attempt to assess the sensitivity of the mucosa in a more objective way. We have recently shown that, as a rule, the frequency of swallowing increases during reflux episodes when compared

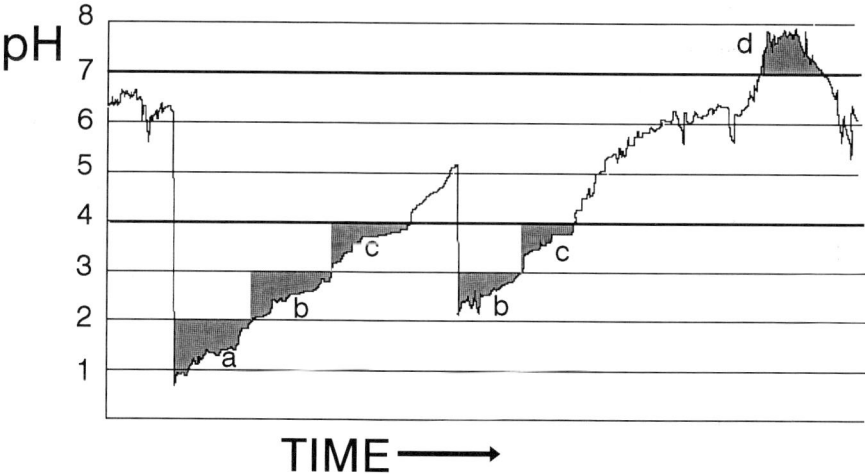

Fig. 2. Method of analysis of esophageal exposure to pH of whole number intervals. Shaded areas show the length of time spent at each interval. These times are summated and expressed as the percentage of the monitored time. a = time at pH 0–2; b = time at pH 2–3; c = time at pH 3–4; d = time at pH 7–8.

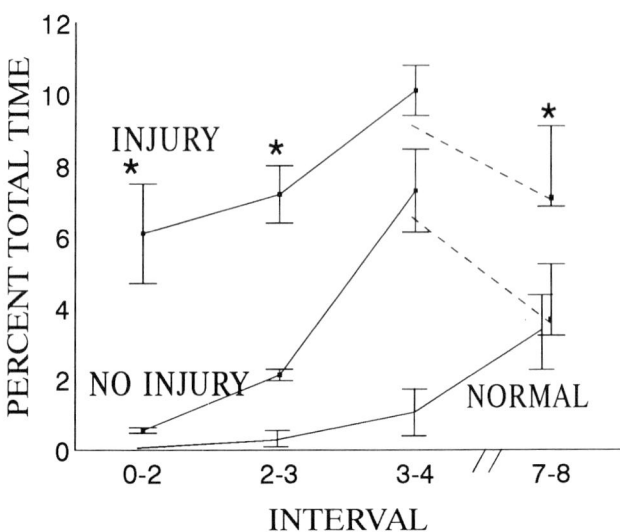

Fig. 3. Mean percent time of esophageal exposure to different pH intervals for normal subjects and patients with normal or injured mucosa. * = p < 0.01 vs. no injury.

to interprandial, nonreflux periods (Fig. 4) [9]. This occurs in normal subjects as well as patients with reflux disease and may represent a subconscious protective mechanism to rapidly clear the esophagus of refluxed material. We have also noted

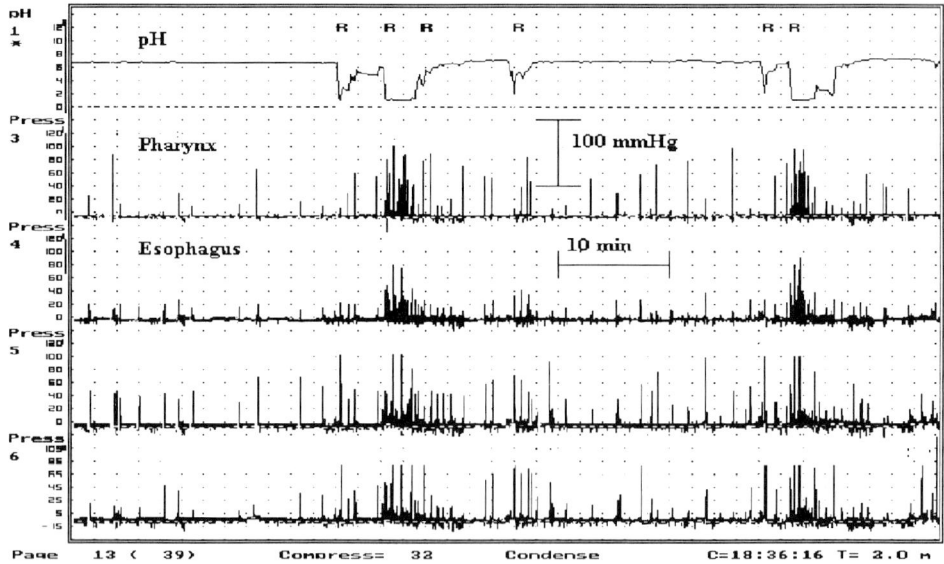

Fig. 4. An example of a simultaneous recording of pharyngoesophageal motility and esophageal pH compressed to show an 80-min time period. Note the increased frequency of swallows during reflux episodes identified by a drop in esophageal pH to below 4.

that some patients with severe reflux disease do not increase their swallowing frequency during reflux, indicating that perhaps these patients have become insensitive to refluxed gastric juice and have lost the protective mechanism. Application of this new technology may provide the first objective method to quantitate the sensitivity of the esophagus to refluxed gastric juice.

References

1. Christensen J. Origin of sensation in the esophagus. Am J Physiol 1984;246:G221–G225.
2. Baldi F, Ferrarini F, Longanesi A et al. Acid gastroesophageal reflux and symptom occurrence. Dig Dis Sci 1989;34(12):1890–1893.
3. Ward BW, Wu WC, Richter JE, Lui KW, Castell DO. Ambulatory 24-hour esophageal pH monitoring: Technology searching for a clinical application. J Clin Gastroenterol 1986;8(suppl 1):59–67.
4. Wiener JG, Richter JE, Coopper JB, Wu WC, Castell DO. The symptom index: A clinically important parameter of ambulatory 24-hour esophageal pH monitoring. Am J Gastroenterol 1988;83(4):358–361.
5. Richter JE, Hewson EG, Sinclair JW, Dalton CB. Acid perfusion test and 24-hour esophageal pH monitoring with symptom index. Dig Dis Sci 1991;36:565–571.
6. Dreuw B, Clark GWB, Hoeft SF, Bremner RM, Burdiles P, Crookes PF, DeMeester TR, Peters JH, Johnson SB, Shibberu H. Correlation between symptoms and reflux episodes in gastroesophageal reflux disease. Gastroenterology 1993;104(4):A72.
7. Smith JL, Opekun AR, Larkai E et al. Sensitivity of the esophageal mucosa to pH in gastroesophageal reflux disease. Gastroenterology 1989;96:683–689.
8. Bremner RM, Crookes PF, DeMeester TR, Peters JH, Stein HJ. The concentration of refluxed acid and esophageal mucosal injury. Am J Surg 1992;164(5):522–528.
9. Bremner RM, Hoeft SF, Costantini M, Crookes PF, Bremner CG, DeMeester TR. Pharyngeal swallowing: The major factor in clearance of esophageal reflux episodes. Ann Surg 1993;218(3):364–370.

How is esophageal sensitivity impaired with age?

D.O. Castell (Philadelphia)

The relationship of aging to esophageal symptomatology has received only occasional attention in the literature, most of it in the past 5 years. The common perception appears to be that esophageal sensitivity may be altered in the aging patient, particularly as it relates to symptoms secondary to gastroesophageal reflux (GER). In a review by Mold and Rankin in 1987, it was noted that there is little evidence that gastroesophageal reflux disease (GERD) increases with age as might be anticipated [1]. These authors quote a prior study by Nano et al., reporting that patients over the age of 60 years with hiatus hernia were more likely to complain of symptoms other than classical retrosternal burning as seen in younger individuals [2]. Mold and Rankin suggest that GERD is actually common in the aging patient, but that underreporting or underrecognition may occur. They suggest the following possible explanations for this phenomenon [1].

1. The refluxed material may be less acidic than in younger patients.
2. Heartburn may not be as severe because of changes in pain perception.
3. Elderly patients may underreport symptoms of GERD.
4. Physicians may underestimate the importance of GERD symptoms in elderly patients who have multiple problems, often seeming more serious.

In 1991, Raiha et al. reported on the characteristics of GERD symptoms in 195 elderly subjects (mean age 74 years). They reported that the occurrence of typical heartburn showed poor correlation with the extent of reflux during pH study and that more common manifestations of GERD in the aged were regurgitation, dysphagia, respiratory symptoms and vomiting [3]. These same investigators subsequently reported the results of a questionnaire completed by 487 subjects age 65 years and over, indicating that typical reflux symptoms were often associated with atypical complaints including abdominal symptoms, chest pain, or respiratory symptoms [4].

A study from the laboratory of Bianchi Porro evaluated a group of 24 elderly patients with typical GERD symptoms (mean age 69 years) compared with 147 symptomatic younger patients (mean age 45 years) [5]. Using prolonged ambulatory pH monitoring and endoscopy, this study showed that the elderly patients had pathologic reflux and esophagitis more frequently than the younger patients. Mean percent time pH < 4 in the elderly patients with esophagitis was 32.5% in 24 h as compared with 12.9% in the younger group. It is possible that decreased sensory awareness to the frequent reflux may be present in this elderly population.

The above observations raise the question of altered sensation to esophageal acid exposure with aging. This phenomenon, however, has not been documented. In our laboratory, we have preliminary information suggesting that altered sensory awareness to stimulation of mechanoreceptors may occur with age. In these studies, four healthy aged volunteers (age 65–86 years; mean 77 years) were compared to 19 younger volunteers (age 19–57 years; mean 29 years). Esophageal balloon distension was performed using a latex balloon (length 30 mm) connected to the central lumen of a multi lumen polyvinyl catheter 4.5 mm in diameter (Wilson Cook Medical, Winston Salem, NC). Rapid balloon inflation was produced by a specially designed pump (Wilson Cook Medical) which moved the plunger of a 30 cc syringe delivering adjustable volumes of air at a rate of 170 cc/s. The balloon was distended with increasing volumes of 2 cc increments (1 s dwell time, 5–10 s intervals of deflation between each increment) through a range of volumes from 6 cc to 30 cc.

All subjects were studied in the supine position after a 6 h fast. The catheter was passed through the nose into the esophagus and positioned with the distal end of the balloon at 5 cm proximal to the lower esophageal sphincter, localized manometrically prior to the placement of the balloon. Pressure was monitored in the balloon throughout the experiment using a 4-way stop clock connected to a pressure gauge. At the beginning of the study, the subjects were given instructions to read informing them how to respond to any sensation which they felt during the study. They were asked to indicate sensation intensity on a 3 point scale: 0 (no sensation); 1 (aware of the balloon, but no pain); 2 (pain or discomfort), without coaxing or active interchange during the study. The results of these studies have demonstrated a major

Table 1.

Elderly (n = 4)	Young (n = 19)
Sensation 1: 20.0 cc	Sensation 1: 8.0 cc
Sensation 2: 28.5 cc	Sensation 2: 17.4 cc

difference in the mean volume for sensory awareness in the elderly subjects compared to the younger volunteers, as shown in Table 1.

References

1. Mold JW, Rankin RA. Symptomatic gastroesophageal reflux in the elderly. J Am Geriatr Soc 1987;35:649–659.
2. Nano M, Ferrara L, Camandona M. Sliding hiatal hernia in the elderly: A clinical entity. J Am Geriatr Soc 1981;29:463–464.
3. Raiha IJ, Heitanen E, Sourander LB. Symptoms of gastro-oesophageal reflux disease in elderly people. Age Aging 1991;20:365–370.
4. Raiha IJ, Impivaara O, Seppala M, Sourander LB. Prevalence and characteristics of symptomatic gastroesophageal reflux disease in the elderly. JAGS 1992;40:1209–1211.
5. Zhu H, Pace F, Sangaletti O, Bianchi Porro G. Features of symptomatic gastroesophageal reflux in elderly patients. Scand J Gastroenterol 1993;28:235–238.

Mucosal protective agents

What is known about the intrinsic properties of resistance of the esophageal mucosa?

R.C. Orlando (New Orleans)

Reflux esophagitis is the most common disorder of the esophagus. It is caused by the frequent and, at times, prolonged contact of gastric acid with the esophageal epithelium [1]. Though common, it is surprising that more people do not have reflux esophagitis, since it is known that virtually everyone has reflux and has it on a daily basis. The reason for the limitation in damaging potential of gastric acid, is that the esophagus comes equipped with a three-tiered system of defenses [1]. These defenses are:
— the antireflux barriers which limit the volume and frequency of reflux;
— the luminal clearance mechanisms which limit the duration of contact between acid with esophageal epithelium; and
— "tissue resistance" which limits the damage during contact of acid with esophageal epithelium (Fig. 1).
Experimental data substantiates both the existence and effectiveness of tissue resistance as a defense against acid injury. It can be shown, for example, that even when the antireflux barriers and luminal acid clearance mechanisms are bypassed, by directly perfusing the esophagus with high concentrations of HCl, the epithelium resists damage even at continuous exposures for one or more hours [2].

DETERMINANTS OF REFLUX INJURY

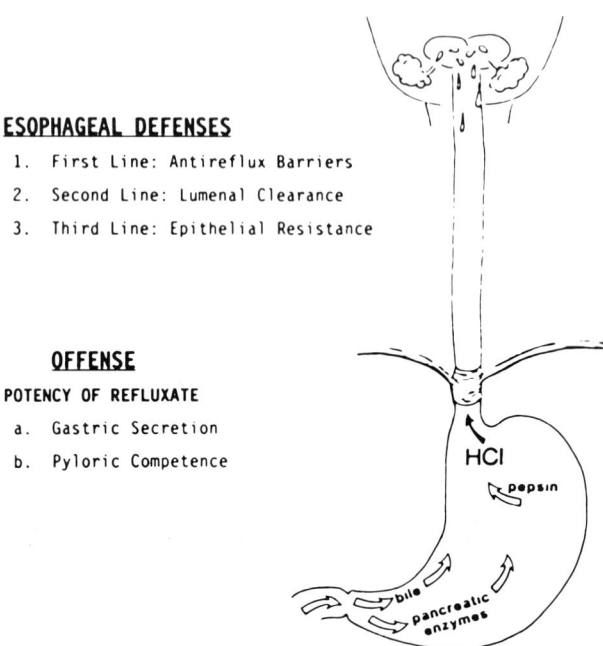

ESOPHAGEAL DEFENSES

1. First Line: Antireflux Barriers
2. Second Line: Lumenal Clearance
3. Third Line: Epithelial Resistance

OFFENSE

POTENCY OF REFLUXATE

a. Gastric Secretion
b. Pyloric Competence

Fig. 1. Diagramatic representation of the three-tiered system by which the esophagus defends itself from damaging agents contained in the gastric refluxate. (Reprinted with permission from Orlando RC. In: Bennett JR (ed) Oesophagitis. London: Current Medical Literature, Ltd. (in press)).

Table 1. Potential esophageal defenses against reflux injury

Pre-epithelial
    1. Mucous layer
    2. Unstirred water layer
    3. Surface bicarbonate ion concentration
Epithelial
    4. Structures (uppermost living cell layer)
        a. cell membranes
        b. intercellular junctional complexes (tight junctions, intercellular glycoconjugates)
    5. Functions
        a. epithelial transport (Na+/H+ exchange, Na-dependent Cl/HCO$_3$ exchange)
        b. intracellular buffers (bicarbonate, phosphate, protein)
        c. extracellular buffers - bicarbonate
        d. epithelial repair - cell replication
Postepithelial
    6. Blood flow
    7. Tissue acid-base status

What comprises the intrinsic properties reflected in the term esophageal mucosal resistance?

Esophageal mucosal resistance is not a single factor, but a group of intrinsic mucosal structures and functions that interact to provide a cohesive defensive system against acid damage. For discussion purposes, the factors comprising this system can be separated into three categories: pre-epithelial; epithelial; and postepithelial defenses (Table 1).

Pre-epithelial defenses

The pre-epithelial defenses are the mucus-unstirred water, layer-bicarbonate complex (Fig. 2). While highly developed as a defense against acid damage to gastric and duodenal epithelium, experimentation in humans does not suggest that this defense is very effective in the esophagus. Thus, the human esophagus only exhibits a pH gradient from lumen to cell surface, of approximately 1 pH unit when the luminal solution is at pH = 2, while the stomach and duodenum can maintain gradients of 3–4 pH units under the same conditions [3]. This limitation in the esophagus is likely to be due to:
— the lack of a well-defined mucous layer;
— the limited permeability to passively diffusing bicarbonate from blood; and
— the lack of surface cells with the capacity to secrete bicarbonate.

Epithelial defenses

The epithelial defenses consist of structures and functions of the stratified squamous epithelial cells themselves (Fig. 3). Key structures include the cell membranes and intercellular junctional complex, the latter being a composite of tight junctions and intercellular glycoconjugate material [4]. The primary method by which these structures protect against acid injury is by limiting the rate of H^+ diffusion into cells

PRE-EPITHELIAL DEFENSES

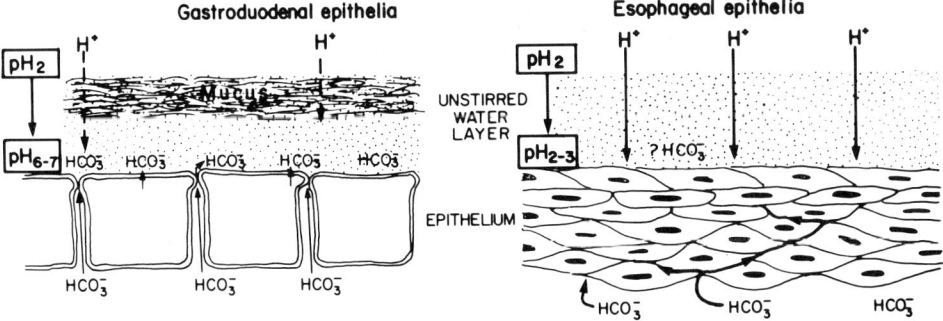

Fig. 2. Pre-epithelial defense. In gastric and duodenal epithelia, but to a far lesser degree in esophageal epithelium, hydrogen ions are substantially reduced in concentration as they diffuse through the mucus-unstirred water layer-bicarbonate barrier before contacting the surface epithelium. (Reprinted with permission from Orlando RC. J Clin Gastroenterol 1991;13(suppl 2)S1–S5 [10]).

EPITHELIAL DEFENSES

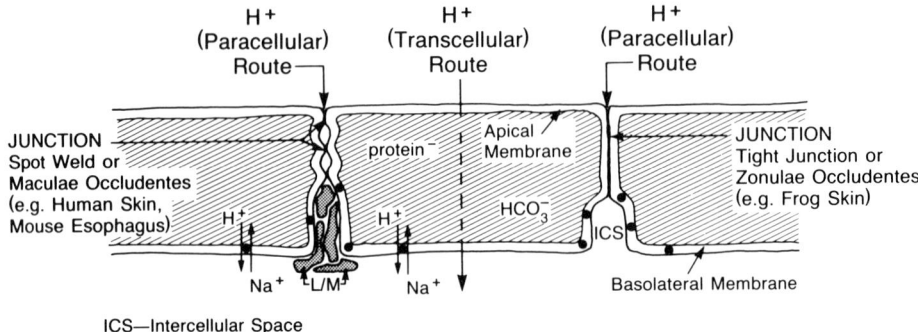

ICS—Intercellular Space
L/M—Lipid/Mucin

Fig. 3. Epithelial defense. Some of the recognized epithelial defenses against acid injury are illustrated. Structural barriers to H⁺ diffusion, include the cell membrane and intercellular junctional complex. Functional components include intracellular buffering by negatively charged proteins and HCO_3- and H+ extrusion processes (e.g., Na^+/H^+ exchange) for regulation of intracellular pH. (Modified from Orlando RC. In: Castell DO, Wu WC, Ott DJ (eds) Gastroesophageal Reflux Disease: Pathogenesis, Diagnosis, Therapy. New York: Futura Publishing Co. Inc., 1985).

and intercellular spaces. Even though the structures themselves are not perfect, the limited quantities of H⁺ that enter, under most circumstances, can be protected against

POST EPITHELIAL DEFENSES

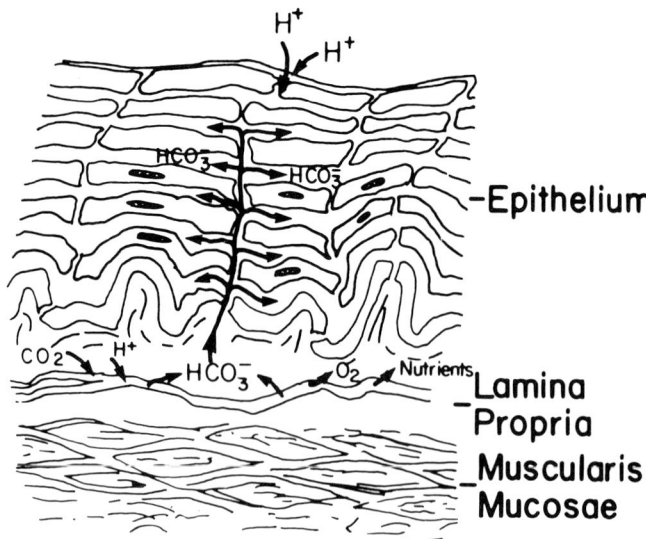

Fig. 4. Postepithelial defense. The major postepithelial defense against acid injury is an adequate blood supply. It provides nutrients and oxygen for cell metabolism and maintains tissue acid-base balance through the delivery of HCO_3^- and removal of H⁺ and CO_2. (Reprinted with permission from Orlando RC. J Clin Gastroenterol 1991;13(suppl 2)S1—S5 [10]).

274

by a variety of buffering processes, intracellular and intercellular (detailed elsewhere in this book by Dr. Tobey, see p. 292). Intracellular buffering of H⁺ can be accomplished by protein, phosphate and bicarbonate and the intercellular buffering of H⁺ entering the paracellular pathway by bicarbonate derived from blood. Furthermore, even after the buffering capacity of the cell is overcome by acid entering the cell, the cell is equipped with two membrane proteins, the Na/H exchanger and Na-dependent Cl/HCO_3 exchanger, that can raise an acidic pH back to normal [5]. The Na/H exchanger operates to alkalinize the cell interior by extruding H⁺ in exchange for extracellular Na⁺ and the Na-dependent Cl/HCO_3 exchanger by transferring HCO_3 from the extracellular fluid into the cell in exchange for Cl. Yet another factor, repair after injury, is an epithelial defense in that repair of minor injury prevents progression to severe injury. In the stomach and duodenum a process known as cell restitution can rapidly heal lesions by cell migration over an epithelial defect; however, this process does not appear to be present within esophagus [6]. Nonetheless, the esophageal epithelium can effectively repair itself by cell replication, a phenomenon recognized by the presence of basal cell hyperplasia on esophageal biopsies from patients with reflux disease [7].

Postepithelial defenses

The major route by which luminal HCl injures the esophageal epithelium, is by altering the permeability of the paracellular pathway so that greater amounts of H⁺ can acidify the intercellular space than normal [8]. As noted above, the buffering of intercellular H⁺ is done by intercellular HCO_3 and this bicarbonate is derived from the primary postepithelial defense — the blood supply (Fig. 4). Esophageal blood flow has been shown to increase during acid exposure, an adaptation that enables more bicarbonate to be delivered to the interstitium for buffering H⁺ [9]. The blood supply also removes excess CO_2 produced by H⁺ neutralization as well as supplying oxygen and nutrients for cell functions, including those for repair of damaged cells and restoration of epithelial architecture [10].

References

1. Orlando RC. Reflux esophagitis. In: Yamada T, Alpers DH, Owyang C, Powell DW, Silverstein FE (eds) Textbook of Gastroenterology. Philadelphia: Lippincott Company, 1991;1123–1147.
2. Salo J, Kivilaakso E. Role of luminal H⁺ in the pathogenesis of experimental esophagitis. Surgery 1982;92:61–68.
3. Quigley EMM, Turnberg LA. pH of the microclimate lining the human gastric and duodenal mucosa in vivo studies in control subjects and in duodenal ulcer patients. Gastroenterology 1987;92:1876–1884.
4. Orlando RC, Lacy ER, Tobey NA, Cowart K. Barriers to paracellular permeability in rabbit esophageal epithelium. Gastroenterology 1992;102:910–923.
5. Tobey NA, Reddy SP, Khalbuss WE, Silvers SM, Cragoe EJ Jr, Orlando RC. Na⁺-dependent and -independent Cl⁻/HCO_3⁻ exchangers in cultured rabbit esophageal epithelial cells. Gastroenterology 1993;104:185–195.
6. Tobey NA, Powell DW, Schreiner VJ, Orlando RC. Serosal bicarbonate protects against acid injury to rabbit esophagus. Gastroenterology 1989;96:1466–1477.
7. Orlando RC. Pathology of reflux oesophagitis and its complications. In: Jamieson GG (ed) Surgery of the Oesophagus. London: Churchill Livingstone, 1988;189–200.
8. Orlando RC. Esophageal epithelial resistance. In: Castell DO (ed) The Esophagus. Boston: Little Brown Inc., 1992; 463–478.
9. Hollwarth ME, Smith M, Kvietys PR, Granger DN. Esophageal blood flow in the cat. Gastroenterology 1986;90:622.
10. Orlando RC. Esophageal epithelial defense against acid injury. J Clin Gastroenterol 1991;13(suppl 2):S1–S5.

What is the role of epidermal growth factor in saliva in protecting the esophageal mucosa?

P.J. Kahrilas (Chicago)

Epidermal growth factor (EGF), also known as epithelial growth factor, urogastrone-EGF, and β-urogastrone, is a single chain polypeptide secreted by the submandibular salivary glands, duodenal Brunner's glands, small intestinal Paneth cells, and other exocrine glands including the pancreas [1]. EGF is found in several body fluids including saliva. Although circulating levels of the peptide are low, high concentrations are found within platelet granules. Transforming growth factor alpha (TGF-α) is a 50 amino acid peptide with 40% homology to EGF that acts on the same receptor. Both EGF and TGF-α are produced extracellularly on the cell membrane as precursor molecules which are then activated by proteolysis [2]. Both peptides are found in many gastrointestinal tissues including the esophagus and stomach. Despite their shared receptor, EGF and TGF-α probably evoke distinct biological effects, by evoking distinct conformational changes in the receptor and activating different secondary messengers [3].

Epidermal growth factor receptor (EGF-R) is an integral plasma membrane glycoprotein. Activation of EGF-R by either EGF or TGF-α is mitogenic in cell culture studies of squamous cells, fibroblasts, and various mucosal tissues [4]. The mitogenic action may be mediated by regulation of the transition rate between G2 phase and mitosis of the cell cycle [5]. Of the two peptides, TGF-α is 10 times as potent mitogenically as well as possessing additional proliferative properties including increased cell ruffling, angiogenesis and megacolony formation [6]. EGF and TGF-α have been invoked as potential causal factors in the development of Barrett's epithelium, dysplasia and carcinogenesis of the esophagus, because of the proliferative effects, although no more than an association has yet been demonstrated [7]. The remainder of this discussion, however, will focus only on the role of salivary EGF on the maintenance of esophageal mucosal integrity.

In vivo actions of EGF in the gastrointestinal tract include promoting wound healing, inducing cellular proliferation, promoting differentiation, and potentially oncogenesis [1]. EGF is immunohistochemically detectable in all layers of the esophageal epithelium, with greatest density in the basal layer compared with the more superficial layers [2]. EGF localizes in the capillary endothelium of the normal esophageal papillae and basal mucosa. However, significantly more EGF positive papillae are found in the normal mucosa as opposed to the inflamed mucosa [2]. This leads to a question of cause and effect, with some investigators hypothesizing that a deficiency of secreted EGF is a cause of erosive esophagitis, whereas other investigators suggest that diminished detection in the mucosa may be an effect of inflammation. The latter hypothesis seems more likely since there are no demonstrable differences in salivary EGF levels among individuals with a normal mucosa, gastritis, or erosive esophagitis [8]. Controversy persists, however, as to whether or not Barrett's epithelium is associated with diminished salivary EGF secretion [8,9].

In part, the above controversy revolves around the origin of EGF found in esophageal tissue. EGF is found in the endothelium of normal capillaries immediately adjacent to the basal cells of the esophageal epithelium and deep esophageal glands. Thus, it is not immediately apparent how luminal EGF contained in saliva could localize to these deep layers of the epithelium. An alternative hypothesis is that EGF is transported to the basal cell layers via platelet EGF; an attractive hypothesis considering where EGF localizes. It has been experimentally demonstrated that EGF administered intravenously exhibits much greater trophic effects than does EGF administered intraluminally [10]. Perhaps, EGF is stored in the endothelial cells of the normal mucosa and is rapidly released and utilized when inflammation occurs. Thus, the observation that mucosal EGF is depleted in peptic esophagitis is better explained by the observation that EGF has a relatively short half life (< 24 h) than by the hypothesis that EGF depletion led to the development of, or susceptibility to esophagitis [11]. However, not all experimental evidence agrees with this hypothesis. There is some experimental evidence supporting the role of salivary EGF in maintenance of the esophageal mucosa. Specifically rats, subject to sialoadenectomy, demonstrate increased mucosal permeability to hydrogen ion and this increased permeability is partially reversed by the intraluminal administration of EGF [12]. Bear in mind, though, that there is more in saliva than just EGF and this experiment might simply be verifying the importance of saliva in mucosal defense.

Another interesting hypothesis regarding the role of salivary EGF is that it acts to stimulate ulcer healing throughout the gut. Areas denuded of normal epithelium would be accessible to luminal EGF and presumably EGF could bind at these sites and stimulate cellular proliferation adjacent to the ulceration. In this capacity, it has also been reported that salivary EGF is bound to sucralfate and bismuth, agents that bind to the base of ulcers and possess "cytoprotective" properties [13,14]. This would then be the explanation for those cytoprotective properties.

References

1. Jankowski J, Coghill G, Tregaskis B, Hopwood D, Wormsley KG. Epidermal growth factor in the esophagus. Gut 1992;33: 1448–1453.
2. Jankowski J, Hopwood D, Wormsley KG. Expression of epidermal growth factor, transforming growth factor alpha and their receptor in gastro-oesophageal disease. Dig Dis 1993;11:1–11.
3. Decker SJ. Epidermal growth factor and transforming growth factor-alpha induce differential processing of epidermal growth factor receptor. Biochem Biophys Res Commun 1990;166:615–621.
4. Todderud G, Carpenter G. Epidermal growth factor; the receptor and its functions. Biofactors 1989;2:11–15.
5. Kinzel V, Kaszkin M, Blume A, Richards J. Epidermal growth factor inhibits transiently the progression from G2 phase to mitosis; a receptor mediated phenomenon in various cells. Cancer Res 1990;50:7932–7936.
6. Burgess AW. Epidermal growth factor and transforming growth factor-alpha. Br Med Bull 1990;45:401–424.
7. Mukaida H, Yamamoto T, Hirai T et al. Expression of human epidermal growth factor and its receptor in esophageal cancer. Jpn J Surg 1990;20:275–282.
8. Maccini DM, Veit BC. Salivary epidermal growth factor in patients with and without acid peptic disease. Am J Gastroenterol 1990;85:1102–1104.
9. Gray MR, Donnely RJ, Kingsworth AN. Role of salivary epidermal growth factor in the pathogenesis of Barrett's columnar lined oesophagus. Br J Surg 1991;78:1461–1466.
10. Goodlad RA, Wilson TJG, Lenton W, Gregory H, McCullagh KG, Wright NA. Proliferative effects of urogastrone-EGF on the intestinal epithelium. Gut 1987;28:37–43.
11. Jankowski J, Austin W, Howat K et al. Proliferation in the esophagus; an index of chronological age. Eur J Gastroenterol

Hepatol 1991;3:675–678.

12. Sarosiek J, Feng T, McCallum RW. The inter-relationship between salivary epidermal growth factor and the functional integrity of the esophageal mucosal barrier in the rat. Am J Med Sci 1991;302:359–363.

13. Konturek SJ, Dembinski A, Warzecha, Bielanski W, Brzozowski T, Drozosowski T. Epidermal growth factor (EGF) in the gastroprotective and ulcer healing actions of colloidal bismuth subcitrate (De-Nol) in rats. Gut 1986;29:894–902.

14. Liu J, Piotrowski J, Tamura S et al. Gastric mucosal EGF and PDGF receptors; effect of sucralfate. Gastroenterology 1991; 100:652 (abstract).

What part do the mucous cells of submucosal mucous glands play in the esophageal pre-epithelial barrier?

J. Sarosiek, Z. Namiot, R. Piascik, D.P. Hetzel, R.M. Rourk, M.C. Edmunds, T.M. Daniel, R.W. McCallum (Charlottesville)

As we well know from the other parts of the alimentary tract, mucosal integrity depends upon the balance between aggressive factors and protective mechanisms. We propose that this also holds true within the esophageal compartment (Fig. 1, panel I). By aggressive factors we mean abnormal esophageal exposure to acid as demonstrated by 24-h pH monitoring study. Approximately 40% of patients with symptomatic gastroesophageal reflux disease (GERD), with abnormal acid exposure time, do not develop reflux esophagitis. The balance, disturbed by excessive aggression of gastroesophageal refluxate in these subjects, is presumably restored by stronger than normal mucosal protective mechanisms, effectively counteracting abnormal reflux (Fig. 1, panel II). Reflux esophagitis (RE) is likely to develop in those in whom the excessive gastroesophageal reflux (GER) cannot be compensated by otherwise normal protective mechanisms (Fig. 1, panel III). Moreover, in approximately 10 to 20% of patients with endoscopic RE, an acid exposure time estimated by 24-h pH monitoring, remains within normal limits. The development of RE in this subset of patients would be mediated by inherently and severely compromised mucosal protection.

In order to develop RE, gastric acid and pepsin require pathogenetic enhancement by at least one of five major abnormalities within the protective mechanisms such as:
— lower esophageal sphincter (LES) incompetence;
— esophageal motility impairment;
— decline in salivary protection;
— compromised esophageal mucosal protection; and
— attenuated mucosal blood flow (Fig. 2).
However, if all five abnormalities overlap, a severe esophagitis (black color) would inevitably develop.

Esophageal mucosal protection is of paramount importance in the maintenance of

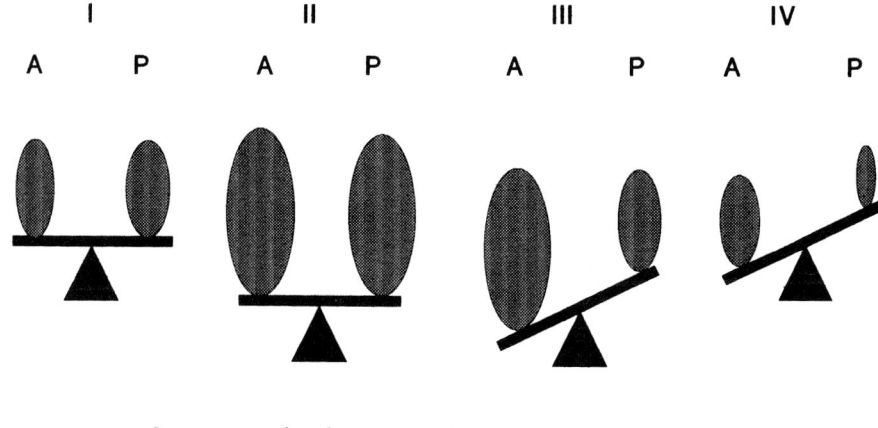

A = aggressive factors   P = protective factors

Fig. 1. The role of aggressive and protective factors in the development of reflux esophagitis.

the mucosal integrity. Esophageal mucosal protection operates at three different but overlapping levels: pre-epithelial, epithelial and postepithelial. Pre-epithelial protection, on the other hand, depends upon the complementary action of salivary and esophageal secretions. Contribution of the submucosal mucous glands secretion to pre-epithelial defense, will currently be focused on.

Human esophageal mucosa, although covered by nonkeratinized squamous epithelium, contains numerous submucosal mucous glands, organized in longitudinal rows with their ducts arranged obliquely in the general direction downward toward the lumen [1—3]. The secretion of such glands, however, has never been explored due to the lack of appropriate methodology. As it has been demonstrated histochemically, the mucous cells within these glands contain neutral, sialylated and sulphated mucins, whereas duct epithelium has been shown to be rich in cytokeratin [4]. One may therefore assume that owing to its content of mucin, the secretion of such glands would exhibit a highly viscous characteristic, typical for all the protective secretions along the alimentary tract. Through perfusion study using a newly developed esophageal perfusion catheter [5], we were able, for the first time in humans, to explore the secretory potential of submucosal mucous glands under the impact of physiological conditions (luminal exposure to saline) and conditions mimicking GER (luminal exposure to acid/pepsin solution).

Subjects and Methods

Subjects

Twenty-one healthy asymptomatic volunteers were investigated and were divided into three groups:
— Group I (7 individuals: 4 males and 3 females; mean age 38) in whom esophageal perfusion with saline alone was conducted during sixteen 2-min perfusion intervals

(consecutive perfusion periods I–IV).

— Group II (7 individuals: 4 males and 3 females; mean age 40) whom esophageal perfusion was performed using NaCl during the first four 2-min perfusion intervals (period I), HCl (0.01 M; pH 2.1) during the next eight 2-min intervals (periods II and III) and again NaCl during the final four 2-min intervals (period IV).

— Group III (7 individuals: 4 males and 3 females; mean age 42) in whom

REFLUX ESOPHAGITIS PATHOGENESIS

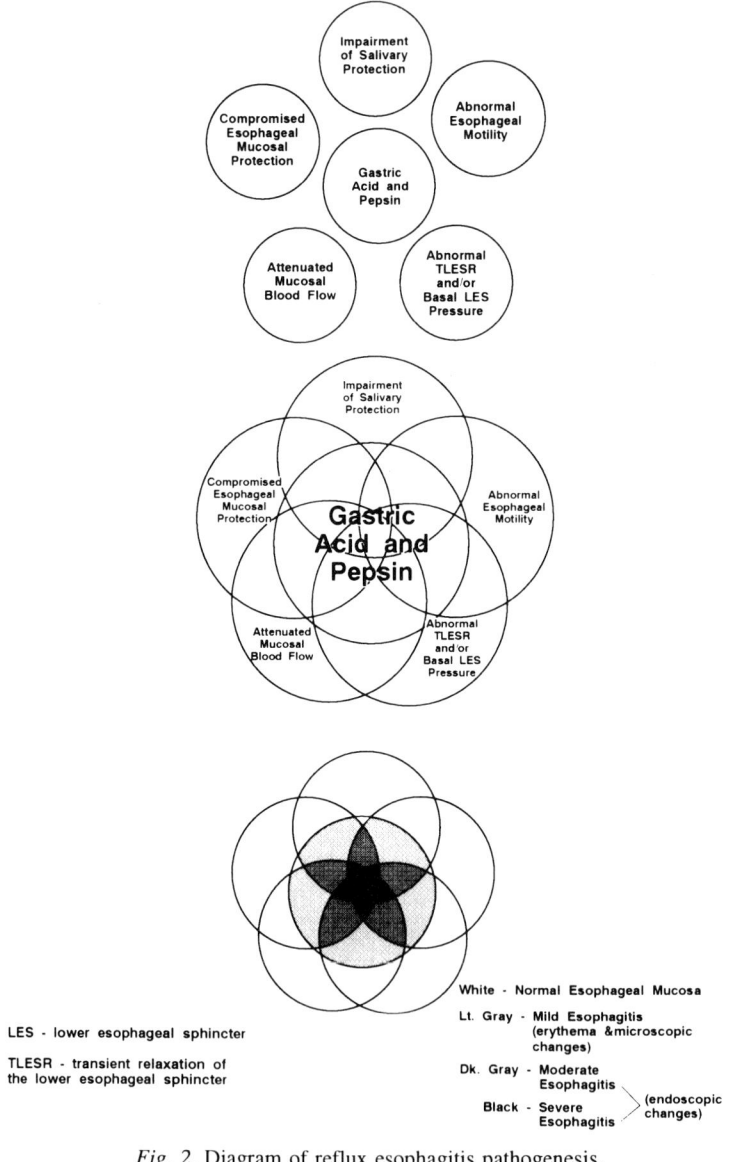

Fig. 2. Diagram of reflux esophagitis pathogenesis.

esophageal perfusion was performed with saline during the first four 2-min perfusion intervals (period I), with HCl (0.01 M; pH 2.1) during the next four 2-min perfusion intervals (period II), with HCl supplemented with pepsin (0.5 mg/ml of 0.01 M HCl) during the next four perfusion intervals (period III) and with saline the final four 2-min intervals (period IV).

All HCl or HCl/pepsin solutions were iso-osmotically equilibrated with NaCl.

Methods

Esophageal perfusion catheter
Esophageal study in humans was performed using our specially designed perfusion catheter [5]. The commercial version of our prototype is now manufactured by the Wilson-Cook Co. (Winston-Salem, NC). The catheter has six channels. The largest diameter channel (3 mm ID) was designated for aspiration of esophageal secretion elaborated during perfusion. The second channel, the longest (1.5 mm ID), served for

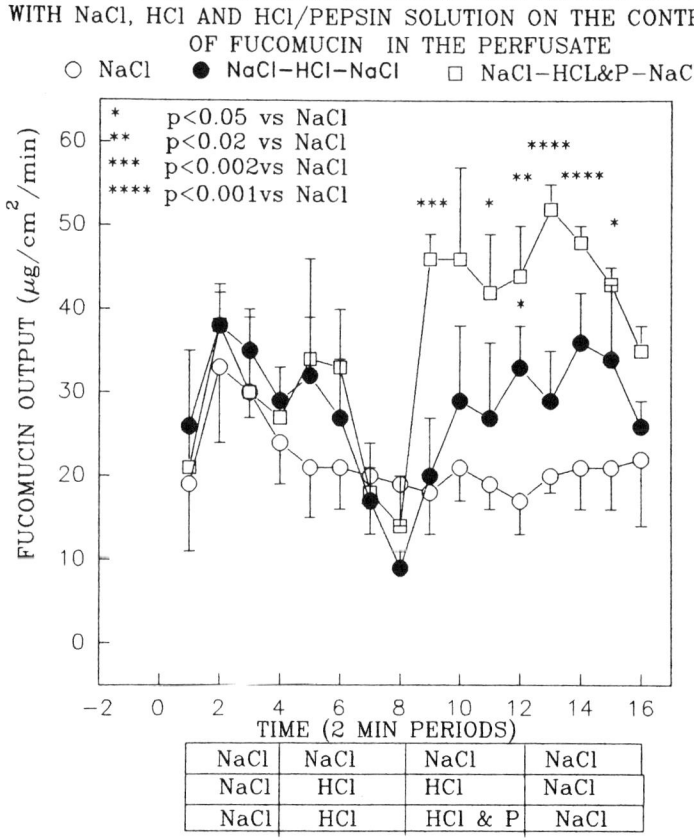

Fig. 3. Secretion of human esophageal fucomucins.

gastric aspiration and subsequent calculation of the rate of recovery of esophageal perfusate. Channels three and four (1 mm ID) were connected directly with the lower and the upper balloons respectively allowing control of both pressure and volume. The fifth channel was designed to aspirate saliva potentially collecting within the esophageal lumen above the upper balloon, if such was accidentally swallowed. The sixth channel served as an air vent for the perfused segment of esophagus. The catheter was equipped with two balloons spaced 75 mm apart. The length of each balloon was 20 mm. An optimal diameter of the inflated lower balloon to secure a very good recovery rate of esophageal perfusate was 25 mm (inflated with 9 cc of air), whereas the optimal diameter of the upper balloon was 20.5 mm (inflated with 5 cc of air). This was determined by looking at the relationship between recovery rates and specific balloons diameters.

Esophageal perfusion model

Our specially designed esophageal perfusion catheter was inserted into the esophagus through the nares so that the distal balloon was located 35–37 cm from the nares and the upper balloon was placed 27.5–29.5 cm from the nares. Such placement of the

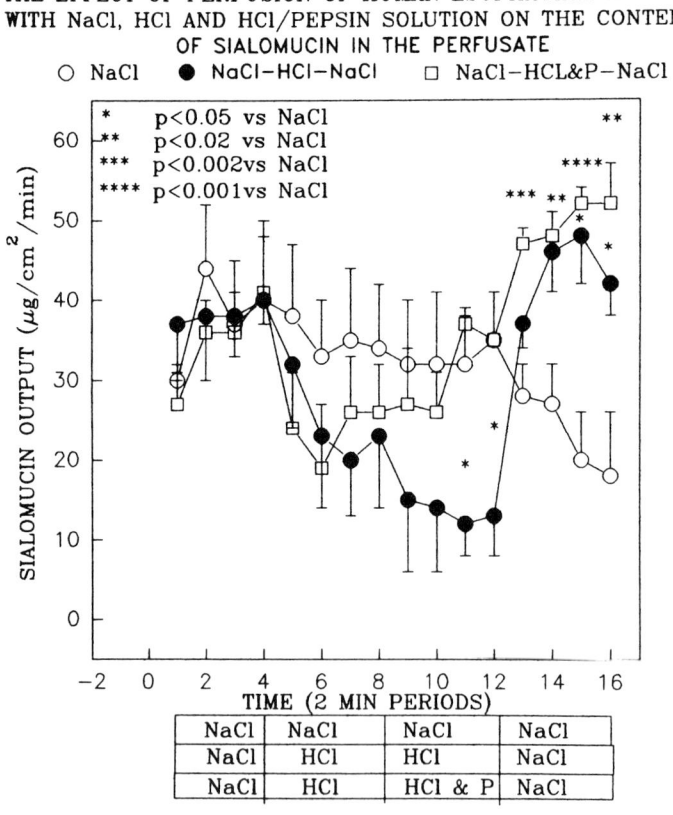

Fig. 4. Secretion of esophageal sialomucins into the esophageal perfusate.

catheter secured isolation of a 7.5 cm segment of the lower esophagus for perfusion. All subjects remained in a semirecumbent position during the study, avoiding straining and coughing which could potentially elevate intra-abdominal pressure. Each subject was advised not to swallow any saliva and to spit salivary secretion into a separate cup every 10 s. Separate analyses were performed on collected saliva. Obtained results will be the subject of a separate manuscript. Furthermore, for potential GER during the study, despite sealing the lower esophagus with a balloon, the pH of the esophageal perfusate was continuously monitored.

Chemical analyses
The measurement of fucomucin, sialomucin and sulfomucin was performed using Alcian Blue methodology [6–8], as previously described [9], with some minimal modification required for the study of esophageal secretion. Total mucin was assessed using periodic acid/Schiff (PAS) methodology [10,11]. The content of total protein was measured by the Lowry method [12]. The viscosity of freshly recovered esophageal perfusates was measured using cone/plate digital viscometer (Brookfield,

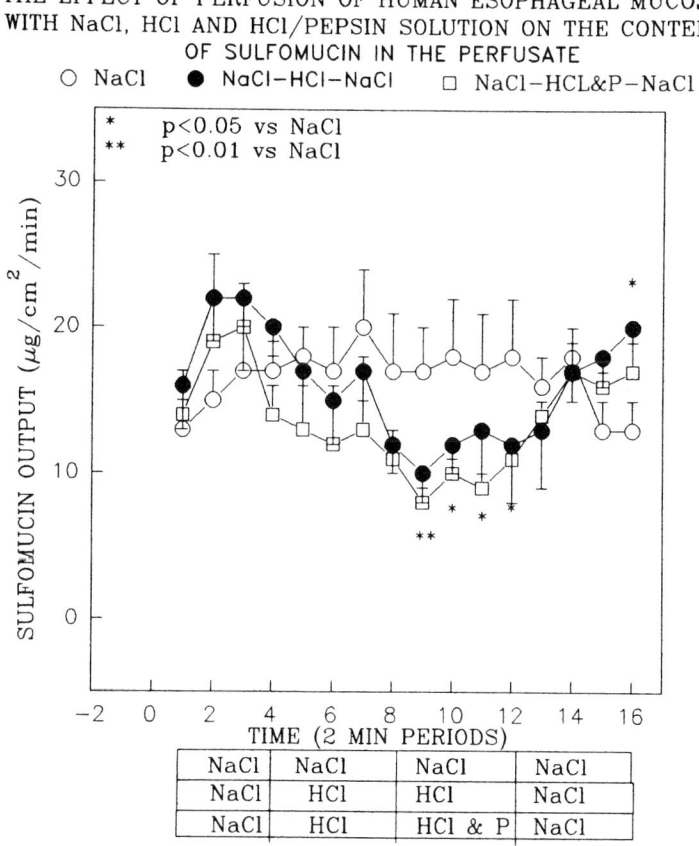

Fig. 5. Secretion of human esophageal sulfomucin under the impact of perfusing solutions.

MA), as previously described [13]. Bicarbonate was measured recording CO_2 and by back-titration [14,15]. Epidermal growth factor (EGF) and PGE_2 were measured using radioimmonoassay (RIA) (Amersham, IL) as previously described [5,16,17].

All results are expressed as means ± SEM. Student's t test was performed using CSS software package for PC.

Results

Esophageal perfusion with saline resulted in a continuous release of fuco-, sialo- and sulfomucins throughout an entire perfusion procedure (Figs. 3,4,5, respectively). Introduction of HCl into the perfusate resulted in a transient inhibition of esophageal fucomucin from 31 ± 6.9 to 21.5 ± 5.2 $\mu g/cm^2/min$ and sulfomucin from 20.2 ± 3.2 to 15.1 ± 2.8 $\mu g/cm^2/min$, whereas secretion of sialomucin was inhibited significantly from 38.2 ± 6.0 to 14.0 ± 6.8 $\mu g/cm^2/min$, p < 0.01. Substitution of HCl with saline resulted in a significant increase in secretion of all types of mucin. Esophageal exposure to HCl/pepsin solution, on the other hand, evoked a significant increase in fucomucin output (44.5 ± 6.9 vs. 25.4 ± 6.3 $\mu g/cm^2/min$; p < 0.01), no change in sialomucin whereas sulfomucin secretion significantly declined (9.1 ± 0.9 vs. 16.7 ± 3.6 $\mu g/cm^2/min$, p < 0.001). Therefore, during perfusion with NaCl sialomucin dominated the total mucin (45%) followed by fucomucin (33%) and sulfomucin (22%) (Fig. 6). During perfusion with acid, however, fucomucin become the predominant component (43%), followed by sialomucin (36%) and sulfomucin (21%).

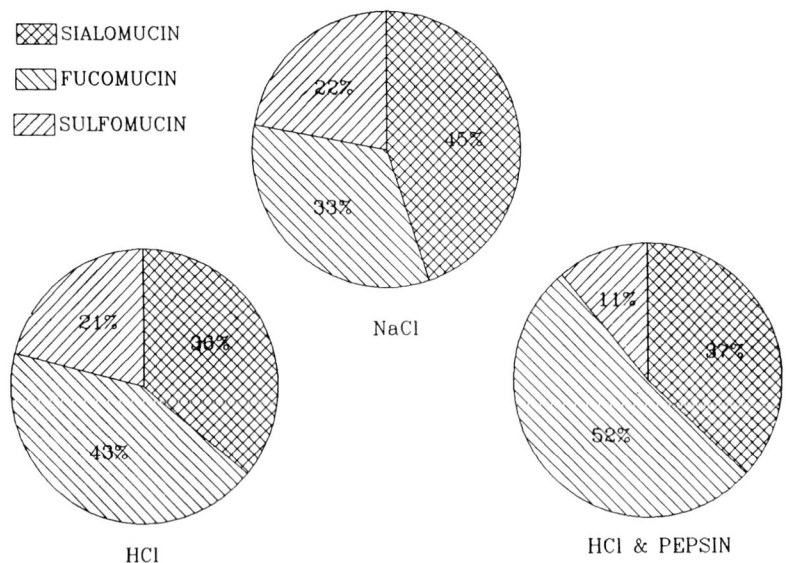

PERCENT CONTENT OF FUCOMUCIN, SIALOMUCIN AND SULFOMUCIN
IN TOTAL ESOPHAGEAL MUCIN

Fig. 6. Composition of human esophageal mucins.

284

During esophageal mucosal exposure to HCl/pepsin solution, fucomucin become the leading mucus glycoprotein within esophageal secretion (52%), while the contribution of sulfomucin declined to 11%. Total mucin output, measured by PAS methodology, declined during exposure to acid from 0.275 ± 0.047 to 0.170 ± 0.045 mg/cm^2/min, but significantly increased during perfusion with acid/pepsin solution (0.320 ± 0.03 vs. 0.170 ± 0.045 mg/cm^2/min, $p < 0.01$) (Fig. 7). Also total protein content in the esophageal perfusate exhibited declining tendency during perfusion with HCl (0.159 ± 0.039 vs. 0.181 ± 16.1 mg/cm^2/min), whereas it significantly increased during exposure to HCl/pepsin solution (0.204 ± 0.018 vs. 0.159 ± 0.039 mg/cm^2/min, $p < 0.05$) (Fig. 8). The viscosity of the esophageal perfusate (Fig. 9) significantly declined under the impact of acid/pepsin solution, perfusion period III (93 ± 15 vs. 157 ± 26, $p < 0.01$) and during subsequent recovery period IV (97 ± 17 vs. 185 ± 33; $p < 0.01$).

During esophageal perfusion with saline human bicarbonate secretion rate varied between 0.097 ± 0.006 and 0.101 ± 0.006 nmol/cm^2/min. Mucosal exposure to acid resulted in an immediate increase in bicarbonate secretion to the value of 841 ± 112 nmol/cm^2/min ($p < 0.0001$ vs. NaCl). Infusion of acid/pepsin solution augmented the rate of esophageal bicarbonate secretion event further to its value of 1078 ± 135 nmol/cm^2/min ($p < 0.0001$ vs. NaCl) (Table 1).

Human esophageal mucosa exhibited an ability to elaborate its own EGF at the basal rate between 10.80 ± 1.46 ng/min and 12.50 ± 1.52 ng/min. Esophageal mucosal exposure to acid resulted in a profound and significant decline of esophageal EGF output to 3.57 ± 0.87 ng/min ($p < 0.001$ vs. NaCl). Esophageal perfusion with

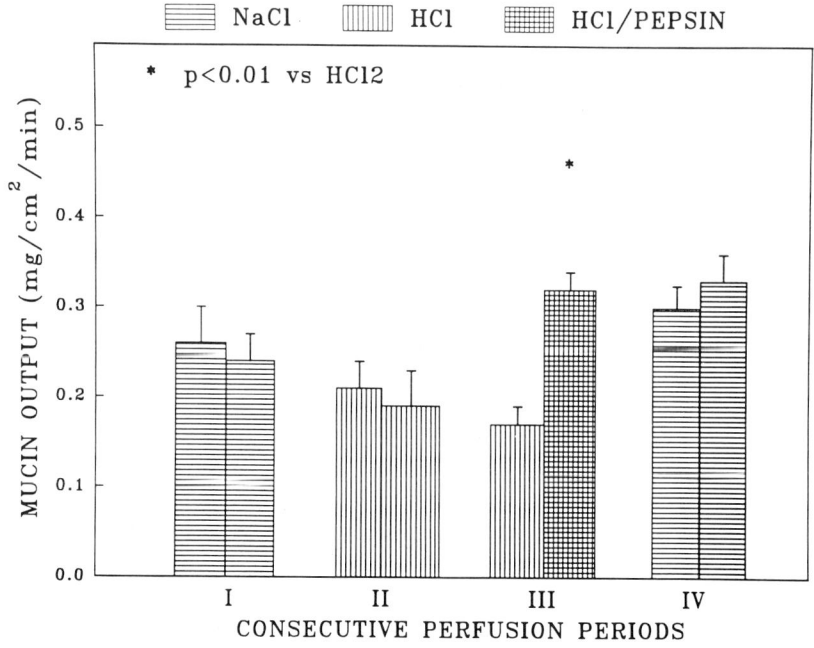

Fig. 7. Total mucin output during esophageal perfusion in humans.

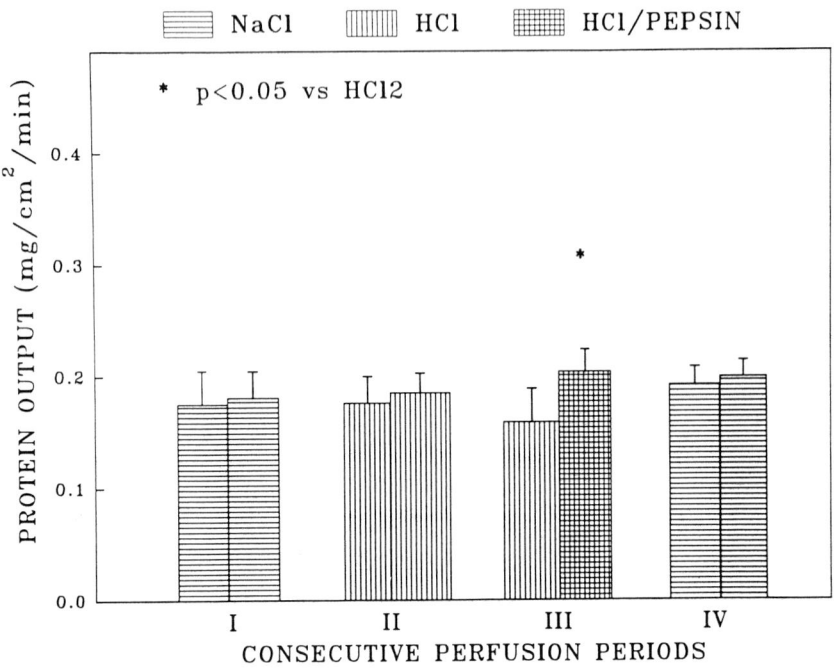

Fig. 8. Luminal release of protein during esophageal perfusion in humans.

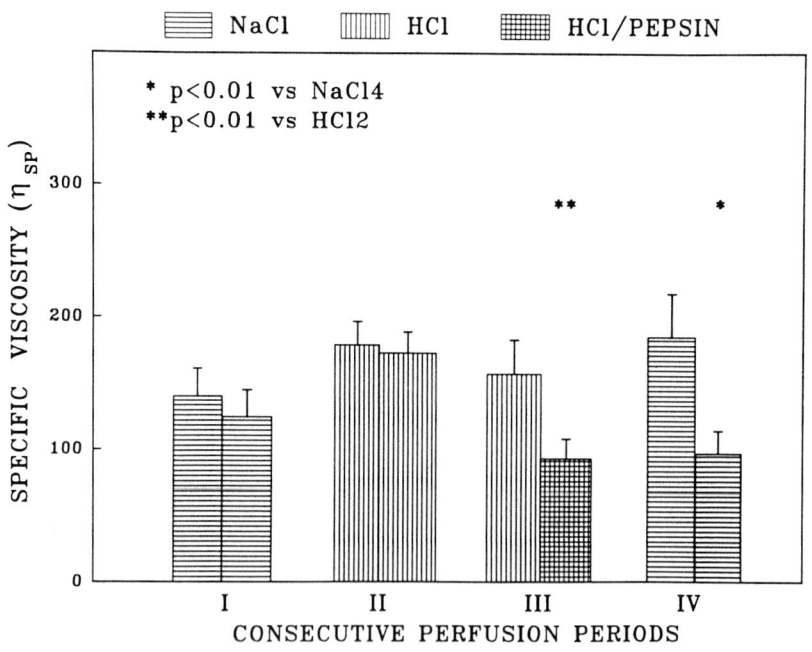

Fig. 9. Specific viscosity of human esophageal secretion.

Table 1. Bicarbonate secretion by human esophageal mucosa during exposure to saline, HCl and HCl/pepsin solutions (mean ± SEM)

Experimental group	Bicarbonate secretion during various modes of perfusion			
Group I (n = 7) nmol/cm^2/min	NaCl 0.098 ± 0.007	NaCl 0.101 ± 0.006	NaCl 0.100 ± 0.005	NaCl 0.097 ± 0.006
Group II (n = 7) nmol/cm^2/min	NaCl 0.091 ± 0.006	HCl 841[a] ± 112	HCl 810[a] ± 92	NaCl 0.104 ± 0.007
Group III (n = 7) nmol/cm^2/min	NaCl 0.102 ± 0.005	HCl 916[a] ± 101	HCl/pepsin 1078[a] ± 135	NaCl 0.112 ± 0.008

[a] $p < 0.0001$ vs. NaCl periods.

Table 2. EGF secretion by human esophageal mucosa during exposure to saline, HCl and HCl/pepsin solutions (mean ± SEM)

Experimental group	EGF secretion during various modes of perfusion			
Group I (n = 7) ng/min	NaCl 11.90 ± 1.83	NaCl 10.80 ± 1.46	NaCl 12.50 ± 1.52	NaCl 12.30 ± 1.63
Group II (n = 7) ng/min	NaCl 11.2 ± 1.83	HCl 6.17[a] ± 1.58	HCl 3.57[c] ± 0.87	NaCl 13.2 ± 1.42
Group III (n = 7) ng/min	NaCl 12.9 ± 1.84	HCl 4.04[c] ± 0.83	HCl/pepsin 9.82[b] ± 1.88	NaCl 13.6 ± 1.52

[a] $p < 0.01$ vs. NaCl; [b] $p < 0.0002$ vs. HCl; [c] $p < 0.001$ vs. NaCl.

Table 3. PGE$_2$ secretion by human esophageal mucosa during exposure to saline, HCl and HCl/pepsin solutions (mean ± SEM)

Experimental group	PGE$_2$ secretion during various modes of perfusion			
Group I (n = 7) pg/min	NaCl 1806 ± 474	NaCl 1823 ± 640	NaCl 1220 ± 433	NaCl 960 ± 369
Group II (n = 7) pg/min	NaCl 1733 ± 469	HCl 1020[a] ± 167	HCl 520[b] ± 71	NaCl 560[b] ± 80
Group III (n = 7) pg/min	NaCl 1880 ± 393	HCl 1010[a] ± 167	HCl/pepsin 1533[c] ± 340	NaCl 1260 ± 220

[a] $p < 0.01$ vs. NaCl; [b] $p < 0.001$ vs. HCl period II and $p < 0.0001$ vs. NaCl; [c] $p < 0.01$ vs. HCl period III (group II).

acid/pepsin solution, on the other hand, evoked increase of luminal EGF output over corresponding values recorded during HCl alone (9.82 ± 1.88 vs. 3.57 ± 0.87; p < 0.0002) (Table 2).

Esophageal perfusion with saline also led to a continuous luminal release of PGE$_2$ at the rate between 1806 ± 474 and 960 ± 369 pg/min. Infusion of acid resulted in a significant decline of PGE$_2$ output to its lowest value of 520 ± 71 pg/min. However, HCl accompanied by pepsin significantly enhanced the luminal release of PGE$_2$ reaching its value of 1553 ± 340 (p < 0.01 vs. HCl in period III, group II) (Table 3).

Discussion

Owing to our recently developed esophageal perfusion model, we are able to demonstrate, for the first time in humans, that the esophageal mucosa exhibits an ability to secrete copious amounts of mucin, nonmucin proteins, polypeptides such as EGF, and prostaglandins. All these mucus components are well known for their protective potential within the gastrointestinal tract. Furthermore, the rate of their secretion is significantly modified by luminal exposure to acid and acid/pepsin solutions, as seen in GERD.

Esophageal exposure to acid resulted in a significant decline of the mucin content in the esophageal perfusate; however, a significant rebound in mucin production occurred when HCl was substituted with saline during the last perfusion period. This may indicate that low pH inhibited mucin secretion from submucosal mucous glands and/or release from the mucus layer by enhancing its viscosity. Evidence that pH does not affect the viscosity of gastric mucus [18,19] seems to support more the former explanation, although an impact of pH on esophageal mucus viscosity still remains to be determined. A transient, pH-dependent increase in esophageal perfusate viscosity, despite a decline in the content of esophageal mucin within the perfusate, may indicate that factors other than mucin and nonmucin protein components of the esophageal secretion could account for this phenomenon. We have previously shown that IgA, prostaglandins, mucus-associated lipids and especially phospholipids affect significantly both viscosity and permselectivity of the gastric mucus and gastric mucus glycoprotein [13,20–22]. Therefore, a potential increase in the luminal release of esophageal phospholipids, under the impact of luminal acid, could potentially enhance the viscosity value of esophageal perfusate. However, the potential modulatory role of lipids in maintaining the protective quality of the human esophageal mucus still requires investigations.

Introduction of pepsin into acidic solutions resulted in a significant increase in luminal mucin release. We also observed that a profound protein release during acid/pepsin perfusion. Since the pH of acid/pepsin solution is the same as that of acid alone, the origin of luminally released mucin could only originate within the mucus components adsorbed to the surface of the mucosa. As it is hard to envisage a potential stimulatory effect of pepsin on the secretory function of submucosal mucous glands, excessive luminal release of mucus component provides indirect evidence for the existence of the mucus layer on the surface of the esophageal epithelium. This layer, however, contains not only mucin but also entrapped other proteins, polypeptides such as EGF and prostaglandins [5,11,16]. Furthermore, this mucus layer may appear to be the major target for acid and pepsin refluxed from the gastric compartment during GER. Therefore, one may assume that the first line of esophageal mucosal defense against refluxed gastric acid and pepsin is the viscous mucus layer, covering the surface epithelium. Furthermore, using dark-field inverted microscopy technique, as we previously described [23], we demonstrated, for the first time in humans, that the thickness of the esophageal mucus gel layer in a surgically resected specimen of the human esophageal squamous mucosa was (mean ± SE) 95 ± 12 μm (unpublished data).

Owing to an ability of the human esophageal mucosa to elaborate bicarbonate, as it has been demonstrated recently in our laboratory and by others [24,25] a mucus-bicarbonate barrier may significantly diminish aggressive potency of the gastroesophageal refluxate. It may also help to protect against other aggressive factors acting from the lumen of the esophageal compartment. Since the mucus layer has perm-selective properties, it may serve to generate a gradient of the damaging factor across the mucus layer with the highest within the lumen and the lowest at the surface of the esophageal epithelium. Such a gradient could help the esophageal epithelium cope with high concentrations of damaging factor and also gradually mobilize intramucosal protective mechanisms by delaying diffusion of the damaging factor.

Therefore, the human esophageal perfusion model provides us with a unique opportunity to explore protective mechanisms within the human esophageal mucosa. It may help in our search for a clue, leading to the development of severe esophagitis with its major complications such as Barrett's esophagus and esophageal stricture.

Conclusion

Human esophageal submucosal mucous glands exhibit a strong secretory potential, highly responsive to esophageal intraluminal stimuli. Owing to the viscous nature of human esophageal secretion, determined by its various components, especially mucin, a layer of the mucus gel on the surface of the esophageal mucosa is continuously maintained. This mucus layer provides the first line of mucosal defense against the action of acid and pepsin present in gastroesophageal refluxate. Therefore, all cellular components of submucosal mucous glands significantly contribute to the maintenance of the integrity of the esophageal mucosa.

Acknowledgements

This study was supported by Jeffress Trust grant J-240, grant from the American College of Gastroenterology and AGA Foundation/SmithKline Beecham award.

References

1. Hamilton SR. Reflux esophagitis and Barrett esophagus. In: Goldman H, Appelman HD, Kaufman N (eds) Gastrointestinal Pathology. Baltimore: William & Wilkins, 1990:11–68.
2. Harmon JW, Rice RP. Esophageal intramural diverticulosis. Ann Thorac Surg 1974;17:260–267.
3. Fenoglio-Preiser CM. The normal anatomy of the esophagus. In: Fenoglio-Preiser CM, Lantz PE, Listrom MB, Davis M, Rilke FO (eds) Gastrointestinal Pathology. New York: Raven Press, 1989:21–31.
4. Hopwood D, Coghill G, Sanders DS. Human oesophageal submucosal glands. Their detection mucin, enzyme and secretory

protein content. Histochemistry 1986;86:107—112.

5. Sarosiek J, Yu Z, Hetzel DP, Rourk RM, Piascik R, Li L, Namiot Z, McCallum RW. Evidence on secretion of EGF by the esophageal mucosa in humans. Am J Gastroenterol 1993;88:1081—1087.

6. Hall RL, Miller AC, Peatfield PS, Richardson I, Williams I, Lampert I. A colorimetric assay for mucus glycoprotein using Alcian blue. Biochem Soc Trans 1980;8:72—73.

7. Corne SJ, Morrissey SM, Woods RJ. A method for the quantitative estimation of gastric barrier mucus. J Physiol (London) 1974;242:116P—117P.

8. Koo MWL, Ogle CW, Cho CW. Effects of verapamil, carbenoxolone and N-acetylcysteine on gastric wall mucus and ulceration in stressed rats. Pharmacology 1986;32:326—334.

9. Bilski J, Sarosiek J, Murty VLN, Aono M, Moriga M, Slomiany A, Slomiany BL. Enhancement of the lipid content and physical properties of gastric mucus by geranylgeranylacetone. Biochem Pharmacol 1987;36:4059—4065.

10. Mantle M, Allen A. A colorimetric assay for glycoprotein based on the Periodic Acid/Schiff stain. Biochem Soc Trans 1978;6:607—609.

11. Namiot Z, Sarosiek J, Rourk RM, McCallum RW. Human esophageal secretion: mucosal response to luminal acid and pepsin. Gastroenterology 1993 (submitted).

12. Lowry OH, Rosenbrough NJ, Farr AL, Randall RJ. Protein measurement with folin phenol reagent. J Biol Chem 1951; 193:265—275.

13. Murty VLN, Sarosiek J, Slomiany A, Slomiany BL. Effect of lipids and proteins on the viscosity of gastric mucus glycoprotein. Biochem Biophys Res Commun 1984;121:521—529.

14. Hamilton BH, Orlando RC. In vivo alkaline secretion by mammalian esophagus. Gastroenterology 1989;97:640—648.

15. Sjovall H, Forsell H, Olbe L. Simultaneous measurement of gastric acid and bicarbonate secretion in man. Scand J Gastroenterol 1989;24:1163—1171.

16. Yu Z, Sarosiek J, Namiot Z, Rourk RM, Hetzel DP, McCallum RW. Impact of acid and pepsin on human esophageal prostaglandins. Am J Gastroenterol 1993 (submitted).

17. Sarosiek J, Namiot Z, Yu Z, Rourk RM, Piascik R, Hetzel DP, McCallum RW. Modulatory effect of esophageal intraluminal mechanical and chemical stressors on salivary prostaglandin E2 in humans. Am J Gastroenterol 1993 (submitted).

18. Allen A. Structure and function of gastrointestinal mucus. In: Johnson LR (ed) Physiology of the Gastrointestinal Tract. New York: Raven Press, 1981:617—639.

19. Neutra MR, Forstner JF. Gastrointestinal mucus: synthesis, secretion, and function. In: Johnson LR (ed) Physiology of the Gastrointestinal Tract, 2nd ed. New York: Raven Press, 1987:975—1009.

20. Sarosiek J, Slomiany A, Slomiany BL. Retardation of hydrogen ion diffusion by gastric mucus constituents: Effect of proteolysis. Biochem Biophys Res Commun 1983;113:1053—1060.

21. Sarosiek J, Murty VLN, Nadziejko C, Slomiany A, Slomiany BL. Prostaglandin effect on the physical properties of gastric mucin and its susceptibility to pepsin. Prostaglandins 1986;32:635—646.

22. Scheiman JM, Kraus ER, Boland CR. Regulation of canine gastric mucin synthesis and phospholipid secretion by acid secretagogues. Gastroenterology 1992;103:1842—1850.

23. Sarosiek J, Marshall BJ, Peura D, Hoffman S, Feng T, McCallum RW. Gastroduodenal mucus gel thickness in patients with Helicobacter pylori: A method for assessment of biopsy specimens. Am J Gastroenterol 1991;86:729—734.

24. Sarosiek J, Hetzel D, Peura D, Piascik R, Feng T, McCallum RW. Human esophageal bicarbonate: The rate of secretion during pension with NaCl, HCl, and HC in pepsin solutions. Gastroenterology 1992;102:A158 (abstract).

25. Meyers RL, Orlando RC. In vivo bicarbonate secretion by human esophagus. Gastroenterology 1992;103:1174—1178.

What is the role of the proliferative capability of the basal layer?

R.H. Riddell (Hamilton)

Like all epithelium, the epithelium in the esophagus is dynamic and has a distinct turnover rate that has been estimated in vitro to be in the vicinity of 5—7 days [1,2].

This can be compared to a car engine idling in that there seems to be a basic rate which seems ideal. Below this, for example in patients given cytotoxic drugs or radiotherapy, the proliferation rate is inadequate for maintaining epithelial integrity and the engine stalls, resulting in ulceration. In practice, it seems likely that the epithelium is not turning over at minimal rate required, as there is continual surface trauma as food and drink are swallowed. Although the experiment appears not to have been done, it seems likely that in the absence of any surface trauma, for example if defunctioned, the turnover rate would probably decrease further.

Conversely, the turnover rate can be increased by a variety of noxious stimuli causing local trauma, whether at a relatively low level as a result of hot food or drink, drink containing chemicals such as acids that are likely to increase the surface degradation of cells, and perhaps most significantly, the reflux of gastric contents into the esophagus (whether acid or alkaline and, if including bile, presumably also including pancreatic enzymes). Such noxious agents can also include medications (antibiotics, quinidine, potassium chloride), and infectious agents, (Candida, Herpes). Whenever cells are removed from the surface, there is a compensatory hyperplasia of activity from the cells in the basal layer, proliferative activity being confined to this layer of glycogen-poor cells that usually constitute the basal 1—3 cell layers in the epithelium. Proliferation of this layer results in a relative thickness of this layer (basal cell hyperplasia) so that it increases to a thickness greater than the usual 15% of the epithelium [3—5]. When epithelial damage is marked, the basal cell layer may actually extend to the surface without maturation. If the capacity to respond is exceeded, ulceration results.

The role of the proliferative capacity of the basal layer is therefore to maintain the integrity of the epithelium by increasing or decreasing the mitotic rate. The feedback in the basal layer required to achieve this has not been elucidated. However, both failure of proliferation, and failure of the epithelium to proliferate at a sufficient rate commensurate with damage occurring in the overlying epithelium, can result in mucosal ulceration.

References

1. Bell B, Almy TP, Lipkin M. Cell proliferation kinetics in the gastrointestinal tract of man. Cell renewal in esophagus, stomach and jejunum of a patient with treated pernicious anemia. J Natl Cancer Inst 1967;38:615—628.
2. Eastwood GL. Gastrointestinal epithelial renewal. Gastroenterology 1977;72:962—975.
3. Ismail-Beigi F, Horton PF, Pope CE II. Histological consequences of gastroesophageal reflux in man. Gastroenterology 1970;58:163—174.
4. Livingstone EM, Sheahan DG, Behar J. Studies of esophageal epithelial cell proliferation in patients with reflux esophagitis. Gastroenterology 1977;73:1315—1319.
5. Weinstein WM, Bogoch ER, Bowes KL. The normal human esophageal mucosa: A histological reappraisal. Gastroenterology 1975;68:40—44.

What part does blood bicarbonate play in the formation of the epithelial barrier?

N.A. Tobey (New Orleans)

Blood bicarbonate (HCO_3^-), which is in equilibrium with interstitial fluid HCO_3^-, can contribute to the esophageal epithelial barrier to acid in four main ways; each through the provision of HCO_3^- for the intracellular or extracellular buffering of hydrogen ions (H^+). These are:

— by serving as a source of HCO_3^- for submucosal gland HCO_3^- secretion;
— by serving as a source of HCO_3^- for the unstirred water layer;
— by serving as a source of HCO_3^- for the paracellular pathway; and
— by serving as a source of intracellular HCO_3 after being transported into the cell on a Na^+-dependent Cl^-/HCO_3^- exchanger [1–4] (Table 1) (Figs. 1 and 2).

Pre-epithelial defenses

Submucosal gland secretion

Like that of the opossum, the human esophagus has submucosal glands that allow it to secrete HCO_3^-, which in turn protect it from (acid) reflux [2,3]. In the opossum, these glands form an extensive network running the entire length of the esophagus and in the submucosa, they also form compound acini which drain to a central duct extending through the muscularis mucosa and epithelium into the lumen [5–8]. Although the gland network in human esophagus is not as extensive as in the opossum, Meyers and Orlando were able to show HCO_3^- secretion by using a double balloon technique that permitted isolation and perfusion of the distal 10 cm of the human esophagus with an unbuffered solution [2]. This secretion probably accounts for the previously suspected nonsalivary component of esophageal acid clearance noted by Helm and Dent et al. [9–11]. The HCO_3^- content within the aspirates was identified and the amounts secreted (75 ± 26 µEq/30 min) were shown to be adequate

Table 1. Blood bicarbonate protective mechanisms

Pre-epithelial defenses
    Submucosal gland secretion
    Unstirred water layer-HCO_3^- complex
Epithelial defenses
    Extracellular buffering
    Intracellular buffering
Postepithelial defenses
    Blood flow

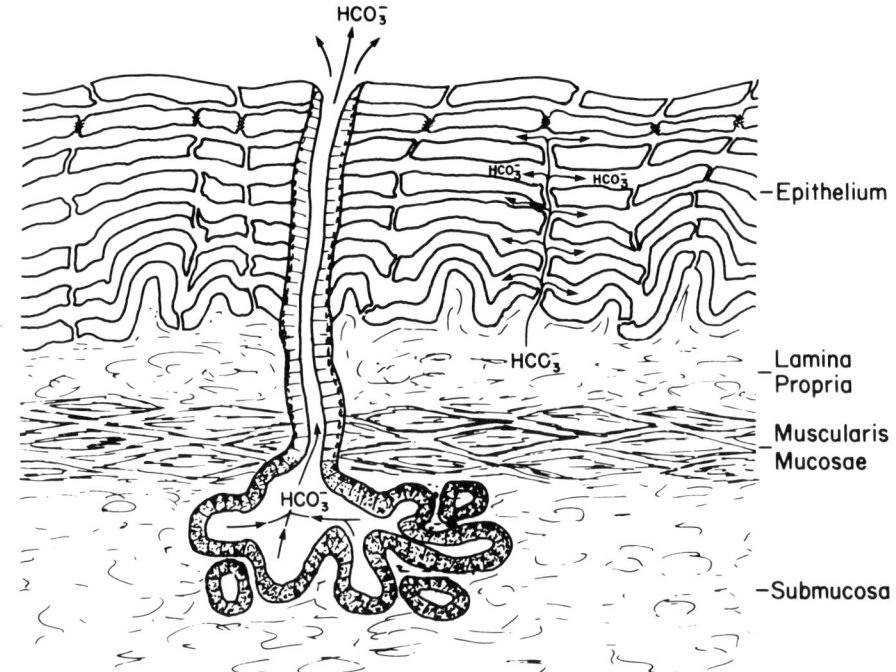

Fig. 1 shows how blood HCO_3^- can result in luminal HCO_3^- (i.e., by secretion from submucosal glands and/or by diffusing between the cells). Note: For HCO_3^- secretion to occur from glands, there must be a HCO_3^- entry mechanism from blood to cell and cell to acinar lumen. (Courtesy of Roy C. Orlando).

for the effective buffering of residual luminal acid, after bolus clearance by peristalsis [10,11]. The mechanism by which HCO_3^- secreted from the glands is derived from blood and interstitium is unknown but presumably occurs in much the same way as HCO_3^- enters the acinus of the salivary gland for secretion into the mouth [12] (Fig. 1).

Unstirred water layer HCO_3^- complex

Once secreted by the submucosal glands, HCO_3^- in the lumen can potentially contribute, by back diffusion, to the HCO_3^- content of the unstirred water layer and there serves as another pre-epithelial defense of the esophagus. This unstirred water layer, by potentially acting as a sink for HCO_3^- secreted from the salivary and esophageal submucosal glands as well as HCO_3^- diffusing from blood, can provide an alkaline microenvironment close to the epithelial surface which can serve to neutralize H^+. The buffering capacity of this layer is suggested by Quigley and Turnberg who demonstrated, with pH electrodes, that the human esophagus maintains a lumen-to-epithelium pH gradient (~1 pH unit) when perfused with acid [13]. However, the pH gradient in human esophagus is much smaller relative to that of stomach and duodenum, suggesting that the HCO_3^- secretion may not be continuous

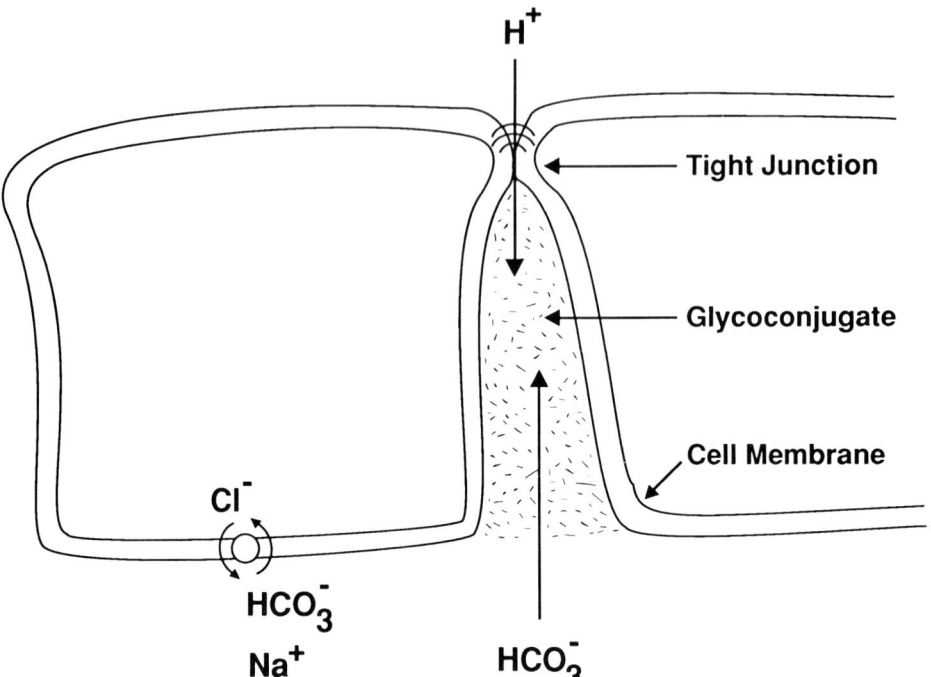

Fig. 2 shows how blood HCO_3^- can buffer within both intracellular and extracellular compartments of the epithelium, the former by entry into cells on the Na^+-dependent Cl^-/HCO_3^- exchanger and the latter by diffusing into the intercellular space. (Modified courtesy of Roy C. Orlando).

or it may not be effectively trapped because of the absence of a well defined layer of mucus.

Epithelial defenses

Extracellular buffering

If acid successfully eludes the more luminal pre-epithelial defenses, the epithelium of the esophagus then provides the next line of defense against back-diffusing H^+ [14]. This lining is a partially keratinized, stratified, squamous epithelium consisting of three layers: the stratum corneum; stratum spinosum; and stratum germinativum. The structural components in the epithelium, which contribute to the barrier, are located predominantly in the stratum corneum and consist of cell membranes and the intercellular junctional complexes. The junctional complex in rabbit esophageal epithelium is composed of tight junctions and intercellular glycoconjugate material, most likely glycoprotein [15] (Fig. 2). These combine to produce an electrically tight tissue with a resistance (R) in the range of 1,000–2,500 $\Omega \cdot cm^2$. Although, tight junctions formed by the interaction of integral membrane proteins from adjacent cell membranes which encircle the cells to seal off the lumen from the intercellular space, are major factors in other tissues and studies suggest that they may be less important in the esophagus. Data support the hypothesis that the primary route for H^+ entry into esophageal epithelium is across the junctions through the paracellular (as opposed to transcellular) pathway (Fig. 2) [1,16]. Therefore, HCO_3^- present in the intercellular spaces, would serve to buffer the incoming H^+ in the paracellular pathway. In vitro studies of rabbit esophageal epithelium, mounted in Ussing chambers, have shown that this is the case [1]. Tissues exposed to luminal acid (HCl, pH 1.1) without the benefit of HCO_3^- (or other buffers) in the serosal medium, sustained severe damage. The damage was evident both functionally and structurally; after washout, potential difference (PD) was abolished, R increased minimally, permeability to mannitol was high and histology showed extensive cell necrosis. Protection by HCO_3^- in the serosal medium was readily demonstrable, in that after washout tissues exposed to HCO_3^- had preserved PD and substantially greater increases in R, relatively low permeability to mannitol and were generally devoid of cell necrosis (Fig. 3). In addition, when

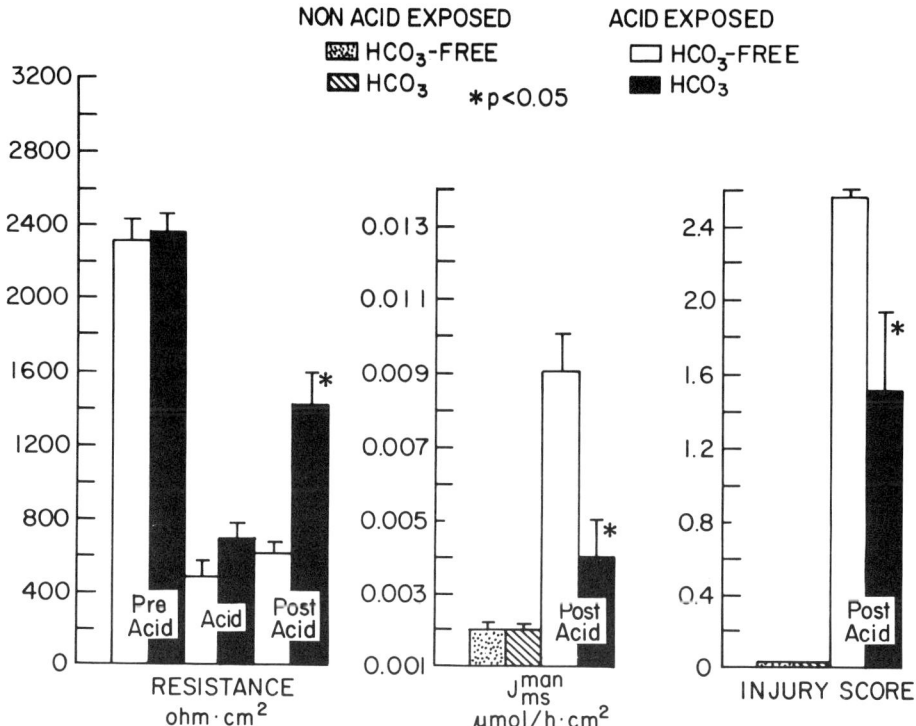

Fig. 3 documents that serosal (blood derived) HCO_3^- can protect esophageal epithelia from luminal acid. The electrical resistance, [^{14}C)mannitol flux (J_{ms}^{man}) and morphologic injury scores are shown for tissues bathed serosally by HCO_3^- or HCO_3^- free solution after exposure to 90 mM HCl (pH 1.1) for 1 h (n = 5–7). * p <0.05 for HCO_3^- vs HCO_3^--free tissues. Injury scoring was as follows: 0 = normal; 1 = intracellular or intercellular edema; 2 = patchy necrosis; 3 = diffuse necrosis; and 4 = transmucosal necrosis (ulceration). (Reprinted with permission from [1]).

HEPES, a large organic buffer impermeable to cells, was substituted for HCO_3^- in the serosal bath, protection almost equal to that of serosal HCO_3^- was provided in tissues exposed to luminal acid (Fig. 4). This observation provides evidence favoring an extracellular site and more specifically within the intercellular compartment, as the locus for protection by serosal (blood derived) HCO_3^- in the rabbit esophagus [1].

Intracellular buffering

An intracellular site for buffering by blood derived HCO_3^- is also present, because studies with primary cultures of rabbit esophageal epithelial cells have shown that HCO_3^- can be transported into the cell from the extracellular fluid by a Na^+-dependent Cl^-/HCO_3^- exchanger [4] (Fig. 2). This exchanger was identified along with two others for pH regulation in rabbit esophageal epithelial cells [4,17–19] (Fig. 5). A Na^+-independent Cl^-/HCO_3^- exchanger was shown to be an acid loader and the above mentioned Na^+-dependent Cl^-/HCO_3^- exchanger, along with a Na^+/H^+ exchanger, were shown to be acid extruders necessary for bringing pH back to neutrality, following

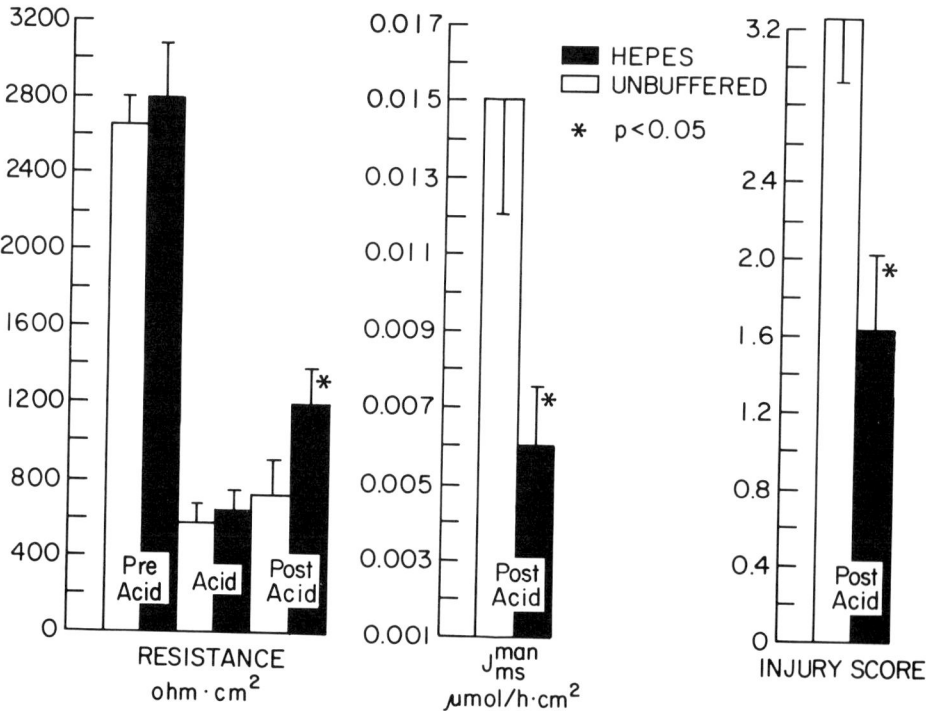

Fig. 4 documents that, serosal HEPES can protect esophageal epithelia from luminal acid. Electrical resistance, (^{14}C) mannitol flux (J_{ms}^{man}) and morphologic injury scores are shown for tissues bathed serosally by either 25 mM HEPES-Ringer's solution or HCO_3^--free Ringers' solution after exposure to 90 mM HCl (pH 1.1) for 1 h (n = 4–9). * p <0.05 for postacid values. Injury scoring was as follows: 0 = normal; 1 = intracellular or intercellular edema; 2 = a patchy necrosis; 3 = diffuse necrosis; and 4 = a transmucosal necrosis (ulceration). (Reprinted with permission from [1]).

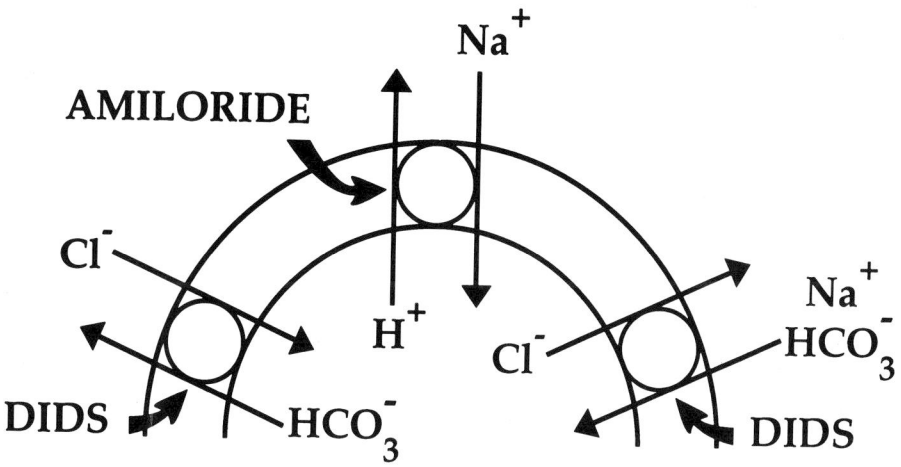

Fig. 5. Shows the three defined exchangers for pH regulation in rabbit esophageal epithelial cells. The Na^+/H^+ exchanger is inhibitable by amiloride and the Na^+-independent and Na^+-dependent Cl^-/HCO_3^- exchangers are inhibitable by the disulfonic acid stilbene, DIDS.

acidification by an ammonium chloride prepulse or acidification by entry of CO_2 following an exchange from a neutral HEPES solution to one containing HCO_3^- and CO_2. The Na^+-dependent Cl^-/HCO_3^- exchanger, as well as the Na^+/H^+ exchanger, is driven by the Na^+-gradient across the membrane and its ability to extrude acid from esophageal epithelial cells is dependent on extracellular HCO_3^- and can be blocked with the disulfonic acid stilbene, DIDS. Although the membrane location has only been established for one of the acid extruders (i.e., the Na^+/H^+ exchanger [20]), it is likely that both exist on the basolateral membrane.

Postepithelial defenses

Blood flow

An adequate flow of blood to the esophagus is important, in that it brings HCO_3^- to the interstitium where it is available through multiple pathways, as discussed above, for the buffering of intracellular and extracellular H^+. An increased blood flow would therefore be desirable to provide HCO_3^- for H^+ neutralization in the event of luminal exposure to H^+. Indeed, in studies where esophageal blood flow was measured in either an in vivo rabbit model of esophagitis with exposure to luminal pH 2 or in the perfused esophagus of the cat with exposure to luminal pH 1.5, brief exposure to acid (5 min) did induce a rapid increase in mucosal blood flow [21–23].

In summary, blood HCO_3^- is important in protecting and so contributing to the epithelial barrier to acid by its capacity for buffering H^+ either in the lumen, at the epithelial surface, within the intercellular space or within the cell. The ability to buffer within the lumen is in part dependent on submucosal gland secretion, while buffering in the intercellular space depends on HCO_3^- diffusion from blood and intracellular protection depends on the presence of basolateral membrane HCO_3^- transport via a mechanism such as the Na^+-dependent Cl^-/HCO_3^- exchanger [4].

References

1. Tobey NA, Powell DW, Schreiner VJ, Orlando RC. Serosal bicarbonate protects against acid injury to rabbit esophagus. Gastroenterology 1989;96:1466—1477.
2. Meyers RL, Orlando RC. In vivo bicarbonate secretion by human esophagus. Gastroenterology 1992;103:1174—1178.
3. Hamilton BH, Orlando RC. In vivo alkaline secretion by mammalian esophagus. Gastroenterology 1989;97:640—648.
4. Tobey NA, Reddy SP, Khalbuss WE, Silvers SM, Cragoe EJ Jr, Orlando RC. Na^+-dependent and -independent Cl^-/HCO_3^- exchangers in cultured rabbit esophageal epithelial cells. Gastroenterology 1993;104:185—195.
5. Boyd DD, Carney CN, Powell DW. Neurohumoral control of esophageal epithelial electrolyte transport. Am J Physiol 1980;239 (Gastrointest Liver Physiol 2):G5—11.
6. Krause WJ, Cutts JH, Leeson CR. The postnatal development of the alimentary canal in the opossum. J Anat 1976;122:293—314.
7. Christensen J, Williams TH, Jew J, O'Dorisio TM. Distribution of vasoactive intestinal polypeptide-immunoreactive structures in the opossum esophagus. Gastroenterology 1987;92:1007—1018.
8. Goetsch E. The structure of the mammalian oesophagus. Am J Anat 1910;10:1—40.
9. Dent J, Dodds WJ, Freedman RH, Sekiguchi T, Hogan WJ, Arndorfer RC, Petri DJ. Mechanisms of gastroesophageal reflux in recumbent asymptomatic human subjects. J Clin Invest 1980;65:256—267.
10. Helm JF, Dodds WJ, Pelc LR, Palmer DW, Hogan WJ, Teeter BS. Effect of esophageal emptying and saliva on clearance of acid from the esophagus. N Engl J Med 1984;310:284—288.
11. Helm JF, Dodds WJ, Hogan WJ, Soergel KH, Egide MS, Wood CM. Acid neutralizing capacity of human saliva. Gastroenterology 1982;83:69—74.
12. Young JA, Cook DI, van Lennep EW, Roberts M. Secretion by the major salivary glands. In: Johnson LR, Christensen J, Jacobson ED, Jackson MJ, Walsh JH (eds) Physiology of the Gastrointestinal Tract, 2nd edn. New York: Raven Press, 1987;773—815.
13. Quigley EMM, Turnberg LA. pH of the microclimate lining the human gastric and duodenal mucosa in vivo studies in control subjects and in duodenal ulcer patients. Gastroenterology 1987;92:1876—1884.
14. Orlando RC. Esophageal epithelial resistance. In: Castell DO, Wu WC, Ott DJ (eds) Gastroesophageal Reflux Disease: Pathogenesis, Diagnosis, Therapy. New York: Futura Publishing Co, Inc. 1985;55—79.
15. Orlando RC, Lacy ER, Tobey NA, Cowart K. Barriers to paracellular permeability in rabbit esophageal epithelium. Gastroenterology 1992;102:910—923.
16. Tobey NA, Orlando RC. Mechanisms of acid injury to rabbit esophageal epithelium: Role of basolateral membrane acidification. Gastroenterology 1991;101:1220—1228.
17. Tobey NA, Reddy SP, Keku TO, Cragoe EJ Jr, Orlando RC. Studies of pH_i in rabbit esophageal basal and squamous epithelial cells in culture. Gastroenterology 1992;103:830—839.
18. Layden TJ, Agnone LM, Schmidt LN, Hakim B, Goldstein JL. Rabbit esophageal cells possess an Na^+/H^+ antiport. Gastroenterology 1990;99:909—917.
19. Lisitza P, Schmidt LN, Goldstein JL, Layden TJ. Isolated rabbit esophageal basal cells possess HCO_3-dependent pH_i regulatory mechanisms. Gastroenterology 1992;102:A114 (abstract).
20. Khalbuss WE, Alkiek R, Marousis CG, Cragoe EJ Jr, Orlando RC. Localization of Na/H exchange to the basolateral membrane of rabbit esophageal epithelial cells. Gastroenterology 1993;104:A116 (abstract).
21. Bass BL, Schweitzer EJ, Harmon JW, Kramer J. H^+ back-diffusion interferes with intrinsic reactive regulation of esophageal blood flow. Surgery 1984;96:404—413.
22. Hollworth ME, Smith M, Kvietys PR, Granger DN. Esophageal blood flow in the cat; normal distribution and effects of acid perfusion. Gastroenterology 1986;90:622—627.
23. Bass BL, Trad KS, Harmon JW, Hakki FZ. Capsaicin-sensitive nerves mediate esophageal mucosal protection. Surgery 1991;110:419—425.

Is it possible to specify the factors of tissue repair during esophagitis?

C.W. Howden (Columbia)

The esophageal mucosa repairs itself principally through the mechanism of increased cell division rather than restitution [1] as occurs, for example, in the gastric mucosa. The increased cell division may be manifested by basal cell hyperplasia as often seen in esophageal mucosal biopsies in patients with gastroesophageal reflux disease (GERD). However, since epithelial cell turnover is rapid in the esophagus as it is in other parts of the alimentary tract, it is difficult to distinguish repair processes from normal maintenance. Acid contact stimulates cell turnover in the esophagus; presumably when the excess acid is removed pharmacologically this increased rate of cell tumor serves to repair any mucosal defects.

Acid exposure of the lower esophagus also stimulates mucosal blood flow. This, too, may ultimately be involved in the healing process by improving the supply of micronutrients to the esophagus and removing acid by-products.

There is no conclusive evidence that prostaglandins exert a useful protective role in the esophagus, although increased production of these compounds in inflamed tissue may play some role in the healing process.

Chronic inflammation implies that the inflammatory process and the healing process continue at the same time in the involved tissue. Therefore, some of the observations made on the esophageal mucosa during healing may reflect either inflammation or healing. This makes it difficult or impossible to "specify" those factors of tissue repair during esophagitis. Some findings may simply be interesting epiphenomena.

Avoidance of certain injurious agents such as cigarettes and alcohol may improve the environment for healing by permitting salivary and esophageal mucosal bicarbonate secretion to return towards normal.

Epidermal growth factor (EGF) levels in esophageal papillae and in capillary endothelium of the esophagus are decreased in GERD patients. Expression of EGF receptors (EGF-R) may be increased in GERD [2].

Serum zinc (Zn) levels have been reported to be slightly reduced in GERD patients, associated with an increased tissue Zn level in the distal esophagus. Treatment of GERD with H_2-receptor antagonists (H_2RA) is associated with a decrease of tissue Zn towards normal levels.

References

1. Livstone et al. Studies of esophageal proliferation in patients with reflux esophagitis. Gastroenterology 1977;73:1315–1319.
2. Jankowski J, Coghill G, Tregaskis B, Hopwood D, Wormsley KG. Epidermal growth factor in oesophagus. Gut 1992;33:1448–1453.

What factors are evidenced by study of the mucins of the esophageal glands during esophagitis?

S.E.A. Attwood (Dublin)

Gastroesophageal reflux disease (GERD) results from damage, due predominantly to acid and peptic damage, to the squamous epithelial lining of the esophagus. Gastroesophageal reflux (GER) is a normal phenomenon, but there are a number of factors which protect the lining of the esophagus from reflux injury.

First, is the barrier to reflux afforded by the lower esophageal sphincter (LES) mechanism. Second, is the luminal clearance mechanism which includes peristalsis for volume removal and salivary bicarbonate secretion. Despite these two mechanisms, the total time that the epithelium of the lower esophagus is exposed to gastric juice is considerable. Even in a normal individual the lower esophagus may be exposed to a pH below 4 for 5% of a 24 h period [1] — a situation which requires a third line of defense to avoid reflux injury. The third and most crucial protection is the esophageal epithelial resistance. This is most clearly seen in experimental studies of perfusion with acid and even continuous exposure over prolonged periods may result in little, if any, morphological injury [2].

The epithelial resistance to reflux injury include pre-epithelial, epithelial and postepithelial mechanisms [3]. The pre-epithelial defenses consist of mucus, the "unstirred water layer" and surrounding surface bicarbonate ions, which minimise or prevent the contact of H^+ ions with the surface. Contact is minimised also because the mucus layer of the esophagus, with its viscoelastic and gel like properties, is a barrier to the penetration of large molecules such as pepsin to the cell surface. The unstirred water layer acts as a sink for HCO_3^-, which creates an alkaline microenvironment adjacent to the cell surface which is capable of neutralizing H^+ as it diffuses towards the tissue.

Microelectrode work in the stomach shows that it is capable of supporting a gradient of pH 7 at the cell surface, to a luminal pH of 2.5. The unstirred water layer has been estimated in the esophagus to be about 0.03 mm thick. Whether this layer in the esophagus is as efficient as that in the stomach is unclear. Studies of the pH with microelectrodes have been performed by Quigley and Turnberg [4] in the esophagus, but their measurements demonstrated a normal luminal to cell surface pH gradient of pH 3.2–4.8, which is not consistent with the usual normal luminal pH of 6.0 in the lower esophagus [1].

The importance of mucus in protecting the esophageal squamous epithelium from peptic injury was first emphasized by Mounier-Kuhn [5], who showed loss of the mucus protective layer in patients with esophageal ulceration. Despite this early clinical observation there have been few studies of the esophageal mucus layer. Martin and Lambert extended these studies to include the mouth and esophagus and demonstrated similarities in the properties of gastric and esophageal mucus composition [6].

Al Yassin et al. have studied the fine structure of the human esophagus and described the structure of the esophageal submucosal glands in detail [7]. Four acinar cell types were identified — mucus cells, subsidiary secretory cells, myoepithelial cells and oncocytes. Within the mucus cells are pale secretion granules, sometimes foamy in nature. The ducts of the glands do not appear to contribute mucus secretion, nor large scale fluid or electrolyte transfer. Innervation is indirect as there are no nerve endings within or around the glands.

Although much has been written about the gastric mucosa and its defense against injury, little is known about this aspect of esophageal mucosa. The glands in the lower esophagus are relatively sparse. The mucus, when mixed with saliva, probably does play a role in protecting the mucosa, giving a protection similar to the unstirred water alkaline fluid layer on the surface of the gastric mucosa cell [8].

The function of sialomucins is to provide physical protection and to buffer H^+ but much less important than that of swallowed saliva or peristaltic clearance [9]. The alkaline secretion of the submucosal glands is a bicarbonate solution in the opossum although its importance in the human has not yet been established [10]. Preliminary results by Meyers and Orlando [11] have indicated that the human lower esophageal glands have the capacity to raise the residual volume of refluxate from a pH of 2.5 to 6.

The study of mucins to date, has concentrated on their differential production in patients with Barrett's esophagus. The Barrett's mucosa, being glandular in nature, produced large amounts of mucin easily stained by Alcian blue, mucimarine, high-iron diamine and borohydide-saponification-periodate. These stains differentiate sulfated from nonsulfated mucins and O-acetylated sialomucins [12,13]. Initially, sulfated mucins were thought to be related to dysplastic change [14,15], but this has not proven to be reliable [16,17]. More recently Lapertosa et al. associated O-acetylated sialomucins with early neoplastic de-differentiation in Barrett's esophagus [13]. Using scanning electron microscope techniques to study the type of mucin production from surface cells, Zwas et al. [18] showed a striking cellular heterogeneity of acid nonsulfated mucins and acid sulfated mucins.

The use of mucin stains may also increase the histological detection of Barrett's type intestinal metaplasia and in the study by Cooper et al. [19] only one of seven children, with a final diagnosis of columnar metaplasia, would have been detected without these stains. Duchatelle studied adults using immunohistochemical techniques (the antimucus antibodies: anti-M1; anti-M3; anti-SIMA; and anti-LIMA) to distinguish sulfomucins in patients with Barrett's esophagus and in reflux esophagitis without Barrett's the presence of anti-LIMA was positivity proposed as a step preceding type III IM in specialized epithelium and may be a precursor to neoplastic change [20].

References

1. DeMeester TR. Definition, detection and pathophysiology of gastroesophageal reflux disease. In: DeMeester TR, Matthews HR (eds) International Trends in General Thoracic Surgery, vol 3, Benign Esophageal Disease. St. Louis, Missouri:

C.V. Mosby, 1987;99–136.

2. Johnson LF, Harmon JW. Experimental esophagitis in a rabbit model. J Clin Gastroenterol 1986;8(suppl 1):26–44.

3. Orlando RC. Esophageal epithelial resistance. J Clin Gastroenterol 1986;8(suppl 1):12–16.

4. Quigley EMM, Turnberg LA. pH of the microclimate lining human gastric and duodenal mucosa in vivo. Studies in control subjects and in duodenal ulcer patients. Gastroenterology 1987;92:1876–1884.

5. Mounier-Kuhn P, Gaillard J, Lafon H, Morgon A, Haguenauer JP. Oesophagites et architecture muqueuse. J Fr Otor Audio Chir Max 1968;17:721–729.

6. Martin F, Lambert R. Role des cellules muqueuses et de leurs sécrétions dans les mecanismes de défense de la paroi gastrique. Acta Gastroenterol Belg 1966;29(3):289–314.

7. Al Yassin TM, Toner PG. Fine structure of squamous epithelium and submucosal glands of human oesophagus. J Anat 1977;123:705–721.

8. Jamieson GG, Duranceau AC. The defense mechanisms of the esophagus. Surg Clin North Am 1983;63:787–799.

9. Helm JF, Dodds WJ, Pelc LR, Palmer DW, Hogan WJ, Teeter BC. Effect of esophageal emptying and saliva on clearance of acid from the esophagus. N Engl J Med 1984;310:284–288.

10. Hamilton BH, Orlando RC. In vivo alkaline secretion by mammalian esophagus. Gastroenterology 1989;97:640–648.

11. Meyers RL, Orlando RC. Bicarbonate secretion by human esophagus. Gastroenterology 1992;102:A126.

12. Lee RG. Mucins in Barrett's esophagus: a histochemical study. Am J Clin Pathol 1984;81(4):500–503.

13. Lapertosa G, Baracchini P, Fulcheri E. Mucin histochemical analysis in the interpretation of Barrett's esophagus. Results of a multicenter study. The Operative Group for the Study of Esophageal Precancer. Am J Clin Pathol 1992;98(1):61–66.

14. Sheahan DG, West AB. Sulfated mucosubstances in Barrett's (columnar cell) esophageal mucosa. Gastroenterology 1981; 80:1282.

15. Peuchmaur M, Potet F, Goldfain D. Mucin histochemistry of the columnar epithelium of the oesophagus (Barrett's oesophagus): a prospective biopsy study. J Clin Pathol 1984;37(6):607–610.

16. Rothery GA, Patterson JE, Stoddard CJ, Day DW. Histological and histochemical changes in the columnar lined (Barrett's) oesophagus. Gut 1986;27(9):1062–1068.

17. Haggitt RC, Reid BJ, Rabinovitch PS, Rubin CE. Barrett's esophagus. Correlation between mucin histochemistry flow cytometry, and histologic diagnosis for predicting increased cancer risk. Am J Pathol 1988;131(1):53–61.

18. Zwas F, Shields HM, Doos WG, Antonioli DA, Goldman H, Ransil BJ, Spechler SJ. Scanning electron microscopy of Barrett's epithelium and its correlation with light microscopy and mucin stains. Gastroenterology 1986;90(6):1932–1941.

19. Cooper JE, Spitz L, Wilkins BM. Barrett's esophagus in children: a histologic and histochemical study of 11 cases. J Pediatr Surg 1987;22(3):191–196.

20. Duchatelle V, Potet F, Bara J, Ma J, Goldfain D. Mucin immunohistochemistry of the columnar epithelium of the oesophagus (Barrett's oesophagus). Virchows Arch Abt A Pathol Anat Histopathol 1989;414(4):359–363.

302

The first endoscopy is of proven prognostic value for the future. How should the endoscopic severity be graded?

G.N.J. Tytgat (Amsterdam)

An adequate answer to the above question and statement will require consideration of various aspects of gastroesophageal reflux disease (GERD).

Role of initial endoscopy in the assessment of the natural history of GERD

The natural history of erosive reflux esophagitis is unclear and rather controversial. Some investigators feel that the degree of reflux induced mucosal damage unrelentingly progresses in time, from initial mild erosions to ultimate ulceration and stenosis, in the majority of the patients [1,2]. Others feel that the initial grade of severity (erosion, ulceration or stricture) determines, at large, the overall long-term severity of the disease. The esophagitis may improve or heal with or without medical or surgical therapy, but will usually not progress to a more severe grade of severity in the majority of the patients [3]. In real life, both pathways are presumably the most likely outcome. In 701 medically treated patients followed in Lausanne, 23% steadily progressed to more severe forms of esophagitis. In contrast, 31% relapsed to similar or milder degrees of mucosal damage, whereas the remaining 46% had no further episodes of esophagitis after the index episode had been healed [4]. It is unclear at present which factors do influence the natural history of reflux esophagitis and the progressive or nonprogressive character of the disease.

The percentage of patients who develop complications, of ulceration or stricture after prior diagnosis of mild, moderate or severe erosive esophagitis, is small and amounts to 11–17% in the Lausanne study [4]. The majority of the patients with complications of ulceration or stricturing present "de novo", because usually no prior endoscopy has been performed despite the presence of occasionally long-standing typical symptoms.

Endoscopy as a predictor of treatment outcome

The presence and severity of esophagitis is the single best predictor of the lowest level of acid suppression which is needed for therapeutic success. There is a significant gradation of percentage esophageal acid exposure from GERD patients without esophageal mucosal damage to patients with severe confluent ulcerative esophagitis [5]. Therapeutic success is closely linked to correction of the esophageal acid exposure values, to within the normal range [6,7]. Many studies have shown that the endoscopic grade of severity is of decisive importance in predicting healing rates with antisecretory therapy, both with H_2 receptor antagonists and proton pump inhibitors. The more severe the esophagitis, the greater and more prolonged is the acid suppressive effect needed to correct pathological esophageal acid exposure [8].

In healing therapy, severity of pretreatment esophagitis has been the most important determinant of success, regardless of the pharmaceutical principle used [9,10]. The more severe the esophagitis, the lower the healing rate.

The endoscopic appearances in reflux disease also give guidance on the appropriate timing of acid suppression through the 24-h period. The contribution of nocturnal reflux to esophageal acid exposure is of minor importance in patients with mild erosive esophagitis or in the absence of mucosal damage [8,11,12]. In contrast, there is considerable nocturnal acid exposure in patients with severe erosive esophagitis or in patients with stricturing and columnar metaplasia [8]. Thus, the endoscopic grading gives an indication of the period of the 24-h cycle, during which acid suppression needs to be most effective.

Role of endoscopy in predicting future relapse

Studies on the natural history of GERD and reflux esophagitis are rare [4,13].

In general, the prevalence of reflux esophagitis ranges from 0.5–23% in the literature of patients referred for endoscopic examination [4]. The prevalence of GERD seems to be increasing [14,4]. There is a clear clinical impression that, in the majority of the patients with GERD, there is a chronically recurrent problem which is especially relentless in patients with more severe esophagitis [15].

The index endoscopy is important as an indicator of the degree of severity of mucosal damage, in case of future relapse. Moreover, the presence and severity of endoscopic reflux esophagitis influences the relapse patterns, as patients who have more severe esophagitis appear to relapse earlier and in greater proportion after withdrawal of medical therapy [16,17], compared to patients with milder disease.

In patients with endoscopy negative reflux disease or only mild erosive esophagitis, it is usual for symptoms and macroscopic esophagitis to persist over periods of several years; although in a minority, symptoms and esophagitis may become intermittent [18]. In more severe esophagitis, there is substantial evidence of the unremitting nature of the reflux disease as spontaneous symptomatic and endoscopic remission is rare [9]. Moreover, medical therapy with limited/moderate acid suppression does not appear to prevent the formation of columnar metaplasia or dysplasia/cancer. Brossard et al. [19], in following 582 patients with recalcitrant esophagitis, noted that 93 of them went on to develop columnar metaplasia. McCallum et al. [20] have reported that almost 20% of patients with columnar metaplasia, initially free of dysplasia, developed dysplasia while on medical therapy and 1.3% developed malignancy.

Grading of reflux esophagitis

How reflux esophagitis should be graded is highly controversial. Over 100 grading systems have been presented in the literature [21]. The main problems encountered in evaluating the various grading schemes are summarized in Table 1.

To reconcile the various systems in a way which is useful to carry out clinical

Table 1. Problems in endoscopic grading of esophagitis

---

* Very problematic is the large number of grading systems expressing lack of agreement on diagnostic criteria (>100 systems published).
* The main difference between the various grading systems is in the definition of grade I disease:
  − American systems accept erythema, color unevenness, fuzzy SCMJ and friability as grade I.
  − European systems require the presence of erosions for grade I disease.
  Inclusion of equivocal abnormalities increases the sensitivity, but markedly compromises the specificity.
* The term "confluence" is poorly defined. Distinction between nonconfluent and confluent erosions is vague.
* Defining circumferential erosion/ulceration is often difficult (does 95% involvement correspond to Savary grade II or III?)
* Diagnosing "circumferential" requires detailed inspection of the total circumference at the SCMJ, which is often difficult due to angulation at the cardia.
* Spots or patches of columnar mucosa may mimic erosions; such columnar islands may become apparent as inflammatory changes resolve.
* The widely accepted Savary-Miller system is often misinterpreted. Lumping all complications in Savary grade IV is a major drawback.
* Endoscopic abnormalities are regularly seen which do not readily fit within the prevailing grading schemes.
* The indistinct boundaries between the grades of esophagitis make the categorical rating more or less arbitrary; reflux mediated damage occurs as a continuous biologic phenomenon.

Table 2. Grading of reflux esophagitis

Grade 0.	No evidence of reflux-induced damage — crisp, sharply delineated SCMJ. No evidence of friability — smooth and shiny squamous mucosa in the distal esophagus.
Grade I.	Mild, patchy or more diffuse erythema at the level of the SCMJ; slight blurring of the SCMJ; minor friability; loss of shininess of the distal squamous mucosa. Such abnormalities are equivocal and cannot be interpreted as genuinely characteristic for reflux induced damage. There is no apparent break in the mucosa.
Grade II.	One or more discrete superficial erosions, seen as red dots or streaks, with or without adherent whitish exudate. Such linear erosions are usually small and often on top of the esophageal folds. They involve less than 10% of the mucosal surface of less than the distal 5 cm of the squamous segment of the esophagus above the gastroesophageal junction.
Grade III.	Confluent but noncircumferential erosions seen as defects that merge either longitudinally or laterally. There may be an additional exudate covering the erosive defects or slough formation. Less than 50% of the overall mucosal surface of the distal 5 cm is involved.
Grade IV.	Circumferential erosions or exudative lesions at the level of the SCMJ, regardless of the extent along the distal esophagus.
Grade V.	Deep ulceration anywhere along the esophagus.
Grade VI.	Various degrees of stricturing, prohibiting passage of a standard (>9 mm) or small caliber (<9 mm) endoscope.

Note: Grades I—VI can be present with/without a segment of columnar metaplasia.

trials and which is simple enough in routine clinical practice, the grading system proposed in Table 2 is presented. In essence, it retains the option of equivocal changes which may occasionally be the end-stage after healing of erosive esophagitis. The grading of erosive damage is rather straightforward and subdivided as mild, moderate and severe. The complications of ulceration and stricture have a separate grading number. All those abnormalities of the squamous mucosa can be diagnosed in the presence or in the absence of a segment of columnar metaplasia. In Table 3, a comparison is given of the currently most prevailing grading systems, the Savary-Miller system [21], the Hetzel grading system [22] used in many trials with proton pump inhibitors and the grading system presented in Table 2.

Concluding remarks

The only way to solve the highly confusing area of grading reflux esophagitis is to create a working party of experts experienced in the field, who should come up with a generally acceptable grading system. This is not a matter of semantics alone. Grading the degree of damage is of importance in selecting the appropriate therapy, estimating the degree of risk and predicting the future outcome. Indeed, the severity of reflux esophagitis is important as an indicator of responsiveness to therapy. Moreover, endoscopic severity is the best and the most practical indicator of disease severity and therefore the best guide to long-term management. Objective grading of the endoscopic appearances is therefore of immense importance.

Although GERD is basically a motor disorder, the symptoms and the degree of esophageal mucosa damage are primarily determined by the duration of esophageal

Table 3. Comparison of commonly used grading schemes

	Savary	Hetzel	Tytgat
Normal	grade 0	grade 0	grade 0
Equivocal changes		grade I	grade I
Mild: nonconfluent erosions; <10%	grade I	grade II	grade II
Moderate: confluent erosions; 10–50%	grade II	grade III	grade III
Severe: circumferent erosions; >50%	grade III	grade IV	grade IV
Ulceration			grade V
Stricture			grade VI

mucosal exposure to gastric acid and pepsin. It is now evident that the more severe the esophageal acid exposure and the more severe the esophagitis, the greater the level of acid suppression required for normalization of esophageal acid exposure values and for healing of esophagitis, if the motor abnormality cannot be corrected. The alternative approach is to attempt to improve the disordered motor pattern thereby decreasing the esophageal acid exposure.

References

1. Palmer ED. The hiatus hernia-oesophagitis-esophageal stricture complex. Am J Med 1968;44:566–579.
2. Savary M, Ollyo JB. L'oesophagite par reflux et ses complications: ulcère, sténose, endobrachy-oesophage. Encycl Med Chir (Paris, France) ORL 1986;20822A10:16.
3. Dedieu P, Gaillard F, Lavignolle A et al. Oesophagites par reflux: aspects épidémiologiques, anatomo-pathologiques et évolutifs (123 cas). Gastroenterol Clin Biol 1981;5:266–274.
4. Ollyo JB, Monnier Ph, Fontolliet C, Savary M. The natural history, prevalence and incidence of reflux oesophagitis. Gullet 1993;3:3–10.
5. Masclee AA, de Best AC, de Graaf R, Cluysenaer OJ, Jansen JBMJ. Ambulatory 24-h pH metry in the diagnosis of GERD. Scand J Gastroenterol 1990;25:225–230.
6. Bate CM, Keeling PWN, O'Morain C et al. Comparison of omeprazole and cimetidine in reflux esophagitis. Gut 1990;31: 968–972.
7. Klinkenberg-Knol EC, Meuwissen SGM. Combined gastric and esophageal 24-h pH monitoring. Aliment Pharmacol Ther 1990;4:485–495.
8. Robertson D, Aldersley M, Shepherd H, Smith CL. Patterns of acid reflux in complicated esophagitis. Gut 1987;28:1484–1488.
9. Bell NJV, Hunt RH. Role of gastric acid suppression in the treatment of gastro-oesophageal reflux disease. Gut 1992;33: 118–124.
10. Tytgat GNJ, Nicolai JJ, Reman FC. Efficacy of different doses of cimetidine in the treatment of reflux esophagitis. A review of three large, double-blind, controlled trials. Gastroenterology 1990;99:629–634.
11. Gudmundsson K, Johnsson F, Joelsson B. The time pattern of GER. Scand J Gastroenterol 1988;23:75–79.
12. DeCaestecker JS, Blackwell JN, Pryde A, Heading RC. Daytime GER is important in esophagitis. Gut 1987;28:519–526.
13. Bianchi Porro G, Santalucia F, Pace F. Natural history of gastro-oesophageal reflux (GOR) disease. Gut 1991;32:845–848.
14. Wienbeck M, Barnert J. Epidemiology of reflux disease and reflux esophagitis. Scand J Gastroenterol 1989;24(suppl 156): 7–13.
15. Spechler SJ. Epidemiology and natural history of gastro-oesophageal reflux disease. Digestion 1992;51(suppl 1):24–29.
16. Koelz HR, Birchler R, Bretholz A et al. Healing and relapse of reflux esophagitis during treatment with ranitidine. Gastroenterology 1986;91:1198–1205.
17. Tytgat GNJ, Anker Hansen OJ, Carling L, De Groot GH, Geldof H, Glise H, Efskind P, Elsborg L, Karvonen AL, Ohlin B, Solhaug OH, Vermeersch B & other Scanedcis trialists. Effect of cisapride on relapse of reflux esophagitis, healed with an antisecretory drug. Scand J Gastroenterol 1992;27:175–183.
18. Pace F, Santalucia F, Bianchi Porro G. Natural history of gastro-oesophageal reflux disease without oesophagitis. Gut 1991;32:845–848.
19. Brossard E, Ollyo JB, Monnier Ph, Fontolliet C, Krayenbuhl M, Savary M. Columnar type epithelium (Barrett's esophagus) develops after healing in 18% of adults with erosive or ulcerative reflux esophagitis. Gastroenterology 1991;100:A36.

20. McCallum RW, Polepalle S, Davenport IS, Boyd S. Role of antireflux surgery against dysplasia in Barrett's esophagus. Gastroenterology 1991;100:A121.
21. Armstrong D, Monnier Ph, Nicolet M, Blum AL, Savary M. Endoscopic assessment of oesophagitis. Gullet 1991;1:63−67.
22. Hetzel DT, Dent J, Reed WD et al. Healing and relapse of severe peptic esophagitis after treatment with omeprazole. Gastroenterology 1988;95:903−912.

Is the gastric mucosa normal in patients with GERD?

J.I. Wyatt, M.F. Dixon (Leeds)

Gastroesophageal reflux disease (GERD) is generally attributed to acid injury to the squamous esophagus, although the role of reflux of alkaline duodenal contents, particularly in the production of Barrett's esophagus, is gaining wider acceptance. In considering the state of the gastric mucosa in patients with GERD, it has to be borne in mind that in most populations at risk there will be a high prevalence of *Helicobacter pylori*-associated chronic gastritis. Thus, one cannot expect the mucosa to be normal in the majority of patients with GERD, and a more pertinent question would be: "Is the pattern of gastritis found in patients with GERD different to that found in a control population?"

One could anticipate two variations to the pattern of gastritis in GERD patients. Firstly, the motility disturbance affecting gastroesophageal competence could also affect antropyloric function and give rise to duodenogastric reflux. Such individuals may exhibit reflux gastritis to a greater degree than control subjects without GERD. Secondly, given that GERD might be more frequently seen in association with increased gastric acid output, it could be anticipated that GERD patients will have the pattern of *H. pylori*-associated gastritis related to hyperacidity − namely an antral-predominant pattern − more frequently than control patients. The data available on both these aspects are strictly limited.

GERD and reflux gastritis

The concept of a distinctive form of gastritis related to reflux of bile and pancreatico-duodenal juice into the stomach is not a new one, but had been poorly documented prior to our 1986 publication [1]. Although originally based on reflux in the postoperative stomach, we have since established that "spontaneous" reflux of bile and the presence of a reflux gastritis can occur in the intact stomach [2]. While "pure" acid reflux could be entirely attributed to gastroesophageal malfunction, alkaline reflux into the esophagus must reflect passage through the stomach which provides an opportunity for damage to the gastric mucosa. Although the existence of pyloric incompetence in patients with GERD [3], the presence of alkaline gastro-esophageal reflux [4] and coexistence of alkaline reflux gastritis and esophagitis [5] have been known for several years, few studies have examined gastric biopsies and none has applied modern diagnostic criteria in the histological interpretation. Thus, Gowen [6] investigated the relationship between spontaneous enterogastric reflux gastritis and esophagitis and found that all 42 patients with intragastric bile reflux and GERD exhibited "chronic gastritis". However, of these 42 subjects, only 11 showed chronic atrophic gastritis and six had chronic active gastritis; the nature of the gastritis in the other 25 patients is not stated.

When we graded esophageal biopsies for the severity of esophagitis in 24 patients whose gastric biopsies revealed the histological changes of reflux gastritis, and compared them with those from 31 subjects whose gastric biopsies were normal, we found no significant difference in histological "esophagitis scores" [Wyatt and Dixon, unpublished observations]. However, the histological picture of reflux gastritis can result from factors other than exposure to bile. We have found identical appearances in patients on long-term aspirin and NSAID treatment and in some individuals who abuse alcohol [2]. Therefore, our findings cannot be used to deny a link between esophagitis in the squamous mucosa and alkaline reflux gastritis.

Thus, while there are theoretical grounds for the coexistence of reflux gastritis and esophagitis, this has not been adequately validated. Given that alkaline reflux is considered to be a more important factor in the pathogenesis of Barrett's esophagus, an association is more likely to emerge if reflux gastritis was sought in these patients.

GERD and *H. pylori*-associated gastritis

It is now clearly established that *H. pylori* infection and the resultant chronic gastritis leads to sustained hypergastrinemia and increased acid output [7]. It could be anticipated, therefore, that patients with symptomatic esophagitis will have a higher prevalence of *H. pylori*-associated gastritis than age-matched controls without esophagitis. However, what little evidence we have is contradictory. In children, Rosioru et al. found the prevalence of biopsy-proven esophagitis to be similar in *H. pylori* positive and negative groups [8].

Koop et al. [9] found a low prevalence of *H. pylori*-associated antral gastritis (24%) in patients with reflux esophagitis refractory to H_2-blockers. A study on gastric acid secretion in GERD patients with and without concomitant duodenal ulcer [10] confirmed that those with coexistent DU had significantly higher gastric acid output than those with esophagitis alone, but did not demonstrate any greater severity of the esophagitis in the former group. While the great majority (if not all) of the DU patients in this study would have been *H. pylori* positive, those with esophagitis alone may or may not have been infected. A higher proportion of *H. pylori* negative patients in the latter group could explain why lower acid production was present, but this does not affect the authors' overall conclusion that acid output is not a major pathogenetic factor in GERD.

Some circumstantial evidence in favour of a relationship between *H. pylori* infection and GERD comes from histological studies. When esophageal biopsies from patients with antral predominant *H. pylori* gastritis (the pattern most closely related to increased acid production) were compared to biopsies from patients with a diffuse *H. pylori* positive pangastritis (a pattern in which normal or subnormal acid secretion occurs), the former group exhibited a higher mean esophagitis score (2.9 vs. 1.53; p < 0.01). However, it should be re-emphasized that histological esophagitis is poorly validated against objective measures of acid reflux such as 24-h pH monitoring, and no acid secretory data was available in this study.

A relationship between *H. pylori*-associated gastritis and GERD could only be properly investigated by studying the effects of eradication treatment on symptoms and acid reflux tests in *H. pylori* positive patients with GERD. Their outcome would be compared with non-eradicated controls. The results of such studies are awaited with interest.

References

1. Dixon MF, O'Connor HJ, Axon ATR, King RFJG, Johnston D. Reflux gastritis: distinct histopathological entity? J Clin Pathol 1986;39:524–530.
2. Sobala GM, King RFJG, Axon ATR, Dixon MF. Reflux gastritis in the intact stomach. J Clin Pathol 1990;43:303–306.
3. Kaye MD, Showalter JP. Pyloric incompetence in patients with symptomatic gastroesophageal reflux. J Lab Clin Med 1974; 83:198–206.
4. Pellegrini CA, DeMeester TR, Wernly JA, Johnson LF, Skinner DB. Alkaline gastroesophageal reflux. Am J Surg 1978;135: 177–184.
5. Little AG, Martinez EI, DeMeester TR, Blough RM, Skinner DB. Duodenogastric reflux and reflux esophagitis. Surgery 1984;96:447–453.
6. Gowen GF. Spontaneous enterogastric reflux gastritis and esophagitis. Ann Surg 1985;170–175.
7. El-Omar E, Penman I, Dorrian CA, Ardill JES, McColl KEL. Eradicating *Helicobacter pylori* infection lowers gastrin-mediated acid secretion by two-thirds in duodenal ulcer patients. Gut 1993;34:1060–1065.
8. Rosioru C, Glassman MS, Halata MS, Schwarz SM. Esophagitis and *Helicobacter pylori* in children: incidence and therapeutic implications. Am J Gastroenterol 1993;88:510–513.
9. Koop H, Stumpf M, Eissele R, Lamberts R, Stöckmann F, Creutzfeldt W, Arnold R. Antral *Helicobacter pylori*-like organisms in different states of gastric acid secretion. Digestion 1991;48:230–236.
10. Zhu H, Pace F, Sangaletti O, Bianchi Porro G. Gastric acid secretion and pattern of gastroesophageal reflux in patients with esophagitis and concomitant duodenal ulcer. Scand J Gastroenterol 1993;28:387–392.

Are control endoscopies necessary in stage II erosive esophagitis?

H.W. Boyce Jr (Tampa)

The question as posed does not indicate the system in question relative to grade II. The response to the question will be based as closely as possible on grade II of the

Savary-Miller system [1]. Grade II is defined as multiple erosive lesions, noncircumferential, affecting more than one longitudinal fold, with or without confluence [1].

Documented healing is defined as complete re-epithelialization of all mucosal defects determined by endoscopy with or without symptoms of gastroesophageal reflux disease (GERD). When complete resolution of all epithelial defects is evaluated as a criterion in research, healing is found to occur in a surprisingly low percentage of patients treated with standard dose H_2-blocker therapy. Johansson et al. evaluated a group of patients unresponsive to phase 1 GERD therapy in a double blind cross-over study comparing ranitidine and placebo [2]. None of the patients with Savary-Miller grade II or III esophagitis had complete healing of esophagitis by endoscopy. Many other studies have confirmed the overall poor healing rates for standard dose up to quadruple dose H_2-blocker therapy. At least 25% of patients with grade II and III disease were unhealed at 8 weeks on ranitidine 300 mg 4 times daily [3].

In one study, improvement occurred in 88% treated with ranitidine 150 mg twice daily, but complete healing occurred in only 18%, none of whom had severe esophagitis at the beginning of the study [4].

When studies that evaluated healing by H_2-blocker therapy are reviewed, one is impressed to find that complete healing occurs in only 27 to 45% of patients with primarily grade I or II disease [5]. Omeprazole was found to have an overall healing rate of 67–92%, again mainly for grades I and II. However, this ATPase inhibitor gave complete healing in 48 to 62% of patients with grade IV disease. Some patients obviously will require double or triple dose omeprazole for complete healing.

One has to be impressed with the recent findings of relatively poor overall healing rates for standard dose H_2-blocker therapy that originally was thought to be the therapeutic solution for patients with erosive esophagitis. Studies to date also have shown that whether higher dose H_2-blockers or standard dose ATPase inhibitors are used, there will be a number of patients who never completely heal erosive esophagitis of grade II or higher. Since the basic pathophysiology of GERD is not changed by acid suppression, the likelihood of recurrence of erosive esophagitis after complete healing will be great when the healing dose of H_2-blocker or ATPase inhibitor is either stopped or reduced. Relapse of erosive esophagitis commonly occurs after stopping treatment. Only about 20% of patients remain in relapse at 6 months with about 50% suffering relapse in less than 8 weeks [5]. Long-term maintenance of healing is improved when either a double dose, higher H_2-blocker therapy or an ATPase inhibitor is used [6].

Armed with this knowledge of the unimpressive healing and low remission maintenance rates for GERD treated by standard dose H_2-blocker therapy, it appears obvious that control endoscopies will be necessary to assure both initial healing and maintenance of healing of esophagitis of grade II and higher. Only a therapeutic program with doses of H_2-blockers and/or ATPase inhibitors that produce complete healing in at least 90% of patients will eliminate the need for control or surveillance endoscopies in patients with grade II esophagitis. Either omeprazole or another ATPase inhibitor will be capable of providing such results. Healing rates of 90–100% with omeprazole in grade I and II esophagitis at 4 weeks, compared to 53–55% with ranitidine clearly indicate the choice of drug therapy needed to reliably assure healing of these grades, so that follow-up or control endoscopy is not needed [6].

The clinical history and pretherapy endoscopic grade of severe esophagitis provide no help in predicting which patients are more prone to relapse during maintenance therapy even with omeprazole [7]. The same situation probably exists in the majority of patients worldwide with grade II esophagitis who are being treated with the less potent acid suppression provided by standard dose H_2-blocker agents.

Another factor that would be important in decisions regarding control endoscopies for grade II esophagitis would be knowledge of the natural history of this stage. Erosive esophagitis has all of the features of a chronic process that recurs in most patients when effective drug treatment is discontinued [8].

Pertinent and yet unanswered questions include:
— What is the natural history of untreated grade II esophagitis?
— Does grade II always progress to grade III?
— Does grade II esophagitis lead to complications of grade IV disease, i.e., ulcer, stricture, columnar-lined esophagus?

Answers to all of these questions could greatly simplify any decision regarding the need for control endoscopies for grade II esophagitis.

The relationship of symptoms to the endoscopic grade of reflux esophagitis is not predictable. It is a well-known fact that grade II, and less often, grade III esophagitis may be associated with very mild or even absent symptoms. Conversely, severe pyrosis may be present in the absence of epithelial injury on endoscopic examination. There is unquestionably a relationship between symptoms and reflux, especially when erosive esophagitis is present [9]. Surprisingly, as many as 85% of acid reflux episodes, as measured by an esophageal pH probe, may not produce symptoms, regardless of the severity of mucosal injury.

The answer then for today is: control endoscopy is necessary to assure healing and remission for grade II erosive esophagitis in all patients not treated by an ATPase inhibitor with maximum suppression of gastric acid secretion.

References

1. Savary M, Miller G. L'oesophage. Manuel et Atlas d'Endoscopie. Solothurn: Verlag Gassmann, 1977.
2. Johansson KE, Boeryd B, Tibbling L. Double blind crossover study of ranitidine and placebo in gastroesophageal reflux disease. Scand J Gastroenterol 1986;21:769—778.
3. Johnson NJ, Mills JG, Wood JR. Acute treatment of reflux esophagitis: a multicenter trial comparing ranitidine 150 mg b.i.d. with ranitidine 300 mg q.i.d. Gastroenterology 1989;96:A242.
4. Goy JA, Maynard JH, McNauton WM, O'Shea A. Ranitidine and placebo in the treatment of reflux esophagitis. Med J Aust 1983;2:558—561.
5. Bell NJV, Hunt RH. Role of gastric acid suppression in the treatment of gastroesophageal reflux disease. Gut 1992;33:118—124.
6. Hetzel DJ, Dent J, Reed WD et al. Healing and relapse of severe peptic esophagitis after treatment with omeprazole. Gastroenterology 1988;95:903—912.
7. Klinkenberg-Knol EC, Meuwissen SGM. Medical therapy of patients with reflux oesophagitis poorly responsive to H_2-receptor antagonist therapy. Digestion 1992;51:44—48.
8. Spechler SJ. Epidemiology and natural history of gastroesophageal reflux disease. Digestion 1992;51(suppl 1):24—29.
9. Baldi F, Ferrarini F, Longanesi A, et al. Acid gastroesophageal reflux and symptom occurrence. Dig Dis Sci 1989;34:1890—1893.

The "MUSE" system

D. Armstrong (Hamilton)
Ph. Monnier, M. Nicolet, A.L. Blum, M. Savary (Lausanne)

The reflux of gastric contents into the esophagus can produce mucosal lesions ranging from esophagitis, which may be evident only on histological examination of biopsies, through erosive esophagitis, ulceration and stricture formation to the development of columnar metaplasia (Barrett's esophagus, endobrachyesophagus). The histological features of esophagitis are still the subject of debate as are the endoscopic features of "early" esophagitis [1], but there is general agreement that mucosal erosions [2,3] constitute unequivocal evidence of esophageal mucosal damage. There is also good evidence that multiple or more extensive erosions are a manifestation of more severe erosive esophagitis and that disease severity is, to a large extent, predictive of the likely response to treatment [4–7]. This evidence is based on semiquantitative assessments of disease severity used to grade esophagitis in the conduct of therapeutic trials. In principle, the use of such grading systems should assist practising physicians in their efforts to tailor treatment regimens to the needs of individual patients and to predict the likelihood that treatment will be successful. Unfortunately, there is now a plethora of grading systems, many attributed to Savary and Miller despite the incorporation of modifications, some more subtle than others, which render them incompatible with the original proposal [3].

The original grading system proposed by Savary and Miller is based on the isolated epithelial erosion or *touche peptique* [2] as the fundamental lesion in grade I reflux esophagitis. Grades II and III are indicative of more extensive, more severe disease whilst grade IV esophagitis includes all complications whether or not they are accompanied by acute erosions (Table 1). Since its initial formulation, however, grade IV has been taken, by some, to indicate only columnar metaplasia with (grade IVb) or without (grade IVa) acute erosive and/or ulcerative changes. On the other hand, a recently-proposed grading system [8], based on the Savary-Miller system, includes discrete erythematous lesions, without further qualification, as a feature of grade I esophagitis. Circumscribed erythematous spots or streaks on mucosal folds are,

Table 1. The Savary-Miller grading system for reflux esophagitis and its complications

Grade I	Single or isolated erosive lesion(s), oval or linear, but affecting only one longitudinal fold
Grade II	Multiple erosive lesions, noncircumferential, affecting more than one longitudinal fold, with or without confluence
Grade III	Circumferential erosive lesions
Grade IV	Complications: columnar epithelium, ulcer(s), stricture(s) and/or short esophagus. Alone or associated with lesions of grades I–III

indeed, very suggestive of erosions and close inspection, using an endoscope with good optics, may reveal a thin, pale film indicative of true erosions. However, erythematous areas may be difficult to distinguish from a nonspecific, age-related finding of diffuse esophageal erythema [9,10]. Such erythema may be transient or noninflammatory [11] and its presence does not predict either the healing rate in response to treatment or the relapse rate after healing [unpublished data]. It is important, therefore, to define precisely those lesions which are pathognomonic of esophagitis, those which are "soft" signs, and those which are irrelevant (Table 2).

The definition of grade IV in the original Savary-Miller classification has also made it difficult to describe accurately the progress of the esophagitis or its response to treatment, since grade IV esophagitis encompasses lesions which can develop and regress independently of each other. Thus, complete healing of active inflammatory lesions may lead to different apparent outcomes depending on the presence of complications: grade III with erosions alone and grade IV with erosions complicated by an ulcer would both become grade 0, whereas grade IV with erosions complicated by a scarred stricture would remain grade IV.

To address the problems which have arisen with current grading systems, a new classification system was developed with the preconditions that it should:
1. differentiate between premalignant lesions (columnar metaplasia), active lesions which might be expected to respond readily to therapy (erosions, ulcers and inflammatory strictures) and active lesions which would be unlikely to respond to medical therapy (scarred strictures);
2. allow the classification of multiple grades of erosive esophagitis and its sequelae as a basis for clinical practice and for clinical trials covering all aspects of esophagitis;
3. employ standard assessment criteria and a standard nomenclature in the interest of an objective and reproducible description of esophagitis severity; and
4. incorporate accepted wisdom, based on the concept of increasingly severe erosive esophagitis in Savary-Miller grades I–III (Table 1) or Hetzel's grades II–IV (Table 3).

Table 2. Endoscopic features of the esophageal mucosa which have been used as signs of esophagitis

Diagnostic criteria for esophagitis		
"Hard"	"Soft"	Irrelevant
Erosions with fibrin deposit	Circumscribed erythema without white film	Generalized diffuse erythema
Junctional ulceration (Wolf or Savary)	Pseudopapilloma at the Z-line	Visible vessels near the cardia
	Cobblestone appearance	Loss of normal vascular pattern
	Mucosal friability	Mucosal edema

Table 3. The Hetzel grading system for reflux esophagitis

Grade 0	No mucosal abnormalities
Grade I	No macroscopic erosions but erythema, hyperaemia or mucosal friability
Grade II	Superficial erosions, involving <10% of the mucosal surface of the last 5 cm of esophageal squamous mucosa
Grade III	Superficial erosions or ulceration involving 10–50% of the mucosal surface of the last 5 cm of esophageal squamous mucosa
Grade IV	Deep peptic ulceration anywhere in the esophagus or confluent erosion of >50% of the mucosal surface of the last 5 cm of esophageal squamous mucosa

Basis for development of the "MUSE" classification system

A detailed, standardized description of the esophagus and all lesions, required in both clinical practice and in clinical research, is best achieved using a formal report form with an accurate diagrammatic representation of all lesions [12] and, in particular, a precise indication of their extent and position in relation to the diaphragmatic hiatus rather than to the teeth (Fig. 1). This approach is particularly important for studies of the long-term progression of columnar metaplasia and dysplasia which necessitate accurate mapping and repeated biopsies. In general, however, the findings of a study must be classified so that only a small number of variables are analyzed and the predefined aims of the study can be tested without loss of statistical power. Thus, for shorter-term studies and multicenter trials with many investigators, reporting is facilitated by pictorial representation of possible lesions (Fig. 2). In general, the findings must then be classified so that only a small number of variables are analyzed statistically: this allows the predefined aims of the study to be tested without loss of statistical power.

Studies of the treatment and progression of esophagitis commonly look at four variables: columnar metaplasia (M), ulceration (U), stricture formation (S) and erosions (E). These variables are related to each other developmentally, the erosion being the primary lesion of reflux esophagitis. However, the variables are also independent in the sense that the presence of one lesion type does not indicate perforce the presence of any other lesion type. For the purposes of a clinical trial protocol, for example it would be essential that these variables be graded independently to permit assessment of the differing responses of each lesion type to therapy. The "MUSE" classification system proposed recently was designed to facilitate the identification and grading of these four independent variables [1]; the initial letter of each lesion type provides the acronym M.U.S.E., upon which to muse when describing the esophagus. In this context, the acronym is simply an *aide memoire*; it does not imply that the lesions of erosive esophagitis will develop in any particular chronological order.

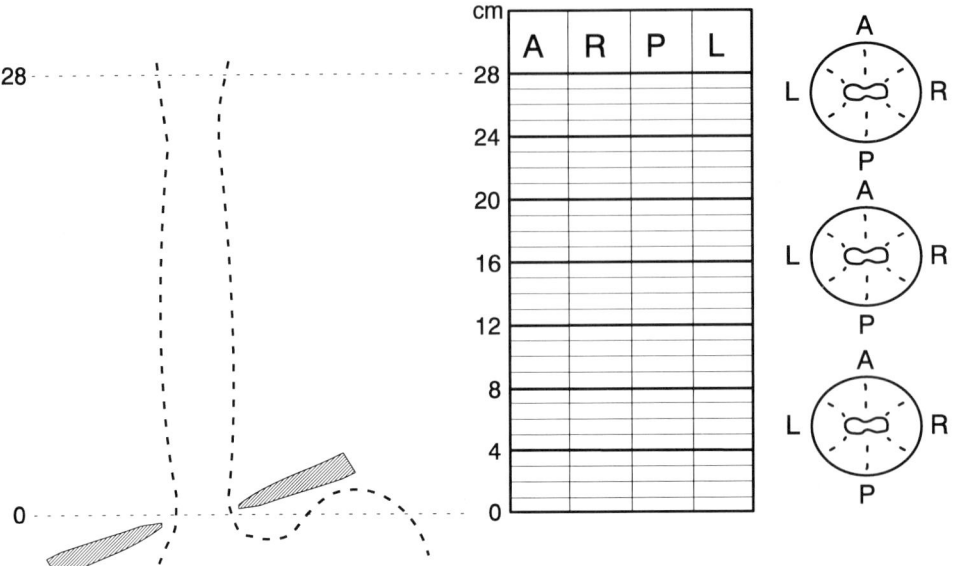

Fig. 1. Endoscopic report form for detailed diagrammatic description of esophageal abnormalities.
Left: pictorial representation of the esophagus, the position and extent of all lesions, including hiatus hernia, may be sketched with reference to the diaphragmatic hiatus; middle: planimetric representation of the esophagus, opened about its longitudinal axis, to show the anterior (A), right (R), posterior (P) and left (L) quadrants, divided vertically into 1 cm segments to allow detailed mapping of metaplastic lesions and an exact record of all biopsy sites; right: axial view of the esophagus at three levels, the endoscopic appearance can be sketched and the level indicated by an arrow to the appropriate level on the middle panel.

At its simplest, the "MUSE" classification system can indicate the presence of a lesion-type with the suffix "⁺" and its absence with "⁻". Thus, a patient with columnar metaplasia, ulceration and erosions would be classified as "M⁺U⁺S⁻E⁺" whereas a patient with only a stricture would be "M⁻U⁻S⁺E⁻". However, in most instances, a more precise assessment of the severity or extent of a lesion is required. In this case, the classification system has been extended, by analogy to the TMN classification of malignant tumors [13], to allow all lesion types to be graded according to their degree of severity. Erosions, for example, are graded as "E_0", (absent), or "E_1", "E_2" or "E_3", corresponding to Savary-Miller grades I–III (Table 1). With four independent classes and four grades of severity (0–III), it is possible, in theory, to classify up to 256 (4^4) different combinations of reflux lesions without providing so many individual categories that the system becomes unwieldy. In practice, there are fewer potential combinations since Barrett's and Savary ulcers, for example, are, by definition, accompanied by columnar metaplasia.

The rationale for the definitions of the different grades in the MUSE classification is as follows:

M: Islands of metaplasia (M_1) may be congenital and may not be premalignant whereas both noncircular metaplasia (M_2) (fingerlike or starlike lesions extending up from the Z-line) and circumferential metaplasia (M_3) are definitely premalig-

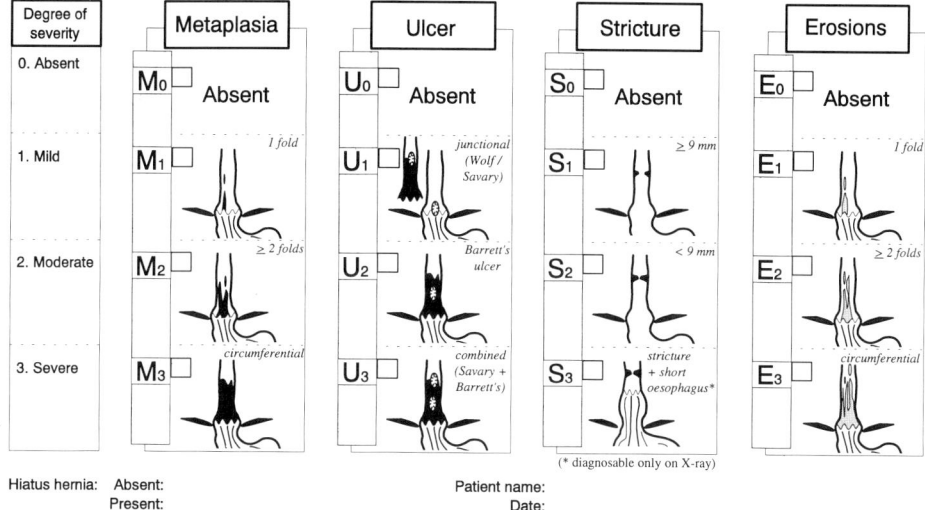

Degree of severity	Metaplasia	Ulcer	Stricture	Erosions
0. Absent	M_0 Absent	U_0 Absent	S_0 Absent	E_0 Absent
1. Mild	M_1 *1 fold*	U_1 *junctional (Wolf/ Savary)*	S_1 *≥ 9 mm*	E_1 *1 fold*
2. Moderate	M_2 *≥ 2 folds*	U_2 *Barrett's ulcer*	S_2 *< 9 mm*	E_2 *≥ 2 folds*
3. Severe	M_3 *circumferential*	U_3 *combined (Savary + Barrett's)*	S_3 *stricture + short oesophagus**	E_3 *circumferential*

(* diagnosable only on X-ray)

Hiatus hernia: Absent:
              Present:

Patient name:
       Date:

Fig. 2. Endoscopy report form based on the "MUSE" esophagitis classification system.
Metaplasia, ulceration, stricture formation and erosions (MUSE) are assessed and graded independently according to the degree of severity: 0: absent; I: mild; II: moderate; III: severe. For each lesion type, the appropriate box is ticked and, if relevant, the extent of a lesion such as columnar metaplasia may be marked with reference to the diaphragmatic hiatus. Examples of some "MUSE" classifications and the corresponding endoscopic features are: $M_3U_0S_1E_3$ — active peptic stricture, diameter >9 mm, situated at the upper pole of a circumferential area of columnar metaplasia; $M_0U_0S_2E_3$ — active junctional stricture, diameter <9 mm, situated at the level of the normal Z-line; $M_3U_3S_0E_0$ — circumferential columnar metaplasia (endobrachyesophagus) with a Barrett's ulcer and a junctional Savary ulcer; $M_0U_0S_0E_2$ — multiple erosions, confluent, affecting more than one longitudinal fold but noncircumferential.

nant [14]; since M_3 indicates more extensive metaplastic change, it is associated with a greater risk of malignancy [15].

U: A junctional ulcer (U_1: Wolf's ulcer or Savary's ulcer) is less likely to bleed than a Barrett's ulcer (U_2) whilst the combination of a junctional ulcer and a Barrett's ulcer (U_3) is the rarest and most severe form of ulceration.

S: The severity of stricturing is difficult to assess, but, pragmatically, an "S_1" stricture may be differentiated from a more severe "S_2" stricture on the basis that the former will allow the passage of a small diameter (9.0–9.2 mm) fiberoptic endoscope. More severe stricturing, leading to a short esophagus (S_3) poses considerable problems for both medical and surgical long-term management.

E: There is good evidence that the severity of erosive esophagitis is correlated with the area of mucosa affected, isolated erosions affecting only one longitudinal fold (E_1) heal more readily than confluent erosions (E_2) and the extensive, circumferential erosive lesions (E_3) often progress to stricturing. A quantitative grading system similar to that used by Hetzel et al. [4] was also considered, but it was decided that it is easier to base a judgement on anatomical features such as mucosal folds than on the percentage of lower esophageal mucosal surface area covered by erosions or ulcers.

With the "MUSE" system, the result of an endoscopy may be written directly with a grade for each lesion type ($M_3U_1S_0E_2$), or it may be recorded by ticking the relevant boxes on a diagrammatic report form (Fig. 2); data recorded in this way can be entered readily into a computerized database and then retrieved for subsequent analysis.

Summary

The "MUSE" system for the endoscopic classification of reflux esophagitis provides a description of the esophagus suitable for clinical practice or research-orientated applications. It differentiates clearly between acute erosive lesions, potentially reversible complications and premalignant changes which have, to date, proved irreversible, and it eschews soft, equivocal signs of esophagitis such as erythema. It provides standardized assessment criteria and a standardized nomenclature which, in the absence of generally-accepted diagnostic criteria derived from an international consensus conference, form the basis for an accurate, objective report format consistent with the original Savary-Miller classification. Finally, an accurate description of esophageal lesions is facilitated by the use of a standardized report form which will permit an accurate, diagrammatic record of all abnormalities.

References

1. Armstrong D, Monnier Ph, Nicolet M, Blum AL, Savary M. Endoscopic assessment of oesophagitis. Gullet 1991;1:63—67.
2. Savary M, Miller G. L'oesophage. Manuel et Atlas d'Endoscopie. Solothurn: Verlag Gassmann, 1977.
3. Savary M. Les hernies hiatales non compliquées. Endoscopie. Maladie peptique oesophagienne et gastrites herniaires. Med Hyg 1968;26:789—791.
4. Hetzel DJ, Dent J, Reed WD, Narielvala FM, MacKinnon M, McCarthy JH, Mitchell B, Beveridge BR, Laurence BH, Gibson GG, Grant AK, Shearman DJC, Whitehead R, Buckle PJ. Healing and relapse of severe peptic esophagitis after treatment with omeprazole. Gastroenterology 1988;95:903—912.
5. Koelz HR, Birchler R, Bretholz A, Bron B, Capitaine Y, Delmore G, Fehr HF, Fumagalli I, Gehrig J, Gonvers JJ, Halter F, Hammer B, Kayasseh L, Kobler E, Miller G, Münst G, Pelloni S, Realini S, Schmid P, Voirol M, Blum AL. Healing and relapse of reflux esophagitis during treatment with ranitidine. Gastroenterology 1986;91:1198—1205.
6. Zeitoun P, Rampal P, Barbier P, Isal JP, Eriksson S, Carlsson R. Oméprazole (20 mg/j) comparé à ranitidine (150 mg 2 fois/j) dans le traitement de l'oesophagite par reflux. Résultats d'un essai multicentrique franco-belge, randomisé en double insu. Gastroenterol Clin Biol 1989;13:457—462.
7. Siewert JR, Ottenjann R, Heilmann H, Neiss A, Döpfer H. Therapie und Prophylaxe der Refluxösophagitis. Ergebnisse einer Multizenterstudie mit Cimetidin. Teil I. Epidemiologie und Ergebnisse der Schubtherapie. Z Gastroenterol 1986;24: 381—395.
8. Colin—Jones DG. Histamine-2-receptor antagonists in gastro-oesophageal reflux. Gut 1989;30:1305—1308.
9. Schüle A, Brändli H, Pelloni S, Koelz HR, Pirozynski WJ, Blum AL. Endoskopische Diagnose der Oesophagitis. Wo liegt der Grenze zum Normalen? Dtsch Med Wochenschr 1977;102:606—609.
10. Leu H, Schüle A, Brändli H, Pelloni S, Blum AL. Glanzverlust, Farbveränderungen und erhöhte Lädierbarkeit der Speiseröhre: altersbedingte Normvarianten. Z Gastroenterol 1978;16:417—421.
11. Monnier Ph, Savary M. Contribution of endoscopy to gastro-oesophageal reflux disease. Scand J Gastroenterol 1984; 19(suppl 106):26—45.
12. Debongnie JC, Macchi H, Mainguet P. Schéma planimétrique destiné à la surveillance de l'oesophage à haut risque. Acta Endoscopica 1981;11:353—356.
13. Hermanek P, Sobin LH. TNM classification of malignant tumors, 4th edn. Berlin: Springer, 1987.
14. Monnier Ph, Fontolliet C, Savary M, Ollyo J—B. Barrett's oesophagus or columnar epithelium of the lower oesophagus. Baillière's Clin Gastroenterol 1987;1:769—789.
15. Ronsom JM, Patel GK, Cliff SA, Womble NE, Read R. Extended and limited types of Barrett's oesophagus in the adult. Ann Thorac Surg 1982;33:19—27.

What are the disadvantages of Savary's classification?

L. Lundell (Gothenburg)

Gastroesophageal reflux disease (GERD) is a common disorder, and the severity by which the disease is clinically expressed varies. A firm diagnosis is of significance not only for the choice of short-term therapy, but particularly so for the long-term therapeutic outcome. To reach that goal, a number of investigations sometimes have to be relied on, since one single test cannot always evaluate all aspects of GERD [1]. The detection and quantification of abnormal acid reflux is carried out by the use of ambulatory pH-metry, whereas esophageal mucosal damage is identified during endoscopy. However, at the most, 50% of patients seeking medical advise for reflux symptoms, present macroscopic peptic lesions in the esophageal mucosa [2,3]. Recent clinical information emphasizes, that the initial severity of the esophageal mucosal lesions not only predicts the outcome of short-term acid inhibitory drug therapy, but the response to maintenance therapy as well [4–8]. In clinical practice it is therefore important to accurately assess the disease severity, giving important clinical guidelines indicating not only the need for therapy, but also the likelihood of relapse after cessation of treatment. Consequently, physicians have become increasingly aware of the necessity to judge the efficacy of various pharmaceutical agents used in GERD, in relation to the degree of severity of reflux induced damage to the esophageal mucosa. However, so many various grading schemes have been used in the literature, that a comparison of the different studies is extremely difficult or even impossible [9,10]. This awareness, however, has not prevented some investigators from proposing even more complicated classification systems. It is vital that future research is based on a formal, standardized classification system to permit a comprehensive estimation of the outcome variables within the trial protocols.

The best known endoscopic grading system is that of Savary-Miller, which despite its widespread acceptance is often misinterpreted (Table 1). Savary's thesis comprised an analysis of 625 endoscopic examinations of the esophagus [11]. This classification scheme suggested grading of reflux esophagitis into four different stages. The original grading, however, did not include the acquired short esophagus, which was added in 1968 [12] and in fact columnar lined esophagus was not included until 1971 [13]. In 1981 further slight modifications were presented, providing a better evaluation of the complicated stages also specifying the association with erosive and/or ulcerative lesions, respectively [14].

One potential problem, that might cause some confusion and risk of misinterpretation, is that the original classification scheme has not been fully published in an English language journal [15]. The fundamental lesion in reflux esophagitis was apparently considered to be the isolated epithelial erosion, whereas subsequent modifications included also discrete erythematous lesions in grade I disease. The problem of using erythema as a diagnostic criteria for esophagitis is obvious, since

Table 1. Description of the Savary grading system

	Savary-Miller (1967–1981)
Stage I	Erythematous or erythemato-exudative erosion (alone or multiple) which can cover several folds (nonconfluent)
Stage II	Confluent but not circumferential erosions
Stage III	Circumferential erosive and exudative lesions
Stage IV	a) Chronic lesions[a] with active inflammation b) Cicatricial stage without active inflammation

[a]Chronic lesion = ulcer, stenosis, brachyesophagus, columnar lined mucosa.

it represents a nonspecific, age related and probably transient lesion even being of noninflammatory nature in some instances [10]. A large number of diagnostic criteria can be established as nonspecific for the disease such as for instance circumscribed erythema, mucosal friability as well as generalized diffuse erythema and mucosal edema. The Savary-Miller grade IV, as defined in 1971 [13], included all complications, such as stricture, ulcers and columnar lined esophagus irrespective of the inflammatory status of the adjacent squamous mucosa. For the general applicability of a similar classification system, this was unfortunate since in clinical practice, as well as within the framework of research protocols, an eventual progression through different severities of the esophagitis would consequently not be corresponded by a progression through the different grades. Thus complete healing of an active, peptic lesion may lead to a different apparent clinical outcome, even in the presence of complications such as stricture and/or columnar lined esophageal mucosa (persistent grade IV).

Another disadvantage of the original Savary classification is that it does not specify the nature of the complication. Although peptic strictures and columnar lined esophagus (Barrett's mucosa) are generally considered to represent complications occurring as a consequence of long-standing severe reflux disease, the short- and long-term impacts for the patients differ significantly between these two separate clinical entities [16,17]. The risk of neoplastic transformation associated with Barrett's esophagus is undisputed. Furthermore, at present it is not clear how accurately endoscopists can distinguish between a chronic lesion (stage IV ulcer) and a circumferential mucosal break (stage III). In general terms the validation of a classification system, by determining the intra- and interindividual variability among endoscopists is not only pertinent for the Savary classification [10].

To be widely used and accepted as a standard in clinical practice, and also as a useful scientific tool, an endoscopic classification system has to comprise relatively few individual grades, enabling the scheme to be easily memorized by the endoscopist. Applicability and acceptance of a classification system are greatly facilitated when the differentiation between the grades of esophagitis is based on a well founded, pathophysiologically sound view on the disease-specific lesions. Another basic requirement is the ease by which it picks up clinical information of significance for the status and the dynamics of the disease, such as complications in the form of strictures, ulcer craters and columnar lined mucosa. Last but not least, all endoscopic classification systems in clinical use today have not been submitted to a validation investigation with the aim of obtaining objective assessment of intra- and inter-individual variations, especially when used by endoscopists with varying levels of experience. The Savary classification suffers from essentially all of these short-comings and a later modification including five gradings still seems to suffer from similar drawbacks [18]. An endoscopic classification system fulfilling all of the above outlined criteria is therefore warranted and should be based on few gradings with the minimal, significant lesion being a mucosal break on the top of the fold. The magnitude of the exposure of noxious material to esophageal mucosa determines the extent of these mucosal breaks on the top of each fold and the breakdown of the mucosal defense in the valleys between the folds, and forms the basis for a circumferential progression of these lesions.

References

1. Armstrong D, Emde C, Inauen W, Blum AL. Diagnostic assessment of gastro-oesophageal reflux disease. What is possible versus what is practical? Hepato-Gastroenterology 1992;39(suppl 1):3.
2. Heading RC. Epidemiology of oesophageal reflux disease. Scand J Gastroenterol 1989;24(suppl 168):33–37.
3. Johnsen R, Bernersen B, Straume B et al. Prevalences of endoscopic and histological findings in subjects with or without dyspepsia. Br Med J 1991;302:749.
4. Sandmark S, Carlsson R, Fausa O, Lundell L. Omeprazole or ranitidine in the treatment of reflux esophagitis. Results of double-blind, randomized, Scandinavian multicenter study. Scand J Gastroenterol 1988;23:625–632.
5. Klinkenberg-Knol EC, Jansen JBMJ, Festen HPM, Meuwissen SGM, Lamers CBHW. Double blind multicentre comparison of omeprazole and ranitidine in the treatment of reflux esophagitis. Lancet 1987;1:349–351.
6. Vantrappen G, Rutgeerts L, Schurmans P, Coenegrachts JL. Omeprazole (40 mg) is superior to ranitidine in the short-term treatment of ulcerative reflux oesophagitis. Dig Dis Sci 1988;33:523–529.
7. Havelund T, Laursen LS, Skoubo-Kristensen E et al. Omeprazole and ranitidine in treatment of reflux oesophagitis: double blind comparative trial. Br Med J 1988;296:89–92.
8. Dent J, Yeomans ND, MacKinnon M et al. Omeprazole versus ranitidine for prevention of relapse in reflux oesophagitis. A controlled double-blind trial. Omeprazole versus ranitidine for prevention of relapse in reflux oesophagitis. A controlled double-blind trial. World Congress of Gastroenterology, Sydney, 1990 FP4.
9. Tytgat GNJ, Nio C, Schotborgh RH. Reflux oesophagitis. Scand J Gastroenterol 1990;25:1–12.
10. Armstrong D, Monnier P, Nicolet M, Blum AL. Endoscopic assessment of oesophagitis. Gullet 1991;1:63–67.
11. Savary M. La séméiologie endoscopique de l'incontinence gastroosophagienne. Thesis. Lausanne (Switzerland), 1967.
12. Savary M. Les hernies hiatales non compliquées. Endoscopie. Maladie peptique oesophagienne et gastrites herniaires. Med Hyg 1968;26:789.
13. Savary M. L'expression endoscopique de l'oesophagite par reflux. XIIIth Congress of International Bronchoesophagological Society, Lyon, 1971. Villeurbanne (France): Ed. Simep, 1971;101.
14. Miller G, Savary M, Monnier Ph. Notwendige diagnostik: Endoskopie. In: Blum AL, Siewert JR (eds) Reflux-therapie. Berlin: Springer-Verlag, 1981;336.
15. Savary M, Miller G. Manuel et Atlas d'Endoscopie. Solothurn (Switzerland): Verlag Gassmann, 1977.
16. Dent J, Bremner CG, Collen MJ, Haggitt RC, Spechler SJ. Working party report to the World Congress of Gastroenterology, Sidney 1990. Barrett's oesophagus. J Gastroenterol Hepatol 1990;6:1–22.
17. Lundell L. Acid suppression in the long-term treatment of peptic stricture and Barrett's oesophagus. Digestion 1992;51(suppl 1):49–58.
18. Ollyo JB, Monnier Ph, Fontolliet C, Savary M. The natural history, prevalence and incidence of reflux oesophagitis. Gullet 1993;(suppl 3):3–10.

E.H. Metman (Tours)

The number of esophagitis classifications proposed in the last 2 decades proves that there is no real consensus in this field. The first comprehensive endoscopic classification of esophagitis came with the main paper from Skinner and Belsey in 1967, based on the large surgical experience upon 1,030 operated patients at Bristol [1].

A four grade classification (Table 1) was correlated with steps of gastroesophageal reflux treatment. This classification was largely used and adapted in France by Moulinier [2] and lead to an international classification with four grades:
— Grade I.   Superficial esophagitis, friability edema.
— Grade II. Erosive esophagitis with or without fibrin.
          Grade IIa. Limited vestibular erosions.
          Grade IIb. Extensive or circumferential erosions.
— Grade III. Erosions with fibrosis and esophageal shortening (brachy-esophagus).
— Grade IV. Stricture with erosions or deep ulcer.
Barrett's esophagus was independent, although it was eventually associated with grades I–V.

The Savary-Miller classification was published in 1977 [3] and was rapidly and widely accepted, because it avoided the equivocal significance of grade I Belsey or "international" classifications, in spite of the questionable incorporation of all complications in grade IV (ulcer as stricture as columnar epithelium).

This criticism brought many authors — mainly for the purpose of clinical trials — to offer new classifications with four [4] to six [5] grades independent of the existence, or not, of columnar epithelium. Unfortunately, these (and other) gradings included grade I equivocal changes, as Belsey's first one.

Monnier and other Lausanne authors [6,7] have subsequently proposed a modification of the grading, called the Savary-Monnier classification. The two main modifications were:
— separate grade V for columnar epithelium;
— modifications of grades I and II: multiple nonconfluent erosions were incorporated in grade II, whereas grade I was restricted to erosions of a single mucosal fold.
Similar criticisms can be addressed to this classification, as columnar epithelium was

Table 1. Results of esophagoscopy and treatment required in type 1 hiatus hernia (adapted from Skinner and Belsey [1])

Esophagitis	Patients	Esophagoscopy	Treatment
None	320	Incompetent cardia	Medical or repair
Grade I	208	Mucosal reddening	Medical or repair
Grade II	146	Superficial ulcer, membrane formation	Surgical repair
Grade III	47	Ulceration, fibrosis, secondary shortening	Repair or resect
Grade IV	158	Mucosa destroyed, fibrosis, shortening stricture	Repeated dilation or resection and reconstruction

one step in the grading. Furthermore, some differences in definitions existing between the first abstract in Gastroenterology [6] and the subsequent papers [8,9] allow easy criticism. In addition, there are apparent discrepancies among authors in using the different types or grades [7,9].

Evidence has also been stated that Barrett's esophagus should not be included as a step in the grading, which now makes Savary-Monnier's classification useless. In Ollyo et al. [8], it was stated that, "the simple classification into five types should be exclusively reserved for epidemiological studies" and that "the detailed classification (i.e., A, B, C, D system, analog to MUSE system), should be the one used in daily practice and for clinical trials".

In opposition to this statement from Ollyo et al., I think that for daily practice, a simple, reliable grading system, and not a complicated one like MUSE (or a similar system) should be used. Moreover, in clinical practice, and particularly in appreciation of surgical indication and choice of procedure, we require a grading in which steps are in accordance with prognostic factors. No classification affords more in this view than Belsey's, which was established on rigid endoscopic examination. I think that it would be simple to change grade I from equivocal reddening to minimal changes specific of early mucosal damage such as red spots, junctional erosion or inflammatory sentinel polyp and fold [10].

In conclusion, actual classifications are questionable because they are numerous, they comprise columnar epithelium as a step of grading (Savary-Miller and Savary-Monnier classifications), or they include a first grade with equivocal changes.

Expert consensus is needed in order to attempt a prognostic classification as simple as possible.

References

1. Skinner DB, Belsey RH. Surgical management of esophageal reflux and hiatus hernia. J Thorac Cardiovasc Surg 1967;53: 33—54.
2. Moulinier B, Ruet D. Aspect fibroscopique des oesophagites. Cah Méd Lyonnais 1974;10:859—862.
3. Savary M, Miller G. L'oesophage. Manuel et Atlas d'Endoscopie. Solothurn (Switzerland): Gassmann, 1977.
4. Hetzel DT, Dent J, Reed WD et al. Healing and relapse of severe peptic esophagitis after treatment with omeprazole. Gastroenterology 1988;95:903—912.
5. Tytgat GNJ. Endoscopy of the oesophagus. In: Cotton PB, Tytgat GNJ, Williams CB (eds) Annual of Gastrointestinal Endoscopy. London: Curr Sci Ltd, 1990;15—26.
6. Ollyo JB, Lang F, Fontolliet Ch, Monnier Ph. Savary-Miller's new endoscopic grading of reflux oesophagitis: a simple reproducible logical and useful classification. Gastroenterology 1990;98:A100.
7. Miller IS. Endoscopy of the esophagus. In: Hennessy TPJ, Cuschieri A (eds) Endoscopy of the Oesophagus in Surgery of the Oesophagus. Oxford: Butterworth Heineman, 1992;89—142.
8. Ollyo JB, Fontolliet Ch, Brossard E, Lang F. Savary's new classification of reflux oesophagitis. Acta Endoscopica 1992;3: 307—320.
9. Ollyo JB, Monnier Ph, Fontolliet C, Savary M. The natural history, prevalence and incidence of reflux oesophagitis. Gullet 1993;3(suppl):3—10.
10. Bleshman MH, Banner MP, Johnson RD et al. The inflammatory polyp and fold. Radiology 1978;128:589—593.

What is the value of the AFP-score in evaluating surgical results?

H. Feussner, J.R. Siewert (Munich)

Whenever the results of different medical and various surgical strategies have to be compared, a precise classification of the stage of the disease is mandatory. This has long been recognized in oncology, leading to the development of the TNM-system. Basically, the same was required for the evaluation of antireflux therapy as well. Bancewicz et al., therefore, created a similar classification system for gastroesophageal reflux disease (GERD). It is a three-dimensional classification system comprising anatomical, pathophysiological (functional) and pathologic aspects [1].

Their first results being most convincing, we adopted this classification system including some slight modifications. The letter A, denoting anatomy, is used to describe the presence and type of hiatal hernia; the letter F, denoting function, codes the findings on 24-h intraesophageal pH measurement; and P, denoting pathology, depicts the presence of mucosal lesions as seen at endoscopy (Table 1). Each of these three elements is graded according to severity.

Table 1. Modified AFP-classification of reflux disease

A = anatomy
    A_0: no hernia present
    A_1: small hiatal hernia
    A_2: large, fixated hernia
    A_3: mixed sliding and paraesophageal hernia or pure paraesophageal hernia

A_{ps} = anatomy after previous surgery
    $A_{ps}0$: normal postoperative anatomy (e.g., cuff in proper position)
    $A_{ps}1$: supradiaphragmatic hernia
    $A_{ps}2$: cuff opened
    $A_{ps}3$: cuff too low or slippage of the wrap (telescope phenomenon)
    $A_{ps}4$: cuff too tight

F = function
    F_0: no pathological reflux on 24-h pH monitoring
    F_1: reflux related to meals
    F_2: upright reflux not related to meals (fasting state)
    F_3: supine reflux with or without upright reflux

P = pathology
    P_0: no macroscopic mucosal abnormality
    P_1: macroscopic esophagitis consisting of singular spotty areas in the distal esophagus
    P_2: linear, longitudinal streaks in the distal esophagus
    P_3: continuous, circular esophagitis
    P_4: reflux esophagitis with complications (penetration, ulcers, strictures, longitudinal fibrosis (short esophagus))

It has to be noted that in this modified system the presence or absence of Barrett's esophagus was not taken into account, since the columnar lined esophagus is considered per se to be a scar resulting from chronic reflux esophagitis. However, this finding can be indicated for the sake of completeness by adding the letters CLE (columnar lined esophagus) to the respective pathological grade.

Furthermore, we felt it necessary to describe the postsurgical results more specifically. Therefore, we defined a special postsurgical grading for the A-group (Table 2).

Table 2. Postsurgical classification of the A (anatomy) element

A_{ps} group 0	proper localization of the fundic wrap
A_{ps} group 1	epidiaphragmatic position of the wrap
A_{ps} group 2	cuff disruption
A_{ps} group 3	cuff too low in relation to the lower esophageal sphincter, or slippage of the cuff
A_{ps} group 4	cuff too tight

The F and P elements are used in the same way as before surgery.

Practical experience with the AFP-system

The modified AFP-system is applied routinely to each patient being referred for antireflux surgery and, likewise, to patients on whom a reoperation has to be performed. After the first series of patients on whom the classification system was tried out [2], it became clear that the number of possible AFP-subgroups is far too high for practical use. If all AFP-subgroups are considered, a total of more than 70 possible combinations (from A_0, F_0, P_0 to A_3, F_3, P_3) can be calculated (Table 3). For practical comparison of two series, a large number of patients was required, which is difficult to obtain in antireflux surgery. Additionally, a long list of subgroups is difficult to interpret. For a more rapid, visual comparison, a 3D plot of the respective elements could be helpful, but this does not facilitate a "quantitative" comparison. The only way to give a quantitative basis for assessing the differences between the patients and to quantify the operative result is to use a score. If it is assumed that all elements of the AFP-system are of equal rank, it is possible to give each patient a score based on the sum of the respective elements (AFP 0 being the best and AFP 10 describing the worst constellation). The score can be calculated for the individual patient as well as for the respective group of patients, according to the formula (A + F + P/n), n being the number of patients and AFP the numerical amount of the respective element. The patients with primary reflux disease prior to fundoplication had an average AFP-score of 5.45, which fell after operation to 1.22. In patients with a failed Nissen fundoplication before surgery, the APSFP value was 7.3, which fell after surgery to 1.07.

Table 3. Distribution of AFP subgroups found in 57 patients prior to fundoplication

AFP subgroup	No. of patients	AFP subgroup	No. of patients	AFP subgroup	No. of patients
$A_0 F_0 P_0$	2	$A_2 F_0 P_4$	1	$A_1 F_1 P_3$	1
$A_1 F_0 P_0$	–	$A_2 F_1 P_4$	4	$A_1 F_2 P_3$	1
$A_2 F_0 P_0$	–	$A_2 F_3 P_0$	5	$A_1 F_3 P_3$	2
$A_3 F_0 P_0$	1				
$A_0 F_1 P_0$	–	$A_2 F_3 P_2$	9	$A_2 F_1 P_1$	–
$A_1 F_1 P_0$	–	$A_3 F_3 P_4$	1	$A_2 F_2 P_1$	–
$A_2 F_1 P_0$	–			$A_2 F_3 P_1$	1
$A_3 F_1 P_0$	–				
$A_0 F_2 P_0$	–	$A_0 F_1 P_1$	–	$A_2 F_1 P_2$	–
$A_1 F_2 P_0$	–	$A_0 F_2 P_1$	–	$A_2 F_2 P_2$	1
$A_2 F_2 P_0$	–	$A_0 F_3 P_1$	–	$A_2 F_3 P_2$	–
$A_3 F_2 P_0$	–				
$A_0 F_3 P_0$	–	$A_0 F_1 P_2$	2	$A_2 F_1 P_3$	–
$A_1 F_3 P_0$	–	$A_0 F_2 P_2$	–	$A_2 F_2 P_3$	–
$A_2 F_3 P_0$	1	$A_0 F_3 P_2$	3	$A_2 F_3 P_3$	3
$A_3 F_3 P_0$	–				
$A_0 F_0 P_1$	2	$A_0 F_1 P_3$	–	$A_3 F_1 P_1$	–
$A_1 F_0 P_1$	–	$A_0 F_2 P_3$	–	$A_3 F_2 P_1$	–
$A_2 F_0 P_1$	–	$A_0 F_3 P_3$	1	$A_3 F_3 P_1$	1
$A_3 F_0 P_1$	–				
$A_0 F_0 P_2$	–	$A_1 F_1 P_1$	–	$A_3 F_1 P_2$	–
$A_1 F_0 P_2$	2	$A_1 F_2 P_1$	–	$A_3 F_2 P_2$	–
$A_2 F_0 P_2$	–	$A_1 F_3 P_1$	1	$A_3 F_3 P_2$	1
$A_3 F_0 P_2$	2				
$A_0 F_0 P_3$	–	$A_1 F_1 P_2$	2	$A_3 F_1 P_3$	–
$A_1 F_0 P_3$	–	$A_1 F_2 P_2$	–	$A_3 F_2 P_3$	–
$A_2 F_0 P_3$	2	$A_1 F_3 P_2$	–	$A_3 F_3 P_3$	–
$A_3 F_0 P_3$	–				
$A_0 F_1 P_4$	2				
$A_1 F_0 P_4$	1				
$A_1 F_1 P_4$	2				

Conclusion

The experience of Bancewicz et al. [1] as well as our own [2], has clearly demonstrated that reflux disease and the results of its treatment cannot adequately be
described by one single parameter. Therefore, the idea of including three elements —
anatomy, function and pathology — allowed for the first time the possibility of giving
a complete picture of the disease before and after therapy. This improved description,
however, is paid for by creating a large number of subgroups making a direct

comparison of small series difficult.

In the TNM system of the UICC [3], the similar problem of too many subgroups was solved by defining tumor stages. In our experience, the use of a cumulative score also reflects the severity of the patient's disease and is as simple and convenient to use. Originally, we were concerned about the fact that scoring systems do neglect drastic changes of a single element if the other ones do not change. Continuous use, however, has clearly shown that isolated changes of only one element are uncommon. Thus, the use of a score system is, once again, confirmed.

References

1. Bancewicz J, Matthews HR, O'Hanrahan T, Adams J. A comparison of surgically treated reflux patients in two surgical centers. In: Little AG, Ferguson MK, Skinner DB (eds) Diseases of the Esophagus, vol II. New York: Mount Kiscoe, 1990.
2. Feussner H, Petri A, Walker S, Bollschweiler E, Siewert JR. The modified AFP Score: An attempt to make the results of antireflux surgery comparable. Br J Surg 1991;78:942–946.
3. TNM Atlas (UICC), 2nd edn. Berlin-Heidelberg: Springer Verlag, 1990.

Critical evaluation of current classification systems for reflux esophagitis?

H.W. Boyce Jr (Tampa)

Accurate endoscopic diagnosis of esophagitis depends upon the existence of visually identifiable changes in the esophageal mucosa that can be confirmed upon biopsy in all cases. Any mucosal alteration that does not precisely correlate with histology is not reliable for a diagnosis that is to be used as a basis for therapeutic decisions, or for evaluation of response to any one or combination of therapies. Many authorities agree that capillary congestion and erythema/hyperemia are visible mucosal changes that do not correlate with histology and therefore should not be used as criteria for endoscopic diagnosis of esophagitis. Prior grading systems for severity of esophagitis that included erythema/hyperemia as endoscopic criteria should not be used.

In past years, the lack of a suitable standard grading system for the lesions of reflux esophagitis has led to confusion in patient care and clinical research studies. The documentation of unequivocal epithelial defects typical for reflux is sufficient for an accurate diagnosis of reflux esophagitis. However, neither the absence of visible mucosal defects nor the complete healing of previously documented mucosal injury confirmed by endoscopy can be considered indicative of normal histology. When either clinical or research requirements dictate the need for documentation of complete mucosal healing, only a biopsy can provide confirmation. The fact that typical symptoms of reflux esophagitis can occur with either microscopic abnormalities or totally normal mucosal histology has been well established. In the absence of unequivocal mucosal defects (erosions), an adequate biopsy is the only method to determine presence or absence of esophagitis.

The accurate diagnosis of reflux esophagitis is possible by endoscopy alone only if there are unequivocal signs of mucosal erosion. The severity of esophagitis by endoscopy or histology does not correlate well with symptoms. An endoscopic grading system for reflux esophagitis can be used only as a measure of the visible extent of mucosal injury, starting at the squamocolumnar mucosal junction and extending proximally into the esophagus either as continuous or "stepping stone" erosions (islands of mucosal erosion surrounded entirely by squamous epithelium). The complications of erosive esophagitis (stricture, ulcer and columnar-lined esophagus) are included in the highest grade of severity. The assumption has been, and it probably is true, that the more extensive the area of mucosal erosion circumferentially about the squamocolumnar mucosal junction, the greater the risk of evolution into stricture, deep ulceration or a columnar-lined esophagus.

A major question is how best to define the degree of erosive disease so that the interpretation of various grades is consistent between endoscopists. The answer may be somewhere between the simple Savary-Miller system proposed in 1977 (Table 1) and the "MUSE" system (M = metaplasia; U = ulcer; S = stricture; E = erosions) proposed in 1992 (Table 3) [1,2].

The need for a grade 0 indicative of normal or no esophageal erosions is uncertain. The only apparent advantage seems to be that it serves to require a definitive response from the endoscopist when grading is a component of the data required for clinical research. Grade 0 serves no purpose for general clinical use in endoscopy reports. Several investigators have also included a grade I indicating hyperemia/erythema with friability (Tables 1 and 2). Interpretation of hyperemia/erythema or friability is subject to wide interobserver variation, and in many cases is overinterpreted. Hence, this definition of grade I does not seem proper for an objective endoscopic grading system.

Most will agree that there is a need for uniformity and precision with any grading system used for evaluating response to therapy in a clinical research protocol. However, is it necessary to apply the same detailed criteria needed for research purposes to the routine clinical diagnosis of esophagitis? Is there a need for general agreement on separate grading systems for clinical and research purposes? It is probably best to have a single grading language to be used between countries, clinicians and investigators. The most objective and simple system would be the best.

The mild, moderate, severe and complicated grades of the original Savary-Miller system seem quite easy to apply for clinical purposes with no obvious need for modification. The proposers of the "MUSE" system (Table 3) state that one of its advantages is that it may be used to predict the response to treatment, the risk of hemorrhage or malignancy, and the need for long-term surveillance [2]. The original Savary-Miller system can be used similarly [1]. The "MUSE" system is also touted as helpful by allowing one to distinguish between the reversible and irreversible sequelae of reflux, i.e., erosions ("E") and complications ("MUS") respectively. Many

Table 1. Grading systems for reflux esophagitis

Scales	Savary-Miller [1] (1977)	Sonnenberg [3] (1982)	Knuff [6] (1984)	Hetzel [4] (1988)
Grade 0		No esophagitis	Normal	Normal mucosa with no abnormalities
Grade I	Single or isolated erosive lesion(s), oval or linear but affecting only longitudinal fold	Mild, isolated round or linear erosions	Mucosal hyperemia, patchy and/or linear	Erythema or hyperemia of the esophageal mucosa with no macroscopic erosion
Grade II	Multiple erosive lesions, non-circumferential, affecting more than one longitudinal fold, with or without confluence	Severe, confluence of the erosions involving the total esophageal circumference	Hyperemia, granularity and/or friability	Superficial ulceration or erosions involving <10% of the last 5 cm of esophageal squamous mucosa
Grade III	Circumferential erosive lesions	Complicated, erosions as described, deep ulcers, peptic stenosis and/or columnar epithelium-lined esophagus	Erosions	Superficial ulceration or erosions involving >10–50% of the last 5 cm of esophageal surface
Grade IV	Complications: columnar epithelium, ulcer(s), stricture(s) and/or short esophagus. Alone or with grades I–III		Stricture or frank ulcer	Deep ulceration anywhere in the esophagus or confluent erosion of >50% of last 5 cm of esophageal squamous mucosa
Grade V				

will disagree that ulcers are irreversible, since healing is often achieved with adequate therapy.

Any detailed system of grading must provide the user with precise definitions of each entity to be graded in order to minimize the degree of interobserver error. The "S" of the "MUSE" mnemonic stands for stricture, but we are not provided with a

Table 2. Grading systems for reflux esophagitis

Scales	Johnson [7] (1989)	Bate [9] (1990)	Tytgat [5] (1990)	Bytzer [8] (1993)
Grade 0	Normal mucosa	Normal esophageal mucosa	No evidence of reflux-induced damage: crisp sharply delineated SCMJ, smooth shiny squamous distal mucosa	No mucosal abnormalities
Grade I	One or more nonconfluent lesions with erythema or exudate above the GE junction	Erythema and friability with spontaneous contact bleeding	Mild, patchy, diffuse erythema at level of SCMJ minor friability, loss of shininess, no mucosal break	One or more of the following: diffuse erythema, edema, mucosal friability isolated round or linear erythema without fibrin
Grade II	Confluent, non-circumferential erosive and exudative lesions	Isolated round or linear erosions affecting the 2 cm of the esophagus and not the entire circumference	Superficial erosions of red dots or streaks with or without exudate. Usually small and on tip of folds. They involve <10% of mucosal surface of the 5 cm above GE junction	Fibrin-covered erosions not involving the entire circumference
Grade III	Circumferential erosive and exudative lesions	Erosions extending above 2 cm or affecting the entire circumference	Confluent, non-circumferential erosions, may be additional exudate covering defects or slough formation. <50% of overall mucosa of distal 5 cm	Confluent erosions extending for the entire circumference or ulceration but without stenosis
Grade IV	Chronic mucosal lesions, i.e. ulceration, stricture or Barrett's esophagus	Frank benign ulcer	Circumferential erosions or exudative lesions at level of SCMJ, regardless of the extent along distal esophagus	Complicated esophagitis: stricture or columnar-lined epithelium >3 cm above the GE junction
Grade V		Stricture	Deep ulceration anywhere or various degrees of stricture	

Table 3. "MUSE" esophagitis classification system

Degree of severity	Metaplasia	Ulcer	Stricture	Erosions
0. Absent	M_0 Absent	U_0 Absent	S_0 Absent	E_0 Absent
1. Mild	M_1 One fold	U_1 Junctional	$S_1 \geq 9$ mm	E_1 One fold
2. Moderate	$M_2 \geq$ Two folds	U_2 Barrett's ulcer	$S_2 < 9$ mm	$E_2 \geq$ Two folds
3. Severe	M_3 Circumferential	U_3 Combined	S_3 Stricture and short esophagus	E_3 Circumferential

Metaplasia, Ulceration, Stricturing and Erosions are assessed and graded independently according to the degree of severity: 0 — absent, 1 — mild, 2 — moderate, 3 — severe. The absence or presence, along with location, of a hiatus hernia is also to be recorded (Adapted from ref. [2]).

precise definition of stricture (due to fibrosis), and how it is to be differentiated from a stenosis which is defined as lumenal narrowing of any etiology (i.e., inflammation, fibrosis or neoplasm). Both inflammatory and cicatricial stenosis occur often with reflux disease, with the former being reversible when due to inflammation alone and the latter, due to intramural fibrosis, is not reversible. This differentiation is difficult to impossible in some cases and will detract from the precision and prognostic potential of the "MUSE" system, if specific criteria for a fibrotic stricture can not be included.

In 1982 Sonnenberg et al. (Table 1) used a modification that incorporated aspects of several previously reported grading systems, including the original Savary-Miller system [4]. They included grade 0 as indicative of no erosions, grade I as mild erosions, grade II as severe erosions and grade III as complicated, which included erosions plus deep ulcers, peptic stenosis and columnar-lined esophagus. Here the generic term stenosis was used rather than the specific term stricture, again creating uncertainty as to the actual pathology present.

The descriptive term "deep" is used in some systems to describe ulcers but is not otherwise defined, thereby reducing the objectivity of assessment [3—5]. How is the endoscopist to differentiate a shallow ulcer and a deep ulcer? Is a shallow ulcer the same as an erosion?

It appears then that the original Savary-Miller system is quite adequate for clinical purposes. When more precision is required for clinical research purposes, as it should be, the MUSE system will provide the best possibility for accurate grading with the least interobserver variation.

References

1. Savary M, Miller G. L'oesophage. Manuel et Atlas d'endoscopie. Solothurn (Switzerland): Verlag Gassmann, 1977.
2. Armstrong D, Monnier Ph, Nicolet M, Blum AL, Savary M. Endoscopic assessment of oesophagitis. Gullet 1991;1:63—67.
3. Sonnenberg A, Lepsien G, Muller-Lissner SA, Koelz HR et al. When is esophagitis healed? Esophageal endoscopy, histology and function before and after cimetidine treatment. Dig Dis Sci 1982;27(4):297—302.

4. Hetzel DT, Dent J, Reed WD, Narielvala FM et al. Healing and relapse of severe peptic esophagitis after treatment with omeprazole. Gastroenterology 1988;95:903–912.
5. Tytgat GNJ. Endoscopy of the oesophagus. In: Colton PB, Tytgat GNJ, Williams CB (eds) Annual of Gastrointestinal Endoscopy. London: Curr Sci Ltd, 1990;15–26.
6. Knuff TE, Benjamin SB, Worsham GF, Hancock JE, Castell DO. Histologic evaluation of chronic gastroesophageal reflux: an evaluation of biopsy methods and diagnostic criteria. Dig Dis Sci 1984;29(3):194–201.
7. Johnson NJ, Boyd EJS, Milis JG, Wood JR. Acute treatment of reflux oesophagitis: a multicenter trial to compare ranitidine 150 mg b.d. with ranitidine 300 mg q.d.s. Aliment Pharmacol Ther 1989;3:259–266.
8. Bytzer P, Havelund T, Hansen JM. Interobserver variation in the endoscopic diagnosis of reflux esophagitis. Scand J Gastroenterol 1993;119–125.
9. Bate CM, Keeling PWN, O'Morain C, Wilkinson SP et al. Comparison of omeprazole and cimetidine in reflux oesophagitis: symptomatic, endoscopic and histological evaluations. Gut 1990;31:968–972.

What type of mild stenoses may reverse with medical therapy only, without dilatation?

J.E. Richter (Birmingham, Alabama)

Peptic esophageal strictures are a sequelae of long-standing reflux esophagitis, with the majority of stricture patients having coexistent reflux esophagitis at the time of diagnosis. Until recently, clinicians paid little attention to the role that coexistent reflux esophagitis plays in the stricturing process and subsequent production of dysphagia. Therapy has centered largely on mechanically relieving the stenosis via bougienage or surgical intervention. Recent studies, however, suggest that coexistent reflux esophagitis may be as important as luminal diameter, in producing dysphagia and determining subsequent need for bougienage.

In one of the earliest clinical trials of medical therapy, Ferguson et al. evaluated the efficacy of cimetidine in 20 patients with symptomatic peptic esophageal strictures and endoscopic esophagitis [1]. Patients received either cimetidine 400 mg 4 times daily or placebo for 6 months, in this double-blind cross-over trial. Significantly greater improvement in esophagitis was seen during cimetidine treatment, compared with placebo. However, no reduction in the frequency of stricture dilatation was seen in either group. In another study with a mean follow-up of 19 months, Starlinger et al. [2] assessed the frequency of dilatation among 28 patients with reflux esophagitis and stricture who were treated with cimetidine 400 mg 4 times daily. Significantly greater improvement in esophagitis was documented among patients taking the cimetidine regularly vs. patients with poor medication compliance. Similar to earlier studies however, there was no difference in the frequency of bougienage between the two groups.

The use of more potent acid suppression regimens has been employed in several recent studies of peptic stricture patients. Koop and Arnold evaluated the efficacy of omeprazole maintenance therapy in 31 patients with H_2 blocker resistant esophagitis (six patients had peptic strictures) [3]. After complete esophagitis healing with omeprazole 40 mg daily, patients were placed on maintenance omeprazole therapy with 20 mg daily. During the follow-up observation period (mean of 24 months), none of the six stricture patients required dilatation. In a short-term study, Ching et al. evaluated 20 patients with dysphagia secondary to peptic stricture and persistent esophagitis refractory to 6 months of medical therapy [4]. All patients were treated with omeprazole 20 mg daily for 8 weeks. Fifteen of the 20 patients had significant improvements in esophagitis grade, with only 2/15 "responders" requiring stricture dilatation during the 8-week observation period. Of the five remaining patients with no improvement in esophagitis, all required stricture dilatation for recurrent dysphagia.

Recently we completed a randomized prospective clinical trial, assessing the therapeutic efficacy of medical antireflux therapy on the healing of esophagitis and frequency of repeated dilatations in patients with peptic strictures [5]. Thirty-two symptomatic patients (i.e., dysphagia occurring at least once a week) with peptic strictures (radiographic diameter <12.5 mm based upon pill retention) and coexistent reflux esophagitis (Savary grades II–IV) were treated with either omeprazole or H_2 blockers. Prior to therapy all patients had their strictures dilated to at least 48 French (16 mm) diameter. Patients then were randomized to omeprazole 20 mg q.AM vs. ranitidine 150 mg b.i.d. (am and 30 min after supper) or famotidine 20 mg b.i.d. If esophagitis was not healed endoscopically within 3 months, drug dosages were doubled and endoscopy repeated at 6 months. Subsequent dilatations were performed only if the dysphagia score was ≥ 2 (≥ 1 episode per week) as determined by a monthly telephone interview by a physician not knowing the patient's drug regimen.

Omeprazole was superior to H_2 blockers in the healing of esophagitis at 6 months (17/17 (100%) omeprazole vs. 8/15 (53%) H_2 blockers, $p < 0.01$) but not at 3 months (11/17 (65%) omeprazole vs. 7/15 (46%) H_2 blockers). Irrespective of specific drug therapy, all seven patients in the nonhealing group required repeat dilatations (23 total; mean 3.3 ± 1.0; SD) while only 11/25 (44%) of the healed group required further dilatations (19 total; mean: 0.8 ± 1.0). Throughout the study, there was a strong trend for fewer patients on omeprazole to require repeat dilatations vs. H_2 blocker treated patients (3 months: 7/18 (39%) omeprazole vs. 12/16 (75%) H_2 blockers, $p = 0.03$; 6 months: 7/17 (41%) omeprazole vs. 11/15 (73%) H_2 blockers, $p = 0.07$). Probably of more clinical importance was the observation that H_2 blocker treated patients required nearly 3-fold more dilatations than patients receiving omeprazole (31 sessions vs. 11 sessions). This difference was present both at 3 months (mean $\pm$ SD sessions: 1.3 ± 0.9 vs. 0.4 ± 0.6, $p < 0.01$) and 6 months (2.1 ± 1.6 vs. 0.6 ± 0.9, $p < 0.05$).

In summary, these data emphasize the key role that active esophagitis plays in producing dysphagia and determining the need for esophageal dilatation. Accordingly, aggressive medical antireflux therapy must be an integral component of stricture therapy. Recent studies consistently show that omeprazole is superior to H_2 blockers in the healing of esophagitis and the reduction in requirement for esophageal dilatations.

References

1. Ferguson R, Dronfield MW, Atkinson M. Cimetidine in treatment of reflux oesophagitis with peptic stricture. Br Med J 1979;2:472–474.
2. Starlinger M, Appel WH, Schemper M, Schiessel R. Long-term treatment of peptic esophageal stenosis with dilation and cimetidine: Factors influencing clinical results. Eur Surg Res 1985;17:207–214.
3. Koop H, Arnold R. Long-term maintenance treatment of reflux esophagitis with omeprazole: Prospective study in patients with H_2 blocker-resistant esophagitis. Dig Dis Sci 1991;36:552–557.
4. Ching CK, Shaheen MZ, Homes GKT. Is omeprazole more effective in the treatment of resistant reflux oesophagitis and associated peptic stricture? Gastroenterology 1990;98:A30.
5. Marks R, Richter JE, Koehler R, Spenney J, Mills T. Does medical therapy improve dysphagia in patients with peptic strictures and esophagitis? Gastroenterology 1992;102:A118.

What is the histology of an esophageal stricture before and after dilatation?

K. Jeyasingham (Bristol)

It has long been established, both by gastroenterologists and esophageal surgeons, that dysphagia of reflux esophagitis can be managed with a conservative medical regime to control the refluxate and the severity of the reflux, combined with intermittent dilatation of the narrowed lumen of the esophagus. Furthermore, it has also been shown that control of reflux by surgery with intermittent dilatation can be applied satisfactorily in patients with gastroesophageal reflux and stricture of the esophagus. It has also been shown in cases where the esophagus is shortened and narrowed, that surgical elongation and antireflux surgery with repeated dilatations can achieve good results. Some patients, however, do require resection for uncontrolled reflux and persistent undilatable stricturing of the esophagus.

Dysphagia is a symptom complex to which the contributory pathological factors are inflammatory edema, esophageal spasm and fibrous infiltration of the wall. Esophageal stricture, on the other hand, is an histopathological entity. When a physician dilates an esophageal stricture successfully and achieves a "good result", he is dealing with the clinical problem of dysphagia contributed to by inflammatory edema and esophageal spasm. He achieves success by stretching the wall and dilating the lumen, whilst controlling the effects of continued action of refluxed material on the esophageal wall with drugs and antireflux measures. When, despite healing the

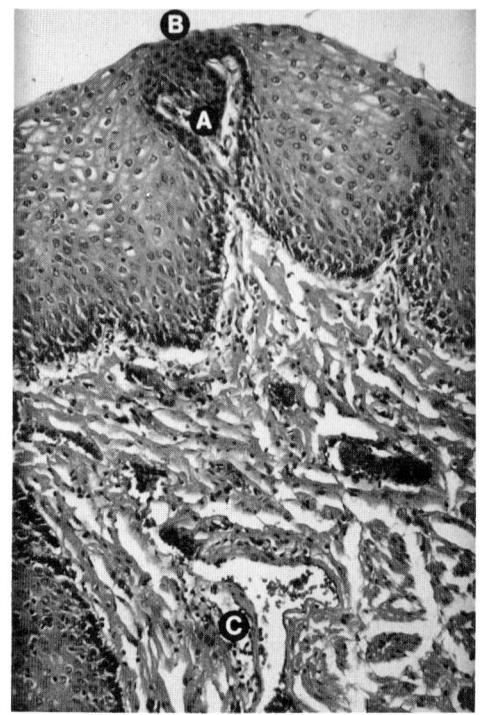

Fig. 1.

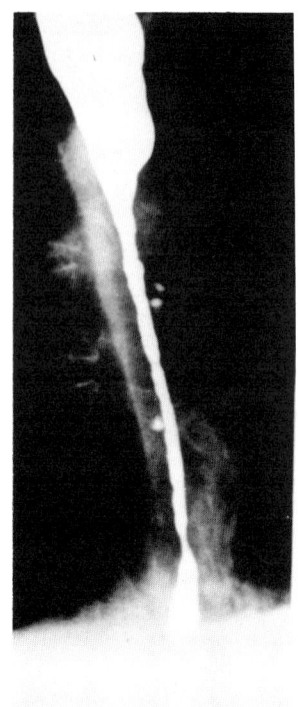

Fig. 2.

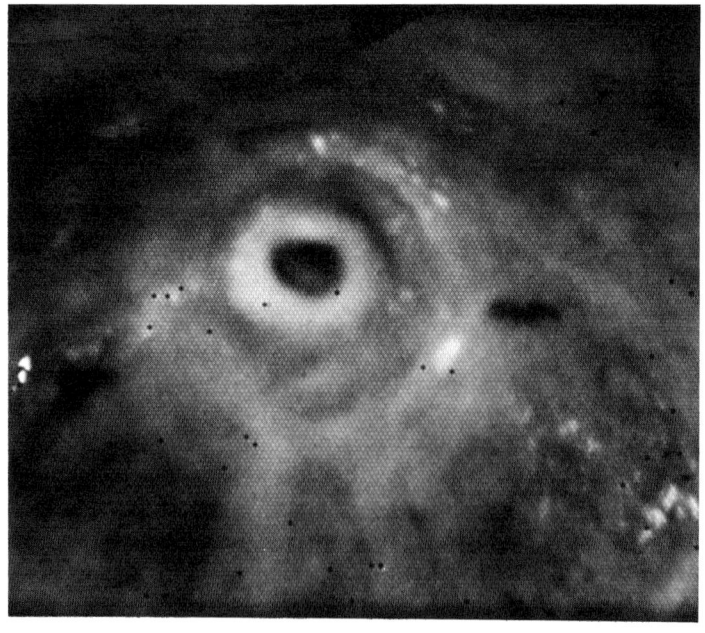

Fig. 3.

endoscopic evidence of esophagitis, the patient returns with dysphagia he is confronted with the third component of the contributory factors — interstitial fibrosis. When repeated dilatations and medical management have failed, the surgeon is confronted with the histopathological entity of chronic esophageal stricture. I confine my remarks to the stricture of chronic gastroesophageal reflux disease.

Wherefrom do we derive histological information on strictures before and after dilatation? The specimen obtained at endoscopy before and after several dilatations must, of necessity, be only superficial. The depth of the biopsy forceps cup only reaches the mucosa and submucosa. Even the rigid esophagoscopic biopsies do not reach the depths required to pick up the deeper layers of the muscularis propria where the pathology lurks. Therefore, one has to depend on surgically resected specimens and specimens removed at post mortem examination to study the histology of structures before and after repeated dilatations.

If one looks at the likely effects of repeated dilatations in a strictured esophagus, one would anticipate seeing mucosal damage in the short term due to surface instrumental trauma. This would be combined with the appearances of pre-existing esophagitis at endoscopy. The lining epithelium shows thickening, the submucosal layers show vascular injection but little fibrous infiltrate and no acute inflammatory cellular infiltration (Fig. 1). This is in reality a successfully dilated esophagus in the stage of acute edema of esophagitis. If, however, the dilatation and drug treatment was not followed by complete healing but resulted in snail track ulceration, then a biopsy in such cases shows that the tissue is only deep enough to show ulceration and submucosal infiltration by chronic inflammatory cells and some fibrous proliferation. When the dilatations have been accompanied by persistent extensive esophagitis and

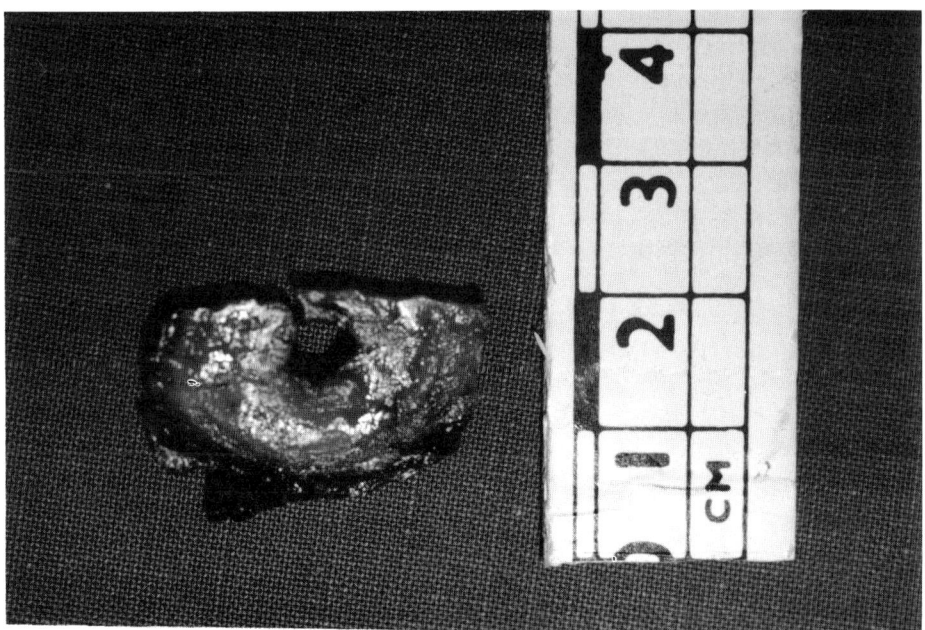

Fig. 4.

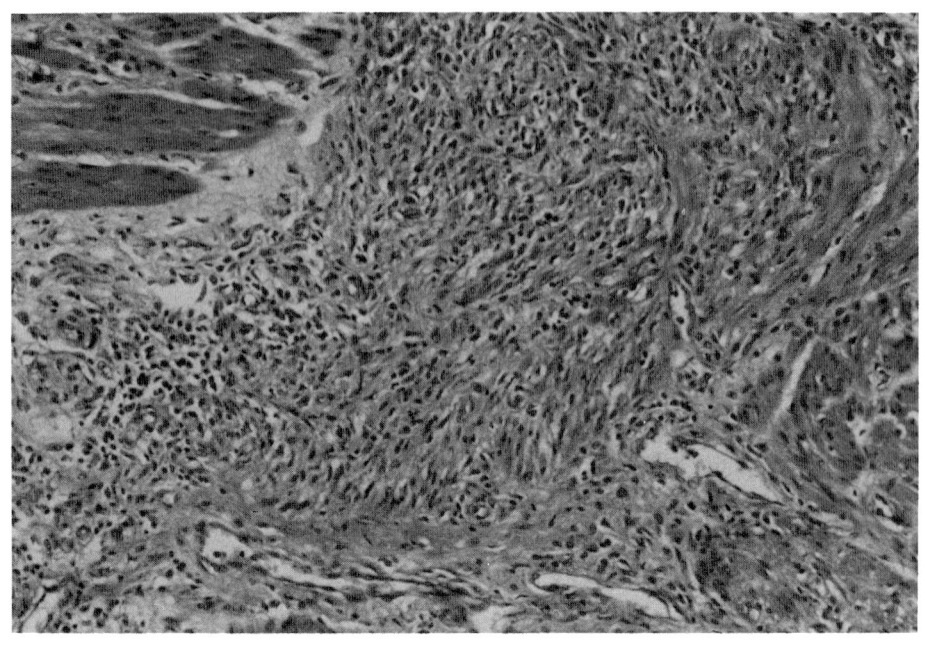

Fig. 5.

ulceration, the histology shows changes in the epithelium and in the submucosa with adjacent ulceration. In the chronic stricture (Fig. 2), repeated dilatations have resulted

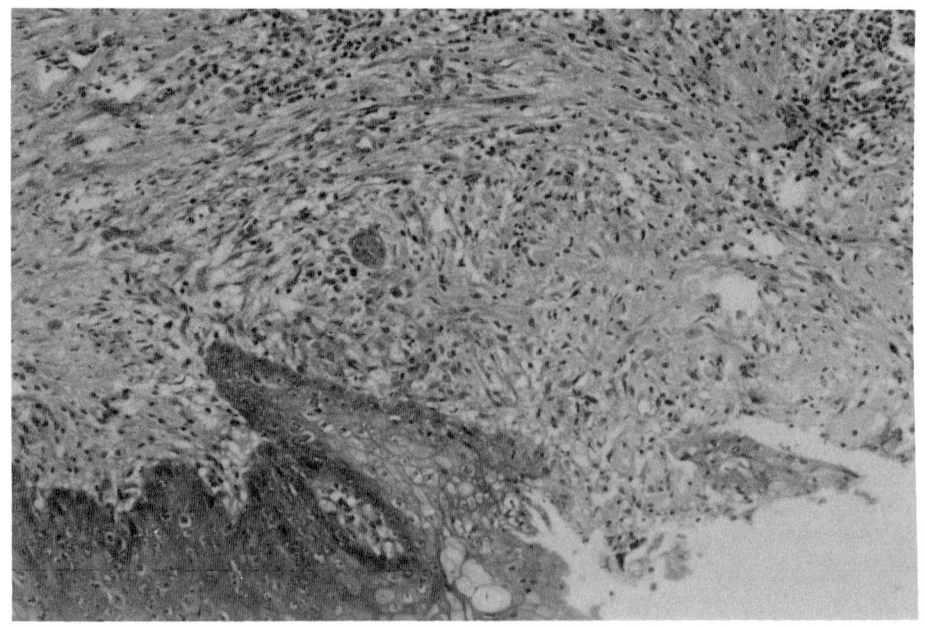

Fig. 6.

in little clinical or radiological improvement with an endoscopic appearance (Fig. 3). A resected specimen usually shows glistening fibrous tissue (Fig. 4). A transverse section of this esophagus at different levels shows varying appearances. Where the lumen is narrow with lining epithelium intact, the epithelial regeneration has produced a surface of hyaline material and there is intense fibrous narrowing of the wall, it shows no acute inflammatory cellular infiltration, but mature fibrous tissue and destruction of the muscularis propria. At a lower level of transection, the lumen is narrowed and ulcerated, with epithelial remnants in areas, but almost total disruption of the muscularis propria and infiltration with mature fibrous tissue. A low power view shows the chronic inflammatory cellular infiltrate with disruption of muscularis propria in one area (Fig. 5), the high power view of the same area shows the appearances of the muscularis propria being infiltrated by mature fibrous tissue undeterred by the repeated dilatations. Elsewhere in the section one can see the ulcerated epithelium with the tall "rete pegs" lining the surface on the interior (Fig. 6).

If one looks at the possible sequence of changes in the histology of the repeatedly dilated chronic peptic stricture (Table 1), one sees a whole spectrum of histological changes ranging from mucosal damage, intramural fibrosis, the persistence of acute reflux esophagitis, regression and healing in areas, metaplasia, dysplasia and malignant change.

Table 1. Histology of chronic stricture after repeated dilatations

Replacement of lining with granulation tissue
Destruction of muscularis mucosae
Interstitial fibrosis
Mucosal regeneration

In summary, the intramural histological picture of the repeatedly dilated chronic peptic stricture is by no means a reversible situation, although the endoscopic appearances may show healing of the surface lining.

Are there histological characteristics that might help in selecting the dilating equipment or dilatation techniques?

H. Aste, M. Conio, M. Picasso (Genoa)

Esophageal strictures may be the result of benign or malignant disorders involving primarily or secondarily the esophagus. A classification of the most common causes

Table 1. Esophageal stenoses

Malignant strictures
— Esophageal tumors
— Extrinsic tumors
Web-rings
Inflammatory strictures
— GERD
— Lye-induced
— Radiations
— Postsurgery
— Post variceal sclerotherapy
Achalasia

of esophageal stenoses is presented in Table 1.

The treatment of esophageal strictures has become one of the most common problems faced by endoscopists. The main goal of this therapy is to re-establish and maintain a patent esophagus with minimal risk and cost to the patient. Whereas the dilatory techniques are readily available, it is important for the endoscopist to have a definite plan of action fixed in their mind before approaching any esophageal stricture.

All stenotic lesions must be located, measured and biopsied. Additional aspects such as narrowness, rigidity, tortuosity, diverticulae, large hernias, signs of extrinsic compression, and the histologic characteristics should be taken into account in selecting the dilatation technique.

Esophageal strictures can be managed with a variety of techniques. Each device for dilatation has its advantages and disadvantages which are important in selecting the appropriate one for each situation (Table 2).

We do not know of controlled comparative studies dealing with histological characteristics of esophageal strictures that might help in selecting dilating techniques.

On the basis of scientific reports and common experience, there are esophageal stenotic lesions for which dilatory procedures are often selected according to the pathological findings.

Malignant strictures

Dilatation of malignant strictures requires frequent repetition unless the tumor is treated with radiation, chemotherapy, laser, Bicap, positioning endoprosthesis or a combination of some of these treatments. Bougie dilatation, by means of tapered

Table 2. Dilatation techniques in esophageal stenoses

1. Mercury-filled bougies (Hurst-Maloney)
2. Graded metal olives (Eder-Puestow)
3. Tapered plastic dilators (Celestin/Savary-Gilliard)
4. Balloon dilators (OTS/TTS)
5. Others (Papillotomy/Laser/Bicap)

plastic dilators of the Celestin [1] or Savary-Gilliard [2] type, appears more effective than balloons in reducing dysphagia and maintaining stricture patency for a longer time where a squamocellular or an adenocarcinoma involvement of the esophagus is concerned [3,4]. However, the absence of symptomatic improvement from dilatation in any histological type of extraesophageal malignant tumor leading to dysphagia is well known.

Esophageal webs and rings

Esophageal webs are thin mucosal folds protruding into the lumen in which an hyperplasia of the squamous epithelium sometimes combined with chronic inflammation, is reported [5].

Schatzki rings develop in the line of junction of esophageal and gastric mucosa, with a slight hyperkeratosis of the squamous epithelium and a mild inflammatory infiltrate in the subepithelial layers [6].

Rupturing of rings and webs with large tapered plastic dilators ("push type" dilators like Savary or Celestin) will usually take care of the problem in one session, although occasionally they may recur [7].

Inflammatory strictures

Inflammatory lesions of the mucosal and submucosal layers of the esophagus whether related to gastroesophageal reflux disease (GERD), lye-induced lesions, radiations or anastomotic reaction after surgery may lead to localized narrowing of the esophagus. Edema, cellular infiltration, vascular changes and progressive fibrotic developments are commonly associated histopathological events.

"Push-type" dilators are well tolerated, easily used, not expensive and offer efficient dilating techniques especially in non-longstanding strictures with a low-grade fibrotic reaction [2,8,9]. In patients with circumferential tight strictures, secondary to extensive fibrotic involvement, dilatations should not be performed in one sitting, and a gradual stepped method will help prevent undue complications. In these cases, radial forces applied by means of balloon dilators appear to be the least dangerous method in the first dilatory sittings [10–13].

Lye-induced strictures are notoriously difficult to treat and often require repeated dilatations for many years [14].

Since the natural history of benign strictures is made of recurrences [15–17], long-term controlled trials will represent the only means to make possible any comparison between balloon measurements and those made with tapered plastic dilators.

Other methods for short fibrous strictures may be employed by experienced endoscopists. They consist in cutting the strictures by papillotomies, electrocautery needles or laser. In experienced hands, these methods have been safely used [18,19].

Achalasia

Esophageal dilatation for achalasia is unique in that it involves forceful disruption of the lower esophageal sphincter by means of radial forces. It is important that an accurate diagnosis be made before dilatation.

Several types of dilators can be used for treating achalasia. More recently, balloons have become available, offering a more reproducible dilatation carried out under endoscopic visual control. These dilators can be attached to a small caliber forward-viewing endoscope (OTS) [20] or passed through the endoscope (TTS) offering a more reproducible dilatation by providing graded sizes in diameter.

The choice of dilators and the technique used should be based on training and experience as there are no comparative studies.

References

1. Celestin LR, Campbell WB. A new and safe system for oesophageal dilatation. Lancet 1981;1:74−75.
2. Monnier Ph, Hsieh V, Savary M. Endoscopic treatment of esophageal stenosis using Savary-Gilliard bougies: technical innovations. Acta Endosc 1985;15:119−129.
3. Heit HA, Johnson CF, Siegel SR, Boyce HW. Palliative dilation for dysphagia in esophageal carcinoma. Ann Int Med 1978;89:629−631.
4. Aste H, Munizzi F, Martines H, Pugliese V. Esophageal dilation in malignant dysphagia. Cancer 1985;56:2713−2715.
5. Shamma'a MH, Benedict EB. Esophageal webs. A report of 58 cases and an attempt at classification. N Engl J Med 1958; 259:378−384.
6. Schatzki R, Gary JE. Dysphagia due to a diaphragm-like localized narrowing in the lower esophagus. AJR 1953;70:911−922.
7. Goff JS. The tight esophagus. Bougies or balloons. Can J Gastroenterol 1990;4:593−595.
8. Cox JG, Winter RK, Maslin SC, Jones R, Buckton GK, Hoare RC, Sutton DR, Bennett JR. Balloon or bougie for dilatation of benign oesophageal stricture. An interim report of a randomised controlled trial. Gut 1988;29:1741−1747.
9. Aste H, Munizzi F, Saccomanno S, Pugliese V. "Splitting" and stretching dilatation of esophageal strictures. Endoscopy 1983;15:41−43.
10. Merrel N, McGray RS. Balloon catheter dilatation of a severe esophageal stricture. Gastrointest Endosc 1982;28:254−245.
11. Graham DY, Tobibian N, Schwartz JT, Smith JL. Evaluation of effectiveness of through-the-scope balloons as dilators of benign and malignant gastrointestinal strictures. Gastrointest Endosc 1987;33:432−435.
12. Kozarek RA. Hydrostatic balloon dilation of gastrointestinal stenoses: A national survey. Gastrointest Endosc 1986;32: 15−19.
13. Abele JE. The physics of oesophageal dilatation. Hepato-Gastroenterol 1992;39:486−489.
14. Browne JD, Thompson JN. Caustic injuries of the esophagus. In: Castell DO (ed) The Esophagus. Boston: Little Brown & Co, 1992;669−685.
15. Ogilvie AL, Ferguson R, Atkinson M. Outlook with conservative treatment of peptic esophageal stricture. Gut 1980;21: 23−25.
16. Glick ME. Clinical course of esophageal stricture managed by bougienage. Dig Dis Sci 1982;27:884−888.
17. Patterson DJ, Graham DY, Smith JL, Schwartz JT, Alpert E, Lanza FL, Cain GD. Natural history of benign esophageal stricture treated by dilatation. Gastroenterology 1983;85:346−350.
18. Venu RP, Geenen JE, Hogan WJ, Kruidenier J, Stewart ET, Soergel KH. Endoscopic electrosurgical treatment for strictures of the gastrointestinal tract. Gastrointest Endosc 1984;30:97−100.
19. Sander R. Benign stenoses. In: Riemann JF, Ell C (eds) Lasers in Gastroenterology. International Experiences and Trends. New York: Georg Thieme Verlag, 1989;44−47.
20. Witzel L. Treatment of achalasia with a pneumatic dilator attached to a gastroscope. Endoscopy 1981;13:176−177.

At what histologic stage are mucosal strictures irreversible?

K. Geboes, J. Mebis (Leuven)

Radiologically, an esophageal stricture is defined as a persistent narrowing that is longer than 1 cm [1]. The most characteristic symptom of an organic narrowing, without complete obstruction, is dysphagia for solids, whereas drinking remains relatively easy. When the stenosis narrows further, even drinking may become difficult. Esophageal strictures can occur in all age groups and have a varied etiology. Especially in the elderly, esophageal stenosis should always arouse suspicion of malignancy. Most benign strictures are the result of chronic inflammation, mainly due to reflux of gastroduodenal contents. Ingestion of caustic agents, drugs, radiation, sequelae of surgical interventions and cutaneous diseases such as pemphigus and benign mucous pemphigoid may also lead to strictures [2].

Narrowing of the esophageal lumen due to inflammatory lesions is the result of a complex process involving inflammation, peristaltic dysfunction and repair. While edema, inflammation and muscle spasm are reversible, repair may lead to an irreversible stricture by inducing fibrosis. The microscopic aspects of esophageal strictures are not very well described and the pathogenesis has not yet been studied in detail. This is explained by the fact that most strictures are treated medically and/or by dilatation, whereas surgery is mainly performed for severe or special cases. Thus the specimens available for thorough pathological examination are mostly from severe, end-stage cases. Microscopic examination of such cases usually reveals erosive or ulcerative epithelial lesions, with a breach in the muscularis propria filled with scar tissue. The ends of the muscle coat are present in the ulcer crater or they merge with the muscularis mucosae at the edges of the lesion. Fibrotic disruption of the musculosa and a disorganization of the smooth muscle coat is common. Neural tissue components are usually still present, but show severe architectural distortion. Prominent nerve fibers are often seen in specimens of caustic esophagitis [3] (Fig. 1).

Inflammation and mucosal strictures

It has been established that the degree of esophagitis is important in determining swallowing ability [4]. In a recent study of 64 patients with benign peptic stricture it was shown that the diameter of the stricture accounted only for 30% of the variation of the dysphagia score, whereas esophagitis and other factors were responsible for the remaining 70%. The dysphagia score was based on nine different items of food, scored according to their solidity. Half of the score was obtained from questioning the patients regarding the items of food which cause dysphagia. The other half of the score was based on the consumption of a test meal [5]. A significant linear association was detected between the dysphagia score and the diameter of the

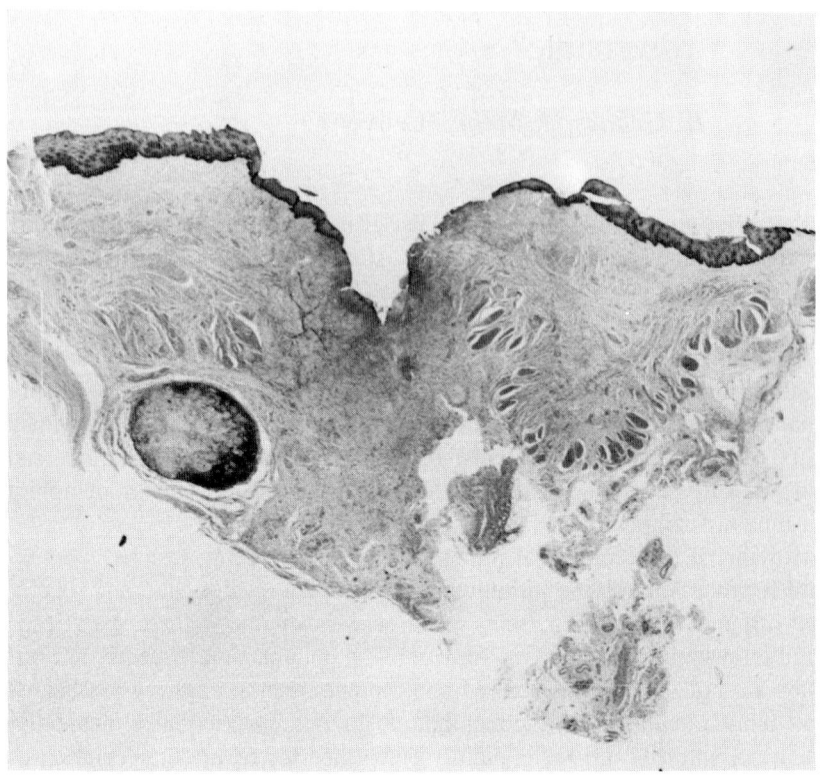

Fig. 1. Transmural esophageal biopsy. The patient was operated for a stricture due to caustic esophagitis. A deep, penetrating ulcer can be seen in the center of the biopsy. The musculosa, outer and inner layer, in the bottom of the ulcer has disappeared and has been replaced by fibrous tissue (H.E. ×20).

stricture (a diameter of 5 mm or less being very important). Dysphagia was clearly worse with increasing severity of esophagitis. The mechanism of esophagitis associated dysphagia remains speculative. Peristaltic abnormalities are probably important but inflammation, by the production of mediators and by injury of the connective and smooth muscle tissue, may also be a major contributing factor [4].

Healing and repair of mucosal strictures

Inflammation in itself is still a reversible condition, whereas damage of muscular or intrinsic nervous components during the process of insult and fibrosis, resulting from healing and repair, may lead to irreversible narrowing. Healing and repair are thus important for the pathogenesis and possible irreversibility of mucosal strictures. This can be concluded from the occurrence of strictures, following the ingestion of caustic agents where injury is massive and usually penetrating.

The cells associated with repair are mononuclear cells such as lymphocytes, plasma cells and cells producing extracellular matrix (ECM) (fibroblasts, myofibroblasts, smooth muscle cells and endothelial cells). Repair has been studied well in the skin and also partially in the stomach (ulcer healing), colon (post polypectomy) and esophagus (caustic lesions) [6,7]. In studies on wound healing in the skin, it has been shown that local infection, early movement and foreign material can impede the healing process by delaying epithelial regeneration and promoting the production of granulation tissue, with the resultant likelihood of larger scars. In the esophagus, factors such as infection and movement are likely to occur. Delayed healing will further be induced by the recurrent nature of the insult, as is the case in reflux esophagitis. Although the esophageal mucosa bears some features which are similar to the skin, the gut is very different because of its contents, its circular structure and the composition of the gut wall (smooth muscle tissue, intrinsic innervation). In the gut, injury can affect the deeper layers. Hence the functional and, therefore, clinical consequences of the insult will also depend on the depth of the injury.

Minimal mucosal injury

Minimal injury to the surface epithelium will result in complete healing, unless the surface of the lesion is very extensive, but even then good functional healing is possible, as shown by a few case reports of patients with benign or idiopathic esophageal casts [8]. Epithelial repair will start from the edge of the lesion while granulation tissue is filling up the defect. Minimal mucosal damage may lead to a slight increase in type III collagen, but rarely an increase in type I collagen, which is the type usually associated with scar tissue [6].

Full thickness mucosal injury and deep penetrating injury

Full thickness mucosal damage and deep ulceration can lead to serious functional disturbances. This type of injury will damage the fibrous tissue of lamina propria and submucosa, the smooth muscle tissue of muscularis mucosae and muscularis propria and the intrinsic nervous tissue. The process of healing will incompletely restore their functional properties.

A classical insult, such as an endoscopic polypectomy in the colon, induces hemorrhage and the formation of a fibrin clot. This clot is stabilized by linking fibronectin to fibrin and factor XII. Fibronectin is chemotactic for fibroblasts and they secrete extracellular matrix (ECM) including proteoglycans and type III collagen providing strength. Fibrosis in and between the muscularis mucosae starts with the formation of collagen III, followed by type I which matures into typical scar tissue. Fibrosis may occur as bands of fibrous tissue in the submucosa, which can extend into the muscularis propria and may affect the latter.

In the esophagus, as in other organs, the composition of the ECM, a component of the intercellular substance, has a role in the biomechanical properties and the functional integrity of the organ. All tissues and organs are composed of cells and intercellular substance. The latter is well developed in the connective tissue, which is quantitatively very important in the gut. The intercellular substance filling up the space between the cells is composed of water, the extravascular pool of plasma proteins, other plasma constituents and the ECM holding the cells and the intercellular substance closely together. The ECM is composed of extracellular matrix proteins, especially collagen and elastin, forming a fibrous network and a ground substance filling up the space in between. Collagens are a family of proteins. There are about 12 types identified, but the most important are type I, which is ubiquitous and a major constituent of scar tissue, type III, which is abundant in the mucosa of the gastrointestinal tract, type IV, a major component of basement membranes, and type V, which is produced by smooth muscle cells. Elastic fibers add to the tensile strength of an organ and its ability to recoil. The ground substance is composed of polysaccharides such as glycosaminoglycans (alternatively mucopolysaccharides) and noncollagenous proteins such as proteoglycans, fibronectin and laminin. Well known glycosaminoglycans are hyaluronic acid, chondroitin-4-sulphate, chondroitin-6-sulphate, dermatan sulphate, keratan sulfate and heparan sulfate. Proteoglycans as glycosaminoglycans are long unbranched molecules, negatively charged and highly hydrophilic.

Fibronectin has been shown to be involved in cell migration. Hyaluronic acid can affect immunological reactions. It can interact with lymphocytes and in high concentrations it inhibits macrophage response to cytokines. In low concentrations it enhances phagocytosis. Collagens, elastins and matrix specialization, in general, are important for the contractile properties of the tissue and disruption, as in deep injury, will lead to loss of mechanical and other properties. A positive correlation can be found with an increase in collagen content and loss of biomechanical properties of the esophageal wall [9].

Adventitial injury

Injury of the deeper layers of the esophageal wall need not necessarily start from the luminal side. Mediastinal infection can affect the connective tissue from the esophageal adventitia and also lead to injury of muscle and nervous tissue and subsequent stenosis [9,10].

Consequences of mucosal stricture

Partial obstruction of the esophageal lumen will further induce alterations of the structure of the esophageal wall, in the segment proximal to the site of obstruction. These alterations are mainly characterized by increased deposition of connective tissue and collagen in the muscularis propria. The increase of collagen content shows a positive correlation with the loss of wall tension and the evolution of other biomechanical properties. These changes may occur after a relatively short period (weeks) as shown in an experimental study in the opossum [9].

Conclusion

Irreversible esophageal mucosal strictures will result from injury, involving the deeper layers of the esophageal wall with damage of connective, (smooth) muscle and nervous tissue and subsequent fibrosis (increased collagen content) in the deeper layers of the wall, at the site of the injury but also in the adjacent proximal segment. The altered composition of the intercellular substance in the submucosal connective tissue and musculosa results in alterations of the biomechanical properties of the wall with subsequent stricture formation.

References

1. Dodds WJ. Esophagus and esophagogastric region including diaphragm. In: Margulis AR, Burhenne HJ (eds) Practical Alimentary Tract Radiology — Year Book. St. Louis: Mosby, 1993;78—118.
2. Vantrappen G, Hellemans J, Geboes K. Etiology and nonsurgical treatment of organic esophageal stenosis. In: Vantrappen G, Hellemans J (eds) Diseases of the Esophagus. Berlin: Springer Verlag, 1974;795—806.
3. Van de Voorde W, Coremans G, Lerut T, Geboes K, Gruwez J, Vantrappen G. Caustic oesophagitis seen through the microscope. Tijdsch Gastroenterol 1989;22:145—150.
4. Triadafilopoulos G. Nonobstructive dysphagia in reflux esophagitis. Am J Gastroenterol 1989;84:614—618.
5. Dakkak M, Hoare RC, Maslin SC, Bennett JR. Oesophagitis is as important as oesophageal stricture diameter in determining dysphagia. Gut 1993;34:152—155.
6. Riddell RH. Healing and repair. In: Snape WJ, Collins S (eds) Effects of Immune Cells and Inflammation on Smooth Muscle and Enteric Nerves. Boca Raton: CRC Press, 1991;11—24.
7. Pelemans W, Hellemans J. Caustic lesions of the esophagus. Etiology and nonsurgical treatment of organic esophageal stenosis. In: Vantrappen G, Hellemans J (eds) Diseases of the Esophagus. Berlin: Springer Verlag, 1974;539—549.
8. Geboes K, Janssens J. The esophagus in cutaneous diseases. In: Vantrappen G, Hellemans J (eds) Diseases of the Esophagus. Berlin: Springer Verlag, 1974;823—833.
9. Little AG, Correnti FS, Calleja IJ, Montag AG, Chow YC, Ferguson MK, Skinner DB. Effect of incomplete obstruction on feline esophageal function with a clinical correlation. Surgery 1986;100;430—436.
10. Gregersen H, Giversen IM, Rasmussen LM, Tottrup A. Biomechanical wall properties and collagen content in the partially obstructed opossum esophagus. Gastroenterology 1992;103;1547—1551.

Is esophageal dilatation easily carried out as an outpatient procedure?

O. Ekberg (Malmö)

Balloon dilatation is an established method in the treatment of esophageal stricture. Dilatation can be made both endoscopically and/or under fluoroscopic control. Overall success rates have been reported to be 67—98%, and rupture rates have been 0—9% in prior studies [1—5]. Using a balloon during dilatation, such esophageal ruptures are virtually eliminated. There are reduced shearing forces for the balloon compared with bougies in vivo and this increases the margin of safety [6]. Balloon dilatation is done with intravenous sedation and/or analgesics and is basically an

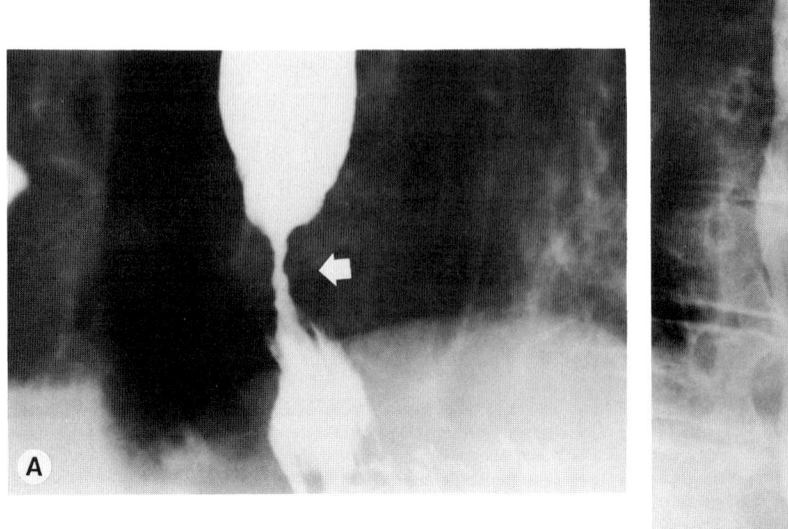

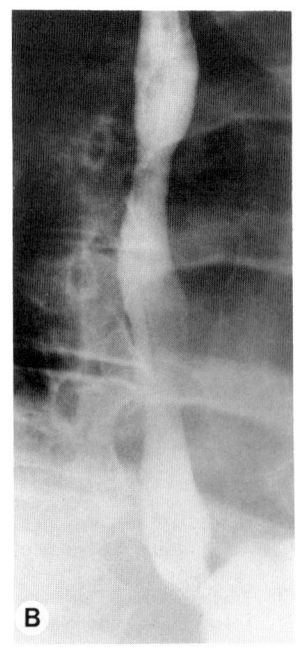

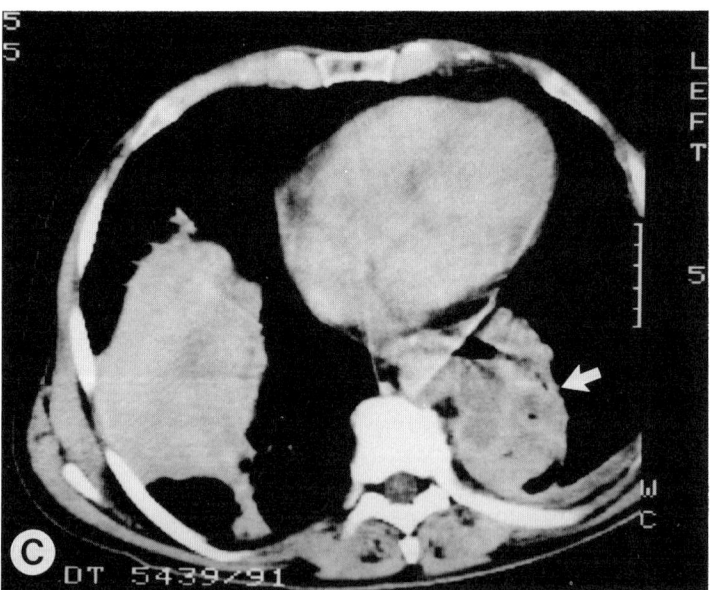

Fig. 1A–C. Severe GERD in a 53 year old male. A) There is a stricture in the distal esophagus (arrow). B) Balloon dilatation was uneventful and a postprocedure gastrografin swallow showed patency of the esophageal lumen. C) The patient was admitted to the hospital 48 h later, with chest pain, shortness of breath and dysphagia. A CT examination of the lower thorax showed a large abcess (arrow) adjacent to the esophagus.

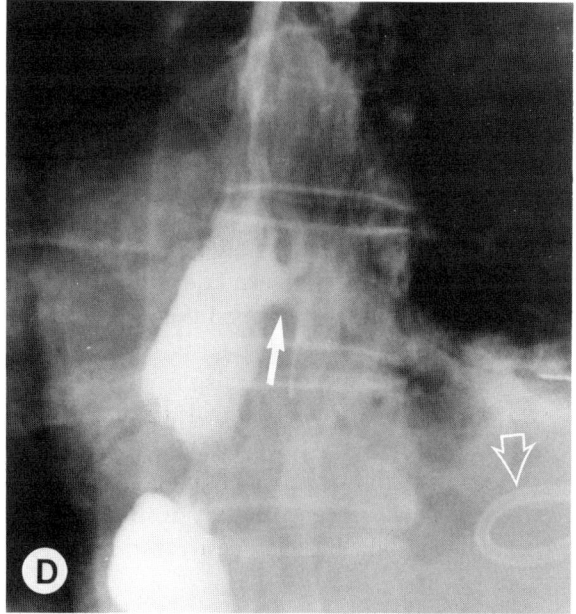
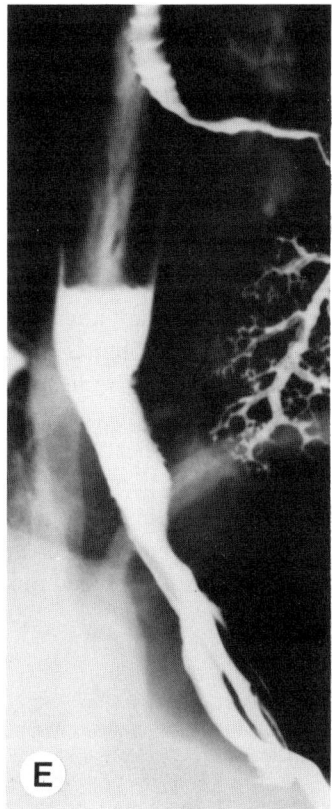

Fig. 1D–E. Severe GERD in a 53 year old male. D) A new gastrografin study showed a leak (arrow) from the proximal area of the dilated stricture and the left thoracic cavity. A percutaneous drainage catheter (open arrow) had been placed under ultrasound guidance. E) After 6 months the patient had recovered. A barium swallow showed only mild narrowing of the distal esophagus. There is, however, aspiration of barium into the airways. The latter was probably not related to the balloon dilatation or its complications.

outpatient procedure. The patient is observed in the recovery area in approximately 4–6 h and then discharged if there is no evidence of chest pain or dysphagia. A postprocedure barium swallow may be added, but is probably not mandatory. However, when major complications occur, i.e., esophageal rupture, prompt and adequate treatment including tracheotomy may be necessary.

Minor complications during the procedure are bleeding and chest pain. There may also be respiratory depression from oversedation. Such minor complications can be handled with the patient in an outpatient setting. Major complication basically means rupture of the esophagus. Such rupture can occur immediately during the procedure, when the patient usually experiences sharp and persistent pain. The symptoms, however, can be insidious and therefore many prefer to regularly do a barium or gastrografin swallow after dilatation. However, the insidious course also includes the possibility of late ruptures. In these patients the rupture may occur hours or even days after the dilatation [7,8]. Therefore, it is necessary to be sure that the patient understands instructions to return immediately when symptoms like chest pain, shortness of breath, and dysphagia occur after dilatation. There does not seem to be any relation between symptoms during the dilatation and whether or not a late rupture will occur, i.e., it is not those patients who had experienced severe pain during the dilatation that will present with late rupture. However, it has been shown that early and late esophageal ruptures do predominantly occur in patients who had undergone several dilatations. Many patients experience immediate symptom relief, i.e., they can eat normally. However, the patient should be instructed to take liquids and only soft food during the day after the procedure and return to solid food the morning after. Some patients get reflux of material cranially to the dilated stenosis. Such reflux of acid material can give heartburn that can be difficult to distinguish from pain due to rupture. Many of these patients, however, are on H_2-blockers and therefore do not experience such heartburn.

Dilatation of peptic strictures of the esophagus is an outpatient procedure that can be safely done in a cooperative patient, who has been carefully instructed about possible late complications and who can reach his physician easily during the next few days after the procedure.

References

1. McLean GK, Cooper GS, Hartz WH, Burke DR, Meranze SG. Radiologically guided balloon dilatation of gastrointestinal strictures. Part I. Technique and factors influencing procedural success. Radiology 1987;165:35–40.
2. de Lange EE, Shaffer HA. Anastomotic strictures of the upper gastrointestinal tract: Results of balloon dilatation. Radiology 1988;167:45–50.
3. Maynar M, Guerra C, Reyes R et al. Esophageal strictures, balloon dilatation. Radiology 1988;167:703–706.
4. Starck E, Paolucci V, Herzer M, Crummy AB. Esophageal stenosis treatment with balloon catheters. Radiology 1984;153: 637–640.
5. Dawson SL, Mueller PR, Ferrucci JT et al. Severe esophageal strictures: Indications for balloon catheter dilatation. Radiology 1984;153:631–635.
6. McLean GK, Le Veen RF. Sheer stress in the performance of esophageal dilatation, comparison of balloon dilatation and bougienage. Radiology 1989;172:983–986.
7. La Berge JM, Kerlan RK, Pogany AC, Ring EJ. Esophageal rupture, complication of balloon dilatation. Radiology 1985; 157:56.
8. Mucci B. Oesophageal ruptures complicating balloon dilatation of strictures, a report of two cases. Br J Radiol 1991;64: 1060–1061.

What factors make it essential to consider resection?

M.B. Orringer (Ann Arbor)

More than 95% of esophageal reflux strictures can be dilated, and if the inflammatory stimulant (i.e., gastroesophageal reflux) that has caused them can be eliminated, the

acute inflammatory component will usually subside sufficiently to permit comfortable swallowing [1]. From experience, if the stricture can be dilated per os to a 40 French size, then intraoperative dilation to a 54–60 French size is usually possible. As a general rule, in order for a patient to swallow normally, an esophageal lumen with a caliber of at least 46 French is necessary, and if it is not possible to achieve this size with dilation, some degree of dysphagia will be present. Therefore, the dilatability of the stricture is not a matter of any size dilator passing through it, but a size sufficient to achieve good relief of dysphagia. Of 81 reflux strictures treated from 1977 through to 1988, the vast majority could be dilated [2]. Sixty-four were treated with intraoperative dilation and the combined Collis-Nissen procedure. Esophageal resection was performed in 17, in 3 because of inability to dilate the stricture or esophageal fracture during attempted dilation, and in the remaining 14 because of associated pathology that in my opinion precluded an antireflux procedure:
— megaesophagus from achalasia;
— severe dysplasia in Barrett's epithelium;
— caustic stricture;
— inability to perform a safe repeat fundoplication after multiple prior repairs.

The development of a reflux stricture in a megaesophagus following a prior esophagomyotomy or balloon dilation is best treated by resection. Dilation of the stricture and a fundoplication will not likely restore comfortable swallowing long term through an atonic end-stage achalasic esophagus, which is also at increased risk for malignant degeneration. The development of severe dysplasia in Barrett's mucosa is a clear indication for resectional therapy. Patients who ingest caustics in childhood may develop esophageal scarring which prevents growth of the esophagus, and as the thorax enlarges with time the esophagogastric junction is pulled into the chest, resulting in a hiatal hernia and gastroesophageal reflux. Thus, reflux esophagitis is superimposed upon the caustic stricture. While an esophageal lengthening procedure combined with a fundoplication is a possibility here, relief of dysphagia associated with panmural caustic stricture is unlikely, the risk of late carcinoma exists and resectional therapy is the best option. When a reflux stricture occurs in a patient who has had multiple prior antireflux operations, a successful outcome with yet another antireflux procedure and dilation of the stricture is not likely. For example, among 10 of our patients with reflux strictures and a history of prior antireflux surgery, treatment with dilation and a combined Collis-Nissen operation produced unsatisfactory results, due to either persistent dysphagia or recurrent reflux in 50%. We therefore regard a history of a prior antireflux operation in a patient with a reflux stricture as a risk factor for recurrence after an antireflux procedure, and we believe these patients are best treated by resection. Similarly, patients with severe strictures (those requiring very forceful dilation preoperatively) are less likely to have a good result from conservative antireflux surgery. The stricture may be dilated, but the established panmural fibrosis persists even if gastroesophageal reflux is controlled and a satisfactory result is not achieved. Resection gives a more reliable result.

While many advocate distal esophagectomy and either a short segment colon or jejunal interposition when a reflux stricture must be resected, my preference is a total thoracic esophagectomy without thoracotomy and a cervical esophagogastric anastomosis [3]. This eliminates heartburn, since without an esophagus there can be no esophagitis and clinically significant gastroesophageal reflux is seldom a problem after a properly performed cervical esophagogastric anastomosis. The functional results after esophageal replacement with stomach have been gratifying [4,5]. An intrathoracic esophagogastric anastomosis after esophageal resection for benign disease should *not* be performed, as the inevitable development of reflux esophagitis may lead to recurrent dysphagia from esophageal stenosis, as bad, if not worse, than the reasons for which the patient was originally operated upon.

References

1. Orringer MB, Stirling MC. Short esophagus and peptic stricture. In: Sabiston DC Jr, Spencer FC (eds) Surgery of the Chest, 5th edn. Philadelphia: W.B. Saunders Company, 1990;930—950.
2. Stirling MC, Orringer MB. The combined Collis-Nissen operation for esophageal reflux strictures. Ann Thorac Surg 1988;45: 148—157.
3. Orringer MB. Transhiatal esophagectomy for benign disease. J Thorac Cardiovasc Surg 1985;90:649—655.
4. Orringer MB, Stirling MC. Cervical esophagogastric anastomosis for benign disease — functional results. J Thorac Cardiovasc Surg 1988;96:887—893.
5. Orringer MB, Marshall B, Stirling MC. Transhiatal esophagectomy for benign and malignant disease. J Thorac Cardiovasc Surg 1993;105:265—277.

What are the residual indications of esophagectomy in reference to the other therapies?

J.M. Collard, M. Kint, J.B. Otte, P.J. Kestens (Brussels)

Esophageal stenosis is, with Barrett's metaplasia, dysplasia and adenocarcinoma, one of the most severe complications of gastroesophageal reflux disease (GERD). It is present in 1.2% of the patients with reflux-induced esophagitis at upper digestive tract endoscopy [1] and in 12 [2] to 30% [3] of those referred to a surgical team for management of reflux-induced esophagitis. Introduction of strong antacid medications such as omeprazole has not reduced the surgical load related to esophageal reflux-induced stenosis in Europe over the past decade [2]. Up to 35% of the patients consult for dysphagia without having any past history of heartburn [2]. A deep disorder of the esophageal body and lower sphincter motility is often detected at esophageal motility study [4].

Different therapeutic modalities may be used for reflux-induced stenosis (i.e., nonsurgical therapies such as antacid medications and endoscopic dilatation, conservative antireflux surgery and esophageal resection). The resection rate in patients operated on for esophageal reflux-induced stenosis varies from one study to another: 2% for Henderson [5], 14.2% for DeMeester [4], 16.8% for Payne [6], 18.2% in a European multicenter study [2] and 30.7% for the team of Peracchia [3].

Nonsurgical therapy

Nonsurgical therapies that are available for the management of esophageal reflux-induced stenosis are antacid medications and endoscopic dilatation.

Medical management alone with H_2-blockers cannot relieve stenosis-related dysphagia, and bougienage needs to be added [7]. Even long-term ranitidine therapy, after initial endoscopic dilatation, fails to reduce the need for subsequent dilatation [8]. However, recent introduction of omeprazole has modified the place of drug therapy in reflux-induced stenosis. So, omeprazole has been shown to be more effective than H_2-blockers in the reduction of the number of endoscopic dilatations needed per year [9]. The high efficacy of omeprazole has been demonstrated in the report of Ching [10] in which 13 of 20 patients with an esophageal stenosis unresponsive to endoscopic dilatation and antacid therapy did not require further dilatation after 40 mg daily omeprazole therapy. Another study [11] has shown that continuation of 40 mg daily omeprazole therapy in association with dilatations after initial successful medical treatment can prevent recurrence of reflux-induced stenosis. Moreover, our own gastroenterologists have evidenced the ability of omeprazole to restore peristalsis in the esophageal body after healing of severe esophagitis [12]. These data, even though preliminary, because of the small number of patients included, already yield to the surgeon the evidence that omeprazole therapy is currently one of the cornerstones of the initial management of esophageal reflux-induced stenosis.

Endoscopic dilatation, either with rubber bougies (Maloney) or with guidewire (Eder Puestow, Savary) or balloon dilators, is the most common mode of therapy of esophageal reflux-induced stenosis. Relief of dysphagia can be achieved in 85 to 100% of the patients [13–17]. Maintenance therapy with antacids and/or repeated dilatations is usually required. In experienced hands, complications such as esophageal perforation and bleeding are uncommon. In an impressive American survey, Silvis et al. [18] reported a perforation rate of 2.4% (59/23,794) and a bleeding rate of 2.3% (57/23,794). In a more recent paper, Tytgat reported a perforation rate ranging from 0 to 1.4% per session of dilatation [19]. Limited extraluminal effusion which remains confined into the mediastinum does not require emergency surgery but can be managed with abstinence of any oral intake, antibiotics and suction in the esophageal lumen [20,21]. On the contrary, prompt surgical management is mandatory in patients with a large perforation into the pleural cavity [21]. Difficulties in suturing chronically inflamed esophageal tissues can lead to esophageal resection.

Conservative antireflux surgery

There are two main indications of antireflux surgery in esophageal reflux-induced stenosis, i.e., healing of stenoses unresponsive to antacid therapy and endoscopic dilatation, and basic treatment of the gastroesophageal reflux disease by restoring effectiveness of the lower esophageal sphincter against reflux.

Different surgical techniques were applied to esophageal reflux-induced stenosis: the subdiaphragmatic Nissen fundoplication [4,22], the intrathoracic Nissen fundoplication [23], the Collis-Nissen fundoplication [24], the Collis-Belsey fundoplication [25], the Belsey fundoplication [22,26], the Toupet hemifundoplication [3] and the Thal-Nissen procedure [27].

Good to excellent results may be achieved in 80 to 100% of the patients following 360° fundoplication. Partial fundoplication seems to be less effective: success rates of 55% after Belsey fundoplication [26], 71% after Toupet hemifundoplication [3] and 76% after Collis-Belsey fundoplication [25] have been reported and in the comparative study of Dilling [22], the Belsey fundoplication has been shown to be less effective on reflux strictures than the Nissen fundoplication. Factors predisposing to failure of conservative antireflux surgery are the existence of an underlying scleroderma [3,24,28], tight stricture [24], prior unsuccessful antireflux surgery [24], shortening of the esophagus [3] and poor response to endoscopic dilatation and poor esophageal body contractility [4]. Moreover, immediate postoperative results tend to deteriorate with time [24].

Duodenal diversion is another approach to esophageal reflux-induced stenosis. Excellent postoperative results have been reported in 72–87% [29] of the patients. Excellent results rate may reach 96% when postoperative bougienage is added during the first year of follow-up [30]. Moreover, duodenal diversion has been shown to be superior to standard Nissen fundoplication as a primary treatment of severe reflux-induced esophagitis in a prospective randomized study [31]. Postoperative mortality is about 2% in large series. Postoperative digestive sequelae may be reduced by limiting the extent of the distal gastric resection. Main indications for this procedure are the existence of a shortened esophagus, bad local conditions secondary to previous surgery such as failed Heller myotomy, unsuccessful antireflux repair and poor general status precluding thoracotomy in complex situations.

Esophageal resection

Esophageal resection should be considered as an ultimate step in the therapeutic process of esophageal reflux-induced stenosis. The latter represented only 1.9% of the indications of esophageal resection in Europe over the past decade [2].

Indications are:
— stenosis unresponsive to antacid medications and dilatations [3,32];
— past history of multiple unsuccessful antireflux operations [33];
— persistent stenosis in spite of effective hiatal repair against reflux which suggests the existence of a transparietal fibrosis [3];

354

- severe motility disorder of the esophageal body and sphincter and poor response to dilatations [4,28];
- long and narrow stenosis [2];
- severe periesophagitis at operation [34];
- concomitant giant Barrett's ulcer [32];
- concomitant Barrett's high grade dysplasia [32];
- suspicion of esophageal carcinoma [35];
- esophageal perforation into the pleural cavity secondary to endoscopic dilatation [21].

Several controversies exist in the surgical literature on the modalities of resection: subtotal vs. distal esophagectomy, transthoracic vs. transhiatal approach, restoration of the digestive continuity using a colon segment vs. a gastric transplant vs. a jejunal loop.

Extent of the esophageal resection

In the past, esophageal resection was mostly limited to the distal part of the esophagus owing to the fact that reflux-induced stenosis usually develops in the lower esophagus, digestive continuity being restored using a jejunal loop [36,37], a short colon segment [37,38], or the stomach [6,39] with intrathoracic esophageal anastomosis. More recently, there was a trend for extending esophageal resection up to the cervical esophagus, probably following the large experience acquired by many surgical teams with subtotal esophagectomy for cancer [35,40–43].

A first advantage of cervical over thoracic esophageal anastomosis is a lower potential for mediastinitis from a cervical anastomotic leak [40], all the more so since intrathoracic anastomosis is often performed with more or less inflamed esophageal tissues [34]. Secondly, acid reflux into the proximal esophagus leading to stricture is a frequent complication of intrathoracic esophago-gastrostomy [39].

Approach to the esophagus

Conflicting opinions exist as to whether subtotal esophagectomy is to be carried out through a thoracic incision [37,39] or a transhiatal approach [35,40]. In many instances, both approaches may certainly be used with the same safety. However, hard periesophagitis can make transhiatal dissection difficult and hazardous. On the other hand, the final decision of esophageal resection is sometimes made at operation only, owing to the presence of close adhesions between an unsuccessful antireflux repair to be taken down and the esophageal wall itself, or evidence of iatrogenic damage to the latter due to multiple previous surgeries. In such complex situations, thoracotomy provides better exposure of the esophagus than does the transhiatal approach. More recently, the thoracic esophagus can be approached thoracoscopically through five 1 cm holes in the chest wall [44]. This new approach seems to be particularly valuable in benign diseases as there is no need for any lymph node clearance, which allows mediastinal dissection to be carried out flush to the esophageal wall far away from the respiratory airways and the descending aorta.

Esophageal substitution

Classically, esophageal surgeons use the colon for benign diseases and the stomach for malignant diseases. The main reason for this attitude is the theoretical potential of colon interposition for providing better alimentary comfort in the long run owing to preservation of the gastric reservoir. Gastric pull-up, an easier and less time-consuming technique of esophageal substitution, is usually reserved for cancer patients owing the short life expectancy of many of them. However, alimentary comfort achieved after colon interposition varies from one team to another [35,42,43,45,46] and nocturnal regurgitation is the most frequent residual complaint in the long run [35,42,43]. On the other hand, several papers have been published over the last few years reporting excellent alimentary comfort with the stomach as well [47,48]. The alimentary comfort is still better when pulling the entire stomach up to the neck rather than a gastric tube [49]. Advantages of the stomach over the colon as an esophageal substitute after esophagectomy are the need for only one anastomosis with the stomach instead of three with the colon, the potential for contamination of the operative field by the colon contents, the individual variations in the vascularity of the mesocolon predisposing to graft necrosis, the possibility of kinking of the colon segment above the diaphragm in the long run and the need for subsequent reoperation due to various problems [46]. On the other hand, the main argument used against the stomach is the high incidence of postoperative dysphagia [50]. However, dysphagia, because it is functional in origin, is usually transient [49] and real anastomotic strictures are quite responsive to a few sessions of endoscopic dilatations [48]. Moreover, anastomotic strictures are less common with the entire stomach than with the gastric tube owing to better blood supply to the anastomotic site in the former [51].

Outcome of esophageal resection

Postoperative mortality after esophagectomy dropped dramatically from a range of 15 to 30% 15 years ago to a few percent today [52]. Technical complications become less frequent while a surgical team gains experience with major esophageal surgery, and general complications such as respiratory failure or cardiovascular problems are less common in patients with a benign disease than in those cancer patients with a history of heavy tobacco and alcohol abuse. Although late functional outcome is far from being optimal in all patients, most of them, however, have a better quality of life after esophageal resection than in their previous situation when they were either taking ineffective antacid medications, were poorly improved by endoscopic dilatations, or were experiencing failure of conservative antireflux surgery.

References

1. Ben Rejeb M, Bouché O, Zeitoun P. Study of 47 consecutive patients with peptic esophageal stricture compared with 3,880 cases of reflux esophagitis. Dig Dis Sc 1992;37:733–736.
2. Collard JM, Triboulet JP, Alvarez A, Chio F. Surgical treatment of esophageal reflux-induced stenosis in Europe (314

cases). 2nd Eurosurgery Meeting, Brussels, Belgium, June 1992, Communication.

3. Bonavina L, Fontebasso V, Bardini R, Baessato M, Peracchia A. Surgical treatment of reflux stricture of the oesophagus. Br J Surg 1993;80:317–320.

4. Zaninotto G, DeMeester TR, Bremner CG, Smyrk TC, Cheng SC. Esophageal function in patients with reflux-induced strictures and its relevance to surgical treatment. Ann Thorac Surg 1989;47:362–370.

5. Henderson RD, Henderson RF, Marryatt GV. Surgical management of 100 consecutive esophageal strictures. J Thorac Cardiovasc Surg 1990;99:1–7.

6. Payne WS. Surgical management of reflux-induced oesophageal stenoses: Results in 101 patients. Br J Surg 1984;71: 971–973.

7. Ferguson R, Dronfield WA, Atkinson M. Cimetidine in treatment of reflux oesophagitis with peptic stricture. Br Med J 1979;2:472–474.

8. Farup PG, Modalsli B, Tholfsen JK. Long-term treatment with 300 mg ranitidine once daily after dilatation of peptic oesophageal strictures. Scand J Gastroenterol 1992;27:594–598.

9. Carr SJ, Wicks AC. Omeprazole and oesophageal stricture. Lancet 1992;339:316.

10. Ching CK, Shaheen MZ, Holmes GTK. Is omeprazole more effective in the treatment of resistant reflux oesophagitis and associated peptic stricture? Gastroenterology 1990;98:A30.

11. Koop H, Katschinski M, Arnold R. Conservative treatment of florid peptic esophageal stenosis. Complete elimination by dilatation and omeprazole in H_2-blocker refractory cases. Med Klin 1991;86:566–568.

12. Fiasse R. Restoration of peristaltic activity in the esophageal body after omeprazole therapy for severe reflux-induced esophagitis. Personal data.

13. Ogilvie AL, Ferguson R, Atkinson M. Outlook with conservative treatment of peptic esophageal stricture. Gut 1980;21: 23–25.

14. Wesdorp ICE, Bartelsman JFWM, Den Hartog Jager FCA, Huibregtse K, Tytgat GNJ. Results of conservative treatment of benign esophageal strictures: A follow-up study of 100 patients. Gastroenterology 1982;82:487–493.

15. Patterson DJ, Graham DY, Smith JL, Schwartz JT, Alpert E, Lanza FL, Cain GD. Natural history of benign esophageal stricture treated by dilatation. Gastroenterology 1983;85:346–350.

16. Bradpiece HA, Galland RB, Spencer J. Esophageal dilation as an outpatient procedure. Surg Gynecol Obstet 1988;167: 45–48.

17. Yamamoto H, Hughes RW, Schroeder KW, Viggiano TR, DiMagno EP. Treatment of benign esophageal stricture by Eder-Puestow or balloon dilators: A comparison between randomized and prospective nonrandomized trials. Mayo Clin Proc 1992;67:228–236.

18. Silvis SE, Nebel O, Rogers G, Sugawa C, Mandelstam P. Endoscopic complications: Result of the 1974 American Society of Gastrointestinal Endoscopy survey. JAMA 1976;235:928–930.

19. Tytgat GNJ. Dilation therapy of benign esophageal stenoses. World J Surg 1989;13:142–148.

20. Wesdorp ICE, Bartelsman JFWM, Huibregtse K, Den Hartog Jager FCA, Tytgat GNJ. Treatment of instrumental oesophageal perforation. Gut 1984;25:398–404.

21. Michel LA, Collard JM. Oesophagus: Perforation, Boerhaave's syndrome and Mallory-Weiss syndrome. In: Oxford Textbook of Surgery. Oxford: Oxford University Press, 1994; in press.

22. Dilling EW, Peyton MD, Cannon JP, Kanaly PJ, Elkins RC. Comparison of Nissen fundoplication and Belsey Mark IV in the management of gastroesophageal reflux. Am J Surg 1977;134:730–733.

23. Collard JM, de Koninck XJ, Otte JB, Fiasse RH, Kestens PJ. Intrathoracic Nissen fundoplication: Long-term clinical and pH-monitoring evaluation. Ann Thorac Surg 1991;51:34–38.

24. Stirling MC, Orringer MB. The combined Collis-Nissen operation for esophageal reflux strictures. Ann Thorac Surg 1988; 45:148–157.

25. Orringer MB, Sloan H. Complications and failings of the combined Collis-Belsey operation. J Thorac Cardiovasc Surg 1977;74:726–735.

26. Orringer MB, Skinner DB, Belsey RH. Long-term results of the Mark IV operation for hiatal hernia and analysis of recurrences and their treatment. J Thorac Cardiovasc Surg 1972;63:25–33.

27. Hollenbeck J, Woodward E. Treatment of peptic esophageal stricture with combined fundic patch-fundoplication. Ann Surg 1975;182:472–477.

28. Mansour KA, Malone CE. Surgery for scleroderma of the esophagus. A 12-year experience. Ann Thorac Surg 1988;46: 513–514.

29. Royston CMS, Dowling BL, Spencer J. Antrectomy with Roux-en-Y anastomosis in the treatment of peptic oesophagitis with stricture. Br J Surg 1975;62:605–607.

30. Salo JA, Ala-Kulju KV, Heikkinen LO, Kivilaakso EO. Treatment of severe peptic esophageal stricture with Roux-en-Y partial gastrectomy, vagotomy and endoscopic dilation. J Thorac Cardiovasc Surg 1991;101:649–653.

31. Washer GF, Gear MWL, Dowling BL, Gillison EW, Royston CMS, Spencer J. Randomized prospective trial of Roux-en-Y duodenal diversion versus fundoplication for severe reflux oesophagitis. Br J Surg 1984;71:181–184.

32. Little AG, Naunheim KS, Ferguson MK, Skinner DB. Surgical management of esophageal strictures. Ann Thorac Surg 1988;45:144–147.

33. Collard JM, DeMeester TR. Symptomatic and functional assessment of failed antireflux procedures. 28th Annual Meeting of the Society of Thoracic Surgeons, Orlando, USA, February 1992, Communication.

357

34. Collard JM, Verstraete L, Otte JB, Fiasse R, Goncette L, Kestens PJ. Clinical, radiological and functional results of remedial antireflux surgery. Int Surg 1993;78:298—306.

35. Negre J, Markkula H. Esophagectomy and colon interposition for benign esophageal stricture. Acta Chir Scand 1984;150: 639—642.

36. Polk HC. Jejunal interposition for reflux esophagitis and esophageal stricture unresponsive to valvuloplasty. World J Surg 1980;4:731—736.

37. Keenan DJM, Hamilton JRL, Gibbons J, Stevenson HM. Surgery for benign esophageal stricture. J Thorac Cardiovasc Surg 1984;88:182—188.

38. Otte JB, Lerut T, Collard JM, Breckx JF, Kestens PJ, Gruwez J. Les plasties coliques de l'oesophage. Acta Chir Belg 1982;82:389—396.

39. Raptis S, Mearns-Milne D. A review of the management of 100 cases of benign strictures of the esophagus. Thorax 1972; 27:599—603.

40. Orringer MB. Transhiatal esophagectomy for benign disease. J Thorac Cardiovasc Surg 1985;90:649—655.

41. Waters PF, Pearson FG, Todd TR, Patterson GA, Goldberg M, Ginsberg RJ, Cooper JD, Ramirez J, Miller L. Esophagectomy for complex benign esophageal disease. J Thorac Cardiovasc Surg 1988;95:378—381.

42. Neville WE, Najem AZ. Colon replacement of the esophagus for congenital and benign disease. Ann Thorac Surg 1983;36: 626—633.

43. Isolauri J. Colonic interposition for benign esophageal disease. Long-term clinical and endoscopic results. Am J Surg 1988;155:498—502.

44. Collard JM, Lengele B, Malaise J, Otte JB, Kestens PJ. En bloc esophagectomy for cancer by thoracoscopy. In: Brown W (ed) Atlas of Thoracoscopic Surgery. St. Louis: Saunders Medical Publishing, 1993; in press.

45. DeMeester TR, Johansson KE, Franze I et al. Indications, surgical techniques and long-term functional results of colon interposition or by-pass. Ann Surg 1988;208:460—474.

46. Curet-Scott MJ, Ferguson MK, Little AG, Skinner DB. Colon interposition for benign esophageal disease. Surgery 1987; 102:568—574.

47. Couraud L, Hafez-Alqudah A, Clerc P, Meriot S. Use of tubular isoperistaltic gastroplasty after total or partial esophagectomy. In: Delarue NC, Wilkins EW, Wong J (eds) International Trends in General Thoracic Surgery, vol 4. St. Louis: The C.V. Mosby Company, 1988;186—189.

48. Collard JM, Otte JB, Reynaert M, Kestens PJ. Quality of life three or more years following esophagectomy for cancer. J Thorac Cardiovasc Surg 1992;104:391—394.

49. Collard JM, Otte JB, Kestens PJ. Gastric pull-up to the neck after total or subtotal esophagectomy. A comparison of two methods of reconstruction. 93rd Congress of the Japan Society of Surgery, Sendai, Japan, April 1993, Communication.

50. Orringer MB, Stirling MC. Cervical esophagogastric anastomosis for benign disease. Functional results. J Thorac Cardiovasc Surg 1988;96:887—893.

51. Collard JM, Otte JB, Kestens PJ. Reconstruction after esophagectomy. In: Steichen F and Welter R (eds) Minimally Invasive Surgery and New Technology. St. Louis: Quality Medical Publishing Inc., 1994;114:629—636.

52. Collard JM, Otte JB, Reynaert M, Michel L, Carlier MA, Kestens PJ. Esophageal resection and by-pass. A 6-year experience with a low postoperative mortality. World J Surg 1991;15:635—641.

Therapeutic strategy

What are the goals of treatment in reflux esophagitis?

J.E. Richter (Birmingham, Alabama)

The goals of treatment in gastroesophageal reflux disease (GERD) are the following:
— relieve the symptoms of GERD;
— heal and prevent the relapse of mucosal lesions (i.e., esophagitis);
— prevent the complications of long-term esophagitis, such as strictures ulcerations, bleeding and columnar metaplasia.
These goals are easy to establish, but efficacy of the therapies and scientific data supporting the obtainability of these goals decrease as we progress from controlling symptoms to preventing complications. Furthermore, these goals are set against a complex background — GERD is a chronic condition that tends to wax and wane in intensity and relapses are common.

Relief of symptoms

From the patient's viewpoint, relief of symptoms is the most important reason for seeking medical attention. Fortunately, the currently available medical and surgical therapies should allow this to be accomplished in all patients both acutely and long term. In patients presenting with reflux symptoms and no esophagitis, this is the only goal. In approximately 20–30% of patients, this may be accomplished by lifestyle changes, antacids or alginic acid [1]. Whether the latter two drugs are better than placebo is controversial, nevertheless this is a rather small point if patients obtain relief of their heartburn. Prokinetics drugs (bethanechol, metoclopramide, domperidone and cisapride) have been shown to produce greater relief of symptoms compared to placebo in controlled studies [2]. Clinically, they are efficacious, but only in mild to moderate reflux disease. The cornerstone of medical therapy for GERD is the H_2-blockers. All are equally effective when used at proper dosages, usually with a twice a day dosing regimen. Overall, 50–70% of symptomatic patients have complete or partial resolution of symptoms with H_2-blockers [3]. Higher dosages of H_2-blockers marginally improve on these results in patients with more severe symptoms. However, I believe the drug of choice in these latter patients are the proton pump inhibitors. Symptomatic responses with omeprazole are seen in 60–95% of cases [3]. Unlike the H_2-blockers where partial symptom relief is the rule, omeprazole usually totally relieves all symptoms allowing the patients to enjoy many previously prohibited foods and sleep without head elevation. To obtain this goal, some patients may require higher doses of omeprazole in the range of 40 to 80 mg per day. Long-term symptom relief is more problematic. Patients with mild symptoms will remain in remission with H_2-blockers or cisapride, usually given b.i.d.. Those with severe symptomatic disease will require omeprazole or antireflux surgery.

Healing of esophagitis

Today most cases of acute reflux esophagitis can be healed. However, this frequently requires marked acid suppression for a prolonged period of time. The key to treating and healing reflux esophagitis is the initial esophagitis grade. The more severe the grade of esophagitis, the stronger the acid suppression and the longer the duration of therapy required to heal the mucosal lesions.

Antacids, alginic acids and most prokinetics drugs have no predicable reliability in healing even mild esophagitis [1,2]. Data with cisapride is more equivocal. European studies show healing of even severe esophagitis after 12 weeks of therapy, while studies in the United States show minimal efficacy primarily in grade II esophagitis [2]. Recent reviews of the literature suggest that healing rates with H_2-blockers rarely exceed 60% after 12 weeks of treatment, even when higher than standard dosages are used [3,4]. Healing rates differ considerably in individual trials and depend mostly on the degree of esophagitis before therapy. Savary grade I esophagitis is reported to heal in 75–90% of patients after most treatments while grade II heals only in 40–50% of patients during treatment with H_2-blockers [5]. Omeprazole has become the drug of choice for treating severe esophagitis or esophagitis unresponsive to H_2-blockers [3]. Five well-designed trials comparing omeprazole 20–60 mg/day with ranitidine 150 mg b.i.d. for healing grade II–IV esophagitis, have uniformly demonstrated significantly better results for the omeprazole treated groups. Healing at 4 weeks in the omeprazole groups ranged from 67–85% vs. 26–45% for ranitidine; healing at 8 weeks in the omeprazole groups ranged from 85–96% vs. 40–66% for ranitidine. Five studies of similar design have evaluated more than 300 patients with esophagitis unresponsive to H_2-blockers and uniformly found that omeprazole 40 mg/day will successfully heal nearly 90% of these patients within 12 weeks.

There is growing awareness that most patients with healed erosive-ulcerative esophagitis will relapse within 6 to 9 months after discontinuation of drug therapy. Therefore maintenance therapy is unanimously recommended, but its efficacy is yet to be conclusively proven. Recent studies suggest that cisapride 20 mg b.i.d. may be superior to placebo in keeping mild grade II esophagitis in remission for up to 6 months [6]. H_2-blockers are also likely to be effective for mild to moderate disease, but require full twice daily dosages regimens. Patients with severe esophagitis will require maintenance therapy with omeprazole. Most will require 20 mg/day, some may be controlled on 10 mg/day, while a smaller group will require at least 40 mg/day [7]. Holiday therapy (3—4 days out of the week) does not seem to be effective.

Prevention of complications

Although it is logical and physiologically sensible, little data is available showing that aggressive medical therapy prevents the development of complicated GERD. Furthermore, many of our patients have well established complicated disease at the time of presentation, which may be beyond relief with either medical or surgical treatments.

Aggressive medical therapy can heal esophageal ulcers and prevent recurrent bleeding [8]. Recent studies in our laboratory suggest that omeprazole can resolve many peptic strictures associated with esophagitis and keep these patients dysphagia free for up to 6 months [9]. However, long-term studies are not available. Barrett's esophagus is more problematic and the major complication that should be prevented. Studies in dogs suggest that severe esophagitis often heals with the development of columnar metaplasia. However, esophagitis, in this animal model, heals with the persistence of squamous mucosa if acid reflux is markedly inhibited [10]. This supports the use of aggressive acid suppression in patients with severe esophagitis, either high dose H_2-blockers or omeprazole. Although formal studies are not available, the clinical experience of most gastroenterologists support these animal observations since Barrett's esophagus rarely develops de novo or progresses after effective control of esophagitis. Having said this, there is little convincing data that either omeprazole or surgery predictably produces regression of Barrett's esophagus once it is established.

References

1. Kitchin LI, Castell DO. Rationale and efficacy of conservative therapy for gastroesophageal reflux disease. Arch Int Med 1991;151:48—54.
2. Ramirez B, Richter JE. Review article: promotility drugs in the treatment of gastroesophageal reflux disease. Aliment Pharmacol Ther 1993;7:5—20.
3. Sontag SJ. The medical management of reflux esophagitis; role of antacids and acid inhibition. Gastroenterol Clin North Am 1990;19(3):683—710.

4. Tytgat GNJ, Nio CY. Medical therapy of reflux esophagitis. Gastroenterology 1987;1:791−807.
5. Koelz HR. Treatment of reflux esophagitis with H_2 blockers, antacids and prokinetic drugs. An analysis of randomized clinical trials. Scand J Gastroenterol 1989;24(suppl 156):25−36.
6. Tytgat GNJ, Anker Hansen OJ, Carling L et al. Effective cisapride on relapse of reflux esophagitis, healed with an anti-secretory drug. Scand J Gastroenterol 1992;27:175−183.
7. Klinkenberg-Knol EC, Jansen JBMJ, Lamers CBHW et al. Use of omeprazole in the management of reflux esophagitis resistant to H_2 receptor antagonists. Scand J Gastroenterol 1989;24:(suppl 116):88−96.
8. Cooper BT, Barbezat GO. Barrett's esophagus: a clinical study of 52 patients. Q J Med 1987;238:97−108.
9. Marks R, Richter JE, Koehler R, Spenney J, Mills T. Does medical therapy improve dysphagia in patients with peptic strictures and esophagitis? Gastroenterology 1992;102:A118.
10. Dent J, Bremner CG, Collen MJ, Haggitt RC, Spechler SJ. Barrett's esophagus. Working party report to the World Congress of Gastroenterology. Sydney, 1990. J Gastroenterol Hepatol 1991;6:1−22.

Should the inadequate effects of antisecretory treatment be related to persistence of the aggressive action of alkaline secretions?

H. Feussner, H.J. Stein, J.R. Siewert (Munich)

It is a well-known fact that some cases of severe reflux esophagitis are refractory to antisecretory treatment, even if ion-pump inhibitors are used. As different groups were able to demonstrate, most of these cases not responding to medical treatment were particularly severe [1,2]. The failure of medical treatment cannot sufficiently be explained by a low compliance of the patient alone. There is some data suggesting that the presence of H^+ ions is not the only aggressive agent leading to severe mucosal damage, since even under a complete elimination of acidity reflux esophagitis does not heal. Based upon experimental observations, bile acids, lecitine and enzymes are considered as auxiliary or additional toxic components of the refluxate. Unfortunately, this could not yet be evaluated under clinical conditions, since no diagnostic tool was available to collect human refluxate and to examine its components. This gap could be closed by the use of a portable suction pump with a specially designed "open flow" aspiration probe.

Ambulatory esophageal reflux aspiration

Ambulatory reflux aspiration is performed using a specially designed double catheter system, which is placed 5 cm above the manometrically determined lower esophageal sphincter (LES) (Fig. 1). The inner aspiration catheter (diameter 6 French) is connected to a portable aspiration pump set to a negative pressure of 100 mmHg (Fig. 2). Suction of the catheter against the esophageal wall is prevented by an outer

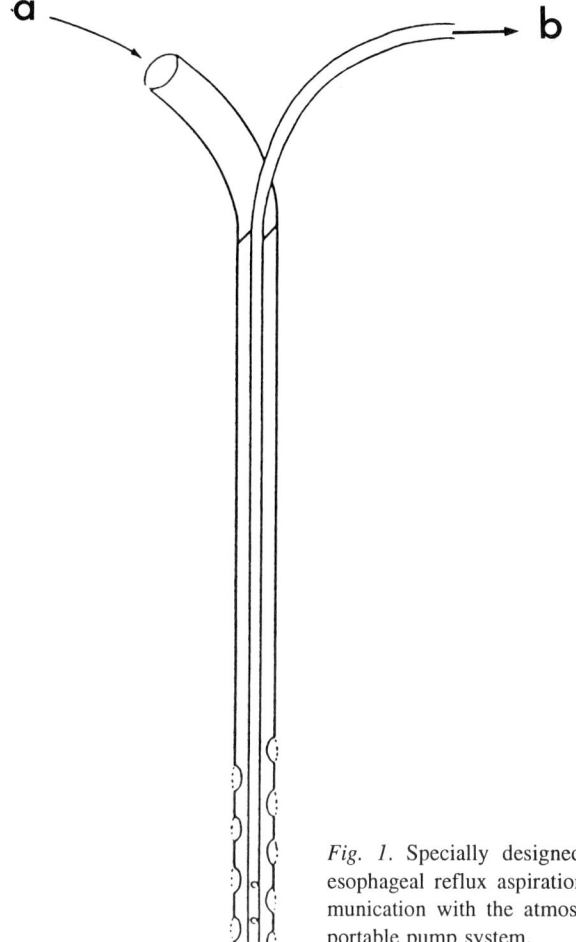

Fig. 1. Specially designed "open flow" suction probe for the esophageal reflux aspiration test; a: Outer hose allows free communication with the atmosphere; b: Inner hose connected to the portable pump system.

perforated 15 French catheter with free communication with the outer atmosphere. Extensive validation studies have shown that this design prevents occlusion of the aspiration catheter by the esophageal mucosa, does not alter the intragastric pressure environment or induce reflux, but leads to aspiration of all liquids that stay in the distal esophagus for more than 6 s and enter the space between the two catheters [3]. Using radiolabeled liquids, it could be demonstrated that less than 1.5% of swallowed food or saliva is collected in the aspiration pump, while reflux episodes lasting longer than 6 s are aspirated at a maximum rate of 1.45 ml/s. This is because full suction is activated only about 4–6 s after contact between the intraesophageal fluid and the aspiration catheter [4].

Reflux aspirates were collected in separate containers during a 3-h postprandial period, an 8-h interdigestive upright period and an 8-h supine sleeping period. Each fraction was assessed for volume, total bile acid concentration and the activity of

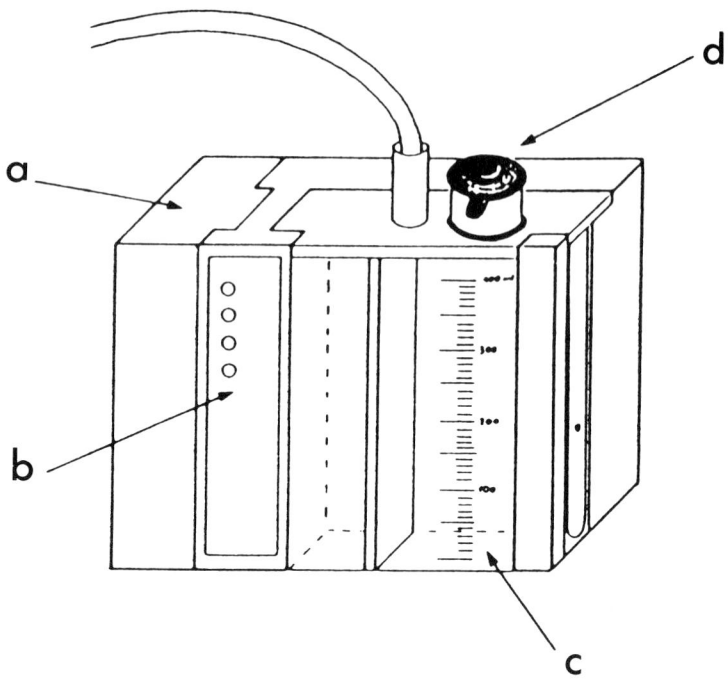

Fig. 2. Portable pump system; a: Rechargeable battery; b: Control panel; c: Exchangeable fluid container; d: Vacuum indicator.

trypsin. The total bile acid concentration in the aspirates was determined enzymatically and considered as increased when it exceeded the 95th percentile of levels measured in normal volunteers (i.e., 88 µmol/l). The activity of trypsin was measured photometrically using a standard test set.

The test system was applied on 43 normal volunteers and 52 patients with gastroesophageal reflux disease (GERD) (proven by pH-monitoring). Endoscopically, no signs of mucosal damage could be found in 14 of the patients, 25 had an erosive esophagitis and 13 of them suffered from reflux esophagitis, complicated by strictures and/or ulceration. The latter conditions were associated with Barrett's esophagus in 10 cases.

Results of long-term pH-monitoring and the ambulatory reflux aspiration test

The mean aspiration volumes, bile acid concentration, and activity of trypsin in the reflux aspirates of the normal volunteers and patients with GERD during the interdigestive upright, postprandial and supine periods were compared. The total bile acid concentration during the postprandial and supine period was significantly increased in patients with GERD. There were no other significant differences between the groups (Table 1).

Table 1. Aspiration volume, bile acid concentration and pancreatic enzymes in the ambulatory esophageal reflux aspirates of asymptomatic volunteers (n = 43) and patients with GERD (n = 52)

	Normal volunteers (n = 43)	Patients with GERD (n = 52)
Aspiration volume (ml/h)		
Upright	7.7 ± 2.0	7.0 ± 1.3
Postprandial	12.7 ± 3.1	15.1 ± 3.6
Supine	3.9 ± 0.7	5.2 ± 0.9
Bile acid concentration (µmol/l)		
Upright	5.2 ± 1.8	12.1 ± 4.8
Postprandial	11.8 ± 4.4	72.3 ± 23.4[a]
Supine	6.7 ± 1.9	107.7 ± 24.6[a]
Trypsine (U/l)		
Upright	3.4 ± 0.7	2.0 ± 0.3
Postprandial	1.7 ± 0.3	2.7 ± 0.6
Supine	0.8 ± 0.3	2.5 ± 0.4

Values are mean ± SEM, [a]$p < 0.05$ vs. volunteers.

In patients with GERD, the total bile acid concentration in the reflux aspirates was highest during the supine period and showed a significant correlation with the extent of the mucosal lesion (Fig. 3). Of the five patients with increased esophageal

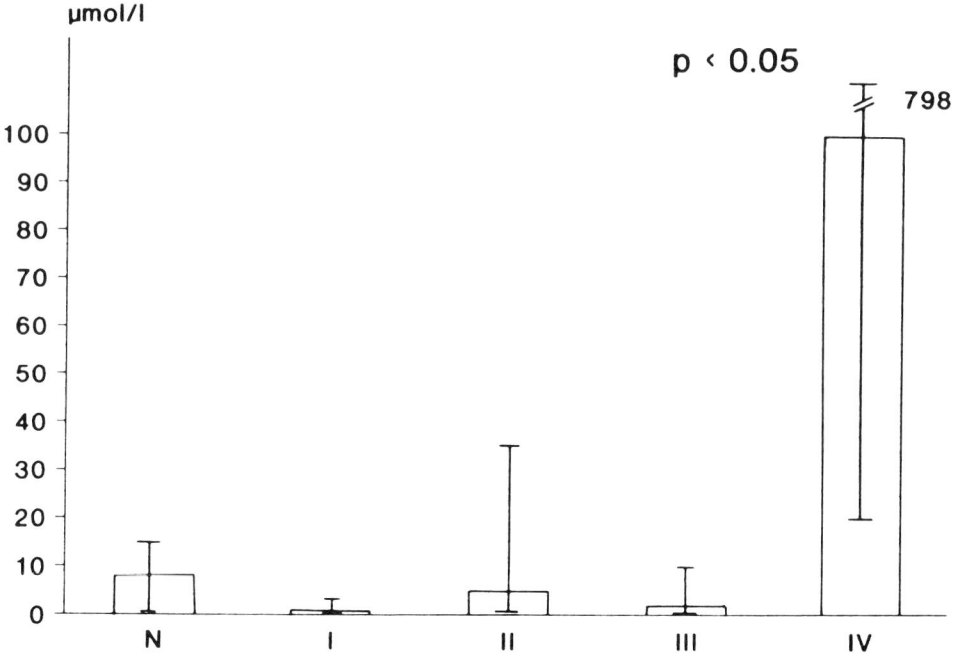

Fig. 3. Total bile acid concentration in normals (N) and patients with different grades of reflux disease (I–IV according to the modified Savary-Miller classification) [5].

exposure to pH > 7, four (80%) had increased bile acid concentration in their reflux aspirates. Of the nine patients with increased bile acid concentration on reflux aspiration, four also had an increased percentage of time pH > 7, on pH-monitoring.

Compared to normal volunteers and patients with no esophageal mucosal injury, the bile acid concentration in the reflux aspirate and the % time pH > 7 on pH-monitoring were particularly increased in patients with stricture or Barrett's esophagus (p < 0.001).

Conclusion

The present data confirm previous reports of an increased esophageal exposure to nonacid factors (in particular bile acids) in patients with severe mucosal lesions. It has to be assumed that conventional antisecretory agents will not be able to protect the mucosa from their detrimental effect, which sufficiently explains why some cases of reflux esophagitis do not heal under medical treatment. In these cases, surgical therapy is the only means to control the disease effectively.

References

1. Hill ADK, O'Donoghue DP. Omeprazole in refractory reflux esophagitis. Gullet 1991;1:81–83.
2. Bardhan KD, Morris P, Thompson M et al. Value of omeprazole in the management of erosive esophagitis refractory to high doses cimetidine. Gut 1987;28:A1375.
3. Feussner H, Weiser HF, Liebermann-Meffert D, Siewert JR. Intestinoösophagealer Reflux nach Gastrektomie. Chirurg 1988; 59:665–669.
4. Stein HJ, Feussner H, Barthlen W, DeMeester TR, Siewert JR. Alkalischer gastroösophagealer Reflux – Quantifizierung und Klinische Relevanz. Langenbecks Arch Chir 1992;377:87–91.
5. Siewert JR, Ottenjann R, Heilmann K, Neiss A, Doepfer H. Therapie und Prophylaxe der Refluxösophagitis. Z Gastroenterol 1986;24:381.

Can the role of acid suppression in the treatment of GERD be accurately precised?

C.W. Howden (Columbia)

Although gastric acid secretion is normal in the majority of patients with gastroesophageal reflux disease (GERD), it is generally accepted that prolonged exposure of the esophageal mucosa to acidic gastric contents is responsible for most of the manifestations of this condition. Therefore, pharmacological inhibition of gastric acid secretion is a common means of treating the condition.

In the treatment of duodenal ulcer, there is a direct relationship between suppression of gastric acidity and healing rates confirmed at endoscopy [1]. This has been fairly simple to demonstrate because of an easily determined treatment end-point (viz., a healed ulcer) and a wealth of published observations from endoscopically-controlled clinical trials.

In the management of GERD the situation is more complex. This is a more heterogeneous condition with gradations in the severity of esophagitis and some disparity of agreement on what constitutes satisfactory healing. However, using results of well-conducted clinical trials of antisecretory medications in the management of GERD, it has been possible to distinguish a relationship between reduction in acidity and healing of erosive esophagitis [2]. Endoscopic healing rates are significantly correlated with reduction in 24-h intragastric acidity and with control of 24-h intraesophageal acid exposure. In turn, these two parameters correlate with each other so that reduction of intragastric acidity is, as might be expected, associated with reduced exposure of the esophageal mucosa to acid.

If intraesophageal pH is only allowed to fall below 4 for 2%, or less, of the 24-h day, healing rates of erosive esophagitis will be maximal. Acid pump inhibitors are more able to achieve this than conventional doses of H_2-receptor antagonists (H_2RA), since the latter are less effective in suppressing daytime gastric acid secretion stimulated by food intake. To date, there have been no controlled trials comparing the efficacy of an acid pump inhibitor with an approved higher dose of an H_2RA.

Increasing degrees of inhibition of acid secretion are associated with higher overall healing rates of esophagitis in GERD [2], as well as with more rapid healing.

References

1. Burget DG, Howden CW et al. Is there an optimal degree of acid suppression for healing of duodenal ulcers? Gastroenterology 1990;99:345—351.
2. Bell NJ, Burget DG, Howden CW, Wilkinson J, Hunt RH. Appropriate acid suppression for the management of gastroesophageal reflux disease. Digestion 1992;51(suppl 1):59—67.

What are the protective effects of sucralfate?

S. Sloan (Chicago)

Sucralfate has been shown to be effective for the treatment of peptic ulcer disease. The importance and effectiveness as an agent for the treatment of erosive esophagitis is not as well established compared to H_2 antagonists or proton pump inhibitors.

Sucralfate is an aluminum salt of sucrose-octasulfate. It is a relatively safe compound and has minimal side effects. Constipation is one of the more common side effects and because of the aluminum hydroxide salt, caution should be used in patients with renal insufficiency.

The mechanism of action for this compound in acid-peptic disease is multifactorial. Sucralfate forms stable complexes with protein. This occurs in damaged mucosa where there is a high concentration of protein, either from fibrinogen, albumin, or globulins from the exudate of an ulcer or from leaky damaged cells. In an acidic environment, sucralfate becomes viscous and partially dissociates into sucrose sulfate and aluminum hydroxide. The sucrose sulfate portion is an anion and thus forms polyvalent bridges with the positively charged proteins in the damaged mucosa [1]. There is evidence that the sucralfate interferes with the action of pepsin [1]. There are numerous mechanisms proposed to account for this. Firstly, sucralfate may form a complex with protein substrates, thus preventing pepsin from digesting them. Secondly, sucralfate may bind to pepsin. Thirdly, sucralfate may provide a barrier to prevent diffusion of pepsin. Finally, sucralfate may restrict the availability of hydrogen ions necessary for the activation of pepsin. This binding action to damaged mucosa has been demonstrated clinically using Technetium labeled sucralfate in detecting erosive esophagitis. This labeling of the esophagus best occurred when there were significant deep lesions and that in lesser degrees of esophagitis there was minimal adherence of the labeled compound [2]. Due to the potential antacid benefit of the hydroxide ion in sucralfate, studies have been done to assess whether the sucrose-octasulfate portion has any therapeutic value in experimental esophagitis models. In an ex-vivo model, rabbit esophagi in isolated tissue preparations were exposed to acid and electrical resistance was continuously measured [3]. Acidification alone decreased the electrical resistance indicating tissue damage, however, when sucralfate was added, the resistance returned to baseline levels. In addition, when aluminum hydroxide was added to the acidified bath the resistance increased along with the luminal pH. This beneficial effect was abolished when the pH was titrated with HCl to maintain pH similar to acid treated control tissue. The sucrose-octasulfate component of sucralfate prevented acid induced decline in electrical resistance. Therefore, it seems that there is a two pronged attack regarding the effects of sucralfate. One is the buffering action of the aluminum hydroxide ion, and the other is the prevention of tissue disruption demonstrated by electrical resistance with the sucrose-octasulfate. Another potential mechanism of sucralfate is that it may provide a barrier for bile salts. Sucralfate is known to stimulate prostaglandin production in the gastric epithelium. This may be a potential secondary effect for sucralfate in the esophagus. The role of prostaglandins in the development of esophagitis is controversial.

Clinical usefulness of sucralfate has been studied. In rabbits, esophagitis induced by acid and pepsin was prevented using sucralfate concurrently [4]. In another animal study, cats pretreated with liquid sucralfate prior to acid infusion were protected against esophagitis [5]. Numerous studies in humans have compared sucralfate to other forms of therapy including alginic acid/antacid, cimetidine and ranitidine. Two separate studies have shown that sucralfate is as effective as Gaviscon with regards to healing of esophagitis and symptomatic improvement [6,7]. The studies involving H$_2$ antagonists also demonstrate equal efficacy compared to sucralfate in treating reflux esophagitis. When directly compared to cimetidine, sucralfate has consistently been equally as efficacious in healing as well as in symptomatic improvement. The healing rates were around 50% for sucralfate and were comparable to cimetidine [8,9]. Most importantly, the higher grades of esophagitis did not respond with regard to healing compared to lower grades of esophagitis. Similarly, in studies comparing the efficacy of sucralfate to ranitidine, there were no significant differences between the two drugs [10,11]. Again, the endoscopic healing was much better when patients started the study with a lower grade of esophagitis. When sucralfate is compared to placebo, there are conflicting data with regard to therapeutic benefit. One report found that after 12 weeks of treatment, sucralfate was superior to placebo in healing esophagitis but not significantly better than placebo in relieving symptoms [12]. In another trial of 8 weeks duration, sucralfate was not significantly different than placebo in healing esophagitis or in relieving symptoms. However, those patients with the most severe esophagitis were in the sucralfate arm and had more endoscopic improvement than the placebo arm [13]. Additionally, in a more recent 12-week trial, sucralfate was found to be superior to placebo in relieving symptoms but not significantly different than placebo in healing esophagitis [14]. Thus there is a discrepancy in the overall effectiveness in the use of sucralfate in patients with reflux esophagitis. It may be that the ineffectiveness of sucralfate is related to the amount of time it is retained in the esophagus. In the Technetium labeled sucralfate study mentioned above, sucralfate is retained within the esophagus for 3 h in less than 50% of the patients with reflux esophagitis [2]. Since an acidic environment is necessary for sucralfate to be effective, ingestion of the drug in a nonacidified esophagus will be rapidly cleared and poorly timed to provide protection against reflux injury [15]. Another use for sucralfate has been, in more specialized instances of esophagitis, either due to pill ingestion, post sclerotherapy ulcers, or bile induced esophagitis. The use in these situations has not been substantiated.

In summary, sucralfate when administered as a treatment for patients with reflux esophagitis should be used in a suspension form. The clinical utility is equivalent to lower dose H$_2$-blocker therapy and Gaviscon with regard to esophagitis healing and improvement of symptoms. Patients with more severe esophagitis may have better adherence of the sucralfate to the damaged mucosa, however, healing rates are poor.

References

1. Nagashima R. Mechanisms of action of sucralfate. J Clin Gastroenterol 1981;3(suppl 2):117−127.
2. Goff JS, Adcock KA, Schmelter R. Detection of esophageal ulcerations with Technetium-99m albumin sucralfate. J Nucl Med 1986;27:1143−1146.
3. Orlando RC et al. Mucosal protection by sucralfate and its componenets in acid-exposed rabbit esophagus. Gastroenterology 1987;93:352−361.
4. Schweitzer EJ et al. Sucralfate prevents experimental peptic esophagitis in rabbits. Gastroenterology 1985;88:611−619.
5. Clark S et al. Comparison of potential cytoprotective action of sucralfate and cimetidine. Am J Med 1987;83(suppl 3B): 56−60.
6. Laitinen S et al. Sucralfate and alginate/antacid in reflux esophagitis. Scand J Gastroenterol 1985;20:229−232.
7. Evreux M. Sucralfate versus alginate/antacid in the treatment of peptic esophagitis. Am J Med 1987;83(3B):48−50.

8. Tytgat GNJ. Clinical efficacy of sucralfate in reflux esophagitis. Comparison with cimetidine. Am J Med 1987;83:38—42.
9. Ros E et al. Healing of erosive esophaitis with sucralfate and cimetidine: influence of pretreatment lower esophageal sphincter pressure and serum pepsinogen levels. Am J Med 1991;91(suppl 2A):107S—113S.
10. Simon B, Mueller P. Comparison of the effect of sucralfate and ranitidine in reflux esophagitis. Am J Med 1987;83(suppl 3B):43—47.
11. Bremner CG et al. Reflux esophagitis therapy: sucralfate versus ranitidine in a double blind multicenter trial. Am J Med 1992;91(suppl 2A);119S—122S.
12. Weiss W et al. Therapie der refluxösophagitis mit sucralfat. Dtsch Med Wochenschr 1983;108:1706—1711.
13. Williams RM et al. Multicenter trial of sucralfate suspension for the treatment of reflux esophagitis. Am J Med 1987; 83(suppl 3B):61—66.
14. Carling L et al. Sucralfate versus placebo in reflux esophagitis. A double-blind multicenter study. Scand J Gastroenterol 1988;23:1117—1124.
15. Orlando RC. Sucralfate therapy and relfux esophagitis: an overview. Am J Med 1991;91(suppl 2A):123S—124S.

What is the cytoprotective action of carbenoxolone?

G.P. Young (Melbourne)

Chemistry of carbenoxolone

Carbenoxolone is a relatively unique compound — hemisuccinate of the natural terpenoid 18β-glycyrrhetic acid (enoxolone) [1]. It is highly lipophilic, crosses cell membranes readily, and has high affinity for plasma proteins.

Oral administration is followed by rapid absorption from stomach and small intestine. Its plasma half-life in normal subjects <65 years old is 15 h. Ninety-eight per cent of a dose is excreted in bile, as glucuronide conjugates.

Mechanism of action

Studies of its mechanism of action have focused primarily on gastric mucosa, even though it has a therapeutic benefit for duodenal ulcer and esophagitis as well [2]. These actions have been reviewed by Parke [1], and fall into three broad categories: effects on mucus, on cell kinetics and on the gastric mucosal barrier.

In 1967, it was shown that carbenoxolone-treated patients had increased mucus in gastric pits [3]. Subsequently, it was shown that carbenoxolone increased mucus synthesis in human gastric mucosa, and some animal species [1]. This was particularly attributed to an increase in the N-acetylneuraminic acid-containing mucoproteins, and was suggested to be due to stimulation of microsomal glycosyl transferases by carbenoxolone.

Carbenoxolone has been shown by a number of investigators in the 1970s [1] to prolong the half-life of gastric mucosal cells by reducing the rate of cell turnover, to decrease DNA synthesis and to diminish epithelial exfoliation. Importantly, this effect is seen in the inflamed mucosa of patients with astrophic gastritis, when biopsies are treated with carbenoxolone in organ culture [4].

Carbenoxolone pretreatment reduces peptic activity and acid secretion in pyloric-ligated rats, and reduces the damaging effect of aspirin on gastric mucosal permeability in humans [5]. Carbenoxolone also reduces net H^+ back diffusion across human gastric mucosa. Thus, in the stomach, carbenoxolone can be considered as a cytoprotective agent.

Carbenoxolone appears to have less marked effects on duodenal than gastric mucus [1], and its action on duodenal epithelial kinetics are unknown. There is no information on its action on esophageal squamous mucosa, although interestingly, it is still available in some countries as an oral preparation (Bioral) for treating oral aphthous ulcers.

Delivering carbenoxolone to the esophagus

The route of action of carbenoxolone has long been considered to be topical on the mucosa. The reasons put forward to support this contention are its lipophilic nature and rapid absorption, its improved efficacy in duodenal ulcer when given in a delayed-release capsule [6], and its lack of effect on gastric mucus secretion when exposure to gastric mucosa is minimized by delivery to duodenum in the delayed-release capsule [7]. The relationship between serum levels and healing of duodenal ulcer does not disprove the concept that it acts topically [6].

The observations that a liquid carbenoxolone preparation without other additives was of inconsistent value in esophagitis [8] led to testing of the possibility that more effective delivery of the drug to the esophagus might be of benefit. Thus a combined alginate/carbenoxolone preparation was developed in an attempt to achieve this by reflux of the viscous carbenoxolone-containing alginate gel [9].

Carbenoxolone in reflux esophagitis

Using a "low-dose" antacid/alginate/carbenoxolone preparation in a single-center controlled trial on 37 patients with reflux esophagitis, carbenoxolone appeared to hasten symptom relief and endoscopic evidence of healing [10]. The number of patients who showed resolution of symptoms was 89% compared to 50% of alginate/antacid-treated controls ($p < 0.025$). Healing occurred endoscopically in 95% vs. 67% ($p < 0.05$). A subsequent uncontrolled study of a large number of patients confirmed these findings [8].

A subsequent formulation of Pyrogastrone® containing 20 mg carbenoxolone, 600 mg alginic acid, 60 mg magnesium trisilicate, 240 mg aluminum hydroxide and 210 mg sodium bicarbonate was released. Tablets were to be chewed before swallowing, one 3 times daily after meals and two at night. This "high-dose" (in terms of antacid and alginate) formulation was compared to antacid/alginate alone in a double-blind multicenter study of 59 patients [8]. Carbenoxolone treated patients showed an 82% improvement in symptom grades over 8 weeks compared to 63% in controls — a 50% faster rate of improvement (p < 0.01). Both groups showed similar significant endoscopic evidence of healing during the first 4 weeks but this improvement was sustained during the second 4 weeks, only in the carbenoxolone-treated group (p < 0.05).

In this study, few side effects occurred. No patient developed edema or renal or hepatic failure. Only one patient on carbenoxolone developed mild hypokalemia. Thus, carbenoxolone in alginate/antacid preparations does offer some therapeutic advantage. In carefully selected and observed patients, the side-effect profile is low.

Carbenoxolone — its role in the 1990s

There have been no direct comparisons of carbenoxolone with H_2-receptor antagonists, proton-pump inhibitors or prokinetic agents in reflux esophagitis. It may be that Pyrogastrone compares well with the earlier, less potent H_2-receptor antagonists, but it seems unlikely that it will compare favorably with the more recent drugs, especially the proton-pump inhibitors. Certainly its side effect profile of mineralocorticoid-like effects (fluid retention, hypokalemia) put it at a disadvantage.

There is some information to suggest that carbenoxolone has an antiviral action (Dr S. Gottfried, personal communication); whether such an effect would be sufficient to be of value in viral esophagitis is completely unknown.

Conclusion

Carbenoxolone is a topically active, cytoprotective agent in the upper gastrointestinal tract. It has a modest but significant effect on symptoms and endoscopic evidence of reflux esophagitis. However, with the advent of more effective and safer agents, it can only be viewed from a historical perspective at this time.

References

1. Parke DV. Some recent advances in the pharmacology of carbenoxolone. In: Jones FA, Langman MJS, Mann RD (eds) Peptic Ulcer Healing. Recent Studies on Carbenoxolone. Lancaster: MTP Press Ltd, 1978;1—8.
2. Jones FA, Langman MJS, Mann RD. Peptic Ulcer Healing. Recent Studies on Carbenoxolone. Lancaster: MTP Press Ltd, 1978;1—151.
3. Goodier TEW, Horwich L, Galloway RW. Morphologic observations of gastric ulcers treated with carbenoxolone sodium. Gut 1967;8:544 547.
4. Klein HJ, Frotz H, Gheorghiu T. Mechanism of action of carbenoxolone. Autoradiographic study of proliferation in vitro of epithelial cells from gastric mucosa of carbenoxolone-treated patients. In: Jones FA, Parke DV (eds) Fourth Symposium on Carbenoxolone. London: Butterworths, 1975;161—170.
5. Hossenbocus A, Colin-Jones DG. Protection of the human gastric mucosa from aspirin by carbenoxolone. In: Jones FA, Parke DV (eds) Fourth Symposium on Carbenoxolone. London: Butterworths, 1975;91—102.
6. Young GP, St John DJB, Coventry DA. Treatment of duodenal ulcer with carbenoxolone sodium: A double-masked endoscopic trial. Med J Aust 1979;1:2—5.

7. Jones FA, Parke DV. Fourth Symposium on Carbenoxolone. London: Butterworths, 1975;125–128.
8. Young GP, Nagy GS, Myren J, Kronborg IJ, Logan KR, Reed PI, Hopper JL. Treatment of reflux oesophagitis with a carbenoxolone/antacid/alginate preparation. A double-blind controlled trial. Scand J Gastroenterol 1986;21:1098–1104.
9. Davies WA, Reed PI. Carbenoxolone treatment of reflux esophagitis. In: Jones FA, Parke DV (eds) Fourth Symposium on Carbenoxolone. London: Butterworths, 1975;215–232.
10. Reed PI, Davies WA. A double-blind comparative study of the use of Pyrogastrone in oesophagitis and oesophageal ulcer. In: Jones FA, Langman MJS, Mann RD (eds) Peptic Ulcer Healing. Recent Studies on Carbenoxolone. Lancaster: MTP Press Ltd, 1978;75–83.

May PGE$_2$ in the esophagus be involved in the pathogenesis of inflammation?

G. Triadafilopoulos (Palo Alto)

Acute and chronic inflammation is the histologic hallmark in reflux esophagitis [1]. This inflammation is characterized by microvascular injury, edema and infiltration by polymorphonuclear leukocytes, which release the vasoactive substances that contribute to these changes [2]. Prostaglandins may be one category of substances that mediate inflammation in the esophagus. Indomethacin, a cyclo-oxygenase inhibitor, appears to prevent the histologic appearance of esophagitis after acid or radiation exposure [3,4]. Prostaglandins and other vasoactive substances produce vasodilation and increased vascular permeability leading to edema, stasis, and migration of neutrophils and eosinophils into the area. Chronic inflammation is characterized by the presence of macrophages and fibroblasts, neovascularization and formation of granulation tissue and strictures [2]. Neutrophils also metabolize arachidonic acid to leukotriene B$_4$ (LTB$_4$), a potent chemotactic agent which induces neutrophils to migrate out of the circulation and into the tissue to further amplify injury [5]. Inhibition of synthesis or inactivation of these inflammatory mediators may in turn bear significant therapeutic potential.

Despite their well established "protective" role in maintaining mucosal integrity in the gastric epithelium, endogenous prostaglandins do not appear to be mediators of esophageal mucosal protection and, in fact, they may be detrimental [6]. For example, in an in vivo cat model of esophagitis, Katz et al. [7] were unable to demonstrate a protective effect of prostaglandin E$_1$ on acid-induced esophagitis, and Harmon et al. [8] could not demonstrate an effect of prostaglandins in preventing bile salt-induced increases in H$^+$ diffusion in an in vivo rabbit perfusion model. Preliminary in vitro studies have also shown that indomethacin has a significant protective effect on H$^+$ ion-induced tissue injury [9]. Prostaglandins may also adversely affect gastroesophageal reflux disease (GERD) by altering smooth muscle function in the body of the esophagus or the lower esophageal sphincter. Experimentally, in both humans and animals, PGE$_1$ and PGE$_2$ diminish esophageal peristalsis and basal LES tone [10,11]. More recently, Stein et al. [12], utilizing homogenates of rabbit esophageal mucosa, have shown that arachidonic acid metabolites were generated to a greater extent via the lipoxygenase pathway than via the cyclo-oxygenase pathway. In an in vivo acid-pepsin-induced model of esophagitis in rabbits, these authors suggest that products of the lipoxygenase pathways and not prostaglandins, may be endogenous mediators of esophageal mucosal protection.

We recently assessed of the role of leukotriene B_4 (LTB_4) and prostaglandin E_2 (PGE_2) in the clinical, endoscopic and histologic manifestations of GERD in a cross-sectional study of 144 consecutive patients with or without reflux who underwent upper endoscopy [13]. In this study, patients were classified as normal symptomatic controls (n = 67), esophagitis with Savary stages I–IV (n = 66), and Barrett's esophagus (n = 11), using clinical, endoscopic, manometric and esophageal 24-h ambulatory pH criteria. Ex vivo LTB_4 and PGE_2 levels were measured by RIA in esophageal mucosal biopsies. In controls, esophageal mucosal LTB_4 levels were 785 ± 58 pg/mg tissue protein. There was a progressive increase in mucosal LTB_4 levels with worsening inflammation (esophagitis stage I: 975 ± 97 pg/mg protein; stage II: 1686 ± 207), followed by relative decline in mucosal LTB_4 levels in the fibrotic stages of the disease (stage III: 1346 ± 181, stage IV: 1569 ± 326 pg/mg protein) (p < 0.05 compared to controls). Highly increased LTB_4 levels (1550 ± 460 pg/mg protein) were observed in Barrett's metaplasia. There was no significant change in mucosal PGE_2 levels among controls, patients with GERD (all stages) or Barrett's esophagus. Mucosal PGE_2 levels in those patients were as follows: controls: 516 ± 59 pg/mg tissue protein; stage I: 502 ± 72 pg/mg protein; stage II: 757 ± 151 pg/mg protein; stage III: 434 ± 153 pg/mg protein; stage IV: 625 ± 247 pg/mg protein; Barrett's esophagus: 505 ± 72 pg/mg protein (Fig. 1). Mucosal PGE_2 and LTB_4 levels correlated highly with symptom severity (r = 0.99 and 0.94, respectively). The highest values were seen in the most symptomatic patients, regardless of endoscopic staging, histology, degree of esophageal acid exposure by ambulatory pH monitoring, or lower

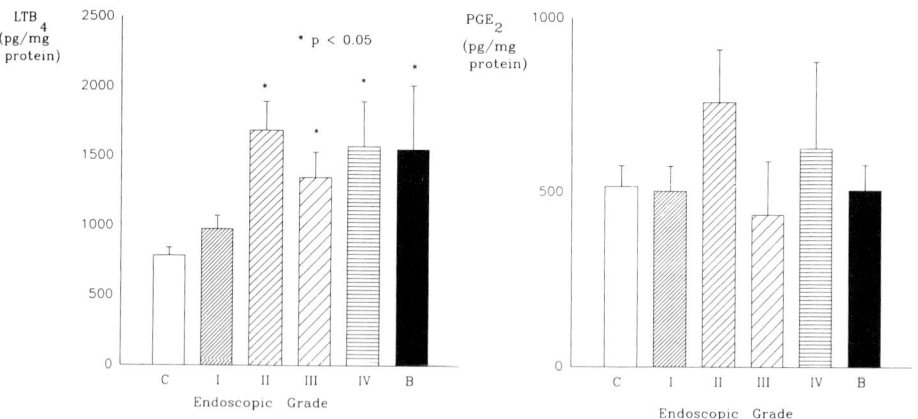

Fig. 1. Esophageal mucosal levels (pg/mg tissue protein) of leukotriene B_4 (LTB_4) and prostaglandin E_2 (PGE_2) in patients with normal esophagus (C), in patients with gastroesophageal reflux disease (endoscopic grades I–IV), and in patients with Barrett's esophagus (B). Results are means ± SEM from a total of 144 patients.

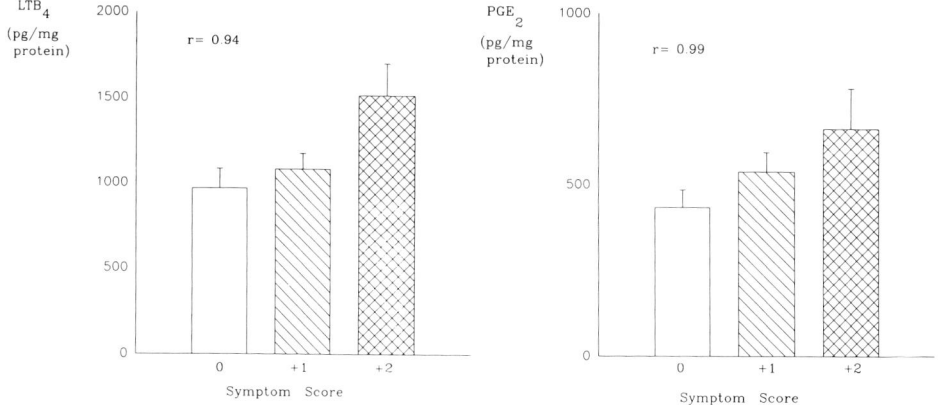

Fig. 2. Relationship between esophageal mucosal levels (pg/mg tissue protein) of leukotriene B_4 (LTB_4) and prostaglandin E_2 (PGE_2) and symptom severity (composite scores 0–2). Results are means ± SEM from a total of 144 patients.

esophageal sphincter resting pressure by esophageal motility (Fig. 2). Treatment with omeprazole 20 mg by mouth daily for 6 weeks significantly reduced both LTB_4 and PGE_2 levels ($p < 0.05$), and was associated with significant improvement of symptoms and endoscopic and histologic appearance of the esophagus in 25 patients (Fig. 3). These results suggest that LTB_4 and not PGE_2 may mediate the inflammatory phenomena of reflux esophagitis, and that both LTB_4 and PGE_2 may play a role in the induction of symptoms in patients with GERD.

Our data are partly in agreement with those noted by Ottignon et al. in their recent study of 19 patients with GERD and esophagitis [14]. Using similar methodology, these investigators noted that in patients with reflux but no esophagitis, PGE_2 levels

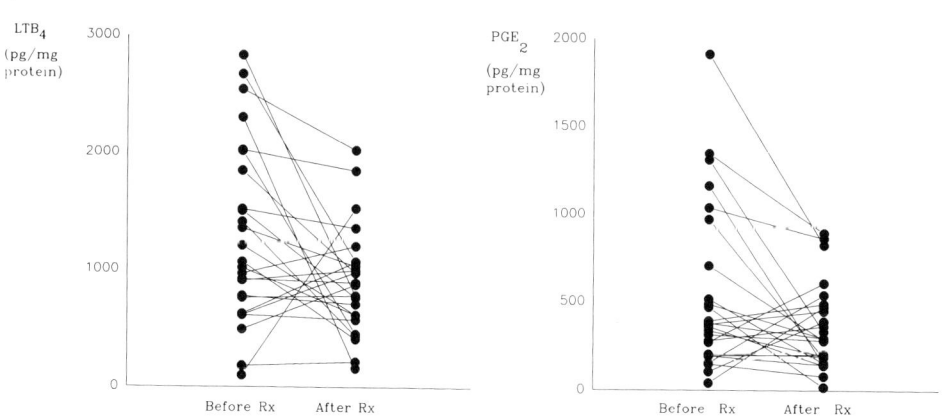

Fig. 3. Effect of treatment with omeprazole 20 mg by mouth daily for 6 weeks on esophageal mucosal levels (pg/mg tissue protein) of leukotriene B_4 (LTB_4) (left panel) and prostaglandin E_2 (PGE_2) (right panel). Individual data from before and after therapy are shown (n = 25). Results are significant at $p < 0.05$ (paired Student's t-test).

were similar to normal volunteer controls, while PGE_2 was significantly increased in patients with endoscopic evidence of esophagitis. In another study, however, there was a statistically significant reduction in mucosal PGE_2 levels in esophagitis patients as compared to controls, suggesting that reduced tissue prostaglandin levels may be related to inflammation and ulceration [15].

The origin and pathophysiology of esophageal symptoms such as dysphagia, chest pain and heartburn in GERD remain elusive [16,17]. Heartburn, the most common clinical symptom of reflux disease, is believed to be caused by acid stimulation of sensory nerve endings located in the deeper layers of the esophageal epithelium. Similarly, the sensation of dysphagia may be related to forceful nonpropulsive motor activity of the esophageal body or luminal distention secondary to acid reflux [18]. In our study, the highly significant correlation noted between PGE_2 and LTB_4 levels and symptoms of GERD raises the intriguing possibility that eicosanoids may play a role in the induction of esophageal symptoms in a fashion similar to joint inflammation and pain in arthritis [19–21].

Clearly, additional studies are required to substantiate these findings and to determine which component(s) of the arachidonic cascade are involved in the maintenance of an effective esophageal mucosal barrier and/or the induction of the inflammatory phenomena of reflux esophagitis. Current knowledge is limited to esophageal PGE_2 and LTB_4 content without obtaining a full profile of all products of the arachidonic acid metabolic cascade(s). The protective or harmful role of other eicosanoid compounds alone or in conjunction to the ones observed in the aforementioned studies remain to be elucidated. Further studies, utilizing specific inhibitors of either the cyclo-oxygenase or the lipoxygenase pathway may elucidate the pathogenetic role and therapeutic potential of eicosanoids in reflux esophagitis.

References

1. Orlando RC. Pathology of reflux esophagitis and its complications. In: Jamieson GG (ed) Surgery of the Oesophagus. Edinburgh: Churchill Livingstone, 1988.
2. Robbins SL, Cotran RS. Inflammation and repair. In: Robbins SL, Cotran RS (eds) Pathologic Basis of Disease, 2nd edn. Philadelphia: W.B. Saunders, 1979.
3. Northway MG, Libshitz HI, Osborne BM et al. Radiation esophagitis in the opposum: Radioprotection with indomethacin. Gastroenterology 1980;78:883–892.
4. Northway MG, Bennett A, Carroll M, Feldman MS, Manuel JJ, Libshitz HI, Szwarc IA, Eastwood GL. Comparative effects of anti-inflammatory agents and radiotherapy on normal esophagus and tumors in animals. Gastroenterology 1980;78:A1229.
5. Zipser RD, Nast CC, Lee M, Kao HW, Duke R. In vivo production of leukotriene B_4 in rabbit colitis. Relationship to inflammation. Gastroenterology 1987;92:33–39.
6. Goyal RK. Deleterious effects of prostaglandins on esophageal mucosa. Gastroenterology 1980;78:1085–1087.
7. Katz PO, Geisinger K, Hassan M et al. Acid-induced esophagitis in cats is prevented by sucralfate but not synthetic prostaglandin E. Dig Dis Sci 1988;33:217–224.
8. Harmon JW, Johnson LF, Maydonovitch CL. Effects of 16,16-dimethyl PGE_2 on bile-induced increases in H^+ permeability in rabbit esophagus. In: Samuelson B, Ramwell PW, Paoletti R (eds) Advances in Prostaglandin and Thromboxane Research. New York: Raven Press, 1980;18:1577.
9. Turjman KA, Powell DW, Orlando RC. Mucosal protective effect of indomethacin against H^+ injury to rabbit esophagus. Gastroenterology 1985;88:A1620.
10. Mukhopadhyay A, Rattan S, Goyal RK. Effect of prostaglandin E_2 on esophageal motility in man. J Appl Physiol 1975;39:479–481.
11. Goyal RK, Rattan S. Mechanisms of the lower esophageal sphincter relaxation. J Clin Invest 1973;52:337–341.
12. Stein BE, Schwartzman ML, Carroll MA, Stahl RE, Rosenthal WS. Role of arachidonic acid metabolites in acid-pepsin

injury to rabbit esophagus. Gastroenterology 1989;97:278–283.

13. Kaczynska MC, Triadafilopoulos G. The role of esophageal mucosal eicosanoid levels in gastroesophageal reflux disease. Gastroenterology 1992;102:A92.

14. Ottignon Y, Alber D, Moussard C, Deschamps JP, Carayon P, Henry JC. Measurement of prostaglandin E_2 in esophageal mucosa in normal subjects and patients with gastroesophageal reflux. (In French). Sem Hop Paris 1988;64:2071–2074.

15. Pugh S, Williams SE, Lewin MR, Barton TP, Salmon PR, Clark CG. Prostaglandin E_2 in normal and abnormal endoscopic biopsies. Gut 1985;26:A560–A561.

16. Hogan WJ, Dodds WJ. Gastroesophageal reflux disease (Reflux esophagitis). In: Sleisenger MH, Fordtran JS (eds) Gastro-intestinal Disease. Pathophysiology, Diagnosis and Management, 4th edn. Philadelphia: W.B. Saunders, 1989;594–619.

17. Cattau EL Jr, Castell DO. Symptoms of esophageal function. In: Castell DO, Johnson LF (eds) Esophageal Function in Health and Disease. New York: Elsevier, 1983:31–46.

18. Triadafilopoulos G. Nonobstructive dysphagia in reflux esophagitis. Am J Gastroenterol 1989;84:614–618.

19. Walter T, Chau TT, Weichman BM. Effects of analgesics on bradykinin-induced writhing in mice presensitized with PGE_2. Agents Actions 1989;27:375–377.

20. Taiwo YO, Levine JD. Prostaglandins inhibit endogenous pain control mechanisms by blocking transmission at spinal noradrenergic synapses. J Neurosci 1988;8:1346–1349.

21. James GWL, Church MK. Hyperalgesia after treatment of mice with prostaglandins and arachidonic acid and its antagonism by anti-inflammatory analgesic compounds. Arzneim Forsch 1978;28:804–807.

Antacids

Antacids and alginate-containing preparations: what is their mechanism of action and their place in the management of GERD?

C. Scarpignato, G. Gimbo (Parma)
S. Bruley des Varannes, J.-P. Galmiche (Nantes)

Although the pathogenesis of gastroesophageal reflux disease (GERD) is multifactorial [1], the damaging power of the refluxed material depends primarily on gastric acid secretion and the nature of refluxate is acid in most of patients with GERD [2]. As a consequence, until the 80s, the medical treatment of GERD consisted mainly of antacids and lifestyle modifications [3]. During the last decade new drugs have been developed, including very potent inhibitors of gastric acid secretion and more effective prokinetic agents [4]. However, in many countries, antacids and alginate containing preparations still remain the mainstay of treatment for patients with heartburn and the so-called "reflux-like dyspepsia".

Antacids are among the most widely used medicines. Often, to be sure, they are taken as a result of self-diagnosis and self-treatment (being available as over-the-counter drugs), and the trigger for buying and taking an antacid is not based on structural abnormalities, but on symptoms. Patients take antacids, as well as alginates, to feel better rather than to heal esophageal lesions.

This paper will summarize the pharmacology of both kinds of preparations and discuss their role in the medical treatment of GERD.

Antacids

Antacids are preparations that are primarily designed to neutralize gastric acid. The proliferation of antacid formulations includes combinations and varying proportions of a number of basic materials, in an attempt to produce improved neutralization characteristics with lowered untoward effects. Currently, the American Hospital Formulary lists over 120 antacid preparations, composed of single ingredients or mixtures, in every conceivable combination. Similarly, the British National Formulary and the French Pharmacopeia contain 58 and 64 formulations, respectively, many of these being very similar.

The chemistry of each antacid is unique [5,6]. On the basis of their biological properties, they can be divided as systemic (i.e., sodium salts), nonsystemic (calcium, magnesium and aluminum salts), and complex antacids (Fig. 1). Most prescribed antacids contain a mixture of aluminum and magnesium salts. Precise methods of preparation and presentation are important because they influence the physico-chemical properties and the therapeutic effects of antacids.

Pharmacological properties of antacids

The pharmacological actions of antacids are summarized in Table 1 [1,7]. Besides the neutralization of hydrogen ions present in gastric secretion, the increase in lower esophageal sphincter pressure (LESP) [8], which is independent of gastrin release [9], could — on theoretical grounds — contribute to the observed reduction of esophageal exposure to acid [10]. An increase in LESP, however, becomes evident only when intragastric pH is kept over 6 [8], a pH level only seldom reached with the common used schedules of antacids. It is worth mentioning that their effect on gastric pH is of short duration; antacids ingested in the fasting state reduce acidity for only approximately 30 min because of their rapid gastric emptying [5]. When antacids (30

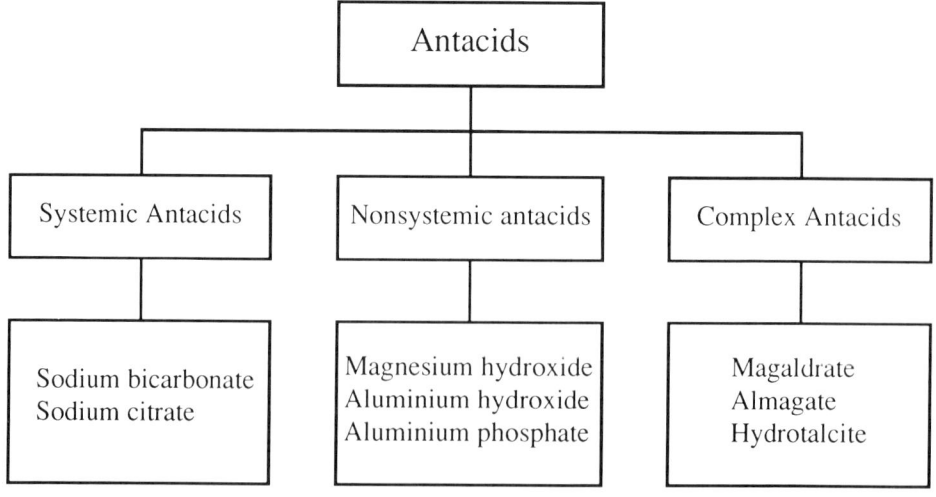

Fig. 1. Classification of antacids.

Table 1. Pharmacological actions of antacids

- *Neutralization of hydrogen ions present in gastric secretion and reduction of their concentration in the refluxed material*
- Mucosal protection
- Adsorption and inactivation of pepsin
- Binding of bile salts
- *Increase of LESP independently from gastrin release*
- Inhibition of gastric emptying rate, mainly dependent on aluminum content

---

ml) are given 1 and 3 h after the meal, gastric pH is kept above 2.0 for only 3 h [11]. The second dose of antacid, given when most of the meal has left the stomach, is slightly less effective than the first one. Moreover, it must be pointed out that acid secretion actually increases while antacids are in the stomach; however, as long as the antacid remains in the stomach, acid can be neutralized. The nocturnal gastric acidity (which normally reaches its peak after midnight) is not adequately controlled by antacids, even when given at bedtime.

Could antacids reduce the esophageal exposure to acids?

Ten years ago, Galmiche's team [12] performed an elegant study comparing an aluminum-magnesium-hydroxide-containing antacid (Dimalan®) with two widely employed histamine H_2-antagonists (cimetidine and ranitidine) in patients with symptomatic gastroesophageal reflux (GER). These were randomly allocated to one of the following therapeutic schedules:
— antacid 15 ml 1 h after meals and at bedtime;
— cimetidine 200 mg after meals and 400 mg at bedtime; and
— ranitidine 150 mg bid.
A standard 3-h postprandial pH test without treatment was also performed in all patients before entering the trial and a postprandial acid reflux score was then calculated. When compared to pretreatment levels of esophageal acidity, the three drugs were found to be almost equally effective in reducing the postprandial pH score. However, comparison of the results from the 20 h pH study showed that during the night H_2-blockers (especially ranitidine) were clearly more efficacious than the antacid, in decreasing the time of exposure of the esophageal mucosa to low pH levels.

Are antacids capable of relieving heartburn?

Although the degree by which acidity must be reduced to relieve heartburn is not yet clearly established [13], a study by Smith and co-workers [14] showed that a solution of pH over 2.5, infused into the esophagus, may not cause pain even if it is of low pH (e.g., pH 3).

The analgesic effect of a liquid antacid (30 ml aluminum and magnesium hydroxides in vitro, buffering capacity 144 µmol) on episodes of heartburn, has been studied by Meyer et al. [15] in 20 chronically symptomatic GER patients (Fig. 2). Their first study compared the effect of single doses of antacid and placebo on two spontaneous heartburn episodes. The second trial compared single doses of the same antacid and placebo on acid induced heartburn. Lastly, antacid and placebo were given on demand for multiple heartburn episodes. In all these studies, antacid and placebo resulted in nonstatistically different degrees of pain relief. Moreover, esophageal pH monitoring during the Bernstein test was not correlated with the degree of pain relief after either antacid or placebo.

Is there any healing effect of antacids on esophageal lesions?

Clinical investigations with antacids on GERD patients concern their effects on both symptoms (heartburn, regurgitation, dysphagia) of GERD and esophageal lesions. As shown in Table 2, there are few published trials [16–19] in which antacids and true placebo were compared. It is evident that a significant symptomatic relief was seldom reported and that an improvement of esophageal lesions was never revealed by endoscopy.

Based on the present knowledge, it should therefore be concluded that antacids are of little, if any, therapeutic value in GERD.

Alginate-containing drugs

These pharmaceutical preparations, of which the most widely known is Gaviscon®, contain alginic acid combined with small doses of antacids. Commercial antireflux

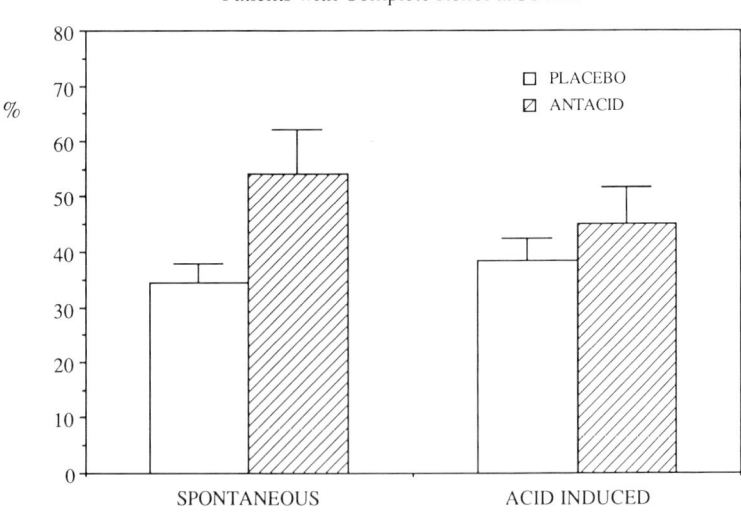

Fig. 2. Effect of antacids on spontaneous and acid-induced heartburn in patients with GERD. Each column represents the percentage of patients symptom-free 30 min after administration of either placebo or antacid (drawn from data in [15]).

Table 2. Placebo-controlled trials with antacid preparations in GERD

Authors	Year	Control therapy	Symptomatic improvement	Endoscopic improvemnt
Furman et al. [16]	1982	Placebo	No	No
Graham and Patterson [17]	1983	Placebo	No	No
Grove et al. [18]	1985	Placebo	Yes	No
Weberg and Berstad [19]	1989	Placebo	Yes	NE

NE = not evaluated.

preparations use a wide range of alginate materials. It is difficult to correlate their properties with those of alginate, since the alginate used is rarely specified by the manufacturer and a wide range of particulates are added to many formulations (e.g., particulate antacids). Even in the same formulation, the composition varies greatly from country to country (Table 3). This is the case with liquid Gaviscon®, which is manufactured under license by different pharmaceutical companies. An interesting study [20] compared four international preparations of liquid Gaviscon® and found that each formulation possesses markedly different raft strength (Fig. 3) and neutralization profiles.

Alginate-containing preparations: how do they work?

Scintigraphic studies have clearly established that Gaviscon® floats on the surface of the gastric pool, providing a mechanical barrier to reflux at the cardia. Using a dual-isotope scintigraphic technique, Malmud and Fisher [21] as well as McKay et al. [22], showed that most of the ingested alginic acid is located in the upper half of the stomach, in both normal subjects and patients with GER (Fig. 4). In those subjects in whom reflux did occur after treatment with alginic acid, the labeled compound refluxed preferentially compared with the liquid contents of the stomach. Therefore, when reflux occurs, this viscous foam first contacts the esophageal mucosa. Compared with antacids, alginate containing preparations float and show a selective retention in the fundus [6].

Optimal dosing in relation to meal intake is needed for alginate to be completely effective (Table 4). To ensure gastric floatation, antireflux agents must indeed be given 30 min after the meal.

Table 3. Composition of the liquid Gaviscon® formulations in various countries [20]

Formulation	U.K.	Canada	U.S.A.	Sweden
Sodium alginate	500 mg	500 mg	267 mg	500 mg
Sodium bicarbonate	267 mg	a	—	170 mg
Aluminum hydroxide	—	200 mg	63.3 mg	1 g
Magnesium carbonate	—	—	275 mg	—
Calcium carbonate	—	—	—	150 mg

a Quoted as 60 mg of sodium/10 ml which is equivalent to 219 mg of sodium bicarbonate/10 ml.

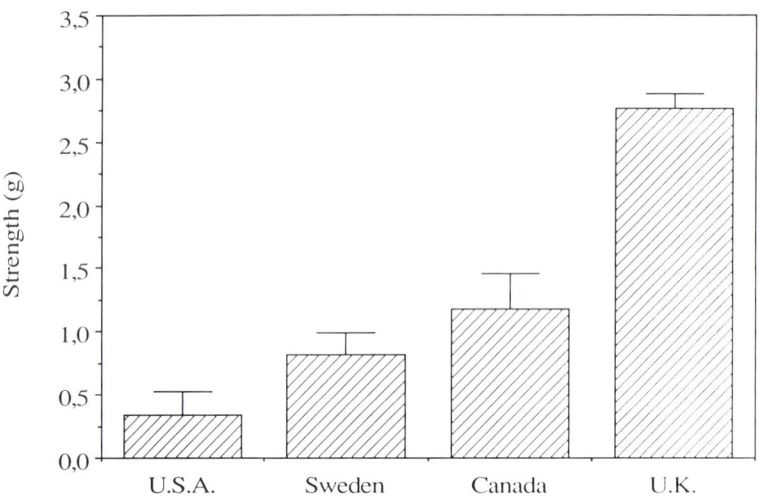

Fig. 3. Raft strengths of the minimum recommended doses of liquid Gaviscon® available in four different countries (from [20]).

Effect of alginate-containing preparations on esophageal exposure to acid

Stanciu and Bennett [23] first showed a significant decrease in the number of reflux episodes and in the percentage time during which the esophageal pH was in the acidic range after the administration of eight tablets per day of an alginate containing preparation (Gaviscon®). Antacid alone (Gaviscon® without alginate) had no effect

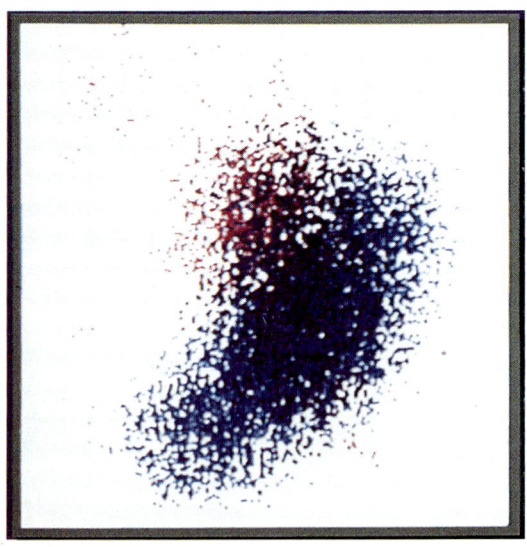

Fig. 4. Dual isotope scintigraphic evaluation of an alginate containing preparation (Algicon®). Patients with symptomatic GERD were given 300 ml ⁹⁹ᵐTc labelled milk (blue) followed by 10 ml suspension of ¹¹³ᵐIn-labeled alginate (red) (from [22]).

Table 4. Alginate-containing preparations: optimal dosing in relation to meals

- Antireflux preparations must be given 30 min after a meal to ensure gastric floatation.
- When the antireflux agent is taken on an empty stomach, the formation sinks to the base of the greater curvature and 50% is emptied within 20 min after administration.
- When the formulation is taken 30 min before, the antireflux agent does not float on a meal ingested subsequently. It will be diluted with the fluid from the meal and thus emptied ahead of the meal without forming a raft.

on esophageal pH. By using postprandial and 24-h intraesophageal pH-metry, respectively, Dudicourt et al. [24], Branicki et al. [25] and Castell et al. [26] confirmed this finding and clearly showed that Gaviscon® is more effective in controlling GER in upright than in supine position (Fig. 5). This finding is not unexpected if one takes into account that gastric emptying of Gaviscon® is strongly influenced by posture. Bennett et al. [27], indeed, demonstrated in healthy volunteers that this raft-forming alginate formulation emptied faster than food in subjects lying on their left sides and slower in subjects lying on their right sides. The recently developed Algicon® behaves quite similarly [28]. More recently, Washington [29] used an esophageal pH probe, coupled with a small γ-detector strapped to the chest wall and, by using a radio-labeled meal, was able to show that 20 ml of liquid Gaviscon®, administered 30 min after the meal, significantly reduced the amount of both acid and food reflux into the esophagus.

Alginate-containing preparations: clinical efficacy in GERD

The clinical efficacy of Gaviscon® has not been definitively established by large placebo-controlled trials [30–32]. The studies in which Gaviscon® appeared superior

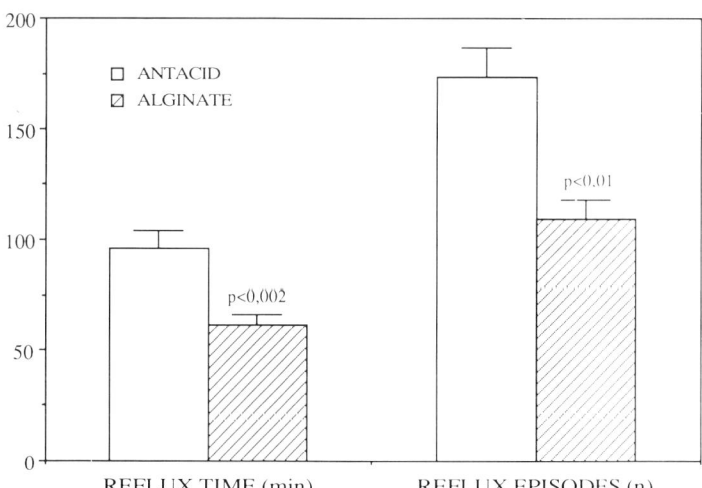

Fig. 5. Upright reflux time (min) and numbers of reflux episodes after a high-fat meal in 10 subjects following administration of an alginic acid-antacid formulation vs. equal strength antacid (redrawn from [26]).

Table 5. Controlled trials with alginate containing preparations

Authors	Year	Control therapy	Symptomatic improvement	Endoscopic improvement
Barnardo et al. [30]	1975	Placebo	Yes	NE
Beeley and Warner [31]	1972	Placebo	Yes	NE
Grossman et al. [32]	1973	Placebo	No	No
Stanciu and Bennett [23]	1974	Placebo	No	NE
McHardy [33]	1978	Antacid	No	No
Scobie [34]	1976	Antacid	No	No
Chevrel [35]	1980	Antacid	Yes	NE
Graham et al. [36]	1984	Antacid	No	No

NE = not evaluated.

to placebo concerned symptoms without information regarding endoscopic or histological findings (Table 5).

In some studies, Gaviscon® was compared with antacids [33–36]. These trials did not show any statistically significant difference between these two drugs, in terms of symptom relief and improvement of lesions [37] but, as pointed out previously, efficacy of antacids themselves remains controversial.

On the whole, clinical experience in general practice suggests that alginates (Gaviscon®) or alginate-antacid preparations (Algicon®) are very effective for the relief of heartburn [38–40], but their efficacy in the healing of esophagitis is at least doubtful.

Antacids and alginates for GERD: are they useful?

In clinical practice, there is generally a consensus to apply a stepwise strategy for the treatment of GERD [4]. In patients with mild symptoms and no lesions at endoscopy (or only an erythema of mucosa), lifestyle modifications and antacids are still recommended as the classical "phase 1" therapy. However, for symptom relief, alginate-containing preparations should certainly be preferred to pure antacids. In France, for instance, a large multicenter trial [38], performed in primary care patients with typical heartburn, showed that about 92% of patients were asymptomatic after a 2-week treatment with an alginate-antacid preparation; moreover, even in those incompletely relieved by treatment, endoscopy showed no or mild esophageal lesions in 60% of them. Antacids or antacid/alginates, however, should not be used alone in severe GERD, when there are persistent or nocturnal symptoms, grade 2 or more esophagitis and/or marked sphincter incompetence with consequent complications.

Acknowledgement

The authors are indebted to Miss Sabina Cavagni for her invaluable help in checking the references and her diligence in the preparation of the manuscript.

References

1. Scarpignato C. Pharmacological bases of the medical treatment of gastroesophageal reflux disease. Dig Dis Sci 1988;6: 117−148.
2. Mittal RK, Reuben A, Whitney JO et al. Do bile acids reflux into the esophagus? A study in normal subjects and patients with gastroesophageal reflux disease. Gastroenterology 1987;92:371−375.
3. Richter JE. Gastroesophageal reflux disease: a review of medical therapy. In: Castell DO, Wu WC, Ott DJ (eds) Gastro-esophageal Reflux Disease: Pathogenesis, Diagnosis, Therapy. Mount Kisco N.Y.: Futura Publishing, 1985;221−241.
4. Scarpignato C, Galmiche JP. Short-term treatment of reflux oesophagitis: A clinical pharmacological approach. In: Tytgat GN (ed) The Medical Management of Oesophageal Reflux Disease. London: Royal Society of Medicine, 1990;60−80.
5. Peterson WL, Richardson CT. Pharmacology and side effects of drugs used to treat peptic ulcer. In: Sleisenger MH, Fordtran JS (eds) Gastrointestinal Disease. Pathophysiology, Diagnosis and Management, 3rd edn. Philadelphia: WB Saunders Company, 1983;708−725.
6. Washington N. Handbook of Antacids and Anti-reflux Agents. Boca Raton: CRC Press, 1991.
7. Scarpignato C, Galmiche JP. Antacids and alginates in the treatment of gastroesophageal reflux disease: How do they work and how much are they clinically useful? In: Scarpignato C (ed) Advances in Drug Therapy of Gastroesophageal Reflux Disease. Basel: Karger, 1992;153−181.
8. Higgs RH, Smyth RD, Castell DO. Gastric alkalinization: effect on lower esophageal sphincter pressure and serum gastrin. N Engl J Med 1974;291:486−490.
9. McCallum LS, Kline M, Sturdevant RAL. Studies on the mechanism of the lower esophageal sphincter pressure response to alkali ingestion in man. Gastroenterology 1975;68:948.
10. Galmiche JP, Scarpignato C. Pharmacodynamic assessment of drugs in gastroesophageal reflux disease: an overview. In: Tytgat GNJ (ed) Medical Management of Esophageal Disease. London: Royal Society of Medicine, 1990;12−33.
11. Deering TB, Malagelada JR. Comparison of an H_2-receptor antagonist and a neutralizing antacid on postprandial acid delivery into duodenum patients with duodenal ulcer. Gastroenterology 1977;73:11−14.
12. Deschalliers JP, Galmiche JP, Touchais JY et al. Ranitidine, cimetidine, antacids and gastroesophageal reflux: results of a 20-h esophageal pH study. Int J Clin Pharm Res 1984;4:217−222.
13. Scarpignato C, Galmiche JP. Antacids and alginates in the treatment of gastroesophageal reflux disease: How do they work and how much are they clinically useful? In: Scarpignato C (ed) Advances in Drug Therapy of Gastroesophageal Reflux Disease. Basel: Karger, 1992;129−152.
14. Smith JL, Opekun AR, Larkai E et al. Sensitivity of the esophageal mucosa to pH in gastroesophageal reflux disease. Gastroenterology 1989;96:683−689.
15. Meyer C, Berenzweig H, Kuljian B et al. Controlled trial of antacid (AA) versus placebo (P) on relief of heartburn. Gastroenterology 1979;76:A1201.
16. Furman D, Mensh R, Winan G et al. A double-blind trial comparing high dose liquid antacid to placebo and cimetidine in improving symptoms and objective parameters in gastroesophageal reflux. Gastroenterology 1982;82:1062.
17. Graham DY, Patterson DJ. Double-blind comparison of liquid antacid and placebo in the treatment of symptomatic reflux esophagitis. Dig Dis Sci 1983;28:559−564.
18. Grove O, Bekker C, Jeppe-Hansen MG et al. Ranitidine and high dose antacid in reflux esophagitis. A randomized placebo-controlled trial. Scand J Gastroenterol 1985;20:457−461.
19. Weberg R, Berstad A. Symptomatic effect of a low-dose antacid regimen in reflux esophagitis. Scand J Gastroenterol 1989; 24:401−406.
20. Washington N, Washington C, Wilson CG et al. What is "Liquid Gaviscon"? A comparison of four international formula-tions. Int J Pharmaceut 1986;34:105−109.
21. Malmud LS, Fisher MS. Scintigraphic detection of gastroesophageal reflux. In: Alavi A, Arger PH (eds) Multiple Image Procedures, vol 3. New York: Grune & Stratton, 1980;97−119.
22. McKay AP, Wraight EP, Hunter JO. The alginate raft: a scintigraphic evaluation. Br J Clin Pract 1989;43(suppl 66):20−24.
23. Stanciu C, Bennett JR. Alginate/antacid in the reduction of gastroesophageal reflux. Lancet 1974;1:109−111.
24. Dudicourt JC, Hemery P, Gignoux C et al. Réduction du reflux gastro-oesophagien postprandial par l'alginate de sodium suspension. Etude pH-métrique multicentrique chez 21 malades. Nouv Presse Méd 1988;17:683−685.
25. Branicki FJ, Evans DF, Jones JA et al. A controlled trial of liquid Gaviscon in gastro-oesophageal reflux using a portable pH-sensitive radiotelemetry system. J Ambul Monit 1988;1:61−72.
26. Castell DO, Dalton CB, Becker D, Sinclair J, Castell JA. Alginic acid decreases postprandial upright gastroesophageal reflux. Comparison with equal-strength antacid. Dig Dis Sci 1992;37:589−593.
27. Bennett CE, Hardy JG, Wilson CG. The influence of posture on the gastric emptying of antacids. Int J Pharmaceut 1984; 21:341−347.
28. Devis G, de Rop H, Peters O. Twenty-four-hour oesophageal pH monitoring of reflux episodes: Effect of Algicon. Br J Clin Pract 1989;43(suppl 66):15−17.
29. Washington N. Investigation into the barrier action of an alginate gastric reflux suppressant, liquid Gaviscon®. Drug Inv 1990;2:23−30.
30. Barnardo DE, Lancaster-Smith M, Strickland ID et al. A double-blind controlled trial of "Gaviscon" in patients with symptomatic gastroesophageal reflux. Curr Med Res Opin 1975;3:388−391.

31. Beeley M, Warner JO. Medical treatment of symptomatic hiatus hernia with low-density compounds. Curr Med Res Opin 1972;1:63–69.
32. Grossman AE, Klotz AP, Rhodes JB et al. Reflux esophagitis: a comparison of old and new medical management. J Kans Med Soc 1973;74:423–424.
33. McHardy G. A multicentric, randomized clinical trial of Gaviscon in reflux esophagitis. Southern Med J 1978;71(suppl 1):16–21.
34. Scobie BA. Endoscopically controlled trial of alginate and antacid in reflux oesophagitis. Med J Aust 1976;1:627–628.
35. Chevrel B. A comparative crossover study on the treatment of heartburn and epigastric pain: Liquid Gaviscon and a magnesium-aluminium antacid gel. J Int Med Res 1980;8:300.
36. Graham DY, Lanza F, Dorsch ER. Symptomatic reflux oesophagitis: a double-blind controlled comparison of antacids and alginate. Curr Ther Res 1977;22:653–658.
37. Tytgat GNJ. Drug therapy of reflux oesophagitis: an update. Scand J Gastroenterol 1989;24(suppl 168):38–49.
38. Bigard MA, Colin R, Galmiche JP, Rampal P, de Meynard C. Evolution des symptômes de reflux gastro-oesophagien (RGO) après 2 semaines de traitement par alginate-antiacide. Facteurs prédictifs et données endoscopiques chez les non-répondeurs. Gastroentérol Clin Biol 1990;14:A110.
39. Ward AE. Comparative study of Algicon versus Gaviscon in symptomatic gastroesophageal reflux. Br J Clin Pract 1989;43(suppl 66):52–55.
40. Maxton DG, Miller JP, Whorwell PJ et al. A study of Algicon, an antacid alginate preparation in patients with reflux oesophagitis. Br J Clin Pract 1988;42:368–371.

What are the most recent data on alginates?

D.O. Castell (Philadelphia)

Sodium alginate is known to act as an antireflux barrier, forming a floating raft on top of the gastric pool [1]. Furthermore, because of its position high in the gastric fundus in the upright position, there is delayed gastric emptying of the alginate [2]. What is the evidence for an effect of alginic acid in the relief of symptoms of gastroesophageal reflux disease (GERD)? The data that provide possible answers to this question come from a variety of sources over a number of years. Earlier studies by Stanciu and Bennett, using stationary pH monitoring, had demonstrated that alginic acid (without antacid) would decrease distal esophageal acid exposure, providing evidence for an antireflux effect [3]. In addition, a multicenter clinical trial reported similar improvement in heartburn and esophagitis with alginic acid alone compared with regular antacid [4]. More recently, alginic acid (without antacid) was found to be superior to placebo in the relief of postprandial symptoms induced by ingestion of a meal consisting of Texas chili, black coffee and a spicy tomato drink [5]. Esophageal acid exposure was not monitored in the latter two studies.

A comprehensive study of the possible effect of alginic acid on reflux, using in-hospital 24-h pH monitoring, revealed no effect for the alginate on 24-h acid exposure [6]. This study did, however, show a trend towards decreased reflux in the upright position with alginic acid, although this effect was not significant. The recent observations by Moss et al. on the flotation ability of alginic acid, suggest a strong potential for an antireflux action primarily in the upright position [2]. This would sup-

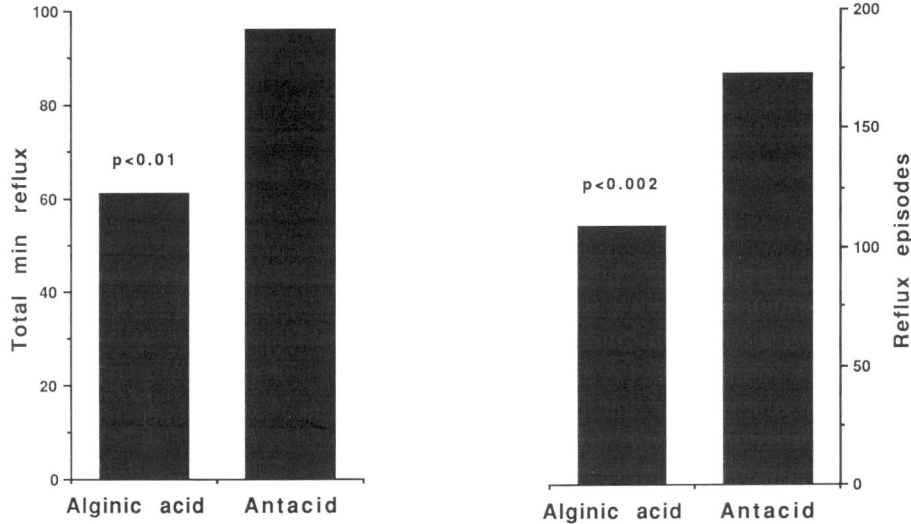

Fig. 1. Total minutes of reflux and total number of reflux episodes following a high-fat meal in the 10 subjects in the upright position during alginic acid-antacid treatment vs. equal strength antacid. There is a significant decrease in upright following alginic acid.

port observations of the symptomatic relief obtained in patients during the daytime.

Recent data from our laboratory indicate that alginic acid/antacid (extra strength Gaviscon) may have an active antireflux effect which is preferentially found in the upright position [7]. We used the technique of promoting reflux in 10 healthy

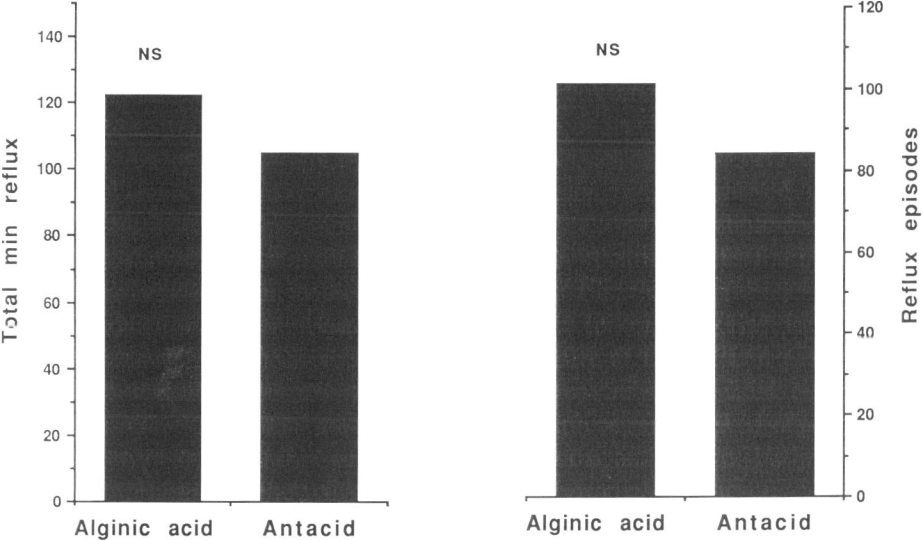

Fig. 2. Total minutes of reflux and total number of reflux episodes, following a high-fat meal in the 10 subjects while in the recumbent position after alginic acid-antacid vs. equal strength antacid. There is no significant difference in the treatment effects.

volunteers with a high-fat (61% fat calories) meal, a method previously reported from our laboratory to promote increased reflux in both the upright and supine position [8]. The alginate-antacid tablets significantly decreased postprandial reflux in the upright position compared to antacid with equal neutralizing capacity (Fig. 1). This effect did not occur in the supine position (Fig. 2). These studies support prior observations of the potential effectiveness of alginic acid to relieve daytime symptoms, particularly those occurring after meals in the upright position. They also suggest a potential role for alginic acid in the treatment of GERD patients having break-through symptoms during the day while receiving therapy with acid-suppressing medications.

References

1. Beckloff GL, Chapman JH, Shiverdecker P. Objective evaluation of an antacid with unusual properties. J Clin Pharm 1972; 12:11–21.
2. Moss HA, Washington N, Greaves JL, Wilson C. Antireflux agents. Stratification or flotation? Eur J Gastroenterol Hepatol 1990;2:45–51.
3. Stanciu C, Bennett JR. Alginate/antacid in the reduction of gastroesophageal reflux. Lancet 1974;1:109–111.
4. McHardy G. A multicenter randomized clinical trial of Gaviscon in reflux esophagitis. Southern Med J 1978; 71(suppl): 16–21.
5. Lanza F, Smith V, Page-Castell J, Castell D. Effectiveness of foaming antacid in relieving induced heartburn. Southern Med J 1986;79:327–330.
6. Johnson LF, DeMeester TR. Evaluation of elevation of the head of the bed, bethanechol, and antacid foam tablets on gastroesophageal reflux. Dig Dis Sci 1981;26:673–680.
7. Castell DO, Dalton CB, Becker D, Sinclair J, Castell JA. Alginic acid decreases postprandial upright gastroesophageal reflux. Comparison with equal-strength antacid. Dig Dis Sci 1992;37:589–593.
8. Becker D, Sinclair J, Castell D, Wu WC. A comparison of high and low fat meals on postprandial esophageal acid exposure. Am J Gastroenterol 1989;84:782–786.

Antisecretory agents

Is it possible to specify the prognostic factors of efficacy of an antisecretory treatment?

G. Cadiot, M. Mignon (Paris)

Factors conditioning the therapeutic response to antisecretory drugs in gastro-esophageal reflux disease (GERD) and esophagitis are not well known. The factors that have been studied are the clinical characteristics of the patients, the characteristics of the disease (clinical, endoscopical, motor and pH-metric) and finally, the gastric secretory characteristics of the patients.

Two multifactorial analyses, the first one in patients treated with ranitidine [1] and the second one in patients with severe esophagitis treated with omeprazole [2], showed that the severity of the esophagitis was the main predictive factor of the therapeutic response. Tobacco consumption negatively influenced healing in the first study [1], but not in the second one [2]. Age, sex, symptom duration, Barrett's mucosa and antisecretory drug dosage were not significant predictive factors of esophagitis healing [1,2].

Esophageal motor abnormalities and low basal pressure of lower esophageal sphincter (LES) did not influence healing in patients, treated with ranitidine [3]. It should be noted in the study by Klinkenberg-Knol and Meuwissen that 18 among the 19 patients who did not heal with omeprazole had basal LES hypotonia and that 63% of them had decreased or virtually absent motility of the esophagus [4]. It is clear, in systemic sclerosis for example, that major motility disorders are responsible for the lack of efficacy of antisecretory drugs given at the "usual" dosage.

Because gastric acid secretion is important in GERD pathophysiology [5] and because antisecretory drugs inhibit acid secretion, some authors looked for prognostic factors of antisecretory drug efficacy among the secretory status, the esophageal acid exposure and the levels of acid output inhibition and esophageal acid exposure by the treatment.

Collen et al. showed that GERD patients in whom symptoms did not disappear after 3 months of treatment with 300 mg/day ranitidine (nonresponders), had significantly higher basal acid output (BAO) than those in whom symptoms disappeared (responders) (11.4 ± 4.4 mEq/h vs. 4.4 ± 3.4, respectively) [6]. Nine among the 12 nonresponders had BAO >10 mEq/h, although on the other hand 1/11 responders only had BAO >10 mEq/h [6]. Such data were not confirmed by Hirschowitz in a nonprospective study [7]. Furthermore, Collen et al. found a correlation (r = 0.81) between BAO measured without antisecretory treatment and the daily dose of ranitidine necessary for the disappearance of the symptoms. This correlation allowed the following equation to be established: daily ranitidine dose = (100 × BAO) − 221 [6]. It should be noted that 10/12 nonresponders and 1/11 responders had Barrett's esophagus [6]. In another study that concerned 42 patients with Barrett's esophagus, the same authors confirmed that most of the patients who did not respond to 300 mg/day ranitidine had basal gastric acid hypersecretion, and that there was a correlation between BAO and ranitidine dosage [8].

In the study by Collen et al. [6], as in others [9], the nonresponders had higher esophageal exposure to acid, assessed with 24-h pH-metry, than the responders. However, this was not confirmed in two other studies [3,10]. The first one compared the symptomatic response to 8 weeks of ranitidine 300 mg/day [10] and the second one, the endoscopical response to 6 weeks of ranitidine, 600 mg/day [3]. In these two studies, the pH-metric parameters measured without treatment were not significantly different between responders and nonresponders [3,10]. This suggests that esophageal pH-metry cannot predict the response to the antisecretory treatment [3,10]. This has also been suggested by Collen et al., who did not find any correlation between the ranitidine dose necessary for the disappearance of the symptoms and the esophageal mucosal acid exposure (r = −0.13) [6].

Insufficient acid secretion inhibition by the treatment is a prognostic factor of inefficacy of the treatment. In patients with esophagitis, as it has been shown in patients with duodenal ulcer, there is a linear correlation between healing rates and percentages of acid inhibition by the antisecretory treatments [11]. Collen et al. showed, when considering the whole group of patients, that one had to diminish BAO (measured under treatment) to 1 mEq/h to obtain the symptomatic response [6]. This threshold is the same one which must be reached in patients with the Zollinger-Ellison syndrome and esophagitis to obtain endoscopical and symptomatical remission [12]. In the study by Johansson and Tibbling, BAO and pentagastrin acid outputs were not significantly diminished by the treatment in nonresponders, whereas they were in responders [10]. In responders, BAO measured under treatment was very low, 0.2 ± 0.3 mEq/h [10] (as in Collen et al. study [6]). In patients treated with omeprazole (20 to 80 mg/day), it has been shown, using combined gastric and esophageal pH-metries, that insufficient gastric acid inhibition was responsible for the treatment "resistance" [4].

392

The study by Klinkenberg-Knol and Meuwissen also suggested that the measurement of gastric acid inhibition (by gastric pH-metry) was more useful than that of residual esophageal acid exposure (by esophageal pH-metry) when looking for the understanding of the mechanisms of antisecretory treatment resistance [4]. Indeed, among the 19 patients who were resistant to omeprazole treatment, seven had normal esophageal pH-metry, whereas gastric pH-metry showed long periods with gastric pH under 4 [4]. In this study, the patients might have acid hypersecretion; however, this was not measured. Johansson and Tibbling showed that pH-metric parameters measured 5 cm above the LES were not modified by the treatment in nonresponders, as well as in responders, whereas acid outputs were diminished in responders only, as mentioned above [10]. In contrast, in the study by Robertson et al., pH-metric parameters (total acid exposure, number of refluxes and mean duration of each reflux episode) were significantly decreased by the treatment in responders (reaching almost normal values), whereas they were not modified in nonresponders [3]. This was not due to differences in esophageal motility [3]. In addition, pretreatment serum gastrin levels were significantly lower in responders than in nonresponders [3]. This might reflect higher acid outputs in nonresponders.

In conclusion, measuring acid output in GERD patients may predict resistance to antisecretoy drugs and the necessity to use higher doses. At an individual level, the determination of the gastric secretory status might be more useful than the knowledge of esophageal exposure to acid for the prediction of antisecretory treatment efficacy. Finally, patients with high grade esophagitis had more frequent resistance to antisecretory drugs. This might be due to higher acid outputs or to lower acid inhibition by the treatments. A multifactorial analysis considering characteristics of the patients and GERD, but also acid outputs without and under treatment, has to be done.

References

1. Koelz HR, Birchler R, Bretholz A et al. Healing and relapse of reflux esophagitis during treatment with ranitidine. Gastroenterology 1986;91:1198−1205.
2. Hetzel DJ, Dent J, Reed WD et al. Healing and relapse of severe peptic esophagitis after treatment with omeprazole. Gastroenterology 1988;95:903−912.
3. Robertson DAF, Aldersley MA, Shepherd H, Lloyd RS, Smith CL. H₂ antagonists in the treatment of reflux oesophagitis: can physiological studies predict the response? Gut 1987;28:946−949.
4. Klinkenberg-Knol EC, Meuwissen SGM. Combined gastric and oesophageal 24-hour pH monitoring and oesophageal manometry in patients with reflux disease, resistant to treatment with omeprazole. Aliment Pharmacol Ther 1990;4: 485−495.
5. Sekera E, Cadiot G, Poitevin C, Vallot T, Vatier J, Mignon M. Sécrétion gastrique de pepsine dans le reflux gastro-oesophagien compliqué ou non d'oesophagite peptique. Gastroenterol Clin Biol 1992;16:141−147.
6. Collen MJ, Lewis JH, Benjamin SB. Gastric acid hypersecretion in refractory gastroesophageal reflux disease. Gastroenterology 1990;98:654−661.
7. Hirschowitz BI. Acid and pepsin secretion in patients with esophagitis refractory to treatment with H₂ antagonists. Scand J Gastroenterol 1992;27:449−452.
8. Collen MJ, Johnson DA. Correlation between basal acid output and daily ranitidine dose required for therapy in Barrett's esophagus. Dig Dis Sci 1992;37:570−576.
9. Bianchi Porro G, Pace F, Sangaletti O. Pattern of acid reflux in patients with reflux esophagitis "resistant" to H₂-receptor antagonists. Scand J Gastroenterol 1990;25:810−814.
10. Johansson KE, Tibbling L. Gastric secretion and reflux pattern in reflux oesophagitis before and during ranitidine treatment. Scand J Gastroenterol 1986;21:487−492.

11. Jansen JBMJ, Lamers CBHW. High doses of ranitidine in patients with reflux oesophagitis. Scand J Gastroenterol 1990;25 (suppl 178):42–46.

12. Miller LS, Vinayek R, Frucht H, Gardner JD, Jensen RT, Maton PN. Reflux esophagitis in patients with Zollinger-Ellison syndrome. Gastroenterology 1990;98:341–346.

Does an increased dosage of an H₂RA have an obvious effect on healing of esophagitis and relief of symptoms?

J.G. Mills (London), *R.H. Murdock* (Glaxo Research Triangle Park, North Carolina)

Ranitidine given 150 mg twice daily, or even as a single 300 mg dose at bedtime is an effective treatment for most patients with reflux esophagitis [1,2]. Nevertheless, a proportion of patients fail to respond. There is some evidence to suggest that patients whose esophagitis does not heal show little or no reduction in acid reflux time [3,4].

Reduction in esophageal acid contact time — a dose response

Ranitidine 150 mg b.d. is associated with a significant reduction in total reflux time. However, this dosage regimen is less effective in controlling daytime than nocturnal acid reflux and does not normalize acid contact time (ACT) in all patients (i.e., reduction of acid contact time (ACT) to ≤4.0%).

Increasing the dose of ranitidine, but more importantly the frequency of dosing, is associated with a further reduction in acid contact time (ACT) [5–7]. A dose-response relationship is most clearly demonstrated by the study of Jansen et al. [5]. The patients studied all had severe erosive esophagitis which had not responded to treatment with 150 mg b.d. However, larger and more frequent doses (up to 4 and 6 times 300 mg) reduced acid contact time (ACT) to within the normal range. A dose-response relationship has been confirmed in studies with other H₂-receptor antagonists. A comparison of famotidine 40 mg nocte, 40 mg b.d. or 20 mg b.d. showed that twice daily administration was significantly more effective than the once daily regimen [8].

Healing of esophagitis — endoscopic assessment

Comparison of the efficacy a ranitidine 300 mg once daily, given after the evening meal or at bedtime, with a twice daily regimen, showed a numerical advantage for ranitidine 300 mg b.d. — cumulative healing of 77% compared to 68% by week 12 — but this difference was not statistically significant [9].

The effects of a higher dose, ranitidine 300 mg q.d.s., were compared with the most usually recommended dosage regimen, 150 mg b.d., in 138 patients with moderate to severe reflux esophagitis, Savary-Miller grades II and III [10]. Data from 122 patients were available for analysis at 4 weeks and from 117 patients at 8 weeks. The results of endoscopic examination are shown in Table 1.

There was a highly significant difference between the two treatment groups. Grade II esophagitis was more likely to have healed than grade III esophagitis after 4 or 8 weeks, irrespective of treatment given. However, the benefit of treatment with the higher dose was most marked in patients with more severe disease.

This study confirmed the benefit of higher dose regimens but did not show whether the benefit is due to the higher dose or shorter dosing interval. Two trials were therefore designed to evaluate the efficacy of ranitidine 150 mg and 300 mg, each given 4 times daily for up to 12 weeks, in a large number of patients with endoscopically confirmed erosive esophagitis [11,12]. In both studies patients with erosive esophagitis, defined as Hetzel grades II–IV, were screened for baseline symptomatology for 7 days and then allocated to one of the three treatment groups. Healing was defined as a normal appearance on endoscopy or erythema only. In each study endoscopically documented healing at 4, 8 and 12 weeks was significantly higher for both ranitidine treatment groups than for placebo. Since the studies were identical with respect to the inclusion criteria, procedures and definition of endoscopic appearance, the results have been combined in Fig. 1 [13].

A total of 670 patients were enrolled in the two studies. After 4 weeks treatment healing of esophagitis was recorded for 48% of patients treated with ranitidine compared to 22% of placebo (p < 0.001). Cumulative healing after 12 weeks was 58, 84 and 82% for placebo, ranitidine 150 mg q.d.s. and 300 mg q.d.s., respectively. There was no difference between the two ranitidine dosage regimens. The benefit of

Table 1.

Esophagitis grade at pretrial visit	Healing							
	4 weeks				8 weeks			
	150 mg b.d.		300 mg q.d.s.		150 mg b.d.		300 mg q.d.s.	
	n	%	n	%	n	%	n	%
II	16/46	35	31/44	70	28/34	65	35/42	83
III	1/13	8	9/19	47	2/13	15	11/19	58
Total	17/59	29	40/63	63[b]	30/56	54	46/61	75[a]

[a]p < 0.01; [b]p < 0.0001 χ^2 test.

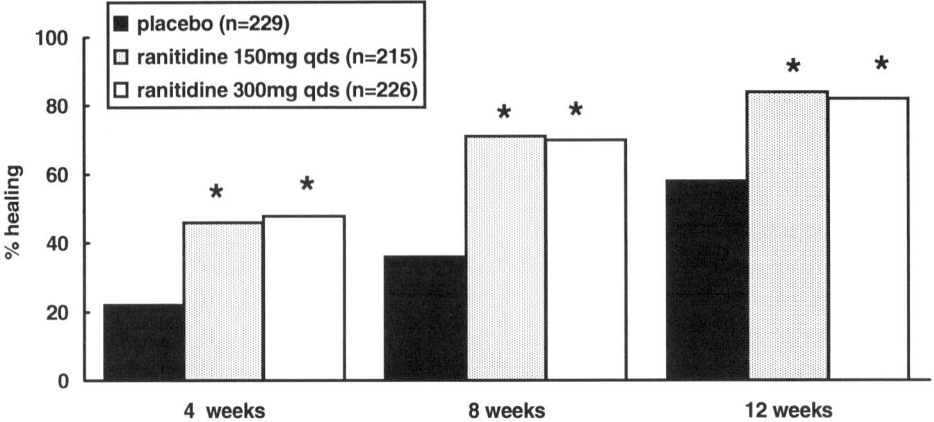

Fig. 1. Healing of reflux esophagitis (*p < 0.001 vs. placebo).

ranitidine was evident in patients with grade II esophagitis and those with more severe disease (grades III and IV).

Symptom relief

After 4 weeks of treatment 46% of patients receiving ranitidine 150 mg b.d. and 67% of those receiving ranitidine 300 mg q.d.s. were completely symptom free [10]. The run-in period incorporated into the design of studies comparing ranitidine 150 mg q.d.s., ranitidine 300 mg q.d.s. and placebo allowed more detailed analysis of the time course of symptom relief. In both studies there was a significant difference in the frequency of heartburn between ranitidine and placebo groups within 24 h of starting treatment (Table 2).

Differences in the frequency and severity of daytime and night-time heartburn were sustained throughout the treatment period.

Conclusions

Increasing doses of ranitidine are associated with an increasing pharmacological response (suppression of intragastric acidity and reduction in esophageal acid contact

Table 2. Mean (SEM) heartburn episodes/day

Time relative to start of treatment	Placebo	Ranitidine 150 mg q.d.s.	Ranitidine 300 mg q.d.s.
One day before	3.3 (0.2)	3.2 (0.2)	3.3 (0.3)
One day after	3.4 (0.2)	1.8 (0.2)[a]	1.5 (0.2)[a]

[a]p < 0.001 vs. placebo.

time). Frequency of dosing is probably more important than an increase in unit dose. Clinical studies provide evidence that higher daily doses are associated with greater healing of esophagitis and rapid relief of symptoms. The best results are achieved with ranitidine 150 mg q.d.s.; a further increase in dose provides no additional benefit.

In this paper we have used ranitidine as an example, but the same general conclusion may be expected from appropriate dosage regimens of other H_2-receptor antagonists.

References

1. Halvorsen L, Lee FI, Wesdorp ICE, Johnson NJ, Mills JG, Wood JR. Acute treatment of reflux oesophagitis: a multi-centre study to compare 150 mg ranitidine twice daily with 300 mg ranitidine at bedtime. Aliment Pharmacol Ther 1989;3: 171–181.
2. Dammann HG. Treatment of gastroesophageal reflux disease with ranitidine. In: Scarpignato C (ed) Frontiers in Gastro-intestinal Research. Basel: Karger, 1992;20:208–230.
3. Robertson DAF, Aldersley MA, Shepherd H, Lloyd RS, Smith CL. H_2-antagonists in the treatment of reflux oesophagitis: can physiological studies predict the response. Gut 1987;28:946–949.
4. Collen MJ, Lewis JH, Benjamin SB. Gastric acid hypersecretion in refractory gastroesophageal reflux disease. Gastro-enterology 1990;98:654–661.
5. Jansen JBM, Baak LC, Lamers CBHW. Are increasing doses of ranitidine helpful in reducing acid exposure of the esophagus in reflux esophagitis? Proc Dutch Soc Gastroenterol, Oct 1988.
6. Barlow A, Watson A, Attwood S, Dixon JS, Johnson NJ. A double-blind crossover comparison of the effects of ranitidine 300 mg q.d.s., 150 mg b.d. and placebo on intragastric acidity and intraoesophageal pH. Gullet 1992;2:63–69.
7. Russell J, Orr WC, King JF, Finn AL. The effects of high doses of ranitidine on oesophageal reflux and symptom severity. Am J Gastroenterol 1988;83:A32.
8. Orr WC, Robinson MG, Humphries TJ, Antonello J, Cagliola A. Dose-response effect of famotidine on patterns of gastro-esophageal reflux. Aliment Pharmacol Ther 1988;2:229–235.
9. Johnson NJ, Laws S, Mills JG, Wood JR. Effect of three ranitidine dosage regimens in the treatment of reflux oesophagitis: results of a multicentre trial. Eur J Gastroenterol Hepatol 1991;3:769–774.
10. Johnson NJ, Boyd EJS, Mills JG, Wood JR. Acute treatment of reflux oesophagitis: a multicentre trial to compare 150 mg ranitidine b.d. with 300 mg ranitidine q.d.s. Aliment Pharmacol Ther 1989;3:259–266.
11. Roufail W, Belsito A, Robinson M, Barish C, Rubin A and Glaxo Erosive Esophagitis Study Group. Ranitidine for erosive esophagitis: a double-blind, placebo-controlled study. Aliment Pharmacol Ther 1992;6:597–607.
12. Euler AR, Murdock RH, Wilson TH, Silver MT, Parker SE, Powers L. Ranitidine is effective therapy for erosive esophagi-tis. Am J Gastroenterol 1993;88:520–524.
13. Euler AR, Murdock RH, Wilson TH, Silver MT, Parker SE. Ranitidine 150 mg and 300 mg four times a day are equally effective for healing erosive esophagitis and relieving heartburn. Hepatogastroenterology 1991; Abstract of the European Digestive Disease Week: A150.

Prokinetic agents

What are the modes of action of prokinetic agents?

L.M.A. Akkermans, A.J.P.M. Smout (Utrecht)

Symptomatic gastroesophageal reflux is a complex syndrome resulting from various defects. In some patients it may be a primary defect of the defense mechanisms of the mucosa, but it is more likely that primary motor disorders of the upper gastrointestinal tract are the main cause [1].

Several motor defects are proposed to play a major role in the pathophysiology of reflux disease. The most important are: 1) mechanisms leading to frequent gastro-esophageal reflux such as, a defective basal lower esophageal sphincter pressure (LESP), an increased frequency of transient lower esophageal sphincter relaxations (TLESR's) and delayed gastric emptying; 2) mechanisms leading to slow esophageal clearance due to esophageal body motor dysfunctions such as disrupted peristaltic contractions with low velocity, duration and amplitude.

Recent excellent reviews give extensive information on gastrointestinal prokinetic agents [2,3]. The purpose of this short communication is to summarize and update the latest results concerning the investigations on the mode of action of established and possible new esophagoprokinetic molecules in gastroesophageal reflux disease (Table 1).

The pharmacological substances which, theoretically, have the potential to correct the above-mentioned motor defects and which may be clinically effective in gastro-esophageal reflux disease can be divided into four groups.

1. The direct cholinergic agonist bethanechol increases LESP when given orally or

Table 1.

Prokinetic agents	

Cholinergic agonists
  bethanechol
	Macrolides
	  erythromycin, erythromycin derivatives

Antidopaminergics
  metoclopramide, clebopride,
  domperidone
	CCK antagonists
	  loxiglumide, devazepine

Substituted benzamides
  metoclopramide, rensapride,
  zacopride, cisapride
	Mixed μ/κ opiate agonists
	  trimebutine, fedotozine

Possible future prokinetics
  compounds aimed to interfere with nonadrenergic
  noncholinergic (NANC)-mediated LES-relaxations
  and esophageal peristalsis	

subcutaneously [4–6]. It also increases the amplitude and duration of the esophageal peristaltic contractions [6]. A major disadvantage of bethanechol is that it increases antropyloroduodenal motility in a non-coordinated way. The consequence of this is that it has only little effect on gastric emptying in patients with gastroesophageal reflux disease [7]. There are also conflicting studies on the possible beneficial effect of bethanechol by increasing salivary flow [8,9]. Bethanechol increases parasympathetic tone which results in enhanced gastric secretion and side effects such as abdominal cramps, flushing, bradycardia, diarrhea and blurred vision.

2. Antidopaminergics (metoclopramide, domperidone) increase LESP [10,11]. Metoclopramide and domperidone have no convincing effects on esophageal peristalsis and also lack a marked effect on esophageal acid clearance [12]. Domperidone improves gastric emptying of liquids and solids by an inhibition of adaptive fundic relaxation, an increase in antral contractility and an improved antroduodenal coordination [13]. Metoclopramide has more convincing effects on gastric emptying but this is probably due to the fact that this drug not only has antidopaminergic properties but also possesses a 5-hydroxy-tryptamine$_4$ (5-HT$_4$) receptor agonist activity, as will be discussed below.

3. Substituted benzamides (metoclopramide, cisapride, renzapride, zacopride) act in the gastrointestinal tract as agonists of the 5-HT$_4$ receptor. The enhanced cholinergic transmission which is induced by stimulation of this 5-HT$_4$ receptor is proposed to be responsible for the prokinetic effects of cisapride and other related benzamides [14,15]. On circular muscular strips of the esophagus of the cat, contractile responses can be induced by electrical stimulation of cholinergic enteric neurons. These responses are enhanced by benzamides such as cisapride and metoclopramide and are mediated by 5-HT$_4$ receptors [16]. Cisapride increases the LESP [17,18]. Intravenous cisapride increases the amplitude of primary

peristaltic contractions. Long-term effects of cisapride on esophageal peristalsis and LESP in patients with gastroesophageal reflux disease have not yet been published. Cisapride decreases the total time of esophageal acid exposure as measured by prolonged intraesophageal pH monitoring [19]. Cisapride (and somewhat less noticeably metoclopramide) enhance antroduodenal coordination and gastric emptying of solid and liquid meals [20,21].

4. Experimental molecules (macrolides, CCK antagonists, mixed μ/κ opioid agonists are currently under investigation. Although macrolides (erythromycin) primarily bind to motilin receptors located in the gastric antrum and proximal duodenum [22], preliminary studies indicate that erythromycin increases the LESP. It has no or only a small effect on esophageal peristalsis and it increases gastric emptying [23–25]. Further studies, with modern gastrointestinal ambulatory motility techniques, are needed to assess the mode of action of macrolides in patients with gastroesophageal reflux disease with and without delayed gastric emptying. The CCK antagonist loxiglumide has no effect on basal LESP but it is able to counteract a high-fat-meal-induced decreased sphincter pressure [26]. Furthermore, loxiglumide can only accelerate gastric emptying of a meal that releases endogenous CCK. This indicates that loxiglumide has no intrinsic effect on gastric emptying [27]. More studies are needed to judge the possible role for CCK antagonists as esophagoprokinetics. Fedotozine, a new synthetic ligand with peripheral selective affinity for κ opioid receptors, has no effect on basal LESP but it decreases the percentage and duration of LES relaxations and increases the duration, amplitude and velocity of peristaltic contractions [28].

Of all the drugs mentioned above, it is clear that cisapride has the most convincing prokinetic effects on esophageal motility and gastric emptying. However, no data are available yet on the effect of these drugs on TLESRs. These studies are urgently needed because abnormally frequent TLESRs are probably the most important mechanism of gastroesophageal reflux [1].

An interesting new area for future research concerning the sensible or sensitized gut is opened with the development of fedotozine. Fedotozine increases the threshold of discomfort to gastric distention [29]. It has been suggested that the peripheral opioid system is involved in the initiation and/or the afferent pathway of gastric visceral sensitivity. It would be very interesting to study fedotozine in the sensitized or "irritable" esophagus. The discovery of nitric oxide (NO) as an important neurotransmitter of nonadrenergic-noncholinergic (NANC) nerves in the enteric nervous system has opened doors to a new area of research [30].

Pharmacological stimulation or inhibition of NANC-excitation or inhibition, or interference with afferent sensory nerves or mechanisms of sensitization will hopefully lead to new therapeutic possibilities in gastroesophageal reflux disease.

Conclusions

Prokinetic drugs which may have beneficial effects in gastroesophageal reflux disease can be divided into four groups: 1) Direct cholinergic agents (bethanechol). Various unwanted effects, such as stimulation of uncoordinated gastroduodenal motility and stimulation of gastric acid secretion, limit their use in clinical practice; 2) Anti-dopaminergics (metoclopramide, domperidone). These drugs only moderately increase lower esophageal sphincter pressure and enhance gastric emptying; 3) Substituted benzamides (metoclopramide, cisapride) increase motility through an indirect potentiation of cholinergic neurotransmission by excitation of presynaptic $5HT_4$ receptors. They increase lower esophageal sphincter pressure, stimulate the amplitude of peristaltic contractions and enhance gastric emptying rate. Furthermore, cisapride is effective in reducing the duration of esophageal acid exposure in 24-h pH monitoring. Cisapride has fewer side effects than metoclopramide. 4) Experimental molecules (macrolides, CCK antagonists and mixed μ- and κ-opioid agonists) are currently under investigation. These drugs directly increase the lower esophageal sphincter pressure (erythromycin and fedotozine) or counteract meal-induced decreased sphincter pressures (CCK antagonists). Gastric emptying is enhanced directly by macrolides. CCK antagonists only increase emptying of a meal that stimulates sufficiently CCK plasma levels.

References

1. Dent J. Gastroesophageal reflux disease: A primary motility disorder. In: Heading RC, Wood JD (eds) Gastrointestinal dysmotility. Focus on cisapride. New York: Raven Health Care Communications, 1992;127–140.
2. Reynolds JC, Putnam PE. Prokinetic agents. Gastroenterol Clin North Am 1992;21:567–597.
3. Ramirez B, Richter JE. Review article: promotility drugs in the treatment of gastro-oesophageal reflux disease. Aliment Pharmacol Ther 1993;7:5–20.
4. Miller WN, Ganeshappa, KP, Dodds WJ et al. Effect of bethanechol on gastroesophageal reflux. Am J Dig Dis 1977;22: 230–234.
5. Farrell RL, Rolig GT, Castell DO. Stimulation of the incompetent lower esophageal sphincter. A possible advance in therapy of heartburn. Am J Dig Dis 1973;18:646–650.
6. Sondheimer JM, Arnold GL. Early effects of bethanechol on the esophageal motor function of infants with gastro-esophageal reflux. J Pediatr Gastroenterol Nutr 1986;5:47–51.
7. McCallum RW, Fink SM, Lerner E et al. Effects of metoclopramide and bethanechol on delayed gastric emptying present in gastroesophageal reflux patients. Gastroenterology 1983;84:1573–1577.
8. Helm JF, Dodds WJ, Pelc LR et al. Effect of esophageal emptying and saliva on clearance of acid from the esophagus. N Engl J Med 1984;310:284–288.
9. Devault KR, Castell DO. Effects of antireflux therapies on salivary function in normal humans. Dig Dis Sci 1987;32: 603–608.
10. Cohen S, Morris DW, Schoen HJ et al. The effect of oral and intravenous metoclopramide on human lower esophageal sphincter pressure. Gastroenterology 1976;70:484–487.
11. Weirauch TR. Evaluation of the effect of domperidone on human oesophageal peristalsis and gastroduodenal motility by intraluminal manometry. Postgrad Med J 1979;55:7–10.
12. Orr WC, Finn A, Wilson T et al. Esophageal acid contact time and heartburn in acute treatment with ranitidine and metoclopramide. Am J Gastroenterol 1990;85:697–700.
13. Johnson AG. Domperidone in the treatment of gastroesophageal reflux disease. Front Gastrointest Res 1992;20:45–53.
14. Bockaert J, Fozard JR, Demuis A et al. The $5-HT_4$ receptor: a place in the sun. Trends Pharmacol Sci 1992;13;141–145.
15. Briejer MR, Akkermans LMA, Meulemans AL et al. Cisapride and a structural analogue, R 76186, are 5-hydroxytrypt-amine$_4$ ($5-HT_4$) receptor agonists on the guinea-pig colon ascendens. Naunyn-Schmiedeberg's Arch Pharmacol 1993;347: 464–470.
16. Schuurkes J. Cisapride and gastrointestinal motility in animal models. In: Heading RC, Wood JD (eds) Gastrointestinal Dysmotility: Focus on Cisapride. New York: Raven Health Care Comm., 1992;1–14.
17. Gilbert, RJ, Dodds WJ, Kahrilas PJ et al. Effect of cisapride, a new prokinetic agent in esophageal motor dysfunction. Dig Dis Sci 1987;32:1331–1336.
18. Smout AJPM, Bogaard JW, Grade AC et al. Effects of cisapride, a new gastrointestinal prokinetic substance, on inter-digestive and postprandial motor activity of the distal esophagus in man. Gut 1985;26:246–251.
19. Rode H, Stunden RJ, Millar AJW et al. Esophageal pH assessment of gastroesophageal reflux in 18 patients and the effect of two prokinetic agents: cisapride and metoclopramide. J Pediatr Surg 1987;22:931–934.

20. Abell TL, Camilliri M, DiMagno EP et al. Long-term efficacy of oral cisapride in symptomatic upper gut dysmotility. Dig Dis Sci 1991;36:616–620.
21. McCallum RW. Gastric emptying in gastroesophageal reflux and the therapeutic role of prokinetic agents. Gastroenterol Clin North Am 1990;19:551–564.
22. Peeters T, Matthijs G, Depoortere I et al. Erythromycin is a motilin receptor agonist. Am J Physiol 1989;257:G470–G474.
23. Dalton CB, Devore MS, Smout AJPM et al. The effect of erythromycin (Ery) and lower esophageal sphincter pressure (LESP) and esophageal motility (EM). Gastroenterology 1990;98:342A.
24. Janssens J, Vantrappen G, Annese V et al. Effect of erythromycin on LES function and esophageal body contractility. Gastroenterology 1990;98:64A.
25. Harrison ME, Ruzkowski CJ, Young MF et al. Erythromycin improves gastric emptying and esophageal motility without affecting gastroesophageal reflux. Gastroenterology 1991;100:80A.
26. Katschinski M, Koppelberg T, Wank U et al. CCK plays a role as a physiological regulator of human esophageal motility. Gastroenterology 1990;98:365A.
27. Meyer BM, Werth VA, Beglinger C et al. Role of cholecystokinin in regulation of gastrointestinal motor functions. Lancet 1989;(2):12–15.
28. Bost R, Bérard H, Bonaz B et al. Effect of fedotozine on esophageal motility in healthy volunteers. Eur J Gastroenterol Hepatol 1991;3(suppl 1):52.
29. Coffin B, Jian R, Lémann M, Fraitag B et al. Fedotozine increases threshold of discomfort to gastric distension in healthy subjects. Gastroenterology 1992;102:A437.
30. Stark ME, Szurszewski JH. Role of nitric oxide in gastrointestinal and hepatic function and disease. Gastroenterology 1992; 103:1928–1949.

Can esophageal acid exposure be reduced by adding a prokinetic agent to an H₂RA?

W. Inauen (Bern)

The effect of adding a prokinetic agent to an H_2-receptor antagonist (H_2RA), was studied in 18 patients with endoscopically proven reflux esophagitis [1]. Each patient was treated with a) placebo; b) ranitidine 150 mg b.i.d.; and c) ranitidine 150 mg b.i.d. + cisapride 20 mg b.i.d.; according to a double-blind, double dummy, within subject, three-way crossover design. Esophageal acidity and motility were monitored under ambulatory conditions over 24 h. Acid reflux was monitored by a pH electrode, located 5 cm above the lower esophageal sphincter (LES). Intraesophageal pressure was simultaneously recorded from 4 transducers placed 20, 15, 10 and 5 cm above the LES. Compared to placebo, the H_2RA ranitidine decreased total reflux (from 10.0% (3.2–32.6) to 6.4% (1.2–22.9), (median (range)), p < 0.01), upright reflux (p < 0.05), supine reflux (p < 0.001) and postprandial reflux (p < 0.01), but did not affect esophageal motility. If the prokinetic agent cisapride was added to ranitidine, cisapride further diminished the acid reflux observed under ranitidine; i.e., cisapride led to an additional reduction of total reflux (from 6.4% (1.2–22.9) to 3.7% (1.0–12.7), p < 0.01), supine reflux (p < 0.05) and postprandial reflux (p < 0.05). In addition, cisapride reduced both the number (p < 0.01) and duration (p < 0.05) of reflux episodes. Cisapride significantly increased amplitude, duration and propagation velocity of esophageal contractions ($p < 0.05$), but did not affect the number of contractions. These findings demonstrate that the 30% reduction of esophageal acid exposure, achieved by a conventional dose of ranitidine (150 mg b.i.d.), can be improved to more than 60% by combination with cisapride (20 mg b.i.d.). The cisapride-induced increase of the esophageal contractile force and propagation velocity appears to enhance the clearance of gastroesophageal reflux (GER). Combination of a histamine H_2RA with a prokinetic agent may therefore provide an alternative treatment of reflux esophagitis.

Introduction

Inhibition of gastric acid secretion has become the traditional medical treatment of reflux esophagitis. The healing rates achieved by a 6—8 weeks treatment of erosive reflux esophagitis are approximately 50% for potent histamine H_2RAs (e.g., ranitidine 150—300 mg b.i.d. [2]) and up to 90% for omeprazole, an inhibitor of $H^+K^+ATPase$ [3,4]. Although these drugs are effective, they do not reduce the reflux of other gastric contents (pepsin, bile) and they do not modify the underlying causes of the disease by restoring LES pressure or improving esophageal clearance and gastric emptying. However, the newest prokinetic agent cisapride, a cholinomimetic drug, has been shown to improve LES function and to improve esophageal and gastric clearance [5]. In addition, cisapride produces healing rates of up to 50% in erosive esophagitis, which is comparable with histamine H_2RAs [6—11]. Since cisapride and histamine H_2RAs exert their effects by affecting different mechanisms, they may have an additive effect and produce higher healing rates than either medication alone. If this is the case, the combination of cisapride and ranitidine should produce a greater diminution in esophageal acid exposure than ranitidine alone.

This hypothesis was tested in patients with proven reflux esophagitis, by performing 24-h ambulatory monitoring of intraesophageal pH and pressure during treatment with placebo, ranitidine and ranitidine combined with cisapride. The use of simultaneous 24-h intraesophageal pH-metry and 4-channel manometry, objective and highly reproducible techniques for assessing acid reflux and esophageal motor function [12], allowed for the determination of whether the effect of treatment on esophageal pH was attributable to changes in esophageal body motility.

Methods

Patients

From the 18 patients (17 males, one female; median age 49.5 years (range 31—72)), three had the endoscopic diagnosis of reflux esophagitis grade I (isolated erosions), 12 patients had reflux esophagitis grade II (linear confluent erosions) and three patients presented with reflux esophagitis grade III (circumferential erosions) [13].

Study drugs and study days

According to a double-blind, double dummy, within subject, three-way crossover design, patients were allocated to receive treatment with: a) placebo (matching ranitidine placebo one tablet b.i.d. + matching cisapride placebo two tablets b.i.d.); b) ranitidine (ranitidine one tablet of 150 mg b.i.d. + matching cisapride placebo two tablets b.i.d.); and c) ranitidine + cisapride (ranitidine one tablet of 150 mg b.i.d. + cisapride two tablets of 10 mg b.i.d.). The study drugs (three tablets each time) were ingested at 9.15 am (before breakfast) and 10.00 pm (bedtime). Each treatment period lasted 4 days and intraesophageal pH and motility was monitored on the 4th day. The treatment periods were followed by a washout period of 10 days, during which the patients were allowed to take antacids.

Patients attended the clinic at 8.00 am, after an overnight fast. After local anesthesia, two catheters (one for pH, one for pressure recording) were inserted transnasally and their tips placed 5 cm above the LES. At 9.00 am, continuous 24-h recording of intraesophageal pH and pressure was started. At 9.15 am, all patients ingested their study medication and received a standard breakfast (bread, butter, marmalade, coffee, tea or milk). At 12.00 pm, a standardized lunch was served, consisting of lasagna (baked layers of noodles, meat, cheese and tomato sauce), bread, salad and cake for dessert. At 4.00 pm, the patients received a snack (tea or coffee with cake), and at 6.00 pm, a standard dinner was served (Swiss style muesli, consisting of cereals, milk, yogurt, fresh fruits). Identical meals were prepared for each study day and they were eaten within 30 min of serving. Free access to water was allowed for drinking. Smoking was permitted, but the number and timing of cigarettes were noted on a diary sheet and had to be similar on all study days. During the study days, the patients were fully ambulatory and could follow their preferred daily routine, except that they had to return to the laboratory for their meals. After dinner, each patient returned home. The times of retiring and getting up, on the following morning, were noted on the diary sheet and marked electronically by pushing the appropriate buttons on the recording unit. At 8.00 am on the following morning, the patients returned to the laboratory and shortly after 9.00 am, the probes and recording equipment were removed.

Statistics

The results are shown as median and range. For statistical comparison, the non-parametric Wilcoxon signed-rank test, for paired observations, was used. P values <0.05 were considered as significant.

Results

Esophageal acid exposure

With placebo treatment, the pH in the distal esophagus (sensor position 5 cm above the LES) remained below 4.0 during 10% (3.2–32.6) of the 24-h recording period

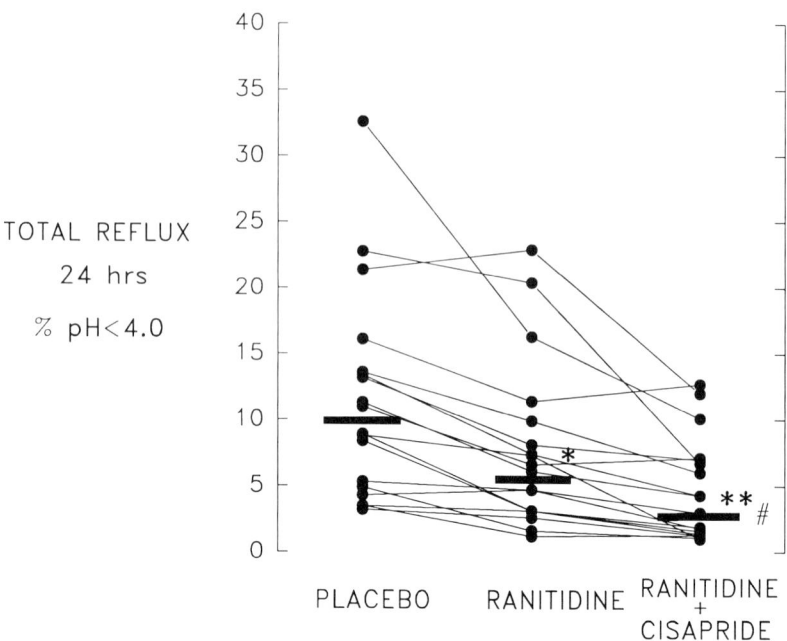

Fig. 1. Esophageal acid reflux (% of time with an intraesophageal pH < 4.0) in 18 patients with erosive reflux esophagitis. Acid reflux is shown for the entire 24-h recording period. Horizontal bars indicate median (n = 18 for all treatments. * p <0.01 / ** p < 0.001 vs. placebo; # p < 0.01 vs. ranitidine).

(Fig. 1). During ranitidine, reflux time fell to 6.4% (1.2–22.9) (p < 0.01 vs. placebo) with a further reduction to 3.7% (1.0–12.7) (p < 0.001 vs. placebo, p < 0.01 vs. ranitidine) during ranitidine plus cisapride. Upright reflux was more than 3 times greater than supine reflux (p < 0.01) (Table 1). Ranitidine reduced both upright and supine reflux and an additional reduction of supine reflux was produced by the combination with cisapride. The highest values for esophageal acid exposure were observed during the postprandial periods. Ranitidine diminished the postprandial reflux observed after breakfast and lunch, but had no effect on postprandial reflux after dinner. The addition of cisapride led to a further reduction of postprandial reflux after lunch. Whereas ranitidine only slightly decreased the number and duration of reflux episodes, the combination of ranitidine plus cisapride reduced the number and maximal duration of reflux episodes during the 24-h upright and supine periods (Table 1).

Esophageal motility

Ranitidine did not affect esophageal motility. As compared to ranitidine, the addition of cisapride led to an increase of contraction amplitude during the upright period (from 28.0 mmHg (14–54) to 32.5 mmHg (13–56), p < 0.05) and the postprandial periods after breakfast (from 27.0 mmHg (14–56) to 33.5 mmHg (12–72), p < 0.05) and lunch (from 27.9 mmHg (15–44) to 35.5 mmHg (19–46), p < 0.05). During the

Table 1. Esophageal acid reflux (defined as intraesophageal pH < 4.0) in 18 patients with erosive reflux esophagitis. Since the duration of the upright and supine periods were different between measurements and individuals, the absolute values for reflux time (min) are shown only for the 24-h period. Values are shown as median and (range) (n = 18 for all parameters)

	Placebo	Ranitidine	Ranitidine + Cisapride
Total reflux (24 h)			
Reflux time (min)	143.5 (45–469)	91.5[b] (17–329)	52.3[ce] (14–183)
pH < 4.0 (%)	10.0 (3.2–32.6)	6.4[b] (1.2–22.9)	3.7[ce] (1.0–12.7)
Reflux episodes >6 s	69.0 (41–572)	64.5 (16–320)	41.5[ce] (14–269)
Reflux episodes >5 min	6.5 (0–13)	3.5 (0–17)	1.0[cf] (0–7)
Mean reflux duration (min)	1.2 (0.6–4.8)	1.2 (0.6–4.2)	0.9[a] (0.4–5.1)
Maximal reflux duration (min)	16.0 (4.7–55.1)	12.2 (3.2–50.7)	6.2[c] (1.8–57.1)
Upright reflux			
pH < 4.0 (%)	13.3 (3.7–35.0)	8.3[a] (1.2–27.1)	5.0[c] (1.6–21.8)
Reflux episodes >6 s	54.5 (36–418)	61.0 (10–297)	39.0[be] (14–211)
Reflux episodes >5 min	4.0 (0–11)	3.0 (0–13)	1.0[ad] (0–7)
Mean reflux duration (min)	1.1 (0.5–3.3)	1.0 (0.5–3.1)	0.9 (0.4–5.1)
Maximal reflux duration (min)	13.9 (3.2–55.1)	10.1 (2.1–50.7)	5.9[a] (1.8–57.1)
Supine reflux			
pH < 4.0 (%)	3.7 (0–37.6)	0.9[c] (0–17.1)	0.0[cd] (0–4.8)
Reflux episodes >6 s	6.5 (1–84)	4.0[c] (0–37)	1.0[cf] (0–29)
Reflux episodes >5 min	1.5 (0–8)	0.0[a] (0–5)	0.0[cd] (0–2)
Mean reflux duration (min)	2.0 (0.1–18.5)	0.6 (0–9.8)	0.1[b] (0–4.2)
Maximal reflux duration (min)	6.7 (0.1–42.1)	1.9 (0–38.0)	0.1[cd] (0–6.5)

[a] $p < 0.05$; [b] $p < 0.01$; [c] $p < 0.001$ vs. placebo; [d] $p < 0.05$; [e] $p < 0.01$; [f] $p < 0.001$ vs. ranitidine.

upright period, cisapride further enhanced the duration of esophageal contractions (from 3.2 s (2.8–4.2) to 3.6 s (3.0–4.4), $p < 0.05$). Cisapride increased the propagation velocity of esophageal contractions (Fig. 2), but had no effects on esophageal contractility (slope of the contraction curve) and on the number of total, propagated and nonpropagated contractions.

Discussion

This study demonstrates that: a) the combination of the histamine H_2RA ranitidine and the prokinetic agent cisapride markedly reduced esophageal acid exposure, and b) the addition of a standard oral dose of cisapride increased amplitude, duration and propagation velocity of esophageal contractions, compared with placebo and ranitidine alone.

The overall reduction of acid reflux by ranitidine (150 mg b.i.d.) was approximately 30% (Fig. 1), which is comparable to the decrease obtained in other 24-h esophageal pH-metry studies [14,15]. Although ranitidine reduced both daytime (upright) and nocturnal (supine) reflux, it led to a more pronounced decrease of nocturnal reflux. These variations reflect the pattern of gastric acid secretion under

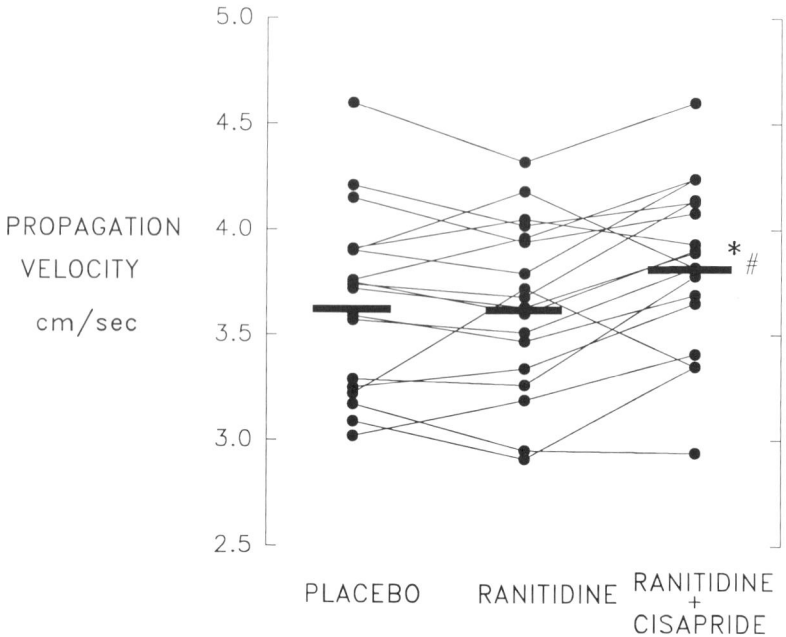

Fig. 2. Propagation velocity (cm/s) of esophageal contractions in 18 patients with erosive reflux esophagitis. Propagation velocity is shown for the entire 24-h recording period. Horizontal bars indicate median (n = 18 for all treatments; * p < 0.05 vs. placebo; # p < 0.05 vs. ranitidine).

treatment with ranitidine and are consistent with the studies measuring the effect of ranitidine on 24-h intragastric acidity, in patients with reflux esophagitis [16,17].

Four-channel manometry of the esophagus, with sensors located at 20, 15, 10 and 5 cm above the LES, permits analysis of contraction characteristics for different parts of the tubular esophagus. The addition of cisapride led to a significant increase of median contraction amplitude and duration, but only in the mid and distal esophagus. This may be explained by the selective cholinomimetic action of cisapride on the smooth muscle in the mid and distal esophagus, whereas the striated muscle of the proximal esophagus has not been affected. The present study confirms reports from short-term stationary manometry studies indicating an increase of contraction amplitude and duration, after intravenous injection of cisapride [18–20]. In contrast to the present study, the available data for oral cisapride do not suggest that cisapride affects esophageal contraction characteristics. These differences might be due to lower doses used in some of these studies [20,21], relatively short measurement periods after oral ingestion which might not have been sufficient to reach effective drug concentrations [18,20], and the fact that esophageal motility was investigated on day 4 (and not day 1) of oral drug treatment.

Although the combination of cisapride and ranitidine significantly increased amplitude, duration and propagation velocity of esophageal contractions, the changes of esophageal motility appear small when compared to the marked reduction of acid reflux. Therefore, additional effects of cisapride on gastroesophageal motility, such as an improvement of LES function [19,20] and an acceleration of gastric emptying [22], might contribute to the reduction of acid reflux. On the other hand, the demonstrated increase of the contractile force of the esophageal body together with an accelerated propagation of the contraction waves may be responsible for the acceleration of acid clearance.

In conclusion, the combination of cisapride with ranitidine leads to a marked and additional reduction of esophageal acid exposure, compared to that achieved by ranitidine alone. Combined treatment, with a histamine H_2RA such as ranitidine and a prokinetic agent such as cisapride, is a promising alternative for medical treatment of reflux esophagitis and should be further tested in clinical trials.

References

1. Inauen W, Emde C, Weber B, Armstrong D, Bettschen HU, Huber T, Scheurer U, Blum AL, Halter F, Merki HS. Effects of ranitidine and cisapride on acid reflux and oesophageal motility in patients with reflux oesophagitis: A 24-h ambulatory combined pH and manometry study. Gut 1993;34 (in press).
2. Koelz HR, Birchler R, Bretholz A et al. Healing and relapse of reflux esophagitis during treatment with ranitidine. Gastroenterology 1986;91:1198−1205.
3. Havelund T, Laursen LS, Skoubo-Kristensen E et al. Omeprazole and ranitidine in treatment of reflux oesophagitis: double blind comparative trial. Br Med J 1988;296:89−92.
4. Lundell L, Backman L, Ekström P et al. Prevention of relapse of reflux esophagitis after endoscopic healing: the efficacy and safety of omeprazole compared with ranitidine. Scand J Gastroenterol 1991;26:248−256.
5. Verlinden M. Review article: a role for gastrointestinal prokinetic agents in the treatment of reflux oesophagitis? Aliment Pharmacol Ther 1989;3:113−131.
6. Baldi F, Bianchi Porro G, Dobrilla G et al. Cisapride versus placebo in reflux esophagitis. A multicenter double-blind trial. J Clin Gastroenterol 1988;10:614−618.
7. Lepoutre L, Van Der Spek P, Vanderlinden I, Bollen J, Laukens P. Healing of grade-II and III oesophagitis through motility stimulation with cisapride. Digestion 1990;45:109−114.
8. Janisch HD, Hüttemann W, Bouzo MH. Cisapride versus ranitidine in the treatment of reflux esophagitis. Hepato-Gastroenterol 1988;35:125−127.
9. Galmiche JP, Fraitag B, Filoche B, Evreux M, Vitaux J, Zeitoun P, Fournet J, Soule JC. Double-blind comparison of cisapride and cimetidine in treatment of reflux esophagitis. Dig Dis Sci 1990;35:649−655.
10. Maleev A, Mendizova A, Popov P et al. Cisapride and cimetidine in the treatment of erosive esophagitis. Hepato-Gastroenterol 1990;37:403−407.
11. Toussaint J, Gossuin A, Deruyttere M, Hublé F, Devis G. Healing and prevention of relapse of reflux oesophagitis by cisapride. Gut 1991;32:1280−1285.
12. Emde C, Armstrong D, Castiglione F, Cilluffo T, Riecken EO, Blum AL. Reproducibility of long-term ambulatory esophageal combined pH/manometry. Gastroenterology 1991;100:1630−1637.
13. Savary M, Miller G. L'oesophage. In: Manuel et atlas d'endoscopie. Solothurn (Switzerland): Gassmann AG, 1977.
14. Johansson KE, Tibbling L. Gastric secretion and reflux pattern in reflux oesophagitis before and during ranitidine treatment. Scand J Gastroenterol 1986;21:487−492.
15. Klinkenberg-Knol EC, Festen HPM, Meuwissen SGM. The effects of omeprazole and ranitidine on 24-hour pH in the distal oesophagus of patients with reflux oesophagitis. Aliment Pharmacol Ther 1988;2:221−227.
16. Mahachal V, Walker K, Thomson ADR. Comparison of cimetidine and ranitidine on 24-hour intragastric acidity and serum gastrin profile in patients with esophagitis. Dig Dis Sci 1985;30(4):321−328.
17. Lind T, Cederberg C, Idstrom JP, Lonroth H, Olbe L, Lundell L. 24-hour intragastric acidity and plasma gastrin during long-term treatment with omeprazole or ranitidine in patients with reflux esophagitis. Scand J Gastroent 1991;26:620−626.
18. Gilbert RJ, Dodds WJ, Kahrilas PJ, Hogan WJ, Lipman S. Effect of cisapride, a new prokinetic agent, on esophageal motor function. Dig Dis Sci 1987;32:1331−1336.
19. Ceccatelli P, Janssens J, Vantrappen G, Cucchiara S. Cisapride restores the decreased lower oesophageal sphincter pressure in reflux patients. Gut 1988;29:631−635.
20. Corazziari E, Bontempo I, Anzini F. Effects of cisapride on distal esophageal motility in humans. Dig Dis Sci 1989;34:1600−1605.
21. Holloway RH, Downton J, Mitchell B, Dent J. Effect of cisapride on postprandial gastro-oesophageal reflux. Gut 1989;30:1187−1193.
22. Maddern GJ, Jamieson GG, Myers JC, Collins PJ. Effect of cisapride on delayed gastric emptying in gastro-oesophageal reflux disease. Gut 1991;32:470−474.

Are the results of the combination of a prokinetic agent with an antisecretory agent affected by tobacco smoking?

B. Fraitag (Paris)

A reduction of tobacco consumption is classically recommended in patients with gastroesophageal reflux disease (GERD) [1], on the basis of enhanced gastric acid secretion [2] and decreased basal pressure of the lower esophageal sphincter (LES) [3] in smokers. However, sizable consequences of these pharmacological effects on the treatment of GERD have not been established. Thus, while healing of esophagitis was delayed in smokers in one study using ranitidine [4], other studies using omeprazole [5], ranitidine [6] and cimetidine [7] have not confirmed this finding. In addition, in a study comparing cimetidine and a placebo [8], symptomatic improvement was better in smokers than in nonsmokers. As a result, the influence of tobacco consumption does not appear to be clear in the above-mentioned studies, using an antisecretory agent as single treatment.

The efficacy of combined prokinetic-antisecretory treatment has been addressed in six studies, the prokinetic being metoclopramide in two [9,10], domperidone in two [11,12] and cisapride in two [13,14]. The combination of metoclopramide and cimetidine proved better than cimetidine alone on healing of endoscopic lesions in one study [10], but not in another one [9]. In both studies using domperidone, combinations of this compound to ranitidine [11] or famotidine [12] did not prove better than any of the two compounds used alone. The combination of cisapride and cimetidine appeared better than cimetidine alone, both on healing of endoscopic lesions and symptomatic improvement [13]. Conversely, the combination of cisapride and ranitidine did not prove better than ranitidine alone in another study [14]; however, in the latter study, cisapride was used at half the dose used in the former one (10 mg b.i.d. vs. 10 mg q.i.d.), providing a potential explanation for the discrepancy between both studies. Thus, while the combination of domperidone and an antisecretory agent cannot be recommended, metoclopramide and particularly cisapride combined to an antisecretory agent seem to offer a significant advantage over the antisecretory alone. To date, no study combining a prokinetic and a proton pump inhibitor has been published; in view of the outspoken efficacy of proton pump inhibitors alone, the improvement brought about by the adjunction of a prokinetic, would be marginal and difficult to demonstrate, requiring a high sample size study.

The influence of tobacco consumption on the results of the combination of prokinetic and antisecretory agents has been assessed in none of the six above-mentioned studies [9–14]. In practical terms, the question raised in the title of this communication will largely remain unanswered. If data obtained from studies using a prokinetic as single treatment were to be extrapolated to the combined treatment, it may be said that, while pharmacological findings favor a negative role of tobacco consumption on the effect of GERD treatment, clinical data do not support this

Table 1. Controlled studies with a combination of prokinetic and antisecretory agents in GERD

Author	No. of patients	Design	Dosage	Duration	Results/ Symptoms	Results/ Endoscopy
Temple et al. [9]	73	Double-blind	MET 10 mg t.d.s/ CIM 400 mg q.d.s. vs. CIM 400 mg q.d.s.	12 weeks	MET/CIM = CIM	MET/CIM = CIM
Lieberman et al. [10]	25	Double-blind	MET 10 mg q.d.s./ CIM 1200 mg/day vs. CIM 1200 mg/day	8 weeks	MET/CIM > CIM/PLA	MET/CIM > CIM/PLA
Masci et al. [11]	45	Double-blind	DOM 20 mg t.d.s. RAN 150 mg b.d.s. DOM/RAN	6 weeks	DOM = RAN = DOM/RAN	DOM = RAN = DOM/RAN
Guslandi et al. [12]	42	Double-blind	DOM 20 mg t.d.s. FAM 40 mg nocte DOM/FAM	8 weeks	DOM = FAM = DOM/FAM	DOM = FAM = DOM/FAM
Galmiche et al. [13]	47	Double-blind	CIS 10 mg q.d.s./ CIS 200 mg 400 mg nocte vs. CIM 200 mg t.d.s. 400 mg nocte	6, 12 weeks	CIS/CIM > CIM	CIS/CIM > CIM
Wienbeck et al. [14]	93	Double-blind	CIS 10 mg b.d./ RAN 150 mg b.d. vs. RAN 150 mg b.d./PLA	6, 12 weeks	CIS/RAN = RAN/PLA	CIS/RAN = RAN/PLA

MET = metoclopramide; CIM = cimetidine; DOM = domperidone; CIS = cisapride; PLA = placebo; RAN = ranitidine; FAM = famotidine; > = significantly better.

411

conclusion (Table 1). The influence of tobacco consumption, thus, cannot be established. Finally, it must be kept in mind that all the above considerations pertain to the acute treatment of GERD and that the effect of tobacco consumption has never been assessed in the maintenance treatment of GERD.

References

1. Richter JE, Castell DO. Current approaches in the medical treatment of esophageal reflux. Drugs 1981;21:283—291.
2. Wright DJ, Pandya A. Smoking and gastric juice volume in outpatients. Can Anaesth Soc J 1979;26:328—330.
3. Castell DO. Physiology and pathophysiology of the lower esophageal sphincter. Ann Otol Rhinol Laryngol 1975;84:569—575.
4. Koelz HR, Birchler R, Bretholz A et al. Healing and relapse of reflux esophagitis during treatment with ranitidine. Gastroenterology 1986;91:1198—1205.
5. Hetzel DJ, Dent J, Reed WD et al. Healing and relapse of severe peptic esophagitis after treatment with omeprazole. Gastroenterology 1988;95:903—912.
6. Berenson MH, Sontag SJ, Robinson MG et al. Effect of smoking in a controlled study of ranitidine treatment in gastroesophageal reflux disease. J Clin Gastroenterol 1987;9:499—503.
7. Siewert JR, Ottenjann R, Heilmann K et al. Therapie und Prophylaxe der Refluxösophagitis. Ergebnisse einer Multicenterstudie mit Cimetidin. Z Gastroenterol 1986;24:381—395.
8. Bennett JR, Buckton G, Martin HD. Cimetidine in gastroesophageal reflux. Digestion 1983;26:166—172.
9. Temple JG, Bradby GVH, O'Connor F et al. Cimetidine and metoclopramide in esophageal reflux disease. Br Med J 1983; 286:1863—1864.
10. Lieberman DA, Keefe EB. Treatment of severe reflux esophagitis with cimetidine and metoclopramide. Ann Int Med 1986; 104:21—26.
11. Masci E, Testoni PA, Passaretti S et al. Comparison of ranitidine, domperidone maleate and ranitidine + domperidone maleate in the short-term treatment of reflux esophagitis. Drugs Exp Clin Res 1985;11:687—692.
12. Guslandi M, Dell'oca M, Molteni V et al. Famotidine vs. domperidone, versus a combination of both in the treatment of reflux esophagitis. Gastroenterology 1989;96:191A(abstract).
13. Galmiche JP, Brandstätter G, Evreux M et al. Combined therapy with cisapride and cimetidine in severe reflux oesophagitis: A double-blind controlled trial. Gut 1988;29:675—681.
14. Wienbeck M. The Ranpride Study Group. Does cisapride added to H₂-receptor-blocking treatment improve healing rates in patients with esophagitis? Digestion 1986;34:144A(abstract).

What are the respective advantages of the different prokinetic agents at the disposal of the gastroenterologist?

D. Couturier (Paris)

Generally, prokinetic agents influence gastrointestinal motility through one or more of the following pathways:
— Promoting cholinergic tone;
— Antagonizing inhibitory neurotransmitters (e.g., serotonin, dopamine);
— Mimicking nonadrenergic noncholinergic compounds that increase motility (e.g., motilin) [1].

Direct cholinergic agonists

Bethanechol is an ester derivative of choline and acts at muscarinic receptors. It enhances the amplitude of contractions throughout the gastrointestinal tract and increases the lower esophageal sphincter (LES) pressure [2]. Side effects from bethanechol have to be taken into account in the treatment of esophageal disease, mainly gastroesophageal reflux (GER). They result from secretion of saliva and gastric acid and from enhancement of parasympathetic tone causing abdominal cramps, diarrhea, salivation, flushing and bradycardia.

Substituted benzamides

These drugs are derivatives of para-aminobenzoic acid. Metoclopramide and cisapride have been extensively evaluated.

Metoclopramide

Although the clinical benefits of metoclopramide (methoxy-2-chloro-5-procainamide) are restricted to the upper intestinal tract, experimental studies demonstrate a significant effect on intestinal smooth muscle. Metoclopramide has both peripheral and central dopamine receptor antagonist effects. The action on the gastrointestinal tract appears to be dependent on the release of acetylcholine from intrinsic cholinergic neurons: atropine antagonizes its effect on the LES. Vagotomy does not reduce the effect of metoclopramide. Metoclopramide has no effect on gastrin acid secretion and serum gastrin level. Metoclopramide's central antidopaminergic effects explain the effective antiemetic action, this benefit in counterpart by some extrapyramidal side effects (akathisia, dyskinesia), more common in children and the elderly.

Cisapride

This drug promotes gastrointestinal motility by indirectly stimulating cholinergic nerves. It causes the release of acetylcholine from enteric neurons, an effect that is antagonized by both tetrodotoxin and corticholinergics. Cisapride acts through several other pharmacological mechanisms whose effects are difficult to evaluate on the esophagus. In clinical trials, a transient increase in stool frequency was the only side effect, which does not limit the use in clinical practice.

Dopamine antagonists

Domperidone is a benzimidazole derivative that specifically antagonizes the inhibitory effects of dopamine, which seems to be an important inhibitory transmitter. It has no cholinergic activity and is not inhibited by atropine. Domperidone has limited ability to cross the blood-brain barrier and therefore acts primarily as a peripheral antagonist. Thus, in contrast to metoclopramide, domperidone rarely causes dystonic or extrapyramidal symptoms and it may increase prolactin levels and occasionally female patients may develop galactorrhea.

Macrolide agents

Recent studies in humans, rabbits and dogs have demonstrated that erythromycin and certain other macrolides stimulate gastrointestinal contractions. The more specific action has been described on small bowel motility. It appears that erythromycin acts through motilin receptors and produces similar motor effects as motilin.

Although gastroesophageal reflux disease (GERD) is often considered a peptic ulcer disease, most of the factors that contribute to the development of reflux esophagitis depend on disorders of esophagus and gastric motility, which produce incompetent LES and impaired esophageal clearance. Incompetent LES may manifest as intermittent inappropriate relaxations or chronically low basal pressure. Effective clearance is dependent on orderly peristaltic contractions with appropriate velocity, duration and amplitude, whose decrease correlates best with delayed acid clearance [3]. On the other hand, delayed gastric emptying also contributes to the risk of reflux.

In theory, prokinetic drugs should be the most recommended agents for the treatment of GERD and esophagitis [4].

Bethanechol increases sphincter pressure and esophageal contractions in a dose-dependent fashion. Some studies suggest that bethanechol reduces reflux symptoms and improves endoscopic findings [5,6]. The overall utility of bethanechol in the treatment of GERD is limited by side effects and concurrent stimulation of acid secretion. Side effects seen in about 15% of patients include abdominal cramps, blurred vision, fatigue and increased micturition.

Metoclopramide has been shown to be more effective than placebo in the treatment of the symptoms of GER [7,8], and as effective as are H_2 antagonists and antacids [9]. A dose of 10 mg orally in an adult is insufficient to improve LES pressure consistently. Although metoclopramide provides symptomatic relief from acid reflux its effectiveness in healing esophagitis lesion is less convincing [7]. The mechanism by which metoclopramide improves symptoms is mainly a dose-dependent increase in LES pressure [10]. Sphincter pressure begins to rise within 20–30 min and peaks approximately 1 h after oral administration.

Cisapride improves both subjective and objective evidence of esophagitis and is at least as effective as either ranitidine or metoclopramide [11]. It is also effective in reducing the duration of acid exposure [12]. In a pediatric series, cisapride appears to be effective in improving endoscopic findings [13]. Cisapride increases the LES pressure, the amplitude of contractions in the distal esophagus, and it enhances the rate of gastric emptying as well. The LES pressure increase is dose-dependent and occurs whether the drug is administered orally or intravenously [14,15].

Domperidone has been shown to be equivalent to ranitidine and superior to placebo in reducing the symptoms of GER and in promoting endoscopic evidence of esophagitis [16]. The effect of domperidone on the motor function of esophagus is inconsistent, and the benefit on esophageal function may be less than that seen with prokinetic agents.

Trials using erythromycin as treatment for gastroesophageal reflux have not yet been reported. Erythromycin significantly increases LES pressure and the duration of peristaltic contractions, acting by stimulation of cholinergic nerves [17]. It has been shown to increase LES pressure in patients with esophageal involvement by systemic sclerosis [18].

Finally, among the available prokinetics drugs, the benefit from treatment with cisapride is well documented. Cisapride improves subjective symptoms as well as endoscopic evidence of mucosal inflammation. The indication of a treatment with metoclopramide is confined to the treatment of nonulcer dyspepsia with or without GER symptoms. Since direct cholinergic agonists increase gastric secretion which is implicated in the pathophysiology of esophagitis, although they have been shown efficient, their clinical use is limited.

Clinical trials, using erythromycin and other motilin-like agonists, are needed as treatment for GER.

References

1. Reynolds JC, Putnam PE. Prokinetic agents. Gastroenterol Clin North Am 1992;21:567–596.
2. Cohen S, Green F. Force velocity characteristics of esophageal muscle effect of acetylcholine and norepinephrine. Am J Physiol 1974;226:1250–1255.
3. Helm JF, Dodds WJ, Pelc LR et al. Effect of esophageal emptying and saliva on clearance of acid from the esophagus. N Engl J Med 1984;310:284–288.
4. Castell DO. Medical therapy for reflux esophagitis: 1986 and beyond. Ann Int Med 1986;104:112–114.
5. Miller WN, Ganeshappa KP, Dodds WJ et al. Effects of bethanechol on gastroesophageal reflux. Am J Dig Dis 1977;22: 230–234.
6. Thanik DK, Chey WY, Shah AN et al. Reflux esophagitis: effect of oral bethanechol on symptoms and endoscopic findings. Ann Int Med 1980;93:805–808.
7. McCallum RW, Fink SM, Winnan GR, et al. Metoclopramide in gastroesophageal reflux disease: rationale for its use and results of a double blind trial. Am J Gastroenterol 1984;79:165–172.
8. McCallum RW, Ippoliti AF, Coon C et al. A controlled trial of metoclopramide in symptomatic gastroesophageal reflux. N Engl J Med 1977;296:354–357.
9. Tonnesen H, Andersen JR, Christoffersen P et al. Reflux esophagitis in heavy drinkers. Digestion 1987;38:69–73.
10. Cohen S, Morris DW, Schoen HJ et al. The effect of oral and intravenous metoclopramide on human lower esophageal sphincter pressure. Gastroenterology 1976;70:484–487.
11. Janisch JD, Hüttemann W, Bonzo MH. Cisapride versus ranitidine in the treatment of reflux esophagiatis. Hepato-Gastroenterol 1988;35:125–127.
12. Rode H, Stunden RJ, Millar AJW et al. Esophageal pH assessment of gastroesophageal reflux in 18 patients and the effects of two prokinetic agents: cisapride and metoclopramide. J Pediatr Surg 1987;22:931–934.
13. Cucchiara S, Staiano A, Capozzi C et al. Cisapride for gastro-oesophageal reflux and peptic oesophagitis. Arch Dis Child 1987;62:454–457.
14. Gilbert RJ, Dodds WJ, Kahrilas PJ et al. Effect of cisapride, a new prokinetic agent on esophageal motor dysfunction. Dig Dis Sci 1987;32:874–880.
15. Smout AJPM, Bogaard JW, Grade AC. Effects of cisapride, a new gastrointestinal prokinetic substance on interdigestive and postprandial motor activity of the distal oesophagus in man. Gut 1985;16:246–251.
16. Masci E, Testoni PA, Pasaretti S et al. Comparison of ranitidine, domperidone maleate and ranitidine and domperidone maleate in the short-term treatment of reflux esophagitis. Drugs Exp Clin Res 1985;19:1–6.
17. Chaussade S, Michopoulos S, Guerre J, Couturier D. Erythromycin (ERY), a motilin agonist, increases the human lower esophageal sphincter pressure (LES) by stimulation of cholinergic nerves. Gastroenterology 1990;98:A335.
18. Chaussade S, Michopoulos S, Samama J et al. Erythromycin, a motilin agonist, increases the human lower esophageal sphincter pressure in patients with systemic sclerosis. Gastroenterology 1991;100:A428.

What effects have prokinetic agents on the amplitude and duration of esophageal contractions?

D. Couturier (Paris)

Esophageal peristaltic function is compromised in patients with peptic esophagitis, with a high incidence of failed peristalsis and hypotensive peristaltic contractions in the esophagus, in comparison with control populations. The incidence of these motor abnormalities increases with the severity of gastroesophageal reflux (GER) disease. Absent or incomplete peristaltic contractions invariably result in little or no volume clearance. It was demonstrated that a minimal regional peristaltic amplitude is required to prevent retrograde escape of gastric content [1,2].

The role of primary and secondary peristaltic contraction in the mechanism of GER and its complications leads one to consider the actions of prokinetic drugs on the amplitude and duration of esophageal contractions.

Prokinetic agents are used for their overall benefit on motility. However, their actions are dependent on the subclass of the drug and on the considered segment of the esophagogastrointestinal tract. In humans their actions on esophageal motility have been mainly studied by manometry.

The most accurately documented effect of direct cholinergic agonist consists in elevating the lower esophageal sphincter (LES) pressure. Cholinergic agonists also increase the amplitude of esophageal contractions and the velocity of esophageal contractions in a dose-dependent fashion [3]. They also enhance transit and the clearance of acid from the esophagus of both normal patients and those with GER. The improvement in esophageal transit, after stimulation of cholinergic receptors by bethanechol, correlates best with the increase in contraction amplitude. However, improvement in clearance seems to be mainly due to increased secretion of saliva, another effect of cholinergic agonist [4].

Cisapride is a benzamide derivate that promotes gastrointestinal motility by indirectly stimulating cholinergic nerves [5]. Cisapride increases LES pressure with the benefit that the lower the basal pressure, the higher the drug-induced increase. It seems to increase esophageal peristalsis, although none of the available results is consistent: cisapride 10 mg i.v. on 12 normal volunteers documented no change in the velocity of transit, but a small increase in distal peristalsis was noted [6] and, in another study conducted on 10 healthy volunteers, no change in amplitude of contraction was observed after 10 mg p.o. t.i.d. of cisapride. Finally, we can consider that esophageal body peristaltic amplitude shows a modest increase after intravenous cisapride, whereas no significant increase occurred after oral administration [7,8].

Metoclopramide is derivative of para-aminobenzoic acid which has both peripheral and central dopamine receptors antagonist effects. Metoclopramide's effect appears to be dependent on the enhanced release of acetylcholine from intrinsic cholinergic neurons. The effect of metoclopramide on esophageal clearance and contractile function is not clear. In first studies it was shown that 10 mg metoclopramide p.o. increases the amplitude of esophageal contractions [9]. Such a response was not seen in subsequent studies, showing that acid clearance was not improved by metoclopramide [10,11].

Like metoclopramide, domperidone, a benzimidazole derivative that specifically antagonizes the inhibitory effects of dopamine on the upper intestinal tract, shows inconsistent effects on the motor function of esophageal body. In children with symptoms of GER, domperidone increases the frequency of peristaltic contractions, but has no effect on the amplitude of contractions [12]. In adults, oral domperidone (80 mg/day) causes a significant increase in LES pressure, however, neither esophageal body motility, duration of esophageal exposure to acid nor esophageal clearance were effected [11].

Erythromycin, a macrolide agent, which mainly acts on small bowel motility as prokinetic agent, increases significantly LES pressure and the duration of peristaltic contractions [13].

Finally, in contrast with the powerful action of the prokinetic drugs on the LES tone, a lack of effect is observed on the esophageal body motility. This might be the purpose for the development of new therapeutic agents for the treatment of GER.

References

1. Kahrilas PJ, Dodds WJ, Hogan WJ. Effect of peristaltic dysfunction on esophageal volume clearance. Gastroenterology 1988;94:73–80.
2. Helm JF, Dodds WJ, Riedel DR, et al. Determinants of esophageal acid clearance in normal subjects. Gastroenterology 1983;85:607–612.
3. Phaosawasdi K, Malmud LS, Tolin RD, et al. Cholinergic effects on esophageal transit and clearance. Gastroenterology 1981;81:915–920.
4. Scarpignato C. Pharmacological bases of the medical treatment of gastroesophageal reflux disease. Dig Dis 1988;6: 117–148.
5. McCallum RW. Cisapride: a new class of prokinetic agent. J Gastroenterol 1991;86:135–149.
6. Case WG, Williams NS. The effect of cisapride upon lower esophageal sphincter pressure (LESP) and primary peristalsis (PP). Dig Dis Sci 1986;31:465S.
7. Gilbert RJ, Dodds WJ, Kahrilas PJ, et al. Effect of cisapride, a new prokinetic agent, on esophageal motor function. Dig Dis Sci 1987;32:1331–1336.
8. Cucchiara S, Staiano A, De Stefano M, Capozzi C, Manzi G, Camerlingo F, Paone FM. Effects of cisapride on parameters of oesophageal motility and on the prolonged intraoesophageal pH test in infants with gastro-oesophageal reflux disease. Gut 1990;31:21–25.
9. Dilawari JB, Misiewicz JJ. Action of metoclopramide on the gastroesophageal function in man. Gut 1973;14:380–382.
10. Behar J, Biancani P. Effect of oral metoclopramide on gastroesophageal reflux in the postcibal state. Gastroenterology 1976;70:331–335.
11. Grande L, Lacima G, Ros E, et al. Lack of effect of metoclopramide and domperidone on esophageal peristalsis and esophageal acid clearance in reflux esophagitis; a randomized, double blind study. Dig Dis Sci 1992;37:583–588.
12. Goethals C. Domperidone in the treatment of postprandial symptoms suggestive of gastroesophageal reflux. Curr Ther Res 1979;26:874–880.
13. Chaussade S, Michopoulos S, Guerre J, Couturier D. Erythromycine (ERY), a motilin agonist, increases the human lower esophageal sphincter pressure (LES) by stimulation of cholinergic nerves. Gastroenterology 1990;98:A335.

What are the modalities of prescription of prokinetics in infancy?

Ch. Dupont (Paris)

The treatment of gastroesophageal reflux (GER) now benefits from numerous improvements in the different classes of drugs available, in their respective potency and therefore in our ability to propose an overall efficient medical treatment, despite the fact that a satisfactory explanation of the pathogenesis of GER is still not available. The beneficial effects of drugs result from a direct reduction of reflux with gastrointestinal prokinetic agents, from using compounds which actively protect the mucosa and from neutralizing or suppressing gastric acid secretion using antacids or H_2-receptor antagonists. Surgery appears as the most efficient way for preventing reflux, but is infrequently required and must be carefully discussed.

Neurotransmitter agonists or antagonists

A consideration of the control of digestive motility suggests that the logical point of attack for pharmacological intervention is the enteric nervous system. Two groups of agents may be used in the treatment of GER and have been extensively reviewed [1]. The first group can be called gastrointestinal motor stimulants such as the muscarinic drug bethanechol, a compound that simply increases smooth motor activity. The second group is composed of the so called prokinetic agents such as metoclopramide, domperidone and cisapride, compounds which restore disordered activity by improving coordinated peristaltic activity.

Bethanechol

Bethanechol (β-methylcholine carbamate) is a stable choline ester with a selective action on muscarinic receptors, which was shown to increase lower esophageal sphincter (LES) pressure and gastric motor activity. Bethanechol improves esophageal clearance but probably not reflux episodes frequency. This improvement of clearance may be due both to an enhanced cholinergic stimulation of salivation [2] and to an increased motility: it has no effect on any motor function of the upper third of the esophagus but increases amplitude and duration of peristaltic contractions of the distal esophagus [3]. Clinical trials indicate, despite some controversial results, the reduction of daily episodes of vomiting and the restoration of weight gain.

Bethanechol is given daily with an average dose of 0.6 mg/kg in three divided doses or subcutaneously with a dose of 0.15–0.2 mg/kg.

Despite the absence of important side effects in the above-mentioned studies, bethanechol exhibits a few drawbacks such as the induction of diarrhea and stimulation of gastric acid secretion. Moreover, it cannot be used in patients who have respiratory symptoms such as children with asthmatic bronchitis or patients with asthma since it has cholinergic effects that may exacerbate bronchospasm [2].

Metoclopramide

Metoclopramide, a dopamine antagonist, is both a stimulant of gastrointestinal smooth muscle and a centrally acting antiemetic drug. Its action on smooth muscle results both from an inhibition of the neurotransmitter dopamine and from an enhancement of acetylcholine release from postganglionic cholinergic nerve terminals. In adults, metoclopramide dose-relatedly increases the resting tone of the LES pressure in normal subjects as well as in patients with GER [4]. The beneficial effect of metoclopramide on LES pressure and esophageal contractions was also shown in children with GER [5]. The effect of metoclopramide occurs 10–20 min after oral ingestion, reaches its maximum at 60 min and lasts at least 120 min [6]. A relationship was shown between plasma concentration 1 h after administration and the reduction of time pH < 4 in esophageal pH metric recordings [7].

The beneficial effect of metoclopramide is likely to occur through its effects on esophageal peristalsis more than on LES tone and perhaps even more through its ability to increase gastric emptying which was demonstrated in preterm babies with persistent intolerance to food and gastric stasis [8] and in infants with gastrointestinal motor disorders [9].

Clinical trials showed a significant reduction in the frequency of regurgitations at a daily dosage of 0.5 mg/kg/day in four divided doses [10], recommended to be taken 10–15 min before meals. However, metoclopramide is more effective at higher doses (1 mg/kg/day), at which the incidence of side effects renders its use hazardous to the child [11].

Indeed, a major drawback in the use of metoclopramide in children is the possible occurrence of extrapyramidal side effects, which have been reported in numerous studies [12]. The symptoms of dystonia may appear even at low dosages but in children are reversible upon arrest of treatment. There have been reports of methemoglobinemia in infants [13].

Domperidone

Domperidone is a benzimidazole derivative with pure dopamine-antagonistic properties which, unlike metoclopramide, is deprived of any cholinergic effects. Domperidone does not readily enter the central nervous system, thus causing no extrapyramidal side effects.

Domperidone augments the contractility of the esophageal body [14] and increases basal LES pressure [15], while also increasing gastric emptying through improvement of antroduodenal motility.

During clinical trials, domperidone induced a significant improvement in occurrence of vomiting, "spitting" and coughing. The efficiency of domperidone in the treatment of GER related respiratory symptoms was recently shown to be associated with a reduction in nocturnal reflux as assessed by pH metric studies [16].

Domperidone has a bio-half-life of 7 h and 30 min. It is given in a dose of 0.3 mg/kg, 3 or 4 times daily before meals and at the start of the night. Domperidone is more effective at doses of 0.5 mg/kg 4 times daily, although side effects have been reported at this dosage rate [17].

Domperidone is normally devoid of the extrapyramidal reactions reported for metoclopramide, although the latter may occur in younger babies, probably due to an incomplete maturation of the blood-brain barrier.

Cisapride

Cisapride is the first drug of a subgroup of substituted benzamides that act on gastrointestinal motor function via indirect cholinergic mechanisms without interfering with dopamine receptors [1]. Cisapride is thought to act only through the enhancement of the physiological release of acetylcholine, selectively in the myenteric plexus. In adults, the motor effects of cisapride have been demonstrated in the esophagus, stomach, and the small and large intestine, so that cisapride is likely to have applications outside of GER [18].

Cisapride significantly improves esophageal peristalsis [19], stimulates gastric emptying, increases LES pressure, but is deprived of any effect on gastric acid secretion.

Cisapride was shown to lower the frequency of long duration reflux episodes, and the percentage of total and nocturnal time spent at pH < 4, as well as to improve esophageal clearance [20,21]. All studies including symptoms evaluation showed the clinical usefulness of cisapride on improvement of repeated regurgitations or vomiting in the vast majority of patients [19], and chronic bronchopulmonary disorders associated with GER [22,23].

The maximal blood level of cisapride is observed 2 h after oral ingestion and its half life is 10—12 h. The doses used in most studies is 0.2 mg/kg, 3—4 times daily by mouth. The side effects reported up to now are limited to rare cases of abdominal cramps and diarrhea.

Management of GER

Management includes, in addition to postural manoeuvres, frequent and thickened fractionated feeds and prokinetic agents, metoclopramide, domperidone or cisapride. According to recent statistics prokinetic agents are likely to be given in up to 10.5% of the whole infant population [24]. The use of antacids such as sodium alginate is commonly indicated in pediatric practice, although some problems may arise from difficulties in feeding infants with bad tasting drugs.

Orenstein [2] recommend the use of H_2-blockers occasionally combined with antacids in patients with documented esophagitis, whereas they use only antacids without an H_2-blocker in patients in whom esophagitis has been suspected but not documented. Management also includes reassurance of parents, since these conservative measures do not always prevent frequent regurgitations and occasional vomiting.

When compared to medical treatment used in earlier studies, the medical treatment of reflux has gained in potency by adaptation of positioning and use of prokinetic drugs. Moreover, when needed, anti-H$_2$ and more recently proton pump inhibitors allow a satisfying control of peptic esophagitis and therefore of the periesophagitis which probably considerably impairs the function of the antireflux barrier.

When started in early infancy, conservative management may be expected to benefit most patients: over 90% will be free of symptoms in 1 year, compared to an estimated 35% in the absence of treatment [25]. In infants with reflux only, reflux is a limited condition that resolves spontaneously as an effective antireflux barrier is gradually established: about 65% of all infants attending hospital with symptoms due to a partial thoracic stomach will become symptom free by 2 years of age if given no treatment [25,26].

There are good reasons for accepting that, in children over the age of 2 years, the course of the reflux disease is not much different from that in adults, where GER seems to be a long lasting problem. In that respect, a major issue concerns the number of patients for whom a long lasting improvement is likely to occur under conservative medical therapy. Based on a long-term follow-up of adults with chronic reflux esophagitis by Lieberman [27], Castell [28] suggests that a long-lasting improvement might be observed in approximately 50% of the patients, with great variations related to the severity of the symptoms. No comparable study is available in the child.

The finding of a hiatus hernia with or without an associated partial thoracic stomach is not in itself an indication for surgery [25]. In children with only digestive manifestations of GER, surgery is restricted to the patients for whom a medical treatment appears either to be needed over a long duration or to be insufficiently effective.

Children with upper or lower respiratory symptoms related to GER do not always exhibit major gastroesophageal abnormalities. In these children the demonstration of GER, mainly through esophageal pH metric recordings, warrants a medical therapy, irrespective of the presence or the absence of digestive symptoms of GER.

Patients with a good response to medical management, obviously more frequently infants than older children, and those with repeated bronchopulmonary diseases without bronchial hyperreactivity more than those presenting a bronchial hyperreactivity, should continue their therapy. Optimal duration of pharmacological therapy is difficult to determine. Discontinuation of the treatment is often followed by relapse of the pulmonary symptoms and surgical fundoplication may be considered as a correct alternative to a prolonged medical therapy.

Patients who do not respond adequately to a maximal medical management, however, present another problem [29]: a more aggressive approach may be needed in some of them.

The patient selection process for surgery therefore still relies mainly on a clinical basis, but the statement of the late 70s that the failure of medical antireflux management does not preclude a favorable response to a subsequent antireflux procedure [30–32] might not remain as valid. It thus seems that surgery becomes more likely to be proposed when the evolution of symptoms under maximal medical treatment suggests a probable good result from surgery.

Conclusion

There is no doubt that current methods of investigation have allowed a better understanding of the nature of GER and of the development of gastroesophageal function in the neonate and infant. The clearer delineation of subgroups of esophageal disorders will enable more specific approaches to management to be developed and objectively evaluated. At the present time, conservative measures are to be recommended in the treatment of children with clinical manifestations of GER. Prokinetic agents exhibit an appropriate rationale so that their use appears in the second place in the decisional tree of the European Society of Pediatric Gastroenterology and Nutrition (ESPGAN) committee on GER treatment. Gastric antisecretory agents must be added in those patients diagnosed to have esophagitis, also in accordance with the same guidelines. It seems that the recent improvement in medical potency might lead to a considerable reduction of indications for surgery.

References

1. Verlinden M, Welburn P. The use of prokinetic agents in the treatment of gastrointestinal motility disorders in childhood. In: Milla PJ (ed) Disorders of Gastrointestinal Motility in Childhood. Chichester, England: John Wiley & Sons Ltd, 1988; 125—140.
2. Orenstein SR, Orenstein DM. Gastroesophageal reflux and respiratory disease in children. J Pediatr 1988;112:847—858.
3. Sondheimer JM, Arnold GL. Early effects of bethanechol on the esophageal motor function of infants with gastroesophageal reflux. J Pediatr Gastroenterol Nutr 1986;5:47—51.
4. Cohen S, Morris DW, Schoen HS, Di Marino AJ. The effect of oral and intravenous metoclopramide on human lower oesophageal sphincter pressure. Gastroenterology 1976;70:484—487.
5. Machida HM, Forbes DA, Gall DG, Scott RB. Metoclopramide in gastroesophageal reflux in infancy. J Pediatr 1988;112: 483—487.
6. Behar J, Biancani P. Effect of oral metoclopramide on the gastroesophageal reflux in the postcibal state. Gastroenterology 1976;70:331—335.
7. Pons G, Duhamel JF, Guillot M, Gouyon JB, d'Athis P, Richard MO, Rey E, Moran C, Bouglé D, Bellissant E, Ement P, Dupont C, Badoual J, Olive G. Dose response study of metoclopramide in gastroesophageal reflux in infancy. Fund Clin Pharmacol 1993;7:161—166.
8. Sankaran K, Yeboak EB, Bingham WT, Ninan A. Use of metoclopramide in preterm infants. Devel Pharmacol Therapeut 1982;5:114—119.
9. Hyman PE, Abrams C, Dubois A. Effect of metoclopramide and betanechol on gastric emptying in infants. Pediatr Res 1985;19:1029—1032.
10. Leung AKC, Lai PCW. Use of metoclopramide for the treatment of gastroesophageal reflux in infants and children. Curr Ther Res 1984;36:911—915.
11. Orenstein SR. Controversies on pediatric gastroesophageal reflux. J Pediatr Gastroenterol Nutr 1992;14:338—348.
12. Low LCK, Gael KM. Metoclopramide poisoning in children. Arch Dis Child 1980;55:310—312.
13. Sutphen JL. Pediatric gastroesophageal reflux. Gastroenterol Clin North Am 1990;19:617—629.
14. Weirauch TR, Förster CF, Krieglstein J. Evaluation of the effect of domperidone on human oesophageal and gastroduodenal motility by intraluminal manometry. Postgrad J Med 1979;55:7—11.
15. Bron B, Massih L. Domperidone: a drug with powerful action on the lower oesophageal sphincter pressure. Digestion 1980;20:375—378.
16. Dupont C, Molkhou P, Petrovic N, Fraitag B. Traitement par motilium du reflux gastro-oesophagien associé à des manifestations respiratoires chroniques. Ann Ped 1989;36:148—150.
17. Clara R. Chronic regurgitation and vomiting with Domperidone: a multicenter evaluation. Acta Paediatr Belg 1979:32: 203—208.
18. Rentjens A, Verlinden M, Aerts T. Development and clinical use of the new intestinal prokinetic drug cisapride (R 51 619). Drug Devel Res, 1986;8:251—265.
19. Cucchiara S, Staiano A, Capozzi C, Di Lorenzo C, Boccieri A, Auricchio S. Cisapride for gastro-oesophageal reflux and peptic oesophagitis in children. Arch Dis Child, 1987;62:454—457.
20. Rode H, Stunden RJ, Millar AJW, Cywes S. Esophageal pH assessment of gastroesophageal reflux in 18 patients and the effect of two prokinetic agents: cisapride and metoclopramide. J Pediatr Surg 1987;22:931—934.

21. Saye Z, Forget P Geubelle F. Effect of cisapride on gastroesophageal reflux in children with chronic bronchopulmonary disease. Pediatric Pulmonology 1987;3:8−12.
22. Saye Z, Forget PP. Effect of cisapride on esophageal pH monitoring in children with reflux-associated bronchopulmonary diseases. J Pediatr Gastroenterol Nutr 1989;8:327−332.
23. Malfroot A, Vandenplas Y, Verlinden M, Piepsz A, Dab I. Gastroesophageal reflux and unexplained chronic respiratory disease in infants and children. Pediatric Pulmonology 1987;3:208−213.
24. Chouhou D, Rossignol C, Bernard F, Dupont C. Le reflux gastro-oesophagien dans les centres de bilan de santé de l'enfant de moins de 4 ans. Arch Fr Pédiatr 1992;49:839−843.
25. Carré IJ. The management of gastro-oesophageal reflux. Arch Dis Child 1985;60:71−75.
26. Carré IJ. The natural history of the partial thoracic stomach ("hiatal hernia") in children. Arch Dis Child 1959;34:344−353.
27. Lieberman D. Medical therapy for chronic reflux esophagitis. Long-term follow-up. Arch Int Med 1987;147:1717−1720.
28. Castell DO. Long-term therapy for chronic gastroesophageal reflux. Arch Int Med 1987;147:1701−1702.
29. Barish CF, Wu WC, Castell DO. Respiratory complications of gastroesophageal reflux. Arch Int Med 1985;145:1882−1888.
30. Jolley SG, Herbst JJ, Johnson DG, Matlak ME, Book LS. Esophageal pH monitoring during sleep identifies children with respiratory symptoms from gastroesophageal reflux. Gastroenterology 1981;80:1501−1506.
31. Shapiro GG, Christie DL. Gastroesophageal reflux in steroid-dependant asthmatic youths. Pediatrics 1979;63:207−210.
32. Ramenofsky ML, Powell MD, Curreri PW. Gastroesophageal reflux. pH probe-directed therapy. Ann Surg 1986;203:531−536.

Why do some patients not respond to combined prokinetic-antisecretory treatment?

W. Inauen (Bern)

Clinical trials indicate that treatment regimens with histamine H_2-receptor antagonists, prokinetic agents, or a combination of both drugs do not achieve healing in all patients with erosive reflux esophagitis. In contrast, most patients with reflux esophagitis can be healed by omeprazole, a proton pump inhibitor. These data indicate that healing of esophagitis is most reliably achieved by a regimen which leads to maximal reduction of esophageal acid exposure. In order to quantify the therapeutic potential of the different treatment modalities, two separate studies were performed. In the first study, the effects of placebo, the H_2-receptor antagonist ranitidine, and a combination of ranitidine with the prokinetic agent cisapride were studied in 18 patients with erosive reflux esophagitis. Compared to placebo, ranitidine (150 mg b.i.d.) reduced 24-h esophageal acid reflux (% time with pH < 4.0) from 10% (3.2−32.6) (median (range)) to 6.4% (1.2−22.9) (p < 0.01). The combination of ranitidine (150 mg b.i.d.) with cisapride (20 mg b.i.d.) further reduced acid reflux from 6.4% (1.2−22.9) to 3.7% (1.0−12.7) (p < 0.01). These results indicate that the 30% reduction of esophageal acid exposure achieved by ranitidine can be improved to 60% by combination with cisapride. In the second study, 24-h intragastric pH-metry was used to investigate whether very high doses of ranitidine (300 mg q.i.d.) could match the reduction of gastric acidity achieved by omeprazole (40 mg mane). Compared to placebo, ranitidine reduced median time with an intragastric pH < 4.0 from 89.8% (79.9−99) (placebo) to 42.2% (4.5−67.4) on day 1, 60.9% (18.5−75.1) on day 2, 70% (32.6–89.9) on day 7, and 74.2% (30–91.7) on day 14. Omeprazole reduced median time with an intragastric pH < 4.0 from 88.7% (83.6–98.1) (placebo) to 52.8% (17.8–96) on day 1, 38.9% (11–78.4) on day 2, 31% (0–56.1) on day 7, and 30.7% (8–56.3) on day 14. These results indicate that on day 1, the high oral dose of ranitidine could match the acid inhibition achieved by omeprazole. However, tolerance, i.e., a significant loss of antisecretory activity, was observed already on day 2 of high-dose ranitidine treatment. On days 7 and 14, median time with intragastric pH < 4.0 was more than 2-fold higher under ranitidine as compared to omeprazole which maintained its high antisecretory effect. Histamine H_2-receptor antagonists, prokinetics, or a combination of both drugs lead to a substantial reduction of esophageal acid exposure which appears to be sufficient in healing mild or moderate degrees of erosive reflux esophagitis in most patients. Due to a rapid development of tolerance, even very high doses of H_2-receptor antagonists cannot match the antisecretory effect of omeprazole. Proton pump inhibitors are therefore the drugs of choice in more severe degrees of reflux esophagitis.

Introduction

Histamine H_2-receptor antagonists and cisapride lead to healing of erosive reflux esophagitis in up to 50% of patients [1–7]. This healing rate can be improved, to 70%, when H_2-receptor antagonists are combined with cisapride [8]. By far the highest healing rates, more than 90%, are achieved by the proton pump inhibitor omeprazole [9–11]. These studies indicate that a marked reduction of esophageal acid exposure is crucial for successful treatment of reflux esophagitis. In order to compare the therapeutic potential of the histamine H_2-receptor antagonist ranitidine, the prokinetic agent cisapride, and the proton pump inhibitor omeprazole, two separate studies were performed. In the first study [12], the effect of ranitidine and the combination of ranitidine with cisapride were tested. Combined treatment with an H_2-receptor antagonist and a prokinetic agent was of special interest, since ranitidine and cisapride exert their effects by affecting different mechanisms and may therefore reduce acid reflux better than either medication alone. In the second study [13], it was investigated whether the antisecretory effect of the proton pump inhibitor omeprazole could be matched by increasing the dose of ranitidine.

Study 1: effect of ranitidine and ranitidine combined with cisapride on esophageal acid exposure [12]

Methods

Eighteen patients (17 males, 1 female, median age 49.5 years (range 31–72)) with reflux esophagitis of grade I (n = 3), grade II (n = 12), and grade III (n = 3) were investigated [14]. According to a double-blind, double dummy, within subject, three-way crossover design, patients were allocated to receive treatment with:

- placebo (matching placebo tablets);
- ranitidine (ranitidine one tablet of 150 mg b.i.d. + matching cisapride placebo two tablets b.i.d.);
- ranitidine + cisapride (ranitidine one tablet of 150 mg b.i.d. + cisapride two tablets of 10 mg b.i.d.).

The study drugs (three tablets each time) were ingested at 9.15 am (before breakfast) and 10.00 pm (bedtime). Each treatment period lasted 4 days and intraesophageal pH and motility were monitored on the 4th day. The treatment periods were followed by a wash-out period of 10 days during which the patients were allowed to take antacids. Patients attended the clinic at 8.00 am after an overnight fast. After local anesthesia, two catheters (one for pH, one for pressure recording) were inserted transnasally and their tips placed 5 cm above the lower esophageal sphincter (LES). At 9.00 am, continuous 24-h recording of intraesophageal pH and pressure was started. At 9.15 am, all patients ingested their study medication and received a standard breakfast (bread, butter, marmalade, coffee, tea, or milk). At 12.00 pm, a standardized lunch was served consisting of lasagna (baked layers of noodles, meat, cheese, and tomato sauce), bread, salad, and cake for dessert. At 4.00 pm, the patients received a snack (tea or coffee with cake), and at 6.00 pm, a standard dinner was served (Swiss style muesli, consisting of cereals, milk, yogurt, fresh fruits). Identical meals were prepared for each study-day and they were eaten within 30 min of serving. Free access to water was allowed for drinking. Smoking was permitted, but the number and timing of cigarettes were noted on a diary sheet and had to be similar on all study-days. During the study-days, the patients were fully ambulatory and could follow their preferred daily routine except that they had to return to the laboratory for their meals. After dinner, each patient returned home. At 8.00 am, on the following morning, the patients returned to the laboratory and shortly after 9.00 am, the probes and recording equipment were removed (see p. 405).

Results

Esophageal acid exposure. With placebo treatment, the pH in the distal esophagus (sensor position 5 cm above the LES) remained below 4.0 during 10% (3.2–32.6) of the 24-h recording period (Fig. 1). During ranitidine, reflux time fell to 6.4% (1.2–22.9) ($p < 0.01$ vs. placebo) with a further reduction to 3.7% (1.0–12.7) ($p < 0.001$ vs. placebo, $p < 0.01$ vs. ranitidine) during ranitidine plus cisapride (see p. 405).

Esophageal motility. Ranitidine did not affect esophageal motility. As compared to ranitidine, the addition of cisapride led to an increase of contraction amplitude during the upright period (from 28.0 mmHg (14–54) to 32.5 mmHg (13–56), $p < 0.05$), and the postprandial periods after breakfast (from 27.0 mmHg (14–56) to 33.5 mmHg (12–72), $p < 0.05$) and lunch (from 27.9 mmHg (15–44) to 35.5 mmHg (19–46), $p < 0.05$). During the upright period, cisapride further enhanced the duration of esophageal contractions (from 3.2 s (2.8–4.2) to 3.6 s (3.0–4.4), $p < 0.05$). Cisapride increased propagation velocity of esophageal contractions (from 3.7 (2.9–4.3) cm/s

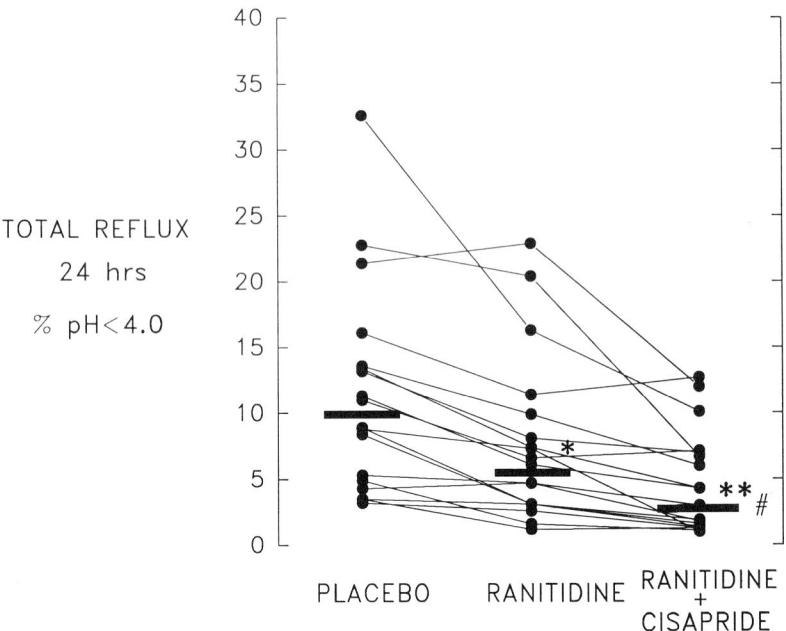

Fig. 1. Effect of ranitidine (150 mg b.i.d.) and ranitidine + cisapride (150 mg b.i.d. + 20 mg b.i.d.) on esophageal acid reflux (% of time with an intraesophageal pH < 4.0) in 18 patients with erosive reflux esophagitis. Acid reflux is shown for the entire 24-h recording period. Horizontal bars indicate median, n = 18 for all treatments. [*]p < 0.01; [**]p < 0.001 vs. placebo; # p < 0.01 vs. ranitidine (Wilcoxon signed rank test).

to 3.9 cm/s (2.9–4.6)), but had no effects on esophageal contractility (slope of the contraction curve) and on the number of total, propagated and nonpropagated contractions (see p. 406).

Discussion

This study demonstrates that ranitidine (150 mg b.i.d.) reduced esophageal acid reflux by approximately 30%. The combination with cisapride (20 mg b.i.d.) further reduced acid reflux by approximately 60%. The cisapride-induced increase of esophageal contractile force and propagation velocity appears to improve esophageal acid clearance.

Study 2: antisecretory effect of high-dose ranitidine and omeprazole treatment [13]

Methods

Twenty-eight healthy *Helicobacter pylori* negative volunteers were randomly assigned to a 2-week treatment with ranitidine or omeprazole. According to a double-blind, double dummy, parallel group study design, subjects were allocated to receive treatment with:

— ranitidine (two tablets of 150 mg q.i.d. + matching omeprazole placebo one capsule mane)
— omeprazole (omeprazole one capsule of 40 mg mane + matching ranitidine placebo two tablets q.i.d.).

The study drugs were ingested at 9.15 am (before breakfast) and 10.00 pm (bedtime). Subjects attended the clinic at 8.00 am after an overnight fast. After local anesthesia, a pH-catheter (glass electrode) was inserted transnasally and the tip placed 10 cm below the pH drop in the esophagogastric junction. At 9.00 am, continuous 24-h recording of intragastric pH was started. At 9.15 am, all subjects ingested their study medication and received a standard breakfast (bread, butter, marmalade, coffee, tea, or milk). At 12.00 pm, a standardized lunch was served consisting of lasagna (baked layers of noodles, meat, cheese, and tomato sauce), bread, salad, and chocolate pudding for dessert. At 4.00 pm, the patients received a snack (cereal biscuit), and at 6.00 pm, a standard dinner was served (bread, butter, cold meat cuts, cheese). A late evening snack (apple) was taken at 10.00 pm. Identical meals were prepared for each study-day and they were eaten within 30 min of serving. Free access to water was allowed for drinking. Smoking was permitted, but the number and timing of cigarettes were noted on a diary sheet and had to be similar on all study-days.

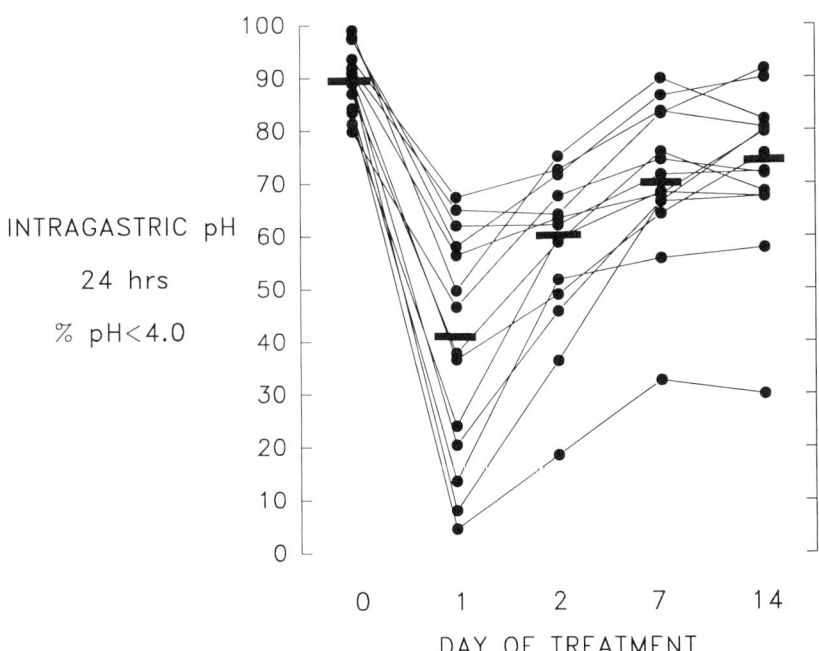

Fig. 2A. Effect of ranitidine (300 mg q.i.d.) on intragastric acidity (% time with an intragastric pH < 4.0) in 14 healthy volunteers. Intragastric acidity was measured for 24 h before (day 0) and on day 1, 2, 7 and 14 of treatment. Horizontal bars indicate median, n = 14 for all measurements.

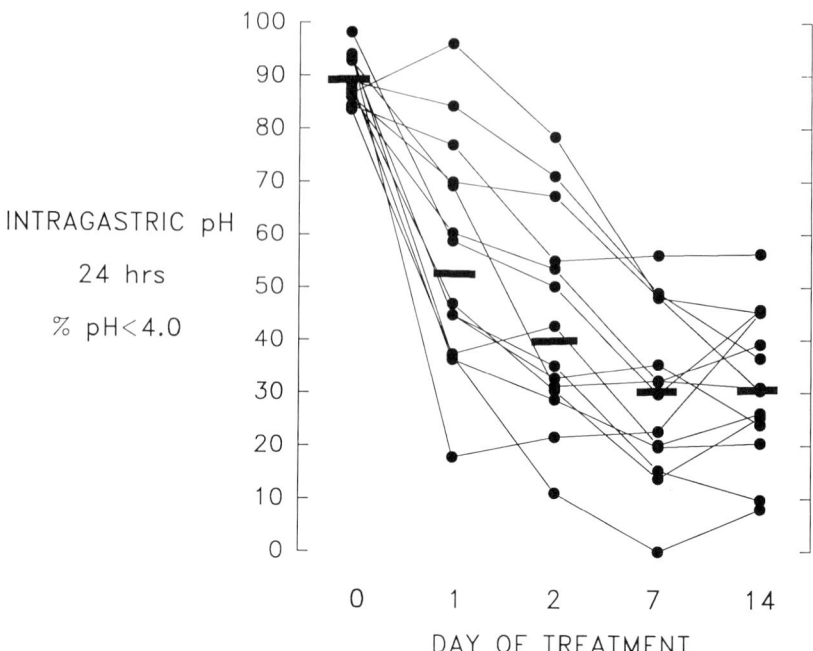

Fig. 2B. Effect of omeprazole (40 mg mane) on intragastric acidity (% time with an intragastric pH < 4.0) in 14 healthy volunteers. Intragastric acidity was measured for 24 h before (day 0) and on day 1, 2, 7 and 14 of treatment. Horizontal bars indicate median, n = 14 for all measurements.

Results

The effect of ranitidine and omeprazole on intragastric acidity (expressed as % time with an intragastric pH < 4.0) is shown in Fig. 2. Ranitidine (300 mg q.i.d.) markedly reduced intragastric acidity on day 1 (Fig. 2A), but the antisecretory effect was less pronounced on treatment days 2, 7, and 14. In contrast, the antisecretory effect of omeprazole (Fig. 2B) was increasing throughout the first week of treatment (days 1, 2, 7) and then remained stable at a high level.

Discussion

These results indicate that on day 1, the high oral dose of ranitidine could match the acid inhibition achieved by omeprazole. However, tolerance (i.e., a significant loss of antisecretory activity) was observed already on day 2 of high-dose ranitidine treatment.

Conclusions

Although combined treatment with histamine H_2-receptor antagonists and prokinetics markedly decreases esophageal acid exposure, they do not achieve the degree of acid reduction obtained by treatment with proton pump inhibitors. Due to rapid development of tolerance, even high doses of histamine H_2-receptor antagonists can not match the antisecretory efficacy of proton pump inhibitors. Whereas the reduction of esophageal acid exposure achieved by histamine H_2-receptor antagonists and prokinetics appears to be sufficient in healing mild or moderate degrees of erosive reflux esophagitis in most patients, proton pump inhibitors are the drugs of choice in more severe degrees of reflux esophagitis.

References

1. Koelz HR, Birchler R, Bretholz A et al. Healing and relapse of reflux esophagitis during treatment with ranitidine. Gastroenterology 1986;91:1198−1205.
2. Janisch HD, Hüttemann W, Bouzo MH. Cisapride versus ranitidine in the treatment of reflux esophagitis. Hepato-Gastroenterol 1988;35:125−127.
3. Galmiche JP, Fraitag B, Filoche B et al. Double-blind comparison of cisapride and cimetidine in treatment of reflux esophagitis. Dig Dis Sci 1990;35:649−655.
4. Maleev A, Mendizova A, Popov P et al. Cisapride and cimetidine in the treatment of erosive esophagitis. Hepato-Gastroenterol 1990;37:403−407.
5. Baldi F, Bianchi Porro G, Dobrilla G et al. Cisapride versus placebo in reflux esophagitis. A multicenter double-blind trial. J Clin Gastroenterol 1988;10:614−618.
6. Lepoutre L, Van Der Spek P, Vanderlinden I et al. Healing of grade-II and III esophagitis through motility stimulation with cisapride. Digestion 1990;45:109−114.
7. Toussaint J, Gossuin A, Deruyttere M, Hublé F, Devis G. Healing and prevention of relapse of reflux esophagitis by cisapride. Gut 1991;32:1280−1285.
8. Galmiche JP, Brandstätter G, Evreux M et al. Combined treatment with cisapride and cimetidine in severe reflux esophagitis: a double blind controlled trial. Gut 1988;29:675−681
9. Havelund T, Laursen LS, Skoubo-Kristensen E et al. Omeprazole and ranitidine in treatment of reflux esophagitis: double blind comparative trial. Br Med J 1988;296:89−92.
10. Lundell L, Backman L, Ekström P et al. Prevention of relapse of reflux esophagitis after endoscopic healing: the efficacy and safety of omeprazole compared with ranitidine. Scand J Gastroenterol 1991;26:248−256.
11. Hetzel DJ, Dent J, Reed WD et al. Healing and relapse of severe peptic esophagitis after treatment with omeprazole. Gastroenterology 1988;95:903−912.
12. Inauen W, Emde C, Weber B et al. Effects of ranitidine and cisapride on acid reflux and oesophageal motility in patients with reflux esophagitis: A 24-h ambulatory combined pH and manometry study. Gut 1993;34:1025−1030.
13. Hurlimann S, Abbühl B, Halter F, Inauen W. Dynamics of tolerance during high dose H_2-receptor antagonist treatment. Gastroenterology 1993;104 (in press) (Abstract).
14. Savary M, Miller G. L'oesophage. In: Manuel et Atlas d'Endoscopie. Solothurn, Switzerland: Gassmann AG, 1977.

Is it possible to distinguish the categories of esophagitis which will benefit more from prokinetic or from antacid treatment?

G.G. Jamieson (Adelaide)

There are several factors which may be important in the pathogenesis of esophagitis. For example:

1. Lower sphincter tone and the capacity of the sphincter to relax to intragastric pressure. The great majority of reflux episodes occur when sphincter tone is at or near to intragastric pressure.
2. The composition of the refluxate. Acid suppression by omeprazole has re-emphasized the fundamental importance of acid in the development of reflux esophagitis. Nevertheless, there is still evidence to suggest that duodenogastric reflux in general, and bile reflux in particular, may play a role in some patients with complicated reflux disease.
3. Esophageal clearance. Reflux episodes are normal events but rely on the esophagus clearing the refluxate back into the stomach.
4. Delayed gastric emptying. This may have an influence by prolonging the postprandial state or may lead to a greater number of lower esophageal sphincter relaxations postprandially.

Agents which lead to acid reduction are active at point 2 whilst prokinetic agents have the potential to act at point 1, 3 and 4. Is it therefore possible to dissect out categories of patients where one or other of these factors predominate? Patients who might be regarded as having the purest form of motility disorder associated with reflux are those with an adynamic esophagus usually associated with a disease such as systemic sclerosis. Even here, though, the picture is a mixed one in that some patients with a totally adynamic esophagus have no symptoms nor endoscopic changes of esophagitis whilst others develop a severe form of the disease often developing stricture formation [1].

The fact that many patients with reflux esophagitis have motility changes in the esophagus has been known since the report of Olsen and Schlegel [2]. Their observations were later confirmed and extended by others. Impaired volume clearance was suggested by Stanciu and Bennett [3] based on observations during standard acid clearance tests. Kahrilas and co-workers [4] defined peristaltic dysfunction as either failed propagated peristalsis or peristaltic sequences with feeble contractions. The vigor of peristalsis required to effect complete volume clearance varies with the esophageal segment, so that quite weak contractions are effective in the proximal part of the esophagus, whereas contractions with a peak of the order of 30 mmHg or more are required for volume clearance from the distal esophagus. It has been suggested that between 25—50% of patients with peptic esophagitis suffer from peristaltic dysfunction, although in a recent study the figure appeared closer to 15% [5]. This may have been partially due to the more restrictive criteria for the definition of defective peristalsis that was used.

Furthermore, it is now well established that about 50% of patients with severe reflux disease have disordered gastric emptying [6—8], particularly of solids. Therefore, if such factors as disordered esophageal motility and delayed gastric emptying are important in the pathogenesis of gastroesophageal reflux disease then prokinetic agents which normalize esophageal and gastric function might be expected to be effective at least in those patients with abnormal function. In fact there have been few studies which have stratified patients according to their esophageal and gastric function.

A prospective randomized trial of metoclopramide and domperidone and placebo was undertaken. No improvement was found with the prokinetic agents compared to placebo regardless of the gastric emptying status of the patient. It is perhaps salutary to note that in this study the placebo and the domperidone and metoclopramide all gave around 40 to 45% improvement in patient's symptoms [9]. The newer agent cisapride has proven more interesting. It has been found to increase esophageal peristaltic amplitude, increase lower sphincter tone and increase gastric emptying in both normal patients and patients with reflux disease [10–12]. In controlled studies it has been found to be at least as effective as ranitidine in the treatment of reflux [13]. Actually, to those of us who treat the severe end of the spectrum of reflux disease this does not say much, as H_2 receptor blockers are largely ineffective in the great majority of patients with severe reflux disease. A recent study has suggested that cisapride is better than placebo alone at maintaining healing once this has been accomplished by other therapy, but relapse rate was still of the order of a third of patients. It seems logical, that if gastric emptying is an important factor in gastro-esophageal reflux disease, then cisapride might exert its beneficial effect best in the group of patients with delayed emptying. This, unfortunately, has not been tested.

In summary, few studies have stratified patients according to their motility disorder in terms of treatment of their reflux disease. In spite of this, prokinetic agents have not yet been demonstrated to show the same efficacy in treatment as the acid lowering agent omeprazole. This suggests that whatever the *cause* of reflux, it is the acid in the reflux which is most often responsible for the patient's symptoms and for the development of esophagitis.

References

1. Maddern GJ, Horowitz M, Jamieson GG, Chatteron BE, Collins PJ, Roberts-Thompson P. Abnormalities of esophageal and gastric emptying in progressive systemic sclerosis. Gastroenterology 1984;87:922–926.
2. Olsen AM, Schlegel JF. Motility disturbances caused by esophagitis. J Thorac Cardiovasc Surg 1965;50:607–612.
3. Stanciu C, Bennett JR. Oesophageal acid clearing: one factor in the production of reflux oesophagitis. Gut 1974;15:852–857.
4. Kahrilas PJ, Dodds WJ, Hogan WJ. Effect of peristaltic dysfunction on esophageal volume clearance. Gastroenterology 1988;94:73–80.
5. Lundell LR, Myers JJ, Jamieson GG. The influence of preoperative oesophageal motor function on the long-term outcome of antireflux surgery. Gullet 1993;3:50–55.
6. McCallum RW, Berkowitz DM, Lerner E. Gastric emptying in patients with gastroesophageal reflux. Gastroenterology 1981;80:285–291.
7. Maddern GJ, Chatterton BE, Collins PJ, Horowitz M, Shearman DJC, Jamieson GG. Solid and liquid gastric emptying in patients with gastro-oesophageal reflux. Br J Surg 1985;72;344–347.
8. Schwizer W, Hinder RA, DeMeester TR. Does delayed gastric emptying contribute to gastroesophageal reflux disease? Am J Surg 1989;157:74–80.
9. Maddern GJ, Kiroff GK, Leppard PI, Jamieson GG. Domperidone, Metoclopramide and placebo – all give symptomatic improvement in gastroesophageal reflux. J Clin Gastro Enterol 1986;8:135–140.
10. Ceccatelli P, Janssens J, Vantrappen G et al. Cisapride restores the decreased lower oesophageal sphincter pressure in reflux patients. Gut 1988;29:631–635.
11. Corazziari E, Scopinaro F, Bontempo et al. Effects of R-51619 on distal esophageal motor activity and gastric emptying. Ital J Gastroenterol 1983;15:185–186.
12. Gilbert RJ, Dodds WJ, Kahrilas PJ et al. Effect of cisapride, a new prokinetic agent, on esophageal motor dysfunction. Dig Dis Sci 1987;32:1331–1336.
13. Janisch JD, Hüttemann W, Bouzo MH. Cisapride versus ranitidine in the treatment of reflux esophagitis. Hepato-Gastroenterol 1988;35:125–127.

Prokinetic agents of the future: do they have any role in the medical treatment of GERD?

C. Scarpignato, G. Gimbo (Parma)
S. Bruley des Varannes, J.-P. Galmiche (Nantes)

Many receptor types are now known to modulate the function of the gut [1,2] and new agents are being developed which enhance gastrointestinal motor function and accelerate transit. Functional alterations of dopaminergic (inhibitory) and muscarinic (stimulatory) receptors are thought to be implicated in the pathogenesis of gut hypomotility. Consequently, gastrointestinal motility has been stimulated through the use of dopamine antagonists (such as metoclopramide, domperidone and L-sulpiride) and by substances which release acetylcholine, such as metoclopramide or cisapride or even directly by cholinergic drugs, which bind and act on muscarinic receptors of the smooth muscle cell (e.g., bethanechol) [3]. Recent evidence strongly suggests that the blockade of cholecystokinin (CCK)-receptors and stimulation of motilin receptors are also promising avenues. Drugs acting on 5-HT receptors, like cisapride, are presently the best available motor stimulating compounds and new derivatives are being developed as prokinetic drugs.

CCK-antagonists

It is well known that minute amounts of CCK are able to affect gastrointestinal motility under all the possible in vivo and in vitro experimental conditions in both animals and humans [4], thus suggesting this action on the gut to be one of the physiological actions of the peptide.

A summary of CCK effects on human gastrointestinal motility is shown in Table 1 [4–6]. CCK was found to reduce lower esophageal sphincter pressure (LESP) in a dose-dependent manner [7] (Fig. 1) and also, to partially inhibit the stimulatory effect of pentagastrin. The fat-induced inhibition of LESP is probably related to CCK release from the duodenum. A recent investigation [8] also showed an increase of postprandial transient LES relaxations (TLESRs) after endogenous CCK (released by high fat meal) (Fig. 2). Gastric emptying of both liquids and solids is significantly delayed by CCK and its synthetic derivatives (e.g., CCK-OP and the amphibian peptide caerulein) [9]. The mechanism through which CCK inhibits gastric emptying probably involves a drop in intragastric pressure, due to relaxation of the proximal stomach, together with a contraction of the antropyloric region, where the peptide decreases the motility index and the basal frequency of the electric rhythm. As far as the small and large intestine are concerned, CCK has a mixture of stimulatory and inhibitory effects on gut motility, although the stimulatory ones are largely predominant. In the first part of the duodenum the peptide has an inhibitory effect on the motility index and basic electric rhythm (BER) frequency, which resembles its

Table 1. Effects of CCK on human digestive motility

- Dose-dependent reduction of LESP
- Inhibition of pentagastrin-induced increase of LESP
- Relaxation of the proximal stomach and contraction of the antropyloric region
- Inhibition of gastric emptying of both solids and liquids
- Inhibition of mechanical and electrical activity of the duodenum
- Stimulation of small bowel and colonic motility

relaxant effect on the sphincter of Oddi.

It is now well established that CCK exerts its physiological effects through binding with specific receptors located on target cells. At least two different receptors mediate CCK biological actions: CCK-A and CCK-B receptors [10,11]. The CCK-A receptor mediates most of the activities of CCK in the gastrointestinal system. It is present on the pancreatic acinar cells, gallbladder as well as alimentary tract muscle, neurones in the myenteric plexus, vagal afferents from the GI tract and also in certain brain nuclei. The CCK-B receptor is mainly a brain receptor and probably modulates the actions of CCK in the central nervous system (CNS). It is worth mentioning that the gastrin receptor is similar to the CCK-B receptor [12] and, to date, no compounds have been described that clearly distinguish between these two receptors.

Eight classes of CCK-antagonists, including hundreds of compounds, have been described [10,11]. These antagonists have been used successfully in animals to confirm the classical actions of CCK, as well as, to explore novel activities, including its role as a neuropeptide. Amongst the compounds characterized as selective CCK-A receptor antagonists, two molecules have reached clinical trials, namely devazepide and loxiglumide (Fig. 3). Since the former was discontinued during early clinical

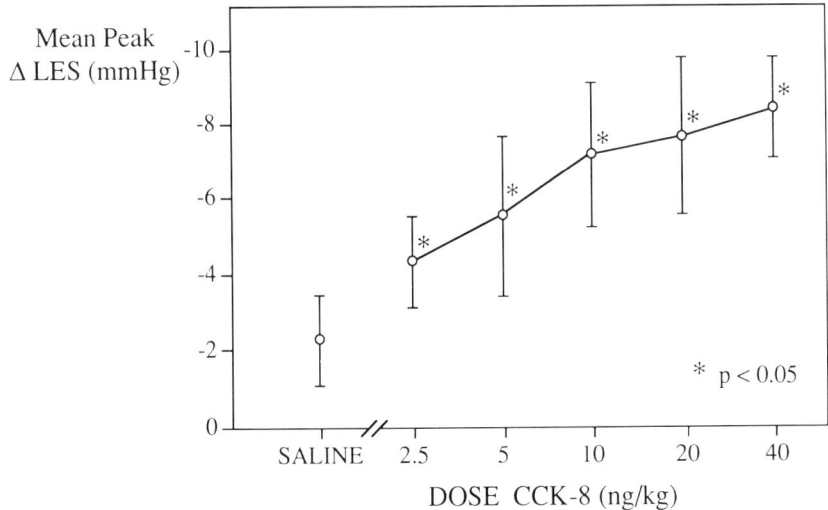

Fig. 1. Dose-dependent reduction of LESP by CCK-8 in humans (redrawn from [7]).

433

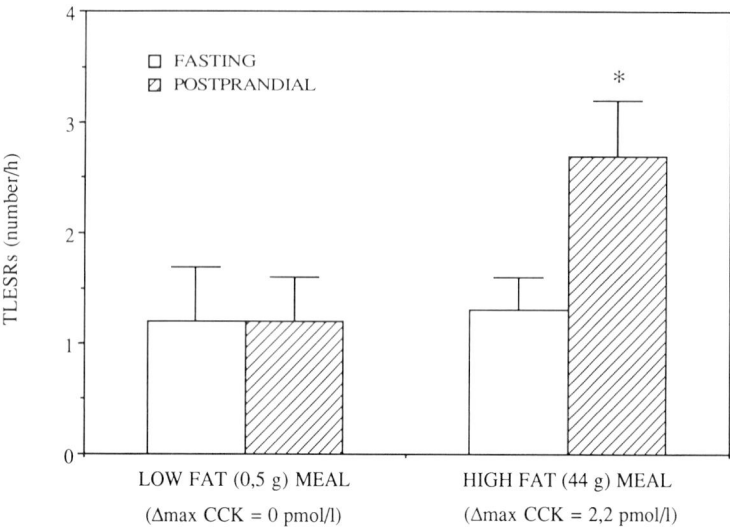

Fig. 2. Increase in the number of transient LES relaxations (TLESRs) during the third postprandial hour by endogenous CCK (released after intake of a high-fat meal) in humans (drawn from data in [8]).

development, almost all the clinical investigations have been performed with loxiglumide.

Effect of loxiglumide on upper digestive motility

Katschinski et al. [13] studied the effect of loxiglumide on esophageal motility in healthy volunteers. The compound was administered intravenously (10 mg/kg/h) in basal conditions and during an intraduodenal infusion of a Lundh test meal. Loxiglumide only slightly affected esophageal peristalsis in the interdigestive state (Table 2) and had no effect in the postprandial period. No effect on basal LESP was

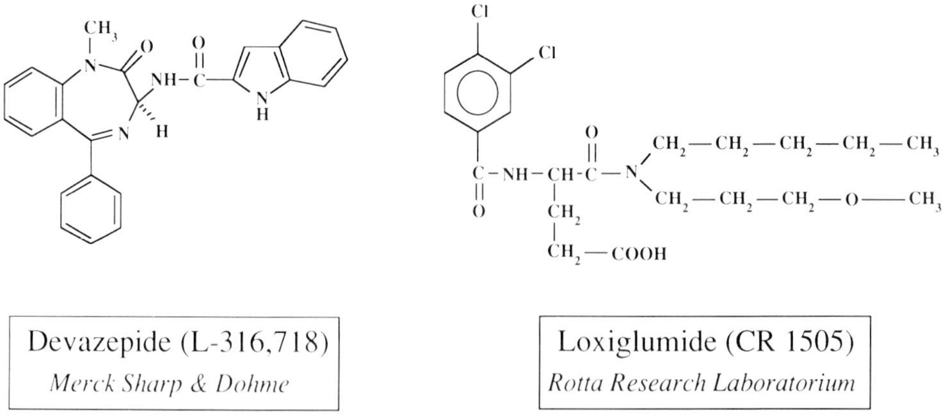

Devazepide (L-316,718)	Loxiglumide (CR 1505)
Merck Sharp & Dohme	*Rotta Research Laboratorium*

Fig. 3. Chemical structure of the CCK-A receptor antagonists available for use in humans.

Table 2. Effect of loxiglumide (10 mg/kg/h) on interdigestive esophageal motility in healthy volunteers [13]

Parameter	Saline	Loxiglumide	Significance
LESP (mmHg)	24.9 ± 2.9	27.2 ± 2.7	NS
Motility index (mmHg × s)	188.1 ± 22.6	210.8 ± 29.5	p < 0.05
Duration of contraction (s)	3.6 ± 0.1	3.9 ± 0.2	p = 0.06
Peristaltic velocity (cm/s)	3.2 ± 0.2	2.8 ± 0.1	p = 0.01

evident, but the compound was able to counterbalance the meal-induced decrease in sphincter pressure (Fig. 4). Provided this action of loxiglumide is also confirmed in patients with GERD, the drug could be useful to prevent or reduce postprandial reflux.

Bearing in mind the inhibitory effect of CCK on gastroduodenal motility, one could predict that CCK-A receptor blockade alone would result in an acceleration of emptying rate. This prokinetic activity of CCK-A antagonists is rarely observed, however, at least in the experimental animals. In fact, while CCK-A receptor antagonists constantly block CCK-induced inhibition of gastric motility [9], their effect on basal gastric emptying is variable and strictly depends on the experimental conditions. Amongst these, the nature (solid or liquid) and composition of the test meal, seem to be the most important ones [14–16].

Results from human studies are in line with those obtained in experimental animals (Table 3). The effect of loxiglumide on gastric emptying in man was first evaluated by means of radio-opaque markers ingested with three different meals [17]. Although loxiglumide significantly accelerated the emptying of the markers after a liquid test meal, no effect was evident when they were ingested with the guar or glucose meals. This apparent contrasting effect can be easily explained, taking into

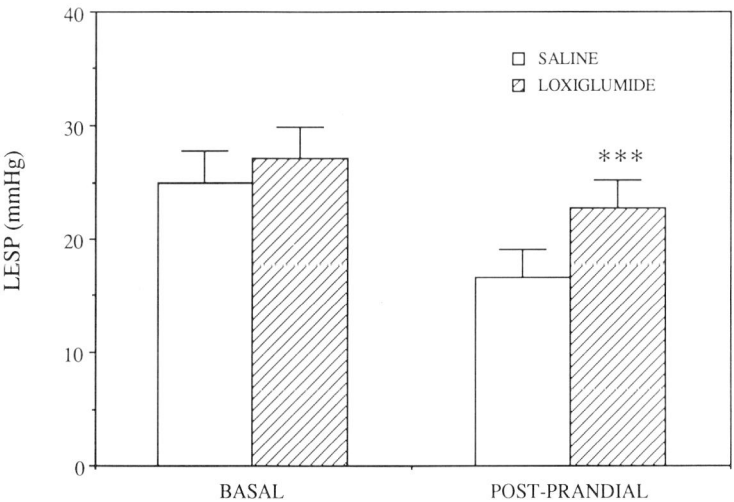

Fig. 4. Effect of loxiglumide (10 mg/kg/h) on basal and postprandial LESP in healthy volunteers (drawn from data in [13]).

Table 3. Effect of the CCK-A antagonists, released for human studies, on basal gastric emptying in healthy subjects

Authors	Type of meal	Antagonist	Dose (mg/kg)	Route of administration	Effect
Meyer et al. [17]	Guar liquid meal	Loxiglumide	30 mg/kg	oral	0
	5% glucose solution	Loxiglumide	30 mg/kg	oral	0
	Mixed liquid meal	Loxiglumide	30 mg/kg	oral	+
Fried et al. [18]	20% glucose solution	Loxiglumide	10 mg/kg/h	i.v.	+
	Mixed liquid meal	Loxiglumide	10 mg/kg/h	i.v.	+
Corazziari et al. [19]	Mixed solid meal	Loxiglumide	800 mg	oral	0
Liddle et al. [20]	Mixed solid/liquid meal	Devazepide	10 mg	oral	0
Cantor et al. [21]	Mixed liquid meal	Devazepide	10 mg	oral	+[a]

Note: i.v. = intravenously; + = acceleration of emptying rate; 0 = no effect on emptying rate; [a]acceleration evident only in the early phase of the emptying process (i.e., the first 75 min).

account that only the mixed meal releases endogenous CCK and show that loxiglumide has no intrinsic effect on gastric emptying. However, Fried et al. [18] were able to evidence with this CCK-A antagonist an acceleration of emptying rate (evaluated by gamma scintigraphy) not only of a mixed liquid meal (Ensure®) but also of a glucose meal. Besides the different technique of gastric emptying measurement (radiography vs. scintigraphy), the different glucose concentration (5 vs. 20%) and caloric content (100 vs. 400 kcal) of the two glucose meals, as well as, the dose (30 mg/kg vs. 10 mg/kg/h) and route (oral vs. intravenous) of administration of loxiglumide may help to explain discrepancies in findings. It is worth mentioning that Corazziari and his coworkers [19], by using another technique (ultrasonographic measurement of the antral volume) and a solid meal, were unable to confirm the gastrokinetic effect of loxiglumide. On the other hand, in one study [20] devazepide (10 mg orally) proved to be unable to modify gastric emptying of both solids and liquids, whereas, in another investigation [21] the same dose was found capable of significantly accelerating the early emptying rate of a liquid mixed meal.

CCK-A receptor antagonists: could they have a role in the treatment of GERD?

Experimental and clinical evidence suggests that CCK-A antagonism results in acceleration of emptying rate under certain experimental and clinical conditions. Due to the delaying effect of CCK on gastric emptying, CCK antagonists may prove to be useful gastrokinetic compounds, not only in patients with (diabetic or idiopathic) gastroparesis or those with motility-like dyspepsia, but also in patients with GERD, whose emptying rate (especially of solid food) is often delayed [22]. In such patients, CCK-A antagonists could also reduce postprandial reflux, due to their ability to counterbalance meal-induced decrease in LESP.

Motilin receptor agonists

Motilin seems to affect mainly, but not exclusively, the proximal part of the gastrointestinal tract [23]. The peptide has no significant influence upon gut contractile activity during the digestive state. Conversely, in the interdigestive state, it induces the cyclic recurrent episodes of caudal moving bands of strong contractions, that move from the lower esophageal sphincter (LES) to the terminal ileum. Exogenous motilin infusion was shown to increase LESP and gastric emptying in humans [23], but this peptide is obviously not suitable for use as a gastrokinetic because of its short half-life and the need of intravenous administration.

Motilin receptors have been identified on gastrointestinal smooth muscle membranes of rabbit [24,25] and isolated guinea pig gastric smooth muscle cells [26].

Effects of motilin agonists on upper digestive motility

Recent studies have shown that erythromycin mimics the effect of motilin on gastrointestinal motility [27]. Erythromycin and related 14-member macrolide compounds inhibit the binding of motilin to its receptors on gastrointestinal smooth muscle membranes and may, therefore, act as motilin agonists [28,29]. The contractile activity of these drugs is similar to that induced by motilin and cannot be blocked by atropine or tetrodotoxin (TTX), thus suggesting a direct effect upon smooth muscle cells [29].

The effect of intravenous erythromycin (150 mg/20 min) on esophageal motility and LESP (measured by a Dent's sleeve) was studied in healthy volunteers [30,31], as well as in scleroderma patients [32]. Compared with placebo, the antibiotic significantly increased LESP, an effect completely blocked by previous administration of atropine (Fig. 5). Erythromycin was also able to augment postprandial LESP [33]. In all these studies, the other esophageal motor parameters were not affected by the drug. Later experiments [34,35] in GERD patients were, however, unable to confirm the LESP enhancing effect of erythromycin (250 mg b.i.d. or q.i.d.), but showed an enhancement of esophageal motility. Despite this, neither investigation detected a reduction in esophageal exposure to acid. Different experimental conditions (healthy volunteers or scleroderma patients vs. GERD patients, i.v. vs. oral administration) may explain differences in findings. Nevertheless, Pfeiffer et al. [36] were able to show that erythromycin completely suppresses postprandial GER induced by white wine in healthy volunteers (Fig. 6). In that study, however, the macrolide was given by intravenous infusion (3.5 mg/kg within 15 min). By this route, the drug effectively increases LESP in humans [30,31]. The fact that in one study [35] a significant improvement of the delayed gastric emptying of solids was documented, may suggest that the different gut regions (namely the esophagus and the stomach) may have different sensitivity to erythromycin. Further studies with different regimens (higher doses and/or more frequent administration) are obviously needed to establish the clinical usefulness of this antibiotic in the treatment of GERD.

At low and microbiologically ineffective doses, intravenous infusion of erythromycin and related macrolides cause a burst of motor activity in the gut, similar to phase III activity [27,37,38] and this event may be accompanied by a rise in motilin levels [37].

The high density of motilin receptors in the stomach and duodenum suggested that

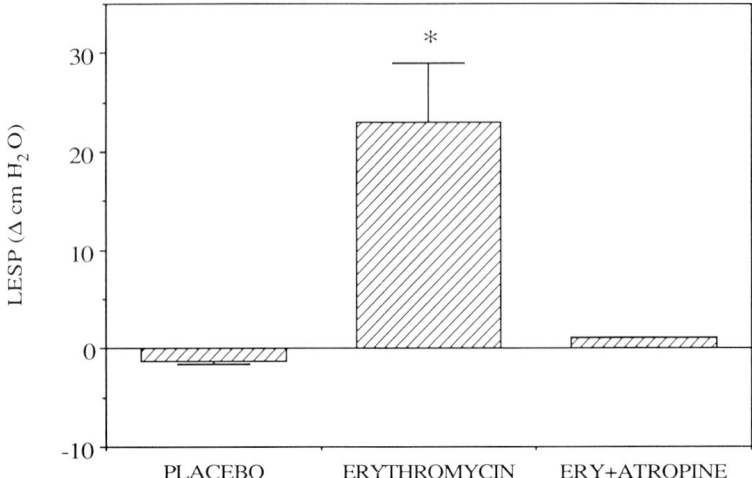

Fig. 5. LESP enhancing effect of intravenous erythromycin (150 mg/20 min) in healthy volunteers (drawn from data in [30]).

erythromycin and related macrolides might increase gastric emptying. As a matter of fact, several papers [39,40] have shown erythromycin to be capable of accelerating emptying rate in diabetic gastroparesis, an effect evident after intravenous [39–41], intraperitoneal [42] and oral [39,41,43] administration. Intravenous erythromycin caused an acceleration of gastric emptying of both solids and liquids, which were emptied at the same rate [43], thus abolishing the physiological discrimination between the different phases of the meal. Similarly, the drug has been successfully employed to treat gastroparesis in a patient with progressive systemic sclerosis [44]. Only recently has the effect of the antibiotic been demonstrated in healthy subjects, where it proved to be capable of accelerating the emptying of both solid and

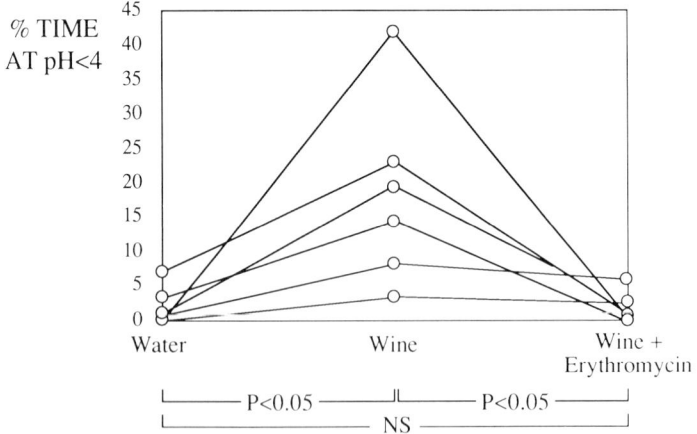

Fig. 6. Inhibition by erythromycin (3.5 mg/kg/15 min) of white wine induced postprandial reflux (redrawn from [36]).

438

hypertonic liquid (50% glucose, Fig. 7) meals [45]. The mechanisms by which erythromycin affects gastric emptying seem to be connected with a strong stimulation of propulsive forces of the human stomach [46] and an increase in proximal, as well as, distal antral pressure activity during the dumping of solids from the stomach [47]. Although the gastrokinetic effect of erythromycin is evident after acute administration, data concerning its long-term effects on idiopathic or diabetic gastroparesis are controversial [41,48]. Further studies are needed, in order to determine how much the frequency of administration or dosage are important for long-term treatment.

Motilin receptor agonists: future drugs for GERD?

Since erythromycin proved to be capable of counterbalancing — under certain experimental and clinical conditions — postprandial GER and accelerating gastric emptying, thus reducing the gastric content available for reflux, its use could be envisaged in the medical treatment of GERD.

Further development of this class of drugs [49], now called motilides, will depend on the synthesis of compounds devoid of antibacterial activity, for instance ME-34

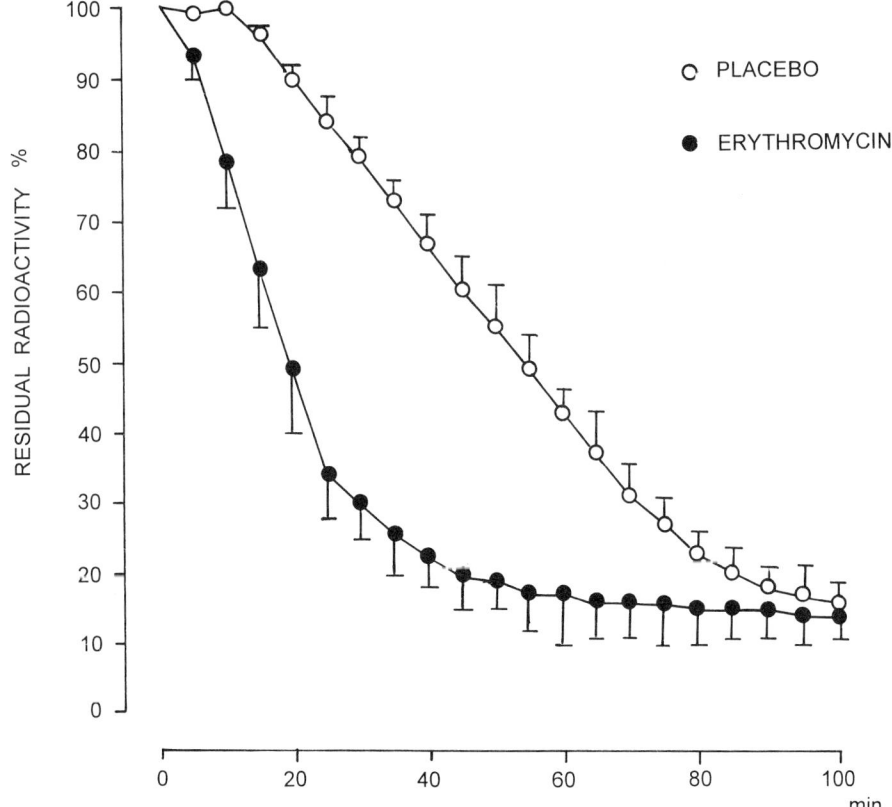

Fig. 7. Gastric emptying of a liquid hypertonic (50%) glucose meal after administration of erythromycin (200 mg intravenously) or placebo in healthy volunteers (from [45]).

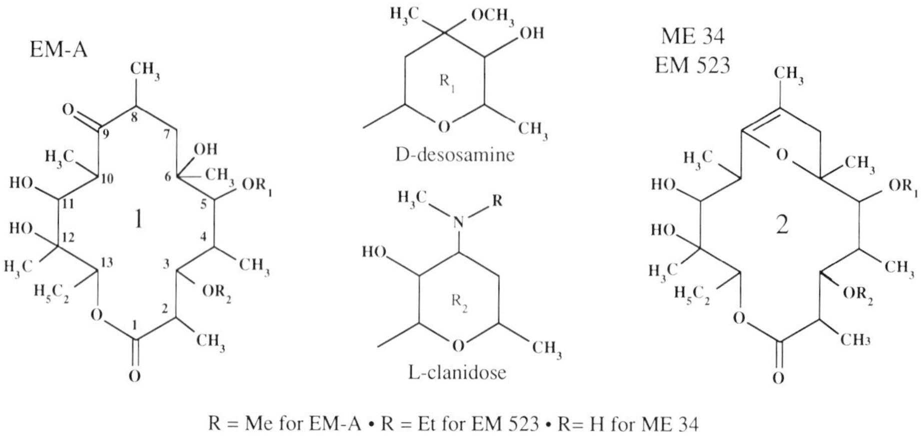

EM-A

D-desosamine

L-clanidose

ME 34
EM 523

R = Me for EM-A • R = Et for EM 523 • R= H for ME 34

Fig. 8. Chemical structure of erythromycin and its derivatives (ME-34 and EM-523) devoid of antibacterial activity.

and EM-523 (Fig. 8) [50–52] or LY-267198 [53] and the absence of fading of the gastrokinetic effect during prolonged administration.

Drugs acting on 5-HT receptors

The use of selective agonists and antagonists allowed the biological actions of 5-hydroxytryptamine (5-HT) to be established as mediated, by at least four types of receptors:
− 5-HT$_1$-like;
− 5-HT$_2$;
− 5-HT$_3$; and
− the recently described 5-HT$_4$ receptor [54].
It is well known that metoclopramide is an effective, albeit weak, antagonist of 5-HT$_3$ receptors which have been found only associated with peripheral autonomic, afferent and enteric neurons [55]. The effectiveness − as antiemetic and motor stimulating compounds − of some selective 5-HT$_3$ antagonists (e.g., ondansetron, granisetron and tropisetron) (Fig. 9), devoid of any effect at dopamine receptors, suggested that blockade of these sites plays an important role in the mechanism of action of metoclopramide [56]. As a consequence, the potential of 5-HT$_3$ antagonists as gastrokinetic drugs has been explored in both animals and humans.

Animal experiments have shown that almost all the available 5-HT$_3$ antagonists are capable of accelerating gastric emptying of either nutrient and nonnutrient meals [57]. In humans, gastric emptying of both solids and liquids (Fig. 10) is accelerated by intravenous [58] and oral [59] administration of tropisetron. Ondansetron, however, proved to be unable to modify emptying rate in healthy volunteers [60].

The effect of tropisetron on esophageal motility was studied in healthy volunteers

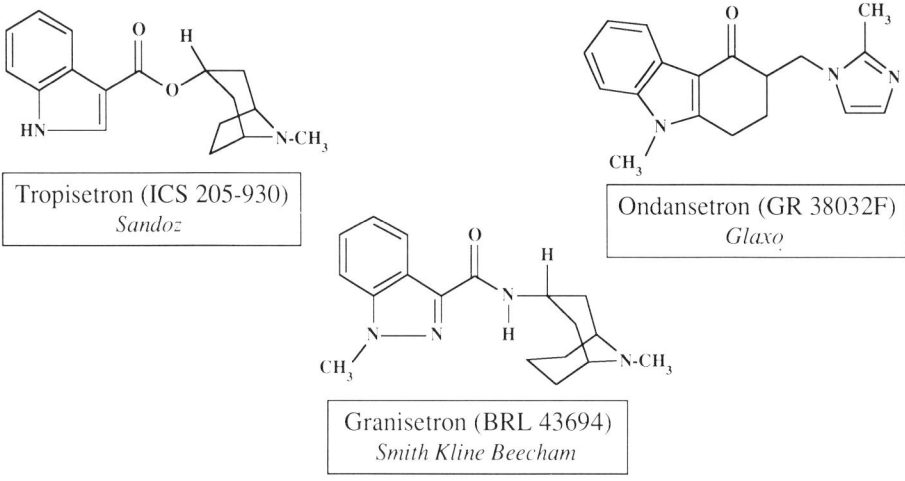

Tropisetron (ICS 205-930)
Sandoz

Ondansetron (GR 38032F)
Glaxo

Granisetron (BRL 43694)
Smith Kline Beecham

Fig. 9. Chemical structure of the selective 5-HT$_3$-antagonists currently available for clinical use.

by Stacher et al. [61], who reported a significant and long-lasting increase of LESP (Fig. 11) after intravenous administration of the compound (20 mg).

The lack of correlation between the potency of these compounds as 5-HT$_3$ receptor antagonists and their ability to stimulate gastrointestinal motility, suggests that mechanisms other than blockade of 5-HT$_3$ receptors should be involved in their motor stimulating activity [62]. Rather, an agonistic activity at level of 5-HT$_4$ receptors, located on nerve terminals of both cholinergic interneurons and motor neurons and whose stimulation increases acetylcoline release, seems to be the key mechanism of established (e.g., cisapride) and new (e.g., renzapride, zacopride, BRL 20627, SDZ

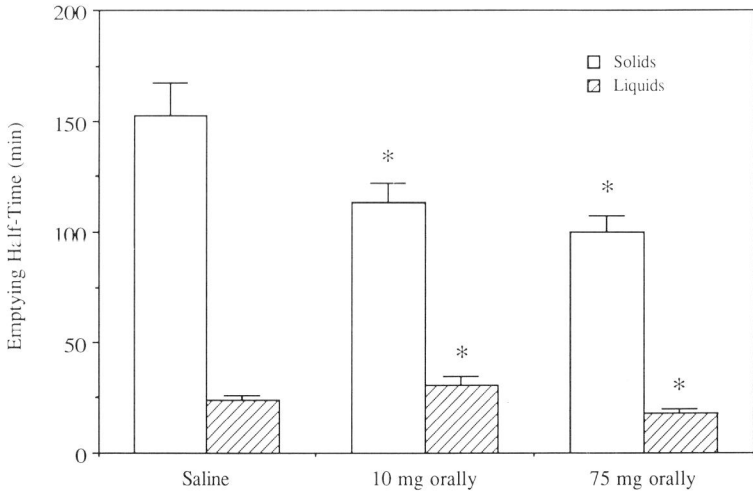

Fig. 10. Acceleration of gastric emptying of both solids and liquids by oral administration of tropisetron in healthy volunteers (drawn from data in [59]).

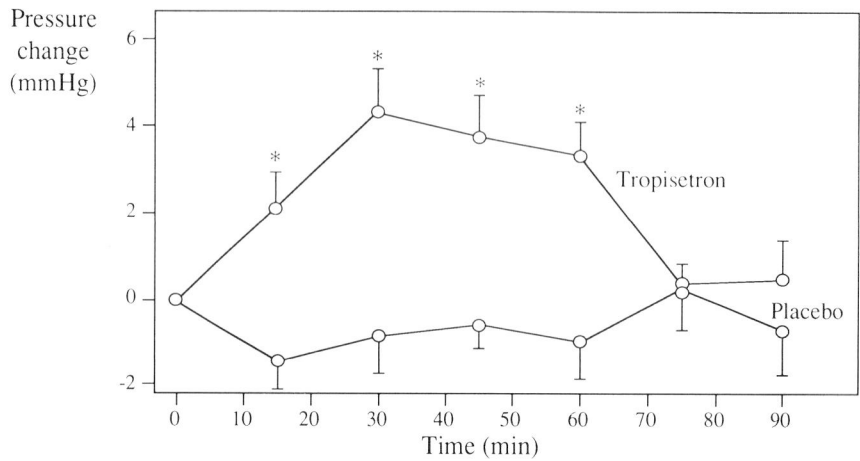

Fig. 11. Effect of tropisetron (20 mg i.v.) on LESP in healthy volunteers (drawn from data in [61]).

HTF 919) gastrokinetic compounds [54,63]. The matter is rather puzzling, since some 5-HT$_3$ antagonists display agonistic properties at the level of 5-HT$_4$ receptors, some are devoid of such an effect, while tropisetron (ICS 205–930) actually behaves (at

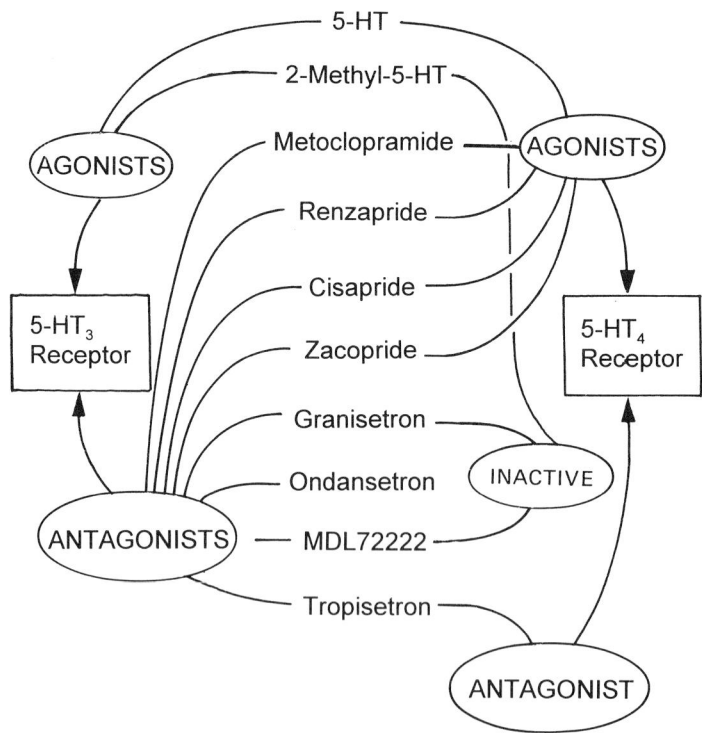

Fig. 12. Activity of some motor stimulating compounds at 5-HT$_3$ and 5-HT$_4$ receptor level [54].

442

high doses) as a 5-HT$_4$ antagonist (Fig. 12). Whatever the receptor subtype involved, drugs acting on 5-HT receptors are capable of affecting upper and lower gastrointestinal motility and, provided their action be confirmed in patients, new gastrokinetic compounds belonging to this class of drugs will be soon available for clinical use.

Perspectives for the future

It is now well established that numerous clinical syndromes may be related to motor abnormalities of the upper gastrointestinal motility. In this context, GERD can be considered a primary motility disorder [64,65] and, as a consequence, gastrokinetic compounds are effective in the medical treatment of the disease [66]. Drugs enhancing gastrointestinal motility and coordination are now available and several new ones are being developed. Further work is needed to determine the predictive value of objective abnormalities for the efficacy of a drug in the individual patient. This is the crucial point in defining a rational strategy in clinical practice, especially when establishing if functional investigation is needed before a gastrokinetic drug is given.

Acknowledgement

We are indebted to Miss Sabina Cavagni for her invaluable help in checking the references and her diligence in the preparation of the manuscript.

References

1. Burks TF, Galligan JJ, Porreca F. Gastrointestinal drug receptors. J Clin Gastroenterol 1983;5(suppl 1):29—36.
2. Ruoff H-J, Fladung B, Demol P et al. Gastrointestinal receptors and drugs in motility disorders. Digestion 1991;48:1—17.
3. Scarpignato C. Pharmacological bases of the medical treatment of gastroesophageal reflux disease. Dig Dis Sci 1988;6: 117—148.
4. Bertaccini G. Peptides: Gastrointestinal hormones. In: Bertaccini G (ed) Handbook of Experimental Pharmacology, vol 59/II. Heidelberg: Springer Verlag, 1982;11—83.
5. Docray GJ. Physiology of enteric neuropeptides. In: Johnson LR (ed) Physiology of the Gastrointestinal Tract, 2nd edn. New York: Raven Press, 1987;41—66.
6. Bruley des Varannes S, Cloarec D, Dubois A et al. Cholécystokinine et ses antagonistes: effets sur la motricité digestive. Gastroentérol Clin Biol 1991;15:794—757.
7. Resin H, Stern DH, Sturdevant RAL, Isenberg JI. Effect of the C-terminal octapeptide of cholecystokinin on lower esophageal sphincter pressure in man. Gastroenterology 1973;64:946—949.
8. Ledeboer ML, Masclee AAM, Batstra M, Lamers CBHW. Effect of cholecystokinin on transient lower esophageal sphincter relaxations. Gastroenterology 1993;104:A539.
9. Scarpignato C, Varga G, Corradi C. Effect of CCK and its antagonists on gastric emptying. J Physiol (Paris) 1993;87: 291—300.
10. Scarpignato C. Cholecystokinin antagonists and motilides: pharmacology and potential in the treatment of gastroesophageal reflux disease and other digestive motor disorders. In: Scarpignato C (ed) Advances in Drug Therapy of Gastroesophageal Reflux Disease. Basel: Karger, 1992;90—128.
11. D'Amato M, Makovec F, Rovati LC. Potential clinical applications of CCK$_A$-receptor antagonists in gastroenterology. Drug News and Perspectives (in press).
12. Lotti VJ, Chang RSL. A new potent and selective nonpeptide gastrin antagonist and brain cholecystokinin receptor (CCK-B) ligand: L-365,260. Eur J Pharmacol 1989;162:273—280.
13. Katschinski M, Koppelberg T, Wank U, Adler G, Rovati L, Arnold R. CCK plays a role as a physiological regulator of human esophageal motility. Gastroenterology 1990;98:A365.

14. Buéno L, Fioramonti J. Drug effects on gastric emptying in animal models depend on the nature of test meals used. Am J Physiol 1988;254:G637.

15. Gue M, Fioramonti J, Buéno L. Influence of stress on gastric emptying depends on the nature of meals, stressors, and animal species. J Gastrointest Motil 1990;2:18—22.

16. Liberge M, Riviere PMJ, Buéno L. Influence of enkephalinase inhibitors on gastric emptying in mice depends on the nature of the meal. Life Sci 1988;42:2047—2053.

17. Meyer BM, Werth BA, Beglinger C, Hildebrand P, Jansen JBMJ, Zach D, Rovati LC, Stalder GA. Role of cholecystokinin in regulation of gastrointestinal motor functions. Lancet 1989;ii:12—15.

18. Fried M, Erlacher URS, Schwizer W, Löchner C, Koerfer J, Beglinger C, Jansen JB, Lamers CB, Harder F, Bischof-Delaloye A, Stalder GA, Rovati L. Role of cholecystokinin in the regulation of gastric emptying and pancreatic enzyme secretion in humans. Gastroenterology 1991;101:503—511.

19. Corazziari E, Ricci R, Biliotti D, Bontempo I, De'Medici A, Pallotta N, Torsoli A. Oral administration of loxiglumide (CCK antagonist) inhibits postprandial gallbladder contraction without affecting gastric emptying. Dig Dis Sci 1990;35:50—54.

20. Liddle RA, Gertz BJ, Kanayama S, Beccaria L, Coker LD, Turnbull TA, Morita ET. Effects of a novel cholecystokinin (CCK) receptor antagonist, MK-329, on gallbladder contraction and gastric emptying. Implications for the physiology of CCK. J Clin Invest 1989;84:1220—1225.

21. Cantor P, Mortensen PE, Myhre J, Gjorup I, Worning H, Stahl E, Survill TT. The effect of the cholecystokinin receptor antagonist MK-329 on meal-stimulated pancreaticobiliary output in humans. Gastroenterology 1992;102:1742—1751.

22. Scarpignato C. Gastric emptying in gastroesophageal reflux disease and other functional esophageal disorders. In: Scarpignato C, Galmiche JP (eds) Functional Investigation in Esophageal Disease. Basel: Karger, 1991;223—259.

23. McIntosh CHS, Brown JC. Motilin: isolation, secretion, actions and pathophysiology. In: Scarpignato C, Bianchi Porro G (eds) Clinical Investigation of Gastric Function. Basel: Karger, 1990;307—352.

24. Bormans V, Peeters TL, Vantrappen G. Motilin receptors in rabbit stomach and small intestine. Regul Peptides 1986;15:143—153.

25. Peeters TL, Bormans V, Matthijs G et al. Comparison of the biological activity of canine and porcine motilin in rabbit. Regul Peptides 1986;15:333—339.

26. Louie DS, Owyang C. Motilin receptors on isolated gastric smooth muscle cells. Am J Physiol 1988;254:G210—G216.

27. Tomomasa T, Kuruome T, Arai H. Erythromycin induces migrating motor complex in human gastrointestinal tract. Dig Dis Sci 1986;31:157—161.

28. Kondo Y, Torii K, Itoh Z. Erythromycin and its derivatives with motilin-like biological activities inhibit the specific binding of ^{125}I-motilin to duodenal muscle. Biochem Biophys Res Comm 1988;150:877—882.

29. Peeters T, Matthijs G, Depoortere I. Erythromycin is a motilin receptor agonist. Am J Physiol 1989;257:G470—G474.

30. Michopoulos S, Chaussade S, Guerre J. Effet de l'erythromycine (ERY) sur la motricité oesophagienne chez l'homme normal. Gastroentérol Clin Biol 1990;14(2bis):44A.

31. Janssens J, Vantrappen G, Annese V, Peeters TL, Tijskens G, Rekoumis G. Effect of erythromycin on LES function and esophageal body contractility. Gastroenterology 1990;98:A64.

32. Chaussade S, Michopoulos S, Kahan A, Samama J, Danel B, Amor B, Menkès CJ, Guerre J, Couturier D. Effets de l'erythromycine (ERY), un agoniste de la motiline, sur la motricité oesophagienne chez des patients presentant une sclerodermie systemique (S.S.). Gastroentérol Clin Biol 1991;15(2bis):A35.

33. Dalton CB, DeVore MS, Smout AJPM, Castell DO. The effect of erythromycin (Ery) on lower esophageal sphincter pressure (LESP) and esophageal motility. Gastroenterology 1990;98:A342.

34. Champion G, Singh S, Nellans H, Richter JE. Erythromycin — from acne to acid reflux? Gastroenterology 1991;100:A41.

35. Harrison ME, Ruzkowski CJ, Young MF, Sanowski RA. Erythromycin improves gastric emptying and esophageal motility without affecting gastroesophageal reflux. Gastroenterology 1991;100:A80.

36. Pfeiffer A, Wendl B, Pehl C, Kaess H. Effect of erythromycin on gastroesophageal reflux. Gastroenterol Clin Biol 1991;15:561—562.

37. Zara GP, Thompson HH, Pilot MA et al. Effects of erythromycin on gastrointestinal tract motility. J Antimicrob Chemother 1985;16(suppl A):175—179.

38. Zara GP, Qin XY, Pilot MA et al. Response of the human gastrointestinal tract to erythromycin. J Gastrointest Motil 1991;3:26—31.

39. Janssens J, Peeters TL, Vantrappen G et al. Improvement of gastric emptying in diabetic gastroparesis by erythromycin. N Engl J Med 1990;322:1028—1031.

40. Pouliquen B, Bizais Y, Murat A, Galmiche JP. L'erythromycine accélère de façon spectaculaire la vidange gastrique (VG) des patients atteints de gastroparesie diabetique (GP). Gastroenterol Clin Biol 1990;14(2bis):47A.

41. Richards RD, Davenport K, McCallum RW. The treatment of idiopathic and diabetic gastroparesis with acute intravenous and chronic oral erythromycin. Am J Gastroenterol 1993;88:203—207.

42. Wadhwa NK, Atkins H, Cabralda T. Intraperitoneal erythromycin for gastroparesis. Ann Int Med 1991;114:912.

43. Urbain JLC, Vantrappen G, Janssens J et al. Intravenous erythromycin dramatically accelerates gastric emptying in gastroparesis diabeticorum and normals and abolishes the emptying discrimination between solids and liquids. J Nucl Med 1990;31:1490—1493.

44. Dull JS, Raufman JP, Zakia MD et al. Successful treatment of gastroparesis with erythromycin in a patient with progressive systemic sclerosis. Am J Med 1990;89:528—530.

45. Mantides A, Xynos E, Crhysos E, Georgopoulos N Vassilakis JS. The effect of erythromycin in gastric emptying of solids and hypertonic liquids in healthy subjects. Am J Gastroenterol 1993;88:198—202.

46. Prather CM, Camilleri M, Thomforde GM, Forstrom LA, Zinsmeister AR. Gastric axial forces in experimenatlly delayed and accelerated gastric emptying. Am J Physiol Gastrointest Liver Physiol 1993;264:G928—G934.

47. Annese V, Janssens J, Vantrappen G, Tack J, Peeters TL, Willemse P, Van Cutsem E. Erythromycin accelerates gastric emptying by inducing antral contractions and improved gastroduodenal coordination. Gastroenterology 1992;102:823—828.

48. Richards RD, Davenport KG, Hurm KD, Wimbish WR, McCallum RW. Acute and chronic treatment of gastroparesis with erythromycin. Gastroenterology 1990;80:A385.

49. Depoortere I, Peeters TL, Matthijs G et al. Structure-activity relation of erythromycin-related macrolides in inducing contractions and in displacing bound motilin in rabbit duodenum. J Gastrointest Motil 1989;1:150—159.

50. Inatomi N, Satoh H, Maki Y et al. An erythromycin derivative, EM-523, induces motilin-like gastrointestinal motility in dogs. J Pharmacol Exp Ther 1989;251:707—712.

51. Inatomi N, Satoh H, Satoh T et al. An erythromycin derivative, EM523, shows motilin-like contractile activity in vivo and in vitro. Eur J Pharmacol 1990;183:2183.

52. Depoortere I, Peeters TL, Vantrappen G. The erythromycin derivatives EM-523 is a potent motilin agonist in man and in rabbit. Peptides 1990;11:515—519.

53. Gidda JS, Prime P, Dieckman D, Greenwood B, Wind JA, Kirst HA, Robertson DW. LY26108: an analog of erythromycin (EM) enhances gastrointestinal motility in anaesthetized and conscious animals. Gastroenterology 1991;100:A444.

54. Costall B, Naylor RJ. 5-hydroxytryptamine: New receptors and novel drugs for gastrointestinal motor disorders. Scand J Gastroenterol 1990;25:769—787.

55. Fernandez AG, Massingham R. Peripheral receptor populations involved in the regulation of gastrointestinal motility and the pharmacological actions of metoclopramide-like drugs. Life Sci 1985;36:1—14.

56. Fozard JR. 5-HT$_3$ receptors and cytotoxic drug-induced vomiting. Trends Pharmacol Sci 1987;8:44—45.

57. Gamse R, Buchheit KH. 5-HT$_3$ receptor antagonists: Pharmacology and potential in the treatment of gastroesophageal reflux disease. In: Scarpignato C (ed) Advances in Drug Therapy of Gastroesophageal Reflux Disease. Basel: Karger, 1992;81—89.

58. Akkermans LMA, Vos A, Hoekstra A, et al. Effect of ICS 205-930 (a specific 5-HT$_3$ receptor antagonist) on gastric emptying of a solid meal in normal subjects. Gut 1988;29:1249—1252.

59. McCallum RW, Mittal RK, Sluss J. Effect of ICS 205-930, a potential prokinetic agent, on upper gastrointestinal motility in normal subjects. Gastroenterology 1989;96:A332.

60. Talley NJ, Phillips SF, Haddad A, Miller LJ, Twomey C, Zinsmeister AR, Ciocola A. Effect of selective 5-HT$_3$ antagonist (GR 38032F) on small intestinal transit and release of gastrointestinal peptides. Dig Dis Sci 1989;34:1511—1515.

61. Stacher G, Steiner G, Gaupmann G et al. Effects of the 5-HT$_3$ antagonist, ICS 205-930, on oesophageal motor activity and on lower oesophageal sphincter pressure: A double-blind crossover study. Hepato-Gastroenterol 1991;37(suppl 2):118—121.

62. Gullikson GW, Loeffler RF, Virina MA. Relationship of serotonin-3 receptor antagonist activity to gastric emptying and motor-stimulating actions of prokinetic drugs in dogs. J Pharmacol Exp Ther 1991;258:103—110.

63. Tonini M, Rizzi CA, Manzo L, Onori L. Novel enteric 5-HT$_4$ receptors and gastrointestinal prokinetic action. Pharmacol Res 1991;24:5—14.

64. Castell DO. Gastroesophageal reflux disease is a motility disorder. In: Scarpignato C (ed) Advances in Drug Therapy of Gastroesophageal Reflux Disease. Basel: Karger, 1992;11—16.

65. Dent J. Gastroesophageal reflux disease: A primary motility disorder. In: Heading RC, Wood JD (eds) Gastrointestinal Dismotility: Focus on Cisapride. New York: Raven Press, 1992;127—140.

66. Ramirez B, Richter JE. Review article: promotility drugs in the treatment of gastro-oesophageal reflux disease. Aliment Pharmacol Ther 1993;7:5—20.

Proton pump inhibitors

 ## Is there a relationship between the degree of inhibition of acid secretion and the degree of endoscopic healing of esophagitis?

S.J. Sontag (Hines, Illinois)

Gastroesophageal reflux (GER) is characterized by upward movement into the esophagus of gastric and/or duodenal contents. The reflux may be physiologic, resulting in no damage to the esophageal mucosa, or pathologic, resulting in erosions, exudate, ulcerations, strictures and/or Barrett's esophagus.

Factors that contribute to esophageal mucosal damage do so by increasing the exposure time of the mucosa to gastric acid and pepsin. Thus, an incompetent lower esophageal sphincter (LES) [1,2], impaired esophageal clearance [3–5], increased frequency of GER episodes [6], delayed gastric emptying [7,8] and the presence of a hiatal hernia [9] all contribute to increased exposure of acid and pepsin.

The role of acid in GER symptoms

Joelsson and Johnsson demonstrated that the frequency of reflux symptoms correlated directly with the percent of time of acid exposure in the esophagus [10]. Symptomatic patients were divided into three groups: occasional symptoms, daily symptoms and almost continuous symptoms. In addition, a group with no symptoms was included. There was complete separation of all four groups throughout the day. The greater the frequency of reflux symptoms, the more esophageal acid exposure throughout the day and night. The correlation between symptoms and acid exposure was present during sleeping hours as well.

A relationship between basal acid output (BAO) and reflux symptoms has also been reported. Collen et al. demonstrated that the dose of ranitidine required to provide complete relief of reflux symptoms was directly related to the pretreatment BAO [11]. Ranitidine 300 mg/day relieved symptoms in most patients with a BAO of less than or equal to 8 mEq/h. The doses of ranitidine required to relieve symptoms in patients with BAO levels above 10 mEq/h ranged from 900 to 1800 mg/day. Overall, patients whose symptoms were relieved had a mean BAO of 5 mEq/h as compared to a mean of 10 mEq/h in patients whose symptoms were not relieved.

The role of acid in esophagitis

The relationship between acid reflux and esophagitis has been established in both animal models and human patients. The results have demonstrated that esophageal mucosal injury is determined by both the pH of the refluxate and the duration of exposure to the acid refluxate. Robertson et al. using esophageal pH testing showed that the percent time pH is less than 4 in the esophagus correlates directly with the grade of esophagitis [12]. Patients with mild esophagitis had about 5% of the total time with pH < 4, whereas patients with severe esophagitis and Barrett's esophagus had about 25% of the total time with pH < 4 [12].

In a meta-analysis of nine independent studies, Bell et al. demonstrated a relationship between healing of esophagitis and reduction of intragastric acidity [13]. Although these studies were done by measuring intragastric (not intraesophageal) pH, the results clearly show that the duration of time that pH is greater than 4 correlates directly with the percentage of patients with healed esophagitis. Measuring intraesophageal acid exposure, Bell also showed that healing of esophagitis was directly related to reduction of intraesophageal acid exposure [13,14]. Seventy to ninety percent of patients with esophagitis healed if the time that the pH was below 4 was reduced to less than 2% of the entire day.

The most impressive and compelling data demonstrating the role of acid in esophagitis comes from maintenance studies in which patients with esophagitis are treated until healed and then maintained on therapy that includes all ranges of acid-suppressing agents [15–24]. Such studies demonstrate that acid reduction during acute therapy leads to complete healing, but that maintenance therapy with dosages less than those required for acute healing may result in recurrence. For instance, Figs. 1–3 show the recurrence of esophagitis during maintenance therapy: month "0" starting points of 100% reflect all the patients that healed during acute therapy (patients who failed to heal during acute therapy are not represented on these graphs). In each figure, the results of daily omeprazole therapy are presented from five separate studies for comparison. Recurrence during daily omeprazole therapy compared with placebo or no maintenance therapy (Fig. 1): after complete healing with omeprazole, 80% of patients recurred within 6 months on no therapy, clearly indicating that

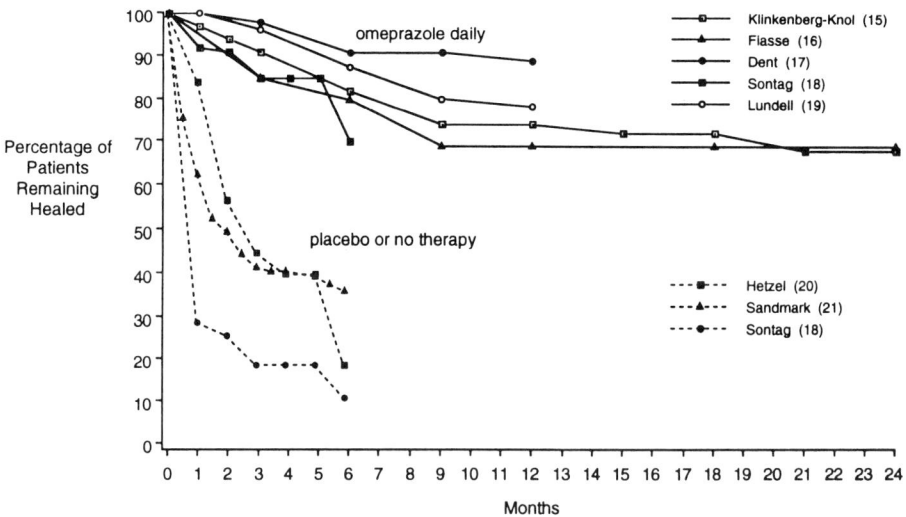

Fig. 1. Recurrence of erosive esophagitis after complete healing. Maintenance: omeprazole 20 mg daily vs. placebo or no therapy.

cessation of acid-suppressing treatment allows recurrence of esophagitis. Recurrence during daily omeprazole therapy compared with interrupted therapy with 20 mg of omeprazole daily on only three consecutive days each week (Fig. 2): omeprazole 20 mg daily on 3 days each week does not prevent recurrence of esophagitis. Indeed, 50—70% of the patients recurred within 6—12 months when maintenance treatment was given only 3 days per week. Recurrence during daily omeprazole therapy

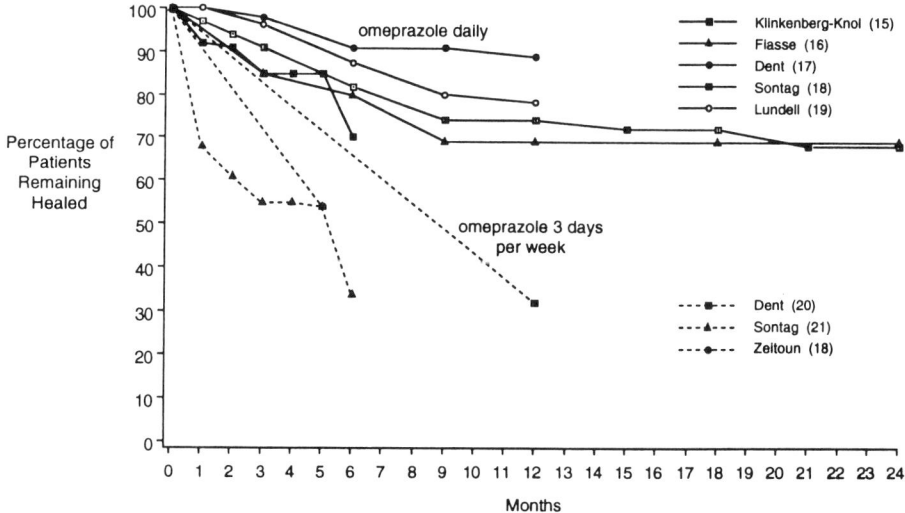

Fig. 2. Recurrence of erosive esophagitis after complete healing. Maintenance: omeprazole 20 mg daily vs. omeprazole 20 mg 3 days a week.

compared with maintenance therapy with H_2-receptor antagonists (Fig. 3): high-dose H_2-receptor antagonists do not prevent recurrence of esophagitis after complete healing, indicating once again that acid-suppressing agents in doses less than those required for healing are ineffective in maintaining healing. Thus, after complete healing of esophagitis with H_2-receptor antagonists or omeprazole, symptomatic recurrences of erosive esophagitis occur in approximately 80% of patients within 6 months if inadequate or no maintenance therapy is given [15–24]. At the end of 2 years, two-thirds of patients receiving daily omeprazole for maintenance therapy remained in remission.

Factors other than acid that influence healing

Overall, up to 20% of patients with severe esophagitis will remain unhealed, regardless of the dose used to suppress acid. Even in doses of omeprazole up to 60 mg/day, 15% of patients will not heal. These findings suggest that factors other than refluxed acid are important in the development of esophagitis. Recent studies show that both cigarette smoking and pretreatment severity of esophagitis are factors that negatively influenced the esophagitis healing rates during H_2-receptor antagonist therapy. Whether these factors also interfere with the effectiveness of omeprazole is currently unknown.

Summary

The results of the numerous studies demonstrate that acid is damaging to the esophageal mucosa, that the frequency of reflux episodes correlates with reflux

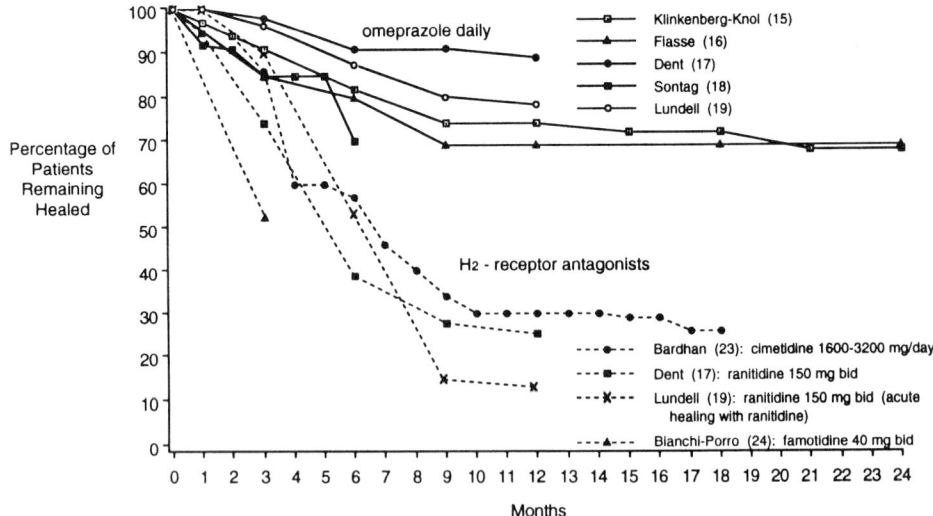

Fig. 3. Recurrence of erosive esophagitis after complete healing. Maintenance: omeprazole 20 mg daily vs. H_2-receptor antagonists.

symptoms and that reduction of gastric acid secretion is associated with improvement in symptoms and esophagitis. Finally, it must be understood that there are no data to indicate that rigorous therapy to achieve and maintain complete esophageal mucosal healing has any advantageous influence on the overall long-term prognosis of the patient. It is quite possible that nonrigorous therapy that relieves reflux symptoms but does not achieve complete mucosal healing may well be an acceptable therapeutic approach. The long-term outcome of nonrigorous therapy needs further study. Finally, the unanswered questions remain: is it really necessary to achieve and maintain complete esophageal mucosal healing? Should maintaining a completely healed esophageal mucosa be the ultimate goal of treatment?

References

1. Dent J, Dodds WJ, Friedman RH, Sekiguchi T, Hogan WJ, Arndorfer RC, Petrie DJ. Mechanism of gastroesophageal reflux in recumbent asymptomatic human subjects. J Clin Invest 1980;65:256−267.
2. Dodds WJ, Dent J, Hogan WJ, Helm JF, Hauser R, Patel GK, Egide MS. Mechanisms of gastroesophageal reflux in patients with reflux esophagitis. N Engl J Med 1982;307:1547−1552.
3. Johnson LF, DeMeester TR. Twenty-four-hour pH monitoring of the distal esophagus: A quantitative measure of gastroesophageal reflux. Am J Gastroenterol 1974;62:325−352.
4. Stanciu C, Bennett JR. Oesophageal acid clearing: One factor in the production of reflux oesophagitis. Gut 1974;15:852−857.
5. Orr WC, Robinson MG, Johnson LF. Acid clearance during sleep in the pathogenesis of reflux esophagitis. Dig Dis Sci 1981;26:423−427.
6. DeMeester TR, Wernly JA, Bryant GH, Little AG, Skinner DB. Clinical and in vitro analysis of determinants of gastroesophageal competence. A study of the principles of antireflux surgery. Am J Surg 1979;137:39−45.
7. Holloway RH, Hongo M, Berger K, McCallum RW. Gastric distention: A mechanism for postprandial gastroesophageal reflux. Gastroenterology 1985;89:779−784.
8. McCallum RW, Berkowitz DM, Lerner E. Gastric emptying in patients with gastroesophageal reflux. Gastroenterology 1981;80:285−291.
9. Kramer P. Does a sliding hiatus hernia constitute a distinct clinical entity? Gastroenterology 1969;57:442−448.
10. Joelsson B, Johnsson F. Heartburn: the acid test. Gut 1989;30:1523−1525.
11. Collen MJ, Gallagher JE. Basal acid output and gastric acid hypersecretion in patients with gastroesophageal reflux disease. Gastroenterology 1990;98:A32.
12. Robertson D, Aldersley M, Shepherd H, Smith CL. Patterns of acid reflux in complicated oesophagitis. Gut 1987;28:1484−1488.
13. Bell NJ, Burget D, Howden CW, Wilkinson J, Hunt RH. Appropriate acid suppression for the management of gastroesophageal reflux disease. Digestion 1992;51(suppl 1):59−67.
14. Bell NJ, Hunt RH. Role of gastric acid suppression in the treatment of gastro-oesophageal reflux disease. Gut 1992;33:118−124.
15. Klinkenberg-Knol EC, Jansen JB, Lamers CB et al. Use of omeprazole in the management of reflux oesophagitis resistant to H₂-receptor antagonists. Scand J Gastroenterol 1989;166:88−93.
16. Fiasse R, Druez P, Coppens JP et al. Omeprazole in the treatment of patients with severe reflux oesophagitis not responding to H₂-receptor antagonists and ineligible for surgery. Acta Gastroenterol Belg 1990;53:573−584.
17. Dent J, MacKinnon M, Reed W, Narielvala F, Hetzel D. Omeprazole prevents relapse of peptic ocsophagitis. International World Congresses of Gastroenterology, Sydney, Australia, 26−31 August 1990;FP4.
18. Sontag S, Robinson M, Roufail W et al. Daily omeprazole is needed to maintain healing in erosive esophagitis: A US, multicenter double-blind study. Am J Gastroenterol 1992;87:A1258.
19. Lundell L, Backman L, Ekström P et al. Prevention of relapse of reflux esophagitis after endoscopic healing: the efficacy and safety of omeprazole compared with ranitidine. Scand J Gastroenterol 1991;26:248−256.
20. Hetzel DJ, Dent J, Reed WD et al. Healing and relapse of severe peptic esophagitis after treatment with omeprazole. Gastroenterology 1988;95:903−912.
21. Sandmark S, Carlsson R, Fausa O et al. Omeprazole or ranitidine in the treatment of reflux esophagitis. Results of a double-blind, randomized, Scandinavian multicenter study. Scand J Gastroenterol 1988;23:625−632.
22. Zeitoun P, Barbier P, Cayphas JP, Isal JP, Carlsson R. Comparison of two dosage regimens of omeprazole − 10 mg once daily and 20 mg weekends − as prophylaxis against recurrence of reflux esophagitis. Hepato-Gastroenterol 1989;36:279−280.

23. Bardhan KD, Morris P, Thompson M et al. Omeprazole in the treatment of erosive oesophagitis refractory to high dose cimetidine and ranitidine. Gut 1990;31:745–749.

24. Bianchi-Porro G, Pace F, Sangaletti O et al. High-dose famotidine in the maintenance treatment of refractory esophagitis: results of a "medium-term" open study. Am J Gastroenterol 1991;86:1585–1587.

What are the pharmacological and morphological consequences of inhibition of acid secretion?

P. Ruszniewski, M. Mignon (Paris)

The availability of potent gastric antisecretory drugs — the proton pump inhibitors (PPIs) — has modified the medical management of reflux esophagitis, for short-term as well as long-term treatment. In the latter situation, the prescription of PPIs for very long periods of time raises the concern about the safety of these drugs (omeprazole, lansoprazole).

Prolonged inhibition of gastric acid secretion is indeed responsible for two kinds of pathophysiological changes. Firstly, it accounts for an antral release of gastrin ("negative feedback mechanism") and hence, for an hypergastrinemia whose consequences must be evaluated. Secondly, achlorhydria (or hypochlorhydria) is responsible for modifications of the gastric ecosystem and a risk of bacterial overgrowth.

The hypergastrinemia and its consequences

Serum gastrin levels

Serum gastrin levels observed during prolonged treatment with omeprazole (20–40 mg/day) are most often moderately elevated, between the upper limit of the normal value and twice this limit (Table 1 [1–7]). However, these are mean or median values and much higher gastrin levels may be encountered in some patients [1,4]. Such elevated serum gastrin levels are usually far below those seen in other clinical conditions presenting with hypergastrinemia, such as chronic atrophic gastritis [8] and Zollinger-Ellison syndrome [9]. Finally, both the number of patients submitted to long-term treatment (about 500 in the literature) and the duration of such treatment (maximum 5–6 years) are still too limited to allow firm conclusions. However, in a recent study from Lamberts et al. [7], 23% of the 74 patients presented a so-called

Table 1. Variations of serum gastrin levels during long-term treatment with omeprazole (daily dosage ≥ 20 mg; duration of treatment ≥ 12 months). N = upper limit normal value. Treatment indication was esophagitis or peptic ulcer

Author	Study characteristics					Serum gastrin levels					Maximal value
	OMZ dosage (mg/day)	N pts included	Median follow up (months)	Maximum follow-up (months)	N pts with max follow-up	Median values					
						3 months	6 months	12 months	24 months		
Jansen 1990 [1]	20–40	31	18	30	3	3.3 N	3.6 N	3.7 N	4.7 N	32 N (24 months)
Brunner 1990 [2]	40	133	19	56	12	2.8 N	2.4 N	2.6 N	2.6 N	unknown
Koop 1991 [3]	20	31	24	42	1	-	N	N	N	11.5 N (12 months)
Haccoun 1991 [4]	20–60	23	24	57	1	-	1.1 N	1.6 N	1.2 N	7.4 N (12 months)
Lind 1991 [5]	20	10	12	12	10	6 N[a]	-	6 N[a]	-	16 N (12 months)
Hendell 1992 [6]	20–80	25	40	63	1	-	N	N	N	6 N (24 months)
Lamberts 1993 [7]	40	74	48	84	3	2.8 N	2.3 N	2.5 N	2.9 N	30 N (6 months)

[a]Integrated 24-h gastrin levels.

453

"severe hypergastrinemia" (≥ 430 pg/ml, N < 60); those patients also presented the highest gastrin values before the long-term treatment with omeprazole (but under acute treatment with H_2-receptor antagonists). Therefore, a correlation exists between pretreatment values and those observed during long-term treatment, helping in defining "high-risk patients".

Consequences of hypergastrinemia on the proliferation of fundic enterochromaffin like (ECL) cells

The trophic effect of gastrin on ECL fundic cells is well established [10,11]. Experimentally, the administration of high doses of omeprazole induces a moderate hyperplasia of ECL cells, according to the international classification of endocrine growths (Table 2 [12]), in several animal species. However, the occurrence of carcinoid tumors has been described in rats (mainly females) receiving very high doses of omeprazole (400 mg/day) during most of their life span [13]. A highly significant correlation between serum gastrin levels and ECL cell density was demonstrated [14]. A peculiar genetic susceptibility of the rat species has been suggested, since identical tumors have been described in aging rats untreated with antisecretory drugs [15].

In man, the evolution of fundic argyrophil cells during long-term treatment with omeprazole has been studied by several groups [4,7,16–17]. Qualitative abnormalities (i.e., an increase in cell density as compared with controls) have been reported (Table 3). Qualitatively (Table 2), hyperplasia has been described in 28–70% of the cases (Table 3). Hyperplasia was of the diffuse type in the majority of the cases; however, the pathological significance of such mild hyperplasia has been questioned [18]. Linear or micronodular hyperplasia has been noted by Solcia et al. in 4.1 and 14.4% of the cases, respectively [17] but these figures were 12.5 and 16.7% in a recent study by Lamberts et al. [7]. No case of carcinoid tumor has ever been reported in a patient submitted to long-term treatment with PPIs. The development of carcinoid

Table 2. International classification of endocrine growths [12]

A. Hyperplasia
    1.   Simple, diffuse
    2.   Linear, chain forming   } ONCOLOGICAL POTENTIAL
    3.   Micronodular   VIRTUALLY ABSENT
    4.   Adenomatoid
B. Dysplasia (< 0.5 mm in size)
    1.   Enlarged micronodules (>150 µm)
    2.   Fused micronodules   } ONCOLOGICAL
    3.   Microinvasive lesions   POTENTIAL
    4.   Nodules with newly formed stroma)
C. Neoplasia
    1.   Intramucosal carcinoids
    2.   Submucosal carcinoids
    3.   Invasive carcinoids
    4.   Metastatic carcinoids

Table 3. Variations of fundic argyrophil cells during long-term treatment with omeprazole (for studies characteristics, see Table 1)

	Quantitative data	Qualitative data	
	ECL cell density	Hyperplasia	Dysplasia
Brunner 1990 [2]	Doubled in 4 years	40%	0%
Lundell 1990 [16]	–	"no significant modification"	"no significant modification"
Haccoun 1991 [4]	Stable; double of controls	73%[a]	0%
Solcia 1992 [17]	–	28%[b]	0%
Lamberts 1993 [7]	Doubled in 5 years	67%[c]	0%

[a]Simple only; [b]Simple: 9.3%, linear: 4.1%, micronodular: 14.4%; [c]Simple: 37.5%, linear: 12.5%, micronodular: 16.7%.

tumors in man could involve, at least in some cases, some genetic factors associated with hypergastrinemia (e.g., carcinoid tumors in Zollinger-Ellison syndrome are observed except in patients with multiple endocrine neoplasia type I (MEN I) [19]. However, the above-mentioned limitations, in the number of patients committed to long-term treatment and in the treatment duration, do not allow one to state that a significant endocrine cell growth cannot occur. Such an event appears improbable according to available data.

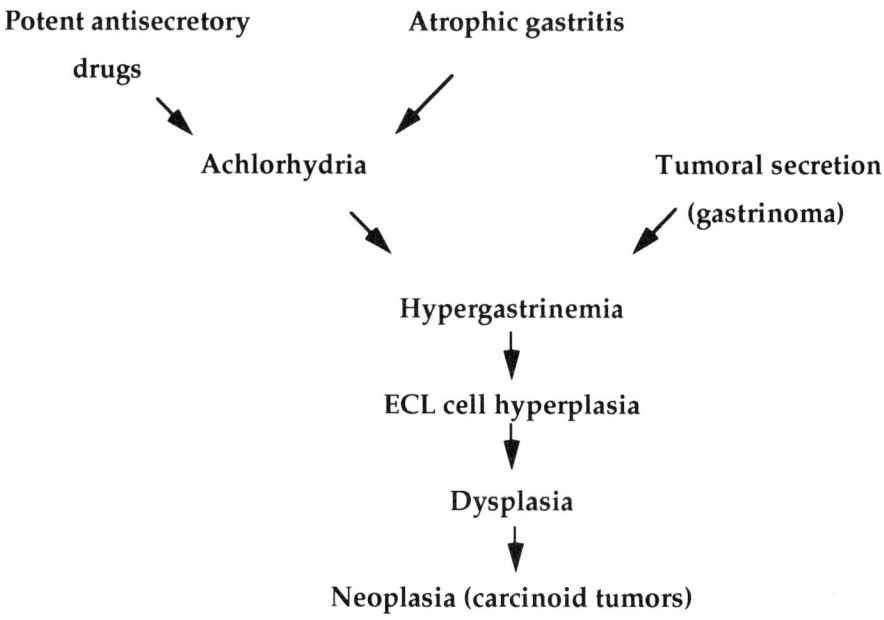

Fig. 1. The gastrin hypothesis.

Should the cause of hypergastrinemia be questioned?

Hypergastrinemia plays a major role in the proliferation of ECL cells: the "gastrin hypothesis" (Fig. 1) accounts for the observed abnormalities. The origin of hypergastrinemia has been challenged, besides drug induced increase in gastrin levels, a more recent approach [7,17,18] underlines the role of the fundic atrophic gastritis (Table 4) that can be observed during the course of "peptic diseases" (duodenal ulcer disease and esophagitis, Fig. 2). However, such an atrophic gastritis is noted in only 9.3% of the patients (Table 4) and its prevalence in a control population is unknown. The respective contribution of antisecretory drugs and atrophic gastritis during the course of peptic diseases should be further studied in order to explain the origin of elevated gastrin levels observed in some patients.

Inhibition of gastric acid and intragastric bacterial proliferation

The stomach is a relatively sterile milieu, nevertheless, gastric bacteria can be found immediately after a meal (Streptococci, Enterobacteria and Bifidobacteria, with total concentrations ranging from 10^2 to 10^5/ml). Gastric acid secretion plays a major bactericidal role and its reduction (in atrophic gastritis or after surgical gastric resection) leads to bacterial overgrowth (10^5–10^7 bacteria/ml; mainly Enterobacteria, Streptococci, Bacteroides). Sustained treatment with antisecretory drugs accounts for the same change: increase in the number of gastric bacteria during treatment with H_2-receptor antagonists [20] or omeprazole [21].

Is such bacterial overgrowth capable of inducing gastric carcinogenesis? Some bacterial species are able to reduce dietary nitrates into nitrites, which can themselves induce the synthesis of N-nitroso compounds whose mutagenic and carcinogenetic properties have been largely demonstrated in numerous animal species [22]. N-nitrosation of nitrites is, however, pH dependent in an inverse fashion of bacterial overgrowth: at high pH values, the latter phenomenon is important but the synthesis

Table 4. Correlation between fundic argyrophil cell hyperplasia and fundic gastritis in 42 patients treated by omeprazole (40 mg/day) during 4 years for upper GI ulcerations (adapted from [7])

	Gastritis (%)					
	None	Mild superficial	Moderate	Interstitial	Atrophic	Total
Argyrophil cell hyperplasia (%)						
None	11.6	18.6	7.0	9.3	–	46.5
Diffuse	9.3	9.3	2.3	–	2.3	23.2
Linear	–	4.7	4.7	2.3	–	11.7
Micronodular	–	2.3	–	**7.0**	**7.0**	**16.3**
Adenomatoid	–	–	–	2.3	–	**2.3**
Total	20.9	34.9	14.0	20.9	**9.3**	

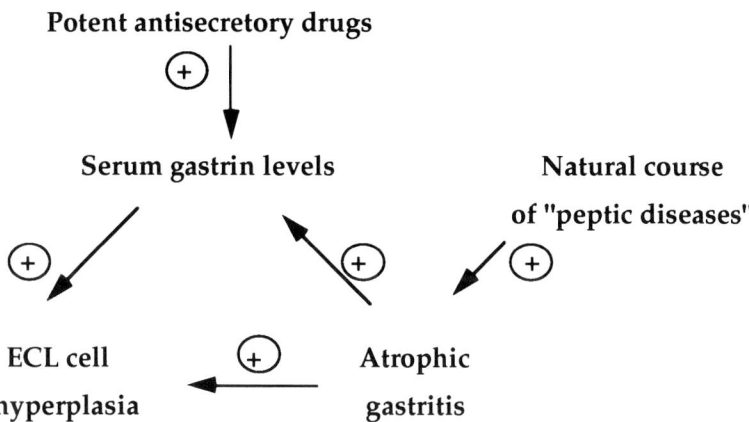

Fig. 2. Relationships between gastrin levels, gastritis, and ECL cells during sustained potent antisecretory treatment.

of N-nitroso compounds is inhibited [22,23]. Moreover, the accuracy of the determination of intragastric N-nitroso compounds is a matter of debate, since numerous shortcomings have been described in their dosage [23].

In summary, the relation between hypochlorhydria, gastric bacterial overgrowth, increase in nitrite concentration and gastric carcinogenesis seems to be well established, and a role for N-nitroso compounds cannot be ruled out. The controversy still exists and the long-term effect of prolonged gastric acid inhibition is not yet fully elucidated.

References

1. Jansen JBMJ, Klinkenberg-Knol EC, Meuwissen SGM, De Bruijne JW, Festen HPM, Snel P et al. Effect of long-term treatment with omeprazole on serum gastrin and serum group A and C pepsinogens in patients with reflux esophagitis. Gastroenterology 1990;99:621–628.
2. Brunner GHG, Lamberts R, Creutzfeldt W. Efficacy and safety of omeprazole in the long-term treatment of peptic ulcer and reflux oesophagitis resistant to ranitidine. Digestion 1990;47(suppl 1):64–68.
3. Koop H, Arnold R. Long-term maintenance treatment of reflux esophagitis with omeprazole. Prospective study in patients with H2-blocker-resistant esophagitis. Dig Dis Sci 1991;5:552–557.
4. Haccoun P, Ruszniewski P, Vissuzaine C, Cadiot G, Combrouze F, Bonfils S, Mignon M. Efficacité et tolérance de l'oméprazole (OMZ) au long cours dans l'oesophagite sévère par reflux (OSR). Gastroenterol Clin Biol 1991;15:A35.
5. Lind T, Cederberg C, Idström JP, Lönroth H, Olbe L, Lundell L. 24-hour intragastric acidity and plasma gastrin during long-term treatment with omeprazole or ranitidine in patients with reflux esophagitis. Scand J Gastroenterol 1991;26:620–626.
6. Hendel L, Hage E, Hendel J, Stentoft P. Omeprazole in the long-term treatment of severe gastro-oesophageal reflux disease in patients with systemic sclerosis. Aliment Pharmacol Ther 1992;6:565–577.
7. Lamberts R, Creutzfeldt W, Strüber HG, Brunner G, Solcia E. Long-term omeprazole therapy in peptic ulcer disease: gastrin, endocrine cell growth, and gastritis. Gastroenterology 1993;104:1356–1370.
8. Cattan D, Roucayrol AM, Launay JM et al. Circulating gastrin, endocrine cells, histamine content and histidine-decarboxylase activity in atrophic gastritis. Gastroenterology 1989;97:586–596.
9. Lehy T, Mignon M, Cadiot G et al. Gastric endocrine cell behavior in Zollinger Ellison patients upon long-term potent antisecretory treatment. Gastroenterology 1989;96:1029–1040.
10. Solcia E, Capella C, Vassallo G. Endocrine cells of the stomach and pancreas in states of gastric hypersecretion. Rendiconti Romani di Gastroenteologia 1970;2:147–158.
11. Larsson H, Carlsson E, Mattsson H et al. Plasma gastrin and gastrin enterochromaffin-like cell activation and proliferation.

Studies with omeprazole and ranitidine in intact and antrectomized rats. Gastroenterology 1986;90:391–399.

12. Solcia E, Bordi C, Creutzfeldt W et al. Histopathological classification of nonantral gastric endocrine growths in man. Digestion 1988;41:185–200.

13. Carlsson E, Havu N, Mattsson H, Ekman L, Riberg B. Gastric carcinoids in rats treated with inhibitors of gastric acid secretion. In: Hakanson R, Sundler F (eds) The Stomach as an Endocrine Organ. Amsterdam: Elsevier, 1991;461–471.

14. Larsson H. Carlsson E, Hakanson R et al. Time-course of development and reversal of gastric endocrine cell hyperplasia after inhibition of acid secretion. Gastroenterology 1988;95:1477–1486.

15. Lee AJ, De Lellis RA, Blount M, Nunnemacher G, Wolfe HJ. Pituitary proliferative lesions in aging male long-evans rats. A model of mixed multiple endocrine neoplasia syndrome. Lab Invest 1982;47:595–602.

16. Lundell L. Prevention of relapse of reflux oesophagitis after endoscopic healing: the efficacy and safety of omeprazole compared with ranitidine. Digestion 1990;17(suppl 1):72–75.

17. Solcia E, Fiocca R, Havu N, Dalväg A, Carlsson R. Gastric endocrine cells and gastritis in patients receiving long-term omeprazole treatment. Digestion 1992;51(suppl 1):82–92.

18. Solcia E, Rindi G, Silini E. Villani L. Enterochromaffin-like (ECL) cells and their growths: relationships to gastrin, reduced acid secretion and gastritis. In: Yeomans ND (ed) Baillière's Clinical Gastroenterology. London: Baillière Tindall, 1993; 149–165.

19. Lehy T, Cadiot G, Mignon M, Ruszniewski P, Bonfils S. Influence of multiple endocrine neoplasia type 1 on gastric endocrine cells in patients with the Zollinger-Ellison syndrome. Gut 1992;33:1275–1279.

20. Ruddell WSJ, Axon ATR, Findlay JM, Bartholomew BA, Hill MJ. The effect of cimetidine on the gastric bacterial microflora. Lancet 1980;i: 672–674.

21. Sharma BK, Santana IA, Wood EC et al. Intragastric bacterial activity and nitrosation before, during and after treatment with omeprazole. Br Med J 1984;289:717–719.

22. Martin F, Martin MS, Lorcerie B. Do antisecretory drugs cause gastric cancer? In: Mignon M, Galmiche JP (eds) Safe and effective control of acid secretion. Paris: John Libbey Eurotext, 1988;115–122.

23. Heatley RV, Sobala GM. Acid suppression and the gastric flora. In: Yeomans ND (ed) Baillière's Clinical Gastroenterology. London: Baillière Tindall, 1993;167–181.

Should gastrin levels be measured during long-term treatment with PPIs?

E.D. Dorval (Tours)

As the Marketing Authorization stipulates no legal requirement to monitor blood gastrin levels, the decision of whether or not to assay gastrin in patients given long-term treatment with PPIs depends on the answers to the following questions:
– Is there a change in blood gastrin levels and if so why?
– Does this change present any risk?
– What are the consequences of this?
– What should be done in practice?

Why?

There is usually an increase in blood gastrin levels during treatment with PPIs. This increase is due to a breakdown in gastrin feedback. This breakdown is only partial because:

458

- In the vast majority of cases the blood gastrin level is not greatly increased (twice the pretherapeutic value and thus very often less than the upper "normal" limit).
- The blood gastrin level remains stable with time (after 1 to 2 months of treatment).
- It remains able to be stimulated by the effects of a meal.
- It returns to its initial value once treatment has been stopped.

The moderate increase in blood gastrin observed during PPI therapy can therefore be seen as the reflection of the PPIs antisecretory capacity and of good patient compliance rather than as undesirable side effects.

In some patients, however, (about 3%), higher levels of gastrin have been observed, sometimes comparable to those found in patients with Biermer's disease or with a Zollinger-Ellison syndrome (ZES). When interpreting these levels it is important to know whether the hypergastrinemia was actually present before the start of treatment with the PPI and if the correct conditions for sampling had been respected: patient fasting, absence of any factors liable to cause gastrin stimulation, correct treatment of the sample and normal laboratory values and method used.

Risks?

Five to 10 year follow-up studies carried out with patients exhibiting marked hypergastrinemia (because of PPI treatment, Biermer's disease or ZES) have shown that there is no risk associated with this prolonged hypergastrinemia, which is in sharp contrast with the results obtained in the laboratory animal. In addition, it is recognized that in man, hyperplasia of enterochromaffin-like cells and of carcinoid tumor cells which may be derived from them, correlates with the severity of the lesions of chronic gastritis and/or associated genetic factors rather than with the degree of hypergastrinemia itself.

In the absence of follow-up data beyond 10 years, it cannot be stated that continuous treatment for more than 10 years is totally free from risk, but if this risk does exist it is probably very small.

As for the extragastric effects of gastrin on tumor induction or growth, these have not been established in man. The increased levels of gastrin observed in subjects with colorectal cancer, rather than being responsible for the tumors, may be due to the secretion of gastrin by the tumors themselves.

Assay of blood gastrin may therefore merely have the effect of identifying patients with major hypergastrinemia in order to evaluate, in these subjects, a potential risk whose nature is not known and which will not become apparent until more than 10 years of follow-up.

Consequences?

The consequences of discovery of major hypergastrinemia during PPI therapy are related to the risk associated with this condition: if there is no risk, there are no consequences and the assay is of no value. If, on the contrary, there is a risk, it must be possible to propose appropriate measures: stop the treatment and replace it with an alternative. If an alternative exists (e.g., antireflux surgery for high grade ulcerated esophagitis) or continue the treatment, on condition that preventive or curative treatment for the risk exists and can be given.

In practice?

Assay of blood gastrin is of no value for short- or medium-term treatment. For long-term treatment (to be given for many years or even for life) the assay is not essential as a routine measure, but will identify those patients (about 3%) with major hypergastrinemia. At present the only thing that can be done when faced with marked hypergastrinemia of this type is to recommend follow-up in order to evaluate the risk. Subsequently, if the long-term follow-up of a large number of patients demonstrates that there really is a risk, surveillance should be directed towards the prevention or correction of this risk.

In practice, a determination of blood gastrin may be considered after a few months of treatment with PPI if this will have to be continued for a very long time. Although there is no set limit, it is probably advisable to follow up the patient if the blood gastrin level is above 400 pg/ml.

References

1. Dent J, Yeomans ND. Acid-related diseases: improving the treatment options. Digestion 1992;(suppl 1)51.
2. MacTavish D, Buckley MT, Heel RC. Omeprazole: an updated review of its pharmacology and therapeutic use in acid-related disorder. Drugs 1991;42:138–170.

Do PPI effects on the cytochrome P_{450} system have implications to significant drug interactions?

A. David Rodrigues (Abbott Park, Illinois), *J.W. Freston* (Farmington, Connecticut)

Various derivatives of imidazole and benzimidazole have been known for years to bind reversibly with varying affinities to the heme of cytochrome P_{450}. This interaction often leads to inhibition and/or induction of cytochrome P_{450}-dependent mono-oxygenase activities. Induction results from the net increase in the levels of the various forms of the enzyme, due to de novo protein synthesis and/or protein stabilization. This may have important pharmacological and toxicological consequences, since the various forms (isoenzymes) of cytochrome P_{450} are the primary locus of metabolism of a large number of exogenous (xenobiotic) and endogenous compounds. There are a number of well documented examples of imidazole-containing drugs that function as inducers and/or inhibitors of cytochrome P_{450}, including clotrimazole, ketoconazole, cimetidine and omeprazole [1–3]. Like omeprazole, lansoprazole is a benzimidazole (H^+, K^+)-ATPase inhibitor. The following is an analysis of the two compounds, with respect to their interactions with cytochrome P_{450}.

Induction

The induction of human cytochrome(s) P_{450} by omeprazole and lansoprazole has been studied in vitro, using primary cultures of hepatocytes or hepatoma (e.g., HepG2) cells [4–7]. Induction by omeprazole (20–60 mg/day/7 days, p.o.) has also been studied in vivo [4,8,9]. The studies indicate that omeprazole and lansoprazole are inducers of the human cytochrome P_{450} (CYP) belonging to the CYP1 gene subfamily (i.e., CYP1A1 and CYP1A2), although the in vivo induction of human CYP1A proteins by lansoprazole remains to be documented.

The concerns associated with induction stem from the fact that CYP1A enzymes are responsible for the "bioactivation" of some aryl hydrocarbons to carcinogens. These compounds are normally found in cigarette smoke, charbroiled food and industrial solvents. In addition, the hepatotoxicity associated with drugs such as acetaminophen and phenacetin has also been linked to their metabolism by CYP1A proteins [4,10].

It has been postulated that inducers of human CYP1A enzymes might theoretically predispose individuals to bioactivate procarcinogens, possibly resulting in malignancies many years after starting therapy, or increase the likelihood of hepatotoxicity with drugs such as phenacetin or acetaminophen [4,10]. However, the significance of such induction remains unclear and controversial. A number of authors have refuted these claims and have suggested that the results obtained are not relevant to the in vivo situation [11,12]. In fact, induction of CYP1A proteins in rodents may actually be protective against some induced malignancies [11,12]. In addition, elevations in the levels of CYP1A proteins, as a result of cigarette smoking or consumption of charbroiled food, has not been shown to potentiate the toxic effects of agents such as phenacetin [11,12]. Finally, there is no evidence that the induction by drugs of other forms of CYP that activate procarcinogens leads to neoplasia. CYP2E1 and CYP3A4 also activate procarcinogens and are induced by widely used agents such as alcohol (CYP2E1), rifampicin, antiseizure medication and glucocorticoids (CYP3A4) [11,12]. Some of these agents, such as the antiseizure medications phenytoin, carbamazepine, and phenobarbital, have been used therapeutically for over 30 years and have demonstrated an acceptable safety profile. This is relevant to omeprazole and lansoprazole which also induce CYP3A4 in cultured human hepatocytes, and thus behave as "mixed" cytochrome P_{450} (CYP1A and CYP3A) inducers [5].

Inhibition

The inhibition of cytochrome P_{450} by omeprazole and lansoprazole has been studied in vitro through clinical drug interaction studies [3,8,13,16] (Table 1), and the use of subcellular fractions (microsomes) prepared from the livers of organ donor subjects. Since both drugs are metabolized by cytochrome P_{450}, they may serve as cosubstrates of the enzyme(s) and thereby inhibit the metabolism of other (coadministered) drugs.

The effect of omeprazole on the pharmacokinetics of a large number of drugs has been studied in vivo, many of which are metabolized by one or more forms of cytochrome P_{450} (Table 1), To date, the only significant interactions with omeprazole have been observed with diazepam and phenytoin. Both of these compounds have been shown to be metabolized by members of the CYP2C subfamily of proteins (S-mephenytoin-4'-hydroxylase or CYP2Cmp and CYP2C9, respectively [3,13,15]. There is no omeprazole interaction resulting in pharmacokinetically significant inhibition of a number of drugs metabolized by CYP3A4 (e.g., cyclosporine, nifedipine, lidocaine and quinidine), CYP2D6 (metoprolol and propanolol) or CYP1A (theophylline and caffeine) [3,14]. Similar studies with lansoprazole have failed to

Table 1. The effect of omeprazole and lansoprazole on the metabolism of compounds with known cytochrome P_{450} pathways

Compound	P_{450} pathway	Omperazole	Lansoprazole
Antipyrine	Not known	None	None
Theophylline	1A2, 2E1,3A4 and others currently undefined	None	Induce[a]
Diazepam	3A and 2C	Inhibit	None
Phenytoin[b]	Possibly 2C9	Inhibit	None
Caffeine	1A2 and others	Induce	Unknown
R-Warfarin	1A2 and 3A4	Inhibit[c]	None
S-Warfarin	2C9	None	None
Indomethacin	2C9	Not known	None
Ibuprofen	2C9	Not known	None
Prednisone	3A	None	None
Triphasil (levonorgestrel and ethinyl estradiol)	3A4	None	None[d]

[a]Increase in theophylline clearance of 10%; decrease in AUC of 13%; both not clinically significant.
[b]Effects on phenytoin may be dose-dependent [17].
[c]A minor but statistically significant increase in concentration of R-warfarin has been reported.
[d]2/20 subjects on triphasil and lansoprazole ovulated in one study (not statistically significant), while no ovulation occurred in any of the nine subjects (including the two who ovulated in the first study) in a subsequent trail. None of the 30 subjects ovulated in the third study.

detect a significant interaction with prednisone (CYP3A4), phenytoin (CYP2C9), diazepam (CYP3A4/CYP2Cmp), warfarin (CYP1A2/CYP3A4/CYP2C9), indomethacin, ibuprofen (CYP2C9) theophylline (CYP1A2) [16]. (Michael D. Karol, personal communications). Additional studies have shown that lansoprazole does not appreciably inhibit the CYP3A4-dependent metabolism of terfenadine in human liver microsomes (unpublished data).

Recent studies with human liver microsomes and cultured hepatocytes have shown both omeprazole and lansoprazole to be primarily metabolized by CYP3A4, although the involvement of polymorphically expressed CYP2Cmp (S-mephenytoin-4'-hydroxylase) in the oxidative metabolism of omeprazole has also been shown [18—20]. Furthermore, both drugs are believed not to be metabolized by CYP1A proteins. The fact that the two drugs are metabolized by CYP3A4 and do not significantly alter the pharmacokinetics and/or metabolism of a number of CYP3A4 substrates, may indicate that their affinity for the enzyme and/or liver concentration is somewhat lower than agents such as nifedipine, diazepam, prednisone, cyclosporine and terfenadine. However, the affinity of omeprazole for CYP2C proteins is sufficient to inhibit the metabolism of diazepam (CYP2Cmp component) and phenytoin in vivo [3,13,15]. Whether or not lansoprazole is metabolized by CYP2Cmp or CYP2C9 remains to be determined. However, the lack of an effect of lansoprazole on the pharmacokinetics of phenytoin, indomethacin, ibuprofen and diazepam in vivo may indicate that a significant interaction with CYP2C proteins is unlikely and that the drug may not exhibit bimodal ("fast metabolizer" vs. "slow metabolizer") pharmacokinetics (c.f., omeprazole) [16]. Consistent with this conclusion is the finding that omeprazole hydroxylation is strongly correlated with S-mephenytoin-4'-hydroxylase (CYP2Cmp) activity in a panel of human liver microsomes, but only weakly correlated with lansoprazole [19,20].

Conclusions

Omeprazole and lansoprazole interact with cytochrome P_{450}. Both drugs are "mixed" (CYP1A and CYP3A) inducers, but the significance of such induction remains unclear and controversial, and it appears that the concerns associated with this effect are unfounded. Both drugs undergo cytochrome P_{450} dependent oxidative metabolism, which is largely mediated by liver microsomal cytochrome P_{450} (CYP3A4), although CYP2Cmp (S-mephenytoin-4'-hydroxylase) is also thought to be involved in the metabolism of omeprazole. Since both drugs fail to inhibit the in vivo and in vitro metabolism of CYP3A4 cosubstrates, it appears that their affinity for the enzyme is relatively low. This is a clinically relevant finding, when one considers that some CYP3A4 substrates, such as terfenadine and cyclosporine, have a relatively narrow therapeutic index. To date, the inhibition of diazepam (CYP2Cmp/CYP3A4-dependent) clearance by omeprazole is the only pharmacokinetically significant interaction described for this class of compounds. The fact that no similar interaction has been observed with lansoprazole, may indicate that the two drugs differentially interact with the CYP2C forms of cytochrome P_{450}.

References

1. Murray M. Mechanisms of the inhibition of cytochrome P_{450}-mediated drug oxidation by therapeutic agents. Drug Metab Revs 1987;18:55–81.
2. Maurice M, Pichard L, Daujat M, Fabre I, Joyeux H, Domergue J, Maurel P. Effects of imidazole derivatives on cytochrome P_{450} from human hepatocytes in primary culture. FASEB J 1992;6:752–758.
3. Anderson T. Omeprazole drug interaction studies. Clin Pharmaco 1991;21:195–212.
4. Diaz D, Fabre I, Daujat M, Aubert BS, Bories P, Michel H, Maurel P. Omeprazole is an aryl hydrocarbon-like inducer of human hepatic cytochrome P_{450}. Gastroenterology 1990;99:737–747.
5. Curi-Pedrosa R, Daujat M, Pichard L, Ourlin JC, Clari P, Gervot L, Lesca P, Domergue J, Joyeux H, Fourtanier G, Maurel P. Gastric pump inhibitors omeprazole and lansoprazole are mixed inducers of CYT1A and CYP3A in human hepatocytes in primary culture. Mol Pharmacol (in press).
6. Quattrochi LC, Tukey RH. Nuclear uptake of the *Ah* (dioxin) receptor in response to omeprazole: transcriptional activation of the human CYP1A1 gene. Mol Pharmacol 1993:504–508.
7. Daujat M, Peryt B, Lesca P, Fourtanier G, Domergue J, Maurel P. Omeprazole, an inducer of human CYP1A1 and 1A2, is not a ligand for the *Ah* receptor. Biochem Biophys Res Commun 1992;188:820–825.
8. Rost KL, Brosicke H, Brockmoller J, Scheffler M, Helge H, Roots I. Increase of cytochrome P_{450}1A2 activity by omeprazole: evidence by the ^{13}C-[N-3-methyl]-caffeine breath test in poor and extensive metabolizers of S-mephenytoin. Clin Pharmacol Ther 1992;52:170–180.
9. McDonnell WM, Schieman JM, Traber PG. Induction of cytochrome P_{450} genes (CYP1A) by omeprazole in the human alimentary tract. Gastroenterology 1992;103:1509–1516.
10. Farrell GC, Murray M. Human cytochrome P_{450} forms. Gastroenterology 1990;99:885–889.
11. Kolars JC, Turgeon DK, Watkins PB. Omeprazole and aryl hydrocarbon hydroxylases: should we be worried? Hepatology 1991;13:197–199.
12. Parkinson A, Hurwitz A. Omeprazole and the induction of human cytochrome P_{450}: a response to concerns about potential adverse effects. Gastroenterology 1991;100:1157–1164.
13. Massoomi F, Savage J, Destache CJ. Omeprazole: a comprehensive review. Pharmacotherapy 1993;13:46–59.
14. Soons PA, van den Berg G, Danhof M, van Brummelen P, Jansen JBMJ, Lamers CBHW, Breimer DD. Influence of single and multiple dose omeprazole treatment on nifedipine pharmacokinetics and effects in healthy subjects. Eur J Clin Pharmacol 1992;42:319–324.
15. Anderson T, Cederberg C, Edvardsson G, Heggelund A, Lundborg P. Effect of omeprazole treatment on diazepain plasma levels in slow versus normal rapid metabolizers of omeprazole. Clin Pharmacol Ther 1990;47:79–85.
16. Lefebvre RA, Flouvat B, Karolac-Tamisier S, Moerman E, van Ganse E. Influence of lansoprazole treatment on diazepam plasma concentrations. Clin Pharmacol Ther 1992;52:458–463.
17. Bachmann K, Sullivan T, Jauregui L, Reese J, Miller K, Lenne L. Br J Clin Pharmacol 1993;36:380–382.
18. Yun CH, Okerholm RA, Guengerich FP. Oxidation of the antihistaminic drug terfenadine in human liver microsomes. Drug Metab Dispos 1993;21:403–407.
19. Chiba K, Kobayashi K, Manabe K, Tani M, Kamataki T, Ishizake T. Oxidative metabolism of omeprazole in human liver microsomes: cosegregation with *S*-mephenytoin 4′-hydroxylation. J Pharmacol Exp Ther 1993;266:52–59.
20. Curi-Pedrosa R, Pichard L, Boufils C, Jacqz-Aigrain E, Maurel P. Major implication of cytochrome P_{450}3A4 in the oxidative metabolism of the antisecretory drugs omeprazole and lansoprazole in human liver microsomes and hepatocytes. Br J Clin Pharmacol 1993;36:156P.

What is the short-term effect of the PPIs compared to other types of treatments in reflux esophagitis?

E.C. Klinkenberg-Knol (Amsterdam)

The aims of medical therapy of gastroesophageal reflux disease (GERD) are to relieve the symptoms, to heal esophageal mucosal damage and to prevent the development of complications [1]. Hence, treatment needs to either prevent the reflux of acidic gastric contents into the esophagus, or to eliminate or reduce the injurious action of acid to a level that will allow healing of the esophageal epithelium.

Motility modulating agents. These may improve GERD by increasing lower esophageal sphincter (LES) pressure, enhancing esophageal peristaltic contractions, and augmenting gastric emptying [2,3]. From a pathophysiological view of gastroesophageal reflux (GER), prokinetic agents are clearly the most logical concept of treating a disorder that is primarily due to disturbed motility.

The prokinetic agents bethanechol, metoclopramide, domperidone and cisapride have all been used for reflux esophagitis, with varying success. Of all the prokinetic drugs cisapride seems to be the most promising. It is significantly better than placebo [4–7] and it compares favorably with ranitidine [8] and cimetidine [9] in patients with erosive reflux esophagitis. It is superior in combination with cimetidine compared to single therapy with cimetidine [10]. The effect on esophageal acid exposure, however, is insufficient to produce a consistently high response rate in the severe grades of GERD.

Antacids/alginate. These provide good immediate relief of reflux symptoms, but improvement of reflux esophagitis has not been demonstrated [11].

Mucosal protective agents

Sucralfate. This polysulfated salt of sucrose offers a unique approach to the treatment of reflux disease [12,13]. In addition to coating damaged mucosa, it binds both bile acids and pepsin. Studies are scarce, but the results indicate that sucralfate is superior to placebo [14,15] and alginate [16], and equally effective compared to H_2-receptor antagonists [17,18]. In one pilot study [19] reflux esophagitis refractory to H_2-blockers was effectively treated with sucralfate. However, in two other studies, sucralfate as adjunctive therapy to cimetidine in reflux esophagitis was unable to improve endoscopical healing [20,21].

The alternative mucosal protective agent, *colloidal bismuth subcitrate* (De-Nol®), reduces peptic injury of the esophagus in rabbits [22]. One placebo-controlled study showed significant symptomatic and endoscopic improvement after 3 weeks of treatment [23], and De-Nol® was statistically superior as adjunctive therapy to cimetidine in the treatment of reflux esophagitis [24]. Thus, sucralfate in particular seems promising for symptomatic relief and mucosal healing of mild reflux esophagitis.

H₂-receptor antagonists

Compared with their uniform success in healing duodenal ulcer, the experience in GERD has been disappointing. A number of authors have reviewed the results of 20 short term placebo controlled studies with cimetidine or ranitidine [1,25,26]. The level of acid suppression reported for later developed H_2-RAs such as famotidine, nizatidine, etintidine and roxatidine, are similar to those of cimetidine and ranitidine; therefore, comparable efficacy in the treatment of GERD might be expected. Healing of macroscopic esophagitis was not significantly better than placebo in half of these trials, although endoscopic improvement occurred more frequently. Studies that directly compare ranitidine with cimetidine (and hence avoid many problems of varying patient severity at entry or variable end point) show no important differences [1]. Complete healing of esophagitis was apparent in 27—45% of patients, and these were mainly patients with grade I—II disease [26].

Some authors have suggested that higher doses may be necessary to treat patients with GERD [27]. With cimetidine, in two or four divided doses up to 1.6 g/day, no major differences between the various regimens have been found [28]. With ranitidine only a very high dose schedule of 300 mg 4 times daily could demonstrate a clear advantage for the high treatment dose in patients with erosive or ulcerative esophagitis, with complete endoscopic healing in 75% of the patients [29]. Long-term pH measurement studies have clearly demonstrated that insufficient suppression of gastric acid secretion during H_2RA therapy is associated with unfavorable symptomatic response [27,30—33].

Proton pump blockade

At present there is plentiful evidence to suggest that a near total acid suppression will produce a greater rate of healing in patients with GERD. Omeprazole, the first of this class of gastric antisecretory drugs to reach clinical use, is a potent and long-acting inhibitor of both basal and stimulated gastric acid secretion [34—36]. Acid suppression is produced by blocking $H^+/K^+ATPase$, the proton pump located on the apical surface of parietal cells. Omeprazole, thus, blocks the final common pathway of acid production. With its pronounced reduction in intragastric acidity and long duration of action [37,38] omeprazole should be a valuable drug in the treatment of reflux esophagitis. Indeed, its effectiveness in reducing the damaging effect of pathological acid reflux on the esophageal mucosa has been proven by the finding that the use of omeprazole, in doses ranging from 20—60 mg once daily, is superior to placebo [39], to ranitidine 150—300 mg b.i.d. and to cimetidine 400 mg q.i.d., in the short-term treatment of reflux esophagitis [39–45] (Table 1).

The major advantage of omeprazole over all other antireflux therapies is the specific efficacy in patients with severe refractory reflux disease, nonhealing Barrett's ulcers or peptic strictures [44,46–50].

What is the basis for the advantage of proton pump inhibitors over H₂-receptor antagonists?

H_2-receptor antagonists are relatively ineffective in reflux disease because these agents cannot easily overcome the integrated meal-stimulated acid secretion [51,52]. They are more effective at reducing intragastric acidity when acid secretion is not otherwise stimulated, and this is probably the basis for their moderate efficacy in

Table 1. Treatment of erosive esophagitis with PPIs: endoscopic healing in double-blind controlled trials [56]

Author	Pts	Treatment regimen	Weeks	Endoscopic healing (%)	
				PPI	Comparator
Hetzel 1988 [39]	63	Ome 20/40, placebo	4	81	6
			8	81	9
	164	Ome 20, Ome 40	4	70	82
			8	79	89
Sontag 1992 [57]	230	Ome 20, placebo	4	39	7
			8	73	14
		Ome 40, placebo	4	45	7
			8	75	14
Klinkenberg-Knol 1987 [40]	51	Ome 60, Ran 300	4	76	27
			8	88	38
Sandmark 1988 [43]	144	Ome 20, Ran 300	4	67	31
			8	85	50
Vantrappen 1988 [42]	61	Ome 40, Ran 300	4	85	40
			8	96	52
Havelund 1988 [41]	88	Ome 40, Ran 300	4	70	26
			8	85	44
Zeitoun 1989 [45]	156	Ome 20, Ran 300	4	81	45
			8	95	66
Dchn 1990 [32]	67	Omc 40, Cim 1600	4	57	29
			8	71	23
Bate 1990 [58]	270	Ome 20, Cim 1600	4	56	26
			8	71	35
Italian Study 1991 [59]	172	Ome 20, Ran 300	4	72	54
			8	90	76
Bardhan 1992 [60]	154	Lan 30, Ran 300	4	84	39
			8	92	53
	152	Lan 60, Ran 300	4	72	39
			8	91	53

Ome = omprazole, Lan = lanzoprazole, Ran = ranitidine, Cim = cimetidine.

GERD. In contrast, proton pump inhibitors effectively suppress gastric acid secretion throughout the day, and can overcome meal-stimulated acid production. Thus, optimal treatment for reflux esophagitis can be achieved by abolishing esophageal acid exposure throughout both the day- and night-time periods. The less effective the LES is in preventing reflux of gastric contents into the esophagus, the more necessary it is to raise the pH of the stomach contents to above 4.0 throughout the 24 h. Combined intraesophageal and intragastric 24-h pH-monitoring studies support the view that an incomplete response to omeprazole is primarily due to inadequate suppression of acid secretion in patients treated with up to 60 mg daily [53]. Bell and others [54] have performed a meta-analysis of treatment trials of reflux esophagitis, in which healing was assessed endoscopically. Results show a correlation coefficient of 0.87 ($p < 0.05$) between the healing rate of esophagitis at 8 weeks and the duration, in hours, that the intragastric pH is maintained above 4.0. The response to antisecretory drugs can therefore be predicted by the duration of suppression of intragastric acidity to above pH 4.0, over a 24-h period, achieved by each treatment regimen.

Conclusion

These results establish proton pump inhibitors as a treatment of unprecedented efficacy for the healing of reflux esophagitis.

Experience so far with omeprazole has shown a good tolerance in clinical trials in 25,000 patients, with a side effect profile no different from placebo or H_2-receptor antagonists [55].

References

1. Tytgat GNJ, Nio CY. The medical therapy of reflux oesophagitis. Balliere's Clin Gastroenterol 1987;1:1−17.
2. Ceccatelli P, Janssens J, Vantrappen G et al. Cisapride restores the decreased lower oesophageal sphincter pressure in reflux patients. Gut 1988;29:631−635.
3. Corazziari E, Bontempo I, Anzini F. Effects of cisapride on distal esophageal motility in humans. Dig Dis Sci 1989;34:1600−1605.
4. Hüttemann W. Cisapride in the treatment of oesophagitis. A placebo controlled trial. In: Johnson AG, Lux G (eds) Progress in the Treatment of Gastrointestinal Motility Disorders: The Role of Cisapride. Amsterdam: Excerpta Medica, 1988;56−63.
5. Baldi F, Bianchi-Porro G, Dobrilla G et al. Cisapride versus placebo in reflux esophagitis. A multicenter double-blind trial. J Clin Gastroenterol 1988;10:614−618.
6. Dodds W, Champion M, Orr W et al. Oral cisapride in GERD: a double-blind placebo-controlled multicenter trial. Gastroenterology 1989;96:A126.
7. Lepoutre L, Bollen J, Vandewalle N et al. Therapeutic effects of cisapride in reflux oesophagitis: a double-blind, placebo-controlled study. In: Johnson AG, Lux G (eds) Progress in the Treatment of Gastrointestinal Motility Disorders: The Role of Cisapride. Amsterdam: Excerpta Medica, 1988;63−65.
8. Janisch HD, Hüttemann W, Bouzo MH. Cisapride versus ranitidine in the treatment of reflux esophagitis. Hepato-gastroenterol 1988;35:125−127.
9. Evreux M, Filoche B, Fournet J et al. Endoscopic and clinical evaluation of cisapride and cimetidine in reflux oesophagitis. Gastroenterology 1988;94:A120.
10. Galmiche JP, Brandstatter G, Evreux M et al. Combined therapy with cisapride and cimetidine in severe reflux oesophagitis: a double-blind controlled trial. Gut 1988;29:675−681.
11. Graham DY, Patterson DJ. Double-blind comparison of liquid antacid and placebo in the treatment of symptomatic reflux esophagitis. Dig Dis Sci 1983;28:559−563.
12. Tytgat GNJ. Clinical efficacy of sucralfate in reflux esophagitis. Comparison with cimetidine. Am J Med 1987;83(suppl 3B):38−42.

13. Simon B, Dammann H-G, Müller P. Sucralfate in the treatment of reflux esophagitis in adults: an update. Scand J Gastroenterol 1989;24(suppl 156):37—41.

14. Weiss W, Brunner H, Büttner G et al. Therapie der refluxosophagitis mit sucralfat. Dtsch Med Wschr 1984;108:1706—1711.

15. Carling L, Cronstedt J, Engqvist A et al. Sucralfate versus placebo in reflux esophagitis. Scand J Gastroenterol 1988;23:1117—1124.

16. Laitinen S, Stahlberg M, Kairaluoma MI et al. Sucralfate versus alginate/antacid in reflux esophagitis. Scand J Gastroenterol 1985;20:229—232.

17. Hameeteman W, Van Den Boomgaard DM, Dekker W et al. Sucralfate versus cimetidine in reflux esophagitis: a single blind multicentre study. J Clin Gastroenterol 1987;9:390—394.

18. Simon B, Beckenbach HP, Daake H et al. Reflux oesophagitis. Wirksamkeitsvergleich von sucralfat und ranitidin. Munch Med Wschr 1988;130:152—154.

19. Ros E, Pujol A, Bordas JM, Grande L. Efficacy of sucralfate in refractory reflux esophagitis. Results of a pilot study. Scand J Gastroenterol 1989;24(suppl 156);49—55.

20. Herrera JL, Shay SS, McCabe M et al. Sucralfate used as adjunctive therapy in patients with severe erosive peptic esophagitis: a randomized double-blind controlled trial. Gastroenterology 1989;96:A207.

21. Schotborgh RH, Hameeteman W, Dekker W et al. Combination therapy of sucralfate and cimetidine, compared with sucralfate monotherapy, in patients with peptic reflux esophagitis. Am J Med 1989;86(suppl 6A):77—80.

22. Tay HP, Chaparala RC, Harmon JW et al. Bismuth subsalicylate reduces peptic injury of the oesophagus in rabbits. Gut 1990;31:11—16.

23. Balan G, Sandulescu E, Cijevschi C et al. De-Nol in the treatment of reflux esophagitis. Rev Med Chir Soc Med Nat Iasi 1989;93:67—70.

24. Borkent MV, Beker JA. Treatment of ulcerative reflux oesophagitis with colloidal bismuth subcitrate in combination with cimetidine. Gut 1988;29:385—389.

25. Sontag SJ. The medical management of reflux esophagitis. Role of antacids and acid inhibition. Gastroenterol Clin North Am 1990;19:683—712.

26. Bell NJV, Hunt RH. Role of gastric acid suppression in the treatment of gastroesophageal reflux disease. Gut 1992;33:118—124.

27. Jansen JBMJ, Baak LC, Lamers CBHW. Effect of increasing doses of ranitidine on exposure of the oesophagus to gastric acid in patients with reflux oesophagitis. Scand J Gastroenterol 1988;23(suppl 154):2—5.

28. Koelz HR. Treatment of reflux esophagitis with H2-blockers, antacids and prokinetic drugs. An analysis of randomized clinical trials. Scand J Gastroenterol 1989;24(suppl 156):25—36.

29. Johnson NJ, Boyd EJS, Mills JG, Wood JR. Acute treatment of reflux oesophagitis: a multicentre trial to compare 150 mg ranitidine b.d. with 300 mg ranitidine q.d.s. Aliment Pharmacol Ther 1989;3:259—266.

30. Robertson DAF, Aldersley MA, Shepherd H et al. H$_2$-antagonists in the treatment of reflux oesophagitis: can physiological studies predict the response? Gut 1987;28:946—949.

31. Orr WC, Robinson MG, Humphries TJ et al. Dose-response effect of famotidine on patterns of gastro-oesophageal reflux. Aliment Pharmacol Ther 1988;2:229—236.

32. Dehn TCB, Shepherd HA, Colin-Jones DG et al. A double-blind comparison of omeprazole (40 mg od) versus cimetidine (400 mg qd) in the treatment of symptomatic erosive reflux oesophagitis, assessed endoscopically, histologically and by 24-h pH monitoring. Gut 1990;31:509—513.

33. Barlow AP, Norris TL, Watson A. Does healing of oesophagitis depend solely on reducing oesophageal acid exposure? Gut 1989;30:A1490.

34. Fellenius E, Berglindh T, Sachs G et al. Substituted benzimidazoles inhibit acid secretion by blocking H$^+$/K$^+$ ATPase. Nature 1981;290:159—161.

35. Lind T, Cederberg C, Haglund U, Olbe L. Effect of omeprazole, a gastric proton-pump-inhibitor, on pentagastrin stimulated acid secretion in man. Gut 1983;24:270—276.

36. Lind T, Cederberg C, Ekenved G, Olbe L. Inhibition of basal and betazole and sham-feeding-induced acid secretion by omeprazole in man. Scand J Gastroenterol 1986;21:1004—1010.

37. Sharma BD, Walt RP, Pounder RE, Gomes M de FA, Wood EC, Logan LH. Optimal dose of oral omeprazole for maximal 24-h decrease of intragastric acidity. Gut 1984,25.957—964.

38. Naesdal J, Bodemar G, Walan A. Effect of omeprazole, a substituted benzimidazole, on 24-h intragastric acidity in patients with peptic ulcer disease. Scand J Gastroenterol 1984;19:916—922.

39. Hetzel DJ, Dent J, Reed WD et al. Healing and relapse of severe peptic esophagitis after treatment with omeprazole. Gastroenterology 1988;95;903—912.

40. Klinkenberg-Knol EC, Jansen JMBJ, Festen HPM, Meuwissen SGM, Lamers CBHW. Double-blind multicentre comparison of omeprazole and ranitidine in the treatment of reflux oesophagitis. Lancet 1987;i:349—351.

41. Havelund T, Laursen LS, Skoubo-Kristensen E et al. Omeprazole and ranitidine in treatment of reflux oesophagitis: double blind comparative trial. Br Med J 1988;296:89—92.

42. Vantrappen G, Rutgeerts L, Schurmans P, Coenegrachts J-L. Omeprazole (40 mg) is superior to ranitidine in short-term treatment of ulcerative reflux oesophagitis. Dig Dis Sci 1988;33:523—529.

43. Sandmark S, Carlsson R, Fausa O, Lundell L. Omeprazole or ranitidine in the treatment of reflux esophagitis. Results from a double-blind, randomized Scandinavian multicenter study. Scand J Gastroenterol 1988;23:625—632.

44. Lundell L, Backman L, Ekström P et al. Omeprazole or high-dose ranitidine in the treatment of patients with reflux

oesophagitis not responding to "standard doses" of H$_2$-receptor antagonists. Aliment Pharm Ther 1990;4:145—157.

45. Zeitoun P, Rampal P, Barbier P, Isal J-P et al. Omeprazole (20 mg o.m.) versus ranitidine (150 mg b.i.d.) in reflux esophagitis. Results of a double-blind randomized trial. Gastroenterol Clin Biol 1989;13:457—462.
46. Brunner G, Creutzfeldt W, Harke U, Lamberts R. Therapy with omeprazole in patients with peptic ulcerations resistant to extended high-dose ranitidine treatment. Digestion 1988;39:80—90.
47. Hameeteman W, Tytgat GNJ. Healing of chronic Barrett ulcers with omeprazole. Am J Gastroenterol 1986;81:764—766.
48. Lee FI, Isaacs PET. Barrett's ulcer: response to standard dose ranitidine, high dose ranitidine, and omeprazole. Am J Gastroenterol 1988;83:914—917.
49. Klinkenberg-Knol EC, Jansen JBMJ, Lamers CBHW et al. Use of omeprazole in the management of reflux oesophagitis resistant to H$_2$-receptor antagonists. Scand J Gastroenterol 1989;24(suppl 166):88—93.
50. Ching CK, Shaheen MZ, Holmes GKT. Is omeprazole more effective in the treatment of resistant reflux oesophagitis and associated peptic stricture? Gastroenterology 1990;89:A30.
51. Hannan A, Chesner I, Mann S, Walt R. Can H$_2$-antagonists alone completely block food stimulated acidity? Eur J Gastroenterol 1991;3:533—537.
52. Merki HS, Wilder-Smith C, Walt R, Halter F. The cephalic and gastric phases of gastric acid secretion during H$_2$-antagonist treatment. Gastroenterology 1991;101:599—606.
53. Klinkenberg-Knol EC, Meuwissen SGM. Combined gastric and oesophageal 24-h pH monitoring and oesophageal manometry in patients with reflux disease resistant to treatment with omeprazole. Aliment Pharmacol Ther 1990;4:485—495.
54   Bell NJV, Burget D, Howden CW, Wilkinson J, Hunt RH. Appropriate acid suppression for the management of gastroesophageal reflux disease. Digestion 1992;51(suppl 1):59—67.
55. Holt S, Howden CW. Omeprazole: overview and opinion. Dig Dis Sci 1991;36:385—393.
56. Hetzel DJ. Medical treatment of reflux oesophagitis. Gullet 1993;3(suppl):60—69.
57. Sontag SJ, Hirschowitz BI, Holt S et al. Two doses of omeprazole versus placebo in symptomatic erosive esophagitis: The US Multicenter study. Gastroenterology 1992;102:109—118.
58. Bate CM, Keeling PWN, O'Morain C et al. Comparison of omeprazole and cimetidine in reflux oesophagitis: symptomatic, endoscopic, and histological evaluations. Gut 1990;31:968—972.
59. The Italian Reflux Oesophagitis Study Group. Omeprazole produces significantly greater healing of erosive or ulcerative reflux oesophagitis than ranitidine. Eur J Gastroenterol Hepatol 1991;3:511—517.
60. Bardhan KD, Long R, Hawkey CJ, Wormsley KG. Lansoprazole, a new proton-pump blocker, vs. ranitidine in the treatment of reflux erosive esophagitis. Gastroenterology 1992;100:A30.

Does the treatment and healing of esophagitis influence the pathophysiology of reflux disease?

D. Armstrong (Hamilton)

The proton pump inhibitors (PPI), omeprazole and lansoprazole, have improved radically our ability to achieve healing and symptomatic relief in patients suffering from reflux esophagitis. This has necessitated a re-evaluation of the roles of medical and surgical therapy in the short- and long-term management of gastroesophageal reflux disease (GERD).

Evidence that treatment with PPIs may influence the pathophysiology of reflux disease can, in principle, be garnered from several sources. However, since there are only limited data concerning the effects of PPIs on esophageal function, some of the potential influences must be inferred from data available regarding the consequences of more established treatment modalities such as antacids, prokinetic drugs, histamine H_2-receptor antagonists (H_2-RAs) and surgery.

To address the question posed in the title, one may ask whether treatment with PPIs is associated with a decreased relapse rate once treatment has stopped. One may also examine whether reduction of esophageal exposure to acid or healing of esophagitis, by whatever means, is associated with a change in any of the parameters considered to be indicative of impaired esophageal function in GERD. These questions will be addressed on the basis of three hypotheses discussed below.

Hypotheses

PPI therapy produces lower relapse rates than other therapies

The pre-eminent effect of PPIs is to reduce the secretion of gastric acid [1] and thereby, to reduce esophageal acid exposure [2,3]; there are no data to indicate that PPIs produce healing of reflux esophagitis by any direct mechanism other than the reduction of esophageal mucosal exposure to acid. However, one may postulate that effective medical therapy breaks the vicious cycle whereby reflux induced esophageal damage impairs esophageal function, such that esophageal exposure to acid is increased and damage is exacerbated still further. If this postulate held true, the recurrence rate would be lower after PPI therapy provided that PPI therapy resulted in more complete esophageal healing than did less effective medical therapy.

In the absence of maintenance treatment, at least half of the patients in clinical trials have relapsed within 6 months of stopping treatment (Fig. 1, [4—14]) and if anything, the relapse rates after PPI therapy are higher than those observed after healing with other medications [13,14]. However, the recurrence rate after omeprazole was not higher than that observed after ranitidine [13] and the higher relapse rates seen after omeprazole are thought to be due to the fact that it produces healing in patients who would not otherwise have healed. In consequence, patients who have severe esophagitis resistant to therapy other than omeprazole are likely to relapse rapidly once treatment stops [15]. Such patients may not be representative of patients with less severe disease in whom motility changes may arguably be reversed by omeprazole. However, there is no evidence that PPIs produce lower relapse rates, after cessation of therapy, than do other therapeutic regimens.

Lower esophageal sphincter (LES) function improves during or after antisecretory therapy

There are numerous reports that LES function is impaired in GERD; the majority have shown that patients with reflux esophagitis have a decreased resting LES pressure [16—18] whilst Dent [19,20] first implicated transient relaxations of the lower esophageal sphincter (TLESRs) in the pathogenesis of GERD. However, it is not immediately obvious which abnormality is the most important in any individual patient. Manometric studies suggest that resting LES pressure is not a major

471

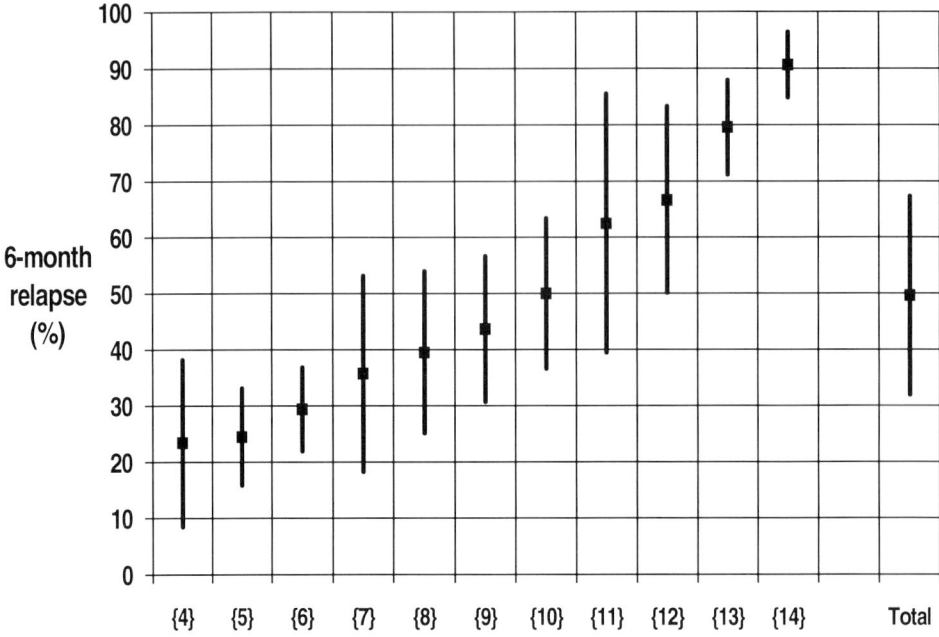

Fig. 1. Relapse rates (with 95% confidence intervals) for reflux esophagitis, 6 months after cessation of therapy with antacids [11], Pyrogastrone [10], H_2-receptor antagonists [4-7,9,10,12,13], cisapride [8] or omeprazole [13,14]. The pooled relapse rate (with 95% confidence intervals), in the absence of active treatment, is shown as the total.

pathogenetic factor in children with reflux esophagitis [21]; the results of another study in adults indicate that TLESRs are equally frequent in controls and patients with reflux esophagitis but that a higher proportion of TLESRs are associated with reflux in patients with reflux esophagitis. However, despite these data and the finding [22] that LES function is poorer in patients with complicated reflux esophagitis (strictures, ulceration or Barrett's esophagus), there are no clear data that LES dysfunction is a consequence rather than a cause of GERD. Certainly, there are no reports that PPIs can improve LES function, although it has been reported that omeprazole therapy does not produce the diminution in LES pressure seen under some circumstances during H_2-RA therapy [23,24].

The notion that LES function might improve with healing of esophagitis receives some support from animal studies showing that acid perfusion of the esophagus or induction of experimental esophagitis are associated with a decrease in basal, resting LES pressure [25,26]. It is clear that LES resting pressure increases in most (Fig. 2A) [27–30] but not all [31] patients following surgery; to a large extent, this is a direct and intended consequence of the surgical procedure, although it is conceivable that the consequent resolution of esophageal inflammation may also contribute to the improvement in LES pressure.

An initial case report did indeed report that LES pressure increased after

472

esophagitis had been healed after treatment with cimetidine and antacids in two patients [32]. However, with the exception of a report that esophagitis healing was followed by an increase in LES pressure during the postprandial period [33], the effect of healing, achieved with acid antisecretory agents, including omeprazole [34], on resting LES pressure has been negligible (Fig. 2B) [2,28,32,33,35–39].

Esophageal body function improves during or after antisecretory therapy

It has been shown in animal studies that esophageal body function is impaired following acid perfusion of the esophagus [40] or induction of experimental esophagitis [41]. Furthermore, there are many reports that esophageal motor function is impaired in patients with GERD [17,18,22,30,35,38,42–44]. However, the exact nature of the defect or defects remains controversial. Impaired esophageal clearance of luminal contents is presumed to be the consequence of esophageal dysmotility; this

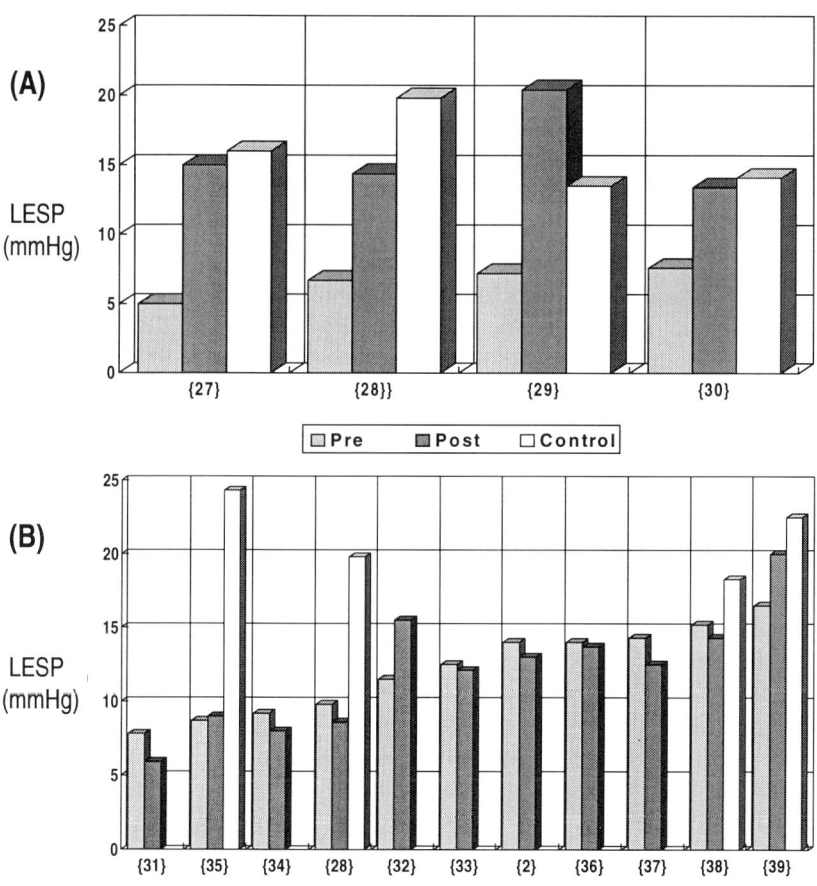

Fig. 2. Basal pressures recorded at the lower esophageal sphincter (LESP) in healthy controls and in patients with reflux esophagitis before (Pre) and after (Post) treatment by surgery (A: upper panel) or acid antisecretory therapy (B: lower panel). The data presented are from studies cited in the reference section.

has been demonstrated using a swallowed radiolabeled bolus [45–47] and also, most elegantly, by Kahrilas and colleagues using manometry and simultaneous video-fluoroscopy of a swallowed barium bolus [48]. The latter group showed that failure to clear barium from the distal esophagus was associated with manometric features of failed primary peristalsis or hypotensive peristalsis in the distal esophagus, previously noted in a substantial minority of patients with peptic esophagitis. One or more features of impaired esophageal body function, including reduced contraction amplitude, reduced contraction duration, reduced propagation velocity of peristaltic contractions and a higher proportion of nonpropagated or incompletely propagated contractions, have been reported to be more prevalent in patients with reflux esophagitis [16–18,22,33, 48–50]. However, it is still not clear which, if any, is the predominant abnormality. More controversial yet, is the nature of the relationship between esophagitis and dysmotility. Several authors have reported that esophageal dysfunction is more marked in patients whose esophagitis is more severe [16,22]. This has been taken to support the hypothesis that esophageal body dysmotility is a consequence of GERD [22] although the alternative hypothesis, that esophageal dysmotility is the primary disorder in GERD, also has its proponents [46,51,52].

The concept that dysmotility is a secondary phenomenon is consistent with the postoperative increases in esophageal contraction amplitude (Fig. 3A) and in the percentage of propagated contractions (Fig. 4A) reported 3 to 30 months after patients have undergone fundoplication [27,29,30]. Improved esophageal motility after surgery is not, however, universal suggesting either that dysmotility is, in some cases, a primary phenomenon which predates the development of GERD or that it is a secondary occurrence which becomes irreversible if inflammation persists or progresses unchecked [22].

If esophageal body dysmotility is, indeed, secondary one might expect that effective medical therapy, leading to healing of reflux esophagitis, would produce improvements in motility comparable to those observed after surgery. The previously mentioned increase in LES pressure following successful medical treatment of reflux esophagitis was accompanied by increases in contraction amplitude and in the percentage of propagated contractions [32]. However, no subsequent papers have reported a clear improvement in esophageal body function — as judged by contraction amplitude (Fig. 3B) or by the percentage of contractions which propagate normally (Fig. 4B) — following medical therapy, either with omeprazole [34,39,53] or with other antisecretory agents [28,32,33,37,38].

Discussion

Despite case reports that improved esophageal function follows healing of esophagitis by medical means [32], subsequent studies have failed to show any change in resting lower esophageal sphincter pressure, in esophageal body contraction amplitude, duration and velocity or in the proportion of esophageal body contractions which is propagated normally. There are limited data on the changes produced by omeprazole, but they do not seem to differ significantly from those seen after treatment with

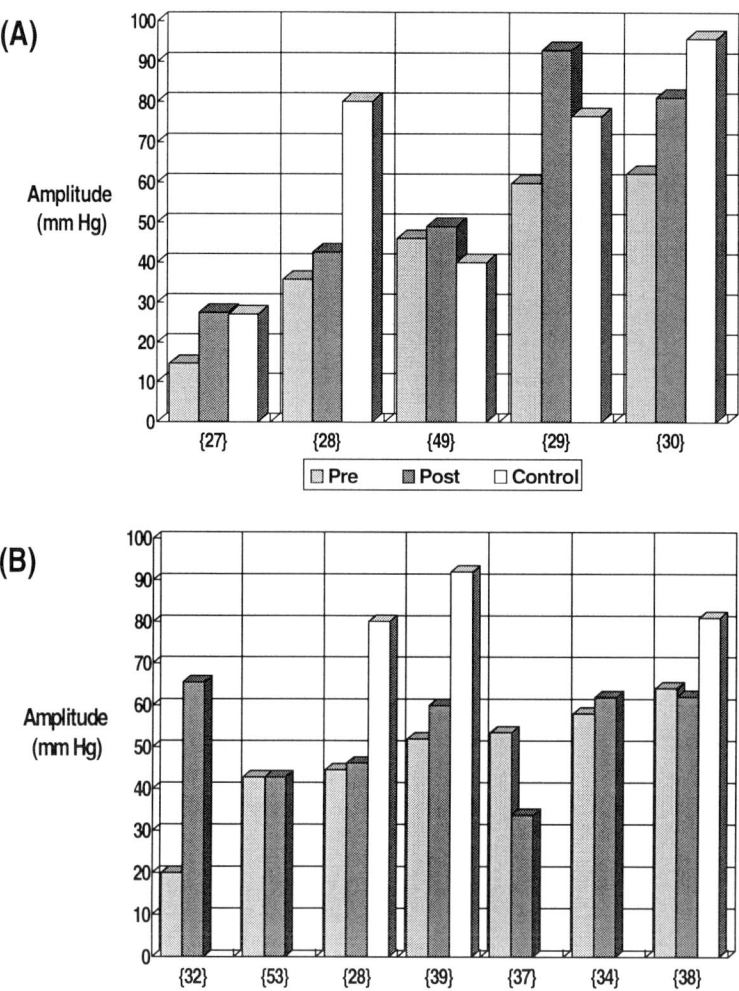

(A)

(B)

Fig. 3. Mean esophageal contraction amplitudes recorded in the distal esophagus in healthy controls and in patients with reflux esophagitis before (Pre) and after (Post) treatment by surgery (A: upper panel) or acid antisecretory therapy (B: lower panel). The data presented are from studies cited in the reference section.

histamine H_2-RAs. Thus, despite their ability to decrease profoundly the secretion of gastric acid, PPIs do not seem to affect the changes in esophageal motility produced by surgery. As mentioned previously, an increase in LESP is to be expected since this is one of the main aims of surgery. However, the major, longer term effect of surgery is to reduce esophageal exposure to acid, similar to the effect of PPIs. It may be argued that surgery also prevents the reflux of acid unrelated gastric contents which may be as injurious under some circumstances as acid and pepsin. However, since there is a clear relationship between gastric acid suppression and the degree and rate

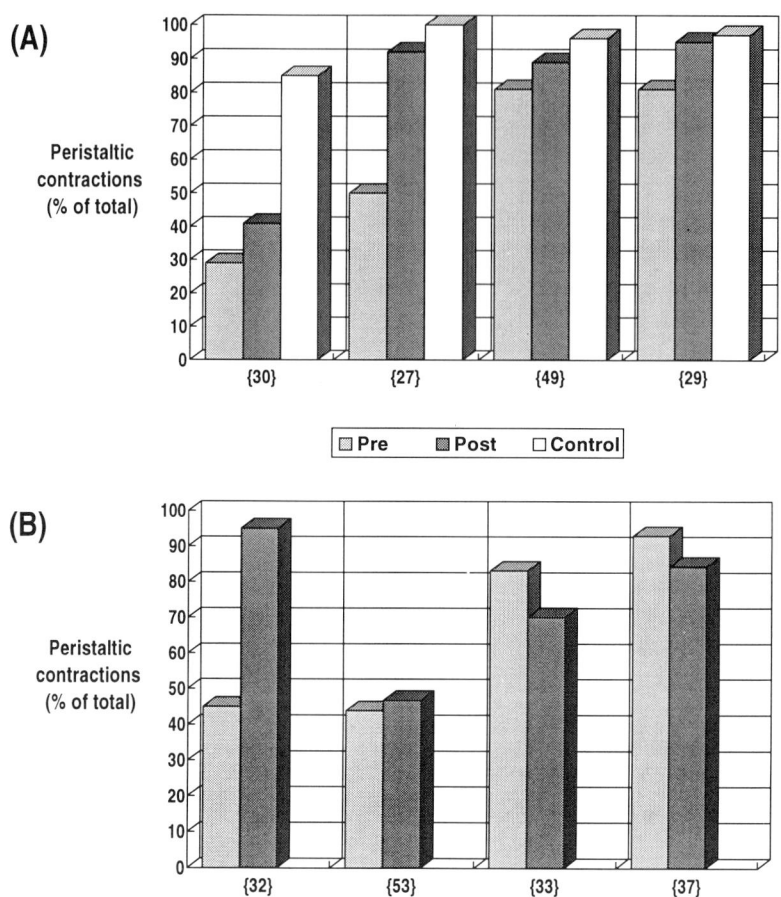

Fig. 4. Peristaltic esophageal contractions recorded, as a proportion of all contractions, in healthy controls and in patients with reflux esophagitis before (Pre) and after (Post) treatment by surgery (A: upper panel) or acid antisecretory therapy (B: lower panel). The data presented are from studies cited in the reference section.

of healing seen with medical therapy in esophagitis [1] and since, furthermore, the majority of patients with esophagitis will heal after treatment with a PPI, it seems probable that acid exposure is the major pathogenetic factor leading to esophageal damage.

One possible explanation for the discrepancy between sequelae of surgery and those of PPI therapy is the difference in duration of treatment prior to esophageal testing in the two groups. In the medical treatment studies, the mean duration of treatment was approximately 2.5 ± 0.1 months, similar to that noted for the four omeprazole treatment groups combined (2.4 ± 0.1 months) [2,34,39,53]. However, the mean time elapsed between surgery and esophageal testing in the studies discussed here is 17 ± 1.1 months. Grande and colleagues [29] showed a clear and steady increase in esophageal contraction amplitude and LES pressure with a progressive

476

increase from pretreatment levels to those seen at 6 months and a further rise between 6 and 12 months (Fig. 5). Thus, the failure to record an effect of medical therapy on esophageal function and hence on the pathophysiology of GERD may be attributable to medical treatment periods which are too short to allow any change to occur. Healing of the esophageal mucosa does not necessarily indicate normalization of esophageal function [35].

Another possible explanation for the increase in esophageal contraction amplitude seen after surgery is that fundoplication produces a degree of obstruction which stimulates esophageal contractility. These changes may be analogous to the increased contraction amplitudes observed in patients with "vigorous" achalasia although the contractions which occur in vigorous achalasia are generally simultaneous [54,55] whilst fundoplication is followed by an increase in the proportion of peristaltic contractions (Fig. 4A).

However, it is highly likely that many other factors also influence the differential, long-term responses of reflux esophagitis to medical and surgical treatment. The pathophysiology of GERD is multifactorial, involving any one or more of the factors shown in Table 1. Barlow et al. [56] found, in a study of 75 patients with an abnormal 24-h pH-metry, that gastric hypersecretion was more common in patients with a normal LES (10/22, 48%) than in patients with impaired LES function (11/54, 20%; p = 0.0244). Thus, in some GERD patients, LES dysfunction is the predominant defect, whereas in other patients gastric hypersecretion is more important. The importance of esophageal body dysmotility remains unclear but, as with other pathogenetic factors, it is unlikely to be the only factor in many patients. Furthermore, a defect in esophageal body motility may be primary in some patients [46,57] but secondary to reflux induced damage [22,57] in other patients. If this is the case,

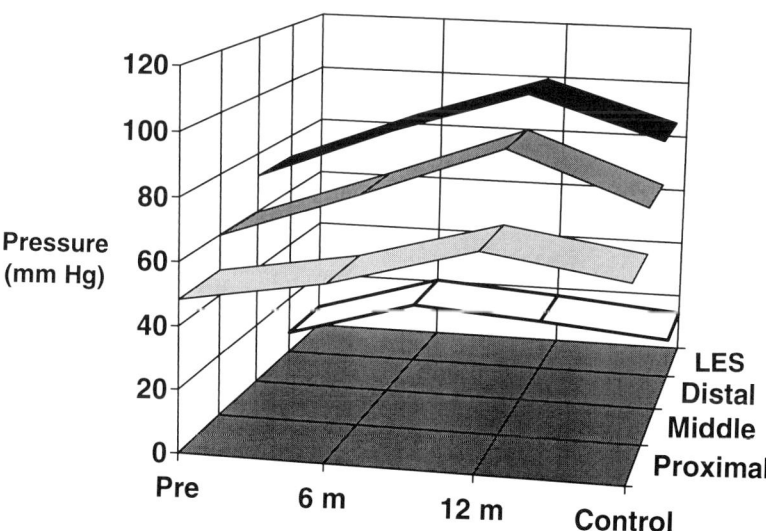

Fig. 5. Contraction amplitudes recorded in the proximal, mid and distal esophagus and basal LES pressure recorded in healthy controls and in patients with reflux esophagitis before (Pre) and 6 and 12 months after the patients had undergone fundoplication [29].

Table 1. The pathophysiology of gastroesophageal reflux disease

Impaired ability of LES to prevent reflux
    Impaired LES function
        Decreased baseline LES resting pressure
        Increased frequency or duration of transient LESRs: appropriate or inappropriate
    Impaired gastric emptying
        Increased (residual) gastric volume

Impaired clearance of refluxed material
    Impaired sensitivity of mucosa to stimulation
    Impaired amplitude of esophageal contractions
    Incoordinated esophageal contraction
    Incompletely propagated esophageal contraction
    Impaired propulsion of luminal contents

Injurious refluxed material
    Increased acidity
    Increased volume
    Increased concentration of other injurious constituents: bile acids, lysolecithin, pepsin, trypsin.

Impaired resistance of esophageal mucosa to refluxed material
    Decreased acid absorption
    Decreased blood flow

the response to therapy, medical or surgical, will be influenced profoundly by predominant defect. For those patients in whom primary dysmotility predominates, no antisecretory medication or surgical treatment is likely to provide any effective change in esophageal function, whereas patients with secondary dysmotility may improve following the reduction of esophageal acid exposure provided irreversible damage has not occurred.

Conclusion

Refutation of the hypothesis that PPIs will influence the pathophysiology of GERD is precluded by the paucity of data. There are some data to indicate that prolonged mucosal healing with or without reduction of esophageal acid exposure, studied for the present only after surgery, may improve some indices of esophageal function. Currently, studies of medical therapy have been too short to allow detection of any treatment effect on esophageal motility. Future studies should also address the problem of defining appropriate markers of esophageal dysfunction relevant to the pathogenesis of GERD. Very low amplitude contractions (<20 mmHg) [48] are ineffective at clearing the esophageal lumen of refluxed acid, but it is not at all clear whether there is a fixed threshold or whether clearance declines progressively as contraction amplitudes decrease. There is, therefore, a need for functional assessments of the esophagus and its ability to clear luminal contents [16,35,39,48,50] if one is to understand the pathophysiology of GERD and its response to treatment.

References

1. Bell NJV, Hunt RH. Role of gastric acid suppression in the treatment of gastro-oesophageal reflux disease. Gut 1992;33: 118—124.
2. Dent J, Downton J, Buckle P, Heddle R, Toouli J, Mackinnon M, Wyman JB. Omeprazole heals peptic oesophagitis by elevation of intragastric pH. Gastroenterology 1985;88:1363(abstract).
3. Ruth M, Enbom H, Lundell L, Lonroth H, Sandberg N, Sandmark S. The effect of omeprazole or ranitidine treatment on 24-h oesophageal acidity in patients with reflux oesophagitis. Scand J Gastroenterol 1988;23:1141—1146.
4. Berlin R, Ebel D, Cook T. Famotidine 20 mg hs and 40 mg hs vs. placebo in the maintenance therapy of reflux esophagitis: results of a double-blind, multicenter trial. Gastroenterology 1989;96:A39 (abstract).
5. Ottenjann R, Siewert JR, Heilman K, Neiss A, Döpfer H. Treatment of reflux oesophagitis. Results of a multicentre study. In: Siewert JR, Hölscher AH (eds) Diseases of the Esophagus. Berlin: Springer Verlag, 1988;1123—1129.
6. Blum AL, Adami B, Bouzo MH, Brandstätter G, Fumagalli I, Galmiche JP, Hebbelin H, Hentschel E, Hüttemann W, Schütz E, Verlinden M and the Italian Eurocis Trialists. Effect of cisapride on relapse of esophagitis. A multinational, placebo-controlled trial in patients healed with an antisecretory drug. Dig Dis Sci 1993;38:551—560.
7. Koelz HR, Birchler R, Bretholz A, Bron B, Capitaine Y, Delmore G, Fehr HF, Fumagalli I, Gehrig J, Gonvers JJ, Halter F, Hammer B, Kayasseh L, Kobler E, Miller G, Münst G, Pelloni S, Realini S, Schmid P, Voirol M, Blum AL. Healing and relapse of reflux esophagitis during treatment with ranitidine. Gastroenterology 1986;91:1198—1205.
8. Toussaint J, Gossuin A, Deruyttere M, Hublé F, Devis G. Healing and prevention of relapse of reflux oesophagitis by cisapride. Gut 1991;32:1280—1285.
9. Armstrong D, Blum AL and the Rezitic Study Group. Full dose H$_2$-receptor antagonist prophylaxis does not prevent relapse of reflux oesophagitis. Gut 1989;30:A1494 (abstract).
10. Maxton DG, Heald J, Whorwell PJ, Haboubi NY. Controlled trial of pyrogastrone and cimetidine in the treatment of reflux oesophagitis. Gut 1990;30:351—354.
11. Behar J, Sheahan DG, Biancani P, Spiro HM, Storer EH. Medical and surgical management of reflux esophagitis. N Engl J Med 1975;293:263—268.
12. Stein DT, Simon TJ, Berlin RG, Berman R, Tornabene L, Kogut D, Rohrfail W. Controlling 24-h esophageal acid exposure in patients with healed erosive esophagitis prevents endoscopic recurrence and symptomatic deterioration: results of a 6-month, randomized, double-blind, US placebo controlled trial comparing famotidine 20 mg b.i.d. and 40 mg b.i.d. Gastroenterology 1991;100:A167 (abstract).
13. Sandmark S, Carlsson R, Fausa O, Lundell L. Omeprazole or ranitidine in the treatment of reflux oesophagitis. Scand J Gastroenterol 1985;23:625—632.
14. Hetzel DJ, Dent J, Reed WD et al. Healing and relapse of severe peptic esophagitis after treatment with omeprazole. Gastroenterology 1988;95:903—912.
15. Klinkenberg-Knol EC, Meuwissen SGM. Temporary cessation of long-term maintenance treatment with omeprazole in patients with H$_2$ receptor antagonist resistant reflux oesophagitis. Scand J Gastroenterol 1990;25:1144—1150.
16. Kahrilas PJ, Dodds WJ, Hogan WJ, Kern F, Arndorfer RC, Reece A. Peristaltic dysfunction in peptic esophagitis. Gastroenterology 1986;91:897—904.
17. Bassotti G, Pelli MA, Miglietti M, Morelli M. Oesophageal motor activity in patients with gastro-oesophageal reflux symptoms and endoscopic oesophagitis. Ital J Gastroenterol 1989;21:263—267.
18. Timmer R, Breumelhof R, Nadorp JHSM, Smout AJPM. Esophageal motility in low-grade reflux esophagitis, evaluated by stationary and 24-h ambulatory manometry. Am J Gastroenterol 1993;88:837—841.
19. Dent J, Dodds WJ, Friedman RH, Sekiguchi T, Hogan WJ, Arndorfer RC. Mechanism of gastroesophageal reflux in recumbent asymptomatic human subjects. J Clin Invest 1980;65:256—267.
20. Dent J, Holloway RH, Toouli J, Dodds WJ. Mechanisms of lower oesophageal sphincter incompetence in patients with symptomatic gastro-oesophageal reflux. Gut 1988;29:1020—1028.
21. Berezin S, Halata MS, Newman LJ, Glassman MS, Medow MS. Esophageal manometry in children with esophagitis. Am J Gastroenterol 1993;88:680—682.
22. Stein HJ, Eypasch EP, DeMeester TR, Smyrk TC, Attwood SEA. Circadian esophageal motor function in patients with gastroesophageal reflux. Surgery 1990;108:769—778.
23. Pedersen SA, Kraglund K, Vinter-Jensen L. The effects of omeprazole on gastro-oesophageal sphincter pressure, intragastric pH and the migrating motor complex in fasting healthy subjects. Scand J Gastroenterol 1987;22:725—730.
24. Smout AJPM, Bogaard JW, van Hattum J, Akkermans LMA. Effects of cimetidine and ranitidine on interdigestive and postprandial lower esophageal sphincter pressures and plasma gastrin levels in normal subjects. Gastroenterology 1985;88:557—563.
25. Eastwood GL, Castell DO, Higgs RH. Experimental esophagitis in cats impairs lower esophageal sphincter pressure. Gastroenterology 1975;69:146—153.
26. Higgs RH, Castell DO, Eastwood GL. Studies on the mechanism of esophagitis-induced lower esophageal sphincter hypotension in cats. Gastroenterology 1976;71:51—57.
27. Ortiz Escandell A, Martinez de Haro LF, Parrilla Paricio P, Aguayo Albasini JL, Garcia Marcilla JA, Morales Cuenca G. Surgery improves defective oesophageal peristalsis in patients with gastro-oesophageal reflux. Br J Surg 1991;78:1095—1097.

479

28. Eckhardt VF. Does healing of esophagitis improve esophageal motor function? Dig Dis Sci 1988;33:161—165.
29. Grande L, Lacima G, Ros E, Pujol A, Garcia-Valdecasas JC, Fuster J, Visa J, Pera C. Dysphagia and esophageal motor dysfunction in gastroesophageal reflux are corrected by fundoplication. J Clin Gastroenterol 1991;13:11—16.
30. Stein HJ, Bremner RM, Jamieson J, DeMeester TR. Effect of Nissen fundoplication on esophageal motor function. Arch Surg 1992;127:788—791.
31. Breumelhof R, Timmer R, Nadorp JHSM, Smout AJPM. Reduction of gastroesophageal reflux by Nissen fundoplication is not caused by changes in the LES or esophageal body function. Gastroenterology 1993;104:A46(abstract).
32. Marshall JB, Gerhardt DC. Improvement in esophageal motor dysfunction with treatment of reflux esophagitis: a report of two cases. Am J Gastroenterol 1982;77:351—354.
33. Baldi F, Ferrarini F, Longanesi A, Angeloni M, Ragazzini M, Miglioli M, Barbara L. Oesophageal function before, during and after healing of reflux oesophagitis. Gut 1988;29:157—160.
34. Howard JM, Frei JV, Flowers M, Bondy DC, Tilbe K, Reynolds RPE. Omeprazole heals esophagitis but does not improve abnormal esophageal motility in reflux esophagitis. Gastroenterology 1990;98:A61 (abstract).
35. Sonnenberg A, Lepsien G, Müller-Lissner SA, Koelz HR, Siewert JR, Blum AL. When is esophagitis healed? Esophageal endoscopy, histology and function before and after cimetidine treatment. Dig Dis Sci 1982;27:297—302.
36. Thor P, Maczka M, Sito E, Oleksy J, Konturek SJ. Gastroesophageal acid reflux, gastric motility and outcome of erosive esophagitis in patients treated with ranitidine and ebrotidine, a novel H₂-receptor antagonist with protective activity. Gastroenterology 1993;104:A211 (abstract).
37. Allen ML, McIntosh DL, Robinson MG. Healing or amelioration of esophagitis does not result in increased lower esophageal sphincter or esophageal contractile pressure. Am J Gastroenterol 1990;85:1331—1334.
38. Katz PO, Knuff TE, Benjamin SB, Castell DO. Abnormal esophageal pressures in reflux esophagitis: cause or effect? Am J Gastroenterol 1986;81:744—746.
39. Singh P, Adamopoulos A, Taylor RH, Colin-Jones DG. Oesophageal motor function before and after healing of oesophagitis. Gut 1992;33:1590—1596.
40. Shirazi S, Schulze-Delrieu K, Custer-Hagen T, Brown CK, Ren J. Motility changes in opossum esophagus from experimental esophagitis. Dig Dis Sci 1989;34:1668—1676.
41. Sinar DR, Fleitcher JR, Cordova CC, Eastwood GL, Castell DO. Acute acid-induced esophagitis impairs esophageal peristalsis in baboons. Gastroenterology 1981;80:1286 (abstract).
42. Baldi F, Ferrarini F, Balestra R, Borioni D, Longanesi A, Miglioli M, Barbara L. Oesophageal motor events at the occurrence of acid reflux and during endogenous acid exposure in healthy subjects and in patients with oesophagitis. Gut 1985;26:336—341.
43. Cucchiara S, Staiano A, Di Lorenzo C, D'Ambrosio R, Andreotti MR, Prato M, De Filippo P, Auricchio S. Esophageal motor abnormalities in children with gastroesophageal reflux and peptic esophagitis. J Pediatr 1986;108:907—910.
44. Jacob P, Kahrilas PJ, Vanagunas A. Peristaltic dysfunction associated with nonobstructive dysphagia in reflux disease. Dig Dis Sci 1990;35:939—942.
45. Roland J, Peters O, Piepsz A, Devis G, Jonckheer M, Ham HR. Evaluation of oesophageal transit in patients with minor peptic oesophagitis. Nucl Med Commun 1989;10:161—165.
46. Eriksen CA, Sadek SA, Cranford C, Sutton D, Kennedy N, Cuschieri A. Reflux oesophagitis and oesophageal transit: evidence for a primary oesophageal motor disorder. Gut 1988;29:448—452.
47. Cunningham KM, Horowitz M, Riddell PS, Maddern GJ, Myers JC, Holloway RH, Wishart JM, Jamieson GG. Relations among autonomic nerve dysfunction, oesophageal dysmotility and gastric emptying in gastro-oesophageal reflux disease. Gut 1991;32:1436—1440.
48. Kahrilas PJ, Dodds WJ, Hogan WJ. Effects of peristaltic dysfunction on esophageal volume clearance. Gastroenterology 1988;94:73—80.
49. Johansson KE, Tibbling L. Esophageal body motor disturbances in gastroesophageal reflux and the effects of fundoplication. Scand J Gastroenterol 1988;23(suppl 155):82—88.
50. Williams D, Thompson DG, Marples M, Heggie L, O'Hanrahan T, Mani V, Bancewicz J. Identification of an abnormal esophageal clearance response to intraluminal distention in patients with esophagitis. Gastroenterology 1992;103:943—953.
51. Russell CO, Pope CE, Gannan RM, Allen FD, Velasco N, Hill LD. Does surgery correct esophageal motor dysfunction in gastroesophageal reflux? Ann Surg 1981;194:290—295.
52. Joelsson BE, DeMeester TR, Skinner DB, Lafontaine E, Waters PF, O'Sullivan GC. The role of the esophageal body in the antireflux mechanism. Surgery 1982; 92:417—424.
53. Timmer R, Breumelhof R, Nadorp JHSM, Smout AJPM. Ambulatory esophageal pressure monitoring before and after healing of reflux esophagitis. Gastroenterology 1993;104:A211 (abstract).
54. Bondi JL, Godwin DH, Garrett JM. "Vigorous" achalasia: its clinical interpretation and significance. Am J Gastroenterol 1972;58:145—154.
55. Vantrappen G, Janssens J, Hellemans J et al. Achalasia, diffuse esophageal spasm and related motility disorders. Gastroenterology 1979;76:450—457.
56. Barlow AP, DeMeester TR, Ball CS, Eypasch EP. The significance of the gastric secretory state in gastroesophageal reflux disease. Arch Surg 1989;124:937—940.
57. Watson A, Jenkinson LR, Norris TL. Reflux oesophagitis and oesophageal transit. Gut 1988;29:1426.

Long-term treatments

 ## What are the clinical effects of long-term maintenance therapy with PPIs?

L.C. Olbe (Gothenburg)

Indications for maintenance therapy

The long-term management of acid related diseases involves several alternatives.

The first hand choice for the treatment of recurrent peptic ulcer disease is eradication of *Helicobacter pylori*. Exceptions are patients with the Zollinger-Ellison syndrome and patients on NSAID medication.

Patients who have had unsuccessful repeated eradication trials, and those who have been reinfected with *H. pylori*, should be managed by a different treatment strategy. Such peptic ulcer patients with infrequent symptomatic episodes (e.g., less than one to two episodes each year) can be easily managed by intermittent antisecretory treatment over 4–6 weeks. Proton pump inhibitors (PPI) are superior to histamine H_2-receptor antagonists (H_2-RA) both with regard to healing rates and fast symptom relief.

Some peptic ulcer patients, who had unsuccessful eradication of *H. pylori*, have a more severe disease with more or less continuous symptoms or repeated complications and may not be suitable for surgery or unwilling to accept surgery. Such patients should be given continuous maintenance treatment.

The situation for patients with gastroesophageal reflux disease and/or reflux esophagitis is more simple. The great majority of patients with daily reflux symptoms or patients with severe reflux esophagitis (grade II–IV) will have relapse of symptoms and esophagitis within a few months of stopping medical treatment. Consequently, almost all of these patients need either continuous maintenance treatment or prophylactic surgery. Surgery may be recommended to relatively young and otherwise fit patients if surgeons well experienced with fundoplication are available and particularly if the surgeons are using the laparoscopic procedure. Otherwise, or if the patient is unwilling to accept surgery, continuous maintenance treatment should be started.

Experience with long-term maintenance treatment for peptic ulcer disease

There is a vast experience of continuous maintenance treatment with histamine H_2-RAs. Traditionally, the maintenance dose has been half the dose used for healing a peptic ulcer. The recurrence rate during half dose maintenance treatment with any of the histamine H_2-RAs has been 25—30% for the first 12 months. This recurrence rate is much lower than that obtained during placebo treatment, but certainly not satisfactory. The same rather poor results have been obtained during half dose maintenance treatment with omeprazole [1,2]. Consequently, there seems to be a case for more potent medical prophylaxis in the maintenance therapy for peptic ulcer (e.g., full dose antisecretory regime).

There are no reports over full dose maintenance treatment with histamine H_2-RAs. There are, however, some reports of full dose maintenance treatment with omeprazole [3,4]. In these studies the recurrence rate during the first 12 months has reached a more satisfactory level of about 10%. This recurrence rate seems to remain stable over a prolonged period of full dose maintenance treatment with omeprazole [3].

Experience with long-term maintenance treatment for reflux esophagitis

In reflux esophagitis patients, antisecretory treatment with PPIs has resulted in far better healing rates and faster symptom relief than treatment with histamine H_2-RAs. This statement is also true for patients with reflux symptoms without severe eso-phagitis, although to a lesser degree [5]. In patients with severe esophagitis, most patients will heal on 20 mg omeprazole daily, but about one quarter of the patients need 40 mg omeprazole to heal and a few patients need even higher daily doses.

Several studies have shown, that omeprazole is very effective in the long-term treatment of reflux esophagitis [6—11]. These studies included almost 1000 patients treated for 6—12 months. Again most patients could be kept in remission on 20 mg omeprazole daily, but about one quarter of patients with severe esophagitis need 40 mg omeprazole daily to stay in remission. The same results have been obtained in long-term maintenance treatment over 2 years [12] and 7 years [3]. There is therefore no doubt that long-term full dose maintenance treatment with omeprazole can keep almost all patients with reflux esophagitis in remission.

In some of the above maintenance studies, treatment with 10 mg omeprazole daily could keep two thirds of the patients with less severe reflux esophagitis (grade II or less) in remission, while only about one quarter of the patients with more severe reflux esophagitis could be kept in remission with that low maintenance omeprazole dose. Since patients with mild reflux esophagitis have a very low risk for severe complications, it might be considered to start maintenance treatment on patients with reflux esophagitis grade 0–II with a 10 mg omeprazole dose. The need for adjustment to a high dose can be easily recognized, since relapse of symptoms and esophagitis during maintenance treatment run in parallel [9].

Experience with long-term maintenance treatment for Zollinger-Ellison syndrome

PPIs are a first hand choice for long-term antisecretory treatment in patients with Zollinger-Ellison syndrome, where the gastrinoma could not be surgically removed. Treatment with omeprazole has now continued up to 5 years [13]. The daily dose has usually been 60–120 mg omeprazole and remained stable over the years [13].

Safety aspects

Safety experience from long-term treatment with omeprazole has been obtained by monitoring adverse events and laboratory data in almost 600 patients treated for more than 6 months and up to 6 years [14]. The adverse event profile for omeprazole during long-term treatment did not differ from that observed during short-term treatment with omeprazole or histamine H_2-RAs. There was no increase with time in the occurrence of any adverse event and there were no serious adverse events that were considered to be casually related to omeprazole. There were no changes in laboratory parameters considered clinically significant. The only laboratory parameter changed was serum gastrin. A moderate increase of serum gastrin of the same magnitude as after vagotomy [15] occurred during the first few months and then remained at that level [3].

The increase of serum gastrin has caused some concern, since the massive hypergastrinemia in the toxicological studies of omeprazole produced enterochromaffine-like (ECL) cell carcinoids in the rat. This is, however, an effect of massive hypergastrinemia in the rat and not an effect of omeprazole, since very high doses of ranitidine and subtotal resection of the acid producing mucosa in the rat will also result in similar frequency of ECL-cell carcinoids [16,17]. In humans ECL-carcinoids have been found in a few percentage of patients with the atrophic fundic mucosa of pernicious anemia and in some Zollinger-Ellison syndrome patients with a primarily normal fundic mucosa. In the Zollinger-Ellison patients, however, the ECL-cell carcinoids seem to develop only in the subgroup of MEN I syndrome and independently of the antisecretory drug used [13]. Thus, the ECL-carcinoid development in a human with a primarily normal fundic mucosa seems to involve not only massive hypergastrinemia, but also the genetic defect of the MEN I syndrome.

Will the moderate hypergastrinemia during omeprazole treatment cause any changes of the ECL-cells? After 4.5 years of continuous treatment with 20–40 mg omeprazole daily, no carcinoids or ECL-dysplasia was observed with the exception of a slight ECL-cell hyperplasia [3]. The same slight ECL-cell hyperplasia was, however, observed during a 4.5 year period in a group of gastric ulcer patients, who had no antisecretory treatment at all [18]. This ECL-hyperplasia seemed to be related mainly to the degree of development of atrophic gastritis. Consequently, long-term full dose maintenance treatment with omeprazole seems to be very safe and no severe adverse events, clinical significant changes in laboratory parameters or histological changes in the gastric mucosa has occurred, at least not during the first 5 years of treatment.

References

1. Lauritsen K, Andersen BN, Laursen LS et al. Omeprazole 20 mg three days a week and 10 mg daily in prevention of duodenal ulcer relapse. Gastroenterology 1991;100:663–669.
2. Bianchi Porro G, Bolling E, Barbara L et al. Maintenance treatment with omeprazole in the prevention of duodenal relapse: A double-blind comparative trial. Gastroenterology 1990;98:A21.
3. Brunner GHG, Lamberts R, Creutzfeldt W. Efficacy and safety of omeprazole in the long-term treatment of peptic ulcer and reflux oesophagitis resistant to ranitidine. Digestion 1990;47(suppl 1):64–68.
4. Goh KL, Boonyapisit S, Lai KH, Chang R, Kang JY, Lam SK. Prevention of duodenal ulcer relapse with omeprazole 20 mg daily – a randomised, double-blind, placebo controlled study. Prevention of duodenal ulcer relapse with omeprazole 20 mg daily – a randomised, double-blind, placebo controlled study. 9th Asian Pacific Congress Gastroenterology 1992:146 (abstract).
5. Havelund T, Laursen LS, Skoubo-Kristensen E et al. Omeprazole and ranitidine in treatment of reflux oesophagitis: a double-blind comparative trial. Br Med J 1988;296:89–92.
6. Laursen LS, Bondesen S, Hansen J et al. Omeprazole 10 or 20 mg daily for the prevention of relapse in gastro-oesophageal reflux disease? A double-blind comparative study. Gastroenterology 1992;102:A109.
7. Lundell L, Backman L, Ekström P et al. Prevention of relapse and reflux oesophagitis after endoscopic healing: the efficacy and safety of omeprazole compared with ranitidine. Scand J Gastroenterol 1991;26:246–256.
8. Isal JP, Zeitoun P, Barbier P et al. Comparison of 2 dosage regimens of omeprazole – 10 mg once daily and 20 mg weekends – as prophylaxis against recurrence of reflux oesophagitis. Gastroenterology 1990;98:A63.
9. Hallerbäck P, Unge P, Carlind L et al. Comparison of omeprazole 20 mg and 10 mg o.d. and ranitidine 150 mg b.i.d. in the long-term treatment of reflux oesophagitis. 9th Asian Congress Gastroenterology 1992:90.
10. Dent J, Yeomans ND, MacKinnon M et al. Omeprazole versus ranitidine for prevention of relapse in reflux oesophagitis. A controlled double-blind trial. World Congress of Gastroenterology 1990:FPY.
11. Sontag SJ, Robinson MG, Roufail W et al. Daily dose of omeprazole (OME) is needed to maintain healing in erosive oesophagitis (EE). Am J Gastroenterol 1992;87:1258 A65.
12. Klinkenberg-Knol EC, Meuwissen SGM. Medical therapy of patients with reflux oesophagitis poorly responsive to H$_2$-receptor antagonist therapy. Digestion 1992;51(suppl 1):44–48.
13. Frucht H, Maton PN, Jensen RT. Use of omeprazole in patients with Zollinger-Ellison syndrome. Dig Dis Sci 1991;36:394–404.
14. Joelsson S, Joelsson IB, Lundborg P, Walan A, Wallander MA. Safety experience from long-term treatment with omeprazole. Digestion 1992;51(suppl 1):93–101.
15. Lind T, Cederberg C, Olausson M, Olbe L. 24-h intragastric acidity and plasma gastrin after omeprazole treatment and after proximal gastric vagotomy in duodenal ulcer patients. Gastroenterology 1990;99:1593–1598.
16. Havu N, Mattsson H, Ekman L, Carlsson E. ECL-cell carcinoids in the rat gastric mucosa following long-term administration of ranitidine. Digestion 1990;45:189–195.
17. Mattsson H, Havu N, Bräutigam J, Carlsson K, Lundell L, Carlsson E. Partial corpectomy results in hypergastrinaemia and development of gastric ECL cell carcinoids in the rat. Gastroenterology 1991;100:311–319.
18. Havu N, Maaroos H-I, Sipponen P. Argyrophil cell hyperplasia associated with chronic corpus gastritis in gastric ulcer disease. Scand J Gastroenterol 1991;26(suppl 186):90–94.

Proton Pump Inhibitors in children

E. Hassall (Vancouver)

Published experience with proton pump inhibitors (PPI) in children has been limited to the use of omeprazole. Our experience with omeprazole in children to date suggests that the drug is invaluable for the treatment of certain children with severe or refractory gastroesophageal (GE) reflux, e.g., children with neurologic handicaps, cystic fibrosis, esophageal atresia postrepair, and those who have failed H_2-blockers and prokinetic agents.

Mild reflux esophagitis may respond to antacids, dietary measures and postural therapy. However, severe reflux esophagitis usually requires more effective exclusion of acid from the esophagus, using antireflux surgery or suppression of gastric acid secretion. More potent acid inhibition has resulted in greater success rates of treatment [1,2].

Studies in adults with erosive esophagitis due to gastroesophageal reflux have confirmed the marked superiority of omeprazole over placebo and also over cimetidine and ranitidine [1–5]. The few early data on the use of omeprazole in children addressed only its short-term (6–8 weeks) use in esophagitis [6] and the treatment of a few patients with peptic ulcer disease [7,8]. However, data in children were lacking regarding the safety and effective dosage range of omeprazole in children. Therefore, we aimed to determine these data in a group of children with GE reflux refractory to other measures [9].

Patients and Methods

The use of omeprazole was evaluated in 15 children (eight boys) with refractory GE reflux. Omeprazole was not first line therapy in any patient; four patients had one or more fundoplications and all had had unsuccessful treatment with H_2-blockers for between 6 weeks to 5 years (mean 9.5 months). In 14 of the 15 patients, courses of prokinetic agents (metoclopramide, domperidone or cisapride) had also failed. Patients ages were 0.8–17 yrs (mean 8.1 years), weights 7.5–30.7 kg (mean 18.6 kg). Clinical features of these children are given in Table 1.

Prior to starting treatment with omeprazole, all patients had barium upper gastrointestinal (UGI) series and UGI endoscopy with serial stepwise esophageal biopsies. Esophagitis by endoscopic examination was graded 0–4 per Hetzel et al. [2]. All patients had CBC and blood urea, creatinine, bilirubin, AST, ALT, alkaline phosphatase, total protein, albumin and fasting serum gastrin levels at baseline, 2, 4, 6, 12 months and then every 6 months.

Before treatment with omeprazole, baseline 24-h intraesophageal pH study was done in 10 patients. In all patients, repeat 24-h intraesophageal pH studies were performed to monitor the degree of acid suppression during omeprazole therapy. In

Table 1. Clinical features of 15 children with refractory esophagitis studied on omeprazole

Patient number	Age (years)	Sex	Gastrointestinal problems	Associated medical condition
1	0.75	M	Hiatal hernia	—
2	2.5	F	Hiatal hernia. G-tube feeding	Cerebral palsy, quadriplegia, seizures
3	4.75	M	Hiatal hernia	—
4	4.5	M	Hiatal hernia	Cerebral palsy secondary to kernicterus, seizures
5	5.25	F	Hiatal hernia. J-tube feeding	Multiple congenital anomalies, delayed development, cleft lip and palate, dysplastic kidneys, renal failure
6	5.75	M	Hiatal hernia	Protracted severe entero-colitis on TPN
7	6.75	F	Hiatal hernia, failed fundoplication, pyloroplasty	Mild gross motor delay
8	6.9	F	T.E. fistula, esophageal atresia, failed fundoplication × 2	—
9	7.9	F	T.E. fistula, esophageal atresia	Portal vein thrombosis, ventricular septal defect
10	8.9	M	Hiatal hernia, failed fundoplication, resection of esophageal stenosis and anastomosis. G-tube feeding	Cornelia-de-Lange syndrome
11	10.25	F	Hiatal hernia. G-tube feeding	Cerebral palsy, seizures
12	11.25	M	Hiatal hernia, failed fundoplication × 2	—
13	14.25	F	Hiatal hernia	Happy Puppet syndrome, seizures
14	14.25	M	Hiatal hernia. Barrett's esophagus. J-tube feeding	Cystic fibrosis
15	17.8	M	Hiatal hernia. Barrett's esophagus. Esophagectomy for multifocal adenocarcinoma of esophagus, gastroesophageal anastomosis. J-tube feeding.	Cerebral palsy

patients with hiatal hernia, care was taken to place the probe 13% above the LES (by convention) [10], as distinct from the more distal diaphragmatic pinchcock, as determined by manometry [11]. Normal value for pH study was ≤6% total time at pH < 4.0 [10].

In patients older than 3 years of age, the starting dose of omeprazole was 20 mg in the morning, which was the smallest capsule commercially available (Astra Hässle, Mölndal, Sweden). Arbitrarily, the starting dose in children less than 3 years of age was omeprazole 10 mg. In patients who could not swallow the gelatin (i.e., enteric coated) capsule whole, it was opened and the granular contents given, according to the manufacturer's instructions, in a weakly acidic vehicle such as orange juice, cranberry juice or yogurt to the fasting patient. Instructions were given that the granules in the vehicle should be swallowed and not chewed. The granules themselves are degraded in the neutral or alkaline pH of the esophagus, but are resistant to gastric acid, therefore when given through gastrostomy tubes, the granules were given in one of the same vehicles. In patients receiving 10 mg, half the granular contents of the capsule were given in the same way. In one patient with renal failure, the granules were dissolved in 5 ml of sodium bicarbonate [12] and given immediately through her jejunostomy tube, according to the manufacturer's instructions.

Twenty-four-hour intraesophageal pH study was repeated after the patient had been receiving omeprazole for 5 days, as maximum acid suppression has occurred and stabilized by that time [12]. If pathologic acid reflux was still present on pH study, the dose was titrated upward until a repeat pH study 5 days after the new dose showed total time pH < 4.0 to be <6%. If adequate daytime acid reflux control was present, but nocturnal reflux was still present during the dose titration, the additional dose was given in the evening. In this way, the adequacy of dosage and timing of dosage in each child were determined by forcetitrating the dose against intraesophageal pH studies.

In nine patients, the starting dose of omeprazole was increased until the pH study was normal before the first follow-up (FU) endoscopy at 2—3 months (FU#1). In the other 6, follow-up pH study was done when the patients were seen for FU#1 at 2—3 months because they lived at a distance from the medical center.

Results

Dose and efficacy

After titrating the dose of omeprazole upward against 24-h intraesophageal pH studies, the dose of omeprazole required to control acid reflux (pH time < 4.0 ≤ 6%) was 20—40 mg (0.7—3.3 mg/kg) in 11 patients, 10 mg in one patient (0.7 mg/kg) and 60 mg (1.9—2.4 mg/kg) in three patients. For the group, the effective dosage range was 0.7—3.3 mg/kg/day (mean 1.9 mg/kg/day).

Symptoms and signs were absent in 70—100% of patients by the time of first follow-up at 2—3 months (FU#1) and all patients were free of symptoms and signs at the second follow-up (FU#2) at 4—6 months from the start of omeprazole therapy (Table 2). Not only were the gastrointestinal features of reflux improved, but persistent and recurrent coughing and wheezing resolved in the 10 patients with these symptoms at presentation. Furthermore, weight velocity improved in all patients.

Pretreatment (baseline) 24-h intraesophageal pII studies showed pH < 4 for 11—88% of monitored time (normal ≤6%) [10]. The last study in each patient was that which showed esophageal acid exposure within the normal range during omeprazole therapy (Fig. 1).

After 3 months of omeprazole treatment (FU#1), six patients had improved from grade II—III esophagitis to grade 0, four patients had improved from grades III—IV to

Table 2. Symptoms and signs pretreatment and at follow-ups

	Baseline	Follow-up #1 (2–3 months)	Follow up #2 (4–6 months)
Vomiting	13	3	0
Chronic respiratory symptoms (coughing, wheezing)	10	3	0
Irritability	8	0	0
Hematemesis	8	1	0
Heartburn	4	0	0
Abnormal weight velocity	11	2	0

Numbers represent the number of patients with that symptom at each evaluation time.

I–II and five patients had no change from grades II–III. After 6 months (FU#2), of the nine patients who had endoscopy, two improved to grade 0 from I, five improved from grade II to grade I and one from grade IV to grade I. One patient had persistent grade I esophagitis, but was asymptomatic with a normal pH on omeprazole therapy. In other words, by 6 months, esophagitis had improved to grade 0 or I in all patients endoscoped (Fig. 2).

Safety

All 15 patients received omeprazole continuously for periods of 5.5–26 months (mean 12.2 months). No major adverse effects were noted. Seven patients had elevations of

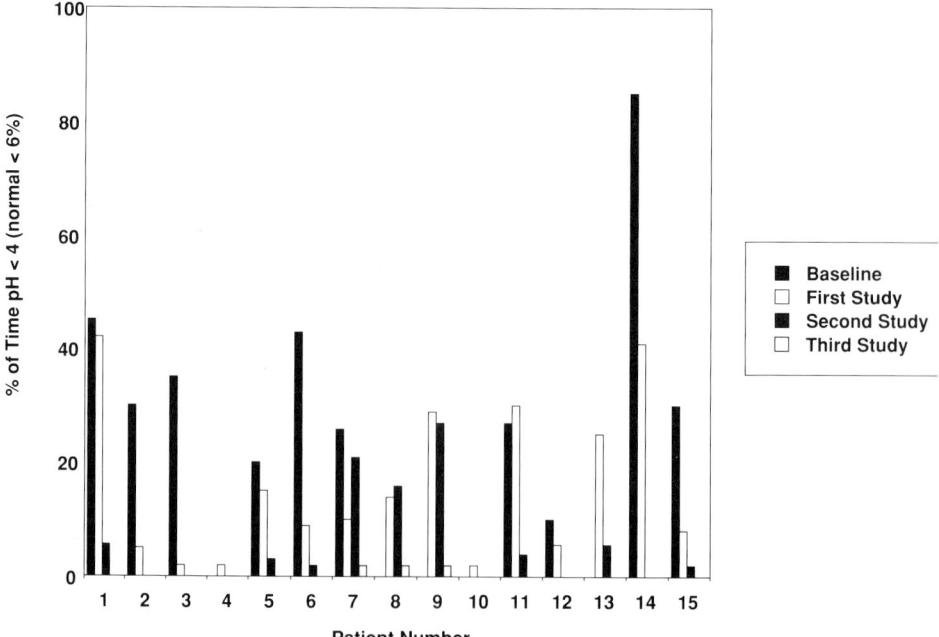

Fig. 1. Changes in 24-h intraesophageal pH studies with omeprazole treatment. Patient numbers correspond to Table 1. Normal range of <6% for time pH < 4 is from Ref. 10.

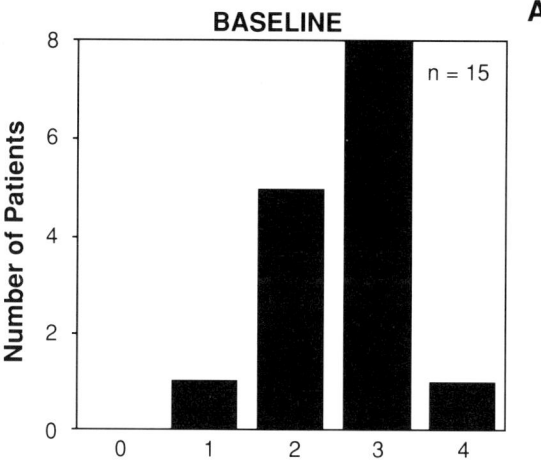

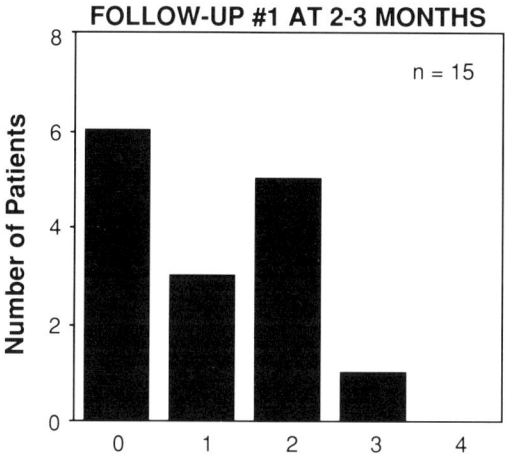

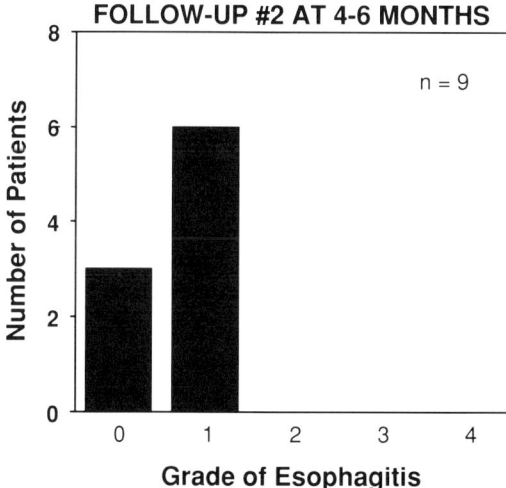

Fig. 2. Grades of esophagitis (0–IV) pretreatment and on omeprazole therapy. A–C show the progressive improvement in grades of esophagitis from baseline values. Esophagitis was graded according to Hetzel et al. [2]. Six patients had complete healing of esophagitis (grade 0) by follow-up #1 and were not re-endoscoped, therefore only 9/15 patients had repeat endoscopy at follow-up #2.

aminotransferase (AST and ALT) values to up to twice normal which were nonprogressive or returned to normal after medication was stopped. Hair loss was reported in one patient after she had been receiving omeprazole for 12 months. This was diagnosed as "telogen effluvium" by a pediatric dermatologist, who considered that omeprazole was unlikely the cause as her hair regrew despite continuing omeprazole at the same dose.

Two patients had elevated fasting serum gastrin levels before starting omeprazole; one had chronic renal failure and the other short bowel syndrome, both recognized causes of hypergastrinemia [13]. In both of these patients, gastrin levels rose further during omeprazole therapy and returned to normal after discontinuation. Three others had elevated gastrin levels within 6 months of starting omeprazole and six patients had elevations after 6 months. In all, 11 patients had hypergastrinemia during omeprazole therapy and four had normal levels. In six of the patients with hypergastrinemia, fasting levels of gastrin 400–700 ng/l were present (upper limit of normal 130 ng/l).

Course

Seven patients are continuing on omeprazole therapy. In eight patients administration of omeprazole was stopped and they were treated as follows: 2 neurologically normal patients underwent fundoplication when the esophagitis was healed; one underwent fundoplication as he had pulmonary aspiration despite previous improvement in esophagitis and resolution of pulmonary symptoms; two had fundoplications because of medication noncompliance; one had pyloroplasty for delayed gastric emptying, and one was switched to cisapride after esophagitis healed. One patient with cystic fibrosis died of pneumonia unrelated to omeprazole therapy.

Discussion

The complications of GE reflux in children are well recognized [14] and include failure to thrive, anemia, pulmonary disease, esophagitis, stricture, Barrett's esophagus [15] and rarely, esophageal adenocarcinoma [16]. Also recognized is that neurologically impaired children, such as many in this study, and children with cystic fibrosis, have an increased predilection to reflux and its complications [14–22], related to a variety of underlying abnormalities. Fundoplication is often highly effective treatment for GER that is refractory to other measures [23–26]. However, even in neurologically normal children, this surgery is usually followed by some undesirable sequelae [27] and there are treatment failures [23,28]. Neurologically-impaired children are usually placed at high risk by such surgery; morbidity and mortality related to antireflux surgery is considerable in these patients [26,28–32], with operative failure rates of 25–28% [28,32] and complication rates up to 59% [26]. A surgical wrap of the lower end of the esophagus in a patient with poor esophageal motility and clearance is attended by the risk of esophageal obstruction by food or secretions, with possible aspiration of esophageal contents.

Many of the children in this study were neurologically impaired and others had major medical problems which placed them at high risk for morbidity or failure of antireflux surgery (e.g., poor esophageal motility due to esophageal atresia). Children with cystic fibrosis are also often placed at high risk by surgical procedures. Due to the failure of H_2 antagonists, prokinetic agents, and surgery in some cases, a trial of omeprazole appeared to be the best therapeutic option for these children.

Reflux esophagitis is due to abnormal reflux of usually acid contents into the esophagus. Therefore we aimed to find the dose of omeprazole necessary to abolish pathologic acid reflux by titrating the dose upward against 24-h intraesophageal studies. That only an 84% improvement in symptoms and signs occurred at 2—3 months could reflect a suboptimal dosage of omeprazole; some patients living at a distance from the medical center could return for repeat pH studies and increase of dose only a few weeks after initial evaluation. The same explanation could apply to the endoscopic follow-up (i.e., quicker resolution of esophagitis might have occurred with more aggressive therapy). The mean effective dose of drug for the group, (1.9 mg/kg/day) appears to be high relative to doses given in adults, in whom a total dose of 20—40 mg daily is usually used. However, 60% of the patients had grade III or IV esophagitis, a group in which "usual" doses of omeprazole in adults have a poor healing rate [2].

In clinical trials of short-term tolerability (<12 weeks), side effects of dyspepsia, flatulence, headache, diarrhea, nausea, abdominal pain, dizziness, fatigue and constipation have occurred in 1—6%, an incidence comparable to that found with ranitidine, cimetidine or placebo [3]. None of these side effects were encountered in our patients, even in the nonhandicapped patients. Minor changes in transaminase values, as occurred in some of our patients and minor changes in hematologic values have been reported but they have been nonprogressive, or normalized on stopping or continuing omeprazole [2,3]. No effects of omeprazole on renal function have been documented in adults or animal studies [3]. Even a patient with renal failure had unchanged values of urea, creatinine and GFR during omeprazole therapy for 7 months. Isolated side effects noted have been peripheral neuropathy, painful gynecomastia, skin rash including lichenoid eruptions, Coombs positive hemolytic anemia and one case of hepatic failure [33].

The tolerability of omeprazole for long-term treatment is an issue of importance, because esophagitis and its complications recur after withdrawal of omeprazole [2]; many patients may require the medication for months, years or indefinitely. In this regard, the issue of hypergastrinemia is important. Omeprazole and high doses of H_2 antagonists may cause profound suppression of gastric acid secretion, resulting in high circulating levels of gastrin, a trophic hormone [3,34]. Some rats given massive doses of omeprazole (14 mg/kg/day) or ranitidine (2 g/day), developed hyperplasia and carcinoids of enterochromaffin-like cells (ECL) (argyrophil cells) of the gastric body as an end-life phenomenon [34]. This was likely due to lifelong sustained hypergastrinemia, as omeprazole itself and its metabolites are nongenotoxic [35]. However, the rat model may not be applicable to humans because of species differences in the nature of ECL cells and their response to gastrin and the duration and doses per kg of omeprazole [34]. With regard to ECL cells, gastric body biopsies from adult humans treated with omeprazole 20–40 mg daily for up to 7 years have shown no qualitative changes beyond hyperplasia [3,34,36]. This information, together with the absence of dysplasia or neoplasia, is reassuring. However, as "developing beings", children may respond differently to the trophic effects of hypergastrinemia and our study patients received larger doses on a per kg basis than adults. More recently, two additional findings have been reported. True gastric polyps developed in four of 11 adults treated with omeprazole 20–40 mg daily for a year [37]. In another study, a retrospective analysis showed pseudohypertrophy of parietal cells in 93% of 198 patients receiving omeprazole [38]. These are preliminary, uncontrolled findings, again without any evidence of malignancy, but they suggest that careful prospective long-term studies in children are warranted.

We conclude that omeprazole is effective for treatment of severe, refractory GE reflux in children. Omeprazole therapy may be an excellent therapeutic alternative to antireflux surgery in children with severe esophagitis or other complications of GE reflux who are at high risk for failure or complications of such surgery, or for children in whom antireflux surgery has failed. The effective dosage range for healing in children is wide; the starting dose should be 0.7 mg/kg/day in a single morning dose and the required dose should be determined by repeated 24-h intraesophageal pH study. A maintenance dose for children also needs to be established. Omeprazole appears to be safe for short-term use, but long-term safety in children should be established by studies in larger numbers of children and by long-term correlation of gastrin levels with gastric histology. Such a study is currently in progress.

Acknowledgements

The authors appreciate the secretarial expertise of Kerrie Glover, the assistance of Barbara Ettinger RN, Head Endoscopy Nurse and Kathi Kinsey RN, GI Nurse Clinician.

References

1. Blum AL. Treatment of acid-related disorders with gastric acid inhibitors: the state of the art. Digestion 1990;47(suppl 1): 3–10.
2. Hetzel DJ, Dent J, Reed WD et al. Healing and relapse of severe peptic esophagitis after treatment with omeprazole. Gastroenterology 1988;95:903–912.
3. McTavish D, Buckley MT, Heel RC. Omeprazole. An updated review of its pharmacology and therapeutic use in acid-related disorders. Drugs 1991;42:138–170.
4. Dent J. Australian clinical trials of omeprazole in the management of reflux esophagitis. Digestion 1990;47(suppl 1):69–71.
5. Sontag SJ, Hirschowitz BI, Holt S et al. Two doses of omeprazole vs. placebo in symptomatic erosive esophagitis: the U.S. multicenter study. Gastroenterology 1992;102:109–118.
6. Karjoo M, Kane RE. Omeprazole treatment in children with peptic esophagitis refractory to ranitidine. Gastroenterology 1992;102:A93.
7. Kato S, Shibuya H, Hayashi Y et al. Effectiveness and pharmacokinetics of omeprazole in children with refractory duodenal ulcer. J Pediatr Gastroenterol Nutr 1992;15:184–188.
8. De Giacomo C, Fiocca R, Villani L et al. Omeprazole treatment of severe peptic disease associated with antral G cell hyperfunction and hyperpepsinogenemia in an infant. J Pediatr 1990;117:989–993.
9. Gunasekaran TS, Hassall E. Efficacy and safety of omeprazole for severe gastroesophageal reflux in children. J Pediatr 1993 (in press).

10. Sondheimer JM. Continuous monitoring of distal esophageal pH: a diagnostic test for gastroesophageal reflux in infants. J Pediatr 1980;96:804—807.

11. Euler AR, Ament ME. Value of esophageal manometric studies in the gastroesophageal reflux of infancy. Pediatrics 1977; 60:59—61.

12. Andersson T. Pharmacokinetics of omeprazole in man. (Monograph). Mölndal: University of Göteborg Press, 1991:8—9.

13. Straus E, Gerson CD, Yalow RS. Hypersecretion of gastrin associated with short bowel syndrome. Gastroenterology 1974; 66:175—180.

14. Boyle JT. Gastroesophageal reflux in the pediatric patient. Gastroenterol Clin North Am 1989;18:315—337.

15. Hassall E. Barrett's esophagus: new definitions and approaches in children. J Pediatr Gastroenterol Nutr 1993;16:345—364.

16. Hassall E. Adenocarcinoma in childhood Barrett's esophagus. Am J Gastroenterol 1993;88:282—288.

17. Sondheimer JM, Morris BA. Gastroesophageal reflux among severely retarded children. J Pediatr 1979;94:710—714.

18. Snyder JD, Goldman H. Barrett's esophagus in children and young adults: frequent association with mental retardation. Dig Dis Sci 1990;10:185—189.

19. Byrne WJ, Campbell M, Ashcraft E et al. A diagnostic approach to vomiting in severely retarded patients. Am J Dis Child 1983;137:259—262.

20. Orenstein SR, Orenstein DM. Gastroesophageal reflux and respiratory disease in children. J Pediatr 1988;12:847—858.

21. Cucchiara S, Santamaria F, Andreotti MR et al. Mechanisms of gastroesophageal reflux in cystic fibrosis. Arch Dis Child 1991;66:617—622.

22. Hassall E, Israel DM, Davidson AGF, Wong LTK. Barrett's esophagus in children with cystic fibrosis: not a coincidental association. Am J Gastroenterol (in press).

23. Fonkalsrud EW, Foglia RP, Ament ME et al. Operative treatment for the gastroesophageal reflux syndrome in children. J Pediatr Surg 1989;24:525—529.

24. Jolley SG, Herbst JJ, Johnson DG et al. Surgery in children with gastroesophageal reflux and respiratory symptoms. J Pediatr 1980;96:194—198.

25. Hassall E, Weinstein WM. Partial regression of childhood Barrett's esophagus after fundoplication. Am J Gastroenterol 1992;87:1506—1512.

26. Byrne WJ, Euler AR, Ashcraft E et al. Gastroesophageal reflux in the severely retarded who vomit: criteria for and results of surgical intervention in 22 patients. Surgery 1982;91:95—98.

27. Harnsberger JK, Corey JJ, Johnson DG, Herbst JJ. Long-term follow-up of surgery for gastroesophageal reflux in infants and children. J Pediatr 1983;102:505—508.

28. Pearl RH, Robie DK, Ein SH et al. Complications of gastroesophageal antireflux surgery in neurologically impaired versus neurologically normal children. J Pediatr Surg 1990;25:1169—1173.

29. Caniano DA, Ginn-Pease ME, King DR. The failed antireflux procedure: analysis of risk factors and morbidity. J Pediatr Surg 1990;25:1022—1026.

30. Jakaite D, Gourley GR, Pellett JR. Erosions of the Angelchik prosthesis in pediatric sized developmentally disabled patients. J Pediatr Gastroenterol Nutr 1991;13:186—191.

31. Spitz L, Kirtane J. Results and complications of surgery for gastroesophageal reflux. Arch Dis Child 1985;60:743—747.

32. Martinez DA, Ginn-Pease ME, Caniano DA. Sequelae of antireflux surgery in profoundly disabled children. J Pediatr Surg 1992;27:267—273.

33. Jochem V, Kirkpatrick R, Greenson J et al. Fulminant hepatic failure related to omeprazole. Am J Gastroenterol 1992;87: 523—525.

34. Berlin RG. Gastrin and gastric endocrine cell data from clinical studies. Dig Dis Sci 1991;36:129—136.

35. Sachs G, Scott D, Reuben M. Omeprazole and the gastric mucosa. Digestion 1990;47(suppl 1):35—38.

36. Lamberts R, Creutzfeldt W, Struber HG, Brunner G, Solcia E. Long-term omeprazole therapy in peptic ulcer disease: gastrin, endocrine cell growth, and gastritis. Gastroenterology 1993;104:1356—1370.

37. Graham JR. Omeprazole and gastric polyposis in humans. Gastroenterology 1993;104:1584.

38. Stolte M, Bethke B, Rühl G, Ritter Omeprazole-induced pseudohypertrophy of gastric parietal cells. M. Z Gastroenterol 1992;30:134—138.

493

In relation to antisecretory agents, what is the proper place of prokinetics in maintenance therapy of reflux?

G.N.J. Tytgat (Amsterdam)

Gastroesophageal reflux disease (GERD) is a chronic relapsing disease for many patients. Symptomatic relapse within 6 months occurs in 40–60% of patients [1]. Endoscopic relapse rates vary widely from 20–82% [2–8]. The high values correspond to patients with severe erosive/ulcerative reflux esophagitis. The usual relapse figures for milder reflux disease vary from 20–36% [1,5].

It is usually stated that mild to moderate lesions most often do not progress over the course of a few years. However, there are exceptions. According to Brossard et al. [9], more severe reflux disease or complications may occur in a third of the patients over the course of 6.5 years of follow-up. Also Schindlbeck et al. [10] found that half of their patients failed to improve, or deteriorated, over 3 years even with medical therapy. As the aims of therapy in GERD include alleviation of symptoms, healing of lesions and prevention of recurrent disease and complications, it would follow that for many patients prolonged medical therapy may be necessary.

Usefulness of prokinetics as maintenance therapy in GERD and reflux esophagitis

Three double-blind trials [6–8] investigated the efficacy of cisapride on the relapse rate after prior healing with antisecretory therapy [6,8] or with cisapride [7].

In the study by Toussaint et al. [7] patients were first healed with cisapride and then treated with 10 mg cisapride b.i.d. versus placebo maintenance therapy. The 6 months symptomatic and endoscopic relapse rates were 20% for cisapride versus 39% for placebo (p = 0.06). The duration of remission tended to be longer for patients with initially milder degrees of esophagitis.

The EUROCIS-trial [6] involved 443 patients with moderate to severe reflux esophagitis who had been healed with prior antisecretory drugs. The majority of the patients were healed initially with H_2-receptor antagonists (H_2-RA) and only 5% received omeprazole. The endoscopic relapse rates at 12 months were 32% for cisapride 10 mg nocte (p = 0.005); 34% for cisapride 10 mg b.i.d. (p = 0.002) and 51% for placebo.

The SCANEDCIS-trial [8] evaluated maintenance treatment with cisapride or placebo over a 6 months period in 298 patients whose reflux esophagitis had been healed with an antisecretory agent. The design of the SCANEDCIS-study was such that equal numbers of patients with grades I, II and III esophagitis were included. Omeprazole was used as healing therapy in 15%, 29% and 54% of patients with grades I, II and III respectively. Of the omeprazole users, no less than 40% received the drug after being unsuccessfully treated with courses of H_2-RAs. Cisapride 20 mg b.i.d. significantly prolonged the time to endoscopic relapse in patients with grade I esophagitis (p = 0.02) and when all patients were combined (p = 0.01). No significant difference between cisapride and placebo was demonstrated for patients with initial grades II and III even though the duration of remission in those patients was 50% longer in the cisapride treated group.

The net therapeutic gain with cisapride can be estimated from these studies at 35–49% in patients with less severe disease and at 10% in a selected population with severe recalcitrant esophagitis. Presumably those patients with GERD who are most likely to respond to prolonged prokinetic therapy include those with mild/moderate disease which responds to H_2-RAs, patients with poor clearing capacity and patients with predominant supine reflux. Yet this has not been established by prospective studies.

Indications for prokinetics in the long-term management of reflux disease

Many algorithms for the long-term management of reflux disease have been published over the last few years. The strategy for long-term treatment of GERD was also the subject of a Working Party [11]. In that study the patients were graded according to severity of reflux disease.

For patients with mild reflux disease, characterized by intermittent reflux symptoms in the absence of mucosal damage, the recommendations centered around implementing lifestyle changes and advising chronic or intermittent therapy with standard dose H_2-RAs or standard dose cisapride. If symptoms improved, reducing the dose was to be attempted, symptoms permitting. It should be realized that this therapeutic strategy has not been evaluated prospectively.

For patients with moderate disease, characterized by more severe recurrent reflux symptoms and/or evidence of mild to moderate erosive esophagitis (solitary or confluent erosions), recommendations centered again around lifestyle modifications and prolonged, if not permanent, therapy with standard dose H_2-RAs or standard dose cisapride. If such therapeutic regimen failed or if symptom suppression was insufficient, long-term therapy with a reduced dose of a pump inhibitor would now be considered to be adequate.

For patients with severe disease, characterized by more severe reflux symptoms or severe reflux esophagitis with confluent erosions or complications and certainly if symptoms proved to be recalcitrant and rather difficult to suppress with other therapies, the advice was to treat those patients with intensifying the lifestyle changes and providing prolonged, if not permanent therapy, with a proton pump inhibitor (PPI), initially in the standard dose and, symptoms and endoscopy permitting, later on a lower dose. In case of intolerance to a PPI, high dose of an H_2-RA together with cisapride could be considered as an alternative. Again proof for the latter statement is essentially lacking.

Concluding remarks

Although inhibition of gastric secretion is currently the mainstay of treatment, improving the competence of the antireflux barrier, improving esophageal clearing capacity, accelerating gastric emptying when delayed and preventing duodenogastric reflux can also be regarded as a valid, physiological way of reducing gastroesophageal reflux. Cisapride has the potential to improve the disturbed motor functions in GERD. Thereby it is capable of relieving symptoms, healing mild/moderate lesions and preventing relapse except in patients with severe recalcitrant disease.

References

1. Bell NJV, Hunt RH. Role of gastric acid suppression in the treatment of gastro-oesophageal reflux disease. Gut 1992;33: 118–124.
2. Hetzel DJ, Dent J, Reed WD et al. Healing and relapse of severe peptic esophagitis after treatment with omeprazole. Gastroenterology 1988;95:903–912.
3. Ottenjann R, Siewert JR, Heilmann K et al. Treatment of reflux esophagitis. In: Siewert JR, Holscher AH (eds) Diseases of the esophagus. Berlin: Springer, 1987;1123–1125.
4. Koelz HR, Birchler R, Bretholz A et al. Healing and relapse of reflux esophagitis during treatment with ranitidine. Gastroenterology 1986;91:1198–1205.
5. Barbara L, Baldi F, Longanesi A et al. Long-term maintenance of healed esophagitis. In: Scarpignato C (ed) Advances in Drug Therapy of Gastroesophageal Reflux Disease. Frontiers in Gastrointestinal Research, vol 20. Basel: Karger, 1992;356–364.
6. Blum AL, Adami B, Bouzo MH et al. Effect of cisapride on relapse of esophagitis. A multinational, placebo-controlled trial in patients healed with an antisecretory drug. Dig Dis Sci 1993;38:551–560.
7. Toussaint J, Gossuin A, Deruyttere M et al. Healing and prevention of relapse of reflux oesophagitis by cisapride. Gut 1991;32:1280–1285.
8. Tytgat GNJ, Anker Hansen OJ, Carling L et al. Effect of cisapride on relapse of reflux oesophagitis healed with an antisecretory drug. Scand J Gastroenterol 1992;27:175–183.
9. Brossard E, Monnier Ph, Ollyo JB et al. Serious complications — stenosis, ulcer and Barrett's epithelium — develop in 21.6% of adults with erosive reflux esophagitis. Gastroenterology 1991;100:A36.
10. Schindlbeck N, Klauser AG, Berghammer G et al. Three-year follow-up of gastroesophageal reflux disease. Gastroenterology 1991;100:A156.
11. Tytgat GNJ, Bianchi Porro G, Feussner H, Pace F, Richter JE, Siewert JR. Long-term strategy for the treatment of gastro-oesophageal reflux disease. Working Team Report. Gastroenterol Int 1991;4:21–32.

Is recurrent esophagitis always symptomatic?

G. Bommelaer (Clermont-Ferrand)

The occurrence of esophagitis of any grade of severity, without any symptom has been documented for years by several authors [1–3].

Moreover, since the discovery of H_2-receptors antagonists (H_2-RA), it is well known that it is possible to alleviate the symptoms of esophagitis in spite of a persistence of mucosal endoscopic lesions [4]. It is therefore not surprising that after complete healing of an esophagitis, an endoscopic relapse could occur without any symptoms. Very few studies however, have specifically addressed this question. Information comes mostly from therapeutic trials comparing H_2 antagonists or proton pump inhibitors (PPI) and placebo in maintenance treatment trials [4–6]. Still, in several such studies, endoscopy was performed only when symptoms recurred, so that asymptomatic recurrences were not assessed [4,5]. On the other hand, some studies which included a systematic endoscopic control several months after healing, do not specify whether the endoscopic recurrences were symptomatic or not [4].

Koelz, in a trial comparing ranitidine 150 mg/day versus placebo in a randomized double-blind maintenance trial, reported one asymptomatic out of 12 recurrences in the ranitidine group and four out of 13 recurrences in the placebo group [7]. Lundell, in his series, reported two asymptomatic recurrences out of 11 in the omeprazole group and two out of 14 in the ranitidine group [6]. In a study on the effects of cisapride on relapse of reflux esophagitis, Tytgat reported that in 77% of all endoscopic relapses, recurrence of symptoms was seen as well, meaning that as much as 23% of recurrences were asymptomatic. The symptom-lesion relationships were similar in the cisapride and placebo group [8]. Accordingly, asymptomatic recurrences of formerly healed esophagitis can occur, either under maintenance treatment or not.

This does not preclude a certain relationship between the severity of symptoms and the risk of endoscopic relapse. It has thus been shown that recurrences are more frequent and more rapid in patients remaining symptomatic after healing of their esophagitis, whether the treatment was medical or surgical [7,9].

References

1. Akdamar K, Ertan A, Agrawal NM, McMahon FG, Ryan J. Upper gastrointestinal endoscopy in normal asymptomatic volunteers. Gastrointest Endosc 1986;32:78–80.
2. Dedieu P, Gaillard F, Lavignolle A, Sugier H, Gibon M, Daveluy P, Perrin D, Miniconi P. Oesophagites par reflux: aspects épidémiologiques, anatomo-pathologiques et évolutifs (123 cas). Gastroenterol Clin Biol 1981;5:266–274.
3. Zeitoun P, Carteret E. Natural history of reflux esophagitis in adults. In: Mignon M, Galmiche JP, (eds) Control of Acid Secretion. Paris: John Libbey Eurotext, 1986:225–238.
4. Sontag SJ. The medical management of reflux esophagitis. Role of antacids and acid inhibition. Gastroent Clin North Am 1990;19:683–712.
5. Hetzel DJ, Dent J, Reed WD, Narielvala FM, MacKinnon M. Healing and relapse of severe peptic esophagitis after treatment with omeprazole. Gastroenterology 1988;95:903–912.
6. Lundell L, Backman L, Ekström P, Enander LK, Falkner S, Fausa O, Grimelius L, Havu N, Lind T, Lönroth H, Sandmark S, Sandzen B, Unge P, Westin IH. Prevention of relapse of reflux esophagitis after endoscopic healing: the efficacy and safety of omeprazole compared with ranitidine. Scand J Gastroenterol 1991;26:248–256.
7. Koelz HR, Birchler R, Bretholz A, Bron B, Capitaine Y, Delmore G, Fehr HF, Fumagalli I, Gehrig J, Gonvers JJ, Halter F, Hammer B, Kayasseh L, Kobler E, Miller G, Munst G, Pelloni S, Realini S, Schmid P, Voirol M, Blum A. Healing and relapse of reflux esophagitis during treatment with ranitidine. Gastroenterology 1986;91:1198–1205.
8. Tytgat GN, Anker Hansen OJ, Carling L, de Groot GH, Geldof H, Glise H, Efskind P, Elsborg L, Karvonen AL, Ohlin B, Solhaug OH, Vermeersch B. Effect of cisapride on relapse of reflux esophagitis, healed with an antisecretory drug. Scand J Gastroenterol 1992;27:175–183.
9. Spechler SJ and the Department of Veterans Affairs Gastroesophageal Reflux Disease Study Group. Comparison of medical and surgical therapy for complicated gastroesophageal reflux disease in veterans. N Engl J Med 1992;326:786–792.

May bacterial treatment directed against *Helicobacter pylori* have an effect on relapse in the small group of antritis due to *H. pylori* combined with reflux?

R.W. McCallum, J. Sarosiek (Charlottesville)

Although the role of esophageal motility impairment and incompetence of the lower esophageal sphincter (LES) in the development of reflux esophagitis (RE) seem to be well established, the pathogenesis of this continuously challenging disease still remains not entirely understood. Detailed analysis of the natural history of RE, its resistance to the treatment with acid suppressing drugs, very high relapse rate despite maintenance therapy, even with proton pump inhibitors, indicates that other factors than acid and pepsin may play the pathogenetic role as well [1–3].

It is generally known that gastroesophageal reflux disease (GERD) quite frequently coexists with a duodenal ulcer (DU) [4]. Since in over 95% of patients with DU *Helicobacter pylori* remains as a causative factor, one may assume that the development reflux-related esophageal mucosal pathology could also be related to this micro-organism.

Among various aggressive factors synthesized and released by this micro-organism (Table 1), the leading damaging potential is frequently assigned to the protease with a strong mucolytic potential [5–8] and phospholipase A_2 [9]. Recently, evidence has been accumulated that ammonia, generated by *H. pylori* due to release of a strong urealytic enzyme, urease, could also significantly affect the metabolism and growth of the gastric mucosal cells in the culture [10,11]. Furthermore, some recent data also indicate that this micro-organism exhibits an ability to elaborate cytotoxins [12,13] and a potent proinflammatory mediator-platelet aggregating factor (PAF) [14].

Insight into the prevalence of *H. pylori* among populations with symptomatology related to GERD provides also some evidence supporting the claim that this micro-organism may contribute to the natural history of reflux esophagitis in a significant fashion. In a retrospective study, McCallum et al. [15] demonstrated that 75% of patients with symptomatic RE (confirmed by histology and/or endoscopy) had evidence of active gastritis as compared to 10% of the normal healthy volunteers (p < 0.005). Sixty percent of RE patients had *H. pylori* identified in a Giemsa stain,

Table 1. Damaging factors elaborated by *H. pylori*

Damaging factor	Reference
Proteases	[5–8]
Phospholipase A_2	[9]
Ammonia	[10,11]
Cytotoxins	[12,13]
PAF	[14]

compared with 5% of the normals (p < 0.02). In another study, Borkent et al. [16] have been able to culture *H. pylori* from esophageal mucosal biopsy specimens in 40% of patients with erosive esophagitis. In 29% of patients with Barrett's mucosa *H. pylori* was isolated from the esophageal mucosa by Walker et al. [17]. Moreover, *H. pylori* was found significantly more frequently (p < 0.05) in stomachs of patients with Barrett's mucosa than in patients with reflux esophagitis not accompanied by intestinal metaplasia within the esophageal mucosal compartment. Also the presence of micro-organisms well correlated with severity of esophagitis [18]. However, an association between *H. pylori* and nonendoscopic (histological only) reflux esophagitis has not been demonstrated [19].

Significant support of proposed hypothetical impact of *H. pylori* colonization within the gastroduodenal compartment on the development of RE could also be found in the literature related to the treatment of endoscopic reflux esophagitis (Table 2). The treatment of erosive reflux esophagitis, cimetidine (800 mg at night) accompanied by bismuth, appeared to be superior to cimetidine alone (p < 0.001) [20].

Table 2. An impact of suppression of *H. pylori* colonization on the outcome of RE treatment[a]

Treatment regimen	Cimetidine (800 mg at night)	Cimetidine and colloidal bismuth (CB) (800 mg at night and CB 120 mg q.i.d.)
Grade of esophagitis		
A) Before therapy		
IV	2	0
III	8	10
B) After therapy; 3 weeks		
IV	0	0
III	6	0
II	3	0
I	1	3

[a]Borkent et al. [20].

In summary, although squamous epithelium, unlike Barrett's mucosa, does not support an attachment and growth of *H. pylori* within the esophageal mucosal compartment, frequent reflux episodes may enormously expose the esophageal epithelium to all *H. pylori*-related enzymes and toxins, present in the gastroesophageal refluxate. Furthermore, even transient presence of *H. pylori* micro-organisms within the esophageal lumen after each reflux episode may further enhance an accumulation of *H. pylori*-related enzymes and toxins on the surface of the esophageal mucosa. Therefore, the potential pathogenetic role of this micro-organism in subsets of patients, especially with erosive and refractory RE, should not be underestimated. In patients with refractory RE (e.g., relapsing while on a standard 20 mg daily dose of omeprazole) the colonization with *H. pylori* should be tested and may result in modification of the treatment regimen. Further vigorous research in this area is worthwhile, including consideration of a trial implementing *H. pylori* eradication.

References

1. Dodds WJ, Dent J, Hogan WJ, Helm JF, Hauser R, Patel GK, Egide MS. Mechanisms of gastroduod nal reflux in patients with reflux esophagitis. N Engl J Med 1982;307:1547−1552.
2. Dodds WJ, Hogan WJ, Helm JF, Dent J. Pathogenesis of esophagitis. Gastroenterology 1981;81:376−394.
3. Hetzel DJ, Dent J, Reed WD, Narielvala FM, MacKinnon M, McCarthy JH, Mitchell B, Beveridge BR, Laurence BH, Gibson GG, Grant AK, Shearman DJC, Whitehead R, Buckle PJ. Healing and relapse of severe peptic esophagitis after treatment with omeprazole. Gastroenterology 1988;95:903−912.
4. Flook D, Stoddard CJ. Gastro-oesophageal reflux and esophagitis before and after vagotomy for duodenal ulcer. Br J Surg 1985;72:804−807.
5. Baxter A, Campbell CJ, Cox DM, Grinham CJ, Pendlebury JE. Proteolytic activities of human Campylobacter pylori and ferret gastric Campylobacter-like organism. Biochem Biophys Res Commun 1989;163:1−7.
6. Sarosiek J, Slomiany A, Slomiany BL. Evidence for weakening of gastric mucus integrity by Campylobacter pylori. Scand J Gastroenterol 1988;23:585−590.
7. Slomiany BL, Bilski J, Sarosiek J, Murty VL, Dworkin B, VanHorn K, Zielenski J, Slomiany A. Campylobacter pyloridis degrades mucin and undermines gastric mucosal integrity. Biochem Biophys Res Commun 1987;144:307−314.
8. Sarosiek J, Peura DA, Guerrant RL, Marshall BJ, Laszewicz W, Gabryelewicz A, McCallum RW. Mucolytic effects of Helicobacter pylori. Scand J Gastroenterol 1991;187(suppl):47−55.
9. Slomiany BL, Nishikawa H, Piotrowski J, Okazaki K, Slomiany A. Lipolytic activity of Campylobacter pylori, effect of sofalcone. Digestion 1989;43:33−40.
10. Langenberg ML, Tytgat GN, Schipper ME, Rietra PJ, Zanen HJ. Campylobacter-like organisms in the stomach of patients and healthy individuals (letter). Lancet 1984;1:1348−1349.
11. Tsujii M, Kawano S, Tsuji S, Fusamoto H, Kamada T, Sato N. Mechanism of gastric mucosal damage induced by ammonia. Gastroenterology 1992;102:1881−1888.
12. Hupertz V, Czinn S. Demonstration of a cytotoxin from Campylobacter pylori. Eur J Clin Microbiol 1988;7:576−578.
13. Leunk RD. Production of a cytotokin by Helicobacter pylori. Rev Infect Dis 1991;13:S686−S689.
14. Denizot Y, Sobhani I, Rambaud JC, Lewin M, Thomas Y, Benveniste J. Paf-acether synthesis by Helicobacter pylori. Gut 1990;31:1242−1245.
15. McCallum RW, DeLuca V, Marshall BJ, Prakash C. Prevalence of Campylobacter-like organisms in patients with gastro-esophageal reflux disease versus normals. Gastroenterology 1987;92:1524.
16. Hazell SL, Markesich DC, Evans DJ, Evans DG, Graham DY. Influence of media supplements on growth and survival of Campylobacter pylori. Eur J Clin Microbiol 1989;8:597−602.
17. Walker SJ, Birch PJ, Stewart M, Stoddard CJ, Hart CA, Day DW. Patterns of colonisation of Campylobacter pylori in the oesophagus, stomach and duodenum. Gut 1989;30:1334−1338.
18. Francoual S, Lamy P, Le Quintrec Y, Luboinski J, Petit JC. Helicobacter pylori: has it a part in the lesion of the gastroesophageal reflux? [letter]. J Infect Dis 1990;162:1414−1415.
19. Cheng EH, Bermanski P, Silversmith M, Valenstein P, Kawanishi H. Prevalence of Campylobacter pylori in esophagitis, gastritis, and duodenal disease. Arch Intern Med 1989;149:1373−1375.
20. Borkent MV, Beker JA. Treatment of ulcerative reflux esophagitis with colloidal bismuth subcitrate in combination with cimetidine. Gut 1988;29:385−389.

How can the cost-effectiveness of PPI treatment be assessed, compared to alternatives?

C.M. Bate (Wigan, Lancashire)

Gastroesophageal reflux disease (GERD) is a common condition: prevalence studies show that at any one time, up to 7% of the population suffer from troublesome reflux symptoms [1]. GERD ranges across a spectrum of severity from heartburn (usually of sufficient severity to cause the patient to consult his General Practitioner (GP), after self-medication with antacids or antacid-alginates has failed), to severe erosive reflux esophagitis (RE). Though usually thought of as a continuum from mild to severe disease, the poor correlation between symptom severity and the severity of lesions detected on endoscopic examination makes this assumption misleading: mild symptoms may coexist with severe mucosal lesions (i.e., high-grade RE) and vice versa [2] such that severe symptoms may be present in the absence of endoscopically detectable lesions [3].

The complications of GERD include stricture formation and the premalignant Barrett's esophagus (columnar-lined esophagus, CLE). The potential for these complications makes GERD an important clinical condition, and in addition its prevalence and tendency to recur (or even be continuous) makes the management of GERD an important condition for pharmacoeconomic evaluation, for healthcare providers and purchasers alike.

Design and standards of pharmacoeconomic evaluations

Most pharmacoeconomic evaluations of GERD have concentrated on retrospective cost-effectiveness analyses in which pairs of drug treatments have been compared in clinical trials in which conventional assessments of clinical efficacy were the primary endpoints. These are probably the most important evaluations for the healthcare purchaser and should be carried out along the principles published by the Australian government for reimbursement of drug costs [4]. Forms of cost-effectiveness evaluation which fail to follow at least the principles in these guidelines should probably be discounted.

In the future, we shall be able to look forward to prospective cost-effectiveness studies, in which clinical trials are designed with the pharmacoeconomic evaluation as their primary objective, rather than relying on retrospective economic analyses from trials. Whether prospective or retrospective economic analyses are carried out, the clinical studies should be adequate in every way, notably in compliance with GCP and with an adequate number of patients included in the study. Although statistical evaluation of pharmacoeconomic studies is currently in its infancy, some assessment of the robustness of the analyses is also highly desirable, even if derived from the primary clinical efficacy variables. A most important consideration is that endpoints

501

should be demanding and rigidly defined: in RE, the endpoint of the study used for pharmacoeconomic evaluation should be both healing (defined by endoscopic examination of the esophageal mucosa, assessed as grade 0 on whatever scale is being used), and complete relief from symptoms for a specific number of days prior to the evaluation. Both healed and symptom free should be demanded since in RE, endoscopic severity of lesions is very poorly correlated with severity of symptoms [2]. Moreover, some clinical trials have reported improvement in symptoms rather than their resolution as an endpoint, and some have accepted grade I esophagitis as healed. Neither is satisfactory. In symptomatic GERD (in general practice studies without endoscopic control) complete resolution of the dominant symptoms over a specified number of days must be regarded as the primary end point.

Treatment options and costs

Treatment options in GERD fall into four groups: 1) antacids, which will almost inevitably have been tried by patients before presentation to their GP; 2) antacid-alginates, which again may have been tried by patients since in at least some countries they are available without prescription; 3) Histamine H_2-receptor antagonists (H_2-RA) such as ranitidine or cimetidine; and 4) omeprazole. It should be noted that of these, only omeprazole is currently licensed in the United Kingdom for continuous use in the management of esophageal reflux disease. The lowest licensed doses and costs of 28 days treatment (recalculated from pack prices as necessary) for the second line treatments following antacids or antacid-alginates are: omeprazole 20 mg (£36.36), ranitidine 150 mg b.i.d. (£27.78) and cimetidine 400 mg q.d.s. (£34.89).

A further consideration is the stage at which a GP refers a patient for either specialist opinion, usually at an outpatient department (OPD) appointment, or for open-access endoscopy. The role of barium meals in diagnosis or confirmation of healing of RE is passé, because of the poor sensitivity and specificity of the examination and the attendant risks of irradiation. In the UK, a fundholding GP may face a charge to his budget of perhaps £200–300 for an esophago-gastroduodeno-scopy (EGDE), representing the cost of around 10 months continuous medical treatment. As most endoscopy units are approaching their capacity [2], it is unrealistic to recommend universal endoscopy for heartburn or dyspepsia and pragmatic guidelines have suggested EGDE for patients with newly-presenting symptoms over an arbitrary age of 45 [5] or 50 [6], but "blind" treatment for younger patients, unless alarm symptoms are present (weight loss, anemia, dysphagia). A predictably effective agent (omeprazole) may also be used as a "therapeutic trial" to confirm or reject the notion that a patient's symptoms are acid-related.

Since the bulk of patients will be managed symptomatically, it is important in selecting a drug that mucosal healing is predictable from symptom relief, since it is to be expected that unhealed lesions, even in the absence of symptoms, will lead to the complications of stricture and CLE. Symptom relief with omeprazole treatment has been shown to be a better predictor of endoscopically-verified mucosal healing than treatment with ranitidine [7].

A final methodological consideration is that if a drug is to be regarded as cost-effective (or more cost-effective than alternative agents), this should be demonstrable over a range of severities of disease and should be apparent in General Practice and hospital treatment alike, since clinical indices are a poor guide on which to base the selection of drugs for GERD [2].

Clinical studies

Several studies, from the British Isles and the USA have demonstrated that in the management of RE, omeprazole 20 mg is more cost-effective than either ranitidine 300 mg/day [7−10] or cimetidine 1.6 g/day [7]. This conclusion is assured since it has been consistent between studies and within studies independent of the clinical endpoints on which the cost-effectiveness analyses were based. Statistical analyses have confirmed the robustness of these findings [11], has also been shown to be more cost effective for the long-term management of RE [8] and in prevention of stricture formation [12].

More recent studies have examined the relative cost-effectiveness of different doses (20 mg and 40 mg) of omeprazole and concluded that in the management of RE, 20 mg is the most cost-effective dose [13].

Furthermore, a recent study in General Practice in the UK, in symptomatic GERD, has shown omeprazole 20 mg to be more clinically effective [14] and so more cost-effective in relieving symptoms than ranitidine 150 mg b.i.d. This latter study has particular importance, since it is in General Practice that the majority of GERD patients are managed. It might thus be expected that GPs would see a milder spectrum of symptoms than hospital physicians and this would result in "convergence" of clinical effectiveness between any pair of drugs, since the milder a condition, the more difficult it is to demonstrate a difference in efficacy between any treatment modalities. If such convergence occurred, a less effective treatment might prove more cost-effective than omeprazole, but in general practice, it costs £65 for each patient successfully relieved of heartburn over 4 weeks treatment with omeprazole 20 mg o.m. compared with £112 over the same period for ranitidine 150 mg b.i.d. (Table 1) [14].

Conclusions

Since omeprazole is more cost-effective than histamine H_2 antagonists in the management of symptomatic GERD and of endoscopically-verified GERD and offers the patient clinical advantages of faster symptom relief and a greater certainty that symptomatic relief will be accompanied by mucosal healing, it is logical to use omeprazole in cases of GERD in which antacids have proved insufficient. The alternative "cascade" treatment in which patients may receive in turn antacids, antacid-alginates, cimetidine, ranitidine, high dose ranitidine and/or motility-enhancing agents and only finally omeprazole, means that some patients have to wait

Table 1.

Results after 4 weeks	Omeprazole 20 mg once daily	Ranitidine 150 mg twice daily
Healing (CV) [7]	57% (£64)	30% (£93)
Symptom relief (CV) [7]	65% (£56)	37% (£75)
Healed and SF (CV) [7]	42% (£87)	17% (£163)
Heartburn relief (CV) [7]	67% (£55)	40% (£70)
Daytime heartburn (DC) [9]	+893d (£4.07)	+265d (£10.48)
Waking at night (DC) [9]	+522d (£6.97)	+252d (£11.02)
SF and no antacids (DC) [9]	+701d (£5.19)	+337d (£8.24)
Heartburn (CV) [13]	56% (£65)	25% (£112)
Asymptomatic (CV) [13]	44% (£83)	20% (£139)

CV = clinic visit assessment; DC = diary card assessment. For details of techniques, see references. Percentages show proportion of patients achieving clinical improvements. Cost refers to the cost of one patient attaining that index of improvement. Diary card data show the number of patient days (d) gained per 100 patients over 1 month and the cost of achieving a symptom free day, SF = symptom free.

for some time before receiving effective treatment; moreover the intervening treatments by their lack of efficacy have been cost-ineffective and symptom improvement without resolution of mucosal lesions may predispose to rapid relapse and the development of complications. When acid suppression is needed to control GERD, omeprazole is the drug of choice.

References

1. Heading RC. Epidemiology of oesophageal reflux disease. Scand J Gastroenterol 1989;168:33—37.
2. Green JRB. Is there such an entity as mild oesophagitis? Eur J Clin Res 1993;4:29—34.
3. Ogorek CP, Cohen S. Gastroesophageal reflux disease: new concepts in pathophysiology. Gastroenterol Clin North Am 1969;18:275—292.
4. Government of Australia. Guidelines for the Pharmaceutical Industry on preparation of submissions to the Pharmaceutical Benefits Advisory Committee. Canberra; Aus. G. Pub. Serv., 1992.
5. Crean G. Causes of dyspepsia and its effective treatment. Prescriber 1992;Jan:29—37.
6. Bate CM, Harvey DJ, McCloy RM et al. In: Scott C (ed) Gastroesophageal Reflux. Update Postgraduate Centre Series. Sutton, Surrey, UK: Reed Healthcare, 1991.
7. Bate CM. Cost-effectiveness of omeprazole in the treatment of reflux oesophagitis. Br J Med Econ 1991;1:53—61.
8. Bate CM, Richardson PDI. A one-year model for the cost-effectiveness of treating reflux oesophagitis. Br J Med Econ 1992;2:5—11.
9. Bate CM, Richardson PDI. Symptomatic assessment and cost-effectiveness of treatments for reflux oesophagitis: comparisons of omeprazole and histamine H₂-receptor antagonists. Br J Med Econ 1992;2:37—43.
10. Hillman AI, Blom BS, Fendrick AM, Schwartz JS. Cost and quality effects of alternative treatments for persistent gastroesophageal reflux disease. Arch Int Med 1992;152:1467—1472.
11. Bate CM, Richardson PDI. Clinical and economic factors in the selection of drugs for gastroesophageal reflux disease. Pharmacoeconomics 1993:3:94—99.
12. Marks R, Rizzo J, Champion G, Mills T, Richter JE. Efficacy and cost-effectiveness of omeprazole in the treatment of patients with peptic strictures and oesophagitis. Gastroenterology 1993;104:A140.
13. Bate CM, Booth SN, Crowe JP, Hepworth-Jones B, Taylor MD, Richardson PDI. Does omeprazole 40 mg daily offer additional benefit over 20 mg daily in patients requiring more than 4 weeks treatment for symptomatic reflux oesophagitis? Aliment Pharmacol Ther 1993 (in press).
14. Hungin APS, Gunn SD, Bate CM, Turbitt ML, Wilcock C, Richardson PDI. A comparison of the efficacy of omeprazole 20 mg once daily with ranitidine 150 mg b.d. in the relief of symptomatic gastro-oesophageal reflux disease in General Practice. Br J Clin Res 1993;4:73—88.

Has the use of PPIs altered the indications for surgery?

J. Barbier (Paris)

Until recently, about 5% of patients with gastroesophageal reflux (GER) underwent surgery.

Have the indications for surgery changed since 1989, when the first proton pump inhibitor (PPI) became available? A survey based on six surgical centers specializing in this type of disease has given discordant results.

— In three centers, the number of operated patients has fallen appreciably from 25 to 75%.

— In the three other centers the percentage has remained the same.

Other authors have reported that, while the number of operations has not changed, the indications have changed. Watson [1] now tends to operate younger patients with more severe esophagitis, with demonstrated incompetence of the lower esophageal sphincter and sometimes with alkaline reflux. These findings justify some comment.

The situation a few months ago

The PPIs heal almost all types of esophagitis and suppress the symptoms, which are closely correlated with the endoscopic lesions, although a dose increase may be necessary.

After healing, the relapse rate at 6 months varies between 25 and 90% according to the author considered. The most optimistic findings were reported by Poynard et al. [2] for 883 patients followed up for 6 months: 76% of these subjects did not relapse, the only treatment being sodium alginate on demand. The relapse rate increases with the severity of the esophagitis and the dose of antisecretory treatment that has to be prescribed [3].

Whatever the relapse rate, maintenance treatment reduces this risk. The dose used must not be less than that of initial treatment. On ranitidine 300 mg/day, however, the relapse rate at 6 months was still 37.5% (150 mg × 2) or 41% (300 mg at night), which was not very different from the rate observed on placebo [4]. Cisapride (10 mg × 2) was found to be better than placebo at 12 months (28% relapse compared with 48.5%) [5].

Omeprazole is much more effective. For 84 patients with severe esophagitis treated with 20 mg/day the relapse rates at 6, 12 and 24 months were 17, 26, and 33%, respectively. The relapse rate is sensitive to dose increases up to 40 or even 60 mg [6].

In contrast, intermittent treatment (3 days a week) is ineffective.

Only a few months ago, these findings could not be turned to practical advantage, as long-term PPI treatment was considered too hazardous. This is why, in global terms, there has been no spectacular fall in the number of indications for surgery.

Current situation

We now have a better understanding of the long-term effects of PPIs. The changes in gastric histology and secretion do not appear to have any clinical repercussions. There is no further increase in blood gastrin levels after the first 2 or 3 months of treatment. The increase in the number of argyrophilic cells is moderate and remains constant after 8 months of treatment, without evidence of dysplasia or neoplasia. In addition, no disorders of iron or vitamin B_{12} absorption have been observed in the long-term studies conducted with patients receiving PPIs [7].

Patients whose esophagitis recurs after treatment can now be given PPI maintenance treatment, either long term or intermittent, on demand, or they can be treated surgically. Both options have their advantages and disadvantages.

The randomized study conducted by Spechler [8] with 247 patients followed up for 1 to 2 years indicated that surgery is more effective, but the medical treatment did not comprise PPIs.

Medical treatment with PPIs

Advantages

— efficacy;
— simplicity (one dose per day);
— safety, which has now been extensively demonstrated;
— possibility of increasing the dose or resorting to surgery should the treatment's efficacy wane.

Disadvantages

— the patient must take an expensive medication daily for years;
— efficacy may diminish in the long term, or currently unknown side effects may develop.

Surgical treatment

Advantages

— efficacy: in the survey conducted by Launois [9] covering 278 patients, surgical treatment gave a good or very good result in 90% of cases. This success rate is confirmed by Stein [10] (91% good results at 10 years) who stresses the importance of patient selection: incompetence of the lower esophageal sphincter without disorders of esophageal clearance. Pope [11] stresses the value of precise clinical evaluation and rating of the various symptoms. The results are considered good if the symptoms of reflux disappear and no further problems arise;

— in principle, surgery is a definitive procedure.

Disadvantages

— the associated mortality rate is extremely low (but not zero);
— the associated morbidity rate (about 10%), with risk of development of new symptoms (dysphagia, difficulties of eructation or vomiting) which are often difficult to treat;
— the operation requires an 8-day period of hospitalization.

Certain complications of reflux (peptic stenosis, Barrett's esophagus) may well result from surgery. In practice, combination of omeprazole and dilatation for stenoses gives the same result as a combination of surgery and dilatation [12]. The regression of Barrett's esophagus after surgery, reported some years ago, has subsequently been extensively contested. However, omeprazole can be successfully used to treat Barrett's esophagus [13].

Aspiration of fluid, which can be the source of pulmonary or ENT complications, may respond poorly to medical treatment and become a good indication for surgery.

Two factors must be taken into account:
— the patient's choice: the patient should be fully informed and allowed to take part in the decision making process;
— the cost of the two therapeutic options: on the whole, 8 days hospitalization on Social Security assistance in a gastrointestinal surgical unit costs 33,000 French francs, which is equivalent to 7 years of treatment with omeprazole.

Coley [14] has suggested that these economic factors should govern the choice so that surgical treatment would automatically be given to patients under 50 years of age and medical treatment would be given to patients over 60 years of age.

The indications for celioscopic surgery, which seems to be associated with a high morbidity rate, remains to be evaluated.

Conclusion

If a patient with recurrent esophagitis is managing well on 20 mg of omeprazole per day, it is believed that it is legitimate to continue this treatment, perhaps occasionally withdrawing it for a few months at a time (the natural history of reflux esophagitis is still poorly understood). It is then always possible to increase the doses or to resort to surgical measures if the symptoms recur despite this treatment.

References

1. Watson A. Surgery for uncomplicated gastro-oesophageal reflux. Gut 1993;34:428–429.
2. Poynard T et Groupe multicentrique. Devenir des patients après guérison d'une oesophagite. Etude prospective pendant 6 mois. Gastroenterol Clin Biol 1992;16(2 bis):A61.
3. Armstrong D, Nicolet M, Monnier Ph, Chapuis G, Savary M, Blum AL. Maintenance therapy: is there still a place for antireflux surgery? World J Surg 1992;16:300–307.

4. Armstrong D, Blum AL, The REZETIC study group. Full dose H_2-receptor antagonist prophylaxis does not prevent relapse of reflux oesophagitis. Gut 1989;30:A1494.
5. Blum AL, Adami B, Bouzo MH, Brandstätter G, Fumagalli I, Galmiche JP, Hebbelin H, Hentschel E, Huttemann W, Schütz E, Verlinden M and the Italian EUROCIS Trialists. Effect of cisapride on relapse of oesophagitis. Dig Dis Sci 1993; 38:551—560.
6. Klinkenberg-Knol EC, Jansen JBMJ, Lamers CBHW, Nelis F, Snel P, Meuwissen SGM. Use of omeprazole in the management of reflux oesophagitis resistant to H_2-receptor antagonists. Scand J Gastroenterol 1989;24 (suppl 166):1888.
7. Festen H, Klinkenberg-Knol EC, Kuipers E, Lamers C, Jansen JB, Biemond I, Tertoolen J, Meuwissen SG. Cobalamir absorption during omeprazole treatment: short- and long-term studies. Gastroenterology 1993;104 (suppl 4):A77.
8. Spechler SJ. Gastro-oesophageal reflux disease study group. Comparison of medical and surgical therapy for complicated gastro-oesophageal reflux disease in veterans. N Engl J Med 1992;326:786—792.
9. Launois B, Paul JL, Teboul F, Bourdonnec P, Cardin JL, Campion JP, Meunier B, de Chateaubriant P. Les résultats fonctionnels du treatment chirurgical du reflux gastro-oesophagien non compliqué. Analyse de 278 observations. Ann Chir 1988;42:191—196.
10. Stein HJ, DeMeester TR. Who benefits from antireflux surgery? World J Surg;16:313—319.
11. Pope CE. The quality of life following antireflux surgery. World J Surg 1992;16:355—358.
12. Ching CK, Shaheen MZ, Holmes GKT. Is omeprazole more effective in the treatment of resistant reflux oesophagitis and associated peptic strictures? Gastroenterology 1990;89:A30.
13. Galmiche JP, Dumas R, Boyer J, Goldfain D, Bury A, Robaskiewicz M, Cadiot G, Diebold MD. Long-term omeprazole effects on Barret's mucosa. Gastroenterology 1993;104 (suppl 4):A85.
14. Coley CM, Barry MJ, Spechler SJ, Wilford WO, Mulley AG. Initial medical vs. surgical therapy for complicated or chronic gastro-oesophageal reflux disease. A cost-effectiveness analysis. Gastroenterology 1993;104(suppl 4):A5.

Indications for surgery

Are motility disturbances secondary to reflux and can improvement be anticipated after effective treatment?

H.J. Stein (Munich), *T.R. DeMeester* (Los Angeles)

The barrier function of the lower esophageal sphincter (LES) and the efficacy of clearance peristalsis of the esophageal body are the major pathogenic factors for gastroesophageal reflux disease (GERD). While a mechanically defective LES predisposes to reflux of gastric contents, impairment of peristalsis prolongs the esophageal exposure time to the refluxate. Using simultaneous manometric and video-fluoroscopic recording of barium swallows, Kahrilas et al. have recently shown that esophageal clearance of a barium suspension depends on the amplitude of esophageal contractions and speed of propagation of the wave along the esophagus [1]. In the distal esophagus a minimum contraction amplitude of approximately 30 mmHg was required to completely occlude the lumen and to propel a bolus. Inadequate amplitude, rapid propagation of contractions (i.e., simultaneous contractions), or an interrupted peristaltic sequence resulted in a failure of clearance [1].

The peristaltic activity of the esophageal body is compromised in a substantial portion of patients with GERD [2–5]. Using standard and ambulatory 24-h manometry of the esophageal body, it was demonstrated that the mean amplitude of esophageal contractions is compromised primarily in patients with a mechanically defective LES and decreases with increasing severity of esophageal mucosal injury (i.e., esophagitis, stricture and Barrett's esophagus) [6,7]. In contrast, an increased frequency of nonperistaltic (i.e., simultaneous, isolated and interrupted) contractions could be demonstrated in patients with GERD independent of the severity of mucosal injury or the presence of a mechanically defective LES [7].

From these studies it remains, however, unclear whether the peristaltic dysfunction in patients with GERD is a primary cause of increased esophageal exposure to gastric juice, or develops secondary to persistent reflux of gastric contents across a mechanically defective LES and progression of esophageal mucosal injury. Evaluation of esophageal motor activity in patients with GERD before and after complete reflux suppression and healing of esophageal mucosal injury could provide an answer to this question. A documentation of recovery of esophageal body function following reflux control and healing of mucosal inflammation would indicate that the loss of esophageal contractility in patients with increased esophageal acid exposure is a secondary phenomenon. In contrast, persistence of esophageal body dysfunction despite reflux suppression and healing of mucosal injury would point towards a primary defect or an irreversible loss of contractility due to permanent transmucosal injury.

Effect of reflux control on LES function

Compared to normal volunteers the resting pressure, overall length and abdominal length, of the LES is decreased in patients with increased esophageal acid exposure [8]. Detailed assessment of the three-dimensional manometric LES pressure profile has shown that a mechanically defective sphincter can be documented in the vast majority of patients with increased esophageal acid exposure [9]. Medical therapy of GERD is aimed primarily at suppressing acid secretion and none of the available drugs has shown any augmenting effect on the compromised barrier function of the LES [2–5]. This explains why symptoms and mucosal injury frequently relapse as soon as medical therapy is discontinued. In contrast, Nissen fundoplication restores the resting pressure, overall length, abdominal length and the three-dimensional manometric pressure profile of the LES to normal thus effectively and definitely prohibiting reflux of any gastric content (Fig. 1) [10].

Effect of reflux control on esophageal body functions

A decreased mean contraction amplitude in the distal esophagus associated with an increased frequency of contractions, with an amplitude below 30 mmHg, isolated contractions, simultaneous contractions and contractions with an abnormal morphology, have repeatedly been described in patients with GERD [2–5]. In a recent study it was shown that reflux control by Nissen fundoplication significantly increases the mean contraction amplitude and reduces the frequency of contractions below 30 mmHg (Fig. 2) [10]. A lack of correlation between postoperative contraction amplitude and LES characteristics indicates that this is not secondary to a compensatory mechanism to overcome the outflow obstruction by the reconstructed LES, but

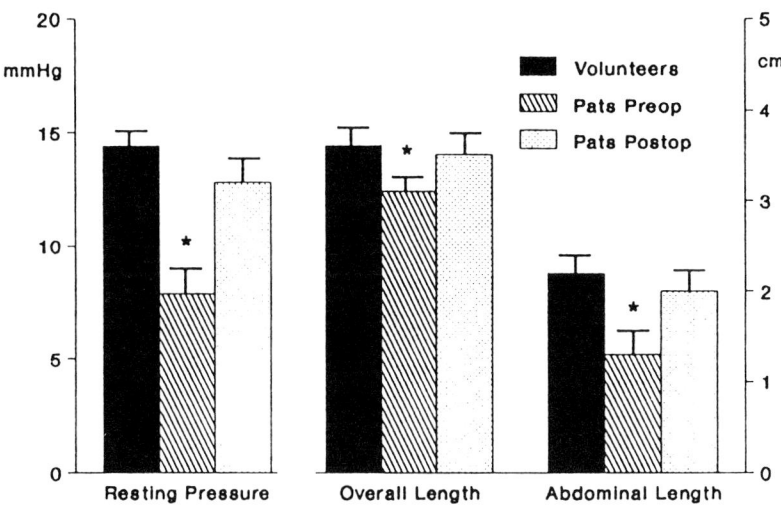

Fig. 1. Characteristics of lower esophageal sphincter function in 40 patients before and after Nissen fundoplication compared to 50 normal volunteers. *: p < 0.01 vs. normal volunteers. From [10] with permission.

represent true recovery of esophageal contractility following abolishment of gastroesophageal reflux and healing of mucosal inflammation.

Recovery of esophageal contractility following a surgical antireflux procedure in patients with GERD has also been reported by other authors [11,12]. Despite

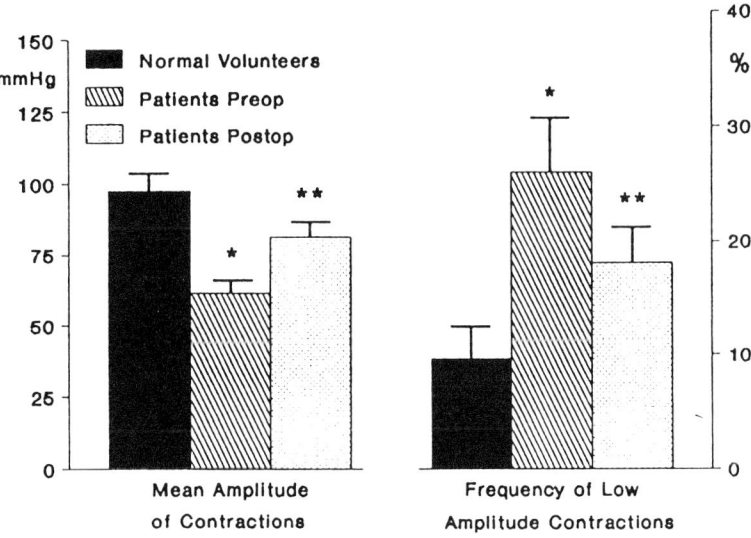

Fig. 2. Mean amplitude of contractions and prevalence of low amplitude contractions (<30 mmHg) in 40 patients with gastroesophageal reflux disease before and after Nissen fundoplication compared to 50 normal volunteers. *: p < 0.01 vs. "normal volunteers"; **: p < 0.05 vs. "normal volunteers" and "patients preop". From [10] with permission.

complete suppression of acid secretion and healing of acute mucosal injury, recovery of esophageal contractility in patients with GERD does, however, not occur with medical management [2–5,13–15]. The reasons for this difference between surgical and medical therapy of GERD are unclear. Incomplete abolishment of reflux and frequent relapse episodes with medical management, in contrast to a durable restoration of the defective LES with complete and permanent abolishment of reflux and reduction of an hiatal hernia with a surgical antireflux procedure may, however, account for this observation [10].

Despite the observed improvement in esophageal contractility after Nissen fundoplication the amplitude of contractions did not return to normal in the study performed [10]. Evaluation of the preoperative and postoperative amplitude of contractions in the distal esophagus in the individual patients showed that an increase in contraction amplitude occurred primarily in patients whose mean preoperative contraction amplitude was above 30 mmHg (Fig. 3). Reflux control and healing of mucosal inflammation with Nissen fundoplication did not result in any improvement of esophageal motor function in patients who had a severely deteriorated contractility with a mean amplitude of contractions below 30 mmHg. This was primarily seen in patients with a stricture or Barrett's esophagus who on histologic studies also have an increase in the submucosal collagen content associated with a loss of muscle fibers in the distal esophagus. These observations suggest that esophageal body in these patients has deteriorated beyond the point of recovery due to permanent transmural injury [7].

The increased frequency of nonperistaltic contractions (i.e., interrupted, isolated and simultaneous contractions) and contractions with an abnormal morphology (i.e.,

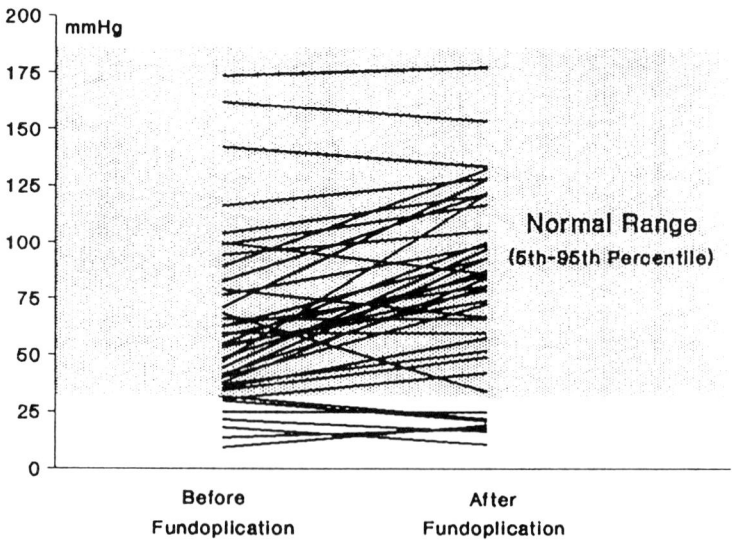

Fig. 3. Mean amplitude of contractions in the distal esophagus of individual patients with gastroesophageal reflux disease before and after reflux control by Nissen fundoplication. No improvement occurred in patients with a mean amplitude of contractions below 30 mmHg before fundoplication. From [10] with permission.

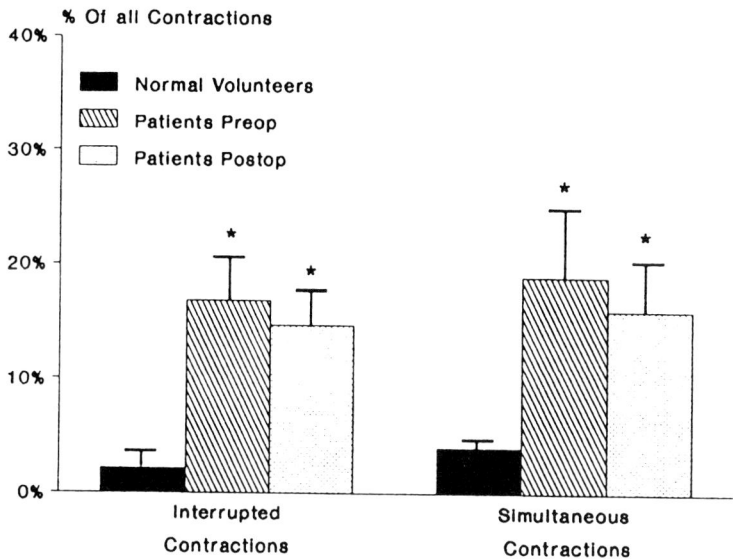

Fig. 4. The prevalence of simultaneous and interrupted contractions in 40 patients with gastroesophageal reflux disease before and after Nissen fundoplication compared to 50 normal volunteers. *: p < 0.01 vs. normal volunteers. From [10] with permission.

contractions with double peaks and prolonged duration) in patients with gastroesophageal reflux is commonly attributed to the irritating effect of refluxed gastric juice on the esophageal mucosa. Surprisingly neither reflux suppression with medications nor antireflux surgery appears to have an effect on the prevalence of these abnormal contractions (Fig. 4) [10].

Conclusion

The question remains whether the observed defects of esophageal function in patients with GERD are primary, or whether they develop secondary to persistent reflux of gastric juice and progression of esophageal mucosal injury. Several studies show that a loss of esophageal contractility rarely occurs in the absence of mucosal injury, whereas a loss of sphincter function is seen in a substantial portion of patients without mucosal injury [9]. A defective sphincter in the absence of inflammatory changes suggests that this is the primary defect and that loss of esophageal contractility follows with the development of complications (i.e., esophagitis, stricture and Barrett's esophagus). This is confirmed by the observation that the loss of contractility in patients with GERD is, at least in part, reversible after reflux control and healing of mucosal inflammation with Nissen fundoplication. However, once esophageal body function has deteriorated to a mean contraction amplitude below 30 mmHg, the defect appears to become irreversible. This would suggest that in patients with increased esophageal exposure to gastric juice, secondary to a defective LES,

513

an antireflux procedure should be performed prior to the deterioration of esophageal body function which may not be reversible.

References

1. Kahrilas PJ, Dodds WJ, Hogan WJ. Effect of peristaltic dysfunction on esophageal volume clearance. Gastroenterology 1988;94:73—80.
2. Katz PO, Knuff TE, Benjamin SB, Castell DO. Abnormal esophageal pressures in reflux esophagitis: cause or effect? Am J Gastroenterol 1986;81:744—746.
3. Kahrilas PJ, Dodds WJ, Hogan WJ, Kern M, Arndorfer RC, Reece A. Esophageal peristaltic dysfunction in peptic esophagitis. Gastroenterology 1986;91:897—904.
4. Eckardt VF. Does healing of esophagitis improve esophageal motor function? Dig Dis Sci 1988;33:161—165.
5. Baldi F, Ferrarini F, Longanesi A, Angeloni M, Ragazzini M, Miglioli M, Barbara L. Oesophageal function before, during, and after healing of erosive esophagitis. Gut 1988; 29:157—160.
6. Zaninotto G, DeMeester TR, Bremner CG, Smyrk TC, Cheng SC. Esophageal function in patients with reflux-induced strictures and its relevance to surgical treatment. Ann Thorac Surg 1989;47:362—370.
7. Stein HJ, Eypasch EP, DeMeester TR. Circadian esophageal motor function in patients with gastroesophageal reflux disease. Surgery 1990;108:769—778.
8. Zaninotto G, DeMeester TR, Schwizer W. The lower esophageal sphincter in health and disease. Am J Surg 1988;155:104—111.
9. Stein HJ, DeMeester TR, Naspetti R, Jamieson J, Perry R. The three-dimensional lower esophageal sphincter pressure profile in gastroesophageal reflux disease. Ann Surg 1991;214:374—384.
10. Stein HJ, Bremner RM, Jamieson J, DeMeester TR. Effect of Nissen fundoplication on esophageal motor function. Arch Surg 1992;127:788—792.
11. Gill RC, Bowes KL, Murphy PD et al. Esophageal motor abnormalities in gastroesophageal reflux and the effects of fundoplication. Gastroenterology 1986;91:364—369.
12. Escandell AO, Martinez de Haro LF, Paricio PP, Albasani JLA, Marcilla JAG, Cuenca GM. Surgery improves defective oesophageal peristalsis in patients with gastro-oesophageal reflux. Br J Surg 1991;78:1095—1097.
13. Allen ML, McIntosh DL, Robinson MG. Healing or amelioration of esophagitis does not result in increased lower esophageal sphincter or esophageal contractile pressure. Am J Gastroenterol 1990;85:1331—1334.
14. Howard TM, Frei JV, Flowers M et al. Omeprazole heals esophagitis but does not improve abnormal motility in reflux esophagitis. Gastroenterology 1990;98:61A.
15. Singh P, Adamopoulos A, Taylor RH, Colin-Jones DG. Oesophageal motor function before and after healing of oesophagitis. Gut 1992;33:1590—1596.

What is the effect of antireflux surgery on the motor function of the esophagus?

G.G. Jamieson (Adelaide)

The function of the esophagus is not universally tested by surgeons prior to antireflux surgery, although some have argued that preoperative detection of severe motility disturbances is important. This is to exclude patients with motility problems from antireflux surgery since such procedures may be followed by obstructive symptoms [1,2].

We have recently followed a group of 131 patients having antireflux surgery and found a significant correlation between failure of peristalsis on manometry and postoperative dysphagia [3]. However, the whole question of the necessity of pre-operative manometry studies revolves around the so far unresolved issue of whether esophageal motor function disorders associated with esophagitis are reversible.

Motor function of the esophagus can be assessed either by a physiological profile, using esophageal manometry, or by a functional profile looking at the ability of the esophagus to clear acid or empty itself of swallowed liquids or solids. Each of these methods has demonstrated abnormalities in patients with gastroesophageal reflux disease (GERD). Thus motility studies have demonstrated failure of transmission of peristaltic sequences, tertiary contractions occurring with swallowing and diminution in amplitude of swallowing waves, particularly in the distal half of the esophagus [4].

Acid clearance has been documented to be poor [5], the clearance of a radioactively labeled liquid swallow to be delayed [6] and the emptying of swallowed solid was shown to be delayed in patients with GERD [7]. At the present time it is not known if these abnormalities are primary or secondary to the reflux disease with both views having adherents.

It now seems well established that some esophageal motility parameters improve after antireflux surgery. Thus three studies have demonstrated that the amplitude of primary peristaltic contractions improves [8–10], although Stein et al. found a subgroup of seven patients with contraction amplitude less than 35 mmHg, who did not achieve improvement following fundoplication [10]. Each of the groups found that tertiary contractions were either unchanged after fundoplication [9,10] or actually increased [8]. There was divided opinion about the effect on failure of peristaltic sequences with no mention [8], no effect [10] and improvement [9] all being suggested. One interpretation of these findings (and the one given by these authors) is that diminution and peristaltic amplitude is a secondary phenomenon consequent on reflux damage, and that prevention of reflux reverses the effect. Stein et al. explained the failure to reverse the effect in their seven patients, with amplitudes less than 35 mmHg, as being due to the more severe reflux disease in these patients having led to irreversible damage. However, none of the authors attempts to explain why peristaltic failure and the increased incidence of tertiary contractions are not reversed by fundoplication. It remains possible and even probable, that the motor defect is a primary phenomenon. When the defect is more severe, one would expect more severe disease, as demonstrated by Stein et al. in their seven cases. This would explain the failure of fundoplication to reverse two of the common three abnormalities seen in reflux. The increased amplitude of contraction would then be explained as a secondary phenomenon to the relative obstruction produced by the fundoplication [11,12], an effect which has been demonstrated experimentally [13]. Lending weight to this interpretation is the fact that studies using liquids and solids to investigate esophageal function have not shown improvement after antireflux surgery. Thus, Hill et al. used a radionuclide-labeled liquid to study patients before and after posterior gastropexy. Their study was of patients in the supine position and they found no improvement in the ability of the esophagus to clear the swallowed liquid after a posterior gastropexy procedure [6]. We studied a group of 18 patients before and at 6 or more months after a total fundoplication. For the test a 10 g piece of radionuclide labeled hamburger was used to measure the ability of the esophagus to empty 95% of the activity. This test was performed in the normal upright eating posture. We found improvement in emptying in five patients, worsening in five, and in eight patients there was no change. With this small group of patients there did not appear to be any obvious improvement in esophageal function following antireflux surgery.

Lending further credence to the view that the motility disorder is primary is the study of Singh et al. which looked at esophageal motor function before and after healing of esophagitis induced by drug therapy. They found no significant change in any of the indices of esophageal function after healing of esophagitis. Thus they came to the conclusion that disordered esophageal motor function in reflux esophagitis is a primary phenomenon [14].

In summary, it has been established beyond doubt that patients with GERD exhibit motor dysfunction of the body of the esophagus, and it appears that the more severe grades of reflux disease are associated with more severely impaired motor function. Most studies of esophageal function have failed to show improvement after antireflux surgery, except in the one parameter of increased amplitude of primary peristalsis. This is probably a secondary effect to the antireflux surgery itself. The evidence for the primacy of esophageal body dysfunction is strong enough to suggest that all patients with GERD should have esophageal manometry before surgery, and in those patients with severe motor dysfunction it may be best to avoid a complete wrap of the lower esophagus.

References

1. Pope CE II. Esophageal motility — who needs it? Gastroenterology 1978;74:1337—1338.
2. Joelsson BE, DeMeester TR, Skinner DB, LaFontaine E, Waters PF, O'Sullivan GC. The role of the esophageal body in the antireflux mechanism. Surgery 1982;92:417—424.
3. Lundell L, Myers JC, Jamieson GG. The influence of oesophageal motor function on the long-term outcome of antireflux surgery. Gullet 1993;3:50—55.
4. Kahrilas PJ, Dodds WJ, Hogan WJ et al. Esophageal peristaltic dysfunction in peptic esophagitis. Gastroenterology 1986;91:897—904.
5. Skinner DB, Booth DJ. Assessment of distal esophageal function in patients with hiatal hernia and/or gastroesophageal reflux. Ann Surg 1970;172:627—637.
6. Russel COH, Pope CE II, Gannan RM, Allen FD, Velasco N, Hill LD. Does surgery correct esophageal motor dysfunction in gastroesophageal reflux? Ann Surg 1981;194:290—296.
7. Maddern GJ, Jamieson GG. Oesophageal emptying in patients with gastro-oesophageal reflux. Br J Surg 1986;73:615—617.
8. Gill RC, Bowes KL, Murphy PD et al. Esophageal motor abnormalities in gastroesophageal reflux and the effects of fundoplication. Gastroenterology 1986;91:364—369.
9. Ortiz Escandell A, Martinez de Haro LF, Parrilla Paricio P, Aguayo Albasini JL, Garcia Marcilla JA, Morales Cuenca G. Surgery improves defective oesophageal peristalsis in patients with gastro-oesophageal reflux. Br J Surg 1991;78:1095—1097.
10. Stein HJ, Bremner RM, Jamieson J, DeMeester TR. Effect of Nissen fundoplication on esophageal motor function. Arch Surg 1992;127:788—792.
11. Kiroff GK, Maddern GJ, Jamieson GG. A study of the factors responsible for the efficacy of fundoplication in the treatment of gastro-oesophageal reflux. Aust NZ J Surg 1984;54;109—112.
12. Ireland AC, Holloway RH, Toouli J, Dent J. Mechanisms underlying the antireflux action of fundoplication. Gut 1993;34:303—308.
13. Mittal RK, Ren J, McCallum RW, Shaffer HA, Sluss J. Modulation of feline esophageal contractions by bolus volume and outflow obstruction. Am J Physiol 1990;258:208—215.
14. Singh P, Adamopoulos A, Taylor RH, Colin-Jones DG. Oesophageal motor function before and after healing of oesophagitis. Gut 1992;33:1590—1596.

Are there physiological parameters that may predict and influence the long-term outcome after antireflux surgery?

L. Lundell (Gothenburg)

Gastroesophageal reflux disease (GERD) is expressed in a variety of clinical manifestations, from severe symptoms without obvious macroscopic lesions in esophagus, to severe complications (columnar lined esophagus) with diffuse and sometimes nonexisting symptoms. Provided, that a proper diagnosis can be established (i.e., by presentation of a typical history with endoscopic evidence of esophagitis in addition to abnormal acid exposure into the esophagus), antireflux procedures have consistently been shown to be effective in controlling reflux, as well as GERD symptoms also when evaluated many years after the operations [1,2]. A number of large, institutional series have presented their long-term results after surgical treatment of the disease, but unfortunately, properly controlled prospective studies, into which a reasonable number of patients have been included with additional long-term follow-up, have so far only rarely been presented [3–7]. The majority of relapses after antireflux surgery seem to occur during the first postoperative year, most likely due to technical failures. Although fundoplication procedures are effective in the long-term control of GERD, no firm conclusions can at present be drawn on the relative merits of the different operative procedures, when these have not been evaluated in controlled, clinical randomized trials. In this context it is, however, relevant to emphasize the cumulative high local complication rates seen after insertion of an Angelchik prosthesis [8].

Considerable information in the literature suggests, that the severity of reflux esophagitis is closely correlated to the magnitude of acid exposure over 24 h. Hence, patients with milder forms of the disease have predominantly daytime acid reflux, whereas those with more severe manifestations suffer from acid reflux over the entire 24-h period. The question has been raised whether patients presenting without endoscopically evident lesions and/or only daytime reflux, would respond less favorably to fundoplication operations than those having more severe forms of the disease [9]. Provided that the GERD diagnosis is firmly established, recent data suggest that patients seem to respond similarly irrespective of the severity of the disease (McCloy et al. to be published). However, more information is needed on the efficacy of different long-term treatment strategies in patients with endoscopy negative disease.

Although antireflux surgery is generally very effective in controlling gastroesophageal reflux, failures are sometimes proven unavoidable. Previous studies have mainly focused on factors responsible for these failures, emphasizing the role of slipping of the wrap, its tightness, dislocation and/or disruption [10–12]. The prevention of reflux alone does not always provide an optimal result for the patients. Persistent postprandial adverse symptoms can mar an otherwise good result in the form of dysphagia, inability to belch and vomit, postprandial fullness, bloating and pain, and sometimes socially embarrassing flatulence. Many of these symptoms have been assembled within the syndrome named, "gas bloat" [13–15]. The question then arises which are the options available to predict patients who would experience adverse symptoms, in the long-term outcome, after antireflux surgery when evaluated in the preoperative setting? Some of the symptoms alleged to be specific for the postfundoplication situation [16] may well reside already before the operation. Few studies have given valid information on this important topic, but a recent study suggested that a significant proportion of GERD patients suffered from similar complaints, also when allocated to and followed up through nonsurgical long-term therapy [17]. Hence investigations of the impact of preoperative diffuse abdominal symptoms (such as flatulence, distension, bloating) on the subsequent outcome after antireflux surgery are warranted. To obtain valid clinical information on this and related topics, it is vital that the study design takes the advantage of an objective assessment of symptoms by an independent, "unbiased" observer who is not too closely involved in the surgical treatment of the patient.

Otherwise, any combination of symptoms or symptom profiles more specifically related to GERD (heartburn, acid regurgitation, aggravated by straining, recumbency etc.) have not so far been found to be of any predictive value in the definition of the outcome of antireflux surgery [13]. It could be anticipated that obstructive symptoms (dysphagia) would have such an impact, especially since similar symptoms are associated with manometric evidence of defective primary peristalsis (see below), but until now no confirmative data are prevailing.

Inability to belch has been reported to occur in about 40% of patients after Nissen fundoplication and inability to vomit in 30–90%. Among patients with a long, tight wrap, half of them complained of increased flatulence and up to 20% reported symptomatic gas bloat of varying severity, whereas the corresponding figures after short, floppy wraps were considerably lower [16,18]. Fundoplication procedures profoundly impairs the ability to belch and relieve bloating also when objectively evaluated [19]. Some studies even report an impressive number of patients being able also to vomit postoperatively especially when interviewed many years after the operation. Similar clinical information should, however, cause concern regarding an eventual disruption of the wrap rather than an example of subsidence of complaints with the passage of time.

Esophageal motor function

The vigor of esophageal peristalsis required to achieve a complete volume clearance varies with the esophageal segment studied, but the consequences of the motility disturbances such as those associated with severe GERD are, among other things, impaired volume clearance [20–22]. Peristaltic dysfunction, has been suggested to affect 25–50% of patients with peptic esophagitis [23–26]. It has been claimed that results of preoperative manometry could be used to predict those who would experience bad results after fundoplication operations, but the messages from similar studies are not consistent [23,27–29]. Data has recently been presented to show that some postoperative complaints, particularly of obstructive nature, could be predicted by the preoperative prevalence of defective primary peristalsis following water swallows [13]. In addition, it has been argued that preoperative detection of severe motility disturbances is important to exclude from antireflux surgery patients, in whom these procedures would invariably be followed by obstructive symptoms. This question, however, relates closely to the so far unresolved issue of whether esophageal motor impairments associated with esophagitis are reversible or not [23–26,29–30]. Evidence against have dominated, whereas recent data indicate that a substantial improvement can occur in some cases, provided that long-term control of reflux is accomplished. However, until these observations have been confirmed in prospective controlled trials comprising a large study population with a well defined disease and a long-term follow-up, firm conclusions cannot be drawn. It is, however, relevant to point out, that patients with a severe reflux disease and concomitant peristaltic dysfunction should be, until proven otherwise, submitted to a fundoplication procedure where the wrap always is short and loose [2,31]. Furthermore, such patients should be warned, that postoperative dysphagia may be a problem.

Esophageal emptying of food as studied by nuclear medicine devices has been shown to pick up a number of motility disturbances in patients with GERD especially when associated with dysphagia. However, a close association between esophageal emptying and the subsequent long-term postoperative outcome has not been established [32–33].

Lower esophageal sphincter function

Patients with severe long-standing GERD often express a low basal pressure in the lower esophageal sphincter (LES) with also frequent transient relaxations associated with reflux of gastric contents [34]. The basal tone of the LES, however, varies continuously when adequate measuring devices are applied [35]. We have studied the relationship between the preoperative basal LES pressure by use of the sleeve device and the capacity of the sphincter to relax after water swallows as well and the subsequent long-term outcome after antireflux surgery [15]. A high preoperative mean sphincter tone predicted postoperative complaints with inability to belch and relieve bloating and distension. No doubt, fundoplication procedures profoundly impairs the ability to belch and relieve bloating and these operations significantly reduces the capacity of the sphincter to relax properly, both as transient events and in response to swallows [19,36].

Gastric emptying

Delayed gastric emptying might be one of many important factors in the genesis of unfavorable postoperative symptoms after fundoplications. It must, however, be remembered that these operations by themselves seem to improve gastric emptying capacity [37]. On the other hand, a combined highly selective vagotomy and a fundic wrap is followed by no clear cut effect on gastric motor function [38]. Therefore, it is relevant to bear in mind that important clinical long-term differences between operations such as fundoplications alone and the combined procedure have not been demonstrated [39], and consequently the role of gastric emptying in the course of postfundoplication symptoms remains to be elucidated. A recent study presented data to suggest that many, if not all, side effects associated with a Nissen fundoplication could be attributed to a failure of the procedure to normalize gastric emptying [40] which, however, probably represents an oversimplification of the problem. We also found that preoperative observations on gastric emptying capacity of solid food items in patients, predicted those who might develop some long-lasting postfundoplication symptoms [41]. The most obvious associations found between gas bloat problems such as postprandial satiety, distension and pain and impaired gastric motor function. The complexity of the mechanisms behind these complaints is, however, obvious and more information is needed before firm clinical recommendations can be taken. Recent data would suggest that the motor capacity of the proximal stomach is of particular importance, not only for the emptying of solid food items in general, but particularly so in patients with reflux disease since the motor function of this part of the stomach might regulate the frequency of transient LES relaxations in the postprandial period [34,41]. Consequently, more data is needed on the role of the emptying capacity of the proximal stomach in relation also to the outcome after antireflux surgery.

To put these observations into a balanced clinical perspective we observed, in our survey, that no relationship at all existed between the gastric emptying parameters and the final clinical outcome after antireflux surgery as scored by the patient [14]. It is always relevant to emphasize that patients may often rate the postprandial symptoms as of nuisance value only and very much less than the preoperative reflux symptoms, which are effectively controlled by the antireflux procedure.

In conclusion, our present state of knowledge strongly supports the view that fundoplications act through more complex mechanisms than just by correcting anatomical defects in the hiatus area and by forming an anatomical and mechanical valve at the gastroesophageal junction [18]. In the preoperative evaluation of patients with severe, long-lasting GERD, important clinical information might be obtained from physiological studies focusing on the function of the tubular esophagus, the LES and on the gastric emptying capacities in order to define the risk profile for those who might phase a high risk of postfundoplication symptoms of predominantly gas bloat nature [42]. Although these complaints might well be of marginal importance compared to the benefit of relieving major reflux symptoms and preventing complications from occurring by the operation, similar complaints can cause significant morbidity to some patients. It should be born in mind, that these complaints deserve to be looked upon as potentially preventable. Defective primary peristalsis in the distal esophagus should lead the surgeon and the patient to the risk of persistent dysphagia postoperatively, and the high preoperative basal tone in the LES indicates an enhanced risk of gas bloat complaints as does delayed gastric emptying of solids. The design of an antireflux procedure, which would avoid many of these drawbacks and subsequently only exceptionally would be associated with severe postoperative complaints [43], will probably never be completed. Instead, high risk patients should preoperatively be informed about the risk of subsequent postoperative complaints, in order to facilitate the clinical decision making process. This is especially important now, when alternative long-term therapeutic strategies can be considered [44].

References

1. Jamieson GG, Duranceau AC, Deschamps C. Surgical treatment of gastroesophageal reflux disease. In: Jamieson GG, Duranceau AC (eds) Gastroesophageal Reflux. Philadelphia: WB Saunders, 1988; Chap. 10.
2. DeMeester TR, Bonavina L, Albertucci M. Nissen fundoplication for gastroesophageal reflux disease. Evaluation of primary repair in 100 consecutive patients. Ann Surg 1986;204:9−20.
3. DeMeester TR, Johnson LF, Kent AH. Evaluation of current operations for the prevention of gastroesophageal reflux. Ann Surg 1974;180:511−525.
4. Washer BF, Gear MWL, Dowling BL et al. Randomised prospective trial of Roux-en-Y duodenal diversion vs. fundoplication for severe reflux oesophagitis. Br J Surg 1984;71:181−184.
5. Gear MWL, Gillison EW, Dowling BL. Randomised prospective trial of the Angelchik antireflux prosthesis. Br J Surg 1984;71:681.
6. Lundell L, Abrahamsson H, Ruth M et al. Lower esophageal sphincter characteristics and esophageal acid exposure following partial or 360° fundoplication: results of a prospective, randomized, clinical study. World J Surg 1991;15:115.
7. Walker SJ, Holt S, Sanderson CJ, Stoddard CJ. Comparison of Nissen total and Lind partial transabdominal fundoplication in the treatment of gastro-oesophageal reflux. Br J Surg 1992;79:410.
8. Deakin M, Mayer D, Tembel JG. Surgery for gastro-oesophageal reflux: the Angelchik prosthesis compared to the floppy Nissen fundoplication. 2-year follow-up study and 5-year evaluation of the Angelchik prosthesis. Ann Roy Coll Surg Eng 1989;71:249.
9. Clark J. Hiatal hernia and reflux oesophagitis. In: Hennessy TPJ, Cuschieri A (eds) Surgery of the Oesophagus. London: Bailliere Tindal, 1986; Chap. 6.
10. Hill LD, Ilves R, Stevenson JK, Pearson JM. Reoperation for disruption and recurrence after Nissen fundoplication. Arch Surg 1979;114:542.
11. Maher JW, Hocking MP, Woodward ER. Reoperations for esophagitis following failed antireflux procedures. Ann Surg 1985;201:723.
12. Siewert JR, Isolauri J, Feussner H. Reoperation following failed fundoplication. World J Surg 1989;13:791.
13. Lundell LR, Myers JC, Jamieson GG. The influence of preoperative oesophageal motor function on the long-term outcome of antireflux surgery. Gullet 1993;3:50−55.
14. Lundell LR, Myers JC, Jamieson GG. Gastric emptying and its relationship to symptoms of "gas bloat" after antireflux surgery. Eur J Surg 1994;160:140.
15. Lundell LR, Myers JC, Jamieson GG. The effect of antireflux operations on lower oesophageal sphincter tone and the postprandial symptoms. Scand J Gastroenterol 1993;28:725.
16. Negre JB. Postfundoplication symptoms. Do they restrict the success of Nissen fundoplication? Ann Surg 1983;198:698.
17. Spechler JS et al. Comparison of medical and surgical therapy for complicated gastro-oesophageal reflux disease in veterans. N Engl J Med 1992;326:786.
18. Little AG. Mechanism of action of antireflux surgery: theory and facts. World J Surg 1992;16:320.
19. Smith D, King NA, Waldron B et al. Study of belching ability in antireflux surgery patients and normal volunteers. Br J Surg 1991;78:32.
20. Kahrilas PJ, Dodds WJ, Hogan WJ. Effect of peristaltic dysfunction on esophageal volume clearance. Gastroenterology 1988;94:73.
21. Kahrilas PJ, Dodds WJ, Hogan WJ et al. Esophageal peristaltic dysfunction in peptic esophagitis. Gastroenterology 1986;91:897−904.
22. Helm JF, Dodds WJ, Riedel DR et al. Determinants of esophageal acid clearance in normal subjects. Gastroenterology 1983;85:607.
23. Gill RC, Bowes KL, Murphy PD, Kingma J. Esophageal motor abnormalities in gastroesophageal reflux and the effects of fundoplication. Gastroenterology 1986;91:364−369.
24. Stanciu C, Bennett JR. Oesophageal acid clearing: one factor in the production of reflux oesophagitis. Gut 1974;15:852.
25. Russel COH, Pope CE II, Gannan RM, Allen FD, Velasco N, Hill LD. Does surgery correct esophageal motor dysfunction in gastroesophageal reflux? Ann Surg 1981;194:290−296.
26. Katz PQ, Knuff TE, Benjamin SD, Castell DO. Abnormal esophageal pressures in reflux esophagitis: cause or effect? Am J Gastroenterol 1986;81:744.
27. Mughal MM, Bancewicz J, Marples M. Oesophageal manometry and pH recording does not predict the bad results of Nissen fundoplication. Br J Surg 1990;77:43−45.

28. Joelsson BE, DeMeester TR, Skinner DB, LaFontaine E, Waters PF, O'Sullivan GC. The role of the esophageal body in the antireflux mechanism. Surgery 1982;92:417–424.
29. Pope CE II. Esophageal motility – who needs it? Gastroenterology 1978;74:1337–1338.
30. Ortiz Escandell A, Martinez de Haro LF, Parrilla Paricio P, Aguayo Albasini JL, Garcia Marcilla JA, Morales Cuenca G. Surgery improves defective oesophageal peristalsis in patients with gastro-oesophageal reflux. Br J Surg 1991;78:1095–1097.
31. Donahue PE, Bombeck CT. The modified Nissen fundoplication – reflux control without gas bloat. Chir Gastroenterol 1977;76:1393.
32. Richter JE, Blackwell JN, Wu WC et al. Relationship of radionuclide liquid bolus transport and esophageal manometry. J Lab Clin Med 1987;109:217.
33. Maddern GJ, Jamieson GG. Oesophageal emptying in patients with gastro-oesophageal reflux. Br J Surg 1986;73:615–617.
34. Holloway RH, Dent J. Lower esophageal sphincter dysfunction in gastroesophageal reflux disease. Gastroenterol Clin North Am 1990;19:517.
35. Dent J, Dodds WJ, Friedman RH et al. Mechanism of gastro-oesophageal reflux in recumbent, asymptomatic human subjects. J Clin Invest 1980;65:256.
36. Ireland AC, Holloway RH, Toouli J, Dent J. Mechanisms underlying the antireflux action of fundoplication. Gut 1993;34:303–308.
37. Maddern GJ, Jamieson GG. Fundoplication enhances gastric emptying. Ann Surg 1985;201:296–299.
38. Jamieson GG, Maddern GJ, Myers JC. Gastric emptying after fundoplication with and without proximal gastric vagotomy. Arch Surg 1991;126:1414–1417.
39. Csendes A, Braghetto I, Korn O, Cortes C. Late subjective and objective evaluations of antireflux surgery in patients with reflux esophagitis: analysis of 215 patients. Surgery 1989;105:374.
40. Hinder RA, Stein HJ, Bremner CG, DeMeester TR. Relationship of a satisfactory outcome to normalisation of delayed gastric emptying after Nissen fundoplication. Ann Surg 1989;210:458–465.
41. Collins PJ, Houghton LA, Read NW et al. Role of the proximal and distal stomach in mixed solid and liquid meal emptying. Gut 1991;32:615.
42. Garstin WI, Hohnston GW, Kennedy TL, Spencer ES. Nissen fundoplication: the unhappy 15%. Royal Coll Surg 1986;31:207.
43. Watson A, Jenkinson LR, Ball CS, Barlow AP, Norris TL. A more physiological alternative to total fundoplication for the surgical correction of resistant gastro-oesophageal reflux. Br J Surg 1991;78:1088.
44. Armstrong D, Nicolet M, Monnier Ph et al. Maintenance therapy: is there still a place for antireflux surgery? World J Surg 1992;6:300–307.

Two examinations seem indispensable:
– pH measurement to confirm doubtful diagnoses
– manometry for choice of technique

J.E. Richter (Birmingham, Alabama)

Prior to any antireflux surgery, the patient's operability has to be evaluated carefully since only minimal operative risk is acceptable for this benign condition. Unfortunately, many physicians believe that the only test necessary prior to surgery is endoscopy. Although this is the best test for defining the presence of reflux esophagitis, it is *not* a test of esophageal function. The best tests for esophageal function are 24-h pH monitoring and esophageal manometry. In most situations, both of these tests should be performed prior to consideration of antireflux surgery.

Ambulatory 24-h pH monitoring is helpful to confirm doubtful diagnoses of gastroesophageal reflux disease (GERD). It is particularly useful in the patient with severe intractable symptoms but no evidence of esophagitis by endoscopy. Ambulatory pH monitoring often will reveal that these patients have acid reflux primarily in the upright position. Chronic atypical symptoms of reflux (e.g., chest pain, chronic cough, recurrent pneumonias, episodes of nocturnal choking, or repeated nausea and vomiting) are also indications for ambulatory 24-h pH monitoring. As these patients usually do not have esophagitis, this may be the only test to confirm that acid reflux is the etiology of the patient's symptoms. If these patients respond to aggressive acid suppression therapy, then a logical and reassuring decision can be made about approaching them with antireflux surgery. Ambulatory 24-h pH monitoring also should be considered in selected patients with esophagitis. The presence of distal erosive esophagitis may not always be related to acid reflux. For example, rare patients with alkaline reflux or achalasia can present with esophagitis. More importantly, older patients with a recent onset of ulcerative esophagitis should be carefully evaluated as studies suggest that approximately 20% of these patients have pill induced esophagitis [1].

Manometry is essential in all patients prior to antireflux surgery. The procedure is not done primarily to evaluate lower esophageal sphincter (LES) pressure as most of these patients, particularly those with erosive esophagitis, will have a sphincter pressure <10 mmHg. Rather, manometry is done to assess the functional motor capacity of the esophagus before deciding whether fundoplication is applicable or not. Some authorities suggest that nonspecific motor disorders, such as low amplitude contractions and intermittent simultaneous contractions, are a contraindication to antireflux surgery. However, more recent studies find that these motility disorders are secondary to reflux disease and do not preclude successful surgery [2,3]. On the other hand, the important manometric abnormality to define is aperistalsis, be it either a manifestation of achalasia, scleroderma esophagus, or severe end stage reflux disease usually associated with a difficult to dilate stricture. As surprising as it may sound, I have seen several patients with unsuspected achalasia who have undergone antireflux surgery [4]. These patients had symptoms of heartburn, nonspecific esophagitis and the "bird beaking" from the hypertensive LES was misinterpreted as a stricture. This can be prevented by all patients having manometry prior to surgery. Fortunately, many patients with scleroderma esophagus and severe esophagitis can now be treated with proton pump inhibitors. Should these patients need antireflux surgery then a floppy Nissen fundoplication or an incomplete wrap, such as a Belsey or Toupet, can be done to prevent worsening of their dysphagia. Another alternative would be to do a vagotomy, antrectomy and Roux-en-Y procedure to prevent reflux of acid, while not risking the production of dysphagia by wrapping the distal esophagus [5]. Strictures that are difficult to dilate return very quickly, and are associated with minimal symptomatic relief, usually identify a subset of reflux patients with a severely damaged esophagus and associated aperistalsis. These patients do poorly with classic antireflux surgery, being best served by distal esophageal resection and esophagogastrostomy and/or colon interposition [6].

References

1. Bonavina L, DeMeester TR, McChesney L. Drug-induced esophageal strictures. Ann Surg 1987;206:173—183.
2. Bancewicz J, Osugi H, Marples M. Clinical implications of abnormal oesophageal motility. Br J Surg 1987;74:416—419.
3. Grande L, Lacima G, Ros E et al. Dysphagia and esophageal motor dysfunction in gastroesophageal reflux are corrected by fundoplication. J Clin Gastroenterol 1991;13:11—16.
4. Mattox HE, Albertson DA, Castell DO, Richter JE. Dysphagia following fundoplication: "slipped" fundoplication vs. achalasia complicated by fundoplication. Am J Gastroenterol 1990;85:1468—1472.
5. Washer GF, Gear MWL, Dowling BL et al. Randomized prospective trial of Roux-en-Y duodenal diverson vs. fundoplication for severe reflux oesophagitis. Br J Surg 1984;71:181—184.
6. Zaninotto G, DeMeester TR, Bremner CG et al. Esophageal function in patients with reflux induced strictures and its relevance to surgical treatment. Ann Thorac Surg 1989;47:362—370.

What are the operative indications in reflux?

T.R. DeMeester (Los Angeles)

Initial therapy

A reasonable protocol for managing patients with gastroesophageal reflux disease (GERD) is shown in Fig. 1. All patients whose symptoms persist despite simple antacid therapy should undergo endoscopy to determine if the complications of reflux disease such as esophagitis, stricture or Barrett's esophagus are present. All are then placed on H_2 blocker or omeprazole therapy. If their symptoms persist while on medication, they should be studied with manometry and 24-h esophageal and gastric pH monitoring. If their symptoms disappear completely after 12 weeks of therapy, the medication should be discontinued and the patient observed. If their symptoms recur within 4 weeks, they should be studied since they are prone to drug dependency. Patients who on repeat endoscopy show persisting complications of the disease, should also be studied. Depending on the results of the tests, therapy may be directed toward the existence of a disease other than GERD, or, if GERD is confirmed, the patient may be considered for surgical therapy if the criteria for an antireflux repair are met. Patients whose symptoms do not reoccur within 4 weeks and are free of complications of the disease should be monitored and treated intermittently when symptoms occur.

Requirements for antireflux surgery

Prior to proceeding with an antireflux procedure, it is necessary to confirm that the patients' symptoms are caused by increased esophageal exposure to gastric juice

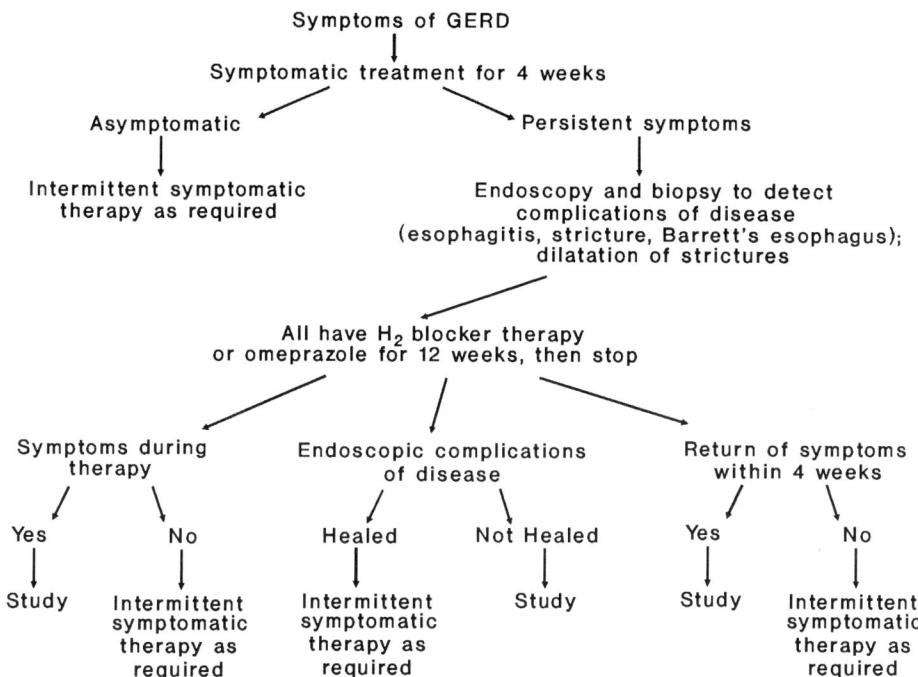

Fig. 1. Algorithm showing medical management and indications for functional studies (i.e., 24-h pH monitoring and manometry) in patients with symptoms of gastroesophageal reflux disease (GERD).

secondary to a mechanically defective lower esophageal sphincter. This requires performing esophageal function studies (i.e., 24-h esophageal pH monitoring and esophageal manometry). A mechanically defective LES is identified by the presence of one or any combination of the following motility abnormalities: a pressure <6 mmHg, an overall sphincter length of <2 cm or an abdominal length of <1 cm. The requirements to proceed with an antireflux procedure are:

— Increased esophageal exposure to gastric juice: 24-h pH monitoring.
— Mechanically defective LES: esophageal manometry.
— Absence of a primary esophageal motility disorder or loss of contractility in the lower half of the esophagus: esophageal manometry.

If 24-h esophageal pH monitoring is normal in a patient with unequivocal endoscopic esophagitis, the possibilities of alkaline, drug-induced, or retention esophagitis should be considered. Patients with increased esophageal exposure to gastric juice in whom the sphincter is manometrically normal, should be evaluated for a gastric abnormality or an esophageal motility disorder. Approximately 40% of these patients will have gastric acid hypersecretion and respond to more aggressive antisecretory therapy. Patients with increased esophageal acid exposure, a mechanically defective sphincter and no complications of the disease should be given the option of surgery if they are drug dependent to control their symptoms.

If the patient responds symptomatically to medical therapy but endoscopic esophagitis persists, surgery should be performed. Without surgery, these patients can progress to develop a stricture or Barrett's esophagus and lose esophageal body function while on therapy, because reflux of alkalized gastric contents continues through the mechanically defective sphincter. In this situation, an antireflux procedure corrects the mechanically defective sphincter, prevents the formation of a stricture or Barrett's.

Factors to consider prior to antireflux surgery

Prior to proceeding with an antireflux operation, several factors should be evaluated.

First, the propulsive force of the body of the esophagus should be evaluated by esophageal manometry to determine if it has sufficient power to propel a bolus of food through a newly reconstructed valve. Patients with normal peristaltic contractions do well with a 360° Nissen fundoplication. When peristalsis is absent, severely disordered, or the amplitude of the contraction is below 20 mmHg, the Belsey two-thirds partial fundoplication is the procedure of choice.

Second, anatomic shortening of the esophagus can compromise the ability to do an adequate repair without tension and lead to an increased incidence of breakdown or thoracic displacement of the repair. Esophageal shortening is identified radiographically by a sliding hiatal hernia that will not reduce in the upright position or that measures larger than 5 cm between the diaphragmatic crura and gastroesophageal junction on endoscopy. When present, the motility of the esophageal body must be carefully evaluated and, if adequate, a gastroplasty should be performed. In patients who have a motility study that shows the absence of contractility or more than 50% interrupted or dropped contractions or a history of several failed previous antireflux procedures, esophageal resection should be considered as an alternative.

Third, the surgeon should specifically query the patient for complaints of epigastric pain, nausea, vomiting and loss of appetite. In the past, these symptoms were accepted as part of the reflux syndrome, but it is now realized that they can be due to excessive duodenogastric reflux which occurs in about one-third of patients with GERD. This problem is most pronounced in patients who have had previous upper gastrointestinal surgery, particularly cholecystectomy, although this is not always the case. In such patients, the correction of only the incompetent cardia may result in a disgruntled individual who continues to complain of nausea and epigastric pain on eating. In these patients, 24-h pH monitoring of the stomach may help to detect and quantitate duodenogastric reflux. The abnormality can also be documented with a ^{99m}Tc-HIDA scan if excessive reflux of radionucleotide from the duodenum into the stomach can be demonstrated. Antireflux surgery may reduce duodenogastric reflux by improving the efficiency of gastric emptying. If the symptoms of duodenogastric reflux persist after antireflux surgery, the administration of sucralfate may relieve the persistent complaint of nausea and epigastric pain. In a few patients this may give inadequate relief and eventually, a bile diversion procedure may be necessary.

Fourth, approximately 30% of patients with proven gastroesophageal reflux on

24-h pH monitoring will have hypersecretion on gastric analysis; 2—3% of patients who have an antireflux operation will develop a gastric or duodenal ulcer. These factors may modify the proposed antireflux procedure in patients with active ulcer disease or documentation of previous ulceration, by the addition of a highly selective vagotomy.

Fifth, delayed gastric emptying is found in approximately 40% of patients with GERD and can contribute to symptoms after an antireflux repair. Usually, however, mild degrees of delayed gastric emptying are corrected by the antireflux procedure and only in patients with severe emptying disorders is there a need for an additional gastric procedure.

References

1. DeMeester TR, Stein HJ. Gastroesophageal reflux disease. In: Moody FG, Carey LC, Jones RS, Kelly KA, Nahrwold DL, Skinner DB (eds) Surgical Treatment of Digestive Disease, 2nd edn. Chicago: Year Book Medical Publishers Inc., 1989;65—108.
2. Crookes PF, DeMeester TR. Reflux oesophagitis. Surgery — Medicine Group Journal 1993;433—444.
3. Peters JH, DeMeester TR. Esophagus and diaphragmatic hernias. In: Schwartz SI (ed) Principles of Surgery, 6th edn (in press).

 L. Tibbling (Linköping)

Respiratory symptoms with cough, chronic bronchitis and bronchial asthma are known to be much more frequent in patients with gastroesophageal reflux disease (GERD) than in controls or in the general population. Gastroesophageal reflux is found in as many as 30—60% of patients with asthma and other bronchial disorders. Various pathways, by which GER may trigger bronchial symptoms, have been suggested such as aspiration, or an esophagobronchial reflex initiated by acid irritation of the esophageal mucosa. Neither of these theories have been convincingly corroborated [1,2].

A new theory

A third theory has recently been tested [3] which implies that pharyngeal dysfunction causes aspiration by partial misswallowing. This theory is based on the idea of co-ordination between the contraction of the longitudinal esophageal muscle, the biodynamic opening of the upper esophageal sphincter and the closure of the larynx to prevent aspiration. For the proper function of any longitudinal muscle, the anchoring at both its ends is necessary. The longitudinal muscle has been shown to contract and stiffen the esophageal wall at swallowing [4] thereby promoting normal transit. In patients with hiatal hernia and GERD, the distal end of the longitudinal muscle of the esophagus has been shortened and dislocated into the thoracic cavity. This shortening impairs contraction of the muscle, which in turn may influence the timing of the rapid pharyngeal phase. The swallowed bolus will then bump against a closed upper esophageal sphincter and hypopharyngeal retention of the bolus may result with increased risk of aspiration. Already in 1967, Urschel and Paulson [5] found in their patients with hiatal hernia that 61% had bronchitis and 16% of these had bronchitis as the only sign of a hiatal herniation.

The theory of pharyngoesophageal incoordination was tested [3] by comparing patients in whom gastroesophageal reflux was treated by omeprazole (n = 78) which inhibits gastric acid secretion, with patients (n = 119) in whom the distal end of the longitudinal muscle was surgically anchored in the abdominal cavity by fundoplication and crural repair. Both groups had an equal rate (30%) of bronchitis. In the medically treated group there was no significant reduction of bronchitis, whereas in the surgical group there was a highly significant reduction of bronchitis.

Misswallowing at meals

The findings support the theory of aspiration due to misswallowing at meals as a cause for the high rate of bronchitis in patients with hiatal hernia. The repeated findings of hiatal hernia in patients with a Zenker's diverticulum [6] provide further support for the idea of impaired coordination between opening of the upper esophageal sphincter and contraction of the longitudinal muscle, when the distal end of the muscle has slipped upwards. Failure for the opening of the sphincter directs the pressure of the bolus to the pharyngeal wall with subsequent diverticular formation.

In a recent article [7], cricopharyngeal dysfunction was reported in patients with chronic obstructive pulmonary disease. The authors assumed that the cricopharyngeal dysfunction leads to occult aspiration of small quantities of oropharyngeal contents. In another study [8], 796 retired people were interviewed about esophageal dysphagia, misswallowing, and coughing when eating. Those having a history of esophageal dysphagia (n = 62) reported intermittent symptoms of getting food down the wrong way and coughing at meals in one third of the cases. Only 5% (p < 0.001) without esophageal problems experienced misswallowings.

Bronchitis can therefore be a strong indication for hiatal hernia surgery, since there is no efficient medical therapy to correct the herniation. Surgeons should be aware of their ability to cure bronchopulmonary problems even in hiatal hernia patients without gastroesophageal reflux.

References

1. Ekström T, Tibbling L. Gastro-oesophageal reflux and triggering of bronchial asthma. A negative report. Eur J Respir Dis 1987;71:177–180.

2. Ekström T, Tibbling L. Esophageal acid perfusion, airway function and symptoms in asthmatic patients with marked bronchial hyperreactivity. Chest 1989;96:995—998.

3. Tibbling L. Wrong-way swallowing as a possible cause of bronchitis in patients with gastroesophageal reflux disease. Acta Otolaryngol 1993;113:405—408.

4. Tibbling L, Ask P, Pope CE II. Electromyography of human oesophageal smooth muscle. Scand J Gastroenterol 1986;21: 559—567.

5. Urschel HC, Paulson DL. Gastroesophageal reflux and hiatal hernia. Complications and therapy. J Thorac Cardiovasc Surg 1967;53:21—32.

6. Hunt PS, Connell AM, Smiley TB. The cricopharyngeal sphincter in gastric reflux. Gut 1970;11:303—306.

7. Stein M, Williams AJ, Grossman F, Weinberg AS, Zuckerbraun L. Cricopharyngeal dysfunction in chronic obstructive pulmonary disease. Chest 1990;97:347—352.

8. Tibbling L, Gustafsson B. Dysphagia and its consequences in the elderly. Dysphagia 1991;6:200—202.

Antireflux valves

 ## What are the factors of increasing LES pressure during dissection of the hiatal orifice?

G. Bommelaer, J. Boulant (Clermont-Ferrand)

Intraoperative measurement of lower esophageal sphincter (LES) pressure was first described by Hill [1]. This new process was proposed as a means of ensuring adequate sphincter pressure during surgery and suggests that, in the operating room [2,3], the surgeon could calibrate the LES pressure. However, the validity of such techniques requires a good correlation between intraoperative and postoperative sphincter pressure [4]. Currently, several studies lead to the conclusion that general anesthesia and laparotomy do not affect preoperative and intraoperative sphincter pressure values. However, there is no significant statistical correlation between the intraoperative pressure after fundoplication, and those obtained postoperatively after 6 or 12 months.

Such intraoperative studies have shown that the mean intraoperative LES pressure after diaphragmatic hiatus dissection is approximately twice the pressure recorded before esophageal manipulation (i.e., values obtained after induction of anesthesia and laparotomy). Orringer and associates [4] found that, in 11 patients, dilatation of peptic strictures or manipulations of the esophagus required for mobilization of the cardia, produced an increase of distal esophagus tone. In our study [5], including patients that only have gastroesophageal reflux without strictures or scleroderma, values recorded after dissection of diaphragmatic hiatus were all significantly increased (1.2 ± 0.8 kPa before dissection, 2.2 ± 1 kPa after dissection ($p < 0.001$)).

These data suggest that intraoperative values obtained at the completion of an antireflux operation not only reflect the increase of distal esophageal pressure resulting from fundoplication, but also a highly variable response of the lower esophageal muscle to dissection of the diaphragmatic hiatus.

However, why does LES pressure increase after dissection of the diaphragmatic hiatus?

First and foremost, the increased LES pressure after dissection of the diaphragmatic hiatus could be due to the operative manipulation. This would indicate that manipulation of the esophagus, like all other smooth muscle organs, causes a certain amount of spasm [4], which is responsible for the high pressure recorded during operation. This spasm could be due to traumatism or partial ischemia secondary to dissection. An argument for this is the rapid decrease in LES pressure [1] observed postsurgically, as compared to values obtained during the operation.

Secondly, the "normalization" of the LES pressure before fundoplication could be explained by the repositioning of the distal esophagus within the abdominal cavity during operation. Nevertheless, Cooper and Orringer [2,3] failed to observe a difference in sphincter pressure with the chest closed or opened. Similarly, Hill failed to observe a difference in the pressure with the abdominal cavity opened or closed, indicating that the positive abdominal pressure had minimal effect on the sphincter pressure. This suggestion is in agreement with the concept that the distal esophageal high pressure zone is not due to the function of a distinct muscle bundle, but more likely to the geometry of the smooth muscle at the cardia. Deficiency of the "cardia" pressure in hiatus hernia with esophageal reflux is also in line with this hypothesis.

Thirdly, it could be suggested that the esophageal dissection would cause a perivascular innervation damage. This neuronal damage due to dissection of the diaphragmatic hiatus could indirectly increase esophageal sphincter pressure by inhibitory innervation impairment. It is well known that the LES pressure is under control of both excitatory and inhibitory mechanisms. Indeed, recent study has proven that esophagitis decreases cholinergic excitation, but leaves intact the neural inhibition to the LES. The suppression of the excitation contribute to the transient LES relaxation and to resting LES hypotension in humans with gastroesophageal reflux. In the presence of esophagitis, the inhibitory mechanisms of the LES pressure remain intact or are effectively increased whereas the excitatory mechanisms are impaired. In contrast diaphragmatic hiatus dissection could impair inhibitory mechanisms.

On the other hand, cholecystokinin causes relaxation of the cat LES by stimulating cholecystokinin receptors on noncholinergic, nonadrenergic inhibitory neurons and causes contraction by stimulating cholecystokinin receptors on the sphincter muscle [6]. Thus, a neuro-hormonal origin of these inhibitory mechanisms could be presumed. Indeed, in agreement with Salapatek et al. [7] we have found (unpublished data) that intravenous injection of cerulatide (Cerulex®), a cholecystokinin analogue, increased significantly and remarkably the LES pressure from 2.2 ± 1 to 7 ± 1 kPa after dissection of hiatus hernia, but not before surgical manipulation. This suggests that inhibitory neurons, could be somehow damaged during surgical manipulation and thus stimulation of intact muscle cholecystokinin excitatory receptors could be unmasked.

Taken together, these different mechanisms could explain the increased LES pressure after dissection of the hiatus hernia. However, other studies should be conducted to prove the involvement of neuro-hormonal inhibitory mechanisms in the pathophysiology of gastroesophageal reflux and in the modifications of LES pressure observed during surgical manipulation. Cholecystokinin, vasoactive intestinal polypeptide or nitric oxide could be the neuromodulators implicated.

References

1. Hill LD. Intraoperative measurement of lower esophageal sphincter pressure. J Thorac Cardiovasc Surg 1978;75:378−382.
2. Cooper JD, Gill SS, Nelems JM, Pearson FG. Intraoperative and postoperative esophageal manometric finding with Collis gastroplasty and Belsey hiatal hernia repair for gastroesophageal reflux. J Thorac Cardiovasc Surg 1977;74:744−751.
3. Noble HG, Christie DL, Cahill FL. Follow-up studies on patients undergoing Nissen fundoplication utilizing intraoperative manometry. J Pediatr Surg 1982;17(5):490−493.
4. Orringer MB, Scheider R, Williams GW, Sloan H. Intraoperative esophageal manometry: is it valid? Ann Thor Surg 1980; 30:13−18.
5. Delasalle P, Boulant J, Dapoigny M, Pezet D, Abergel A, Ferrier C, Chipponi J, Bommelaer G. Per operative manometry of lower esophageal sphincter (LES): effects of Toupet and Nissen fundoplicature. European Digestive Disease Week Amsterdam 20−26 October 1991. Eur J Gastroenterol Hepatol 1991;3:S11.
6. Rattan S, Goyal RK. Structure activity relationship of cholecystokinin receptors in the cat esophageal sphincter. Gastroenterology 1986;90:94−102.
7. Salapatek AM, Diamant NE. Assessment of neural inhibition of the lower esophageal sphincter in cats with esophagitis. Gastroenterology 1993;104:810−818.

What is the definition of brachyesophagus?

J. Testart (Rouen)

Brachyesophagus (BE) means a short esophagus. This term, first applied to infants, was used also for grown-ups by Resano [1] and Lortat-Jacob [2]. Being only descriptive, it implies no particular cause. To define BE is to draw its frontiers with an esophagus of normal length.

Akerlund in 1926, when classifying hernias through the diaphragmatic esophageal hiatus, already set apart the short esophagus from sliding hernias and paraesophageal hernias [2]. However, neither Akerlund nor Resano nor Lortat-Jacob gave any definition. Among 35 papers dealing with BE, the short or the shortened esophagus, only one gives a definition: "when the cardia is fixed at a point more than 4 cm above the diaphragm we speak of a second degree shortening of the esophagus" [3].

However, Resano, in 1950, had already given some indications that could be used in a definition "mistake than attempting a surgical reduction" "7th thoracic vertebra" "34 cm from the teeth". But in 1950 the endobrachyesophagus was still unknown. It is indeed nonsense to define the BE without drawing its frontier with the endobrachyesophagus as well as with the normal esophagus above a sliding hernia.

Endobrachyesophagus (Barrett's esophagus) was clearly described and defined by Lortat-Jacob in 1957 as the "outside aspect of a quite normal esophageal musculus but with a gastric fundic mucosa on some centimeters" [4]. At the OESO Meeting in 1988, Lortat-Jacob [5] confirmed the definition of the endo-BE as an "esophagus whose external morphology is normal or appreciably normal with preservation of an abdominal esophagus and its relations with the gastric fundus, while internally the malpighian mucosa does not occupy the entire length of the esophagus. A certain length of the lower esophagus may be clothed on its inner aspect with a gastric mucosa of fundal type or a metaplastic, even intestinal mucosa". There he also confirmed that it was synonymous with the "lower esophagus lined by columnar epithelium", described in 1950 [6] and interpreted in 1957 by Barrett [7]. Precisely in 1950, Barrett had considered only the mucosa to differentiate esophagus and gaster and he had described the endo-BE as a tubular stomach below a congenitally short esophagus [6]. Therefore, it was only in 1957 that the endo-BE was distinguished from the BE. The only addition that appeared since in its definition is the need to have the gastric mucosa at least 3 cm circularly above the cardia [8].

However, if it is easy to validate the gap between the mucosa and the muscularis frontiers, it is much more difficult to situate the muscular frontier relative to the anatomical marks.

Usually the cardia is situated at the level of the 10th thoracic vertebra, just above the celiac arterial truncus. However, due to physiological pressure measurements and surgical explorations, the position of the cardia must be evaluated relative to the diaphragm. Normally there are 2 cm of esophagus in the esophageal hiatus of the diaphragm and 2.5 ± 1 cm below. Surgically, four more centimeters can be easily lowered [9].

No matter how high the cardia may be in a hiatus hernia, as long as it can be lowered below the diaphragm, the term BE can not be used.

However, what if this can only be obtained by strong pulling after extensive mobilization up to the aortic arch, sometimes with truncal vagotomies and slits of the external longitudinal muscularis layer of the esophagus?

Hill and Mercer [10] noted that they "have yet to encounter a so called short esophagus except in a small number of patients who have had perforation or repeated bougienage with complete destruction of the esophagus". Hill is afraid of a diagnosis leading to "surgical treatment... by complex and formidable operations" instead of the conservative operation he described. Indeed, it would be insincere not to admit that, besides this definition of BE, lies the problem of the lowering of the inferior sphincter of the esophagus below the diaphragm inside the abdominal pressure zone. This appears obvious in the Henderson's paper about "irreducible cardia" [9]. He then noticed that the true shortening of the esophagus was more difficult to judge through a transthoracic than through an abdominal approach. The abdominal approach allows longitudinal pulling of the esophagus. Moreover, the abdominal approach allows an easier dealing with the diaphragm: 1) it can be pushed upwards with the help of curarization; and 2) the esophagus can be forced forwards in the hiatus, taking advantage of the obliquity of the diaphragm.

However, can such forced lowering of "irreducible cardia" be maintained even by a tight anchoring?

An accurate definition of BE or "irreducible cardia" must take into account the strength that must be used in order to lower the esophagus after its mobilization to a definite mark.

When operating through an abdominal approach, we measured the strength used when pulling on an elastic lace placed around the esophagus. The maximal force attempted was 1 kg. However, from 0.3—1 kg the lowering gain was small. High strength is not very useful there. While the upward pushing of the diaphragm often allows to place the cardia below it, the problem is to find a technique that maintains this position after anesthetic relaxation wears off.

Therefore, it is proposed to keep the term BE when a 0.3 kg traction cannot give 2 cm of esophagus below the frontal edge of the hiatus without pushing up the diaphragm.

Now, is it possible to diagnose a BE before operating upon it? Endoscopy shows only the Z-line. Echoendoscopy cannot situate the muscular frontier. Only X-rays can sometimes suspect or affirm the BE. At first, the cardia can be situated when the stomach is saccular and then the muscular junction can be easily recognized; then the cardia is high (T 7 or 8) and the esophagus above tight. Conversely, when the stomach is like a funnel and the esophagus loose, the BE cannot be diagnosed before operating, although we think, with Henderson [9], that the BE is nearly always associated with ulceration or stenosis that help to situate the Z-line on X-ray.

We also agree with Henderson in that "there is no absolute preoperative test of esophageal length" [9], and a definition of the BE is impossible outside an operation.

References

1. Resano JH. Etude clinique et chirurgicale du brachy-oesophage. Sem Hop Paris 1950;26:932—944.
2. Lortat-Jacob JL. Chirurgie de l'oesophage. Paris: Editions Medicales Flammarion, 1951.
3. Petrovsky BV, Kanshin NN. The problem of the surgical treatment of sliding hiatus hernias and a shortened esophagus. In: Nyhus LM, Harkins HN (eds) Hernia. Chicago: Lippincott Company, 1964;513—521.
4. Lortat-Jacob JL. L'endo-brachy-oesophage. Ann Chir 1957;11:1247—1255.
5. Lortat-Jacob JL. What is the definition of Barrett's esophagus? In: Giuli R, McCallum RW (eds) Benign Lesions of the Esophagus and Cancer. Berlin: Springer Verlag, 1988;619—620.
6. Barrett NR. Chronic peptic ulcer of oesophagus and "oesophagitis". Br J Surg 1950;38:175—182.
7. Barrett NR. The lower esophagus lined by columnar epithelium. Surgery 1957;41:881—886.
8. Skinner DB, Walther BC, Riddell RH, Schmidt H, Iascone C, DeMeester TR. Barrett's esophagus comparison of benign and malignant cases. Ann Surg 1983,198.554—565.
9. Henderson RD. How can a conservative procedure be considered in view of a stenosis on an irreducible cardia? In: Giuli R, McCallum RW (eds) Benign Lesions of the Esophagus and Cancer. Berlin: Springer Verlag, 1988;459—462.
10. Hill L, Mercer CD. Surgery for peptic esophageal stricture. In: Hill LD, Kozarek R, McCallum RW, Mercer CD (eds) The Esophagus. W.B. Saunders, 1988;139—147.

Should intraoperative motility be assessed?

G.G. Jamieson (Adelaide)

The idea of assessing the lower esophagus manometrically during surgery arose from the desire to improve upon good, but not perfect, results being achieved with antireflux surgery. Lucius Hill and his colleagues used a single side hole perfusion technique intraoperatively and several times postoperatively to assess the pressure in the lower sphincter region following posterior gastropexy. They found that the pressure was very high intraoperatively and fell to about half by the time of the postoperative reading. They stated that a pressure below approximately 40 mmHg intraoperatively was associated with recurrent reflux and a figure greater than approximately 60 mmHg was associated postoperatively with dysphagia. Unfortunately no data was provided to demonstrate how they came to these conclusions [1]. Orringer and his group similarly measured sphincter pressures using a perfused side hole technique measuring pressures preoperatively, intraoperatively and postoperatively. They found that the variable intraoperative lower esophageal sphincter (LES) values obtained were not reliable predictors of the values obtained at 6 and 12 months postoperatively and furthermore, had no relationship to the patients outcome. They concluded that intraoperative manometry was not helpful [2].

Since the usefulness of the technique had not been established it was decided to measure LES pressure with a sleeve device preoperatively, intraoperatively before and after a total fundoplication and postoperatively [3]. The aim was to see if intraoperative pressures correlated with outcome. No attempt was made to alter the lower sphincter pressure once the fundoplication had been constructed. In other words the wrap was not calibrated in the way Hill et al. advocated. Our results did not show any correlation between intraoperative or postoperative sphincter pressures and outcome (Table 1). Due to the belief that fundoplication may work at least in part by preventing full sphincter relaxation [4,5], we designed a further study to investigate the variables influencing intraoperative measurement of LES pressure and also to evaluate a new method of assessing the effect of the fundic wrap on LES function in 13 patients undergoing a fundoplication [6]. The effect of the fundic wrap independent of LES pressure was assessed by inducing sphincter relaxation with esophageal balloon distension. We found once again that LES pressure increased after mobilization of the proximal stomach and distal esophagus (11.1 ± 1.5 mmHg to 19.8 ± 2 mmHg, p < 0.005). We found that LES relaxation was elicited with 16 of 33 distensions after mobilization of the esophagus, but only five of 33 distensions after completion of the wrap. Furthermore, it was found that residual LES pressure following sphincter relaxation was increased before mobilization of the esophagus over preoperative values, and then increased further after mobilization of the esophagus, although these increases were not statistically significantly different from the preoperative value. Their trend was all in the same direction suggesting that further numbers may have led to a different statistical result.

Table 1. Relationship between manometric pressures in lower esophageal sphincter and symptomatic outcome

Parameter assessed	No of pts	Median lower sphincter pressure at completion of operation (range)	p[a]	Median lower sphincter pressure at >6 months postoperatively (range)	p[a]
Standard acid reflux test normal	27	27 (12–60)	NS	21 (6–43)	NS
Standard acid reflux test abnormal (>3 reflux episodes)	7	24 (12–44)	NS	14 (8–22)	NS
Absence of postprandial bloating	15	26.5 (12–52)	NS	21.5 (10–55)	NS
Postprandial bloating	19	28 (12–60)		18 (6–38)	
No dysphagia	29	29 (12–57)	NS	17 (6–43)	
Dysphagia	4	22 (17–38)	NS	20 (15–24)	

[a]Mann-Whitney U test; NS = not significant.

This study led us to conclude that anaesthesia and intraoperative manipulation have significant effects on LES function which will detract from the validity of intraoperative assessment of antireflux operations.

A systematic study of the use of intraoperative manometry during myotomy for achalasia does not appear to have been reported, although we have used it in order to be sure of adequately attenuating lower sphincter tone. At an anecdotal level, it can be said that the technique is useful in this setting.

At present, the usefulness of intraoperative manometry has not been proven in antireflux surgery. However, more sophisticated ways of using manometry, which will allow control of such variables as manipulation of the sphincter and anaesthesia may yet allow tailoring antireflux operations to esophageal function. Therefore, we believe it is justified to continue to study the problem.

References

1. Hill LD. Intraoperative measurement of lower esophageal sphincter pressure. J Thorac Cardiovasc Surg 1978;75:378–382.
2. Orringer MB, Schneider R, Williams GW, Sloan H. Intraoperative manometry: is it valid? Ann Thorac Surg 1980;30:13–18.
3. Jamieson GJ, Myers JC. The relationship between intraoperative manometry and clinical outcome in patients operated on for gastroesophageal reflux disease. World J Surg 1992;16:337–340.
4. Kiroff GK, Maddern GJ, Jamieson GG. A study of factors responsible for the efficacy of fundoplication in the treatment of gastro-oesophageal reflux. Aust NZ J Surg 1984;54:109–112.
5. Ireland AC, Holloway RH, Toouli J, Dent J. Mechanisms underlying the antireflux action of fundoplication. Gut 1993;34: 303–308.
6. Johnsson F, Ireland AC, Jamieson GG, Dent J, Holloway RH. Effect of intraoperative manipulation and anaesthesia on lower oesophageal sphincter function during fundoplication. Br J Surg (in press).

Is it legitimate to consider "standard" antireflux procedures in the presence of stricture?

A.G. Little (Las Vegas)

The ideal management of a patient with gastroesophageal reflux disease (GERD) would involve antireflux surgery before stricture development. This means the willingness of the patient and the treating physician to acknowledge that conservative treatment is unsuccessful when persistent symptoms or esophagitis are documented, despite a reasonable trial of medical management. Unfortunately, some GERD patients present for the first time with developed fibrous strictures and in others, strictures are allowed to develop before surgical evaluation.

These patients with strictures can be subdivided into two pathogenetic categories. One type includes patients with a typical reflux or peptic stricture which is found in the distal esophagus and is the result of the natural progression from erosive reflux esophagitis, with the damage being caused by the combination of pepsin and acid [1,2] to fibrous stricture. The second type of patient is a patient with a Barrett's esophagus in which the distal portion of the esophagus is lined with columnar epithelium. Although the exact pathophysiology is not fully elucidated, one of the benign complications of Barrett's esophagus is stricture formation at the squamocolumnar junction. In these patients, the stricture is usually found in the middle part of the esophagus. Whether this stricture is a result of continuing inflammation caused by reflux, or is simply part of the abnormal epithelial degeneration, is not known.

The key to patients with esophageal stricture is to individualize treatment to fit the disease and the patient. The approach should always involve serial, graded dilations of the stricture. During the time the esophagus is being dilated, there should be intensive medical management of the reflux to prevent continuing damage from acid/pepsin reflux through the opened stricture. When the stricture can accommodate serial dilations to a sufficient size, usually greater than a size 40 French bougie, then a standard reflux operation can usually be accomplished. Obviously, patients with a Barrett's esophagus should also undergo careful endoscopic examination of the abnormal epithelium with biopsy documentation of the absence of dysplasia. If severe dysplasia is present, then esophagectomy is an appropriate consideration as the majority of these patients will have carcinoma in situ or invasive cancer in the final specimen.

If the patient does not respond adequately to dilation, then resection of the diseased esophagus and reconstruction is the only reasonable surgical approach. The choices for reconstruction are use of either the colon or jejunum for an intrathoracic reconstruction with the possibility of colon or tubularized stomach for reconstruction with an esophagogastrostomy in the neck. All these procedures are accompanied by a significant morbidity which emphasizes the benefits of timely antireflux procedures prior to stricture development.

An experience reported by the University of Chicago group in 1988 suggests that when patients are able to be dilated, then a standard reflux operation is able to be accomplished and is successful [3]. The choice between a Nissen fundoplication or a Belsey Mark IV procedure does not seem to be important and should be made according to the experience of the surgeon. Since publication of this article, my own practice has evolved somewhat: I am still not reluctant to perform a standard antireflux procedure when the stricture can be dilated and at surgery there is no difficulty in reducing the completed repair beneath the diaphragm. However, if any difficulty is anticipated with this essential aspect of antireflux surgery, I am not reluctant to add a Collis gastroplasty which I combine with either a Nissen or a Belsey type antireflux procedure. I think that this does decrease vertical tension on the esophagus and the repair and this is likely to improve long-term results. I also prefer to operate on these stricture patients through a thoracotomy rather than a laparotomy which is my choice for patients without stricture or prior antireflux surgery. The thoracic approach allows the surgeon to easily mobilize the esophagus up to the aortic arch, to construct a Collis gastroplasty and to resect and replace the diseased esophagus if necessary.

References

1. Little AG, Martinez EI, DeMeester TR, Blough RM, Skinner DB. Duodenogastric reflux and reflux esophagitis. Surgery 1984;96:447–454.
2. Evander A, Little AG, Riddell RH, Walther B, Skinner DB. Composition of the refluxed material determines the degree of reflux esophagitis in the dog. Gastroenterol 1987;93:280–286.
3. Little AG, Naunheim KS, Ferguson MK, Skinner DB. Surgical management of esophageal strictures. Ann Thorac Surg 1988; 45:144–147.

What disparities may be observed between clinical improvement and antireflux effectiveness?

A.J.P.M. Smout, R. Breumelhof, L.M.A. Akkermans, A. Jansen
(Utrecht)

Surgical treatment of gastroesophageal reflux disease (GERD) usually results in significant reduction of esophageal acid exposure, improvement of reflux symptoms and healing of reflux esophagitis [1–4]. However, reflux symptoms may persist after antireflux surgery. Other symptoms such as dysphagia and gas bloating are thought to be caused by esophageal and gastric motor disorders brought about by the procedure, but may in part be pre-existent [5,6]. Usually symptoms are taken as reliable indicators of the success of an antireflux procedure. However, objective evidence to support this concept is lacking. We therefore undertook a study in order to investigate the relationships between symptoms, gastroesophageal reflux (GER), and lower esophageal sphincter (LES) function after Nissen fundoplication.

Methods

Thirty-eight patients who had undergone Nissen fundoplication for therapy resistant GERD 3–10 years previously, entered the study. These patients (14 women, 24 men) had a mean age of 51.3 years, all were younger than 56 years. The symptoms heartburn, regurgitation, dysphagia, gas bloating, angina-like chest pain and epigastric pain were assessed, using a symptom score of 0 to 3. Zero indicated complete absence of symptoms, 3 indicated severe symptoms interfering with normal daily activities. In all patients, stationary esophageal manometry was carried out using a water perfused system. The stationary pull-through technique was used to study the LES. Twenty-four-hour combined esophageal pH and pressure monitoring was carried out using a portable system [7]. A glass pH electrode with built-in reference (Ingold, Urdorf, Switzerland) and a solid-state catheter with two miniature pressure transducers (PPG Hellige, Best, the Netherlands) were used. The pH electrode and the distal pressure transducer were positioned at 5 cm above the LES.

Results

Based on the subjective symptoms, the patients were divided into three subgroups. Group 1 (13 patients) consisted of patients who were completely free of symptoms. Group 2 (14 patients) consisted of patients who suffered from reflux symptoms (heartburn, acid regurgitation or both). Some of these patients also had dysphagia. Group 3 (11 patients) consisted of those patients who had nonreflux symptoms such as dysphagia, epigastric pain or bloating.

The patients with reflux symptoms had significantly lower resting LES pressures (2.3 ± 0.29 kPa) than the patients without symptoms (3.8 ± 0.44 kPa). However, patients with nonreflux symptoms had similar LES pressures (2.4 ± 0.56 kPa).

In the patients with nonreflux symptoms (group 3) the amplitude of esophageal peristaltic waves (5.2 ± 1.19 kPa) was significantly lower than that in group 2 and in group 1. Similar findings were made using the ambulatory manometry technique. Twenty-four-hour pH-monitoring showed that in group 1, GER was completely absent (i.e., the time with pH < 4 was 0%, in five patients, while in the other eight patients reflux was minimal (0.1–2.2%). As shown in Fig. 1, reflux occurred more frequently (p < 0.02) in group 2 than in group 1, but 8 out of 14 patients in this group had a nonpathological pH profile. In the patients with an abnormal profile, reflux was pathological in the supine position only. In group 3, none of the patients had typical

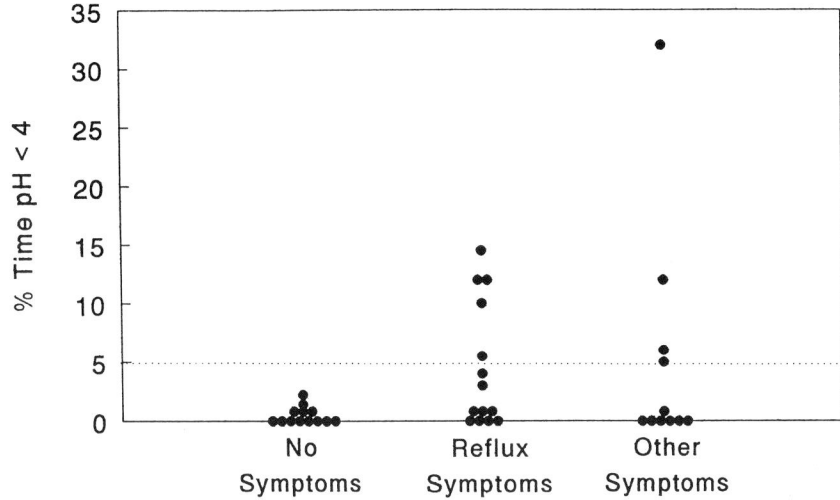

Fig. 1. Esophageal acid exposure (% of time with pH < 4) in the three subgroups of patients who underwent Nissen fundoplication. Although the patients with persisting reflux symptoms have significantly (p < 0.02) higher acid exposure, nine out of 14 patients with reflux symptoms had nonpathological reflux.

reflux symptoms, but 4 of these patients were shown to have a pathological pH profile (time with pH < 4: 5.9–32.5%). Two of these patients had supine reflux only, one had upright reflux and one had reflux in both positions. Endoscopy showed that macroscopic esophagitis was present in 3 out of the 6 patients with a pathological reflux profile. In group 3, one of the patients had macroscopic esophagitis, with a normal reflux profile.

Discussion

Although a good correlation was found between objective reflux variables and the symptoms heartburn and acid regurgitation, less than half of the patients with persisting reflux symptoms after antireflux surgery (42.8%) have a pathological profile, especially in the supine position. About one-third of the patients with nonreflux symptoms have pathological reflux. These findings are in agreement with observations made by others [3,5]. Apparently, symptoms and reflux do not necessarily run parallel after antireflux surgery. This is not too surprising since symptoms also appear to be rather unreliable indicators of reflux disease in patients not operated upon [8]. These findings emphasize that for the objective assessment of the success of an antireflux procedure, the patient's symptoms alone are insufficient. In addition to endoscopy, 24-h esophageal pH-monitoring should be carried out.

References

1. DeMeester TR, Johnson LF. Evaluation of the Nissen antireflux procedure by esophageal manometry and twenty-four-hour pH monitoring. Am J Surg 1975;129:94—100.
2. Shirazi SS, Schulze K, Soper RT. Long-term follow-up for treatment of complicated chronic reflux esophagitis. Arch Surg 1987;122:548—552.
3. Johnsson F, Joelsson B, Gudmundsson K, Floren CH, Walther B. Effects of fundoplication on the antireflux mechanism. Br J Surg 1987;74:1111—1114.
4. Breumelhof R, Smout AJPM, Schyns MWRJ, Bronzwaer PWA, Akkermans LMA, Jansen A. Prospective evaluation of the effects of Nissen fundoplication on gastroesophageal reflux. Surg Gynecol Obstet 1990;171:115—119.
5. Luostarinen M, Isolauri J, Laitinen J, Koskinen M, Keyriläinen O, Markkula H, Lehtinen E, Uusitalo A. Fate of Nissen fundoplication after 20 years. A clinical, endoscopical, and functional analysis. Gut 1993;34:1015—1020.
6. Breumelhof R, Fellinger HW, Vlasblom V, Jansen A, Smout AJPM. Dysphagia after Nissen fundoplication. Dysphagia 1991;6:6—10.
7. Smout AJPM, Breedijk M, Van Der Zouw C, Akkermans LMA. Physiological gastroesophageal reflux and esophageal motor activity with a new system for 24-h recording and automated analysis. Dig Dis Sci 1989;34:372—378.
8. Klauser AG, Schindlbeck NE, Müller-Lissner SA. Symptoms in gastro-oesophageal reflux disease. Lancet 1990;335:205—208.

How can one reach a compromise between the efficiency of a valve, its deterioration with time, and the digestive comfort of the operated patient?

A. Sicular (New York)

The normal esophagogastric valve permits the propulsion of esophageal liquid and solid contents through a compliant barrier into the higher pressure stomach and impedes regurgitation of food and acid between swallows. This apparently simple valvular function has been intensely studied over the years, dissecting its components which permit competent aboral uphill flow. Factors include intrinsic esophageal restraint with extrinsic modulation by the pinchcock diaphragm and subjacent mediastinal high pressure zone to permit efficiency of such a valve in preventing reverse flow from the high pressure abdominal cavity.

Thanks to the precise work of DeMeester through holographic computerized simulation of individual patient valve functions (Fig. 1), base line parameters necessary for efficient valve function are now understood [1].

Simultaneous cinefluorographic and manometric patient analyses by Kahrilas et

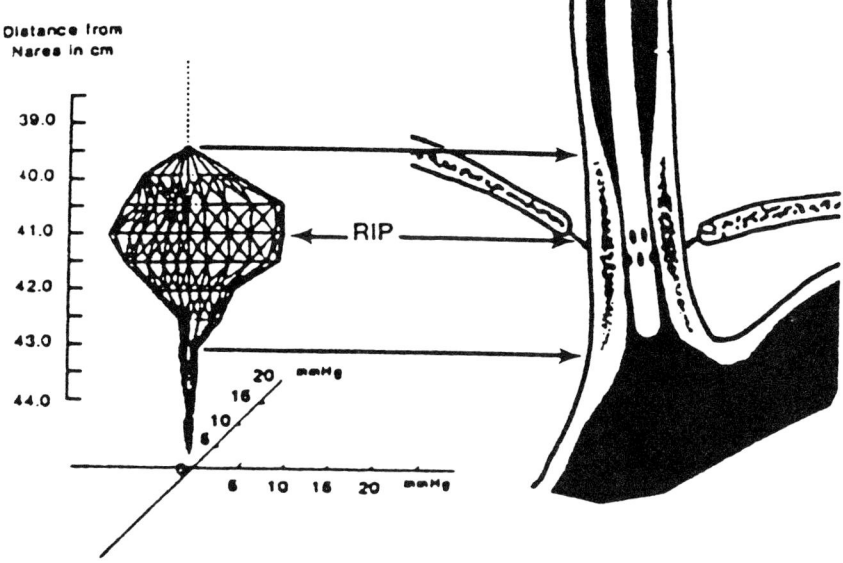

Fig. 1. Computerized three-dimensional imaging of lower esophageal sphincter. A catheter with four to eight radial side holes is withdrawn through the gastroesophageal junction. For each level of the pullback, the radially measured pressures are plotted around an axis representing gastric baseline pressure. When a stepwise pullback technique is used, the respiratory inversion point (RIP) can be identified.

al. [2] have further defined precise mechanisms both reinforcing valve competency in a normal location and interference of valve function by the sliding hernia and the nonreducible hernia in the chest (Fig. 2). Kahrilas has shown that hiatal hernia compromises competent sphincter function during swallows or abdominal pressure increase [3]. In the cardial emptying of patients with hernia prolonged distal acid exposure, the reflux event increases the vulnerability to reflux between swallows with concomitant low lower esophageal sphincter (LES) pressure. This impairment deteriorates with further sliding of the hernia over time.

Thirdly, the normal esophageal stripping wave propels an ingested bolus through the site of LES which is receptively open through neurotransmitter and mechanical functions, permitting immediate passage of the bolus into the stomach. Conversely, cessation of the peristaltic wave is rapidly followed by closure of the competent lower sphincter.

With the aging process, changing physical parameters compromise this valve, namely the lengthening and widening of the phrenoesophageal moorings constraining the stomach in the abdomen. Both the pulling of the longitudinal esophageal muscles and abdominal pressure differential displace the LES into the chest. Additionally with aging, loss of stripping wave strength or integrity may leave the unfortunate patient with inability to empty esophagus, except by pharyngeal contraction and the force of gravity.

The history of corrective antireflux surgery has focused on two mechanisms:

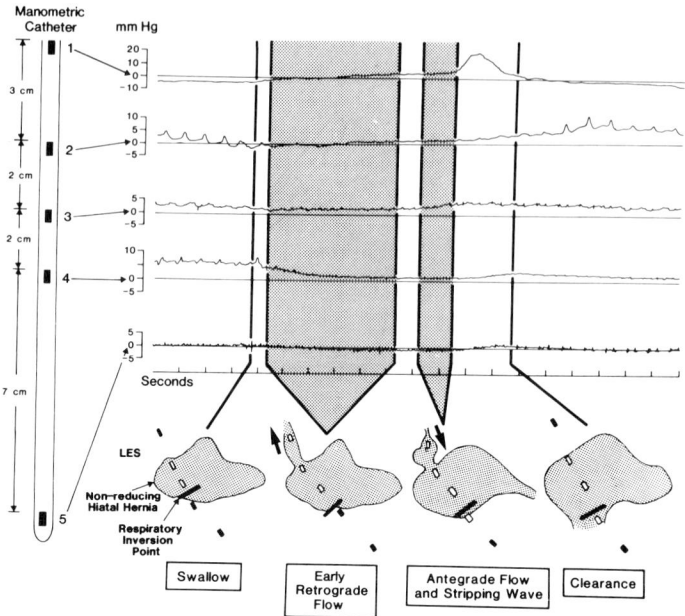

Fig. 2. Concurrent manometric and video recording of a 10-ml barium swallow characterized by early retrograde flow in a subject with a nonreducing hiatal hernia. Tracings from the video images are below the manometric record and correspond to the times on the manometric tracings intersected by the vertical lines. The schematic diagram to the left depicts the relative spacing of the pressure sensors, the tracings of which are depicted. The arrows next to the video image indicate the direction of barium flow. The first video image to the far left shows a barium-filled hiatal hernia at the time the swallow is initiated with sensor 1 in the distal esophagus, sensor 2 in the LES, sensor 3 within the hernia, sensor 4 measuring crural contractile activity, and sensor 5 within the abdominal stomach. The second image was about 1 s after the swallow and depicts the onset of retrograde flow; intrahernial pressure was 2 mmHg and LES pressure 0 mmHg. Retrograde flow continued for 5 s until the peristaltic contraction reached the distal esophagus. The third image depicts antegrade flow with the stripping wave progressing down the esophagus, and LES pressure increasing to equal intrahernia pressure (~4 mmHg). The final image to the far right shows barium cleared from the esophagus with the LES pressure now exceeding intrahernial pressure.

firstly, the construction of a substitute valve to restore lower esophageal incompetence and, secondly, the restoration of infradiaphragmatic position of the lower esophageal valve below the pinchcock of the diaphragm in a high pressure milieu.

The partial wrap perfected by Sir Ronald Belsey has achieved nondysphagic and relatively competent valve function. The circumferential gastric wrap of Nissen (Fig. 3) and his followers has the additional advantage of servomechanistic function responding to gastric contraction and intra-abdominal pressure increase with *pari passu* valve compression, so that the wrap function is not disturbed by these phenomena. However, deterioration with time may lead to failures. Too high a wrap may induce dysphagia; too low a wrap may trap acid in a thoracic fundus and lead to rapid stasis ulceration. Too tight a wrap may overcome the esophageal stripping mechanisms; too loose a wrap may permit reflux through failure of esophageal

544

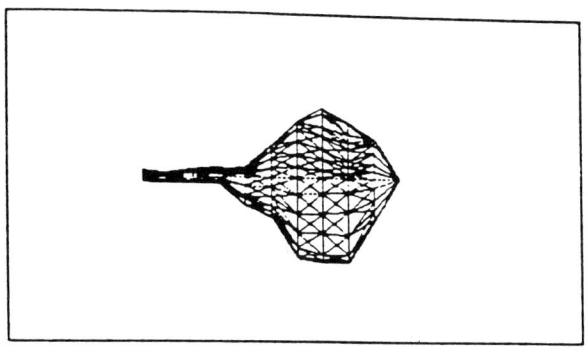

Normal

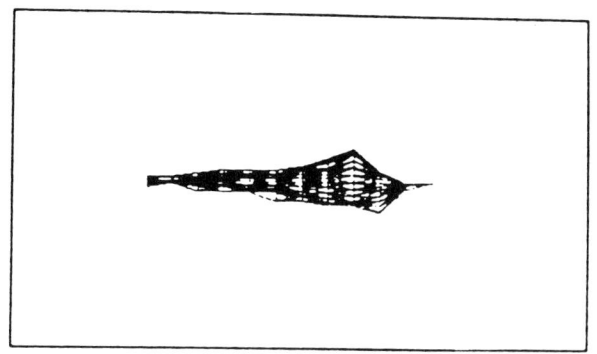

Barrett's Preop

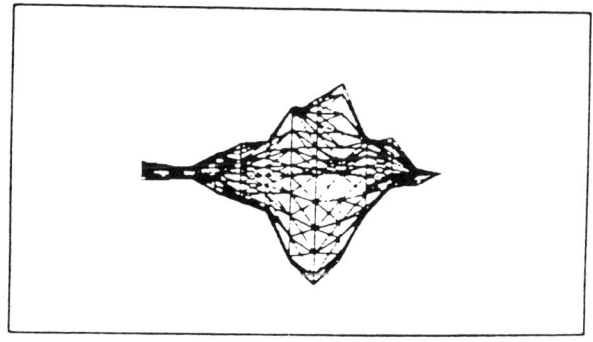

After Nissen

Fig. 3.

channel coaptation. Thus, the surgical art of valve construction is critical.

Circumferential plastic esophageal compression ring valves are deficient in multiple ways: 1) these plastic rings are not compliant; 2) they are not servo-

545

mechanistically responsive to gastric pressure change; 3) they induce fibropseudo-capsule formation leading to long-term dysphagia; 4) nonreactive plastic rings may migrate or perforate through the esophageal gastric junction.

The second surgical maneuver is the reconstruction of a competent subdiaphrag-matic pinchcock milieu by correcting the stretched hiatus and building a posterior buttress using sturdy nonabsorbable sutures fixing the gastric wrap to the buttress or diaphragm. This again requires surgical precision to avoid a too tight or too loose reconstruction leading to dysphagia or recurrent herniation.

Surgical experience and skill in both aspects of repair have achieved success rates approaching 90%, persisting over decades of follow-up study.

The infant surgical manipulations of laparoscopy and thoracoscopy are being studied now in anticipation for reconstructing both types of repair through keyhole instrumentation, whereas early literature and experience is promising, clinical follow-up status only exists for a year or two and the numbers of expert individual repairs with variation are, for the most part, in their teens [4]. Hinder has published more than a 120 cases with good early results. In 3 to 5 years, long-term follow-up will show that what one can do through an incision, one can reproduce through a pinhole.

The third factor, mainly reproduction of efficient valvular receptive relaxation, has not yet been duplicated in a circumferential valve formation. This may be simulated by the appropriate reconstruction of phreno-esophageal ligaments to distract the cardial esophagus as a direct function of contraction of the longitudinal muscles [5]. With this third surgical manipulation, it may be possible to recreate the normal sensation, ease and efficiency of swallowing after the valve reconstruction in a positive pressure milieu.

References

1.   DeMeester T. Surgical therapy for motility disorders of the esophageal body and sphincters. SSAT State of the Art Address, March 18, 1993.
2.   Sloan S, Rademaker W, Kahrilas P. Determinants of gastroesophageal junction incompetence: hiatal hernia, lower esophageal sphincter, or both? Ann Int Med 1992;117(12):977—982.
3.   Sloan S, Kahrilas P. Impairment of esophageal emptying with hiatal hernia. Gastroenterology 1991;100:596—605.
4.   Cuschieri A, Shimi S, Nathanson L. Laparoscopic reduction, crural repair, and fundoplication of large hiatal hernia. Am J Surg 1992;163(4):425—430.
5.   Boutelier P. A new method of surgical treatment of gastroesophageal reflux. Retroesophageal fundoplication associated with peritoneal tying of the cardia. Chirurgie 1990;116(8—9):597—601.

May vagal injury be related to certain poor results?

H.G. Gooszen, J.M.L.M. Horbach, A.A.M. Masclee, C.B.H.W. Lamers (Leiden)

Since there is a close relationship between the distal part of the esophagus and the vagal nerves, an antireflux operation may jeopardize these nerves. Only few studies exist which have investigated the role of the vagal nerves in antireflux surgery. Generally, it is thought that additional truncal vagotomy during antireflux surgery is adversely affecting the surgical outcome [1,2] in terms of reflux control, and some patients report symptoms suggestive for vagal nerve damage. In these patients vagal nerve damage has often not been notified or reported. The exact incidence of accidental vagotomy during antireflux surgery is therefore not well known, but is thought to be approximately 2% [3,4].

Measurement of plasma pancreatic polypeptide (PP) response to insulin-induced hypoglycemia provides an indirect method to test the integrity of the vagal nerve. Hypoglycemia strongly stimulates PP secretion. The PP response to hypoglycemia, however, is mediated through efferent vagal activity as indicated by its abolition by truncal vagotomy and its inhibition during administration of atropine [5,6]. With an intact vagus nerve and a normally functioning pancreas, hypoglycemia leads to a distinct rise in the plasma PP level. An impaired plasma PP increment to insulin hypoglycemia indicates a complete or partial interruption of the vagal innervation to the pancreas, as observed in patients with truncal vagotomy or in patients with diabetic neuropathy [7–9].

We have prospectively evaluated the effect of antireflux surgery on vagal nerve integrity. In addition, this study focuses on the relation between the change in plasma PP response as induced by operation and clinical symptoms well known to occur as a result of vagal nerve damage. It is also investigated whether the decrease in plasma PP response is transient, based upon the assumption that manipulation and traction during operation temporarily interferes with vagal nerve conduction ("neuropraxia").

Materials and Methods

The effect of antireflux surgery on the plasma PP response to insulin-induced hypoglycemia, was prospectively investigated in 22 patients who were selected for operative treatment. Twenty-six patients had medically intractable gastroesophageal reflux disease (GERD) and seven had type II hiatal hernia as the indication for surgery. Antireflux surgery was performed through a left sided thoracotomy according to the technique described by Belsey [3]. The group consisted of 11 men and nine women with a median age of 40 years and a range from 25 to 70 years.

Basal plasma PP levels and the PP response to insulin-induced hypoglycemia were measured before and at 3 months after antireflux surgery. Reaction to insulin-induced hypoglycemia was expressed as plasma PP peak response and as the incremental plasma PP response (ΔPP). Details of the test have been described previously [9,10]. In a randomly selected subgroup of nine patients, PP increments to insulin-induced hypoglycemia were also studied 14 days after fundoplication. None of the patients had pancreatic disease or previous thoracic or abdominal surgery, except for one patient who had cholecystectomy in the past. In addition, 20 age-matched healthy individuals without previous upper abdominal surgery (14 men, six women; median age 45 years; range 21–77 years), and a group of 11 patients who had undergone truncal vagotomy for different indications (truncal vagotomy with pyloroplasty in eight and colon interposition in three; four men, seven women; median age 45 years; range 27–74 years) were studied as negative and positive control groups for vagotomy. Informed consent was obtained from each individual. The study had been approved by the Ethics Committee of the Leiden University Hospital.

Before and over 3 months after antireflux surgery, the effect of operation on reflux-related symptoms were scored by a standardized questionnaire. Retrosternal pain, regurgitation and dysphagia were scored for severity and frequency [11]. Subjective success of surgery was defined as complete relief or major improvement of symptoms without further need for medical treatment and without interfering with normal daily life.

To analyze whether antireflux surgery had induced truncal vagotomy-related symptoms, epigastric fullness and diarrhea were included in the questionnaire. Epigastric fullness was defined as an uncomfortable filled-up feeling in the upper abdomen, shortly after each regular meal and diarrhea was defined as passage of three or more loose watery stools per day with a frequency of at least 1 day per month. Results are expressed as mean ± SEM. Statistical analysis was done using the Chi square test and the Fisher exact probability test, as well as the Wilcoxon signed rank test for paired results. Differences were scored as significant with $p < 0.05$.

Results

In 20 patients studied before antireflux surgery, a distinct rise in plasma PP response to insulin-induced hypoglycemia was observed from a mean ± SEM basal level of 37 ± 5 pM to a mean peak increment of 185 ± 24 pM ($p < 0.0005$) before operation.

At 14 days after surgery, the mean basal PP level of 38 ± 5 pM was stimulated to a mean peak increment of 114 ± 22 pM ($p < 0.05$). The PP peak increment at 14 days was significantly lower than was observed before the operation ($p < 0.01$). At 3 months after surgery the mean basal level was 36 ± 5 pM and the peak increment was 124 ± 13 pM ($p < 0.0005$). The difference between peak increment before and 3 months after surgery was significant ($p < 0.05$). No significant difference was found between the PP increment response at 14 days and the results scored over 3 months after antireflux surgery ($p = 0.17$). The plasma PP-increment level in the patient group prior to surgery was not significantly different from the plasma PP increment

548

level observed in the control group (n = 20). The group of 11 patients with truncal vagotomy had a basal plasma PP level which was not different from controls and patients before and after antireflux surgery. The mean plasma incremental PP response after truncal vagotomy, however, was only 9 ± 4 pM. All test results with an incremental plasma PP response of over 94 pM, the lowest value in the group of healthy controls, were considered to be normal. Test results below the level of 47 pM, the upper limit in truncally vagotomized patients, were considered to represent proven truncal vagotomy. With this subdivision, three patients after fundoplication had a response pattern compatible with truncal vagotomy. One of these fell in the range between normal and the truncal vagotomy level.

At 14 days after operation, two out of the nine patients studied at that interval had a plasma incremental PP response <47 pM. One of these was still at the truncal vagotomy (<47 pM) level more than 3 months after operation while the other showed an increase in PP response, back to the normal range (>94 pM). Three of the nine patients examined at 14 days had normal plasma PP response, which remained normal during follow-up. The remaining four patients had an intermediate response with plasma peak increment levels <94 pM and >47 pM at 14 days after operation; two of them returned to a PP increment level >94 pM, one was still in the intermediate range and the remaining one showed a further decrease to a level compatible with truncal vagotomy at 3 months after surgery.

In the whole group of 20 patients who were tested at 3 months after surgery, 15 patients had a normal plasma PP response <94 pM, three patients with a response compatible with truncal vagotomy and two patients with an intermediately disturbed incremental response.

Two patients had low (<94 pM; 58 and 78 pM with hypoglycemia levels of 1.6 and 1.7 mmol/l, respectively) plasma PP increment levels before operation. One patient had a neurological disease of unknown origin, with paraplegia, nystagmus, dyskinesia of facial musculature and abnormal esophageal manometry (decreased amplitude and simultaneous contractions without propulsive activity). The second patient did not have neurological, muscular or metabolic disease, particular pancreatic disease, potentially leading to a disturbed PP response, but was significantly overweight. Prior to antireflux surgery endocrinological causes for her overweight were excluded.

Effect of surgery on gastroesophageal reflux-related symptoms

Sixteen patients were scored as subjectively successful, and four patients had recurrence or persistence of symptoms after surgery. Of the failures, two had esophagitis grade II on endoscopy and the other had unchanged Barrett's esophagus on short-term follow-up. One patient had no esophagitis. Of the patients with esophagitis one had a postoperative plasma PP increment response <94 pM, two <47 pM as well.

Of the 16 patients with successful outcome, 16 had a normal incremental PP response and two were listed as intermediately disturbed (<94 pM), with none of the patients in the truncal vagotomy range; one out of four patients who were classified as unsuccessful had a truncal vagotomy type incremental PP response (<47 pM: p < 0.05); the other three had a PP response below normal, but >47 pM. Retrosternal pain was the dominating symptom in these patients.

Effect of surgery on vagotomy-related symptoms

Epigastric fullness

Epigastric fullness was reported by 10 patients before the operation. The complaint disappeared after surgery in seven and remained unchanged in three patients at 3 months after surgery. Two other patients acquired this symptom. Hence, epigastric fullness was not reported more frequently after surgery than before. Patients with plasma PP increment <94 pM did not have higher incidence of postoperative epigastric fullness (0/10) than patients with a normal postoperative PP response (5/14) (p = 0.19).

Diarrhea

Diarrhea was reported by one patient before and after operation. After surgery four other patients newly acquired this symptom and three of them had a PP increment level <94 pM, one of them with an incremental PP response <47 pM. Two other patients with a PP increment level <47 pM did not experience any change in bowel habit. A trend was observed towards more frequent occurrence of diarrhea after antireflux surgery in patients with plasma PP increment levels <94 pM (p = 0.09).

Discussion

We have previously reported that after the operation, according to Nissen, about 30% of the patients had a plasma PP response below normal [8]. It is not clear whether the decreased plasma PP response observed in that retrospective study should be ascribed to the Nissen fundoplication or be considered as an epiphenomenon of GERD. Although it has been suggested that vagal nerve function is impaired in patients with GERD [12,13], this suggestion is not supported by present data on insulin-induced PP stimulation in GERD patients before operation, which show no difference in incremental response between normal controls and nonoperated patients with GERD. In order to obtain an adequate stimulus for PP secretion we agreed, as in other studies, that i.v. insulin should induce a decrease in blood glucose level <2.5 mmol/l [10,14]. If not, a false positive indication for vagal nerve damage may be obtained. Apart from three patients, all nonoperated GERD patients had plasma PP increment levels >94 pM, which is the lowest level in controls. In one patient, no underlying cause for the abnormally low preoperative incremental PP response was observed other than moderate obesity. In the second patient with a BMI of 37 kg/m^2, the severe obesity was held responsible for the low preoperative incremental PP response. Obesity is a well documented cause for a decreased PP response to insulin-induced hypoglycemia [15,16]. In the third patient the abnormal PP response may well be associated with his neurological disease.

This study also shows that antireflux surgery by the Belsey Mark IV procedure affects the plasma PP response and leads to a decreased incremental response compatible with truncal vagotomy in 15%. None of the patients had troublesome diarrhea, as described in 1–2% after truncal vagotomy [17]. In none of the patients was intraoperative damage to one or both major vagus nerve branches notified.

We observed no relationship between a decrease in incremental PP response and the occurrence of epigastric fullness after antireflux surgery, as a manifestation of vagotomy-related decreased gastric emptying. Even if antireflux surgery induces a delay in gastric emptying through vagotomy, this may be unnoticed, especially by those patients who already had epigastric fullness and nausea prior to surgery. In our group of operative candidates, epigastric fullness was reported in 30% before and in 15% of patients after surgery. These data stand in contrast to those of Spechler [18], who reports a similar incidence of "early satiety" in GERD patients before surgery, but a rise of 58% after Nissen fundoplication. These data not only suggest that "postprandial epigastric fullness" or "early satiety" are a GERD-related symptom, but also that postoperative epigastric fullness is more a degree of fundoplication-related than a (partial) vagotomy-related symptom.

Symptoms like "increased abdominal girth" and "abdominal fullness" were reported by about 50% of GERD patients on medical treatment, and of these symptoms the frequency after Nissen fundoplication fell in the same range (53 and 56% respectively). The incidence of diarrhea, however, decreased in their study from 40% on medical treatment to 25% after Nissen fundoplication. We cannot explain why the incidence of diarrhea in our study is lower before and higher after fundoplication. The higher incidence of postoperative diarrhea may be due to dissection of the vagi free from the distal esophagus to prevent encroaching of the nerves in the fundoplication. This manoeuvre, which is not carried out as part of a standard Nissen fundoplication, carries a risk of vagal nerve lesion.

There is a significant relationship between the effect of surgery on GERD-related symptoms and a decreased plasma PP response postoperatively. All patients who described their surgery as unsuccessful because they experienced persistent retrosternal pain had a plasma PP response <94 pM. One of these patients had esophagitis grade III. From the 15 patients tested before, 14 days and over 3 months after surgery, three patterns of plasma PP response to insulin-induced hypoglycemia could be recognized. The first pattern is a decrease in PP response 14 days after surgery, recovering to the normal response level after 3 months. This recovery could be due to manipulation, compression or traction during surgery with reversible abnormal vagal nerve conduction and dysfunction. The second pattern is a decrease in plasma PP increment at 14 days after surgery, to a level compatible with truncal vagotomy, without recovering at 3 months after surgery. This finding suggests persistent vagal nerve damage due to surgery, although a prolonged nerve recovery from traction damage longer than 3 months cannot be excluded at 1 month. The third pattern is a gradual decline in incremental plasma PP response from 14 days to 3 months after surgery. This reaches either a level >94 pM or a level <94 pM. This pattern may be the result of scar tissue formation at the level of the hiatus due to the operation, encroaching up on the vagal nerves.

In summary, antireflux surgery affects the insulin-induced plasma PP response. At 14 days 47% and at 3 months 20% show an abnormal response with 20 and 15% at the truncal vagotomy level respectively. The effect may be transient, but not in all patients. Five percent of patients with a normal insulin-induced PP response before surgery had a decreased PP response after surgery, compatible with complete vagal cholinergic denervation. Direct surgical trauma during operation and later damage, caused by scar tissue formation, both may play a role. Vagotomy-related symptoms are not significantly associated with a decreased incremental PP response after antireflux surgery, but the subjective success of antireflux surgery in terms of reflux symptoms is adversely associated with an abnormal PP response due to yet unresolved mechanisms.

Acknowledgements

The authors gratefully acknowledge the technical assistance of J.P. Gilliams and the secretarial support of Ms P.G. Kruize.

References

1. Vansant JH, Payne RL, McAlpine RE. Vagotomy and pyloroplasty in the management of hiatal hernia. Ann Surg 1967;165: 888–892.
2. Pearson FG, Stone RM, Parrish RM, Falke RE, Drucker WR. Role of vagotomy and pyloroplasty in the therapy of symptomatic hiatus hernia. Am J Surg 1969;117:130–133.
3. Belsey RHR. Transthoracic partial fundoplication (Belsey repair). In: Jamieson GG (ed) Surgery of the Oesophagus. London: Churchill Livingstone; 1988.
4. Low DE, Mercer CD, James EC, Hill LD. Post-Nissen syndrome. Surg Gynecol Obstet 1988;167:1–5.
5. Schwartz TW. Pancreatic polypeptide: a hormone under vagal control. Gastroenterology 1983;85:1411–1425.
6. Schwartz TW, Holst JJ, Fahrenkrug J et al. Vagal, cholinergic regulation of pancreatic polypeptide secretion. J Clin Invest 1978;61:781–789.
7. Hilsted J, Madsbad S, Krarup T, Tronier B, Galbo H, Sestoft L, Schwartz TW. No response of pancreatic hormones to hypoglycemia in diabetic autonomic neuropathy. J Clin Endocrinol Metab 1982;54:815–819.
8. Kennedy FP, Go VLW, Cryer PE, Bolli GB, Gerich JE. Subnormal pancreatic polypeptide and epinephrine responses to insulin-induced hypoglycemia identify patients with insulin-dependent diabetes mellitus predisposed to develop over autonomic neuropathy. Ann Int Med 1988;108:54–58.
9. Jansen EH, Horbach JMLM, Klamer M, Jansen JBMJ, Hopman WPM, Gooszen HG, Lamers CBHW. Plasma pancreatic polypeptide responses to insulin hypoglycemia after Nissen fundoplication. Scand J Gastroenterol 1989;24(suppl 171): 9–12.
10. Lamers CBHW, Diemel CM, Van Leer E, Van Leusen R, Peetoom JJ. Mechanism of elevated serum pancreatic polypeptide concentrations in chronic renal failure. J Clin Endocrinol Metab 1982;55:922–926.
11. Horbach JMLM, Cnossen MH, Jansen JBMJ, Lamers CBHW, Zwinderman AH, Terpstra JL, Gooszen HG. A prospective study of the effects of Belsey Mark IV antireflux surgery on endoscopic esophagitis, lower esophageal sphincter pressure and 24-h pH measurements. Relation to symptom improvement. Dig Dis Sci (in press).
12. Ogilvie AL, James PD, Atkinson M. Impairment of vagal function in reflux oesophagitis. Q J Med 1985;54:61–74.
13. Cunningham KM, Horowitz M, Riddell PS, Maddern GJ, Meyers JC, Holloway RH, Wishart JM, Jamieson GG. Relations among autonomic nerve dysfunction, oesophageal motility, and gastric emptying in gastro-oesophageal reflux disease. Gut 1991;32:1436–1440.
14. Floyd JC, Fajans SS, Pek S, Chance RE. A newly recognized pancreatic polypeptide: plasma levels in health and disease.

Recent Prog Horm Res 1977;33:519–570.

15. Marco J, Angeles Zulueta M, Correas I, Villanueva ML. Reduced pancreatic polypeptide secretion in obese subjects. J Clin Endocrinol Metab 1980;50:744–747.

16. Lassman V, Vague P, Vialettes B, Simon MC. Low plasma levels of pancreatic polypeptide in obesity. Diabetes 1990;29: 428–430.

17. Blake G, Kennedy TL, McKelvey STD. Bile acids and postvagotomy diarrhoea. Br J Surg 1983;70:177–179.

18. Spechler SJ. Comparison of medical and surgical therapy for complicated gastroesophageal reflux disease in veterans. N Engl J Med 1992;326:787–792.

Can an undiagnosed achalasia be held responsible for some of the poor results?

E.H. Metman (Tours)

Side effects of antireflux surgery include inability to belch or vomit, gas-bloat syndrome with abdominal fullness, meteorism and delayed gastric emptying due to disturbed vagus nerve function and dysphagia.

Transient dysphagia following Nissen fundoplication, probably related to vagal denervation, occurs in many patients. Persistent dysphagia occurs in 3–24% of patients according mainly to the length of the wrap [1].

There have been a number of reports of patients with postoperative dysphagia following Nissen fundoplication in whom esophageal manometry has revealed poor peristalsis [2,3]. As a consequence, many authors recommend that all patients should have preoperative manometry and, if poor peristalsis is found, a partial fundoplication should be performed instead of a Nissen procedure [4].

Many reports of antireflux surgery being performed for misdiagnosed achalasia have stated that symptoms of achalasia could be misinterpreted. This is particularly true when a careful therapeutic trial with antireflux medications is not performed. If a patient does not have esophagitis at endoscopy, it is essential that esophageal manometry and a gastroesophageal X-ray examination are performed if antireflux surgery is considered [5].

Author's personal experience

Our experience consists of nine dysphagic patients who were referred for dilatation after a history of immediate acceleration in the development of dysphagia following Nissen fundoplication. Each had had extensive evaluation, and all but one exhibited narrowing of the distal esophagus and manometric failure of LES relaxation.

— Three patients had stricture requiring difficult bougienage at 15 mm diameter; three were reoperated for overtightened crural repair with or without modification of fundoplication, with good results. Preoperative manometry showed intermittent failure of peristalsis in one patient with dysautonomia.

— Two patients had an aperistalsis with a tight wrap, and were treated by pneumatic dilatation, with good results. No definitive diagnosis was possible between hypoperistalsis secondary to gastroesophageal reflux disease (GERD) and achalasia.

— Two patients were previously reoperated: they underwent a Heller myotomy 1 and 2 years after Nissen; they had persistent dysphagia (and heartburn) 3 and 23 years later; the final diagnosis was primitive achalasia in one case, and suspicion of GERD associated aperistalsis in the other.

— Two patients underwent reoperation because of improper initial location of the wrap around the stomach with twisting of the body of the stomach.

Evaluation of patients with postoperative dysphagia

It is important to discern clearly whether postoperative dysphagia following antireflux surgery relates directly to technical failures or to misdiagnosed previous motility disorders.

Mattox et al. proposed criteria to differentiate dysphagia due to slipped Nissen from dysphagia due to misdiagnosed achalasia [6], the former with progressive dysphagia several months/years after an asymptomatic interval following surgery, the latter with immediate worsening of dysphagia after surgery. However, other technical problems, such as overtightened crural repair or wrap, induce immediate postoperative dysphagia. In our experience this is more frequent than unrecognized achalasia. Moreover, after Nissen fundoplication, the diagnosis of achalasia could be difficult if not impossible:

— Incomplete relaxation is frequently seen after fundoplication, being the rule for fundoplication without mobilization of gastric fundus [7].

— Aperistalsis can be related to reflux disease itself in a proportion of 5–12.5% of esophagitis [8,9] or to postsurgical distal obstruction [10].

— Good results of pneumatic dilatation for postoperative dysphagia can be regarded as a hallmark for achalasia, as stated by Mattox et al. [6], but pneumatic dilatation can be successful in dysphagia due to a too tight wrap.

— Pharmacologic tests: Nifedipine or nitrates manometric relaxative tests [11] or isosorbide dinitrate X-ray test [12] are mandatory to differentiate achalasia from mechanical obstruction. In mechanical obstruction, due to tight repair or tight wrap, no enhancement of the narrowed distal esophagus appeared after isosorbide dinitrate contrary to the results for achalasia [12].

— When mechanical obstruction is apparent, a differentiation between overtightened crural repair and too tight wrap may be obtained with high diameter bougienage. In three patients with overtightened crural repair, we observed that bougienage was difficult with a 15 mm diameter dilator (and impossible in one patient with

18 mm diameter). Dilatation led to no improvement and surgical revision was mandatory in these three patients. This was not the case in two patients with a too tight wrap, in whom bougienage was easy and subsequent pneumatic dilatation afforded good results.

Should Nissen fundoplication be avoided in patients with poor peristalsis or aperistalsis?

Many authors recommend that when low peristalsis is found at manometry, a partial fundoplication should be performed instead of a Nissen procedure. However, others have reported improvement of esophageal motility following Nissen fundoplication [13–17].

The major factor is whether the fundoplication produces distal obstruction: in this case postoperative dysphagia will occur or be worsened in patients with altered peristalsis. Two reports failed to demonstrate that manometry could predict bad results of fundoplication on an individual basis [18,19]. This is not in agreement with a previous assertion of Joelsson et al. [20].

The important thing in Nissen fundoplication is to make sure that the wrap is short and floppy [4,21] and thus unlikely to cause obstruction, regardless of the quality of peristalsis, provided that primitive achalasia had been excluded or treated with concomitant Heller procedure [22]. Moreover, the crural repair should not be overtightened, regardless of the peristalsis.

In conclusion, the role of nondiagnosed achalasia in postfundoplication failure exists, but is less frequent than technical failures due to overtightened crural repair, too tight wrap or improper initial location of the wrap around the body of the stomach. All these technical problems lead to immediate worsening of dysphagia after surgery more often than misdiagnosed achalasia itself.

References

1. DeMeester TR, Stein HJ. Minimizing the side effects antireflux surgery. World J Surg 1992;16:335–336.
2. Pope CE. Esophageal motility — who needs it? Gastroenterology 1978;74:1337–1338.
3. O'Brien CJ, Collins S, Collins BJ, McGuigan J. Aperistaltic oesophageal disorders unmasked by severe postfundoplication dysphagia. Postgrad J Med 1990;66:1047–1049.
4. DeMeester TR. Surgical management of gastroesophageal reflux In: Castell DO, Wu WC, Ott DJ (eds) Gastroesophageal Reflux Disease. Pathogenesis, Diagnosis, Therapy. New York: Futura Publishing Co. Inc., 1985;243–280.
5. Bancewicz J. What is the place of surgery in the therapy of reflux oesophagitis? Gullet 1993;3(suppl):85–91.
6. Mattox HE, Albertson DA, Castell DO, Richter JE. Dysphagia following fundoplication: "slipped" fundoplication vs. achalasia complicated by fundoplication. Am J Gastroenterol 1990;85:1468–1472.
7. DeMeester TR, Bonavina L, Albertucci M. Nissen fundoplication for gastroesophageal reflux disease. Evaluation of primary repair in 100 consecutive patients. Ann Surg 1986;204:9–20.
8. Kahrilas PJ, Dodds WJ, Hogan WJ et al. Esophageal peristaltic dysfunction in peptic esophagitis. Gastroenterology 1986;91:897–904.
9. Meshkinpour H. Esophageal aperistalsis and gastroesophageal reflux disorder. Gastroenterology 1993;104:A146.
10. Siewert JR, Feussner H. The options for surgical therapy of reflux esophagitis. Gullet 1993;3(suppl):76–84.
11. Wong RKH, Maydonovitch CL, Garcia JE, Johnson LF, Castell DO. The effect of terbutaline sulfate, nitroglycerine and aminophylline on lower esophageal sphincter pressure and radionuclide esophageal emptying in patient with achalasia. J Clin Gastroenterol 1987;9:386–389.
12. Metman EH, Scotto B, Rifaat M, Dorval E, Picon L, Codjovi Ph. Lower esophageal sphincter relaxation is incomplete in

atypical achalasia with apparently normal manometric relaxation. Use of isosorbide dinitrate X-ray test. Gastroenterology 1992;102:A484.

13. Gill RC, Bowes KL, Murphy PD et al. Esophageal motor abnormalities in gastroesophageal reflux and the effects of fundoplicatlon. Gastroenterology 1986;91:364—369.

14. Johansson KE, Tibbling L. Esophageal body motor disturbances in gastroesophagoal reflux and the effects of fundoplication. Scand J Gastroenterol Suppl 1988;155:82—88.

15. Grande L, Lacima G, Ros E, Pujol A, Garcia-Valdecasas JC, Fuster J, Visa J, Pera C. Dysphagia and esophageal motor dysfunction in gastroesophageal reflux are corrected by fundoplication. J Clin Gastroenterol 1991;13:11—16.

16. Escandell AO, Martinez de Haro LF, Parilla Paricio P, Aguayo Albasini JL, Garcia Marcilla JA, Morales Cuenca G. Surgery improves defective oesophageal peristalsis in patients with gastro-oesophageal reflux. Br J Surg 1991;78:1095—1097.

17. Baldi F, Longanesi A, Ferrarini F, Michieletti G, Morselli-Labate AM. Oesophageal motor function and outcome of treatment with H₂-blockers in erosive oesophagitis. J Gastrointest Motil 1992;4:165—171.

18. Mughal MM, Bancewicz J, Marples M. Oesophageal manometry and pH recording does not predict the bad results of Nissen fundoplication. Br J Surg 1990;77:43—45.

19. Lundell LR, Myers JC, Jamieson GG. The influence of preoperative oesophageal motor function on the long-term outcome of antireflux surgery. Gullet 1993;3:50—55.

20. Joelsson BE, DeMeester TR, Skinner DB, Lafontaine E, Waters PF, O'Sullivan GC. The role of the esophageal body in the antireflux mechanism. Surgery 1982;92:417—424.

21. Ellis FH Jr, Crozier RE. Reflux control by fundoplication: a clinical and manometric assessment of the Nissen operation. Ann Thorac Surg 1984;38:387—392.

22. Donahue PE, Samelson S, Schlesinger PK, Bombeck CT, Nyhus LM. Achalasia of the esophagus. Treatment controversies and the method of choice. Ann Surg 1986;203:505—511.

How may new symptoms appearing after surgical relief be related to the different techniques?

L. Lundell (Gothenburg)

Antireflux surgery is generally very effective in controlling gastroesophageal reflux. However, some failures have proven unavoidable and a substantial number of studies have focused on causative factors for these failures such as slipping, tightness, dislocation or disruption of the wrap [1—5]. It should, however, be borne in mind that prevention of reflux alone does not always provide an optimal result for the patient. Persistent postprandial adverse symptoms can mar an otherwise excellent result in a small, but significant group of patients after similar procedures in the form of dysphagia, inability to belch and vomit, postprandial fullness, bloating and pain and sometimes socially embarrassing flatulence [6—9]. Except for dysphagia, these complaints have been assembled under the clinical syndrome named "the gas bloat". It should always be kept in mind, that patients very often rate these postprandial symptoms as of nuisance value only, and very much less than the preoperative reflux symptoms. One basic requirement for the prevention of similar symptoms after antireflux surgery would be to elucidate the mode of action of the actual procedures, which subsequently would allow an understanding of the mechanisms also behind the postfundoplication symptoms. During recent years, data have emerged [10,11], which

556

allows some speculations, but still our knowledge is far from complete.

Inability to belch has been reported to occur in about 40% of patients after Nissen fundoplication and inability to vomit in 30–90%. Some studies report an impressive number of patients being able to vomit also postoperatively, especially when interviewed after many years [7,12–15]. Similar clinical information should, however, cause concern regarding an eventual disruption of the wrap rather than an example of subsidence of complaints with the passage of time. Among patients with a long, tight fundic wrap, half of them had increased flatus and up to 20% reported symptomatic gas bloat of varying severity. No doubt, fundoplication procedures profoundly impair the ability to belch and relieve bloating also when objectively evaluated [16]. In fact, these operations have been shown to effectively diminish the capacity of the lower esophageal sphincter (LES) to relax properly, an important mechanism for belching in man [17–18]. Another significant clinical observation is, that postfundoplication symptoms in general and also gas bloat symptoms improve with the passage of time.

A fundamental question is, how frequent these so-called gas bloat symptoms are recorded already at the preoperative evaluation of patients? Few studies have given valid information on this important topic, but a recent one suggests a significant proportion of patients suffer from similar complaints already at the time of preoperative evaluation, symptoms which were maintained on subsequent nonsurgical therapy [19]. It would definitely be of clinical importance to know to what extent the existence of these symptoms preoperatively would affect a subsequent postoperative outcome.

Since effective treatment of established, severe postfundoplication symptoms is lacking, prevention is a primary concern. A number of technical considerations have been focused on and alleged to counteract some of these problems [20–22]. The aim of this presentation is to summarize the information that can be obtained from controlled clinical studies, where the outcome of different antireflux procedures have been studied in patients with severe long-standing gastroesophageal reflux disease (GERD). A similar analysis would allow an evaluation of the impact of technical factors on the occurrence of postfundoplication symptoms of various kinds and severities.

Control of major reflux symptoms

The pioneers within the field of surgical treatment of hiatal hernia, with or without an association with reflux disease, focused on the anatomical repair of the hiatus hernia only, a surgical approach that was not followed by any success [23,24]. Nissen popularized the fundoplication procedure, which has subsequently become the most widely used form of antireflux surgery [25]. The efficacy of this operation has been established by clinical and endoscopic follow-up and by esophageal pH-monitoring as well [15,20–21,26–29]. It is clear, that the overwhelming majority of reports quote a success rate in the order of 80% or better. Provided that information is extracted from controlled clinical trials, it cannot, however, be concluded that, among the different antireflux procedures which have been and are still extensively used in clinical practice, there is any clear-cut difference in efficacy with regard to long-term control of reflux symptoms. In this context, it is relevant to point out that, attention has to be paid to technical details in order to minimize complications and failures. Each surgeon uses the procedure which works best in his or her hands, but it seems as if not every exponent of a technique is as satisfied with the results as the originator. GERD is a common disorder, and consequently it is impossible for every patient to be attended by an expert, and this is one reason for some of the poor results. Excellent control of GER symptoms can be obtained with a total fundic wrap, a 270° fundoplication, 180° fundoplication or Hill posterior gastropexy [30–34], provided that each operation involves the reduction of hiatal hernia coupled with the construction of a valve mechanism to re-establish gastroesophageal competence. It must be emphasized that these success rates should be achieved with negligible mortality and morbidity. The problem is, however, that published results usually represent the best results in the field of antireflux surgery and the local level of expertise can vary considerably. Accordingly, it is reasonable to propose that antireflux surgery should be performed only in centers, where there is particular interest in this area and where an expertise has been assembled in the management of GERD as well as in the essential diagnostic facilities. Data are now accumulating to show that the short-term outcome after laparoscopic fundoplications is as advantageous as that following open surgery. A technique which largely eliminates the intersurgeon variation in technique is the introduction of the Angelchik prosthesis. This operation has been shown to be an effective operation for controlling reflux. In controlled, clinical trials presented so far, this procedure has been shown to be as effective as a Nissen fundoplication in preventing reflux symptoms [35–37]. The disadvantages with the prosthesis are, however, obvious [38–39] and are referred to below.

Dysphagia

If a patient does not have reflux in the first place, then obviously it is unlikely that an antireflux operation will cure whatever is causing this patient's symptoms. Achalasia is perhaps the single most common nonreflux disorder that unfortunately is sometimes treated as reflux. For example, Hill et al. [1] reported one such case in 25 failed fundoplications, whereas in other series four out of 25 failed operations and one case out of 24 operated patients have been reported to suffer from achalasia [2–4]. The situation with an adynamic esophagus is not quite so clear-cut. There is little doubt that the potential for creating a relatively too tight wrap in a patient with an adynamic esophagus is quite high [40]. It seems not unreasonable, however, to accept that a very floppy complete wrap can be advocated, although others state that a partial fundoplication is preferred in these circumstances [41].

The usual problem is, however, the construction of a wrap which is too tight, therefore producing obstruction to a normally functioning esophagus. Shirazi et al. [14] reported that, by increasing the bougie, around which the fundoplications were

558

constructed, from <40 to 60 Fr, they could decrease the incidence of dysphagia significantly. In an early randomized, prospective clinical trial comparing Nissen, Hill and Belsey antireflux procedures [42], it was shown that Nissen fundoplication was effective in controlling reflux as assessed subjectively by the relief of symptoms, and objectively with the standard acid reflux test and 24-h pH monitoring. This effect was, however, accomplished at the expense of a temporary mild postoperative dysphagia. In 100 consecutive cases DeMeester et al. [21] performed three technical modifications of the Nissen procedure: they increased the caliber of the esophageal bougie used at operation from 36 to 60 Fr gauge and reported a reduction in the incidence of painful swallowing from 83 to 39%, and shortening the length of the fundoplication allegedly reduced dysphagia. Division of the short gastric vessels to achieve further mobilization of the fundus was claimed to increase the incidence of complete distal esophageal sphincter relaxation on swallowing from 31 to 71%. Clearly, there are many variables that may contribute to a good clinical result after a Nissen fundoplication [11,20].

The few prospective, randomized trials so far presented have not given persistent results which would advocate one technique over the other. The total fundic wrap has been argued to control reflux better than other techniques, by providing the greatest increase in high pressure zone in LES area and by localizing a larger part of the sphincter in the abdomen. This goal may, however, be achieved at the expense of a higher frequency of temporary postoperative dysphagia. We observed mild dysphagia to occur more frequently 3 months postoperatively after a total fundic wrap than in those having a semifundoplication according to Toupet. This difference did, however, disappear when the patients were reassessed some months later [30]. When these patients were subsequently evaluated more than 3 years after the operation by an independent observer, no difference at all could be observed in the frequency of obstructive symptoms (Lundell et al., to be published).

The use of the silicone Angelchik prosthetic device was initially complicated by reports of migration of the implant, erosion into the gastrointestinal tract and postoperative dysphagia necessitating subsequent removal. The technical modifications that were instituted might have reduced the rate of migration and the survey of surgeons in the UK, who had implanted a total of 1,113 devices, reported severe postoperative dysphagia in 66 patients, erosion in nine and migration in seven patients [43]. Persistent postoperative dysphagia necessitated removal of prosthesis in 5.1%. The incidence of dysphagia increases with the length of follow-up and preoperative dysphagia is apparently a contraindication to implantation of this prosthesis. Trials with short-term follow-up comparing fundoplication with Angelchik prosthesis have shown that the latter is a quicker operation with a shorter inpatient stay, with controlled reflux proven equivalent to that after fundoplication, but with dysphagia being a more prominent problem in patients allocated to insertion of this prosthesis. In fact, one randomized trial comparing Nissen fundoplication with Angelchik prosthesis has been abandoned prematurely because of a 20% dysphagia rate following the latter procedure, despite initially reported success with the device [37,44].

Gas bloat syndrome

When Nissen fundoplication was introduced in clinical practice, it was thought that a successful operative treatment for pathological reflux would result in a super-competent valve at the gastroesophageal junction [10]. A similar valve would allow food and drink to pass into the stomach, but prevent any reflux of air and liquid gastric contents into the lower part of the esophagus. The creation of a super-competent antireflux barrier caused, however, dysphagia and gas bloat due to the tightly wrapped fundoplication. For instance, Negre [8] found that nearly half of the patients had these secondary symptoms after a 10 year follow-up period. Bombeck and colleagues [20] have argued that it is essentially impossible to make a fundoplication too loose and pathological reflux could be eliminated by any wrap, no matter how loose. They subsequently reported a 1—8 year follow-up in 71 patients, with diverse side effects reported in only two patients (one with gas bloat and one with inability to belch or vomit) [20]. When similar techniques have been applied in controlled, prospective trials also comparing various technical modifications, the significance of making a wrap floppy and short has been confirmed [21,28,29,31,42]. At the moment it is, however, unclear whether semifundoplication procedures are associated with less gas bloat symptoms than total fundic wraps. A clear tendency has been reported in two series, but data from long-term follow-up in a large group of patients are still warranted [30,32].

It has been suggested that delayed gastric emptying might contribute to an unfavorable postoperative outcome after antireflux surgery. In this context it ought to be remembered that a fundoplication operation by itself seems to improve gastric emptying [45], whereas the combined highly selective vagotomy and fundic wrap procedures exert more unpredictable or no effects [46]. Important differences in clinical results between these two procedures have not been demonstrated [47,48] and therefore the role of gastric emptying in the cause of postfundoplication symptoms remains to be elucidated. A retarded gastric emptying of solid food items, when evaluated in the preoperative situation, might predict those who develop some long-lasting postfundoplication symptoms, particularly of gas bloat character [49]. The most obvious associations were found between gas bloat problems such as postprandial satiety, distension and pain and impaired preoperative gastric motor function. At the present time, the predictive value of gastric emptying studies is not strong enough to allow operations to be tailored. In this context it is relevant to point out that clinical reports, in which essentially no postfundoplication symptoms are prevailing after modified fundoplication procedures [13,21—22], are not totally trustworthy. This is especially so, since similar studies do not take the advantage of an independent observer in the symptom scoring of patients during the postoperative follow-up [6] in evaluating these symptom complexes, which are also notoriously difficult to analyze, depending on the high degree of subjectivity.

Failure of antireflux operations

The fact that many failure associated problems became apparent only months after the operative procedure strongly suggests that these failures are dependent on technical inadequacies. In general terms, about half of the failures after antireflux surgery are not strictly related to recurrent reflux, but instead to other mechanical problems [1–5,50,51].

Inappropriate surgery has been referred to in cases of an adynamic esophagus and inadequate diagnosis of GERD. It is still a matter of debate as to the wisdom of carrying out a total fundic wrap in patients with failed primary peristalsis of the esophagus following water swallows [52].

The slipping of a wrap is a quite frequent technical failure. This is especially true, since it is impossible to know if, for instance, a gastric Nissen was fashioned in the first place or after fundoplication has slipped down from around the esophagus to lie around the stomach, or if the longitudinal muscle of the esophagus has pulled the distal stomach through the fundoplication. The symptom complexes presented by patients suffering from the consequences of technical failures are difficult to comprehensively analyze, but those of obstructive nature are to be taken most seriously.

All patients who present with recurrent reflux probably have breakdown of their repair to some degree. The reasons why a repair should break down with time are conjectural. It might be expected that a loose wrap should be less likely to break down than a wrap constructed under some tension. However, there is no evidence from the literature that one type of repair is more likely to break down than the other. The fact that many of the repairs seem to break down early in the postoperative course again emphasizes the importance of adherence to technical perfection.

In conclusion, it can be summarized that recurrent reflux has not been shown to be more frequently associated with one type of antireflux procedure compared to another, provided that the technique is designed to reconstruct the gastroesophageal competence. Obstructive symptoms occur frequently after insertion of an Angelchik prosthesis, and data would support that, in cases of severe esophageal motility disturbances, a loose and short fundoplication can be recommended and perhaps a semifundoplication should be preferred. The occurrence of gas bloat complaints might be more common in patients being operated on with a total fundic wrap.

However, the most important issue is: how to prevent these adverse complaints from occurring? Important prognostic information may be hidden within the patients specific functional parameters, as well as in a comprehensive analysis of preoperative symptom profiles. At the moment, it cannot be argued that the design and construction of one antireflux procedure has reduced the problem of postfundoplication symptoms to the level of being clinically insignificant.

References

1. Hill LD, Ilves R, Stevenson JK, Pearson JM. Reoperation for disruption and recurrence after Nissen fundoplication. Arch Surg 1979;114:542–548.
2. Leonardi HK, Crozier RE, Ellis FH. Reoperation for complications of the Nissen fundoplication. J Thorac Cardiovasc Surg 1989;81:50–56.

3. Skinner DB. Surgical management after failed antireflux operations. World J Surg 1992;16:359.
4. Siewert RJ, Isolauri J, Feussner H. Reoperation following failed fundoplication. World J Surg 1989;13:791.
5. Maher JW, Hocking MB, Woodward ER. Reoperations for oesophagitis following Nissen antireflux procedures. Ann Surg 1985;201:723.
6. Pope CE. The quality of the life following antireflux surgery. World J Surg 1992;16:355.
7. Jamieson GG, Duranceau AC, Deschamps G. Surgical treatment of gastroesophageal reflux disease. In: Jamieson GG, Duranceau AC (eds) Gastroesophageal Reflux. Philadelphia: WB Saunders, 1988;Chap 10.
8. Negre JB. Postfundoplication symptoms. Do they restrict the success of Nissen fundoplication? Ann Surg 1983;198:698.
9. Garstin WI, Johnston GW, Kennedy TL, Spencer EF. Nissen fundoplication: the unhappy 15%. J R Coll Surg Edinb 1986; 31:207.
10. Little AG. Mechanism of action of antireflux surgery: theory and facts. World J Surg 1992:16;320.
11. DeMeester TR, Stein HJ. Minimizing the side-effects of antireflux surgery. World J Surg 1992;16:335—336.
12. Rossetti M, Hell K. Fundoplication for treatment of gastro-oesophageal reflux disease in hiatal hernia. World J Surg 1977;1:439.
13. Low DE, Anderson RP, Ilves R, Ricciadelli E, Hill LD. 15—20 years results after the Hill antireflux operation. J Thorac Cardiovasc Surg 1989;98:444.
14. Shirazi SS, Schulze K, Soper RT. Long-term follow-up for treatment of complicated chronic reflux esophagitis. Arch Surg 1987;122:548—552.
15. Negre SB, Markkula HT, Keyrilainen O, Matikainen M. Nissen fundoplication. Am J Surg 1983;146:635.
16. Smith D, King NA, Waldron B et al. Study of belching ability in antireflux surgery patients and normal volunteers. Br J Surg 1991;78:32.
17. Ireland AC, Holloway RH, Toouli J, Dent J. Mechanism underlying the antireflux action of fundoplication. Gut 1993;34: 303—308.
18. Dent J, Holloway RH, Toouli J, Dodds WJ. Mechanisms of lower oesophageal sphincter incompetence in patients with symptomatic gastro-oesopnageal reflux. Gut 1988;29:1020.
19. Spechler JS et al. Comparison of medical and surgical therapy for complicated gastro-oesophageal reflux disease in veterans. N Engl J Med 1992:326:786—792.
20. Donahue PE, Samelson SL, Nyhus LM, Bombeck CT. The floppy Nissen fundoplication. Arch Surg 1985;120:663—668.
21. DeMeester TR, Bonavina L, Albertucci M. Nissen fundoplication for gastroesophageal reflux disease. Evaluation of primary repair in 100 consecutive patients. Ann Surg 1986;204:9—20.
22. Watson A, Jenkinson LR, Ball CS, Barlow AP, Norris TL. A more physiological alternative to total fundoplication for the surgical correction of resistant gastro-oesophageal reflux. Br J Surg 1991;78:1088—1094.
23. Allison BR. Hiatus hernia: a 20-year retrospective survey. Ann Surg 1973;178:273.
24. Woodward ER, Thomas SHF, McAlhany JC. Comparison of crural repair and Nissen fundoplication in the treatment of oesophageal hiatus hernia with peptic oesophagitis. Ann Surg 1971;173:782.
25. Nissen R. Eine einfache Operation zur Be-einflussung der Refluxösophagitis. Schweiz Med Wochenschr 1956;86:590.
26. Breumelhof R, Smout AJPM, Schyns MWRJ, Bronzwaer PWA, Akkermans LMA, Jansen A. Prospective evaluation of the effects of Nissen fundoplication on gastro-oesophageal reflux. Surg Gyneacol Obstet 1990;171:115—119.
27. Mughal MM, Bancewicz J, Marples M. Oesophageal manometry and pH recording does not predict the bad results of Nissen fundoplication. Br J Surg 1990;77:43—45.
28. Matikainen M. Nissen-Rossetti fundoplication for the treatment of gastro-oesophageal reflux. Acta Chir Scand 1982; 148:173.
29. Feussner H, Petri A, Walker S et al. The modified AFP-score: an attempt to make the results of antireflux surgery comparable. Br J Surg 1991;78:942.
30. Lundell L, Abrahamsson H, Ruth M, Sandberg N, Olbe L. Lower esophageal sphincter characteristics and esophageal acid exposure following partial or 360° fundoplication: results of a prospective, randomized, clinical study. World J Surg 1991;15:115,
31. Johansson J, Johnson F, Joelsson BE, Florén CH, Walther B. Outcome from 5 years after 360° fundoplication for gastro-oesophageal reflux disease. Br J Surg 1993;80:46.
32. Walker SJ, Holt S, Sanderson CJ, Stoddard CJ. Comparison of Nissen total and Lind partial transabdominal fundoplication in the treatment of gastro-oesophageal reflux. Br J Surg 1992;79:410.
33. Johansson K-E, Tibbling L. Maintenance treatment with ranitidine compared with fundoplication in gastro-oesophageal reflux disease. Scand J Gastroenterol 1986;21:779.
34. Thor KBA, Silander T. A long-term randomized prospective trial of the Nissen procedure vs. a modified Toupet technique. Ann Surg 1989;210:719.
35. Stuart RC, Dawson K, Keeling P, Byrne PJ, Hennessy TPJ. A prospective randomized trial of Angelchik prosthesis vs. Nissen fundoplication. Br J Surg 1989;76:86.
36. Gear MWL, Gillison EW, Dowling BL. Randomized prospective trial of the Angelchik antireflux prosthesis. Br J Surg 1984;71:681.
37. Deakin M, Mayer D, Tembel JG. Surgery for gastro-oesophageal reflux: the Angelchik prosthesis compared to the floppy Nissen fundoplication. Two-year follow-up study and a five-year evaluation of the Angelchik prosthesis. Ann Royal Coll Surg (UK) 1989:71:249.

38. Wale RJ, Royston CMS, Bennett JR, Buckton GK. Prospective study of the Angelchik antireflux prosthesis. Br J Surg 1985;72:520.

39. Durrans D, Armstrong CP, Taylor TV. The Angelchik antireflux prosthesis — some reservations. Br J Surg 1985;72:525.

40. Siewert JR, Feussner J. Collagen diseases. Chapter 54. In: Jamieson GG (ed) Surgery of the Oesophagus. Edinburg: Churchill Livingstone, 1988.

41. Duranceau A, Topart P, Deschamps G, Taillefer R. Reflux control in operated scleroderma patients. Abstract # SP-080, 5th World Congress of International Society of Diseases of the Esophagus, 1992.

42. DeMeester TR, Johnson LF, Kent AH. Evaluation of current operations for the prevention of gastro-oesophageal reflux. Ann Surg 1974;180:511.

43. Morris DL, Robertson CS, Hardcastle JD. National survey of use of the Angelchik antireflux prosthesis. Br Med J 1987; 295:308.

44. Kimiot WA, Kirby RM, Akinola D, Temple G. Prospective randomised trial of Nissen fundoplication and Angelchik prosthesis in the surgical treatment of medically refractory gastro-oesophageal reflux disease. Br J Surg 1991;78:1181.

45. Maddern GJ, Jamieson GG. Fundoplication enhances gastric emptying. Ann Surg 1985;201:296.

46. Jamieson GG, Maddern GJ, Myers JC. Gastric emptying after fundoplication with and without proximal gastric vagotomy. Arch Surg 1991;126:1414.

47. Oester MJ, Csendes A, Funch-Jensen P, Casalnuovo CA, Hanberg Soerensen F, Amdrup E. PCP and modified Hill procedure as surgical treatment of reflux esophagitis: results in 108 patients. World J Surg 1982;6:412.

48. Csendes A, Braghetto I, Corn O, Cortes C. Late subjective and objective evaluation of antireflux surgery in patients with reflux esophagitis: analysis of 215 patients. Surgery 1989;105:374.

49. Lundell LR, Myers JC, Jamieson GG. Gastric emptying and its relationship to symptoms of "gas bloat" after antireflux surgery. Eur J Surg 1994;160:140.

50. O'Hanrahan T, Marples M, Bancewicz J. Recurrent reflux and wrap disruption after Nissen fundoplication: detection incidence and timing. Br J Surg 1990;77:545—547.

51. Maddern GJ, Jamieson GG, Chatterton BE, Collins PJ. Is there an association between failed antireflux procedures and delayed gastric emptying? Ann Surg 1985;202:162.

52. Lundell LR, Myers C, Jamieson GG. The influence of preoperative oesophageal motor function on the long-term outcome of antireflux surgery. Gullet 1993:3;50—55.

Which is the best clinical application for long-term follow-up of operated cases?

C.O.H. Russell (Melbourne)

Major advances in pharmacology, refinement of surgical techniques and the advent of laparoscopic surgery have greatly enhanced the therapeutic options available to treat reflux disease. It would be appropriate to know which therapeutic option was the most appropriate and cost effective in a given set of circumstances. To achieve this knowledge, patients must be grouped by rigid criteria, randomized and then treated by standard protocols. There should then be a prolonged period of follow-up (e.g., 10 years) with regular review and assessment of the subjective and objective indices of reflux disease. If the patient grouping, treatment and follow-up are not standardized, then any study is not truly comparative. Attempts have been made to perform comparative studies [1,2] and these probably reflect the realities of clinical research rather than the ideals. It is relatively easy to standardize therapeutic and follow-up protocols, although it is not always easy to ensure the compliance of the subjects involved. Selection of the patient groups and assessment of the clinical parameters of reflux disease is somewhat more illusory.

Parameters for assessment

Patient characteristics

— age;
— habitus (e.g., obese);
— smoking habits;
— alcohol consumption;
— medications especially aspirin, NSAIDs
— other coexisting problems (e.g., cholelithiasis, irritable bowel syndrome).

Disease characteristics

Subjective symptoms
— description and duration of complaint;
— frequency;
— severity;
— response to medications.

Objective
— hiatus hernia (size, type);
— esophageal motility;
— LES function;
— gastric emptying;
— prolonged pH monitoring;
— grading of esophagitis including presence and extent of columnar lined esophagus (CLE).

Costs of treatment

The true costs of initial and subsequent treatments should be calculated.

Complications of treatment

All complications should be recorded. All of these parameters are important in reflux disease but their inclusion in any scoring system, like the "TNM" classification would be impractical (and involve the entire alphabet) and require very large trials to demonstrate any clinical benefit. The other more practical option is to select predefined groups of patients and use a scoring system to assess the disease characteristics (subjective and objective). The AFP score developed by Bancewicz [1] and its modification by Siewert [2] are genuine attempts to standardize assessment. These methods could be enhanced by OESO, and an international standard developed.

References

1. Bancewicz J, Matthews HR, O'Hanrahan T, Adams J. A comparison of surgically treated reflux patients in two surgical centres. In: Little AG, Ferguson MK, Skinner DB (eds) Diseases of the Esophagus, vol II. New York: Mount Kiscoe, 1990;177—180.
2. Feussner H, Petri A, Walker S et al. The modified AFP score: an attempt to make the results of antireflux surgery comparable. Br J Surg 1991;78:942—946.

How should the manometric findings after antireflux surgery be interpreted?

J. Bancewicz, T. Ismail, J. Barlow (Manchester)

Despite much investigation, the mode of action of antireflux operations remains a matter of debate. It is common practice in published follow-up studies to measure the lower esophageal sphincter pressure (LESP), show that this has risen and claim that this indicates that the operation has been successful. However, close examination of the literature indicates that this is a false assumption.

The ability of an antireflux operation to control reflux is most accurately assessed by 24-h pH recording. In virtually all studies of pH recording and manometry after antireflux operations, there is a significant increase in LESP in the group of patients whose reflux is corrected. However, there is not a one to one correlation between increased LESP and successful reflux control in individual subjects [1—4]. Our own studies carried out following Nissen fundoplication showed good reflux control in 16 of 29 patients in whom LESP decreased postoperatively [4]. There was also a poor correlation between the length of the intra-abdominal segment of the LES and control of reflux. These observations suggest that the change in the manometric characteristics of the LES following operation may be an artefact of the operation rather than the means by which reflux is controlled.

The lack of correlation between manometric characteristics and reflux control should not be surprising. Most antireflux operations involve fundoplication and this alters the nature of pressure transmission from stomach to esophagus. The altered pressure relationship is greatest following a full 360° fundoplication, and least following insertion of an Angelchik prosthesis or a Narbona sling operation. Following a very loose fundoplication there is no reason why lower esophageal pressure should increase. If the fundoplication is tight, intraesophageal pressure will certainly be increased. Overtightening of the hiatus can have the same undesirable effect. Thus the surgeon may manipulate tissues at operation to increase LES pressure in an artefactual manner that has no particular value in controlling reflux. By contrast, it may be essential that LES pressure is increased for a Narbona sling to be successful, since this operation acts in a different way.

It has recently been suggested that Nissen fundoplication may prevent reflux by reducing the triggering of transient lower esophageal sphincter relaxations (tLESR) and by maintaining a minimum baseline pressure during transient or swallow-induced relaxations [5]. This suggestion requires careful investigation. However, there are two significant problems with the hypothesis. First, there is some evidence that tLESR may not be the most important factor in the genesis of GERD [6] and it is difficult to imagine how a simple surgical manoeuvre might produce a complex neuromuscular change. Second, it is the stomach that is full of gas or food that is most at risk of reflux [6,7] and a small residual pressure in the relaxed LES seems unlikely to have much to do with stopping reflux. Assessment of the collapsed, fasted stomach, such as is done in most manometric studies, is almost certainly not the best way to assess the antireflux action of fundoplication.

We have been interested in the measurement of yield pressure which has been described as a simple means of assessing the competence of the cardia [8,9]. The yield pressure can be measured by endoscopy or by manometry, and there is an inverse linear relationship between yield pressure and esophageal acid exposure. There was no relationship between yield pressure and the pressure and length of the

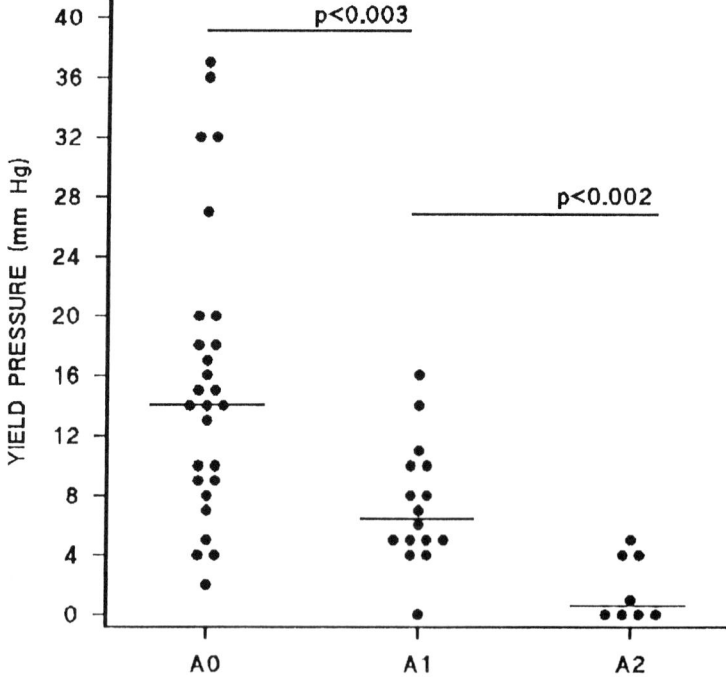

Fig. 1. Relationship between hiatus hernia and yield pressure.

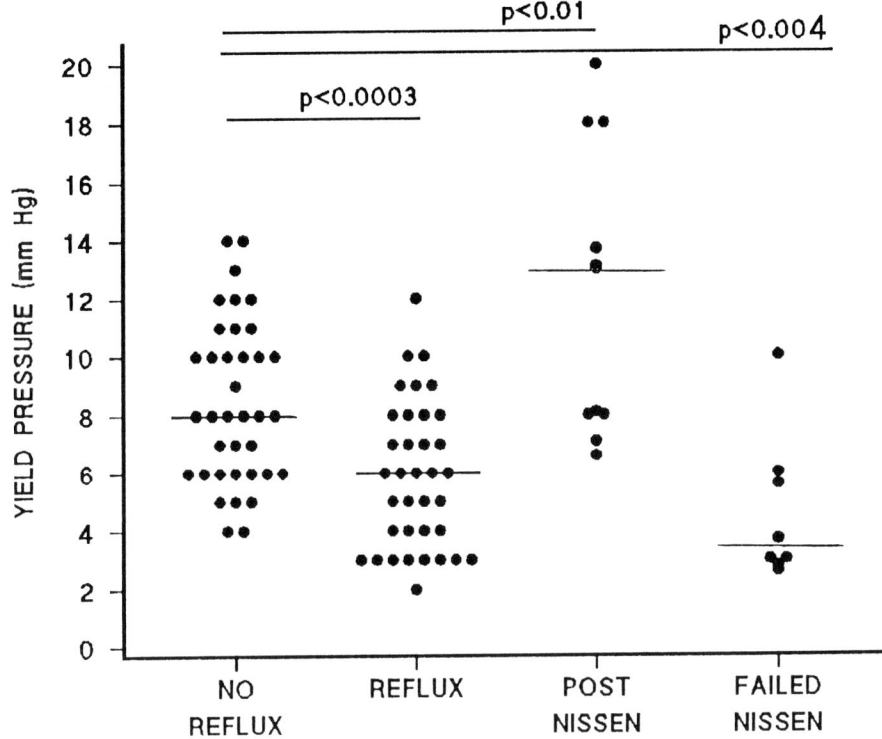

Fig. 2. Yield pressure measurement by manometry.

LES, even if vector volume analysis was used, suggesting that these measure different aspects of the continence mechanism of the cardia. Yield pressure was also related to the structure of the cardia, decreasing with the presence and size of a hiatal hernia [10] (Fig. 1).

Following floppy Nissen fundoplication yield pressure increased to supranormal values, despite normal LES pressure and length [10,11]. There was perfect discrimination between successful and failed fundoplication (Fig. 2) with one exception in a complex patient who had periesophageal fibrosis following an Angelchik prosthesis and then subsequently sustained a disrupted fundoplication. Vector volume analysis failed to make the discrimination as consistently as yield pressure. As far as is known, yield pressure is the only measure that reliably identifies successful or failed fundoplication and documents the slight overcompetence of the cardia that is characteristic of even a floppy Nissen fundoplication.

Since yield pressure is related to the anatomical structure of the cardia and to the presence of an intact fundoplication, it is tempting to suggest that it is a measure of the flap valve component of the cardia. It is believed that yield pressure measurement is the best single measure of the competence of the cardia following antireflux surgery.

References

1. Bjerkeset T, Nordgard K, Schjonsby H. Effect of Nissen fundoplication on the competence of the lower esophageal sphincter. Scand J Gastroenterol 1980;15:213–217.
2. Donahue PE, Samelson S, Nyhus LM, Bombeck CT. The floppy Nissen fundoplication. Effective long-term control of pathologic reflux. Arch Surg 1985;120:663–668.
3. Gill RC, Bowes KL, Murphy PD et al. Esophageal motor abnormalities in gastroesophageal reflux and the effects of fundoplication. Gastroenterology 1986;91:364–369.
4. Bancewicz J, Mughal M, Marples M. The lower oesophageal sphincter after floppy Nissen fundoplication. Br J Surg 1987;74:162–164.
5. Ireland AC, Holloway RH, Toouli J, Dent J. Mechanisms underlying the antireflux action of fundoplication. Gut 1993;34:303–308.
6. Bardhan CP, Gotley DC, Miller R, Mills A, Alderson D. Pressure events surrounding oesophageal acid reflux episodes and acid clearance in ambulant healthy volunteers. Gut 1993;34:444–449.
7. Holloway RH, Hongo M, Berger K, McCallum RW. Gastric distension: a mechanism for postprandial gastroesophageal reflux. Gastroenterology 1985;89:779–784.
8. Smiddy FG, Atkinson M. Mechanisms preventing gastro-oesophageal reflux in the dog. Br J Surg 1960;47:680–687.
9. McGouran RCM, Galloway JM, Spence DS, Morton CP, Marchant D. Does measurement of yield pressure at the cardia during endoscopy provide information on the function of the lower oesophageal sphincter mechanism? Gut 1988;29:275–278.
10. Ismail T, Bancewicz J. Anatomy of the cardia and gastro-oesophageal reflux. Gut 1992;33(suppl 2):S62.
11. Ismail T, Bancewicz J, Barlow J. The gastric cardia – valve or sphincter. Irish J Med Sci 1992;161(suppl 11):5.

Can the results of a technique be assessed purely clinically?

C. Gautier Benoit (Lille)

Since DeMeester [1] has compared in a randomized trial three surgical procedures: Belsey Mark IV, Nissen and Hill procedures, with endoscopy, manometry and pH metry as follow-up criteria, it is customary to use those criteria to compare surgical procedures used to cure gastroesophageal reflux (GER). Nevertheless, follow-up in this study was only four months.

Today, any treatment for GER should be estimated with a follow-up period of up to 2 years. Therefore, late recurrence of symptoms could be demonstrated for several techniques like the Lortat-Jacob's or Toupet's procedure [2,3].

Shirazi [4], in a retrospective study including 350 patients with a follow-up from 1–20 years, observed that patients without symptoms many years after surgery do not willingly undergo investigations. We made the same observation subsequently, with a mean length of 8 years follow-up. Patients do not understand the utility of investigations, like endoscopy or manometry.

Is it possible to estimate the results of therapy with only a clinical estimation?

Firstly, it must be pointed out that surgery of GER has a functional aim. Consistently, the functional result must be appreciated, and new symptoms are more important for evaluating a surgical procedure than improvement or recurrence of reflux symptoms.

Secondly, correlation between clinical estimation and so-called "objective tests" is diversely estimated. The correlation is good according to Teboul [5], but incomplete for Brandt [6]. However, it has never been demonstrated that patients having no clinical symptoms, but having mild endoscopic or histologic symptoms of esophagitis, will have a poorer long-term result than patients without any endoscopic or histologic symptoms.

Last but not least, Fuchs and DeMeester [7] evaluated specificity, sensitivity and positive value of various objective tests (esophagoscopy, standard acid reflux test, manomctry and pH monitoring), in a population composed of patients with classic symptoms of reflux and others who never experienced these symptoms. Therefore, clinical symptoms appear to be a kind of "gold standard".

Some authors grade their results using clinical criteria, as excellent, good, fair or poor.

Hill [8] summarizes the results of the Hill's repair as follows:

— excellent for asymptomatic patients;
— good for patients without symptoms of GER but with other symptoms from surgery; and
— poor for patients with aggravation or recurrence of reflux symptoms.

Visik's classification is also used, but it seems preferable to assign grades to specific symptoms like dysphagia, heartburn or postoperative symptoms, with emphasis being given to their intensity and frequency.

Pope [9] proposed a composite score giving an overall impression of the patients; he thinks that it is useless to confirm the score by objective tests. As he reported [9], a patient who suffers from severe heartburn does not care whether the postoperative lower esophageal sphincter pressure will rise or not, the important thing being that the heartburn cease postoperatively.

In reality, the answer must be full of nuances. In a study of long-term follow-up, it cannot be seriously envisaged to classify, as a good result, a patient who suffers from any clinical symptom. However, the objective tests are useful to make a precise evaluation of a patient still being symptomatic, for example, in differentiating atypical symptoms of reflux from other postoperative symptoms. Indeed, such a differentiation is necessary, not only to estimate the results, but also to treat symptomatic patients.

References

1. DeMeester TR, Johnson LF, Kent A. Evaluation of current operations for the prevention of gastroesophageal reflux. Ann Surg 1974;180:511—525.
2. AURC. Traitement chirurgical du reflux gastro-oesophagien. Etude prospective contrôlée multicentrique comparant les interventions de Nissen, Toupet et Lortat Jacob. Ann Chir 1987;41:561 (abstract).
3. Galmiche JP, Téniere P, Ducrotté P, Denis P, Colin R, Testart J. Traitement du reflux gastro-oesophagien acide par hémi-fundoplicature postérieure. Résultats cliniques et pH métriques. Gastroenterol Clin Biol 1983;7:385—391.
4. Shirazi SS., Schulze K, Soper RT. Long-term follow-up for treatment of complicated chronic reflux esophagitis. Arch Surg 1987;122:548—552.
5. Teboul F. Cure du reflux gastro-oesophagien chez l'adulte par fundoplicature complète (Nissen) et cardiopexie postérieure (Hill). Thèse, Lyon, 1985.

6. Brandt DL, Eastwood TR, Martin D, Carter WP, Pope CE. Esophageal symptoms manometry and histology before and after antireflux surgery. Gastroenterology 1979;76:1393.

7. Fuchs KH, DeMeester TR, Albertucci M. Specificity and sensitivity of objective diagnosis of gastroesophageal reflux disease. Surgery 1987;102:575–580.

8. Russell COH, Hill LD. Gastroesophageal reflux. In: Ravitch MM (ed) Current Problems in Surgery, vol XX. Chicago: Year Book Medical, 1983;vol XX:4.

9. Pope CE. The quality of life following antireflux surgery. World J Surg 1992;16:355–358.

10. Gautier-Benoit C, Bugnon PY, Pinchon-Marsy S, Meignie Ph. Résultats éloignés de la gastropexie postérieure de Hill dans le traitement du reflux gastro-oesophagien non compliqué de l'adulte. Chirurgie 1988;114:566–57..

Early recurrences seem due more often to poor selection than to poor surgery

C. Iascone, D. Castiglia, M. Barreca (Rome)

Gastroesophageal reflux disease (GERD) is a multifactorial pathology, where lower esophageal sphincter (LES) competence, esophageal body clearing capacity and gastric function play an important role. The development of complications of GERD is related to the presence of a mechanically defective LES. This indicates that a mechanically defective sphincter is the major factor in the pathogenesis of complications [1]. All antireflux valves aim to restore LES competence, which is impaired in 92% of patients with GERD [2]. It is reasonable to think that antireflux procedures can achieve the best results in those patients with proven GERD on 24-h pH monitoring of the esophagus, who only present a mechanically defective LES on manometry [3]. According to these criteria DeMeester et al. [4] performed Nissen operations in 100 consecutive patients with an actuarial success rate of 91% over a 10-year period. In our overall experience obtained with the Belsey Mark IV operation, the incidence of failure is 4.2% in patients with normal motor activity of the body of the esophagus, and 33% in those with altered motility [5]. Mughal et al. [6] failed to find any difference in the outcome of Nissen fundoplication in subsets of patients with or without LES competence impairment or motor abnormalities on manometry preoperatively. However, when the motor function of the esophagus is highly impaired, the results of surgery are often unsatisfactory. Experimental data suggest that alkaline reflux can damage the mucosa of the esophagus [7]. Recently, Stein et al. [1] showed that severe mucosal injuries of the esophagus are directly related to an increased esophageal exposure to both acid and alkaline reflux. Gastric antrectomy and Roux-en-Y reconstruction reduce acid production and divert biliopancreatic secretions. In a randomized prospective trial, Washer et al. [8] found that in patients with complicated reflux disease, this operation appeared to be superior to the Nissen fundoplication. Fayek et al. [9] found that the success of Belsey procedure diminishes steadily as the severity of esophagitis increases. When local conditions of gastroesophageal junction are compromised due to severe inflammation, so that performing a fundoplication may be hazardous, gastric resection and Roux-en-Y reconstruction may be the best treatment, especially in those patients with nonacid reflux. Approximately 30% of patients with proven GERD will have hypersecretion on gastric juice analysis; 2—3% of subjects who have antireflux procedure will develop a gastric or duodenal ulcer. These factors may modify the proposed antireflux procedure by the addition of a highly selective proximal vagotomy [3]. Delayed gastric emptying has been implicated in the pathogenesis of reflux disease. Maddern et al. [10] demonstrated that patients with recurrent reflux symptoms have delayed gastric emptying compared with normal controls and prefundoplication values. They suggest that delayed gastric emptying, either before or after surgery, may be of value in predicting patients likely to have poor outcomes. Hinder et al. [11] found that side effects associated with Nissen fundoplication, rather than due to technical details, are due to the failure to normalize gastric emptying. Further investigations and long-term follow-up studies are needed to clarify whether the parameter of gastric emptying can be used to predict the clinical outcome after fundoplication. If the importance of delayed gastric emptying is demonstrated for the outcome of surgery, it would be justified to add a gastric drainage procedure to the fundoplication in this subset of patients. As GERD is a multifactorial pathology, surgery should be also adapted to the different physiopathologic patterns of the disease in order to achieve the best results. Long-term results are also influenced by the physiologic derangement of antireflux procedures as time goes by, so that an accurate selection of patients can improve the short-term more than the long-term results.

References

1. Stein HJ, DeMeester TR, Perry RP. The development of complications in gastroesophageal sphincter, esophageal acid and acid/alkaline exposure, and duodenogastric reflux. Ann Surg 1992;216:35.
2. Zaninotto G, DeMeester TR, Schwizer W. The lower esophageal sphincter in health and disease. Am J Surg 1988;155: 104—111.
3. Stein HJ, DeMeester TR. Who benefits from antireflux surgery? World J Surg 1992;16:313—319.
4. DeMeester TR, Bonavina L, Albertucci M. Nissen fundoplication for gastroesophageal reflux disease. Ann Surg 1986; 204:9—20.
5. Stipa S, Fegiz GF, Iascone C, Paolini A, Moraldi A, De Marchi C, Addario Chieco P. Belsey and Nissen operations for gastroesophageal reflux. Ann Surg 1990;208:583—589.
6. Mughal MM, Bancewicz M, Marples A. Oesophageal manometry and pH recording does not predict the bad results of Nissen fundoplication. Br J Surg 1990;77:43—45.
7. Salo JA, Kivilaakso E. Role of bile salts and trypsin in the pathogenesis of experimental alkaline esophagitis. Surgery 1983;93:525.
8. Washer GF, Gear MWL, Dowling BL, Gillison EW, Roystone CMS, Spencer J. Randomized prospective trial of Roux-en-Y duodenal diversion versus fundoplication for severe reflux esophagitis. Br J Surg 1984;71:181—184.
9. Fayek DS, Graham L. Long-term results of Belsey Mark IV antireflux operation in relation to the severity of esophagitis. J Thorac Cardiovasc Surg 1985;202:162.
10. Maddern GJ, Jamieson GG, Chatterton BE, Collins PJ. Is there an association between failure of antireflux procedures and delayed gastric emptying? Ann Surg 1985;202:162.
11. Hinder RA, Stein HJ, Bremner CG, DeMeester TR. Relationship of a satisfactory outcome to normalization of delayed gastric emptying after Nissen fundoplication. Ann Surg 1989;210:458—465.

Are late recurrences often associated with evolutive tissular dysplasia or persistent delay in gastric emptying?

K. Geboes, M. Tshibassu (Leuven)

Surgical correction for gastroesophageal reflux disease (GERD) is usually considered when an adequate trial of medical management has not brought satisfactory results after a 6-month period, and when good evidence of gastroesophageal reflux (GER) remains. In the late seventies, surgical antireflux procedures were indicated in 5—10% of the patients with GERD, but the development of more successful medical treatment, most notably with omeprazole, has greatly challenged the pre-eminence of surgical therapy in the long-term management of GERD [1].

Yet a patient, especially a young one, who continues to have troublesome symptoms despite safe medical treatment should consider surgery [2]. Surgery is also indicated for patients who develop complications (including stricture, bleeding, Barrett's ulcer).

The different antireflux operations available, regardless of the modifications, prevent reflux adequately and provide patient satisfaction in the majority of the cases, although limited data on the effect of antireflux surgery on ulceration and stricture formation are available [3]. Failures of surgical therapy are uncommon but, when they occur, they are difficult to treat medically or with further surgery. Failures are more likely to occur in difficult settings, such as aperistalsis of the esophagus. In such cases, gastric contents that reflux into the esophagus cannot be effectively cleared and this leads to an increased incidence of complications. A related situation is encountered when patients have coexistent gastroparesis and GERD. Careful preoperative assessment and intraoperative manometry can help as a useful check for the operator and prevent postoperative problems.

Major causes of postoperative problems are thus underlying motility disorders of the esophagus and stomach, such as delayed emptying of the stomach and changes in the tissular composition of the esophageal wall. The latter can be either of inflammatory nature or show features of degeneration. Motility studies were performed in a group of patients after dilatation to a 60-F size followed by a Nissen fundoplication. Patients with either relief of dysphagia after dilatation, adequate motility, or both, had excellent relief of dysphagia in 86% and good relief in 14% of patients. Four patients who had persistent dysphagia after dilatation and inadequate motility were found to have transmural fibrosis on pathologic examination of the resected esophagus [4].

In a retrospective study of 117 patients operated following the Belsey Mark IV procedure, good results, assessed symptomatically, were seen in patients without severe esophagitis at the time of operation [5]. However, in a long-term follow-up study of 600 patients treated by Nissen fundoplication, it was shown that severe histologic changes of esophagitis require many months to revert to normal, even though relief of symptoms occurs almost immediately [6]. Therefore, it remains to be proven that severe inflammatory changes will affect the long-term outcome of the operation. Recurrent reflux after Nissen fundoplication was seen in 12 of 125 (9.6%) patients in association with a Nissen wrap disruption, not necessarily due to previous tissular abnormalities.

Barrett's esophagus presents a special problem. Antireflux surgery is being recommended as a means for preventing esophageal cancer in patients with Barrett's esophagus. However, little has been published on the effect of antireflux surgery on dysplasia in Barrett's metaplasia. The few data available suggest that dysplasia (defined as an unequivocally neoplastic lesion) is as likely to progress as to regress in severity after such operations. Furthermore, there are numerous reports of patients who developed a carcinoma in Barrett's esophagus following antireflux surgery [7,8].

References

1. Richter JE, Castell DO. Gastroesophageal reflux: pathogenesis, diagnosis and therapy. Ann Int Med 1982;97:93−103.
2. Gelfand DW. Gastroesophageal reflux disease. Med Clin N Am 1991;75:923−940.
3. Richardson JD, Kuhns JG, Richardson RL, Polk HC. Properly conducted fundoplication reverses histologic evidence of esophagitis. Ann Surg 1983;197:763−770.
4. Zaninotto G, DeMeester TR, Bremner CG. Esophageal function in patients with reflux-induced strictures and its relevance to surgical treatment. Ann Thorac Surg 1989;47:362−370.
5. Salama FD, Lamont G. Long-term results of the Belsey Mark IV antireflux operation in relation to the severity of esophagitis. J Thorac Cardiovasc Surg 1990;100:517−519.
6. David J. Advocate's look at antireflux procedures. In: Society for Surgery of the Alimentary Tract, Postgraduate Course. San Francisco, 1983;1−15.
7. Spechler SJ. Columnar-lined (Barrett's) esophagus. Curr Opin Gastroenterol 1991;7:557−561.
8. Williamson WA, Ellis FH, Gibb SP, Shahiau DM, Aretz HT. Effect of antireflux operation on Barrett's mucosa. Ann Thorac Surg 1990;49:537−542.

What are the results of antireflux valves?

A. Del Genio, G. Izzo, V. Maffettone, L. Fei,
N. Di Martino, A. Cosenza, A. Martella, G. Angilletta
(Naples)

Today the surgical therapy of gastroesophageal reflux disease (GERD) has a very important role. It has to treat selected patients, such as the "no responders" to medical therapy and/or those affected by serious complications.

Fundoplication (partial 180°−270° fundoplication: Dor, Toupet, Hill and Belsey Mark IV; total 360° fundoplication: Nissen) is more used than anatomical surgical procedures (Allison, Lortat-Jacob, Boerema). The great number of antireflux procedures proves that there is no perfect operation, which is able to treat gastroeso-phageal reflux (GER), preventing disturbances correlated to the anatomo-functional modifications caused by the operation itself.

The results published in literature during the last 10 years are reported in the tables: in Tables 1 and 2 there are the data concerning a review by Inaspettato et al. [1] in 1988.

In Table 3, are found the global long-term clinical results, not always defined with objective criteria. Table 4 shows the same results in relation to the persistence of GER symptoms, Table 5 in relation to pH-metric GER recurrence, Table 6 in relation to esophagitis persistence; Table 7 reports the incidence of transitory dysphagia; Table 8 reports the incidence of persistent dysphagia, occasional or not; Table 9 shows the incidence of transitory or permanent gas bloat syndrome. Finally, Tables 10 and 11 concern death and morbidity rates.

Authors' personal experience

Of the 648 patients affected by abnormal GER, 85 (13.1%) have been operated since 1985. Among them, 71 were operated with laparotomic (ChLt) and 14 with laparo-scopic (ChLs) procedures.

In all cases we performed Nissen fundoplication modified by Rossetti [30]. Its characteristics are: 1) the use of the only anterior wall of the gastric fundus to make the wrap; 2) no short blood vessels section; 3) no opening of the little omentum; and 4) no diaphragmatic pillars treatment. The fundoplication was performed with the use of the intraoperative esophageal manometry (IEM) [31–33]; it allowed for the calibration of the wrap reaching pressure values included between 20 and 40 mmHg [34]. These values were classified into:

- sufficient (20–40 mmHg) in 83.5% (71/85: 39/71 = 83% ChLt; 12/14 = 85.7% ChLs); and
- not sufficient in 16.5% (14/85: 12/71 = 16.9% ChLt; 2/14 = 14.2% ChLs).

In these last patients, in order to increase pressure values, a second and sometimes a third layer was made (ChLt patients), or other single stitches were set (ChLs patients). So, the following intraoperative pressure values were reached: 1) 24.46 ± 5.22 mmHg for a length of 2.87 ± 0.42 cm in ChLt and; 2) 26.04 ± 5.72 mmHg for a length of 2.68 ± 0.52 cm in ChLs. The values obtained are greater than preoperative values (7.02 ± 3.46 mmHg) and than those of 15 healthy subjects (15.20 ± 2.45 mmHg) (p < 0.001).

Therefore, high intraoperative pressure values (hypercalibrated Nissen: 20–40 mmHg), compared to those of a normal sphincter, derived from the fact that we observed GER appearance in 23.8% of the treated patients with normal pressure values (normocalibrated Nissen fundoplication: 10–20 mmHg).

Death and morbidity rates were 0%. Laparoscopy lasted from 45 min to 2 h, with a decrease in the postoperative pain.

Deambulation started again in the evening, when the infusive therapy was suspended. The day after the operation, patients began to eat again. Hospitalization lasted 3.2 ± 0.8 days vs. 7.3 ± 1.34 days after laparotomy.

The clinical follow-up, made on all 85 patients (46.8 ± 14.6 months, 71 ChLt patients; 9.06 ± 5.20 months, 14 ChLs patients), showed transitory dysphagia in four patients (4.7%) (3 ChLt and 1 ChLs) and transitory gas-bloat syndrome in three ChLt patients (4.2%); both the complications disappeared spontaneously in 3 months. Light and occasional dysphagia (once or twice a week) was found in seven patients (8.2%) (6 ChLt and 1 ChLs). The patients thought that the result was good and did not use medication. A ChLt operated patient showed epigastric pain, caused by herniated Nissen fundoplication; it was treated with laparoscopic hyatoplasty. Another patient showed pyrosis with disrupted Nissen and pH-metric GER recurrence; it was treated with another antireflux fundoplication. Twenty-four hour combined pH-monitoring performed on 41 patients (37 ChLt: 32.8 ± 3.14 months, 4 ChLs: 7.2 ± 2.12 months) documented a Nissen fundoplication hypercompetence. At the same time, no refluxes, even postprandial ones, were observed, except for the one patient with pyrosis.

Manometry showed that, in all patients, the new HPZ pressure values were lower than the intraoperative ones (13.46 ± 4.84 mmHg ChLt; 12.84 ± 3.76 mmHg ChLs). In 6 months, the values came near to those found in healthy subjects. The dynamic study of new HPZ demonstrated postdeglutitive relaxations of 74.82 ± 15.26% (ChLt) and of 77.42 ± 8.44% (ChLs), lower than those obtained in a control group (95.53 ± 3.99% $p < 0.001$). Endoscopy showed no esophagitis (39 ChLt; follow-up 36.2 ± 4.36 months).

Discussion

The difficulties in comparing the results obtained with different methods are due to: a) lack of homogeneity in the group of patients; b) different parameters examined; c) frequent subjective modifications brought in the single operations; d) subjective evaluation of the results; e) follow-up differences; and f) different numbers of patients treated by the authors. Nevertheless, the good results obtained prove the effectiveness of the antireflux surgical therapy, although no method can be considered as the "gold standard". Anatomical operations (Allison, Boerema, Lortat-Jacob) are not used any more, although some good results were reported (Table 1). In 1988, Inaspettato et al. [1] showed that in 10,203 operations performed until 1977, GER recurrence ranged from 0.3% (Boerema) to 14% (Lortat-Jacob).

Table 1. Results of surgical therapy for GER: literature review 1956–1977 (10,203 patients) [1]

Procedure	Hiatal hernia recurrence (%)	Reflux recurrence (%)	Hiatal hernia and reflux recurrence (%)
Allison	10	9	4
Belsey	2.3	6.5	5
Boerema	6	0.3	6.9
Hill	—	3.7	1
Lortat-Jacob	6.6	14	3.7
Nissen	1.5	0	0.5

Table 2. Results of surgical therapy for GER: Belsey, Nissen and Hill operations [1]

Procedure	Year	Pts.	Recurrence(%)	Range (%)
Belsey	1988	892	11.5	5.9–14.6
Nissen	1975–1988	1,048	7.8	0.2–19
Hill	1988	1,860	3.2	1.5–5

In Table 2, the same author reports the results obtained in 3,800 operated patients until 1988. Among Hill, Belsey and Nissen procedures, the former was the most frequently performed with the best results (GER recurrence = 3.2% on 1,860 cases).

In our review, we found poor contributions concerning partial fundoplication: Dor procedure is used only to prevent GER after Heller's myotomy. Narbona procedure [4,9] showed good results, although today it is not often performed.

Table 3. Surgery for GER: long-term clinical results

Authors	Year	Pts.	Operation	F-up (year)	F-up (pts.)	Excellent No.	Excellent %	Good No.	Good %	Poor No.	Poor %
Ellis [2]	1984	92	Nissen	5.7	82	32	39	23	28	27	33
DeMeester [3]	1986	100	Nissen[a] I-II-III-IV	1–13	100	83	83	10	10	7	7
Narbona [4]	1988	1491	Cardiopexy with round ligament	5–20	998	702	70	161	16	96	10
Low [5]	1989	447	Hill	9–20	167	112	67	35	21	20	12
Rossetti [6]	1989	377	Nissen-Rossetti	2–20	377	326	86	41	11	10	3
Henderson [7]	1989	127	270° posterior valve	10	125	79	63.2	22	17.5	24	19.2
Hill [8]	1989	1300	Hill	5–15	1300	1015	78	221	17	65	5
Flament [9]	1989	76	Cardiopexy with round ligament and Toupet	5	76	72	94.8	–	–	4	5.2
Ellis [10]	1989	157	Floppy Nissen	6	157	152	90.2	–	–	5	9.8
Mughal [11]	1990	126	Floppy Nissen	–	126	67	53.3	38	30.1	21	16.7
Stipa-Fegiz [12]	1990	30	Belsey	5–10	28	19	67.9	6	21.4	3	10.7
Stipa-Fegiz [12]	1990	32	Nissen	5–10	30	16	53.3	10	33.3	4	13.3
Rohr [13]	1992	117	Floppy Nissen	> 1	99	75	75.7	10	10.1	14	14.1
Bjerkeset [14]	1992	82	Floppy Nissen-Rossetti	6	82	65	79.2	14	17	3	3.6
Del Genio [15]	1993	85	Nissen-Rossetti (IEM)	4	85	76	89.4	7	7.2	2	2.3

[a]I-II-III-IV: four types of Nissen performed by author. Pts. = Patients; F-up = Follow-up; No. = Number.

576

Table 4. Surgery for GER: symptoms following surgery

Authors	Year	Pts.	Operation	F-up (year)	F-up (pts.)	GER symptoms	
						No.	%
Ellis [2]	1984	92	Floppy Nissen	> 1	82	8	9.8
Donahue [16]	1985	77	Floppy Nissen	4	62	0	0
DeMeester [3]	1986	100	Nissen[a] I-II-III-IV	1—13	100	3	3
Lorenzini [17]	1986	36	Dor	> 1	36	0	0
Bancewicz [18]	1987	61	Floppy Nissen	3—6	61	3	4.9
Narbona [4]	1988	1491	Cardiopexy with round ligament	5—20	998	39	4
Seineldin [19]	1989	78	Nissen	> 1	78	9	11.5
Low [5]	1989	447	Hill	15—20	167	20	4.4
Rossetti [6]	1989	377	Nissen-Rossetti	2—20	377	42	11.1
O'Hanrahan [20]	1989	125	Floppy-Nissen	> 1	125	19	15.2
Hill [8]	1989	1300	Hill	5—15	1300	65	5
Flament [9]	1989	76	Cardiopexy with round ligament and Toupet	5	76	2	2.7
Ellis [10]	1989	157	Floppy Nissen	> 1	157	8	5
Breumelhof [21]	1990	27	Nissen	—	27	10	37
Mughal [11]	1990	126	Floppy Nissen	—	126	10	7.9
Stipa-Fegiz [12]	1990	30	Belsey	5—10	28	3	10.7
Stipa-Fegiz [12]	1990	32	Nissen	5—10	30	4	13.3
Kmiot [22]	1991	25	Angelchik	2	25	2	8
Kmiot [22]	1991	25	Nissen	2	25	1	4
Grande [23]	1991	117	Floppy Nissen	> 1	35	2	6
Rohr [13]	1992	117	Floppy Nissen	—	117	22	18
Bjerkeset [14]	1992	82	Floppy Nissen-Rossetti	6	82	2	2.4
Del Genio [15]	1993	85	Nissen-Rossetti (IEM)	4	85	1	1.1

[a]I-II-III-IV: four types of Nissen performed by author. Pts. = Patients; F-up = Follow-up; No. = Number.

Nissen fundoplication is the most commonly used. Tables 3, 4, 5 and 6 show no significant differences in the results of the various methods.

Long-term results (Table 3) seem to be satisfactory (excellent-good) in percentages ranging from 83.2 [11] to 97.6% according to our personal experience [15]; on the contrary, in 1984, Ellis reported poor results in 32.9% of cases [2].

Table 4 shows that GER symptoms are present in percentages ranging from 0 [16] to 15.2% [20] after floppy Nissen procedure; nevertheless, Breumelhof [21] reported persistent GER symptoms in a high percentage (37%) after Nissen fundoplication.

Table 5 shows that the results of pH-metric GER recurrence are different: 0.6 and 30% according to Ellis [10] and Rohr [13], respectively, after floppy Nissen; 51.8% according to Breumelhof [21] after Nissen fundoplication.

Esophagitis (Table 6) is reported in percentages ranging from 0 (personal data) [15] to 30% [13]; it generally occurs after floppy Nissen. DeMeester reports that the fundoplication is able to control abnormal GER in 91% of cases (10-year follow-up) [3]. However, this value decreases to 3% in patients with upright reflux, or with lower esophageal sphincter (LES) competence, or with serious diffuse motor abnor-

Table 5. Surgery for GER: pH metric recurrence of reflux

Authors	Year	Pts.	Operation	F-up (years)	F-up (pts.)	Recurrence of reflux	
						No.	%
Ellis [2]	1984	92	Floppy Nissen	> 1	25	5	20
Donahue [16]	1985	77	Floppy Nissen	4	62	2	3.2
DeMeester [3]	1986	100	Nissen[a] I-II-III-IV	1—13	100	6	16.6
Lorenzini [17]	1986	36	Dor	> 1	13	1	7.6
Bancewicz [18]	1987	61	Floppy Nissen	3—6	36	4	11.1
Shirazi [24]	1987	350	Nissen	20	350	17	4.8
Ackermans [25]	1987	290	Nissen	10	290	39	13.1
Narbona [4]	1988	1491	Cardiopexy with round ligament	5—20	998	32	4
Rossetti [6]	1989	377	Nissen-Rossetti	2—20	377	42	11.1
O'Hanrahan [20]	1989	125	Floppy Nissen	> 1	125	12	9.6
Flament [9]	1989	76	Cardiopexy with round ligament and Toupet	5	76	2	2.7
Ellis [10]	1989	157	Floppy Nissen	> 1	157	1	0.6
Breumelhof [21]	1990	27	Nissen	—	27	14	51.8
Bancewicz [26]	1990	126	Floppy Nissen	> 1	76	12	15.7
Mughal [11]	1990	126	Floppy Nissen	—	126	7	5.5
Stipa-Fegiz [12]	1990	30	Belsey	5—10	28	2	7.1
Stipa-Fegiz [12]	1990	32	Nissen	5—10	30	3	10
Kmiot [22]	1991	25	Angelchik	2	25	2	8
Kmiot [22]	1991	25	Nissen	2	25	1	4
Rohr [13]	1992	117	Floppy Nissen	> 1	26	8	30
Del Genio [15]	1993	85	Nissen-Rossetti (IEM)	4	41	1	2.4

[a]I-II-III-IV: four types of Nissen performed by author. Pts. = Patients; F-up = Follow-up; No. = Number.

malities (DMA) of the esophageal body (nonpropagating waves >50%).

Other authors documented that after 18—24 months, recurrence does not increase any more [21]. We observed that only one patient (1.1%) had pyrosis and GER pH-metric recurrence, caused by disrupted Nissen after four months.

There are some postoperative consequences which are difficult to accept in the treatment of a benign disease. After fundoplication, the most common are transitory or persistent dysphagia, gas-bloat syndrome, and inability to belch and vomit.

Transitory dysphagia (Table 7), is commonly reported in fundoplication, with percentages ranging from 0.8 [13] and 62.8% [23] after floppy Nissen. It disappears within 2—12 months. This disturbance is due to postoperative DMA of the esophageal body [18] that are transitory. According to Grande [23] and to our own experience, on the contrary, transitory dysphagia disappears when new HPZ pressure values decrease.

Persistent dysphagia (Table 8) is a serious postoperative disturbance which sometimes requires a reoperation. It is more frequent after Nissen fundoplication (up to 40%) [21] than after floppy Nissen (0—11% according to Donahue and Grande, respectively) [16,23]. Dysphagia is usually occasional and, most of the times, light. Besides, we documented that 8.2% of the patients who complained of this symptom,

Table 6. Surgery for GER: persistence of esophagitis

Authors	Year	Pts.	Operation	F-up (years)	F-up (pts)	Esophagitis No.	Esophagitis %
Donahue [16]	1985	77	Floppy Nissen	3	62	7	11.2
Lorenzini [17]	1987	36	Dor	> 1	13	1	7.6
Bancewicz [18]	1987	61	Floppy Nissen	–	36	1	1.6
O'Hanrahan [20]	1989	125	Floppy Nissen	> 1	125	8	6.4
Breumelhof [21]	1990	27	Nissen	–	19	2	10.5
Rohr [13]	1992	117	Floppy Nissen	> 1	26	8	30
Bjerkeset [14]	1992	82	Floppy Nissen-Rossetti	6	79	2	2.5
Del Genio [15]	1993	85	Nissen-Rossetti (IEM)	4	41	0	0

Pts. = Patients; F-up = Follow-up; No. = Number.

could eat normally, without drug consumption.

The incidence of gaseous disturbances (Table 9), is reported at different rates. It is caused by: 1) a hypercorrection of the antireflux valve; 2) lesions of the vagus nerve fibers [35]; and 3) an excessive length of the wrap (>4 cm) [3,28,36,37].

According to numerous authors [3,14], postoperative gaseous disturbances are due to aerophagy and to preoperative gastric difficulties.

In his study on 82 patients treated with floppy Nissen-Rossetti, Bjerkeset reported that 30% of those who showed postoperative gaseous disturbances (6/20) had

Table 7. Surgery for GER: temporary dysphagia

Authors	Year	Pts.	Operation	F-up (pts)	Temporary dysphagia No.	Temporary dysphagia %	Duration (months)
Donahue [16]	1985	77	Floppy Nissen	77	8	10.3	–
DeMeester [3]	1986	100	Nissen[a] I-II-III-IV	100	50	50	3
Lorenzini [17]	1986	36	Dor	36	15	41.6	1
Bancewicz [18]	1987	61	Floppy Nissen	61	16	26.2	12
Narbona [4]	1988	1491	Cardiopexy with round ligament	998	4	0.4	1
Low [5]	1989	447	Hill	447	28	6.3	3
Hill [8]	1989	1300	Hill	1300	260	20	–
Flament [9]	1989	76	Cardiopexy with round ligament and Toupet	76	14	18.6	6
Kmiot [22]	1991	25	Angelchik	25	0	0	–
Kmiot [22]	1991	25	Nissen	25	1	4	3
Grande [23]	1991	35	Floppy Nissen	35	22	62.8	2
Rohr [13]	1992	117	Floppy Nissen	117	1	0.8	4
Del Genio [15]	1993	85	Nissen-Rossetti (IEM)	85	4	4.7	1

[a]I-II-III-IV: Four types of Nissen performed by author. Pts = Patients; F-up = Follow-up; No. = Number.

580

Table 8. Surgery for GER: persistent dysphagia

Author	Year	Pts	Operation	F-up (years)	F-up (pts)	Persistent dysphagia No.	Persistent dysphagia %
Donahue [16]	1985	77	Floppy Nissen	1—8	62	0	0
DeMeester [3]	1986	100	Nissen[a] I-II-III-IV	1—13	100	14	14
Bancewicz [18]	1987	61	Floppy Nissen	3—6	61	3	4.9
Shirazi [24]	1987	350	Nissen	20	350	10	2.8
Ackermans [25]	1987	290	Nissen	10	290	32	11.3
Narbona [4]	1988	1491	Cardiopexy with round ligament	5—20	998	0	0
Seineldin [19]	1989	78	Nissen	>1	78	10	12.8
O'Hanrahan [20]	1989	125	Floppy Nissen	>1	125	7	5.6
Ellis [10]	1989	157	Floppy Nissen	>1	157	1	0.6
Breumelhof [21]	1990	27	Nissen	>1	27	11	40
Mughal [11]	1990	126	Floppy Nissen	—	126	6	5.7
Kmiot [22]	1991	25	Angelchik	2	25	5	20
Kmiot [22]	1991	25	Nissen	2	25	0	0
Grande [23]	1991	35	Floppy Nissen	>1	35	4	11.4
Rohr [13]	1992	117	Floppy Nissen	>1	99	4	4
Bjerkeset [14]	1992	82	Floppy Nissen-Rossetti	5	82	0	0
Del Genio [15]	1993	85	Nissen-Rossetti (IEM)	4	85	7	8.2

[a]I-II-III-IV: Four types of Nissen performed by author. Pts = Patients; F-up = Follow-up; No. = Number.

generally undergone another operation, in addition to Nissen fundoplication, for gastric ulcer. According to the author, the inability to belch is due to the fact that patients swallow air to clear their esophagus of the refluxed acid.

Table 10 shows death-rates according to Hill (0—1.9%) [8]; thromboembolism is the most common cause of death. Morbidity (Table 11) is high after Floppy Nissen (up to 30.7%) [13]; it is generally due to splenic and esophageal lesions. These consequences are in contrast with the good results of GER surgical therapy. To reduce the occurrence of these symptoms, several surgeons selected patients carefully, modified surgical techniques and used intraoperative functional tests such as electromanometry. This has been proposed since 1972 in order to calibrate fundo-plication [31—33].

DeMeester argues that patient screening can be carried out on the basis of: a) LES competence; b) different types of reflux; c) presence of disordered motor activity [3]. As a matter of fact, patients exposed to the risk of GER recurrence and of postoperative consequences are: those with LES pressure >5 mmHg, with intra-abdominal LES length >1.5 cm and/or with total LES length >2.5 cm; those with abnormal upright reflux and/or with simultaneous postdeglutitive waves (>50%).

Siewert also asserts that dysphagia is almost an unavoidable event in patients with esophageal peristaltic deficit [28]. These patients should not undergo surgery, such as those with scleroderma, other collagenopathies, or with diabetic neuropathy. On the contrary, other authors documented no correlation between clinical results and preoperative DMA, or between clinical results and LES competence [18,26,38].

Table 9. Surgery for GER: gas-bloat syndrome

Authors	Year	Pts	Operation	F-up (years)	Gas-bloat syndrome		Impossibility to belch and/or to vomit	
					No.	%	No.	%
Ellis [2]	1984	92	Nissen	> 1	—	—	15	19.7
Donahue [16]	1985	77	Floppy Nissen	4	1[b]	1.2	1	1.2
DeMeester [3]	1986	100	Nissen[a] I-II-III-IV	1—13	15	15	63	63
Lorenzini [17]	1986	36	Dor	> 1	4	11.1	0	0
Shirazi [24]	1987	350	Nissen	20	20	5.7	—	—
Ackermans [25]	1987	290	Nissen	10	0	0	0	0
Narbona [4]	1988	1491	Cardiopexy with round ligament	5—20	30[b]	3	—	—
Seineldin [19]	1989	78	Nissen	> 1	6	7.6	17	21.7
O'Hanrahan [20]	1989	125	Floppy Nissen	> 1	1	0.8	—	—
Ellis [10]	1989	157	Floppy Nissen	> 1	1	0.6	—	—
Mughal [11]	1990	126	Floppy Nissen	> 1	1	1.5	—	—
Stipa-Fegiz [22]	1990	30	Belsey	5—10	8	28.6	2	7.1
Stipa-Fegiz [22]	1990	32	Nissen	5—10	12	40	3	10
Kmiot [22]	1991	25	Angelchik	> 1	0	0	—	—
Kmiot [22]	1991	25	Nissen	2	1[b]	4	—	—
Rohr [13]	1992	117	Floppy Nissen	> 1	11	9	14	12
Bjerkeset [14]	1992	82	Floppy Nissen-Rossetti	6	20	24	5	6
Del Genio [15]	1993	85	Nissen-Rossetti (IEM)	4	3[b]	4.2	0	0

[a]I-II-III-IV: Four types of Nissen performed by author; [b]Transient; Pts = Patients; F-up = Follow-up; No. = Number.

Patients with upright reflux must not be operated upon, as they can develop gas-bloat syndrome. They often suffer from aerophagia, delayed gastric emptying and/or duodeno-gastric reflux.

In 1985, Donahue proposed floppy Nissen procedure which is the most commonly used technical variation of the traditional Nissen fundoplication [16]. According to him, in order to have better results, it was necessary to prevent Nissen wrap from being a permanent mechanical obstruction to the esophagogastric transit. Therefore, he performed this operation, mobilizing the gastric fundus widely and dividing the short blood vessels; moreover, he set a big probe along the esophagus, so that the Nissen was floppy. Some authors do not confirm Donahue's good results; at the same time, he reports a persistent esophagitis in 11% of cases, which can be due to a poor GER control.

Other authors argue that the best results can be obtained with a very floppy Nissen fundoplication [3,28,39], unlike those [23,26,41] who argue that, in order to increase LES pressure, Nissen fundoplication is the most effective procedure.

McGouran says that a 360° valve controls reflux by itself [39], but as a matter of fact, there is no sure correlation between new HPZ pressure and clinical results [26,28]. In normal conditions, the contraction of gastric oblique fibers prevents the effect of the gastric wall straining on the LES. In patients with abnormal reflux, this

Table 10. Surgery for GER: mortality and morbidity (30 days)

Author	Year	Pts	Operation	Mortality		Morbidity	
				No.	%	No.	%
Ellis [2]	1984	92	Nissen	0	0	8	8.8
Donahue [16]	1985	77	Floppy Nissen	1	1.2	8	10.3
O'Rourke [27]	1985	105	Nissen	0	0	8	7.6
DeMeester [3]	1986	100	Nissen[a] I-II-III-IV	1	1	13	13
Lorenzini [17]	1986	36	Dor	1	2.7	9	25
Shirazi [24]	1987	350	Nissen	0	0	71	20.2
Gouge [28]	1987	81	Nissen	0	0	14	17.2
Siewert [29]	1987	88	Nissen	0	0	10	11.3
Narbona [4]	1988	1491	Cardiopexy with round ligament	15	1	298	20
Low [5]	1989	447	Hill	6	1.3	83	18.5
Rossetti [6]	1989	377	Nissen-Rossetti	2	0.5	–	–
O'Hanrahan [20]	1989	125	Floppy Nissen	0	0	–	–
Hill [8]	1989	1300	Hill	24	1.9	–	–
Flament [9]	1989	76	Cardiopexy with round ligament and Toupet	1	1.3	16	21
Breumelhof [21]	1990	27	Nissen	0	0	2	7.4
Stipa-Fegiz [22]	1990	30	Belsey	0	0	4	13.3
Stipa-Fegiz [22]	1990	32	Nissen	0	0	2	6.2
Rohr [13]	1992	117	Floppy Nissen	1	0.8	36	30.7
Del Genio [15]	1993	85	Nissen-Rossetti (IEM)	0	0	0	0

[a]I-II-III-IV: Four types of Nissen performed by author. Pts = Patients; No. = Number.

mechanism is insufficient, so the gastric wall tension has a negative effect on LES, with its consequent relaxation and with GER occurrence.

According to McGouran, by modifying the gastric fundus, Nissen fundoplication prevents the negative effects on LES due to the gastric tension. Moreover, DeMeester reported that he had obtained his best results with a floppy Nissen: he mobilized the gastric fundus widely, introduced a 60 F probe into the esophagus and performed a very short valve (1 cm) [3]. Therefore, by increasing the esophageal probe caliber ($36 \rightarrow 60$ F) he reduced the incidence of temporary swallowing discomfort ($83 \rightarrow 39\%$) and of persistent dysphagia ($21 \rightarrow 3\%$).

This result was obtained by reducing the length of the wrap from 4 to 1 cm, and the wide mobilization of the gastric fundus allowed a better postdeglutitive new HPZ relaxation ($31 \rightarrow 71\%$).

According to the author, the stronger effectiveness of this operation on abnormal GER demonstrates that it does not create any esophageal obstruction. This modified fundoplication does not alter the total number of reflux episodes, but reduces the number of episodes lasting more than 5 min, compared to the traditional Nissen fundoplication, as it does not influence the esophageal clearing.

Traditional Nissen fundoplication would alter esophageal clearing for two reasons: 1) the interference of the esophageal body on motor activity; and 2) the incomplete new HPZ postdeglutitive relaxation of a Nissen which is too short or too long.

Table 11. Surgery for GER: morbidity (30 days)

Authors	S-I		E-P		G-P		W-I		W-D		P-C		V-T		Other	
	No.	%	No.	%	No.	%	No.	%	No.	%	No.	%	No.	%	No.	%
Ellis [2]	—	—	—	—	—	—	4	4.4	—	—	—	—	—	—	4	4.4
Donahue [16]	3	3.9	1	1.2	—	—	3	3.9	1	1.2	—	—	—	—	—	—
O'Rourke [27]	—	—	—	—	—	—	3	2.8	—	—	5	4.7	—	—	—	—
DeMeester [3]	1	1	1	1	—	—	1	1	—	—	5	5	2	2	3	3
Lorenzini [17]	—	—	—	—	—	—	—	—	—	—	9	25	—	—	—	—
Shirazi [24]	30	8.5	—	—	—	—	14	4	—	—	21	6	—	—	6	1.6
Gouge [28]	6	7.4	—	—	—	—	—	—	—	—	5	6.2	—	—	3	3.7
Siewert [29]	2	2.2	—	—	—	—	4	4.4	—	—	4	4.4	—	—	—	—
Low [5]	37	8.3	2	0.4	—	—	9	2	1	0.2	10	2.2	4	0.4	20	4.4
Flament [9]	5	6.5	—	—	—	—	11	14	—	—	—	—	—	—	—	—
Stipa-Fegiz [22]	—	—	—	—	—	—	—	—	—	—	4	13	—	—	—	—
Stipa-Fegiz [22]	2	6.2	—	—	—	—	—	—	—	—	—	—	—	—	—	—
Rohr [13]	15	13	1	0.8	1	0.8	11	9.1	—	—	4	3.4	4	3.4	—	—

S-I = splenic injury; E-P = esophageal perforation; G-P = gastric perforation; W-I = wound infection; W-D = wound dehiscence; P-C = pulmonary complication; V-T = venous thrombosis.

With regard to floppy Nissen, we think that the anatomical variations in performing traditional Nissen procedure are not sufficient to reach good results; these are connected to the new HPZ basal pressure [15,23,40].

In a previous work we reported that, after normocalibrated Nissen, GER recurrence was found 23.8% of cases, and in one patient with persistent dysphagia, the usual postoperative decrease of the new HPZ pressure had not occurred. Therefore, in functional esophageal surgery, one is unable to estimate the intraoperative functional results. They can be different for every patient and are correlated to the tone of the gastric fundus.

Intraoperative manometry is the only test that can document the functional variations occurring during the operation. It allows for a good calibration of the fundoplication reaching the required values. At the same time, it reduces the consequences due to the mechanical obstruction (too tight Nissen) and can control GER.

Hypercalibrated Nissen (20–40 mmHg) determines the so-called "valve hyper-competence", characterized by a total absence of refluxes, even the physiological postprandial refluxes. It is due to an incomplete postdeglutitive new HPZ relaxation (75%), with a residual pressure gradient opposing GER in every situation. The hypercompetence is very useful for patients with serious peristaltic deficit, because, even if there are light refluxes, they can be responsible for persistence or worsening of the esophagitis.

In our experience, there was no report of any correlation between DMA of the esophageal body and the clinical results. So, the surgical indication and the type of operation are independent of the presence (or absence) of nonpropagating esophageal body motor activity [3,28].

Our surgical procedure does not create obstruction to the esophagogastric transit, as the new HPZ relaxes during swallowing, altering the esophageal body motor activity [41]. The good results obtained in achalasia and scleroderma patients, prove this as well [42–44].

In order to achieve good results, partly from the use of IEM, the operation should be as conservative as possible. We do not mobilize the gastric fundus nor do we open the little omentum in order to prevent dangerous splenic and esophageal lesions, gastric innervation and vagal fibers injuries.

In our patients' follow-up, there were no splenic or esophageal lesions; gas-bloat syndrome and gaseous disturbances were significantly reduced and transitory, compared to floppy Nissen results.

In conclusion, after hypercalibrated Nissen fundoplication, we reported occasional persistent light dysphagia in seven patients (8.2%). A high percentage of patients showed a good GER control (98.9%), and the global results were satisfactory (97.6%).

Finally, noninvasive surgery must be considered. In our experience, laparoscopy [45,46] showed results which were very similar to those of traditional surgery [45,47]. The advantages of laparoscopy are: 1) absence of postoperative pain; 2) absence of surgical scars; 3) precocious mobilization and eating; 4) rapid return to work; and 5) short hospitalization. On the basis of all these advantages, it is evident that noninvasive surgery is going to become the prevalent procedure in therapy of gastroesophageal reflux disease.

References

1. Inaspettato G, Laterza E, Rodella L et al. Trattamento delle recidive della chirurgia nella malattia da reflusso (MKGE). Chir Ital 1990;42:191–197.
2. Ellis FH, Crozier RE. Reflux control by fundoplication: a clinical and manometric assessment of the Nissen operation. Ann Thorac Surg 1984;38:387–392.
3. DeMeester TR, Bonavina L, Albertucci M. Nissen fundoplication for gastroesophageal reflux disease. Evaluation of primary repair in 100 consecutive patients. Ann Surg 1986;204:9–20.
4. Narbona B. The sling approach to the treatment of reflux peptic esophagitis (the cardiopexy with the round ligament). In: Nyhus-Condon (ed) Hernia, 3rd edn. Philadelphia: Lippincot, 1988.
5. Low DE, Anderson RP, Ilves R, Ricciardelli E, Hill LD. Fifteen to twenty year results after the Hill antireflux operation. J Thorac Cardiovasc Surg 1989;98:444–450.
6. Rossetti M. Results of the Nissen procedure. In: Giuli R, McCallum RW (eds) Benign Lesions of the Esophagus and Cancer. Berlin: Berlin, Heidelberg: Springer-Verlag, 1989;403.
7. Henderson RD. Partial fundoplication. In: Giuli R, McCallum RW (eds) Benign Lesions of the Esophagus and Cancer, Berlin, Heidelberg: Springer-Verlag, 1989;407–409.
8. Hill LD, Thor KBA. The Hill procedure. In: Giuli R, McCallum RW (eds) Benign Lesions of the Esophagus and Cancer. Berlin, Heidelberg: Springer-Verlag, 1989;427–430.
9. Flament JB, Plet H, Palot JF, Delattre JF, Rives J. Cardiopexy with umbilical ligament. In: Giuli R, McCallum RW (eds) Benign Lesions of the Esophagus and Cancer. Berlin, Heidelberg: Springer-Verlag, 1989;375–383.
10. Ellis FH. Results of the Nissen procedure. In: Giuli R, McCallum RW (eds) Benign Lesions of the Esophagus and Cancer. Berlin, Heidelberg: Springer-Verlag, 1989;397–399.
11. Mughal M, Bancewicz J, Marples M. Oesophageal manometry and pH recording does not predict the bad results of Nissen fundoplication. Br J Surg 1990;77:43–45.
12. Stipa S, Fegiz GF, Iascone C et al. Belsey and Nissen operation for gastroesophageal reflux. Ann Surg 1990;208:583–599.
13. Rohr S, Banzaoui H, De Manzini N, Dai B, Meyer Ch. Valeur du "Floppy" Nissen dans le traitement du reflux gastro-oesophagien. A propos de 117 cas. Ann Chir 1992;46:578–583.

14. Bjerkeset T, Edna TH, Fjosne U. Long-term results after "Floppy" Nissen-Rossetti fundoplication for gastroesophageal reflux disease. Scand J Gastroenterol 1992;27:707−710.

15. Del Genio A, Izzo G, Maffettone V et al. Reflusso Gastroesofageo (RGE). Relazione al 95° Congr Soc Ital Chir, Milano 17−20 October 1993. Proceedings of Congress, in press.

16. Donahue PE, Samelson S, Nyhus LM, Bombeck CT. The floppy Nissen fundoplication. Arch Surg 1985;120:663−668.

17. Lorenzini L, Lorenzi M. La fundoplicatio secondo Dor net trattamento chirurgico del reflusso gastroesofageo. Min Chir 1986;41:1409−1412.

18. Bancewicz J, Mughal M, Marples M. The lower oesophageal sphincter after floppy Nissen fundoplication. Br J Surg 1987;74:162−164.

19. Seineldin S. Results of the Nissen procedure. In: Giuli R, McCallum RW (eds) Benign Lesions of the Esophagus and Cancer. Berlin, Heidelberg: Springer-Verlag, 1989;399−403.

20. O'Hanrahan T, Marples M, Bancewicz J. Recurrent reflux and wrap disruption after Nissen fundoplication: detection, incidence and timing. Br J Surg 1989;77:545−547.

21. Breumelhof R, Smout AJPM, Schyns MWRJ, Bronzwaer PWA, Akkermans LMA, Jansen A. Pospective evaluation of the effects of Nissen fundoplication on gastroesophageal reflux. Surg Gynecol Obstet 1990;171:115−119.

22. Kmiot WA, Kirby RM, Akinola D, Temple JG. Prospective randomized trial of Nissen fundoplication and Angelchik prosthesis in the surgical treatment of medically refractory gastroesophageal reflux disease. Br J Surg 1991;78:1181−1184.

23. Grande L, Lacima G, Ros E et al. Dysphagia and esophageal motor dysfunction in gastroesophageal reflux are corrected by fundoplication. J Clin Gastroenterol 1991;13:11−16.

24. Shirazi SS, Schulze K, Soper RT. Long-term follow-up for treatment of complicated chronic reflux esophagitis. Arch Surg 1987;122:548−552.

25. Ackermann CH, Margreth L, Muller C. Symptoms 10 to 20 years after fundoplication. In: Siewert JR, Hölscher AH (eds) Diseases of the Esophagus. New York: Springer-Verlag, 1987;1198−1202.

26. Bancewicz J, Osugi H, Marples M. Clinical implications of abnormal oesophageal motility. Br J Surg 1987;74:416−419.

27. O'Rourke IC. Fundoplication for gastroesophageal reflux. Aust NZ J Surg 1985;55:347−354.

28. Gouge TH. The complete, loose fundoplication: results of operation for severe reflux esophagitis 1975−1985. In: Siewert JR, Hölscher AH (eds) Diseases of the Esophagus. Berlin: Springer-Verlag, 1987;1226−1229.

29. Siewert JR, Feussner H. Early and long-term results of antireflux surgery: a critical look. In: Tytgat GNJ (ed) Baillière's Clinical Gastroenterology. London: Baillière Tindall-WB Saunders, 1987;821−842.

30. Lanzara A, Del Genio A. La fundoplicatio sec. Nissen. Arch Atti Soc Ital Chir 1979;I:813−826.

31. Del Genio A. La nostra esperienza in tema di elettromanometria esofagea. Acad Scien Med Palermo 1978;12(suppl 1): 59−69.

32. Del Genio A, Di Martino N, Fei L et al. Manometria esofagea intraoperatoria. Relazione al Sanitec '87. Simposio su "I disordini della motilità esofago-gastroduodenale: aspetti di fisiopatologia, diagnosi e cenni di terapia", Turin 10 May 1987. Proceedings pp. 99−105.

33. Di Martino N, Amato G, Maffettone V, Landolfi V, Ambrosio A. Effetto della d-tubocurarine sullo sfintere esofageo inferiore (LES): studio elettromanometrico intraoperatorio. Min Chir 1986;41:1−7.

34. Del Genio A, Amato G, Maffettone V et al. Surgical treatment of esophageal achalasia according our experience: Heller and Nissen fundoplication. Second International Polydisciplinary Congress of the OESO, Paris 24−27 June 1987:11 (abstract).

35. Goldstein P, Butterfield W. Modified Nissen fundoplication and the gas bloat syndrome as measured by the possibility to vomit: an experimental study. Am J Surg 1970;126:89−92.

36. Boutelier Ph, Chipponi J. Le traitement chirurgical du reflux gastro-oesophagien de l'adulte. Paris: Masson, 1989.

37. Siewert JR, Feussner H, Walker J. Fundoplication: how to do it? Peri-esophageal wrapping as a therapeutic principal in gastroesophageal reflux prevention. World J Surg 1992;16:326−334.

38. Del Genio A, Fei L, Izzo G, Di Martino N, Maffettone V, Ambrosio A, Amato G. Indicazioni e limiti dell'intervento di Nissen. Atti IX Incontri di Chirurgia a Foggia. Gerni Edn., 1989:49−61.

39. McGouran RCM, Galloway JM, Wells FC, Hendrie ORS. Is yield pressure at the cardia increased by effective fundoplication? Gut 1989;30:1309−1312.

40. Touchais JY, Lerebours E, Sauger F et al. Analyse des différents facteurs conditionnant les resultats du traitement chirurgical du reflux gastro-oesophagien. Gastroenterol Clin Biol 1985;9:712−718.

41. Di Martino N, Izzo G, Maffettone V et al. Gastro-esophageal reflux (GER): esophageal disordered motor activity (DMA), clearing and severity of mucosal lesions. Proceedings 11th world Congress of Collegium Internationale Chirurgiae Digestivae, New Delhi 3−7 November 1990, PW9-124.

42. Del Genio A, Maffettone V, Izzo G et al. Acalasia dell'esofago. Atti dei Seminari Irpini di Gastroenterologia, 1986:5−38.

43. Di Martino N, Maffettone V, Fei L et al. La fundoplicatio sec. Nissen associata a cardiasmiotomia sec. Heller per acalasia esofagea. Comunic. al VIII Congresso Nazionale della Sezione Italiana del Collegium Internationale Chirurgiae Digestivae, Bologna 19−21 May 1987. Proceedings Tomo I:443−449, 1987.

44. Del Genio A, Fei L, Amato G et al. Il trattamento dell'acalasia esofagea mediante Heller e Nissen. Relazione all'VIII Congresso Nazionale della Sezione Italiana del Collegium Internationale Chirurgiae Digestivae, Bologna 19−21 May 1987. Proceedings Tomo I:429−434, 1987.

45. Del Genio A, Landolfi V, Martella A, Angilletta G, Cedrangolo L, Albino V. La Nissen "calibrata" per via laparoscopica. Giorn Ital Chir 1992;XLVI:190−193.

46. Zucker KA. Laparoscopia chirurgica. Ed. Medical Books, 1991;1–35.
47. Del Genio A, Di Martino N, Landolfi V, Ambrosio A, Maffettone V, Martella A. Laparoscopic Nissen fundoplication for the cure and prevention of gastroesophageal reflux (GER). Video "3rd IGSC Joint Meeting of Surgeons and Gastroenterologist", Padua June 24–27, 1992. Proceedings 434.

What constitutes the need for intervention following any failed antireflux operation?

C.A. *Hiebert* (Portland, Maine)

The Belsey adage, "diagnosis precedes treatment", alerts us to be wary. Were the symptoms that prompted the first operation related to gastroesophageal reflux disease (GERD), or was the original culprit gallstones or narrowed coronaries? Indeed, in the second century, Galen named the uppermost portion of the stomach the "cardia" because he thought its proximity to the heart should result in overlapping symptoms. Years may have elapsed since the original procedure; the recrudescence of symptoms, that, either correctly or incorrectly, were once ascribed to a hiatal hernia may now represent the distress signal of a different organ.

The decision to operate for adult GERD is ordinarily based on the presence of one or more of the following: 1) severe reflux symptoms that defy response to medical measures; 2) the presence of complications, including biopsy proven esophagitis, stricture, bleeding and/or aspiration; 3) massive herniation, a circumstance that, even with few symptoms, has lethal potential from unheralded ulceration, hemorrhage, or strangulation. Objective verification requires pH testing, motility studies, esophago-scopy, and an upper GI series. A Bernstein test may supply additional evidence. I have also found that amelioration of heartburn with a swallow of 5 ml of viscous 2% xylocaine is equally sensitive.

It is important to recognize that the once-operated patient is a different patient. Dysphagia from the start may be the result of an overly tight repair, but the insidious appearance of swallowing problems, months or years later, may represent a reflux stricture, motility change, or the development of carcinoma. In contrast to a large growth in the same location, a small tumor at the cardia may stop reflux before the obstruction is appreciated, thereby lulling both patient and doctor to erroneously ascribe the improvement to medicines or good fortune.

Other esophageal corruptions may have been missed on the original workup or else developed in the interim. These include cricopharyngeal achalasia, pharyngo-esophageal diverticula, Barrett's esophagus and the spectrum of motility disorders. Hiatal hernia keeps company with both congenital and developmental maladies of the entire foregut and it is often difficult to know whether the diverticulum or motility malfunction, for example, is of primary or secondary importance.

586

The patient's general condition may also have changed. The fit 69-year-old patient, who experienced no difficulty with her first repair, may have become obese, hypertensive, and decrepit 10 years later. Finally and most importantly, what are the patient's wishes? A previously satisfied individual who has been relieved of the need to diet, sleep with the head of the bed elevated and ingest expensive medicines may willingly accept the incremental risk for the prospect of returning to the unalloyed pleasures of eating and drinking that should be a compensatory hallmark of one's later years. The wise doctor will recognize this, even as he or she is sobered by the fact that secondary operations at the hiatus are amongst the most difficult in the entire repertoire of the esophageal surgeon.

Nissen fundoplication

What is the mode of action of fundoplication?

L. Lundell (Gothenburg)

Almost 40 years ago when Allison reported his technique for hiatal hernia repair, surgical attention was on the anatomical defect at the hiatus rather than the problems of a physiological incompetence in the reflux preventing mechanisms operating on the gastroesophageal junction [1]. Subsequently, operations which anatomically repaired the hiatal hernia without incorporating the technical features designed to restore the reflux preventing barrier, were not followed by any success [2,3]. Nissen discovered that a fundic wrap prevented reflux when he studied a patient many years after partial esophagectomy, where the initial aim was not to prevent reflux, but rather to protect the anastomotic area [4]. Fundoplication has subsequently become the most widely used form of antireflux surgery, the efficacy of which has been established by clinical and endoscopic follow-up and by esophageal pH-monitoring as well [5–7]. Despite this fact, these methods have developed largely on an empirical basis rather than on a conceptional view of the alleged mode of action. However, one basic requirement for the designation of a proper operation for gastro-esophageal reflux disease (GERD) is a comprehensive understanding of the patho-physiology of the disease. Although information has been collected over the years on the role of the lower esophageal sphincter (LES) in the pathogenesis of GERD [8], other factors have emerged, forming a multifactorial pathophysiological model. The aim of this article is to focus on the mode of action of fundoplication operations, with particular emphasis on the influence of these procedures on central pathogenetic mechanisms operating within the gastroesophageal junction.

Lower esophageal sphincter

Although encircling the esophageal circumference to different extents, all fundo-plication procedures seem to enhance the basal pressure recorded in the LES region, when determined by pull through manometric techniques. However, LES pressure varies continuously, even when studied over a limited time period [9]. This sphincter prevents reflux of gastric content into the esophagus by maintaining a basal tone between swallows to counteract the pressure gradient between the high intragastric and the low intrathoracic pressure [10]. Irrespective of the techniques used to establish the high pressure zone, antireflux surgery creates an external compression on the LES region, which may explain the transient dysphagia that ensues. It remains to be established whether the inability of the sphincter region to relax fully after antireflux surgery is closely paralleled by clinical complaints of obstructive nature [11]. However, despite the high basal tone in the sphincter area, water swallows are being variably followed by a profound relaxation in patients after a fundoplication, although the residual pressure after swallows did not usually reach the preoperative level [11,12]. Whether a shorter or partial fundic wrap would lead to a lower residual pressure (Nadir pressure) is not yet known [13]. However, in patients with an Angelchik prosthesis, the corresponding relaxation was less complete [11]. By use of conventional manometric techniques, a total fundic wrap has repeatedly been reported to enhance and "normalize" the basal pressure in the region of the LES, but a somewhat lower basal pressure can be recorded when a partial fundic wrap is performed [13–17]. It has also to be established whether patients having a partial fundic wrap are more prone to relax their sphincter as a response to gastric mechano-stimulation in the form of air insufflation. By use of the sleeve device to continuously record LES pressure, it has recently been shown that not only an increase in basal sphincter tone ensues on fundoplication, but also that the full relaxation of the sphincter was impaired [11]. Consequently, periods of absence of basal tone are prevented from occurring: episodes which have been suggested to be of particular importance in the genesis of gastroesophageal reflux [8].

Some evidence has been presented to suggest that the improvement in LES pressure in patients is, in part, due to an increased efficacy of the anatomic sphincter. A careful analysis of patients undergoing antireflux surgery indicated that a partial improvement in the native smooth muscle function was observed, which could be separated from the functional performance of the gastric smooth muscle of the wrap, when the responses to cholinergic stimulation, protein meal and swallowing were analyzed [17]. Speculatively, the operation might alter the length-tension properties of the LES smooth muscle. On the other hand, it has been shown that the increase in LES pressure created by surgery can be obtained completely independent of the presence of a native LES, emphasizing that the role of the gastric muscle constituting the fundic wrap is of paramount importance [18,19].

Laboratory studies, as well as human investigations, have demonstrated the importance of the length of the LES to obtain reflux control and the longer the artificial sphincter was constructed, the lower is the pressure required to establish competence [20]. Several investigations have subsequently shown that the length of the LES, as well as the pressure magnitude, are increased by surgery. Another alleged mechanism has been revealed by analyzing the determinants of gastric wall tension, which show that, on increasing the sphincter length, the importance of gastric wall tension decreases in the opening of the sphincter [21–23]. This means that more gastric distension can occur before an opening pressure is reached. Although the establishment of an intra-abdominal segment of the esophagus has a theoretical role in an effective antireflux operative strategy, in practice it does not appear to be crucial. Nissen fundoplications, which are left in the chest, are absolutely devoid of an intra-abdominal esophageal segment, but are definitely competent [24-25].

Transient LES relaxations

Combined manometric and pH recordings have, during the last decades, shown that virtually all reflux episodes in healthy subjects and most reflux episodes in patients with reflux disease occur during transient LES relaxation periods, during which the high pressure zone at the gastroesophageal junction is abolished [8]. A recent study confirmed not only the potent antireflux effect of a fundoplication, but showed that this effect was associated with a substantial reduction in the rate of transient LES relaxations as well as the proportion of these relaxations accompanied by reflux [12]. The mechanism(s) by which fundoplications interfere with the triggering of transient LES relaxations has, however, to be defined. A well founded hypothesis is that this is a result of changes in the distensibility of the gastric cardia because of the fundic wrap. The trigger zones for transient LES relaxations are concentrated in the area around the cardia, when studied in dogs. Similar studies have found that distension of the cardia by banding reduces the rate of belching associated with a decline in the rate of transient LES relaxations during gas insufflation [26,27]. Fundoplication may also alter the pattern of the LES relaxations by altering the neural signals to the sphincter area.

Vector-volume determination

LES characteristics have recently been assessed by use of a new computerized manometric device, which considers the effects of the pressures exerted over the entire sphincter length and integrates the parameters of pressure and length into a figure defined as sphincter vector-volume [28–30]. The overall LES vector-volume is significantly increased by the surrounded gastric wrap in patients, compared to controls. The relevance of the fundoplication in increasing the LES vector-volume is demonstrated by the observation that LES vector-volume is augmented only in its abdominal part, where the wrap actually surrounds the intra-abdominal esophagus. It may be inferred that these operations correct abnormal gastroesophageal reflux, partly by restoring sphincter function by modifying the shape of the high pressure zone, resulting in a more homogenous distribution of the pressures over the sphincter length.

Gastroesophageal valve

On a theoretical basis, the angle between the esophagus and the gastric fundus would result in a more oblique entry of the esophagus into the stomach, creating a barrier against reflux operating primarily in response to increased intraluminal pressure in the stomach [10]. The validity of this theory has so far been unclear. Clinical experience obtained by just simply suturing the left lateral esophagus to the fundus has been unsuccessful [31]. However, recent data would strongly support the importance of these mechanisms in establishing control of reflux, especially when these procedures are performed within the chest. It has recently been shown that a semifundoplication constructed above and around an intrathoracic esophagogastrostomy, after esophageal resection, controlled reflux effectively without creating a demonstrable high pressure zone above the anastomosis [32]. At endoscopy, however, a clear mucosal valve could be demonstrated, and a competent antireflux barrier was established by use of ambulatory dual point 24-h pH-metry.

Gastric emptying

Many patients with GERD have delayed gastric emptying, but the relative proportion of these patients remains a controversial issue [33–35]. Data have been presented to show that delay in solid gastric emptying in patients with reflux disease is associated with retention of food in the proximal portion of the stomach [36,37]. Whether this retention is due to a failure of the antrum to accept or pass on food, or a consequence of primary disorder of the fundus and body, remains to be elucidated. From a pathophysiological point of view, it is interesting to note that in cases of delayed gastric emptying, acid and pepsin rich fluids are retarded in the stomach for longer periods of time than normal, inducing a greater stomach volume with subsequent distension, and thereby triggering an increased number of transient LES relaxations [8]. In fact, Holloway et al. recently observed a substantial increase in the rate of relaxations after a meal only in patients with GERD, whereas no change was found in the control subjects [38]. We have also observed significant increase in the rate of transient LES relaxations following meal ingestion. When the stomach emptying pattern was broken down into proximal and distal gastric emptying, the closest association was observed between proximal gastric emptying and the postprandial frequency of transient LES relaxations [39].

Fundoplication not only effectively controls pathological gastroesophageal reflux, but also improves gastric emptying [40]. The significance of changes in these motor events for the success of this operation has, however, not been fully elucidated. Delayed gastric emptying has previously been reported in a group of patients with failed antireflux procedures, but the role of such delay as a cause of the defect has not been established [41]. One study suggested that essentially all side effects associated with Nissen fundoplication could be attributed to a failure of the procedure to normalize gastric emptying, as evaluated by use of ^{99m}Tc (technetium) labeled oatmeal [42]. This conclusion is probably an oversimplification of the problem and is not supported by the excellent long-term results observed after a combined highly selective vagotomy and fundoplication, especially since the latter operation does not at all affect solid gastric emptying [43,44].

The mechanism by which fundoplication operations affect gastric emptying is unknown, but it is conceivable to assume that a reduction in the size of the proximal gastric reservoir contributes. Similar restrictive consequences of these procedures might thus constitute the common denominator for the effects on the proximal stomach emptying, as well as on the triggering mechanisms for the postprandial increase in transient LES relaxations.

References

1. Allison BR. Reflux oesophagitis, sliding hiatal hernia and the anatomy of repair. Surg Gynecol Obstet 1951;92:419.
2. Santos GH. Is hiatus hernia responsible for reflux? Chest 1983;84:242.
3. Woodward ER, Thomas SHF, McAlhany JC. Comparison of crural repair. A Nissen fundoplication in the treatment of oesophageal hiatus hernia with peptic oesophagitis. Ann Surg 1971;173:782.
4. Nissen R. Eine einfache Operation zur Beeinflussung der Refluxösophagitis. Schweiz Med Wochenschr 1956;86:590.
5. Jamieson GG, Duranceau AC, Deschamps C. Surgical treatment of gastroesophageal reflux disease. In: Jamieson GG, Duranceau AC (eds) Gastroesophageal Reflux. Philadelphia: WB Saunders, 1988;Chapt 10.
6. Feussner H, Petri A, Walker S et al. The modified AFP-score: an attempt to make the results of antireflux surgery comparable. Br J Surg 1991;78:942—946.
7. DeMeester TR, Bonavina L, Albertucci M. Nissen fundoplication for gastroesophageal reflux disease. Evaluation of primary repair in 100 consecutive patients. Ann Surg 1986;204:9—20.
8. Holloway RH, Dent J. Lower esophageal sphincter dysfunction in gastroesophageal reflux disease. Gastroenterol Clin N Am 1990;19:517.
9. Dent J. A technique for continuous sphincter pressure measurement. Gastroenterology 1976;71:261.
10. Little AG. Mechanism of action of antireflux surgery: theory and facts. World J Surg 1992;16:320.
11. Lundell LR, Myers JC, Jamieson GG. The effect of antireflux operations on lower oesophageal sphincter tone and the postprandial symptoms. Scand J Gastroenterol 1993;28:725.
12. Ireland AC, Holloway RH, Toouli J, Dent J. Mechanisms underlying the antireflux action of fundoplication. Gut 1993;34:303—308.
13. Lundell L, Abrahamsson H, Ruth M et al. Lower esophageal sphincter characteristics and esophageal acid exposure following partial or 360° fundoplication: results of a prospective, randomized, clinical study. World J Surg 1991;15:115.
14. Fischer RS, Malmud LS, Lobis IF, Maier WP. Antireflux surgery for symptomatic gastro-oesophageal reflux: mechanism of action. Am J Dig Dis 1978;23:152.
15. Bjerkeset T, Nordgard K, Schjonsby H. Effect of Nissen fundoplication operation on the competence of the lower esophageal sphincter. Scand J Gastroenterol 1980;15:213—217.
16. Bancewicz J, Mughal M, Marples M. The lower oesophageal sphincter after floppy Nissen fundoplication. Br J Surg 1987;74:162—164.
17. Higgs RH, Castell DO, Farrell RL. Evaluation of the effect of fundoplication on the incompetent lower oesophageal sphincter. Surg Gynecol Obstet 1975;140:571.
18. Moossa AR, Hall W, Wood RA et al. Effect of pentagastrin infusion on gastro-oesophageal manometry and reflux status before and after oesophagogastrectomy. Am J Surg 1977;133:23.
19. Condon RE, Kraus MA, Woolheim D. Cause of increase in lower oesophageal sphincter pressure after fundoplication. J Surg Res 1976;2:445.
20. Stein HJ, DeMeester TR. Who benefits from antireflux surgery. World J Surg 1992;16:313.
21. DeMeester TR, Wernly JA, Bryan GH et al. Clinical and in vitro analysis of determinants of gastro-oesophageal competence: a study of the principles of antireflux surgery. Am J Surg 1979;137:39—46.
22. Pettersson GB, Bombeck CT, Nyhus LM. The lower oesophageal sphincter: mechanisms of opening and closure. Surgery 1980;88:307—314.
23. Pettersson GB, Bombeck CT, Nyhus LM. Influence of hiatal hernia on lower oesophageal sphincter function. Ann Surg 1981;193:214.
24. Bennell TC. Supradiaphragmatic correction of oesophageal reflux. Ann Surg 1981;173:775.
25. Richardson JD, Larson GM, Polk HC. Intrathoracic fundoplication for shortened oesophagus: treacherous solution to a challenging problem. Am J Surg 1982;143:29.
26. Franzi SJ, Martin CJ, Cox MR, Dent J. Response of canine lower esophageal sphincter to gastric distension. Am J Physiol 1990;259:G380.

27. Strömbeck DR, Griffen DW, Harrold D. Eractation of the gastro-oesophageal sphincter before and after limiting distension of the gastric cardia or infusion of a beta-adrenergic amine in dogs. Am J Vet Res 1989;50:751.
28. Bombeck CT, Waz O, De Salvo J, Donahue PE, Nyhus LM. Computerised axial manometry of the oesophagus. A new method for the assessment of antireflux operations. Ann Surg 1987;206:465.
29. Stein HJ, DeMeester TR, Naspetti R, Jamieson J, Perry RE. Three-dimensional imaging of the lower oesophageal sphincter in gastro-oesophageal reflux disease. Ann Surg 1991;214:374.
30. Costantini M, Bremner RM, Hoeft SF, Crookes PF, DeMeester TR. A new method for the evaluation of the lower oesophageal sphincter: slow motorised pull through. J Gastrointest Motil 1992;4:215A.
31. Aldau ES, Goldsmith HS. Efficacy of fundoplication in preventing gastric reflux. Am J Surg 1973;126:322.
32. Liedman B, Ruth M, Sandberg S et al. Prevention of reflux after oesophageal resection and reconstruction with a gastric tube. Diseases of the Esophagus 1993 (in press).
33. McCallum RW, Berkowitz DM, Lerner E. Gastric emptying in patients with gastroesophagael reflux disease. Gastroenterology 1981;80:285—291.
34. Collins PJ, McFarlane RJ, O'Hare MT, Shore C, Buchanan KD, Lowe AHG. Gastric emptying of a solid/liquid meal and gastrointestinal hormone responses in patients with erosive oesophagitis. Digestion 1986;33:61.
35. Maddern GJ, Chatterton BE, Collins PJ, Horowitz M, Shearman DJC, Jamieson GG. Solid and liquid gastric emptying in patients with gastro—oesophageal reflux. Br J Surg 1985;72:344.
36. Collins PJ, Horowitz M, Chatterton BE. Proximal, distal and total stomach emptying of a digestible solid meal in normal subjects. Br J Radiol 1988;61:12.
37. Myers JC, Collins PJ, Dehnt CB, Maddern GJ, Horowitz M, Jamieson GG. Which part of the stomach is responsible for delaying gastric emptying of solids in patients with gastro-oesophageal reflux disease (GORD)? J Gastroenterol Hepatol 1988;3:20.
38. Holloway RH, Kocian K, Dent J. Provocation of transient lower oesophageal sphincter relaxations by meals in patients with symptomatic gastro-oesophageal reflux. Dig Dis Sci 1991;36:1034.
39. Lundell L, Anvari M, Myers JC et al. The association between gastric emptying, gastric distension and transient lower oesophageal sphincter relaxations in patients with gastro-oesophageal reflux disease. Gastroenterology 1991;102:A478.
40. Maddern GJ, Jamieson GG. Fundoplication enhances gastric emptying. Ann Surg 1985;201:296.
41. Maddern GJ, Jamieson GG, Chatterton BE, Collins PJ. Is there an association between failed antireflux procedures and delayed gastric emptying? Ann Surg 1985;202:1162.
42. Hinder RA, Stein HJ, Bremner CG, DeMeester TR. Relationship of a satisfactory outcome to normalization of delayed gastric emptying after Nissen fundoplication. Ann Surg 1989;210:458.
43. Csendes A, Braghetto I, Korn O, Kortes C. Late subjective and objective evaluations of antireflux surgery in patients with reflux oesophagitis: analysis of 215 patients. Surgery 1989;105:374.
44. Jamieson GG, Maddern GJ, Myers JC. Gastric emptying after fundoplication with and without proximal gastric vagotomy. Arch Surg 1991;126:1414—1417.

Suture of the cuff to the esophagus seems essential to prevent its invagination into the stomach

T.P.J. Hennessy (Dublin)

The classical Nissen fundoplication [1] involved: division of the upper part of the gastro-hepatic ligament, division of the upper short gastric vessels and division of the connective tissue binding the upper part of the posterior wall of the stomach to the posterior abdominal wall. This extensive mobilization was considered necessary to allow equal proportions of the anterior and posterior gastric wall to be incorporated into the fundoplication.

Apart from the other undesirable sequelae, such as division of the hepatic branch of the vagus with consequent dilatation of the gallbladder, the extensive mobilization outlined above rendered the fundoplication unstable and, despite attempts at securing the wrap to the esophageal wall, slipping of the fundoplication, either in a proximal or a distal direction, became a recognized complication. As a result, modifications were made to the classical operation.

For fundoplication to achieve its objective and control reflux, the wrap must be stable and maintain its anatomical relationship to the abdominal esophagus. This can be achieved to a considerable extent by minimizing dissection around the abdominal esophagus.

It is sufficient to mobilize the esophagus to the extent that a wrap 2 cm in depth can be constructed around its lower end. The dissection should be limited inferiorly on the right side of the esophagus by the thickened portion of the gastro-hepatic omentum containing the hepatic branch of the anterior vagus nerve. The gastro-hepatic ligament should not be divided.

The gastro-phrenic ligament is divided to the left of the abdominal esophagus, but the short gastric vessels should be preserved.

However, in order to ensure that the fundoplication maintains its position permanently, relative to the abdominal esophagus, some method of fixation is necessary. This may be achieved in various ways.

The classical fundoplication procedure of Nissen consists of suturing equal proportions of the posterior and anterior walls of the stomach in front of the esophagus. In order to prevent the cardia from slipping back in eversion and producing the so-called telescope effect, at least one of the fundoplication sutures is passed through the wall of the esophagus. While passage of all sutures in the fundoplication through the esophageal wall will clearly provide more stability than the use of the most superior suture only, it should be recognized that the muscular wall of the esophagus possesses little ability to hold stitches. This is evident from the frequency of disruption of partial fundoplication with the passage of time, and it seems fairly certain that sutures passed through the esophageal wall will tear out sooner or later.

In the Rossetti-Hell [2] modification of Nissen's fundoplication, the anterior wall of the stomach is passed around the back of the abdominal esophagus and sutured to the stomach in front of the esophagus as a loose wrap. The authors emphasize that the fundoplication should not be sutured to the esophagus. Instead, they recommend that the inferior border of the fundoplication should be fixed to the anterior wall of the stomach with stabilizing sutures.

In the Rossetti-Hell modification of the Nissen procedure, the preservation of the hepatic branch of the vagus and the preservation of the short gastric vessels add further stability to the wrap. Thus, neither telescoping of the esophagus nor slippage of the wrap distally should occur.

Condon [3] is also opposed to fixation of the fundoplication by placing sutures through the esophageal wall. He recommends fixation of the wrap, in relation to the esophagus, by passing the most distal suture of the fundoplication through the fibrous tissue at the gastroesophageal junction. He also recommends passing the most superior stitch of the fundoplication through the central tendon of the diaphragm.

In summary, fixation of the fundoplication in relation to the abdominal esophagus is essential to its proper function. Migration proximally or distally will give rise to symptoms including dysphagia. Use of the muscular wall of the abdominal esophagus is probably inadequate to establish stability because of the tendency of such sutures to cut out. Fixation of the fundoplication by sutures securing the inferior edge of the wrap to the stomach wall is much more reliable in preventing wrap migration. Alternatively, stabilization can be achieved by fixing the wrap to the cardia, using the most distal suture of the wrap. Added stability is provided by limiting dissection to division of the gastro-phrenic ligament on the left and division of the peritoneum above the hepatic branch of the vagus on the right.

References

1. Nissen R. Gastropexy as the lone procedure in surgical repair of hiatus hernia. Ann J Surg 1956;92:389–392.
2. Rossetti M, Hell K. Fundoplication for the treatment of gastroesophageal reflux in hiatal hernia. World J. Surg 1977;1:439–444.
3. Condon RE. Intraoperative dilatation and fundoplication for benign peptic oesophageal stricture. In: Jamieson GG (ed) Surgery of the Esophagus. New York: Churchill Livingstone, 1988:341–349.

Do we know why only certain antireflux valves come undone?

H.J. Stein, J.R. Siewert (Munich)

Recurrent reflux is the most common cause of failure of antireflux procedures. This is usually due to a partial or complete breakdown of the repair. There are at least three causes for disruption of an antireflux repair during the postoperative course:

1. Choice of operation: partial fundoplications (e.g., the Toupet procedure) are more prone to disruption than a complete 360° wrap (i.e., the Nissen fundoplication). This is because the construction of a partial fundoplication requires significantly more abdominal length of the esophagus than a complete wrap, and the integrity of the wrap in the partial fundoplications depends on sutures to the esophageal wall.

2. Inadequate suture technique: taking inadequate bites of tissue when constructing the wrap and the use of flimsy or quickly absorbable suture material predispose to wrap disruption. Consequently, we recommend that nonabsorbable suture material is used to prevent disruption of the cuff with time.

3. Esophageal shortening: unrecognized esophageal shortening and insufficient

mobilization of the distal esophagus lead to tension and may eventually cause wrap disruption.

In our experience, partial or total breakdown of an antireflux repair is, in most instances, due to insufficient mobilization of the fundus and the use of absorbable sutures during the initial operation.

The endoscopy should be performed by the surgeon, especially in recurrences

H.J. Stein, J.R. Siewert, H.-J. Dittler (Munich)

Persistent, recurrent or emerging new symptoms after an antireflux procedure may be due to a myriad of causes including wrap disruption, a too tightly constructed wrap, a slipped wrap, a wrap that has been placed too low, development of a stricture, the presence of a motor disorder of the esophageal body, or a combination of the above. A thorough diagnostic work-up is essential in each patient who complains of symptoms after an antireflux procedure. In addition to a detailed symptomatic assessment, contrast radiography and functional studies, an upper gastrointestinal endoscopy is an essential part of this work-up.

Endoscopic inspection of the esophagus will provide information on the presence and severity of esophageal mucosal injury. In addition, biopsies can be taken and assessed for histologic alterations of the esophageal mucosa. Inspection of the distal esophagus may also show residuals from the previous surgical procedure (i.e., scars, sutures, a narrowing or deformities). An esophageal stenosis can be identified by the inability to pass the endoscope with ease.

Inspection of the gastroesophageal junction from below is accomplished by inversion or retroflexion of the endoscope. This allows assessment of the anatomy of the fundus and the status of a previous antireflux procedure. An intact Nissen fundoplication is characterized by a pronounced "nipple" visible on retrograde view of the fundus. This "Nissen-nipple" disappears when the fundoplication disrupts [1]. Paraesophageal hernias, or the so-called "riding ulcers", may also be detected on retrograde inspection of the gastroesophageal junction.

Assessment of the stomach and duodenum are essential parts of the endoscopic examination in patients who complain of upper gastrointestinal symptoms after a previous antireflux procedure. Residual food or a gastric bezoar indicate delayed gastric emptying as a sequela of vagal during the antireflux procedure. Endoscopic assessment of the stomach and duodenum may also show mucosal injury (i.e., inflammatory changes or ulcerations) which can explain the patients' complaint. Excessive duodenogastric reflux, which is frequently associated with gastroesophageal reflux, may also account for symptoms after an antireflux procedure. Incompetence of the pylorus and a bile lake in the stomach on endoscopy can indicate excessive duodenogastric reflux [2].

Upper gastrointestinal endoscopy in experienced hands thus can make a valuable contribution in assessing the reasons for failure of an antireflux procedure and is essential to identify patients that need further surgical intervention [3,4]. Endoscopic examination in patients with upper gastrointestinal symptoms after a previous antireflux procedure should therefore be carried out by a surgeon who has sufficient experience with antireflux surgery, rather than an endoscopic consultant.

References

1. O'Hanrahan T, Marples M, Bancewicz J. Recurrent reflux and wrap disruption after Nissen fundoplication: detection, incidence, timing. Br J Surg 1990;77:545−547.
2. Stein HJ, Smyrk TC, DeMeester TR, Rouse J, Hinder RA. Sensitivity and specificity of endoscopy and histology in the diagnosis of excessive duodenogastric reflux. Surgery 1992;112:796−804.
3. Siewert JR, Feussner HJ. The options for surgical therapy of reflux esophagitis. Gullet 1993;3:76−84.
4. Siewert JR, Isolauri J, Feussner H. Reoperation following failed fundoplication. World J Surg 1989;13:791−797.

What are the indications for reoperation after antireflux surgery?

A. Peracchia (Milan)

A successful antireflux operation eliminates symptoms due to an incompetent cardia and results in healing of endoscopic esophagitis, if present, without causing adverse effects such as dysphagia or bloating [1]. It is not yet clear to what extent antireflux surgery may affect the natural history of the columnar epithelium lining the esophagus and the occurrence of dysplasia or Barrett's carcinoma.

Current reports indicate that reflux is controlled in about 90% of patients undergoing physiological antireflux operations (Nissen, Belsey, Hill, Toupet). Similar success rates can be achieved with the antireflux prosthesis designed by Angelchik. However, 10−25% of the operated patients develop complications not necessarily related to reflux. Dysphagia is the most common complaint, requiring reoperation in the majority of cases [2,3].

The incidence of failure is probably similar for all current types of antireflux operation. The surgeon's experience plays a key role; the high failure rates reported for the Nissen fundoplication certainly reflect the fact that this is the most commonly performed operation.

The need for reoperation may occur early during the postoperative period, or later in the follow-up. Early complications requiring reoperation are the perforations of the distal esophagus and splenic hematoma [4].

The most common causes of persistent or recurrent symptoms after antireflux surgery are: disruption of the crural repair (causing anatomic recurrence of the hiatal hernia), disruption of the wrap (causing incompetency of the lower esophageal sphincter (LES)), and inadvertent damage to the vagal nerves (causing gastric outlet obstruction). On the other hand, a tight or a slipped repair produces dysphagia, a disabling side effect [5–10]. Patients with Barrett's esophagus should be followed closely after a successful fundoplication, since progression to dysplasia and cancer has been observed [11].

Redo surgery for failure of an antireflux operation represents a surgical challenge. The indications for reoperation should be based on the analysis of clinical history, radiological and endoscopic findings and tests of esophageal and gastric function (manometry, 24-h pH-monitoring, scintigraphy). These investigations can dictate the type of reoperation to be performed, although the final decision can be made only in the operating room when the dissection is complete. The reoperation should be carried out by an expert surgeon, familiar with all types of esophageal procedures. Indications for reoperation are as follows:

— persistent or recurrent reflux symptoms and/or esophagitis due to breakdown of the repair;
— intractable dysphagia with progressive esophageal dilation;
— paraesophageal hernia;
— wrap dislocation (slipped Nissen);
— severe gastric outlet obstruction;
— severe dysplasia or adenocarcinoma in Barrett's esophagus.

Since 1976, 52 patients with previous antireflux surgery have undergone reoperation in our institution. There were 30 males and 22 females, mean age 46 (15–71 years). Seventeen of these patients had been operated upon by us and this represents a reoperation rate of 6.5% out of a total number of 260 antireflux operations. During the same study period, 38 patients were treated conservatively (pharmacologic therapy

Table 1. Previous operations and major complaints in 52 patients

Operation	Patients	Reflux	Dysphagia	Asympt.
Nissen	18	5	12*	1
Toupet	11	7	4	
Dor	6	6	—	
Lortat-Jacob	6	6	—	
Belsey Mark IV	5	4	1	
Angelchik	4	1	3	
Vankemmel	1	1	—	
Anterior gastropexy	1	1	—	

* 1 laparoscopic fundoplication.
Four patients had undergone two previous operations.

Table 2. Classification of the failures

	Patients	%
LES incompetency	27	51.9
Esophageal dysmotility	9	17.3
Delayed gastric emptying and/or duodenogastric reflux	8	15.4
Esophageal stricture	7	13.5
Barrett's adenocarcinoma	1	1.9

and/or endoscopic dilation). The previous operations in the 52 patients are listed in Table 1.

Thirty-two patients (61.5%) presented with reflux symptoms and 20 patients (36.5%) with dysphagia as the major complaint. The patient with Barrett's adenocarcinoma was asymptomatic and without objective evidence of gastroesophageal reflux (Table 1). Based on the results of the diagnostic work-up, patients were recognized as failures for the reasons listed in Table 2. The operations performed on the 52 patients are listed in Table 3.

There was no operative mortality. Morbidity consisted of: splenic lesion in one patient, bowel obstruction in two patients and wound infection in two patients. The mean follow-up is 55 months (6–183 months). Two patients presented, at 6 and 8 months after fundoplication, with recurrent reflux (slipped Nissen). Another patient required a transthoracic vagotomy because of a marginal ulcer after total duodenal diversion. Long-term results are satisfactory (Visick 1–2) in 44 of the 52 patients (84.6%). An interesting point is that in patients with esophageal dysmotility, the success rate was lower (57%) than in patients with isolated LES incompetency (73%).

We conclude that reoperation after failed antireflux repair is indicated when medical therapy has failed, undilatable esophageal stricture is present, or a mechanical complication of the wrap occurs. The occurrence of severe dysplasia or adenocarcinoma arising from Barrett's mucosa is another indication to reoperative surgery. The operation is technically demanding and should be undertaken only after precise identification of the cause of the unsuccessful outcome.

Table 3. Reoperative surgery in the 52 patients

Operation	Patients
Redo fundoplication	26
Esophageal resection	12
Total duodenal diversion	12
Crural repair	2

References

1. DeMeester TR, Bonavina L, Albertucci M. Nissen fundoplication for gastroesophageal reflux disease. Evaluation of primary repair in 100 consecutive patients. Ann Surg 1986;204:9–20.
2. Leonardi HK, Ellis BH. Complications of the Nissen fundoplication. Surg Clin North Am 1983;63:1155–1165.

3. Skinner DB. Surgical management after failed antireflux operations. World J Surg 1992;16:359—363.
4. Baulieux J, Janody P, Mondesert C, Peix J. Chirurgie iterative du reflux gastroesophagien. A propos de 41 cas. Lyon Chir 1985;81:370—374.
5. Giuli R, Clot P, Estenne B, Richard C, Lortat-Jacob JL. Les interventions iteratives au cours des maladies peptiques de l'oesophage. Ann Chir 1974;28:13—19.
6. Hill LD, Ilves R, Stevenson JK, Pearson JM. Reoperation for disruption and recurrence after Nissen fundoplication. Arch Surg 1979;114:542—548.
7. Ancona E, Zaninotto G, Costantini M et al. Reoperations after complications or failure of antireflux surgery. In: Siewert JR, Hölscher AH (eds) Diseases of the Esophagus. Berlin: Springer Verlag, 1986.
8. Siewert JR, Isolauri J, Feussner H. Reoperation following failed fundoplication. World J Surg 1989;13:791—797.
9. Joost M, Horbach M, Jansen E et al. Incidence and clinical relevance of postfundoplication vagal nerve damage. In: Little AG et al. (eds) Diseases of the Esophagus, vol 2. New York: Futura Publishing Co., 1990.
10. Bonavina L, Fontebasso V, Bardini R, Baessato M, Peracchia A. A Surgical treatment of reflux stricture of the esophagus. Br J Surg 1993;80:317—320.
11. Williamson WA, Ellis FH, Gibb P et al. Effect of antireflux operation on Barrett's mucosa. Ann Thorac Surg 1990;49: 537—542.

How can one compare the results of an operation which may be performed with so many variations?

J. Isolauri (Tampere)

Nissen fundoplication, with modifications, has been a widely used antireflux procedure for 30 years, with abolition of reflux symptoms reported in 81—97% of patients [1—4] and normal findings at pH-monitoring in 90% [5]. Disturbing post-operative symptoms, such as dysphagia, gas bloat and epigastric pain have been described as occurring, sometimes in a substantial number of patients [4,6,7]. Recurrences of reflux have been reported in 2—19% of patients [3,4].

The original procedure presented by Rudolf Nissen was plication between the posterior and the anterior wall of the gastric fundus. The gastro-hepatic ligament was divided [1]. Rossetti's modification of the procedure is based on plication between the anterior walls of the fundus [2]. The floppy Nissen modification includes mobilization of the fundus by dividing the short gastric vessels [8]. The fundic wrap may be fixed to the esophagus or to the gastric cardia. The original fundic wrap constructed by Nissen was 6 cm long but, currently, there is a trend towards shorter (1.5—3 cm long) fundoplications.

Reoperations in cases of recurrent reflux or other severe disturbing postoperative symptoms are more difficult and potentially more dangerous than primary fundoplication, and the results may not he equally good. The procedures proposed include repeat Nissen fundoplication, Belsey Mark IV procedure, Nissen or Belsey Mark IV procedures with gastroplasty, conversion Nissen to Hill operation and antrectomy with Roux-en-Y reconstruction.

Author's experience

Patients

At Tampere University Hospital, 760 Nissen fundoplications have been performed from 1963 to 1991. By 1991, reoperation had been performed in 23 cases (3%). The indication for reoperation was recurrent reflux in 18 cases, persistent esophageal stricture despite cure of reflux in three cases and epigastric pain without subjective or objective recurrence of reflux in two cases. Repeat Nissen fundoplication was done in all of the 18 cases. Subtotal esophageal resection with colon interposition was used in four cases of esophageal stricture (operations performed before endoscopic dilatation for esophageal strictures had become a routine procedure in the institution). In one patient, the fundic wrap was simply taken down, because of severed fundic circulation that would have made repeat fundoplication too dangerous. Fifteen consecutive patients with one previous Nissen fundoplication between 1972 and 1989 comprised the study group. Nissen-Rossetti type anterior wall plication was used in the primary operation in 14 cases, and classic Nissen fundoplication in one. Nonabsorbable suture material had been used in all cases. The wrap was fixed to the cardia in seven cases and to the esophagus in eight. All the primary operations were carried out, or directly supervised, by senior surgeons.

Indications to reoperations

The median symptom-free time after the primary operation was 6 (range 0–92) months. Symptoms recurred during the first 2 years in 73% of the patients. The median time between the first and second operations was 55 (range 8–149) months. All the 15 patients had recurrent heartburn and regurgitation as the main complaints before the operation. Endoscopic esophagitis of Savary-Miller grade II–III was observed in 10 patients, and grade IV in one patient. Ten wraps were slipped and five disrupted. All the reoperations were done through transabdominal route. A Nissen-Rossetti fundoplication was redone, using three or four nonabsorbable sutures, with the lowermost fixed to the gastric cardia. A 32 F tube was inserted in the esophagus during the plication.

The median observation time after repeat fundoplication was 18 (range 5–152) months. The follow-up examination included endoscopy, manometry and 24-h pH monitoring.

Results

There were no deaths. Postoperative complications occurred in six patients. None of the complications had long-term consequences. Nine of the 15 patients (60%) were unsatisfactorily classified in Visick grades I and II, six (40%) in grade III and none in grade IV. Postoperatively, dysphagia was a clinical problem in one patient, who needed successive dilatations for esophageal stricture. All the other patients ate normal meals. Increased flatus was reported by six patients and mild bloating by three.

At follow-up endoscopy, fundic wrap was intact in 12 cases and slipped in three. Esophageal mucosa was abnormal in six cases: endoscopic esophagitis (grade II–IV) in four patients and Barrett's metaplasia in three. Two of the four patients with esophagitis had an intact wrap, and two a slipped one. In six of the fourteen 24-h pH recordings, the total reflux time was more than 4.2%. Only one of these six had normal esophageal mucosa. Three had a slipped wrap, and three an intact one at endoscopy.

Discussion

Twenty-three of the 760 patients (3%) who underwent primary Nissen fundoplication at our institution had undergone reoperation (Table 1). This number of reoperations is reliable, because the hospital is the only one in the catchment region where reoperations are undertaken. The 3% reoperation rate of our institution is acceptable. Centers which perform antireflux surgery frequently have a failure rate of 3–5% [9]. All reoperations described here are redo Nissen procedures. We do not have any experience of other kinds of reoperations, except esophageal resections for strictures, at the time when endoscopic dilatation was not used. Furthermore, we do not have any experience with second or third reoperations after failed Nissen procedure. The transabdominal route has always been used in refundoplications.

In an extensive study of 61 reoperations for failed antireflux operations, Little et al. divided the operations into three groups based on the number of previous

Table 1. Reoperations after 760 primary fundoplications

Indications for reoperation	Number of cases
Recurrent reflux	18
slipped wrap	13
disrupted wrap	4
paraesophageal hernia	1
Epigastric pain	2
paraesophageal hernia	1
partially disrupted wrap	1
Persistent esophageal stricture (no recurrent reflux)	3
Total	23 (3%)

operations [9]. Thirty-four patients had only one previous operation, 19 patients had two, and eight patients had three. Nissen fundoplication was the first operation in 43 cases. The reoperation was a Nissen fundoplication in 18 cases, Belsey procedure in 22, Hill in five and resection with interposition in 14. Two patients underwent simple exploration. The authors prefer thoracic route for the first reoperation and use is exclusively after multiple antireflux procedures. They state that patients with one prior operation and recurrent gastroesophageal reflux are similar to those with no prior operation and that the results of repeat antireflux operations deteriorate with increasing number of operations, due to impaired esophageal function and progressive tissue destruction.

Our results of the first reoperations are not as good as those of primary operations. Morbidity is higher, and only 60% of the patients have excellent or good subjective results (Visick grade I or II) with a median follow-up of 18 months, compared to 77% with a follow-up of 77 months after primary Nissen fundoplication [4]. There was no mortality, even though other series have been reporting 30 days hospital mortality up to 17.6% after reoperations for failed antireflux procedures [10–12].

Most of these series do not give the outcome of the different types of reoperations. In a study of 87 reoperations, Stirling and Orringer, however, reported excellent or good results in 62% (13 patients) after Collis-Belsey procedures, in 67% (55 patients) after Collis-Nissen and in 65% (23 patients) after esophagectomy [13]. In a study of Little et al., excellent or good results were reported in 85% of cases after first reoperation and in 66 and 42% after second and third operation, respectively [9]. The authors did not, however, indicate the results of different types of reoperations.

From our experience, Nissen fundoplication can be redone through the abdominal route for the first reoperation. Siewert et al., in a study of 50 reoperations for failed Nissen fundoplication, were able to perform refundoplication in 42 cases (84%) [14]. The results after reoperations are not as good as those after primary operations in most reports. Technically, the procedures are much more demanding than the primary operations, and should therefore be undertaken in specialized units only. The patients should undergo endoscopy, esophageal radiogram, manometry and 24-h pH monitoring before the decision is made, in order to exclude patients with severe esophageal motility disorders or symptoms caused by diseases other than recurrent reflux or otherwise failed antireflux surgery. There are not many data comparing the results of the different types of reoperations, such a comparison being difficult since different types of reoperations are used for different stages of disease. The purpose of reoperations should, however, be similar to that of primary operations: to lessen gastroesophageal reflux to normal ranges, and put an end to the symptoms caused by it, without any new adverse effects. Mortality and morbidity should be acceptable. Redoing the operation that the surgeon is familiar with is a reasonable solution for the first reoperation in cases where severe motility disturbances do not provide any other kind of solution.

References

1. Nissen R. Eine einfache Operation zur Beeinflussung der Refluxösophagitis. Schweiz Med Wochenschr 1956;86:590–592.

2. Rossetti M, Hell K. Fundoplication for treatment of gastroesophageal reflux in hiatal hernia. World J Surg 1977;1:439–444.
3. DeMeester TR, Bonavina L, Albertucci M. Nissen fundoplication for gastroesophageal reflux disease. Ann Surg 1986;204: 9–20.
4. Luostarinen ME. Nissen fundoplication for reflux esophagitis. Long-term clinical and endoscopic results in 109 of 127 consecutive patients. Ann Surg 1993;217:329–337.
5. O'Hanrahan T, Marples M, Bancewicz J. Recurrent reflux and wrap disruption after Nissen fundoplication: detection, incidence and timing. Br J Surg 1990;77:545–547.
6. Low DE, Mercer CD, James EC, Hill LD. Post-Nissen syndrome. Surg Gynecol Obstet 1988;167:1–5.
7. Negre JB. Postfundoplication symptoms: do they restrict the success of Nissen fundoplication? Ann Surg 1983;198:689–700. Surg 1993;217:329–337.
8. Donahue PE, Samelson S, Nyhus LM, Bombeck TC. The floppy Nissen fundoplication. Arch Surg 1985;120:663–668.
9. Little AG, Ferguson MK, Skinner DB. Reoperation for failed antireflux operations. J Thorac Cardiovasc Surg 1986;91: 511–517.
10. Maher JW, Hocking MP, Woodward ER. Reoperations for esophagitis following failed antireflux procedures. Ann Surg 1985;201:723–727.
11. Hill LD. Management of recurrent hiatal hernia. Arch Surg 1971;102:296–302.
12. Zucker K, Peskin GW, Saik RP. Recurrent hiatal hernia repair. Arch Surg 1982;117:413–414.
13. Stirling MC, Orringer MB. Surgical treatment after failed antireflux operations. J Thorac Cardiovasc Surg 1986;92:667–672.
14. Siewert JR, Isolauri J, Feussner H. Reoperation following failed fundoplication. World J Surg 1989;13:791–797.

How can one distinguish patients who would benefit from another type of procedure?

A. Duranceau (Montreal)

Nissen fundoplication remains the most popular repair for correction of pathologic reflux disease. When compared prospectively with partial fundoplication operations [1], this procedure provides best relief for symptoms, returns the postsurgical patient to normal 24-h pH values and better increases the distal esophageal sphincter pressures. Despite these excellent results, the total fundoplication operation may fail just as its partial fundoplication counterpart. Reports on reoperative surgery for gastroesophageal reflux bear witness to these failures [2–5].

When the proper indication exists and no technical errors are made, the failed fundoplication may be due to fundoplication disruption. More often there is tension on the repair caused by esophageal inflammation and shortening. In this situation, eversion of the fundoplication over the gastric body may occur, especially if the hiatus was repaired snugly above the fundoplication, or the fundoplication may simply ascend into the posterior mediastinum through a wider hiatus. Partial fundoplications fail to control reflux and reflux damage in a high proportion of patients when used in patients with strictures [6].

Short esophagus

Thus, the first strong indication to opt for another type of antireflux operation than the Nissen is when the severity of esophagitis is known to cause transmural inflammation resulting in potential shortening. This is seen mostly in patients with a stricture or with an extensive circumferential columnar lined esophagus covering their distal esophagus. Other risk factors that predispose to recurrent reflux after standard hiatal hernia repairs are suggested: obesity, periesophagitis from other antireflux operations or chronic obstructive pulmonary disease. The large paraesophageal hernia with chronic shortening may well be responsible for a short esophagus as well. In these patients, four choices of repair are available: 1) the Collis gastroplasty associated with a partial or total fundoplication; 2) a total fundoplication; 3) the intrathoracic fundoplication; and 4) the intrathoracic Thal-Nissen repair.

The Collis elongation operation, when a partial fundoplication is made around it with the remaining gastric fundus, forms the Collis-Belsey operation. It was used extensively by Pearson [7] and recent results have been reported by Waters [8]. Control of reflux symptoms was noted in 76% of the operated group. However, when pH studies were added, esophageal acid exposure was documented in up to 46% of operated patients [9,10]. When a Collis gastroplasty is wrapped by a total fundoplication [11–13], objective acid reflux control measurement by pH studies still reveals 25% of their 55 patients having esophageal acid exposure. Ellis reported that a majority of his Collis Nissen gastroplasties succeeded in controlling reflux disease in patients with stricture and short esophagus. Piehler and Payne [14], as well as Demos [15], reported their early experience with a 3 cm uncut gastroplasty, claiming good symptomatic results in 94% of their patients.

Maher et al. [16] propose as an alternative a total fundoplication which is left in a supradiaphragmatic position. They used this operation in 44 patients with strictures difficult to dilate preoperatively but dilatable at operation, with failed previous antireflux operations and in patients with acquired esophageal shortening without previous surgery. Clinically, they report a 7.5% mortality with two in hospital deaths and one late death. Sixty-eight percent of their patients show excellent results, 14% good results and 5% poor results.

Woodward [4], instead of resection or elongation, prefers a Thal-Fundic patch covered with a split thickness skin graft from the chest wall, combined with a Nissen fundoplication. They report on 68 patients with a 4% mortality and 65% of their group showing good clinical results.

Leaving a total fundoplication in the chest, either as an intrathoracic wrap above the diaphragm or as a Thal-Nissen operation, may result in causing potentially lethal complications from the operation. The three categories of complications reported by Richardson [17] and Mansour [18] are diaphragmatic hernias, gastric ulcerations and gastric fistulas with surrounding structures.

Reoperative surgery

Reoperative surgery for correction of reflux damage may be a second indication for choosing another type of repair than the standard Nissen fundoplication. Maher [19] opted for transthoracic repair in all but three of his 55 patients. In 12 patients he preferred to perform a Thal repair. Hill et al. [3] reported on 114 patients with a failed Nissen fundoplication.

Most of these patients presented with recurrent reflux symptoms and dysphagia. They transformed the first operation into a Hill posterior gastropexy. They report satisfactory results in 80% of the patients with a 2% mortality. Leonardi and Ellis [20], however, reported on 54 failed operations and only three patients with strictures had to be reoperated through the chest: two had a Collis-Nissen gastroplasty with excellent results, one required a resection. Ellis [20] observed excellent reflux control and a normal recreation of a high pressure zone amplitude when using a gastroplasty with a total fundoplication for patients with a strictured esophagus.

Alkaline esophagitis

Esophagitis resulting from reflux disease in patients who had previous gastric resections, whether partial or total, should be treated by total bile diversion. A Roux diversion with a 50–60 cm limb and a bilateral truncal vagotomy should ensure full protection for the esophageal mucosa.

Reflux esophagitis of peptic origin with a significant alkaline component of the refluxate may be responsible for significant esophageal damage. If present with an intact stomach, such damage is better treated with conventional antireflux operations: a Nissen fundoplication, if minimal or erosive damage exists, or an elongation gastroplasty with a total fundoplication if the damage is more severe. Bile diversion with gastric resection and vagotomy should not be proposed in this situation, with the possible perspective of having to use the stomach as a replacement organ if, in the future, more damage or complications were to occur in the esophagus.

The atonic esophagus

The esophagus is rendered atonic by esophageal myotomy performed for primary idiopathic motor disorders. Adding an antireflux operation below a myotomized segment may result in the esophagus being unable to properly empty its content. Gastroplasties, with either partial or total fundoplication, will result in obstructive symptoms [10]. The use of a Nissen fundoplication, even if made loose and short, creates enough functional obstruction over time to warrant reoperation in nearly 50% of patients treated with this operation [21]. The use of a partial fundoplication to protect the myotomized esophagus from potential reflux seems to reach its goal while allowing satisfactory emptying of the esophagus.

Scleroderma causes atony and poor propulsion in a majority of patients affected by this condition when referred for reflux symptoms. A standard Nissen repair in this situation may become obstructive. In our experience of 14 patients treated for that condition, 12 had a total fundoplication although modified by being made short (2 cm) and over a large bougie. Our observations showed that these patients had symptoms of slow emptying and only one showed episodes of dysphagia. Poor emptying was seen on esophageal scintigram. Esophageal exposure to acid was still documented in 50% of the group in spite of the total fundoplication. Thus, the ideal operation in the scleroderma patient may not be a total fundoplication, but, for the time being, it provides significantly better comfort for these patients, even with the imperfect results.

In summary, it seems that it is the extent of damage and the type of damage that will dictate best the choice of an antireflux operation other than the Nissen fundoplication. Previous gastric surgery and the atonic esophagus following myotomy for motor disorders will also dictate an alternative procedure.

References

1. DeMeester TR, Johnson LF, Kent AH. Evaluation of current operations for the prevention of gastroesophageal reflux. Ann Surg 1974;180:511—525.
2. Leonardi HK, Ellis FH. Reoperative surgery for gastroesophageal reflux. In: Jamieson GG (ed) Surgery of the Oesophagus. London: Churchill Livingstone, 1988;291—298.
3. Thor K, Mercer CD, James E, Hill LD. Post-Nissen syndrome. In: Siewert JR, Holscher DH (eds) Diseases of the Esophagus. Berlin: Springer-Verlag, 1988;1203—1205.
4. Maher JW, Hocking MP, Woodward ER. Reoperations for esophagitis following failed antireflux procedures. Ann Surg 1985;201:723—727.
5. Orringer MB. Management of failed antireflux procedures. Surgery 1987;181—195.
6. Orringer MB, Skinner DB, Belsey RH. Long-term results of the Mark IV operation for hiatal hernia and analyses of recurrences and their treatment. J Thorac Cardiovasc Surg 1972;63:25—33.
7. Pearson FG, Henderson RD. Long-term follow-up of peptic strictures managed by dilatation, modified Collis gastroplasty and Belsey hiatus hernia repair. Surgery 1976;80:396—404.
8. Waters PF, Piazza D, Cooper JD, Patterson GA, Todd TR, Pearson FG. Gastroplasty and partial fundoplication in patients with peptic esophagitis and acquired shortening: results in long-term follow-up. In: Siewert JR, Holscher AH (eds) Diseases of the Esophagus. Berlin: Springer Verlag, 1988;1286—1290.
9. Orringer MB, Sloan H. Collis-Belsey reconstruction of the esophagogastric junction. J Thorac Cardiovasc Surg 1976;71:295—303.
10. Orringer MB, Sloan H. Complications and failings of the combined Collis-Belsey operation. J Thorac Cardiovasc Surg 1977;74:726—735.
11. Henderson RD. Reflux control following gastroplasty. Ann Thorac Surg 1977;24:206—214.
12. Orringer MB. Combined Collis gastroplasty Nissen reconstruction of the esophagogastric junction. Ann Thorac Surg 1978;25:16—21.
13. Orringer MB. The combined Collis-Nissen operation. In: Jamieson GG (ed) Surgery of the Oesophagus. London: Churchill Livingstone, 1988; 327—335.
14. Piehler JM, Payne WS, Cameron AJ. The uncut Collis-Nissen procedure for esophageal hiatus hernia and its complications. Problems in General Surgery 1984;1:1—14.
15. Demos NJ. Stapled uncut gastroplasty for hiatal hernia: 12 years follow-up. Ann Thorac Surg 1984;38:393—399.
16. Maher JW, Hocking MP, Woodward ER. Long-term follow-up of the combined fundic patch fundoplication for treatment of longitudinal peptic strictures of the esophagus. Ann Surg 1981;194:64—69.
17. Richardson JD, Larson GM, Polk HC. Intrathoracic fundoplication for shortened esophagus: treacherous solution to a challenging problem. Am J Surg 1982;143:29—35.
18. Mansour KA, Burton HG, Miller JL Jr. Complications of intrathoracic Nissen fundoplications. Ann Thorac Surg 1981;32:173—178.
19. Maher JW. Intrathoracic fundoplication for shortened esophagus. In: Jamieson GG (ed) Surgery of the Esophagus. London: Churchill Livingstone, 1988;321—326.

20. Ellis FH Jr., Leonardi HK, Dabuzhsky L, Crozier RE. Surgery for short esophagus with stricture: an experimental and clinical manometric study. Ann Surg 1978;188:341–350.
21. Topart P, Deschamps C, Taillefer R, Duranceau A. Long-term effects of total fundoplication on the myotomized esophagus Ann Thorac Surg 1992;1046–1052.

Are ulcers of the antireflux valve characteristic of the Nissen procedure?

C.G. Bremner (Los Angeles)

Gastric ulceration following the Nissen fundoplication occurs either distal to the wrap, proximally within the wrap, or in the chest associated with an intrathoracic Nissen fundoplication. Krupp and Rossetti first described an antral ulcer and two fistulae near the wrap in a series of 524 Nissen fundoplication operations [1]. Sifers et al. reported on ten gastric ulcers in a series of 381 operations which they described as the reefing method of fundoplication [2]. Specific attention was drawn to the association of gastric ulcer after the Nissen fundoplication by Bushkin et al. [3] and Bremner [4,5]. Since then, numerous reports have appeared.

Gastric ulceration occurring distal to the wrap of a Nissen fundoplication (Table 1)

Gastric ulcer occurring distal to a Nissen fundoplication has been reported in approximately 2.8% of 1,756 operations [1–14]. The ulcer is usually on the lesser curve of the stomach or in the antrum, but there is one report of a greater curve ulcer following the procedure. The interval between the Nissen fundoplication operation and the first symptoms of the ulcer is variable and is between 1 month and 7 years, with a median interval of 15 months from reported series [3,4,7]. There is no agreement as to the possible pathogenesis of these ulcers. Bushkin et al. suggests that the prime problem was gastric stasis with hypergastrinemia, because four of their patients had gas bloat [3]. Bremner found alkaline duodenal gastric reflux in his patients and could not show evidence of delayed gastric emptying or hypergastrinemia [4]. It is also possible that these patients would have developed ulceration despite the Nissen operation. No studies have been reported, for example, of a possible association with *Helicobacter pylori*. Herrington suggested that vagal entrapment could be a cause, but gave no objective evidence that such an event altered gastric physiology or secretion [7]. In his article, he gives a detailed description of how to avoid incorporation of the vagal trunks in the Nissen fundoplication. Unrecognized truncal vagotomy would also lead to gastric stasis and possible ulceration. Anti-inflammatory drugs were the cause of antral ulceration after

Table 1. Gastric ulceration occurring distal to the wrap of a Nissen fundoplication

Author(s)	Date	Number gastric ulcerations	Number antireflux operations
Krupp, Rossetti [1]	1966	3	524
Sifers [2]	1976	10	381
Bushkin [3]	1976	5	160
Bremner [4]	1977	4	43
Maher [6]	1982	2	
Herrington [7]	1982	5	158
Campbell [8]	1983	13	
O'Rourke [9]	1985	5	
Fleming [10]	1986	23	
Low [11]	1988	6	
Tissot [12]	1989	1	
Bonaldi [13]	1989	1	
Houdelette [14]	1989	1	

a supradiaphragmatic Nissen in Maher's series [6]. Treatment of these cases poses a particular problem. Medical treatment has been used successfully in some reported cases, but antrectomy, wedge resection and wrap take-down with pyloroplasty and partial gastrectomy have all been reported [3,4,7,18]. Tissot (see p. 622) suggests that the treatment should be total gastrectomy if medical treatment fails [12]. One patient in the author's series perforated a lesser curve gastric ulcer about 4 years after the Nissen operation and the attending surgeon in another district operated and oversewed the ulcer. The patient has subsequently been symptom- and ulcer-free for a further 5 years. Of interest, this patient had histological gastritis prior to the Nissen operation.

Gastric ulceration occurring within the wrap of an intra-abdominal Nissen fundoplication (Table 2)

Ulceration occurring within the wrap of a Nissen is reportedly less common than ulceration occurring distal to the wrap, and it occurred in 16 reported cases [15–19]. These ulcers may fistulate and develop several days after surgery, suggesting a

Table 2. Gastric ulceration occurring within the wrap or proximal to an intra-abdominal Nissen fundoplication

Author(s)	Date	Number of cases	Number in series	Proposed causes
Launois [15]	1990	8		Gastric stasis, alkaline reflux
Pennell [16]	1981	3	200	
Burnett [17]	1977	1		
Scobie [18]	1979	3	100	Mechanical
Deschamps [19]	1990	1		Ischemia

610

different pathogenesis such as ischemia, handling of the stomach with forceps, or devascularization of the fundus. Suturing the wrap with silk sutures has a potential for ulceration. Such ulcers may present with pain and bleeding and may be difficult to diagnose [8]. Double contrast radiological studies and endoscopy usually confirm the diagnosis [20]. A double-lumen esophagus was evident at endoscopy in one patient who had developed an esophagogastric fistula [10]. No clear guidelines are included in the literature as to how these cases should be treated. Conservative management has resulted in healing in a few reported cases, but gastric resection may be necessary. One of Scobie's cases relapsed after medical healing and required resection [18].

Gastric ulceration occurring in the intrathoracic Nissen fundoplication [21—28]

It is evident from several reports that the intrathoracic Nissen wrap is subject to serious complications such as gastropleural, gastrobronchial, gastropericardial fistula formation and intracardiac rupture [17]. Both Mansour [28] and Richardson [21] argue strongly against the continued use of this operation. On the other hand, Maher et al. [6] have reported on excellent results following a series of 44 intrathoracic Nissen operations. They did experience two antral ulcers following this procedure, but no intrathoracic problems occurred. It is suggested that variations in operative technique may be responsible for poor results reported by others. In a personal communication with Woodward some years ago, the explanation given was that a tight hiatus leads to stasis and that this should be guarded against when performing the intrathoracic procedure. Collard also noted that complications following the intrathoracic wrap were decreased by enlarging the hiatus [24]. This explanation seems plausible, because the perforation occurs at an early stage, suggesting an ischemic basis for the complication.

Not included in the published series of gastric ulcers after Nissen fundoplications are the cases reported by personal communication to Herrington [7]. Polk had experience with two cases in 600 plication procedures; DeMeester had two cases in a series of 200 fundoplications. Menguy and Bombeck had not encountered gastric ulcer as a complication in 150 and 165 cases respectively. Of interest, Hill reported

Table 3. Gastric ulceration occurring in the intrathoracic Nissen fundoplication

Author(s)	Date	Number of cases	Number in series	Complications
Richardson [21]	1982	4	600	
Parikh [22]	1991	1	55	Pericardial fistula
Bianchi [23]	1991	1		Intracardiac fistula
Collard [24]	1991	5	31	Gastrobronchial fistula
Chong [25]	1990	1		Gastrobronchial fistula
Gaensler [26]	1988	1		Gastrobronchial fistula
Gianello [27]	1985	7		
Mansour [28]	1981	3		Perforation (2 deaths)

to Herrington that he had not encountered a gastric ulcer in his large series of posterior gastropexy antireflux procedures. Bushkin found that gastric ulcer was exclusive to the Nissen procedure and he had also performed 120 Allison operations, 60 Hill procedures, and 13 others [3]. Yuen [20] described four proximal gastric ulcers in a series of 100 Belsey Mark IV procedures and Mullen [29] reported an esophagogastric fistula following a Belsey operation in a patient with scleroderma. Yuen concluded that local ischemia and mechanical trauma are important in the development of the ulceration which can occur as early as 1 week after fundoplication.

Conclusions

Gastric ulceration after antireflux procedures is characteristic of the Nissen operation, although five cases have been reported after the Belsey Mark IV procedure. No cases have been reported after the Hill operation, which suggests that technical factors may be important in the pathogenesis of this complication. Gastric ulceration distal to the wrap probably has a different cause to ulceration and perforation within the wrap and following the intrathoracic procedure. Possible causes of distal ulceration are ischemia, vagal nerve entrapment, duodenal gastric reflux, or a combination of these factors. Ulceration and fistula within the wrap are likely to be due to ischemic factors, whereas fistulation from the intrathoracic Nissen may be related to entrapment of the stomach by a tight hiatus which could cause ischemia. The latter operation should be discontinued in favor of a lengthening procedure (Collis) combined with a Nissen fundoplication.

References

1. Krupp S, Rossetti M. Surgical treatment of hiatal hernia by fundoplication and gastrectomy (Nissen repair). Ann Surg 1966;106:927.
2. Sifers EC, Taylor TL, Rick GG et al. The role of gastrin in the treatment of sliding hiatal hernia with reflux using the reefing method of fundoplication. Surg Gynecol Obstet 1976;143:376—380.
3. Bushkin FL, Woodward ER, O'Leary JP. Occurrence of gastric ulcer after Nissen fundoplication. Ann Surg 1976;42: 821—826.
4. Bremner CG. Gastric ulceration after the Nissen fundoplication. A complication of alkaline reflux. S Afr Med J 1977; 51:791—793.
5. Bremner CG. Gastric ulceration after a fundoplication. Surg Gynecol Obstet 1979;168:62—66.
6. Maher JW, Hocking MP, Woodward ER. Supradiaphragmatic fundoplication. Long-term follow-up and analysis of complications. Am J Surg 1984;147:181—186.
7. Herrington JL, Meacham PW, Hunter RM. Gastric ulceration after fundic wrapping. Vagal nerve entrapment, a possible causative factor. Ann Surg 1982;195:574—581.
8. Campbell R, Kennedy T, Johnston G. Gastric ulceration after Nissen fundoplication. Br J Surg 1983;70:406—407.
9. O'Rourke IC. Fundoplication for gastro-oesophageal reflux. Aust NZ J Surg 1985;55:347—354.
10. Fleming JL, DiMagno EP. Double lumen esophagus: presentation of esophagogastric fistula, a rare complication of fundoplication. Dig Dis Sci 1986;31:106—108.
11. Low DE, Mercer CD, James EC, Hill LD. Post-Nissen syndrome. Surg Gynecol Obstet 1988;167:1—5.
12. Tissot E, Naouri A, Gabriele S, Tissot-Favre A. Ulcer of the gastric fundus after abdominal fundoplication. A peculiar entity? J Chir (Paris) 1989;126:379—381.
13. Bonaldi U, Riva R, Ribera M. Spontaneous esophagogastric perforation after fundoplication. Minerva Med 1989;80:729—732.
14. Houdelette P, Kunkel K, Moreau X, Dumotier J. Subcardial ulcer and the Nissen technique. A propos of a case of recovery by partial release of the fundoplication. Ann Chir 1989;43:282—284.

15. Launois B, Bardaxoglou E, Meunier B, Campion JP, Lebeau G, Chasseray V, Corbel L. Severe and late complications after Nissen's procedure. Chirurgie 1990;116:667−672.
16. Pennell TC. Supradiaphragmatic correction of esophageal reflux strictures. Ann Surg 1981;193:655−665.
17. Burnett HF, Read RC, Morris WD, Campbell GS. Management of complications of fundoplication and Barrett's esophagus. Surgery 1977;82:521−530.
18. Scobie BA. High gastric view after Nissen fundoplication. Med J Aust 1979;1:609−610.
19. Descamps OS, Donckier JE, Collard JM, Michel JM, Trigaux L, Melange M, Buysschaert M. Recurrent pleuro-pericarditis due to gastrodiaphragmatic fistula. Acta Clin Belg 1990;45:126−129.
20. Yuen ML, Somers S, McGrath FPA. Gastric ulceration after fundoplication. Can Assoc Radiol J 1992; 43:40−46.
21. Richardson JD, Larson GM, Polk HC. Intrathoracic fundoplication for shortened esophagus: Treacherous solution to a challenging problem. Am J Surg 1982;143:29−35.
22. Parekh D, Tas PK. Results of fundoplication in a UK paediatric centre. Br J Surg 1991;78:346−381.
23. Bianchi A, Ubach M. Giant gastric ulcer penetrating into the heart as a late complication of Nissen fundoplication. Eur J Surg 1991;157:61−62.
24. Collard JM, Dekoninck XJ, Otte JB, Fiasse RH, Kestens PJ. Intrathoracic Nissen fundoplication: Long-term clinical and pH monitoring evaluation. Ann Thorac Surg 1991;51:34−38.
25. Chong WK, Constant OC. Gastrobronchial fistula. Clin Radiol 1990;41:141−142.
26. Gaensler EH, Jeffrey RB Jr, Noonan CD. Gastrobronchial fistula: an unusual complication of Nissen fundoplication. Gastrointest Radiol 1988;13:6−8.
27. Gianello P, Baulieux J, Maillet P. Esophageal and gastric fistulas following surgery of the esophagogastric junction. Acta Chir Belg 1985;85:167−178.
28. Mansour KA, Burton HG, Miller JI Jr, Hatcher CR Jr. Complications of intrathoracic Nissen fundoplication. Ann Thorac Surg 1981; 32:173−178.
29. Mullen JT, Burke EL, Diamond AB. Esophagogastric fistula. A complication of combined operations for esophageal disease. Arch Surg 1975;110:826−828.

Can one envisage the role of partial devascularization of the fundus and gastroesophageal junction?

B. Launois, E Bardaxoglou, B. Meunier, S. Landen (Rennes)

Rationale for the surgical management of gastroesophageal reflux was brought forward by Behar [1] in 1974, before the advent of H_2-blockers. The study showed the superiority of surgery over medical treatment. Another study by DeMeester indicated that the Nissen fundoplication was the best antireflux operation, judging by postoperative esophageal pH monitoring and manometry [2]. This technique became the intervention of our own choice for treating GERD. With time, however, late and severe complications developed in our series, as observed in other centers.

Materials and Methods

A total of 11 severe complications were observed among eight patients having undergone a Nissen procedure. Seven patients had been operated on in the department and one patient in a neighboring city. Technical details of our surgical procedure have already been published [3].

One single patient had been under medication that may have altered the gastric mucosa. All patients had undergone gastric fibroscopy prior to the Nissen fundoplication. There were three women and five men with a mean age of 42 ± 11 years (range 25–61 years). Complications occurred within a mean delay of 4 years, 7 months ± 3 years, 10 months (range 0.75–11.25 years). Five patients had been included in a previous study [3], and had at that time presented only two complications, instead of seven in the present review.

Diagnosis (Table 1)

Clinical pictures were of two sorts:

Perforated ulcer (n = 5)
Three of five patients experienced premonitory symptoms that included gastric fullness (n = 1), epigastric pain (n = 4), retrosternal pain (n = 3), left upper quadrant pain (n = 1), dysphagia (n = 1) and unexplained fever (n = 2) several weeks or months before the complication occurred.

At the start, symptoms are acute, including retrosternal pain (n = 3) and left upper quadrant pain (n = 2) that are relieved in the supine position. Other symptoms varied with the site of perforation: cardiac tamponade (n = 1), subcutaneous emphysema in the right subclavian region (n = 1), purulent pleurisy (n = 1), fever (n = 2) and septic shock (n = 1). The chest X-ray is often essential in establishing the diagnosis. Three of five patients had signs of pneumopericardium, pneumomediastinum or purulent pleurisy. Gastrograffin swallow shows the site of perforation. Gastric fibroscopy is most often useless, and may even be hazardous because of the greatest difficulties encountered in examining the mucosa within the wrap.

Bleeding ulcer (n = 6)
In complete contrast with the previous clinical picture, premonitory symptoms were

Table 1. Characteristic features of perforated and bleeding gastric ulcers following Nissen fundoplication

	Perforated ulcers	Bleeding ulcers
Clinical signs		
Premonitory symptoms	+	0
Acute symptoms	+	+
Diagnosis		
Chest X-ray	+	0
Gastrograffin swallow	+	0
Gastric fibroscopy	0	+
Pathology		
Infracardial ulcer	0	+
Chronic ulcer situated on the wrap	+	0

Table 2. Operative findings

	Perforated ulcers (n = 5)	Bleeding ulcers (n = 6)
Extensive devascularization of the greater curvature[a]	5	5
Chronic ulcers	3	2
Nonabsorbable sutures	3	1
Thoracic ascension	4	0
Delayed gastric emptying	2	1
Alkaline reflux	1	

[a]One patient had been secondarily referred.

usually absent with the exception of one patient who had unexplained fever and unrelenting hiccups. Presenting features included either hematemesis, melaena, or unexplained bleeding syndrome. Three patients had severe hemorrhagic shock requiring 36, 19 and 38 blood packs and 37, 16 and 17 fresh frozen plasma units, respectively.

In such cases, gastric fibroscopy was essential, revealing a bleeding cardial ulcer (n = 4) or a gastric ulcer centered around suture material in one case.

Multiple complications

Two patients experienced multiple complications. One patient underwent laparotomy for a bleeding ulcer 4 and 6 years following the initial procedure. Another patient was operated on 3 times for ulcer perforations into the mediastinum against the right crural sling after 14 months, then into the left diaphragmatic sling after 28 and 52 months, the latest episode being accompanied by an acute hemorrhage. Between the last two operations, the patient had undergone a pyloroplasty because of delayed gastric emptying.

Serum gastrin dosages and gastric acid output measurements were normal in all patients. Mean BAO was 3.17 mmol and mean PAO was 7.41 mmol. The patient having presented successive perforations underwent, at the time of the third perforation in the left crural sling, a partial gastrectomy and a short Belsey-type interposition coloplasty. He subsequently developed two ulcers on the colonic segment, but pH-metry and manometry failed to show acid reflux, esophageal motility anomalies or increased intraluminal pressure at the site of the two anastomoses. However, HIDA and technetium scans showed numerous episodes of prolonged alkaline reflux, and the patient underwent duodenal diversion.

Associated gastric emptying abnormalities

Two patients presented a small bowel obstruction requiring a laparotomy. One patient developed gastric hemorrhage 8 days later, due to a bleeding ulcer. The second patient had laparotomy for bowel obstruction shortly after undergoing a pyloroplasty for delayed gastric emptying.

Operative findings (Table 2)

Perforated ulcer
The perforation involved the pericardium (n = 1), mediastinum and diaphragmatic crura (n = 2), pleura (n = 1) and diaphragmatic crural sling (n = 1). Three of five lesions were chronic ulcers freshly perforated into the right (n = 1) or left crural sling (n = 2).

Punched-out or punctiform, the ulcers were situated in the posterior (n = 3) or anterior (n = 2) portion of the fundic wrap. The ulcer was centered around nonabsorbable suture material in three cases and was associated with athoracic ascension of the wrap in four cases.

Bleeding ulcer
Bleeding ulcers were most frequently situated just below the cardia (n = 4) or on the posterior portion of the fundic wrap (n = 2). Thoracic ascension was never observed. One ulcer contained suture material and pathological examination revealed two chronic ulcers.

Results

Incidence of complications (Table 3)

Seven of 134 (5.2%) patients having undergone a Nissen procedure experienced a total of 10 late complications.

Surgical management

— All perforated ulcers were treated by simple suture.
— For bleeding ulcers, the treatment was adapted to each individual situation. There were two direct sutures and one excision-suture. One Nissen procedure was converted to a 3/4 circumference wrap (Toupet), and H_2-blockers were administered. In one case a giant infracardial ulcer with the left gastric artery bleeding in

Table 3. Incidence of gastric ulcers

Author	Year	Number	Nissen	%	Suspected etiology
Sifers [7]	1976	10	384	2.6	Hypergastrinemia
Bremner [8,9]	1977/9	5	90	5.6	Bile reflux
Bushkin [10]	1979	5	160	3	Gastric distension
Polk [11]	1981	3	600	0.3	Vagus nerve injury
DeMeester [12]	1981	2	200	1	Vagus nerve injury
Woodward [13]	1981	10	300	3.3	Delayed gastric emptying
Launois [18]	1990	7[a]	134	5.2	Multifactorial

[a] 10 complications among seven patients.

the crater required a total gastrectomy. For the last patient, who presented three recurrent ulcers, the only possible solution was to undergo resection of the gastric fundus followed by interposition of a short segment of the colon (Belsey).

Morbidity and hospital mortality

There was no operative mortality or morbidity, but two patients had recurrent ulcers.

Etiology

In 10 patients, extensive devascularization of the greater curvature had been performed to obtain adequate mobilization and a tension free wrap. There were five chronic ulcers, of which four were centered around nonabsorbable suture material. The wrap had ascended into the thorax 4 times. Delayed gastric emptying was noted 3 times and alkaline reflux was noted once.

Discussion

The frequency and severity of gastric perforation in patients undergoing intrathoracic Nissen procedures have been previously documented [6], but complications associated with the abdominal wrap were until now considered to be sporadic. With a follow-up of at least 8 years for all patients in this series, we were able to show for the first time that serious and potentially life-threatening complications may arise with a delay of up to 11 years from the Nissen procedure.

Complications fall into two opposing categories. Perforations occur in ulcers situated anteriorly or posteriorly on the fundic wrap, and are associated with a thoracic ascension of the antireflux mechanism, as was the case in four of five patients, even though approximation of the crural slings had been performed. The etiopathogeny would then appear to be similar to that observed in thoracic Nissen fundoplication. In three of five patients they were the result of long-standing evolution of a chronic fibrotic ulcer that often contained nonabsorbable suture material.

Sifers, in 1976, was the first to report the development of gastric ulcers in 10 of 384 patients having undergone fundoplication. Likewise, Bremner (1977) and Bushkin (1979) reported incidences of 4/43 and 5/150 gastric ulcers respectively. Among 600 patients operated, Polk noted three ulcers associated with a recurrence of a hiatal hernia and two ulcers without. DeMeester and Woodward reported incidences of gastric ulcers of 2/200 and 10/300, respectively.

Perforated ulcers described here for the first time represent 3.7% of Nissen procedure performed in our patient group.

The etiology of these ulcers remains uncertain. It is tempting to incriminate delayed gastric emptying, as was observed in three of the patients. Entrapment of the vagus nerves has also been put forward as a possible explanation [14]. Herrington suggests that the wrap should be passed between the esophagus and vagus nerves. In the presence of pre-existent anomalies of gastric emptying, he considers that the added trauma to the vagus nerves could trigger the release of gastrin and subsequent ulcer formation. It is a fact that 57% of patients with gastroesophageal reflux exhibit delayed gastric emptying for solids and liquids [15]; Herrington suggests that the wrap could alter gastric emptying, and estimates that the height of the wrap should not exceed 3—4 cm, and should never lie below the esophago-gastric junction [16].

The possible role of alkaline reflux was put forward by Bremner. This appears to be the mechanism responsible for three ulcer recurrences in one of our patients who then had a partial gastrectomy and a Belsey-type interposition gastroplasty. New ulcers developed on the colon, and were managed successfully with a duodenal diversion procedure. Bremner believes that alkaline reflux is present initially, but is aggravated postoperatively because of pyloric dysfunction. Herrington suggests that patients be assessed in a fasting state for alkaline reflux, including dosage of bile acids, before undergoing an antireflux operation [14].

Finally, another possible factor of gastric ulceration may be the compression and venous stasis caused by the wrap itself [17]. Partial devascularization of the gastric fundus and esophago-gastric junction could play a role, and the presence of non-absorbable sutures within the ulcer corroborates this hypothesis. This complication appears to be specific to Nissen fundoplication. Indeed, among 144 patients who underwent other types of antireflux procedures (Hill, Lortat-Jacob) during the period of the study, none developed such complications.

Among the six bleeding ulcers, two were on the posterior portion of the wrap, and their pathogeny may be likened to perforated ulcers. Completely different are the four other bleeding ulcers, some of which were giant which were situated just below the cardia and eroded the left gastric artery. They could be considered similar to ulcers reported after supraselective vagotomy, but the lesser curvature had never been devascularized during fundoplication.

Conclusions

The etiology of these complications is probably multifactorial. While devascularization of the greater curvature is likely to play a role, other factors, such as delayed gastric emptying and the use of nonabsorbable sutures, are probably implicated as well.

References

1. Behar J, Sheahhan DG, Biancani P, Spiro HM, Storer EH. Medical and surgical management of reflux esophagitis, a 38-month report on a prospective clinical trial. N Engl J Med 1975;293:263—268.
2. DeMeester TR, Johnson LF, Kent AH. Evaluation of current operations for the prevention of gastroesophageal reflux. Ann Surg 1974;180:511—525.
3. Launois B, Paul JL, Teboul F, Bourdonnec P, Cardin JL, Meunier B, de Chateaubriant P. Les résultats fonctionnels du traitement chirurgical du reflux gastro-oesophagien. Analyse de 278 observations. Ann Clin 1988;42:191—196.
4. Negre FB. Postfundoplication symptoms. Do they restrict the success of Nissen fundoplication? Ann Surg 1983;198:698—700.
5. Skinner DB. Pathophysiology of gastro-oesophageal reflux. Ann Surg 1985;202:546—556.

6. Saubier EC, Gouillat C. Traitement des sténoses peptiques de l'oesophage par fundoplicature intra-thoracique avec dilatation per-opératoire de la sténose. Chirurgie 1983;109:494–500.
7. Sifers EC, Taylor TL, Rick GG, Hartmann CR. The role of gastrin in the treatment of sliding hiatal hernia with reflux using the reefing method of fundoplication. Surg Gynecol Obstet 1976;143:376–380.
8. Bremner CG. Gastric ulcer after the Nissen fundoplication, a complication of alkaline reflux. S Afr Med J 1977;51:791–793.
9. Bremner CG. Gastric ulceration after the fundoplication operation for gastro-oesophageal reflux. Surg Gynecol Obstet 1979;148:62–66.
10. Bushkin FL, Woodward ER, O'Leary JP. Occurrence of gastric ulcer after Nissen fundoplication. Ann Surg 1976;42:821–826.
11. Polk HC. Personal communication 1981 in 14.
12. DeMeester TR. Personal communication 1981 in 14.
13. Woodward ER. Personal communication 1981 in 14.
14. Herrington JL Jr, Meacham PW, Hunter RM. Gastric ulceration after fundic wrapping vagal nerve entrapment, a possible causative factor. Ann Surg 1982;195:574–581.
15. McCallum RW, Berkovitz DM, Lerner E. Gastric emptying in patients with gastroesophageal reflux. Gastroenterology 1981;80: 285–291.
16. Herrington JL Jr. Invited commentary of Maher JW, Cerda JJ. The role of gastric stasis in the genesis of gastric ulceration following fundoplication. World J Surg 1982;6:797–799.
17. Scobie BA. High gastric ulcer after Nissen fundoplication. Med J Austr 1979;1:609–610.
18. Launois B, Bardaxoglou E, Meunier B, Campion JP, Lebeau G, Chasseray V, Corbel L. Complications sévères et tardives après interventions de Nissen. Chirurgie 1990;116:667–672.

May the etiologic factors possibly differ,
— in early ulcers
— and in late ulcers?

E. Tissot (Lyons)

Potential benefits of Nissen fundoplication in the treatment of gastroesophageal reflux must be weighed against significant morbid complications from 13 to 20% [1].

Early or delayed gastric ulcer are rare complications that reflect etio-pathogenesis problems and especially in the management of particularly high situated gastric ulcers.

Sifers [2] and Bushkin et al. [3] described the first cases of gastric ulcer following fundoplication in 1976. Different studied series have found ulcer frequencies from 1–5% (Table 1).

The characteristics of postplication gastric ulcers are particular:
— the interval of occurrence of the lesions is very variable, ranging from 2 months after operation to 11 years [12];
— the locations of the ulcers are always gastric, but it can be differentiated into prepyloric ulcers and high situated ulcers, in which the ulcer can be found on subcardiac curvature or at the level of the valve itself [13];
— these ulcers are mostly large, exacerbated, and with major tendency of complica-

Table 1. Frequency of gastric ulcer after Nissen procedure

Author	Number of ulcers		Number of Nissen procedures	
	Year	Number	Number	%
Sifers [2]	1976	10	384	3.84
Woodward [4]	1977	10	300	3.00
Bushkin [3]	1979	5	150	3.00
Bremner [5]	1979	5	90	5.50
Scobie [6]	1979	10	300	3.00
Peix [7]	1981	1	107	0.90
Herrington [8]	1982	5	158	3.20
Campbell [9]	1983	8	170	4.70
DeMeester [10]	1986	2	200	1.00
Saubier [11]	1986	6	112	5.30
Gossot [1]	1987	1	96	1.04

tions [14,15] such as: severe digestive bleeding, perforation in abdominal viscus organs or into the abdominal cavity. Sometimes when the Nissen reascended in the thorax, gastrobronchial fistula, gastropericardiac or gastroaortic fistula could be found [16].

Several different etio-pathogenetic mechanisms have been proposed

Bushkin [3] suggested that, because of the valvuloplastic mechanism, trapped gastric air may cause distension of the antrum and stimulate gastrin release. Gastrin increases gastric acid secretion. Gastrin also decreases gastric emptying. This cycle of gastric distension, gastrin release and delayed gastric emptying may play a role in the production of the gastric ulcer. However, in this series no patient demonstrated evidence of high gastrin levels.

According to Maher [17], secondary vagal dysfunction after surgery or pre-existing with delayed gastric emptying and hypergastrinemia have been incriminated. This finding was demonstrated in two of his observations.

Herrington [8] also agreed that operative injury to vagus nerves is a contributing factor and tends to meticulous surgical technique by isolating and protecting the vagus nerves from the fundic wrap.

Bremner [5] reported that gastritis, probably induced by bile reflux, is an important factor in the development of gastric ulcer. He reported that alkaline reflux was present in all of his six cases and felt that gastric ulcer resulted from bile reflux. In his study, there was no evidence of hypergastrinemia, acid hypersecretion or gastric emptying dysfunction. He suggests preoperative routine assessment to detect biliary reflux or delayed gastric emptying and to perform a duodenal diversion when diagnosis of biliary reflux is documented.

Mechanical theory has been suggested by Scobie [6] and Campbell et al. [9]. The fundic wrap could induce ischemia by direct compression and venous congestion.

Scobie suggested that the angulation at the upper curve is an important contributing factor.

Partial gastroesophageal junction devascularization, ligation of one or two short gastric vessels, sometimes needed during mobilization of the fundus, could be another supporting factor and subcardial ulcer seems to be similar to necrosis occurring after supraselective vagotomy [12]. Campbell [9] had seen three cases of acute lesser curve necrosis after proximal gastric vagotomy and all occurred in patients having concomitant fundoplication. He believed that they were probably due to a combination of ischemia and gastric distension.

In fact, the etiology of gastric ulceration following plication remains unclear. It appears reasonable to postulate that multiple factors, as outlined, may be involved (ischemia, anatomical distortion, bile reflux, vagal dysfunction, hypergastrinemia). These factors should be given careful consideration in the evaluation of preoperative patients.

References

1. Gossot D, Sarfati E, Azoulay D, Celerier M. Facteurs de morbidité de l'intervention de Nissen. J Chir 1987;124:367–371.
2. Sifers EC, Taylor TL, Rick GG, Hartmann CR. The role of gastrin in the treatment of sliding hiatal hernia with reflux using the reefing method of fundoplication. Surg Gynecol Obstet 1976;143:376–380.
3. Bushkin FL, Woodward ER, O'Leary JP. Occurrence of gastric ulcer after Nissen fundoplication. Am J Surg 1976;42:821–826.
4. Woodward ER. Surgical treatment of gastroesophageal reflux and its complications. World J Surg 1977;1;453–461.
5. Bremner CG. Gastric ulceration after a fundoplication operation for gastro-oesophageal reflux. Surg Gynecol Obstet 1979;168;62–64.
6. Scobie BA. High gastric ulcer after Nissen fundoplication. Med J Aust 1979;1:609–610.
7. Peix JL, Baulieux J, Boulez J, Donne R, Maillet P. Complications et séquelles des fundoplicatures. Lyon Chir 1981;77:6–9.
8. Herrington JL, Meacham PW, Hunter RM. Gastric ulceration after fundic wrapping. Ann Surg 1982;195:574–581.
9. Campbell R, Kennedy T, Johnston G. Gastric ulceration after Nissen fundoplication. Br J Surg 1983;70:406–407.
10. DeMeester TR, Bonavina L, Albertucci M. Nissen fundoplicature for gastroesophageal reflux disease. Ann Surg 1986;204:9–20.
11. Saubier EC, Gouillat C, Teboul F. Traitement du reflux gastro-oesophagien par fundoplicature complète de Nissen. Chir 1986;112:123–131.
12. Launois B, Bardaxoglou E, Meunier B, Campion JP, Lebeau G, Chasseray V, Corbel L. Complications sévères et tardives après intervention de Nissen. Chir 1990;116:667–672.
13. Tissot E, Naouri A, Gabriele S, Tissot-Favre A. Ulcère de la grosse tubérosité gastrique après fundoplicature abdominale. Une entité particulière. J Chir 1989;126:379–381.
14. Edelmann G, Boutelier Ph, Champault G. Les ulcères du pôle supérieur de l'estomac. Problèmes chirurgicaux. Lyon Chir 1974;70:299–302.
15. Jensen HE, Hoffmann PDJ, Wille-Jourgensen P. High gastric ulcer. World J Surg 1987;11:325–332.
16. Low DE, Mercer CD, James EC, Hill LD. Post-Nissen syndrome. Surg Gynecol Obstet 1988;167:1 5.
17. Maher JN, Cerda JJ. The role of gastric stasis in the genesis of gastric ulceration following fundoplication. World J Surg 1982;6:794–799.

# Is it not reasonable to consider a total gastrectomy for an ulcer of the fundus resistant to medical treatment?

E. Tissot (Lyons)

Medical management is rarely sufficient [1]. Eight patients were treated by Campbell [2] all the ulcers healed, but four later recurred.

Surgical revision according to various modalities is generally unavoidable.

Simple closure of perforation has been suggested for perforated ulcers [3], as well as inferior partial gastrectomy distal or involving the ulcer in case of lower localization [2,4].

Surgical difficulties are markedly observed in cases of highly situated complicated ulcers.

Hemostasis suture for bleeding ulcer, associated with vagotomy and pyloroplasty or wedge excision of the ulcer with pyloroplasty, are often exposed to recurrent bleeding. They required an emergency total gastrectomy [5,6].

Take-down of the previous Nissen wrap, with constitution of another antireflux procedure has been successfully performed, especially in cases of perforated intra-thoracic ulcer [7].

However, in the case of a giant ulcer and repeated bleeding, it seems to be necessary to realize total gastrectomy rather than a proximal esogastrectomy [3,5,6].

Conclusion

In case of failure of medical treatment, when takedown of the fundoplication and reconstruction seem to be hazardous, total gastrectomy at the first onset can be recommended.

References

1. Houdelette P, Kunkel K, Moreau X, Dumotier J. Ulcère sous-cardial et technique de Nissen. A propos d'une observation de guérison par décomplètement de la fundoplicature. Ann Chir 1989;43:282–284.
2. Campbell R, Kennedy T, Johnston G. Gastric ulceration after Nissen fundoplication. Br J Surg 1983;70:406–407.
3. Launois B, Bardaxoglou E, Meunier B, Campion JP, Lebeau G, Chasseray V, Corbel L. Complications sévères et tardives après intervention de Nissen. Chir 1990;116:667– 672.
4. Gossot D, Sarfati E, Azoulay D, Celerier M. Facteurs de morbidité de l'intervention de Nissen. J Chir 1987;124:367–371.
5. Tissot E, Naouri A, Gabriele S, Tissot-Favre A. Ulcère de la grosse tubérosité gastrique après fundoplicature abdominale. Une entité particulière. J Chir 1989;126:379–381.
6. Teboul F, Partensky C. Une complication exceptionnelle de l'opération de Nissen: l'ulcère gastrique fistulisé dans l'artère splénique. A propos de deux observations. Lyon Chir 1987;83:411.
7. Low DE, Mercer CD, James EC, Hill LD. Post-Nissen syndrome. Surg Gynecol Obstet 1988;167:1–5.

What is the degree of obstruction to swallowing created by the Nissen valve?

A. Del Genio, G. Izzo, V. Maffettone, N. Di Martino, L. Fei,
P. Zampiello, A. Allaria, A. Nuzzo (Naples)

Surgical therapy of gastroesophageal reflux disease (GERD), with a 360° fundoplication, is a very interesting subject. Numerous problems are connected to it, the most important being the estimate of the degree of obstruction which can be determined by Nissen fundoplication.

Several authors [1—4] show some reserve towards this procedure: it can provoke serious obstructive complications that cannot be considered as normal consequences in the treatment of a benign pathology. Dysphagia is the most common and frequent symptom of these obstructions; it can be transitory or persistent, light or heavy, so that a new operation could be necessary.

From the data in the literature, it is clear that dysphagia is present in percentages ranging from 0.8 [5] to 62.8% [6], but the mean value is about 10—20% [7—10]. Persistent dysphagia, on the contrary, is present in percentages ranging from 0% [7,11] after floppy Nissen to 40% [12], reported by Breumelhof after traditional Nissen fundoplication. However, the values range generally from 5 to 10% [5,6,8,9,13—17].

Personal experience

Since 1985, we have performed 191 Nissen fundoplications, 85 for the therapy of GER and 106 in patients with achalasia after Heller cardiasmyotomy. Among them, 156 were operated through laparotomy (ChLt) (71 GER, 85 achalasia), and 35 by means of laparoscopy (ChLs) (14 GER, 21 achalasia).

Nissen fundoplication was performed in the same way for every patient [18,19]: 1) using only the anterior wall of the gastric fundus; 2) with stitches that remain extramucosal; 3) without cutting the short blood vessels; 4) without opening the little omentum; and 5) without approximating the diaphragmatic pillars. The operation was performed with the use of intraoperative esophageal manometry [20—22] which, after Heller, allowed documentation of LES pressure decrease to zero in all of the the achalasic patients, and calibration of the Nissen wrap to the required pressure values.

In our experience, the calibration should achieve pressure values between 20 and 40 mmHg. Such high intraoperative pressure values (hypercalibrated Nissen), compared to those obtained in a group of 15 healthy subjects (15.20 ± 2.45 mmHg), derived from the fact that GER was observed in 23.8% of those patients who were treated with calibrated fundoplication with normal pressure values (normocalibrated Nissen fundoplication) of 10—20 mmHg.

After the first intraoperative control, intraoperative esophageal manometry (IEM) after Heller showed the persistence of a high pressure zone in 28.3% of cases (30/106): this was due to an incomplete myotomy in 12.2% (13/106) and to the compression by the diaphragmatic pillars in 16% (17/106). In all 30 patients, IEM documented the decrease of the pressure to zero after divarication of the diaphragmatic pillars, or section of the residual muscle fibers; they were found at the lower part of the myotomy in seven cases, at the higher part in two cases, and more in depth in four cases.

During the operation, a lesion of the mucosa occurred in nine patients (5 ChLt, 4 ChLs), and was sutured. A conversion into laparotomy was necessary in two of the four ChLs patients.

The manometric control after Nissen fundoplication showed the following values: "sufficient" (20–40 mmHg) in 82.19% (157/191) (71 GER, 86 achalasia) and "not sufficient" (<20 mmHg) in 16.23% (31/191) (14 GER, 17 achalasia). In order to increase the pressure values in these last patients, a second layer, and sometimes a third layer, was made. In the other three patients (1.5%) who also suffered from achalasia, the intraoperative values were high (>40 mmHg). Therefore, it was necessary to redo the fundoplication, after cutting the previous stitches.

The pressure values were: 1) 25.32 ± 5.73 mmHg for a length of 2.81 ± 0.46 cm in patients with an abnormal GER; and 2) 24.71 ± 4.92 mmHg for a length of 2.88 ± 0.56 cm in those who suffered from achalasia. These values are higher (p < 0.001) than the preoperative ones in patients with GER (7.02 ± 3.46 mmHg) and in healthy subjects.

The death rate was 1% (2/191): the first patient died because he vomited the complete meal he had eaten the day after the operation (Boheraave syndrome); the second one, a cirrhotic patient, died of hepatic failure, due to portal thrombosis.

The clinical follow-up made on 85 patients suffering from an abnormal GER (44.6 ± 15.09 months) and on 104 with achalasia (43.39 ± 14.25 months), showed a transitory dysphagia in 10 patients (5.2%) (four GER, six achalasia), and a gas bloat syndrome (transitory too) in four (2.1%) (three GER, one achalasia); both consequences disappeared spontaneously in 3 months.

A light persistent dysphagia was found in 26 patients (13.7%) (seven GER, 19 achalasia). However, they considered that the result was good, because the symptom did not hinder a normal alimentation and did not require any consumption of drugs. Three patients (1.5%) reported a chest pain; two of them were part of a group of 11 persons who were affected by "vigorous achalasia" (*achalasia vigorosa*), the third patient suffered from GER and showed a "herniated Nissen", which was treated with ChLs hyatoplastic operation. Only one female patient, who had been operated for GER, showed pyrosis which was correlated to GER recurrence caused by "disrupted Nissen", and necessitating a new Nissen fundoplication.

The combined esophago-gastric 24-h pH-monitoring, made on 89 patients (41 GER, 48 achalasia) (follow-up 31.82 ± 5.36 months), documented that only the patient with pyrosis showed GER recurrence. In the other 88 patients, the test documented that refluxes were completely absent, even the postprandial ones (hypercompetent Nissen).

The esophageal manometry (follow-up 30.94 ± 5.48 months) also documented a new HPZ pressure decrease in all cases compared to the intraoperative values (13.39 ± 4.92 mmHg, GER, 12.46 ± 4.76 mmHg achalasia, p < 0.001). In 6 months, it reached pressure values which were very close to those of our control group values and to the postoperative ones observed by others [6–9,17].

The dynamic study of new HPZ documented a postdeglutitive relaxation of 75.91 ± 14.37% in patients with abnormal reflux and of 73.22 ± 16.04% in those ones with achalasia. These results are in accordance with those of Lind (1965, 1969) and Siewert (1973, 1976) on the capability of relaxation of the anterior wall of the gastric fundus during swallowing. This relaxation was less significant than that of a control group (95.53 ± 3.99%) showing the persistence of a residual pressure gradient. This observation was also reported by DeMeester et al. [8].

The study of the esophageal body in patients with abnormal reflux did not show significant modifications, compared to preoperative motor activity.

In fact, after Nissen fundoplication new serious disturbances of the esophageal body were observed. In six patients with achalasia, the reappearance of the peristaltic waves in 46% of the postdeglutitive motor activity was documented. The endoscopic follow-up (40.24 ± 6.47 months) showed no esophagitis.

Discussion

The analysis of the results is not easy because it is necessary to estimate: 1) the obstruction caused by a Nissen fundoplication; 2) the preoperative existence (or absence) of serious motor disturbances of the esophagus.

Transitory dysphagia is commonly reported after every Nissen procedure and disappears spontaneously in 2–12 months [6,7]. It seems to be related to the postoperative occurrence of disordered motor activity [9], which disappears within several weeks. Two cases were observed (one of whom had been operated on by us) of an aperistaltic acute megaesophagus; both of them disappeared after a medical therapy with cholinergic drugs. According to Grande et al. [6], and to our experience, transitory dysphagia disappears as the new HPZ pressure value decreases.

Persistent dysphagia is reported more frequently after traditional Nissen fundoplication (10–40%) [12,14], than after floppy Nissen (0–11.4%) [6,7]. It can be light, as happened in our experience, or it can be very severe as Low et al. reported [1], in analyzing the data of the literature from 1962 to 1986.

They report that Nissen fundoplication is the antireflux operation which is the most affected by postoperative obstructive consequences. Among 305 patients who suffered from failure of the antireflux procedure, 38% (116) had been operated with Nissen fundoplication. Persistent dysphagia was the most common symptom of this failure, as it was present in 69 of the 116 patients operated, and in 60 of them it was severe enough to require reoperation.

According to Leonardi et al. [24], persistent dysphagia was the most frequent cause of failure of Nissen fundoplication (14/25 patients). This disturbance of swallowing is due to: 1) a too tight Nissen, with partial obstruction of the esophagus (3.3%) [1]; 2) the incomplete postdeglutitive relaxation of the new HPZ and/or the occurrence of disordered motor activity (DMA) of the esophageal body (14%, 33%, 100%) [6,8,13]; and 3) an anatomical complication of the Nissen procedure, such as slipped Nissen (93.3%) [1] or herniated Nissen (16.6%) [13].

According to many authors, it is possible to reduce the occurrence of these symptoms of esophageal obstruction by a careful selection of patients. As a matter of fact, DeMeester [8] argues that patients who risk postoperative obstructive consequences are those with lower esophageal sphincter (LES) pressure >5 mmHg, with an intra-abdominal length >1.5 cm and a total LES length >2.5 cm, or with an upright reflux and/or with nonpropagating postdeglutitive motor activity, in a percentage higher than 50%.

Siewert [23] agrees with this theory: he thinks that in those patients with a serious peristaltic deficit, dysphagia is almost an unavoidable event. These patients should not be operated, such as those affected by scleroderma or other collagenopathies and diabetic neuropathy.

In our experience and in others [9,13], no correlation was found between 1) the clinical results and the presence of serious preoperative disordered motor activity (DMA); 2) the clinical results and the manometric parameters of the LES competence.

Low reported that 39.78% of the cases in which Nissen procedure had failed, showed serious, but not specific DMA, such as the presence of tertiary waves, sometimes with a high amplitude and peristaltic waves characterized by an increased duration [1]. The Nissen procedure would provoke these disturbances (DMA), not only due to the partial obstruction of the esophagus, but also because fundoplication implicates the posterior dissection of the stomach, with a consequent loss of its anchorage. So, would the conditions be met to determine a slipped Nissen, which seems to be responsible for 93.3% of the cases of permanent dysphagia.

In order to reduce the esophageal-obstruction disturbances caused by a 360° total fundoplication, several authors have modified this operation.

Floppy Nissen is an interesting modification: its first results were reported by Donahue in 1985 [7]. The procedure includes a wide mobilization of the gastric fundus with section of the short vessels and setting a big Maloney probe near the esophagus.

After this operation, there were neither serious swallowing disturbances nor slipped or herniated Nissen. However, the author reported a pH-metric GER recurrence in 3.2% of the cases and a moderate esophagitis in 11.2%, but no patient showed any persistent symptoms of GER. In conclusion, Donahue had succeeded in controlling the esophageal obstruction symptoms, but GER control was not so successful.

In 1986, DeMeester [8] defined the "technical rules" that must be observed, so that Nissen fundoplication can control GER and, at the same time, avoiding swallowing disturbances. The author divided his patients into four groups operated on with Nissen procedure, but with different technical modalities for every group; he reports that the best results were obtained with floppy Nissen.

He mobilizes the gastric fundus widely, setting a 60 F probe into the esophagus and making a wrap of 1 cm in length. In order to perform the plication, he uses stitches in the esophageal wall and strengthened with four small teflon patches, two on the stomach and two on the esophagus.

With this method, he reduced the incidence of transitory dysphagia from 83 to 39% and the incidence of persistent dysphagia from 21 to 3%. This last result was determined by a better new HPZ postdeglutitive relaxation (from 31 to 71%), correlated to: 1) the wide mobilization of the gastric fundus; and 2) the reduction of the length of the wrap (from 4 to 1 cm).

According to the author, the effectiveness of this operation on abnormal GER demonstrates that it does not create any esophageal obstruction. This modified fundoplication does not alter the total number of reflux episodes, but it reduces the number of those longer than 5 min when compared to traditional Nissen fundoplication, as it does not influence esophageal clearing.

Traditional Nissen fundoplication would alter esophageal clearing for two reasons: 1) the interference of the esophageal body on motor activity; and 2) the incomplete new HPZ postdeglutitive relaxation of a Nissen which is too short or too long.

These results were partly confirmed by others, such as Siewert [23], who notices a reduction of transitory dysphagia from 83.3 to 38.8%, using a 60 F probe instead of a 36 F one. However, gaseous disturbances were still present in the same percentages (gas bloat syndrome 11%, increased flatus 30%, inability to belch 36%) [8], and not related to the Nissen obstruction, but to aerophagy and/or to gastric disorders.

Results show that, from the experience of those who succeeded in preventing swallowing disturbances [5,7], Nissen fundoplication does not control GER perfectly. On the contrary, those who could control GER [8] observed a high incidence of gaseous disturbances.

In our opinion, this happens as it is impossible to obtain a perfect calibration of the valve, for the anatomomorphological reasons that were examined above. In fact, long-term results are strongly correlated to the functional ones derived from the operation: they cannot be accurately predicted, they are highly conditioned by several factors, such as the tone of the gastric muscle fibers, even if the same fundoplication had been performed each time.

So, the fundoplication should be calibrated with per-operative functional test, enabling one to evaluate the results obtained. Since 1972, intraoperative esophageal manometry (IEM) was proposed to allow calibration of the plication, and to reach the pressure values which are required in each case.

If the team is efficient, no more than 10 min are necessary for the IEM, the pressure values of which are not influenced by anesthetic drugs [25,26]. The use of IEM allowed control of GER in 99.4% of the patients (188/189), the exception being the patient in whom a disrupted Nissen occurred. None of the 189 patients showed GER symptoms; moreover, none of them showed endoscopic esophagitis or reflux episodes on 24-h pH-monitoring.

Swallowing disturbances resulted: 1) transitory in 10 patients (5.2%) (four GER, six achalasia); 2) persistent in 26 patients (13.7%) (seven GER, 19 achalasia); they were occasional (once or twice a week) and light, so that patients could eat normally. These results seem to be very satisfactory, associating a perfect GER control with light swallowing disturbances.

A long-term GER control is the most important aim; it can be obtained only with a hypercompetent Nissen fundoplication. Otherwise, even if the refluxes are light, they could cause serious esophagitis in patients with abnormal esophageal clearing, such as those suffering from severe esophagitis or achalasia.

From our experience, hypercalibrated Nissen fundoplication with IEM, performed routinely and independently of the type of motor activity of the esophageal body, does not determine serious esophageal obstructions; good results are evident in patients with achalasia [27,28]. Persistent dysphagia regressed in 85 patients (81.7%), persisting in a light degree and only occasionally in 18.2% (19 patients). At the same time, GER prevention was total in 100% of the cases that had been studied after the operation, with 24-h pH-monitoring and esophagoscopy.

Moreover, the reappearance of the peristaltic activity of the esophageal body, observed in six of the 48 patients with achalasia (12.5%), is the proof that IEM functional calibration prevents Nissen fundoplication from being a significant obstruction. As a matter of fact, it relaxes during swallowing without altering the motor activity of the esophageal body.

This last observation is in contrast with Low's [1] literature review; and we think that the serious postoperative DMA observed by the author in patients with post-Nissen dysphagia are not correlated to the fundoplication, but to slipped Nissen.

These complications can be prevented by performing a no-tension Nissen fundoplication after preparing the mediastinal esophagus.

Moreover, with regard to DeMeester's experience [18] concerning gaseous disturbances, it is thought that they are correlated to the wide mobilization of the gastric fundus, with consequent gastroenteric denervation.

In conclusion, Nissen procedure should be as conservative as possible: 1) without sectioning the short blood vessels, and b) without opening the little omentum.

Therefore, dangerous splenic, gastric and esophageal lesions, due to a wide mobilization of the gastric fundus, may be prevented.

References

1. Low DE, Mercer CD, Jones EC, Hill LD. Post-Nissen syndrome. Surg Gynecol Obstet 1988;167:1—5.
2. Hill LD, Thor KBA. The Hill procedure. In: Giuli R, McCallum RW (eds) Benign Lesions of the Esophagus and Cancer. Berlin, Heidelberg: Springer-Verlag, 1989;427—430.
3. Narbona B. The sling approach to the treatment of reflux peptic esophagitis (the cardiopexy with the round ligament). In: Hernia, 3rd edn. Philadelphia: Lippincot, 1988.
4. Flament JB, Plet H, Palot JP, Delattre JF, Rives J. Cardiopexy with umbilical ligament. In: Giuli R, McCallum RW (eds) Benign Lesions of the Esophagus and Cancer. Berlin, Heidelberg: Springer-Verlag, 1989;375—383.
5. Rohr S, Banzaoui H, De Manzini N, Dai B, Meyer Ch. Valeur du "floppy" Nissen dans le traitement du reflux gastro-oesophagien. A propos de 117 cas. Ann Chir 1992;46:578—583.
6. Grande L, Lacima G, Ros E et al. Dysphagia and esophageal motor dysfunction in gastroesophageal reflux are corrected by fundoplication. J Clin Gastroenterol 1991;13:11—16.
7. Donahue PE, Samelson S, Nyhus LM, Bombeck CT. The floppy Nissen fundoplication. Arch Surg 1985;120:663—668.
8. DeMeester TR, Bonavina L, Albertucci M. Nissen fundoplication for gastroesophageal reflux disease. Evaluation of primary repair in 100 consecutive patients. Ann Surg 1986;204:9—20.
9. Bancewicz J, Mughal M, Marples M. The lower oesophageal sphincter after floppy Nissen fundoplication. Br J Surg 1987; 74:162—164.

10. Kmiot WA, Kirby RM, Akinola D, Temple JG. Prospective randomized trial of Nissen fundoplication and Angelchik prosthesis in the surgical treatment of medically refractory gastroesophageal reflux disease. Br J Surg 1991;78:1181–1184.
11. Bjerkeset T, Edna TH, Fjosne U. Long-term results after "floppy" Nissen-Rossetti fundoplication for gastroesophageal reflux disease. Scand J Gastroenterol 1992;27:707–710.
12. Breumelhof R, Smout AJPM, Schyns NWRJ, Bronzwaer PWA, Akkermans LMA, Jansen A. Prospective evaluation of the effects of Nissen fundoplication on gastroesophageal reflux. Surg Gynecol Obstet 1990;171:115–119.
13. Mughal MM, Bancewicz J, Marples M. Oesophageal manometry and pH recording do not predict the bad results of Nissen fundoplication. Br J Surg 1989;77:43–45.
14. Shirazi SS, Schulze K, Soper RT. Long-term follow-up for treatment of complicated chronic reflux esophagitis. Arch Surg 1987;122:548–552.
15. Ackermann CH, Margreth L, Muller C. Symptoms 10 to 20 years after fundoplication. In: Siewert JR, Hölscher AH (eds) Diseases of the Esophagus. New York: Springer-Verlag, 1987;1198–1202.
16. O'Hanrahan T, Marples M, Bancewicz J. Recurrent reflux and wrap disruption after Nissen fundoplication: detection, incidence and timing. Br J Surg 1989;77:545–547.
17. Ellis FH: Results of the Nissen procedure. In: Giuli R, McCallum RW (eds) Benign Lesions of the Esophagus and Cancer. Berlin, Heidelberg: Springer-Verlag, 1989:397–399.
18. Lanzara A, Del Genio A. La fundoplicatio sec. Nisse. Arch Atti Soc Ital Chir 1979;1:813–826.
19. Rossetti M. Results of the Nissen procedure. In: Giuli R, McCallum RW (eds) Benign Lesions of the Esophagus and Cancer. Berlin, Heidelberg: Springer-Verlag, 1989;403–409.
20. Lanzara A. Manometria esofagea intraoperatoria: 10 anni di esperienza personale. Min Chir 1983;38:1673.
21. Del Genio A. La nostra esperienza in tema di elettromanometria esofagea. Acad Scien Med Palermo. 1978;12(suppl 1): 59–69.
22. Del Genio A, Di Martino N, Fei L et al. Manometria esofagea intraoperatoria. Relazione al SANITEC 1987. Simposio su "I disordini della motilità esofago-gastro-duodenale: aspetti di fisiopatologia, diagnosi e cenni di terapia", Torino 10 maggio 1987. Proceedings: 99–105.
23. Siewert JR, Feussner H. Early and long-term results of antireflux surgery: a critical look. In: Tytgat GNJ (ed) Baillière's Clinical Gastroenterology. London: Baillière Tindall-WB Saunders, 1987;821–842.
24. Leonardi HK, Crozier RE, Ellis FH. Reoperation for complications of the Nissen fundoplication. J Thorac Cardiovasc Surg 1981;51:50–56.
25. Del Genio A, Izzo G, Maffettone V et al. Reflusso Gastro-esofageo (RGE). Relazione al 95° Congr Soc Ital Chir, Milano 17–20 ottobre 1993. Congress Proceedings (in press).
26. Del Genio A, Fei L, Izzo G, Di Martino N, Maffettone V, Ambrosio A, Amato G. Indicazioni e limiti dell'intervento di Nissen. Atti IX Incontri di Chirurgia a Foggia. Gerni Edn., 1989:49–51.
27. Del Genio A, Maffettone V, Izzo G et al. Acalasia dell'esofago. Atti dei Seminari Irpini di Gastroenterologia, 1986:5–38.
28. Di Martino N, Maffettone V, Fei L et al. La fundoplicatio sec. Nissen associata a cardiasmiotomia sec. Heller per acalasia esofagea. Comunic. al VIII Congresso Nazionale della Sezione Italiana del Collegium Internationale Chirurgiae Digestivae, Bologna 19–21 maggio 1987. Proceeding Tomo I:443–449, 1987.

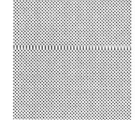

What are the risk factors for morbidity in Nissen's operation?

M. Celerier (Paris)

Nissen's operation is the most effective procedure for the treatment of gastroesophageal reflux (GER) [1–4] but it still retains a significant morbidity [5].

More important risk factors can be deduced from analysis of a personal series of 201 patients and of other major series of conventional surgical operations.

The arrival of laparoscopic surgery, however, may well upset our near-certainties.

629

Will this procedure be a copy of the operation which is accepted as the best possible? Whether or not does it carry an unacceptable mortality? What is its morbidity? Can pneumoperitoneum cause a flare-up of mediastinitis after perioperative perforation of the esophagus or stomach? Persistent rumours give rise to a sense of urgency. Clearly, conclusions about long-term results cannot be drawn from the current literature, but operative morbidity was very small (2%) in an impressive series of 197 patients over the period of less than 2 years [6].

This study will be confined to the knowledge gained from conventional surgery.
— Operative mortality: 0%
— Operative morbidity: 10% (12%) [7]
   · gastroesophageal tears
   · tears of the spleen
   · subphrenic abscess
   · complications of associated procedures
— Long-term morbidity:
   The list is long, and the incidence is high:
   · Dysphagia: 21—44% [1,3,7]
   · Inability to vomit: 31—63% [1,7], or belch: 19—36% [1,7]
   · Epigastric distension: 21% [1], and flatulence: 50% [1]
   · Persistent esophagitis: 25% [9—11], either found after operation or as Barrett's esophagus
   · Changes in the valve ranging from displacement towards the body of the stomach: 25% [11—14], to complete disruption: 8—9% [10,15]
   · Intrathoracic migration of the site of fundoplication [5,13,16,17]
   · Gastric ulcers and fistulas: 3—9% [5,18—22].
What, then, are the risk factors and, once identified, how can they be obviated?

Operative morbidity

Esophageal tears

Esophagitis because the esophagus may become fragile as a result of inflammation around it. This is becoming rare because patients are only referred to a surgeon now after considerable delay for effective treatment with antacids.

Short esophagus may also cause problems, but in practice this risk must be very small in the light of the extensive series carried out purely through the abdomen. It could be overcome by elongating the esophagus by section/stapling of the fundus of the stomach.

Reoperation. The risk of esophageal tears is certainly increased by reoperation [23,24]. Nevertheless, it is better to use the abdominal route again [25,26] because of the lower morbidity. Complete diversion of the duodenum may be very helpful.

Tears of the stomach

Reoperation increases the risk once again.

"Gas-bloat" syndrome may lead to tearing over the sutures in fragile valves [12,17]. It is wise to avoid this by leaving a gastric tube in place until normal transit through the bowel is re-established [5].

Tears of the spleen

The incidence of about 7% in some series is always surprising [17]. There were three cases in our series of 201 patients (1.5%). Release of the fundus from below upwards and from the front backwards under the left ribs makes this accident unusual. A small tear does not involve splenectomy.

Possible role of associated procedures

Vagotomy. This is debatable as a supplementary procedure to an antireflux valve, but it may be considered if there is also an ulcer. The risk of "gas-bloat syndrome" may be increased. Highly selective vagotomy which impairs the blood supply to the lesser curvature carries the risk of gastric necrosis. Truncal vagotomy with pyloroplasty or gastroenterostomy may be preferred.

Perioperative dilation of a peptic stenosis may be a risk factor [7,27,28]. There is now agreement that premedical treatment is preferable with progressive preoperative dilations.

Late morbidity

The long-term results depend on the reason for operation after failure of medical treatment for at least 6 months:
— established lesions of the esophageal mucosa, and/or;
— pathological reflux on 24-h pH-recording, incompetence of the lower sphincter;
— Barrett's esophagus (large sliding or paraesophageal hernias with symptoms, surgical reduction of which may lead to incompetence of the sphincter) [29].
The elapsed time since operation is a very important factor, and 5 years must pass before "definitive" results can be established using appropriate criteria [30–32].

Dysphagia

There appear to be two determining factors: 1) a valve which is too long, 2) a valve which is too tight (Nissen-Rossetti).
   A too-tight valve is caused by inadequate mobilization of the fundus; a large part of the stomach must be loosened in order to relieve the tension in the sutures [1]. The

calibre of the esophagus should be 40 French [23,26,33] to 60 French [1]. In our experience the valve is 6~1.5 cm in length. Temporary dysphagia has been shown [1] to have decreased from 83 to 39%, and persistent dysphagia from 14 to 3%.

Inability to vomit or belch

Epigastric distension and flatulence

Epigastric distension and flatulence appear to respond in a manner which is inversely proportional, as might be expected.

Few patients, however, complain of difficulty with eructation when they recall the symptoms of reflux which they had before the operation. The risk factors are the same as for dysphagia.

Esophagitis

This is found more frequently on endoscopy as the period of monitoring extends — which does not make it a risk factor (18%) [7]. The basic reason for finding it appears to be breakdown of the fundoplication [7].

Barrett's esophagus

At present, it is not possible to ensure that this improves after a Nissen operation. It may be that the risk of deterioration is reduced. In any event, when severe dysplasia is found during preoperative investigations, the operation required is no longer a Nissen procedure, but esophagectomy with esophagoplasty.

Changes in the valve

Migration towards the body of the stomach may occur in Barrett's esophagus, and if the valve is not fixed to the anterior aspect of the esophagus.

Total breakdown which is a complication of "gas-bloat" syndrome in the post-operative period is caused by the use of absorbable suture material and sutures under tension. It is important to emphasize the importance of the sutures in the valve. Our technique is to use sutures *supported* by four Teflon strips [1].

Movement into the chest

This is the result of failure to close the crura correctly. This procedure may be difficult. It may thus be associated with fixation of the fundoplication to the diaphragm.

Gastric ulcers and fistulas

Ulcers of the body of the stomach are due to stasis following injury to the vagus nerves [18] or alkaline reflux [20]. Bronchial or aortic fistulas occur more commonly when there is intrathoracic fundoplication or following surgery for relapse [19,22].

Conclusion

Nissen's operation, through the abdominal approach with a short complete valve attached to the anterior aspect of the esophagus and sutured without tension but with strips, is certainly the best way of preventing gastresophageal reflux at present.

The future will reveal whether laparoscopic surgery will alter the current situation as far as mortality and morbidity are concerned.

References

1. DeMeester TR, Bonavina L, Albertucci M. Nissen fundoplication for gastroesophageal reflux disease. Ann Surg 1986;204:9–20.
2. Donahue PE, Samelson S, Nyhus LM et al. The floppy Nissen fundoplication. Arch Surg 1985;120:663–668.
3. Ackermann Ch, Margareth L, Muller C et al. Symptoms 10–20 years after fundoplication. In: Siewert JR, Hölscher AH (eds) Diseases of the Esophagus. Berlin Heidelberg: Springer Verlag, 1988;1198–1202.
4. Negre JB, Markkula HY, Keyrilainen O et al. Nissen fundoplication: results at 10-year follow-up. Am J Surg 1983;146:635–638.
5. Gossot D, Sarfati E, Azoulay D, Celerier M. Facteurs de morbidité de l'intervention de Nissen. J Chir (Paris) 1987;124:367–371.
6. Dallemagne B, Weerts JM, Jehaes C, Markiewicz S, Lombard R. Techniques and results of endoscopic fundoplication. Endosc Surg 1993;1:72–76.
7. Luostarinen ME. Nissen fundoplication for reflux esophagitis. Ann Surg 1993;217:329–337.
8. Negre JB. Postfundoplication symptoms: do they restrict the success of Nissen fundoplication? Ann Surg 1983;198:689–700.
9. Johnsson F, Joelsson B, Gudmundsson K et al. Effects of fundoplication on the antireflux mechanism. Br J Surg 1987;74:1111–1114.
10. O'Hanrahan T, Marples M, Bancewicz J. Recurrent reflux and wrap disruption after Nissen fundoplicaiton: detection, incidence and timing. Br J Surg 1990;77:545–547.
11. Thor K, Silander T. A long-term randomized prospective trial of the Nissen procedure versus a modified Toupet technique. Ann Surg 1989;210:719–724.
12. Menguy R. A modified fundoplication which preserves the ability to belch. Surgery 1978;84:301–307.
13. Skinner DB. Complications of surgery for gastroesophageal reflux. World J Surg 1977;1:485–491.
14. Hill LD, Ilves R, Stevenson JK, Pearson JM. Reoperation for disruption and recurrence after Nissen fundoplication. Arch Surg 1979;114:542–548.
15. Feussner H, Petri A, Walker S et al. The modified AFP score: an attempt to make the results of antireflux surgery comparable. Br J Surg 1991;78:942–946.
16. Leonardi HK, Ellis FH. Complication of the Nissen fundoplication. Surg Clin North Am 1983;91:371–378.
17. Polk HC. Fundoplication for reflux esophagitis: misadventures with the operation of choice. Ann Surg 1976;183:645–650.
18. Buskin FL, Woodward ER, O'Leary JP. Occurrence of gastric ulcer after Nissen fundoplication. Am J Surg 1976;42:821–826.
19. Campbell R, Kennedy T, Johnston GW. Gastric ulceration after Nissen fundoplication. Br J Surg 1983;70:406–407.
20. Bremner CG. Gastric ulceration after a fundoplication operation for gastroesophageal reflux. Surg Gynecol Obstet 1979;148:62–64.
21. Low DE, Mercer CD, James EC et al. Post-Nissen syndrome. Surg Gynecol Obstet 1988;167:1–5.
22. Richardson JD, Larson GM, Polk HC Jr. Intrathoracic fundoplication for shortened esophagus: treacherous solution to a challenging problem. Am J Surg 1982;143:29–35.
23. Henderson RD, Marryat GV. Total fundoplication gastroplasty (Nissen gastroplasty): five-year review. Ann Thorac Surg 1985;39:74–79.
24. Little AG, Ferguson MK, Skinner DB. Reoperation for failed antireflux operations. J Thorac Cardiovasc Surg 1986;91:511–517.
25. Baulieux J, Janody P, Mondesert C, Peix JL. Chirurgie itérative du reflux gastro-oesophagien. A propos de 41 cas. Lyon Chir 1985;81:370–374.

26. Saubier EC, Gouillat C, Teboul F. Traitement du reflux gastro-oesophagien par fundoplicature complète de Nissen. Résultats de 112 observations. Chirurgie 1986;112:123−131.
27. Mercer CD, Hill LD. Surgical management of peptic esophageal strictures. Twenty year experience. J Thorac Cardiovasc Surg 1986;91:371−378.
28. Watson A. The role of antireflux surgery combined with fiberoptic endoscopic dilatation in peptic esophageal stricture. Am J Surg 1984;148:346−349.
29. Kaul BK, DeMeester TR, Oka M. The cause of dysphagia in uncomplicated sliding hiatal hernia and its relief by hiatal herniorraphy. Ann Surg 1990;211:410−415.
30. DeMeester TR, Johnson LF, Joseph GJ et al. Patterns of gastroesophageal reflux in health and disease. Ann Surg 1976; 184:459−470.
31. Visick AH. Measured radical gastrectomy. Review of 505 operations for peptic ulcer. Lancet 1948;1:505−510.
32. DeMeester TR, Johnson LF. The evaluation of objective measurements of gastroesophageal reflux and their management. Surg Clin North Am 1976;56:39−53.
33. Vankemmel M. Etude comparée schématique de quatre procédés de correction du reflux gastro-oesophagien par voie abdominale. J Chir 1982;119:295−301.

What factors, other than mechanical ones, are involved in the syndrome of gastric distension?

G.G. Jamieson (Adelaide)

The syndrome of gastric distension (also called the gas bloat syndrome when it occurs after surgery) has not been much studied. For this reason, perhaps, the syndrome has not been well characterized. It is usually regarded as comprising symptoms such as early postprandial satiety, a feeling of postprandial bloatedness and sometimes ill-defined postprandial discomfort and/or pain.

Gastric distension can be caused by gas, liquids or solids. There is no doubt that some patients with reflux disease swallow air more frequently than normal. The finding that patients with reflux disease often have disordered secondary peristaltic mechanisms lends some weight to this fact [1]. Thus when reflux episodes occur, instead of clearing them by secondary peristalsis, the patient has to initiate a swallow which may clear the esophagus but also leads to the swallowing of air. When solids and liquids are ingested, it has been found that some patients with reflux disease have delayed gastric emptying of both solids and liquids, which can lead to a sense of fullness after eating [2−4]. Changes in gastric motor function are of interest as transient relaxations of the lower esophageal sphincter may be triggered from the distended stomach [5] leading to gastroesophageal reflux. Fundoplication not only effectively controls pathological gastroesophageal reflux, but also improves gastric emptying [6−8]. The significance of changes in these motor events for the success of these operations has not been established. However, disturbances in gastric emptying may be involved in the genesis of postfundoplication symptoms and influence the risk of failure after fundoplication [7,9]. This issue is of clinical significance, but more knowledge of the mechanisms behind postfundoplication symptoms is needed.

Recently, we investigated gastric motor function by determining the emptying of a labeled mixed solid and liquid meal in 81 patients with long-standing severe gastroesophageal reflux disease before antireflux surgery. The study was repeated postoperatively in 47 of the patients. The gastric emptying parameters were analyzed in relation to the clinical outcome of operation, in order to determine if they had any predictive value for the development of postfundoplication symptoms.

Preoperative delayed gastric emptying of solids predicted persistent postoperative complaints of "gas bloat" type, with the predominant symptoms being postprandial satiety and pain. Liquid emptying was correlated only with transient postoperative complaints. Odynophagia and inability to belch and relieve bloating were associated with persistent prolonged emptying after operation. These results demonstrate that preoperative gastric motor function may influence the outcome of antireflux surgery. Preoperative gastric emptying studies may help predict those patients with gastro-esophageal reflux disease who will suffer from postfundoplication complaints of a "gas bloat" nature. Although these correlations were significant, they contributed only about 25% of the influence on the symptoms of gas bloat, so clearly other unidentified factors must play an important role in this syndrome.

References

1. Schoeman MN, Tippett M, Dent J, Holloway RH. Integrity and characteristics of secondary peristalsis in patients with gastroesophageal reflux disease. Gastroenterology 1981;80:285–291.
2. McCallum RW, Berkowitz DM, Lerner E. Gastric emptying in patients with gastroesophageal reflux. Gastroenterology 1981;80:285–291.
3. Maddern GJ, Chatterton BE, Collins PJ, Horowitz M, Shearman DJC, Jamieson GG. Solid and liquid emptying in patients with gastro-oesophageal reflux. Br J Surg 1985; 72:344–347.
4. Schwizer W, Hinder RA, DeMeester TR. Does delayed gastric emptying contribute to gastroesophageal reflux disease? Am J Surg 1989;157:74–81.
5. Holloway RH, Dent J. Lower esophageal sphincter dysfunction in gastroesophageal reflux disease. Gastroenterol Clin North Am 1990;19:517–535.
6. Maddern GJ, Jamieson GG. Fundoplication enhances gastric emptying. Ann Surg 1985;201:296–299.
7. Hinder RA, Stein HJ, Bremner CG, DeMeester TR. Relationship of a satisfactory outcome to normalization of delayed gastric emptying after Nissen fundoplication. Ann Surg 1989;210:458–465.
8. Jamieson GG, Maddern GJ, Myers JC. Gastric emptying after fundoplication with and without proximal gastric vagotomy. Arch Surg 1991;126:1414–1417.
9. Maddern GJ, Jamieson GG, Chatterton BE, Collins PJ. Is there an association between failed antireflux procedures and delayed gastric emptying? Ann Surg 1985;202:1162–1165.

What are the causes of failure of Nissen's operation?

H.J. Stein, J.R. Siewert, H. Feussner (Munich)

Nissen fundoplication has become the most popular of the antireflux procedures in patients with gastroesophageal reflux disease. Recent series show a long-term success rate of over 90% with this procedure. This is superior to any currently available medical treatment option [1,2].

Failure of Nissen fundoplication occurs when the patient, after the repair, experiences persistent or recurrent reflux symptoms, is unable to swallow normally, or suffers from upper abdominal discomfort or other gastrointestinal symptoms. The assessment of these symptoms and the selection of patients who need further surgery remains a challenging problem.

Recurrence or persistence of reflux symptoms (i.e., heartburn and regurgitation) and postoperative persistent dysphagia are the most common indicators for failure of Nissen fundoplication. Recurrent or persistent reflux symptoms and/or dysphagia occur in about 8% of patients after Nissen fundoplication. In a series of 50 patients who required reoperation after a failed Nissen fundoplication, heartburn and regurgitation were the most common presenting symptoms [3]. The prevalence of persistent dysphagia showed a marked decrease after 1983 (Fig. 1). This may reflect a change in the operative techniques and a subsequent change in the reasons for failure of the antireflux procedure in the past 20 years. Weight loss and the so-called gas bloat syndrome were a rare cause of failure before and after 1983 (Fig. 1).

The quality, intensity and time course of the patients' symptoms cannot be used frequently to determine the cause of failure. A thorough diagnostic work-up is essential in each patient. This includes contrast radiography and endoscopy of the upper gastrointestinal tract as well as functional tests. Contrast roentgenography may identify the presence, status and location of the wrap. In general, motion-recording contrast radiography (i.e., cine- or video fluoroscopy) is preferable to standard barium swallows to delineate alterations in anatomy caused by the previous surgical procedure. Endoscopy with biopsy is essential to assess the presence of esophagitis. In addition, the state of the fundoplication can be determined by observing the typical

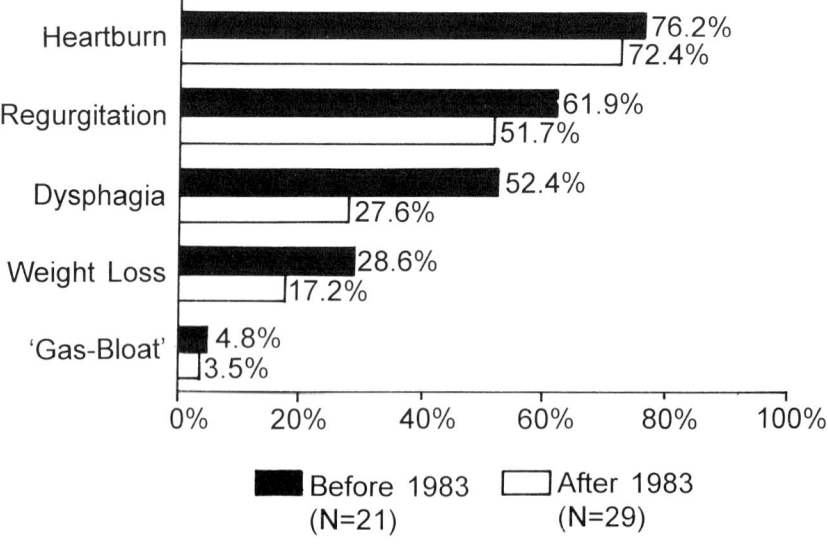

Fig. 1. Presenting symptoms of patients requiring a redo antireflux procedure before and after 1993.

"Nissen nipple" on retroflexion of the endoscope [4]. Manometry and 24-h esophageal pH monitoring are required to evaluate the function of the lower esophageal sphincter, assess motor abnormalities of the esophageal body and objectively quantitate the presence and amount of gastroesophageal reflux. Gastric denervation and emptying disorders should be evaluated with scintigraphic techniques [5].

Persistent or recurrent postoperative reflux symptoms are usually due a breakdown of the repair and can be treated by a repeat antireflux procedure or acid suppression therapy. In contrast, postoperative dysphagia or a combination of dysphagia and reflux symptoms may be due to a myriad of causes which include a too tightly constructed wrap, a slipped wrap, a wrap that has been placed too low around the proximal stomach, development of a stricture, the presence of a motor disorder of the esophageal body, or a combination of these factors (Fig. 2). These situations frequently can not be solved by a simple redo fundoplication [3].

Wrap disruption has become the most common cause of failure in the past 10 years [3]. It frequently occurs early during the postoperative course [4]. This reflects the widespread use of absorbable suture material when creating the wrap. Inadequate suture technique (i.e., taking inadequate bites of tissue) and insufficient mobilization of the fundus may also contribute to wrap disruption.

The creation of a too tight or too long wrap is manifested by persistent dysphagia starting immediately after the antireflux procedure. Postoperative manometry in these patients shows a high-pressure sphincter which does not relax on swallowing.

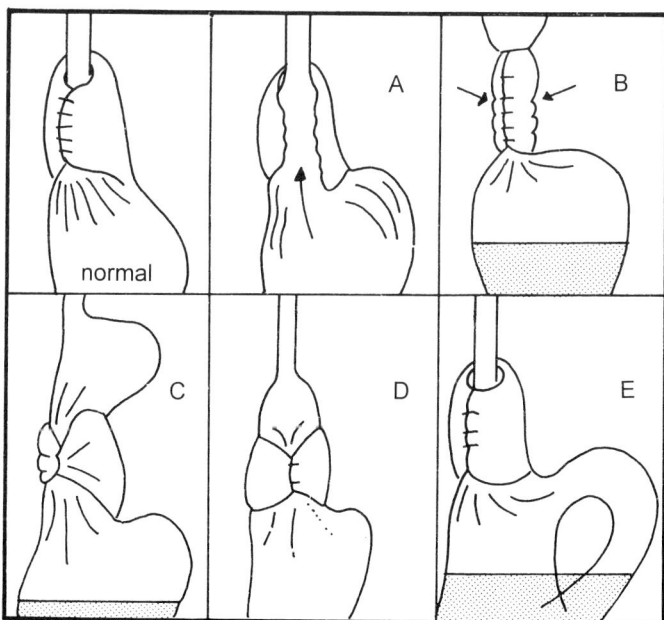

Fig. 2. Schematic representation of the reasons for failure of Nissen fundoplication: A) wrap disruption; B) too tight and too long wrap; C) "slipped Nissen"; D) wrap around the stomach; E) gastric denervation.

Manometry occasionally may also demonstrate simultaneous contractions in the esophageal body in these patients. Creation of a too tight or too long wrap was a common cause of failure prior to 1983. This was due to a misperception of the mechanism of action of a fundoplication. An increased awareness of the principles of constructing a fundoplication (i.e., careful fundic mobilization and construction of a short and loose wrap around a large bougie) has resulted in a marked decrease of too tight or too long wraps in the past years [6,7].

The so-called telescope phenomenon or "slipped Nissen" develops when the proximal part of the stomach slides through the wrap [8]. A predisposition for the telescope phenomenon to occur is most often created at the time of surgery when the fundus of the stomach is not mobilized, or when unrecognized esophageal shortening and inadequate mobilization of the esophagus lead to a wrapping of stomach around stomach, rather than stomach around the lower esophagus. In this situation, dysphagia and heartburn are present immediately after surgery because of a partial obstruction and reflux from the acid producing proximal stomach which lies above the wrap.

Slipping of the wrap can also occur gradually during the postoperative period if the sutures are not passed through the esophageal wall or cardia. These patients usually complain of heartburn and dysphagia occurring after a symptom free postoperative interval.

Gastric denervation symptoms (i.e., abdominal fullness, meteorism, delayed emptying and/or diarrhea) result from damage to the vagus nerve during antireflux surgery. With meticulous surgical technique, vagal injury can be avoided completely.

Inappropriate patient selection will also lead to dissatisfaction of the patient postoperatively [9]. This most often occurs when the operation has been performed for symptoms in the absence of objective documentation of the disease, or when the presence of a severe esophageal motor disorder (i.e., achalasia) is not realized. Careful assessment with 24-h esophageal pH monitoring and manometry in all patients, prior to considering antireflux surgery, will minimize the incidence of such problems.

This analysis of the reasons for failure of Nissen fundoplication indicate that several factors are essential for a successful outcome after fundoplication. These are: 1) the identification and careful selection of patients who might benefit from antireflux surgery; 2) a meticulous surgical technique; and 3) a sound understanding of the principles of antireflux surgery. Attention to these factors will avoid failures in most instances.

References

1. Nissen R. Eine einfache Operation zur Beeinflussung der Refluxoesophagitis. Schweiz Med Wochenschr 1956;86:590–592.
2. Siewert JR, Feussner H, Walker SJ. Fundoplication: how to do it? Peri-esophageal wrapping as therapeutic principle in gastroesophageal reflux prevention. World J Surg 1992;16:326–334.
3. Siewert JR, Isolauri J, Feussner H. Reoperation following failed fundoplication. World J Surg 1989;13:791.
4. O'Hanrahan T, Marples M, Bancewicz J. Recurrent reflux and wrap disruption after Nissen fundoplication: detection, incidence, timing. Br J Surg 1990;77:545–547.
5. Stein HJ, DeMeester TR, Hinder RA. Outpatient physiologic testing and surgical management of foregut motility disorders. Cur Probl Surg 1992;29:415–555.
6. Donahue PE, Samelson S, Nyhus LN, Bombeck CT. The floppy Nissen fundoplication. Arch Surg 1985;120:663–668.

7. DeMeester TR, Stein HJ. Minimizing the side effects of antireflux surgery. World J Surg 1992;16:335–336.
8. Siewert JR, Lepsien G, Weiser HF, Schattenmann G, Peiper HJ. Das Teleskop-Phänomen Chirurg 1979;48:640.
9. Stein HJ, DeMeester TR. Who benefits from antireflux surgery? World J Surg 1992;16:313–319.

What are the causes of motor disorders after a failed Nissen procedure?

C. Iascone (Rome)

Despite Nissen fundoplication being the most popular antireflux procedure, there are still unsatisfactory results in 10–15% of the patients. They may be attributable to misdiagnosis, errors in technical execution and patient selection. Manometry can distinguish the various types of esophageal motor disorders in this group of patients. We performed a manometric study according to the technique described by Winans et al. [1] in 13 symptomatic patients after a Nissen antireflux procedure (group A). The results were compared with a group of 10 normal subjects (group B). The lower esophageal sphincter (LES) pressure was 10.7 ± 8.1 mmHg in group A, and 13.5 ± 5.7 mmHg in group B ($p = $ N.S.). Six out of the 13 patients (46%) had LES pressure below 6 mmHg in group A and zero out of the 10 in group B ($p < 0.04$). Abnormal motor activity in the body of the esophagus (peristaltic waves <70% and/or low amplitude waves >40%) was present in five out of the 13 patients (38%) in group A, and zero out of the 10 subjects in group B ($p = $ N.S.). Two patients had both LES hypotension and peristalsis derangement: one patient had Barrett's esophagus at endoscopy and the other had hyperemic esophagitis with disabling heartburn and regurgitation, in spite of intensive therapy with H_2-antagonists and prokinetics. According to Skinner et al. [2], we found that LES incompetence, esophageal dysmotility and the association of both findings are often present in patients with a failed Nissen procedure. The causes of sphincter mechanism failure are considered as technical, and related to surgery. Commonly, the placement of sutures too shallow in the esophageal wall, or under tension because of inadequate mobilization of the esophagus leads to the disruption of the antireflux valve. Valve disruption was present in 75% of patients with recurrent reflux after Nissen procedure in the series of O'Hanrahan et al. [3]. These data confirm that recurrence of reflux is mainly due to the failure of Nissen fundoplication to restore competence of gastroesophageal junction and consequently prevent reflux of gastric juice into the esophagus [4]. Low et al. [5] found evidence of nonspecific motor abnormalities, which, in most instances, were not present prior to the fundoplication, in 40% of a large series of 116 patients requiring reoperation after failed Nissen procedures. They suggest that there may be two causes of dysmotility. A tight Nissen fundoplication may partially obstruct the esophagus, resulting in high amplitude and nonperistaltic or tertiary contractions. Furthermore, as a consequence of dissection of the normal posterior attachment of the distal esophagus required to perform the fundoplication, the esophagus, no longer anchored, may contribute to disrupted motility. The most common cause of a combined failure is the slipped Nissen, which was present in 48% of patients in the series of Low et al. [5]. A part of the stomach is then located above the slipped wrap that acts as an obstruction, so that acid pools and refluxes freely in the esophagus. The impairment of esophageal motor activity, probably due to the obstruction, makes reflux worse so that the patients with this pattern will have very severe clinical disturbances, as we saw in two subjects with both LES incompetence and esophageal motor abnormalities. Most of these patients require reoperation [6]. The potential for Nissen fundoplication to cause esophageal clearance failure is confirmed by the study of Skinner et al. [6], where 25 out of 29 patients had clearance failure after Nissen antireflux procedure, compared to 16 out of 49 patients having this problem after other antireflux operations (p < 0.001). In our opinion the Belsey Mark IV procedure is the most suitable operation in these subjects, as it is looser than the Nissen wrap and easier to perform, as transthoracic approach gives an adhesion-free operative field.

References

1. Winans CS, Harris LD. Quantitation of lower esophageal sphincter competence. Gastroenterology 1967;52:773–778.
2. Skinner DB, Klementschitsch AG, DeMeester TR, Belsey RH. Assessment of failed antireflux repairs. In: DeMeester TR and Skinner DB (eds) Esophageal Disorders: Pathophysiology and Therapy. New York: Raven Press, 1985;303.
3. O'Hanrahan T, Marples M, Bancewicz J. Recurrent reflux and wrap disruption after Nissen fundoplication: detection, incidence and timing. Br J Surg 1990;77:545–547.
4. Goodall RJR, Temple JG. Effect of Nissen fundoplication on competence of the gastroesophageal junction. Gut 1980;21:607.
5. Low DE, Mercer CD, James EC, Hill LD. Post-Nissen syndrome. Surg Gynecol Obstet 1988;167:1–5.
6. Skinner DB. Surgical management after failed antireflux operations. World J Surg 1992;16:359.

Can the valve itself interfere with gastric emptying?

A. Moraldi, C. Iascone, P. Ginevri, C.U. Casciani (Rome)

Eleven years ago, at the Second International Symposium on Esophageal Disorders held in Chicago, May 1983, we presented a paper on the role of gastric emptying (GE) in patients with gastroesophageal reflux (GER). At that time, it was concluded that delayed GE could be present both in patients with proven GER, as well as in those symptomatic patients with negative 24-h pH-monitoring or absence of esophagitis at endoscopy. These patients, with equivocal symptoms of GER, may present an underlying functional pathology of the stomach which is difficult to assess and must be carefully studied [1].

In fact, a few years later we showed that, in patients with GER and associated gastric pathology, there was a higher incidence of delayed GE with more frequent and severe symptoms than in patients without gastric disorder [2].

In physiological conditions, the proximal stomach is responsible for gastric emptying of liquids, while the distal stomach plays a major role in emptying of solids. More recently, however, it has been shown that, in patients with GER and delayed gastric emptying for solids, the delay is due to retention in the proximal stomach and slow transit of solids from proximal to distal stomach [3]. These results support the concept that the fundus and body of the stomach may play a more fundamental role in emptying of solids than is usually acknowledged.

At present, it can be said that delayed gastric emptying occurs with equal frequency in patients with and without reflux, and that GER is not associated with delayed gastric emptying. In fact, even if 30–40% of patients with GER show a delayed GE, the mean gastric emptying curve in all patients with reflux lies well within the limits of normal GE.

Still controversial is the point whether a delayed GE may or may not be associated with reflux esophagitis, some investigators having reported this association [4,5], and others not [6,7], raising the question whether delayed emptying plays any role in the pathophysiology of GER disease.

Patients with GER resistant to medical therapy are successfully treated by fundoplication and it is interesting to note the resolution, in most cases, of other nonspecific symptoms of reflux such as nausea, early satiety, vomiting or bloating. Now the question is: is there any relationship between fundoplication and gastric emptying? If yes, how does the fundoplication work?

It is known from physiology that before a bolus of food enters the stomach from the esophagus, relaxation of the proximal stomach occurs. This relaxation is followed by a more prolonged "accommodation" in response to gastric distension [8].

After fundoplication, this capacity of accommodation and receptive relaxation of the proximal stomach will be abolished, similar to the situation with proximal gastric vagotomy, thus causing a pressure increase. This increase in pressure of the fundus of the stomach will accelerate both the emptying of solids and liquids, either for a greater gastric wall tension or for the promotion of antral peristalsis.

In our opinion, there are at least three reasons why fundoplication interferes with gastric emptying:
— the diminution in capacity of the proximal stomach (with fundoplication) will enhance antral peristalsis and accelerate gastric emptying;
— peristaltic contractions in the presence of a mechanically competent sphincter will increase intragastric pressure, favoring gastric emptying;
— reduction of the radius of the proximal stomach by fundoplication increases the rate of gastric emptying, a mechanism that could be explained by Laplace's law.

Since 1985, some investigators assessed GE before and after fundoplication [9]. They concluded that GE of both solids and liquids tended to be increased following fundoplication, this enhancement of emptying possible being a further mechanism by which this procedure achieves its good results.

In fact, as confirmed by a following study from the same authors [10], patients with recurrence of reflux symptoms after surgery showed a significant delay in GE of both solids and liquids, compared to a control group of patients who had undergone a standard fundoplication. The authors did not know whether the delayed emptying in the failed operative group was responsible for the failure of antireflux surgery, but certainly delayed GE before or after surgery could be of value in predicting patients likely to have poor outcomes.

The importance of the normalization of gastric emptying after fundoplication with absence of symptoms and, on the other hand, the persistence of symptoms only in those patients with pre-existing gastric disturbances, is stressed by other investigators [11].

They report that, in those patients with recurrence of symptoms, gastric emptying was abnormal after surgery, due to a concomitant gastric pathology in most of the cases.

The importance of the integrity of the gastric mucosa on the emptying of the stomach was observed some years before by McCallum et al. [12] who have reported that the slow GE of solids in the population of GER patients could be correlated with the degree and severity of antral gastritis: the more severe the gastritis, the slower the gastric emptying.

Some controversies still exist on the effect of proximal gastric vagotomy associated with fundoplication on the gastric emptying.

Whereas some clinical results suggest that vagotomy is unlikely to cause delayed GE in patients with GER disease and can actually speed up gastric emptying [11], other studies support the concept that proximal vagotomy interferes with reflux pathways involved in the acceleration of solid gastric emptying after fundoplication; if delayed solid GE plays any role in the development of recurrent reflux disease, then proximal vagotomy may be seen as having a negative effect [13]. At present the following conclusions can be drawn:

- impairment (delay in most cases) of gastric emptying is a common feature in patients with GER disease, but its interpretation has still to be defined: coincidence of two frequent disorders, or physiopathologic relationship between gastric stasis and GER?
- Patients who undergo antireflux surgery improve their clinical status, and clinical results suggest that fundoplication enhances gastric emptying. Even specific symptoms of delayed emptying such as bloating, epigastric fullness, nausea or vomiting are in most cases cured. One-third of our own patients operated on for GER showed a delayed GE; after Belsey Mark IV repair, specific symptoms of delayed emptying disappeared in 92% of cases.
- Those patients complaining of recurrence of symptoms after surgery are likely not to have had their gastric emptying normalized by the operation. In these patients, with often more severe symptoms and more delayed gastric emptying, a concomitant gastric pathology must be excluded to avoid surgical failure.

642

References

1. Moraldi A, Iascone C, Caputo V, Ziparo V, Zerilli M, De Vito G, Camerino C. The role of radioisotopic gastric emptying in patients with gastroesophageal reflux. In: DeMeester TR, Skinner DB (eds) Esophageal Disorders. Chicago: Raven Press, 1985;87–90.
2. Iascone C, Moraldi A, Zerilli M, Addario Chieco P, Caputo V, Ginevri P, Sleiter B, Stipa S. Reflusso gastro-esofageo e gastropatia. Min Diet Gastr 1987;33:129.
3. Myers JC, Collins PS, Dehn TBC, Maddern GJ, Horowitz M, Jamieson GG. Which part of the stomach is responsible for delay in gastric emptying of solids in patients with gastroesophageal reflux disease? J Gastroenterol Hepatol 1988;3:988.
4. Mattioli S, Stanghellini V, Pilotti V, Corbelli C, Felice V, Gozzetti G. Influence of hiatus hernia on gastric emptying of solids and liquids in patients affected by GER esophagitis. Fifth World Congress of I.S.D.E., Kyoto, 1992:160(abstract).
5. Maddern GJ, Chatterton BE, Collins PJ, Horowitz M, Shearman DJC, Jamieson GG. Solid and liquid gastric emptying in patients with gastroesophageal reflux. Br J Surg 1985;72:344.
6. Schwizer W, Hinder RA, DeMeester TR. Does delayed gastric emptying contribute to gastroesophageal reflux disease? Am J Surg 1989;157:74.
7. Shay SS, Eggli D, McDonald C, Johnson LF. Gastric emptying of solid food in patients with gastroesophageal reflux. Gastroenterology 1987;92:459.
8. Horowitz M, Collins PJ, Shearman DJC. Disorders of gastric emptying in humans and the use of radionuclide techniques. Arch Int Med 1985;145:1467.
9. Maddern GJ, Jamieson GG. Fundoplication enhances gastric emptying. Ann Surg 1985;201:296.
10. Maddern GJ, Jamieson GG, Chatterton BE, Collins PJ. Is there an association between failed antireflux procedure and delayed gastric emptying? Ann Surg 1985;202:162.
11. Hinder RA, Stein HJ, Bremner CG, DeMeester TR. Relationship of a satisfactory outcome to normalization of delayed gastric emptying after Nissen fundoplication. Ann Surg 1989;210:458.
12. Fink SM, Barwick K, De Luca V, Sanders FJ, Kandathil M, McCallum RW. The association of histologic gastritis with gastroesophageal reflux and delayed gastric emptying. J Clin Gastroenterol 1984;6:301.
13. Jamieson GG, Maddern GJ, Myers JC. Gastric emptying after fundoplication with and without proximal gastric vagotomy. Arch Surg 1991;126:1414.

What technical procedures are available to prevent vagal inclusion in the valve?

B. Launois, E. Bardaxoglou, B. Meunier, S. Landen (Rennes)

The Nissen procedure is associated with potential long-term complications involving the development of gastric ulceration, the etiology of which remains controversial. One may speculate that, in the presence of pre-existent anomalies of gastric emptying, the added operative trauma to the vagus nerves could trigger the release of gastrin and subsequent ulcer formation. A number of authors consider vagus nerve injury to be a major contributing factor [1]. Various technical artifices have been devised to avoid such trauma.

Isolation and exclusion of the vagus nerves

The vagus nerves are separated from the esophagus at the hiatus and reclined to the right, along with the hepatic plexus. Dissection is begun at the hiatus, down to and not beyond the level of the esophago-gastric junction, where the vagus trunks become the anterior and posterior nerves of Latarjet.

The initial step consists in the ligation of the short gastric vessels at the upper aspect of the greater curvature. This will allow the mobilization of the stomach pouch to produce a tension free wrap. The abdominal segment of the esophagus is encircled with a tape, and the hernia sac is excised. The left vagus nerve is dissected from the esophagus, at the level of the hiatus, and great care is taken not to damage the hepatic branch which runs across the upper portion of the lesser omentum. The small direct nervous branches to the esophagus are severed from the hiatus down to the esophago-gastric junction, along with the terminal branches of the left gastric artery. More distally, the left branch of the vagus nerve runs parallel to the lesser curvature and becomes the anterior nerve of Latarjet. It is not unusual to find an early division of the anterior vagus nerve into two branches that run at the anterior aspect of the esophagus. The right vagus nerve is found posteriorly to the right of the esophagus. It is encircled with a vessel loop, and followed in the direction of the celiac ganglion. A large posterior branch arises from the main trunk, runs parallel and gives small branches to the esophagus, originating from the nerve at a right angle, and then descending towards EG junction. More distally, the posterior branch follows its course on the posterior part of the lesser curvature and constitutes the posterior gastric nerve of Latarjet.

At this level, the right and left vagus nerves along, with the hepatic branches are reclined a few centimeters to the right of the esophagus. The diaphragmatic crural slings are approximated posteriorly using 2–3 interrupted sutures. The posterior vagus trunk is carefully secured at the level of the hiatal orifice. The gastric pouch is then wrapped around the abdominal esophagus to constitute a valve that is 2–3 cm wide, and that should not lie below the esophago-gastric junction. The right and left margins of the wrap should be approximated with sutures anchored to the anterior aspect of the esophagus.

Isolation of the anterior vagus trunk

The anterior trunk is not dissected away from the esophagus and is included in the wrap.

Supraselective vagotomy [2]

When associated to Nissen fundoplication, this procedure obviously implicates denervation of the upper part of the fundus, but the vagus nerves are carefully preserved, as is antro-pyloric function.

Discussion

The etiology of gastric ulceration after Nissen fundoplication remains controversial. If vagus nerve injury is suspected to play a role, then avoiding entrapment into the gastric wrap appears logical. Several authors make reference to such measures, but fail to be explicit on the technical details of the procedures. Herrington [1] was the first to propose measures aimed at avoiding vagus nerve damage. Indeed, it is conceivable that the anterior branch may be injured if included in the bites taken on the anterior esophageal wall while anchoring the wrap. Likewise, the posterior branch may be damaged while approximating the crural sling fibers. Supraselective vagotomy may be considered, in some views, as the best technical artifice to prevent damage to the nerves, but the technique described by Herrington appears to induce a greater traumatism than when the nerves are included in the wrap. However, as of yet there are no randomized studies that prove this.

References

1. Herrington JL Jr, Meacham PW, Hunter RM. Gastric ulceration after fundic wrapping. Ann Surg 1982;195:574–581.
2. Jordan PH Jr. Parietal cell vagotomy facilitates fundoplication in the treatment of reflux esophagitis. Surg Gynecol Obstet 1978;147:593.

Can alkaline gastritis be implicated in postoperative complaints?

P. Burdiles, C.G. Bremner (Los Angeles)

Gastroesophageal reflux disease (GERD) is one of the most common causes for medical consultation in adult populations in the western world. Its diagnosis can be made on the basis of typical symptoms such as heartburn and regurgitation, as well as on the presence of atypical symptoms such as noncardiac chest pain, asthma, chronic laryngitis etc. The occurrence of serious esophageal complications (esophageal ulcers, strictures and Barrett's esophagus) contribute to more alarming symptoms, such as dysphagia, loss of weight and anemia, together with a risk of cancer [1].

The variety of symptoms is the consequence of reflux events and its chronic mucosal injury. The pathophysiology of the disease considers several factors including the antireflux barrier of the lower esophageal sphincter (LES), the ability of the esophagus to clear the reflux episodes, the amount of gastric content available for reflux and the injurious agents contained in the gastric content. For a more rational approach to the disease, all of these factors should be kept in mind when the diagnosis of GERD has been considered. The presence of a mechanically defective LES has been extensively studied and is found in 60% of these patients [2]. In addition, a hiatal hernia is present in up to 60% of patients with GERD and intermittent epigastric pain and dysphagia are frequently found in this group [3,4]. Gastric acid hypersecretion is present in 20% of GERD patients with a defective LES and this figure rises to 48% in GERD patients with normal LES [5]. Although esophageal motility is progressively impaired in the more severe degrees of GERD esophagitis [6], it is controversial whether this finding is a consequence of chronic reflux or due to an intrinsic motility defect of the esophageal body and LES function.

In contrast, few studies have assessed the importance of other factors such as duodenogastric reflux (DGR) and gastric emptying in the pathogenesis of GERD [7]. The reflux of duodenal content into the stomach is a normal event and occurs intermittently [8]. Experimentally, it has been demonstrated that bile salts and pancreatic enzymes cause severe damage to gastric [9] and esophageal epithelium [10] and severe esophagitis can occur in some patients after total gastrectomy [11]. In addition, combined ambulatory 24-h pH gastric and esophageal monitoring have shown increased alkaline exposure (pH > 7) in the lower esophagus and abnormal profiles of gastric alkalinization in patients with complicated GERD and in patients with Barrett's esophagus, suggesting abnormal duodenogastric reflux in these groups [12]. However, reflux of mixed gastric juice and duodenal content, assessed by quantitation of bile salts and pancreatic enzymes in the esophageal lumen, also occurs when the esophageal pH is below 7, suggesting that this event is more frequent than was assumed [13]. In addition, a history of cholecystectomy, a well-known cause of increased DGR [14], is consistently reported in a proportion of patients with GERD esophagitis [12,15,16] providing further evidences for DGR as a factor in the pathogenesis of GERD. What, then, causes a physiologic event (DGR) to become a pathologic condition? Delay in gastric emptying has been proposed as an associated condition for the development of symptoms and gastric or esophageal mucosal damage when excessive DGR is present [7,17].

What is the importance of these considerations from a clinical point of view?

Diagnostic work-up for GERD is focused on excluding other organic foregut diseases (peptic ulcer, cancer etc.) and to confirm the presence of esophagitis; it usually considers esophago-gastroduodenoscopy, X-ray evaluation of the foregut and occasionally, manometric evaluation and ambulatory 24-h pH esophageal monitoring [18]. Assessment of DGR and disturbances in gastric emptying are infrequently reported in the medical literature of GERD.

When therapeutic considerations for GERD are made, the initial steps are oriented to decreasing the volume of gastric content, changing dietary habits and reducing the esophageal acid exposure by elevating the head of the bed, suppressing gastric acid secretion and using prokinetic drugs [19,20]. Surgical antireflux procedures seek to restore the functional competence of the LES as an antireflux barrier and to repair anatomical abnormalities such as hiatal hernia and shortened esophagus, avoiding any disturbance in the already impaired esophageal motility.

Among these surgical procedures, the Nissen fundoplication operation is a very satisfactory curative procedure for GERD and long-term follow-up for as long as 10 years has shown good symptomatic control in up to 91% of patients [4]. Poor results in symptomatic control are due largely to technical problems which can be prevented by careful surgical procedure [21,22]. Those failures include recurrent reflux in about

10% [23], dysphagia, gas bloat, recurrent hiatal hernia or the development of paraesophageal hernia. The results of reoperation on these patients are satisfactory in about 92% of patients [24]. There remains a hard core of patients with unsatisfactory results which do not fit into any of the above categories and this group is ill defined. Gastric ulcer following the Nissen fundoplication operation has been the subject of much debate and the cause is unknown. Herrington [25] suggests that it is related to vagal nerve entrapment, but there is no physiological or objective support for this hypothesis. Gastric stasis, gas bloat and hypergastrinemia is a further theory [26] which is not supported by all [27]. Duodenogastric reflux is a possible cause, and this may have existed prior to the procedure because the Nissen fundoplication does not affect duodenogastric reflux in the experimental model [28].

It is well known that DGR causes gastritis in humans [29], however, two important considerations should be mentioned. The first is the lack of a "gold standard" for the diagnosis of DGR since radiologic or isotopic studies take place over too short a duration (1–2 h), aspiration studies are cumbersome and performed on an intermittent basis, and continuous intragastric pH monitoring shows good sensitivity for severe DGR but poor specificity [30]. The second problem is that Ritchie's clinical criteria [31] for the diagnosis of DGR only considers patients who are extremely symptomatic with severe pathology. The prevalence of DGR and its severity after the Nissen operation are not known but may represent a secondary effect of the surgical procedure which decreases the gastric emptying time [32,33]. From reported analyses of failures after antireflux surgery, there is a striking lack of information regarding the presence or prevalence of "alkaline" gastritis. The term "alkaline" is misleading, because it assumes that the damage (gastritis) is related to an alkaline pH and that this in turn is caused by DGR. However, it has been demonstrated that bile salts can be also present when the pH in the stomach is acidic [34], suggesting that DGR may occur in severe degrees without any important change the intragastric pH. Furthermore, in vitro tests have demonstrated minor changes in gastric pH when hydrochloric acid at pH 1.0 is mixed with duodenal content at pH 7.7, even at the point where the mixture contained 50% of each component, the pH of the solution remained below 2. This finding supports the idea that continuous pH monitoring in the stomach is very sensitive in detecting patients with extremely abnormal DGR, but is not specific for reliable monitoring of those events.

The development of a new spectrophotometric system may allow a direct and continuous assessment of duodenogastric reflux on an ambulatory basis, using the specific optical absorbance of bilirubin as an indicator of bile reflux into the gastric and esophageal lumen [35].

The surgeon must be aware of those patients with atypical GERD because other minor complaints may be underestimated by the patient or by the physician. A history of chronic epigastric pain in patients with GERD, and particularly if there is a history of cholecystectomy in the past, should alert the clinician to the possibility of DGR, and specific diagnostic studies should be considered. If these symptoms are ignored, an underlying DGR may become evident only after a successful surgical procedure for gastroesophageal reflux disease, impairing the clinical results and giving rise to some questions about the benefits of surgical therapy in GERD.

At present, the "alkaline gastritis" syndrome is reported infrequently after antireflux surgery. The development of new technology for DGR assessment may help towards a better understanding of the characteristics of this event and improve the preoperative recognition of pathologic DGR. In symptomatic patients after antireflux surgery, it will contribute to a better diagnosis when organic postoperative complications or failed antireflux procedures have been excluded.

References

1. Klinkenberg-Knol EC, Castell DO. Clinical spectrum and diagnosis of gastroesophageal reflux disease. In: Castell DO (ed) The Esophagus. Boston: Little, Brown, 1992;441–448.
2. Zaninotto G, DeMeester TR, Schwizer W, Johansson KE, Cheng SC. The lower esophageal sphincter in health and disease. Am J Surg 1988;155:104–111.
3. Code CF, Kelley ML, Schlegel JF, Olsen AM. Detection of hiatal hernia during esophageal motility tests. Gastroenterology 1962;43:521–531.
4. DeMeester TR, Bonavina L, Albertucci M. Nissen fundoplication for gastroesophageal reflux disease. Ann Surg 1986;204:9–20.
5. Barlow AP, DeMeester TR, Ball CS, Eypasch EP. The significance of the gastric secretory state in gastroesophageal reflux disease. Arch Surg 1989;124:937–940.
6. Stein HJ, Eypasch EP, DeMeester TR, Smyrk TC, Attwood SEA. Circadian esophageal motor function in patients with gastroesophageal reflux disease. Surgery 1990;108:769–778.
7. Dubois A. Clinical relevance of gastroduodenal dysfunction in reflux esophagitis. J Clin Gastroenterol 1986;8(suppl 1):17–25.
8. Keane FB, DiMagno EP, Malagelada JR. Duodenogastric reflux in humans: its relationship to fasting antroduodenal motility and gastric, pancreatic and biliary secretion. Gastroenterology 1981;81:726–731.
9. Lawson HH. The production of chronic gastritis under experimental conditions. Scand J Gastroenterol 1981;16(suppl 67):91–98.
10. Johnson LF, Harmon JW. Experimental esophagitis in a rabbit model. J Clin Gastroenterol 1986;8(suppl 1):26–44.
11. Helsingen N. Oesophagitis following total gastrectomy. A follow-up study on 9 patients 5 years or more after operation. Acta Chir Scand 1959/1960;118:190–201.
12. Stein HJ, Barlow AP, DeMeester TR, Hinder RA. Complication of gastroesophageal reflux disease. Role of the lower esophageal sphincter, esophageal acid and acid/alkaline exposure, and duodenogastric reflux. Ann Surg 1992;216:35–43.
13. Gotley DC, Appleton GVN, Cooper MJ. Bile acids and trypsin are unimportant in alkaline esophageal reflux. J Clin Gastroenterol 1992;14:2–7.
14. Warshaw AL. Bile gastritis without prior gastric surgery: contributing role of cholecystectomy. Am J Surg 1979;137:527–531.
15. Hyvärinen H. Relationship of previous cholecystectomy to esophagitis and gastroduodenal ulcers. Hepato Gastroenterol 1987;34:74–80.
16. Jazrawi S, Walsh TN, Byrne PJ, Hill AD, Li H, Lawlor P, Hennessy TPJ. Cholecystectomy and oesophageal reflux: a prospective evaluation. Br J Surg 1993;80:50–53.
17. Mackie C, Hulks G, Cuschieri A. Enterogastric reflux and gastric clearance of refluxate in normal subjects and in patients with and without bile vomiting following peptic ulcer surgery. Ann Surg 1986;204:537–542.
18. Armstrong D, Emde C, Inauen W, Blum AL. Diagnostic assessment of gastroesophageal reflux disease: what is possible vs. what is practical? Hepato Gastroenterol 1992;39(suppl 1):3–13.
19. Johnson DA. Medical therapy for gastroesophageal reflux disease. Am J Med 1992;92(suppl 5A):88S–97S.
20. Bell NJV, Hunt RH. Role of gastric acid suppression in the treatment of gastro-oesophageal reflux disease. Gut 1992;33:118–124.
21. O'Hanrahan, Marples T, Bancewicz J. Recurrent reflux and wrap disruption after Nissen fundoplication: detection, incidence and timing. Br J Surg 1990;77:545–547.
22. Ellis FH, Crozier R. Reflux control by fundoplication: a clinical and manometric assessment of the Nissen operation. Ann Thorac Surg 1984;38:387–392.
23. Ellis FH, El-Kurd MF, Gibb SP. The effect of fundoplication on the lower esophageal sphincter. Surg Gynecol Obstet 1976;143:1–5.
24. DeMeester TR, Stein HJ. Minimizing the effects of antireflux surgery. World J Surg 1992;16:335–336.
25. Herrington JL, Meacham PW, Hunter RM. Gastric ulceration after fundic wrapping. Vagal nerve entrapment, a possible causative factor. Ann Surg 1982;195:574–581.
26. Bushkin FL, Woodward ER, O'Leary JP. Occurrence of gastric ulcer after Nissen fundoplication. Ann Surg 1976;51:791–793.
27. Bremner CG. Gastric ulcer after a fundoplication. Surg Gynecol Obstet 1979;168:62–66.

28. Reipton CMS, Dowling BL, Spencer J. Antrectomy with Roux-en-Y anastomosis in the treatment of peptic oesophagitis with stricture. Br J Surg 1975;62:605–607.
29. DuPlessis DJ. Pathogenesis of gastric ulceration. Lancet 1965;1:974.
30. Stein HJ, Hinder RA, DeMeester TR, Lloyd BA, Fuchs KH, Attwood SEA, Gupta NC. Clinical use of 24-h gastric pH monitoring vs. O-diisopropyl iminodiacetic acid (DISIDA) scanning in the diagnosis of pathologic duodenogastric reflux. Arch Surg 1990;125:966–971.
31. Ritchie WP. Alkaline reflux gastritis: an objective assessment of its diagnosis and treatment. Ann Surg 1980;192:288–298.
32. Maddern GJ, Jamieson CG. Fundoplication enhances gastric emptying. Ann Surg 1985;201:296–299.
33. Hinder RA, Stein HJ, Bremner CG, DeMeester TR. Relationship of a satisfactory outcome to normalization of delayed gastric emptying after Nissen fundoplication. Ann Surg 1989;210:458–465.
34. Brown TH, Holbrook I, King RF, Ibrahim K. 24-h intragastric pH measurement in the assessment of duodenogastric reflux. World J Surg 1992;16:995–999.
35. Bechi P, Falciai R, Baldini F, Cosi F, Pucciani F, Boscherini S. A new fiberoptic sensor for ambulatory entero-gastric reflux detection. Proc SPIE 1992;1648:130–135.

Hill operation

Does Vansant's method facilitate the learning of Hill's technique?

C. Gautier-Benoit (Lille)

The posterior gastropexy described by Hill consists of anchoring of the phrenoeso-phageal bundles to the preaortic fascia and the median arcuate ligament. This technique implies two dangers.

The first one arises when the surgeon is dissecting the median arcuate ligament, located immediately above the celiac trunk, a thick nervous plexus masks the artery. If an injury of the vessel occurs, it may be difficult to place a stitch.

The second danger is injury to the celiac trunk, or even the aorta, when sutures are passed through the full thickness of the median arcuate ligament.

To avoid these dangers, Hill [1] has suggested passing a Goodell dilatator beneath the ligament. However, while introducing the dilatator, it is still possible to injure the artery.

In 1976, Vansant [2] proposed another artifice now recommended by Hill himself.

Vansant's artifice avoids the difficult dissection of the celiac trunk. The fibroareolar tissue overlying the aorta is simply divided by sharp dissection in the esophageal hiatus. The index finger is then passed beneath the preaortic fascia down to the celiac trunk to stop its downward movement. The sutures are placed through the median arcuate ligament without danger to the aorta, and the celiac artery is protected by the finger aligned in the plane between the aorta and the ligament.

One hundred and twenty operations, of which one-third were performed by surgeons in training, were achieved without any vascular injury [3].

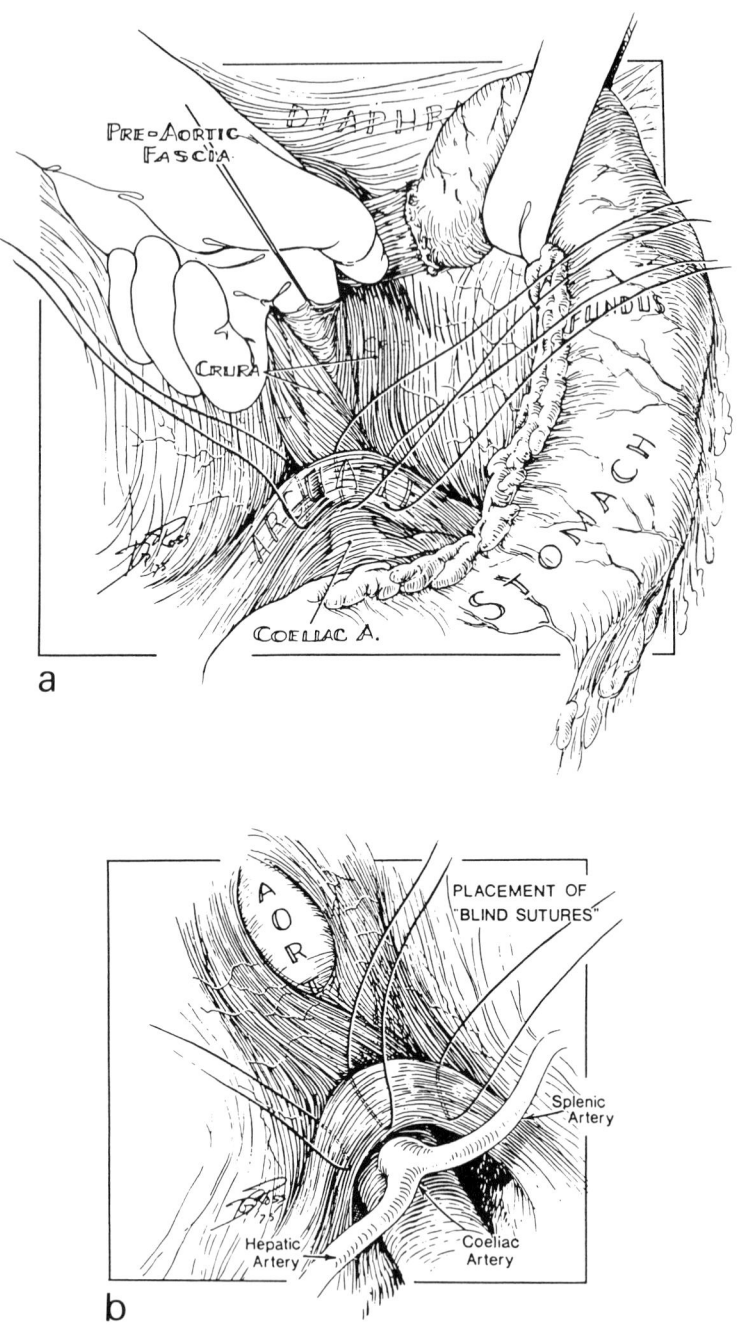

Fig. 1. a) Three sutures of braided No. 1 silk are accurately placed through the median arcuate ligament without danger to the aorta and celiac artery which are protected by the index finger in the plane between the aorta and the median arcuate ligament. b) The relationship of the origin of the celiac artery to the median arcuate ligament and the accurate blind placement of the median arcuate sutures are shown [2, with permission].

In my opinion, Vansant's artifice is useful to learn Hill's procedure with minimal danger to the patients.

References

1. Hill LD. Résultats éloignés de la gastropexie postérieure de Hill dans le traitement du reflux oesophagien non compliqué de l'adulte. In: The Esophagus. Philadelphia: WB Saunders, 1988.
2. Vansant JH, Baker JW, Ross DG. The esophagus. Surg Gynecol Obstet 1976;143:637–642.
3. Gautier-Benoit C, Bugnon PY, Pinchon Marsy S, Meignie Ph. Modification of the Hill technique for repair of hiatal hernia. Chirurgie 1988;114:566–571.

Are the functional sequelae of Hill's operation associated with the constraint imposed on the cardia?

S.J.M. Kraemer (Munich), *L.D. Hill* (Seattle)

Complications of gastroesophageal reflux (GER) or reflux symptoms intractable to medical therapy may require surgical treatment. In general, the primary goal of any antireflux procedure is to make the cardia competent again by improving its function. Different antireflux procedures employ different techniques to achieve this function. What are the anatomical and functional consequences of the tension imposed on the cardia in the Hill repair?

GER is one of the most common abnormalities of the upper gastrointestinal tract. It is due to a malfunction of the gastroesophageal antireflux barrier (GEARB) of the gastroesophageal junction (GEJ). The GEARB is an effective barrier consisting of:
— the crura of the diaphragm;
— the lower esophageal sphincter (LES);
 the abdominal segment of the esophagus; and
— the gastroesophageal flap valve mechanism (GEV).
The "anatomical arrangement" of the GEJ leads to the assumption that it is not arbitrarily organized. This combination of anatomical features indicates that another very "complex biovalve" mechanism is being dealt with here, of which there are a number in the human body, where liquids are transported such as the ileocecal valve etc. A partial or complete loss of the GEARB, mostly associated with hiatal hernia, has been identified as a cause for gastroesophageal reflux disease (GERD), which may lead to such complications from heartburn, esophagitis, ulceration, dysphagia, stricture, upper gastrointestinal bleeding, chronic aspiration, to Barrett's esophagus and, ultimately, even to esophageal cancer.

In most patients with a hiatal hernia, the GEJ slides through the widened esophageal hiatus into the posterior mediastinum, and thereby eliminates the angle of His and the GEV. The abdominal segment of the esophagus is lost. Over time, a dilatation of the LES can be found in a great number of these patients, allowing free reflux of gastric juice into the esophagus.

— During endoscopy, a pinch-cock effect of the diaphragm on the esophagus can be observed. It has been demonstrated that LES pressure is elevated during diaphragmatic contraction [1,2].

— The LES is not well-defined anatomically. Different studies seem to show that a circular constrictor of the cardia does not exist, except an asymmetric muscle thickening above the angle of His and below the diaphragm. However, it is well defined manometrically, the manometrically-defined high pressure zone being located in this area of muscle thickening [3,4].

— Loss of the abdominal segment leads to a loss of competence of the cardia. The shorter the abdominal length, the greater the muscle tone required to maintain competence [5].

— The GEV consists of a musculomucosal fold at the side of the lesser curve of the stomach. It is created by the angle of His (or esophagogastric angle) and the oblique angle in which the esophagus enters the stomach [6]. It is a 180° one-way flap-valve, which closes effectively against the lesser curve of the stomach. In a healthy subject it presents no obstruction to the downward flow of esophageal contents, but it effectively resists any reflux of gastric contents.

This valve, however, can be eliminated by the diaphragm depressing the fundus of the stomach, which eliminates the angle of His, thus converting the GEJ into a funnel. This happens when a person belches or vomits under synchronous opening of the esophageal sphincters. Similarly, the GEV is also lost and the GEJ transformed into a funnel in patients with severe GERD and/or those patients with a hiatal hernia. This valve, its aspects and different functions have been repeatedly described in the past [7—10].

With the Hill repair the GEARB is restored [11]: first the hiatal hernia is reduced and the enlarged hiatus is narrowed; then the "repair stitches" are passed one by one through the dissected anterior and posterior phrenoesophageal bundle, carefully preserving the vagus nerves, and then down to the preaortic fascia. These sutures are tied down under manometric control, approximating the phrenoesophageal bundles to each other and to the preaortic fascia. This maneuver brings the GEJ caudally, thereby bringing the esophagus down to its original attachments, thus regaining the abdominal segment of the esophagus. A length of 2 cm or more of abdominal esophagus has been shown to allow maintenance of competence of the cardia over a wide range of changes in intra-abdominal pressures.

By adjusting the pressure on the stitches manometrically, the "high-pressure zone" of the GEJ is calibrated to the desired intraoperative pressure, including the LES. Intraoperative manometry allows careful calibration of the high pressure zone of the GEJ to the specific requirements of the patients disease.

The tension imposed on the collar sling musculature approximates the angle of His. This, in turn, automatically restores the GEV, closely matching the appearance of the physiological anatomical valve in normal volunteers [12]. In patients with GERD and a normal esophageal motility, a physiological GEV of 3—4 cm length can be created and the barrier pressure can be brought up to normal values. In those patients with GERD and an additional motility disorder, an adequate and competent GEV can be restored with a barrier pressure of 0 mmHg, with little or no obstruction to downward flow of esophageal contents, but, at the same time, effectively resistant to any GER.

Anchoring or posterior fixation of the GEJ to the preaortic fascia efficiently prevents the GEJ from being forced back up into the hiatus, and the length of abdominal esophagus from being reduced, when the intra-abdominal pressure increases. Furthermore, it upholds the propulsive power of the esophageal motility, as it reduces the relative shortening occurring during esophageal contractions resulting in nonpropulsive motility.

It is important to point out, once more, that the Hill repair is not a fundoplication. The phrenoesophageal bundles are imbricated together, and there is actually no stomach wrap around the lower esophagus.

With the tension imposed on the cardia through the repair stitches of the Hill operation, the major anatomical and functional features of the GEARB of the GEJ are restored all at once, without any major anatomical or functional manipulations at the site of the GEJ. This makes the Hill repair a highly effective antireflux procedure [13], which is now performed laparoscopically as well, in accordance with the same established principles [14].

References

1. Mittal RK, Fisher MJ. Electrical and mechanical inhibition of the crural diaphragm during transient relaxation of the lower esophageal sphincter. Gastroenterology 1990;99(5):1265—1268.
2. Mittal RK, Rochester DF, McCallum RW. Electrical and mechanical activity in the human lower esophageal sphincter during diaphragmatic contraction. J Clin Invest 1988;81:1182—1189.
3. Sontag SJ, Schnell TG, Miller TQ, Nemchausky B, Serlovsky R, O'Connell S, Chejfec G, Seidel UJ, Brand L. The importance of hiatal hernia in reflux esophagitis compared with lower esophageal sphincter pressure or smoking. J Clin Gastroenterol 1991;13(6):628—643.
4. Liebermann-Meffert D, Allgöwer M, Schmid P, Blum AL. Muscular equivalent of the lower esophageal sphincter. Gastroenterology 1979;76(1):31—38.
5. DeMeester TR, Wernly JA, Bryant GH et al. Clinical and in vitro determinations of gastroesophageal competence: a study of the principles of antireflux surgery. Am J Surg 1979;137:39—46.
6. Allison PR. Reflux esophagitis, sliding hiatal hernia and the anatomy of the repair. Surg Gynecol Obstet 1951;92:419—431.
7. von Gubaroff A. Über den Verschluß des menschlichen Magens an der Cardia. Arch Anat Physiol 1886:395.
8. Braune W. Topographisch-anatomischer Atlas nach Durchschnitten an gefrorenen Cadavern. Leipzig: Kleine Ausgabe, 1878:113—114.
9. Barrett NR. Hiatus hernia: a review of some controversial points. Br J Surg 1954;42:231—243.
10. Hill LD. An effective operation for hiatal hernia: an 8-year appraisal. Ann Surg 1967;166:681—692.
11. Kraemer SJM, Aye RW, Hill LD. The Hill-repair. A definitive antireflux procedure. In: Nyhus LM (ed) Surgery of the Esophagus, Stomach and Small Intestine, 5th edn (in press).
12. Kraemer SJM, Hill LD, Kozarek RA, Aye RW, Pope CE II. Does retroflexed endoscopic examination of the cardia allow prediction of reflux status? In: Giuli R, Tytgat GNJ, DeMeester TR, Galmiche JP (eds) The Esophageal Mucosa, O.E.S.O., 1994:126—131.
13. Low DE, Anderson RP, Ilves R, Riccardelli E, Hill LD. Fifteen- to twenty-year results after the Hill antireflux operation. J Thorac Cardiovasc Surg 1989;98(3):444—450.
14. Kraemer SJM, Aye RW, Kozarek RA, Hill LD. The laparoscopic Hill-repair. Gastrointest Endosc (in press).

The results of Hill's operation

L.D. Hill, S.J.M. Kraemer, C.E. Pope, R.A. Kozarek (Seattle)

The Hill Repair is an operation designed to restore the function of the antireflux barrier. The normal gastroesophageal junction (GEJ) is a highly competent barrier against reflux of gastric contents into the esophagus. With the development of a hiatal hernia, the GEJ slides into the posterior mediastinum and the barrier is lost, resulting in reflux.

Gastroesophageal reflux with its complications of esophagitis, heartburn and pneumonitis is the most common abnormality of the upper gastrointestinal (GI) tract. Despite the frequency of gastroesophageal reflux (GER), the components of the antireflux barrier have been poorly understood until recently. For antireflux surgery to be effective, the components of the antireflux barrier must be clearly understood in order that they may be restored by an operation.

The antireflux barrier

The antireflux barrier consists of the gastroesophageal valve (GEV), the lower esophageal sphincter (LES), the diaphragm [16], posterior fixation of the GEJ and esophageal clearance.

With our ability to measure the lower esophageal sphincter pressure (LESP) [5], the GEV has been overlooked. The LES generates a pressure of around 15–18 mmHg in the resting state and can generate pressures up to 100 mmHg or more. However, it is a weak sphincter and cannot alone withstand the large pressures exerted against the GEJ with heavy lifting, straining and trauma.

The GEV can be readily viewed in the cadaver through a gastrostomy. In the living person it can be seen with the retroflexed endoscope. We have also viewed the GE valve in patients through a gastrostomy. When seen through a gastrostomy without an endoscope through the valve, it has essentially the same structural appearance as that seen through the retroflexed endoscope. The valve is created by the angle of entry of the esophagus into the stomach and is an intragastric musculo-mucosal fold that, in the normal subject, adheres to the endoscope through all phases of respiration. It opens with swallowing, belching and vomiting, and closes promptly.

In our series using cadavers with no premorbid evidence of hiatal hernia or esophageal disease, we have shown that a measurable gradient of approximately 15 cm of water exists across the GE junction [28]. This gradient can be eliminated effectively by depressing the fundus of the stomach 45°. This maneuver causes the angle of His to become obtuse, which eliminates the GE flap valve, converts the ostium of the esophagus into a funnel and results in free reflux. Since there is no lower esophageal sphincter (LES) function in the cadaver, the presence of a gradient

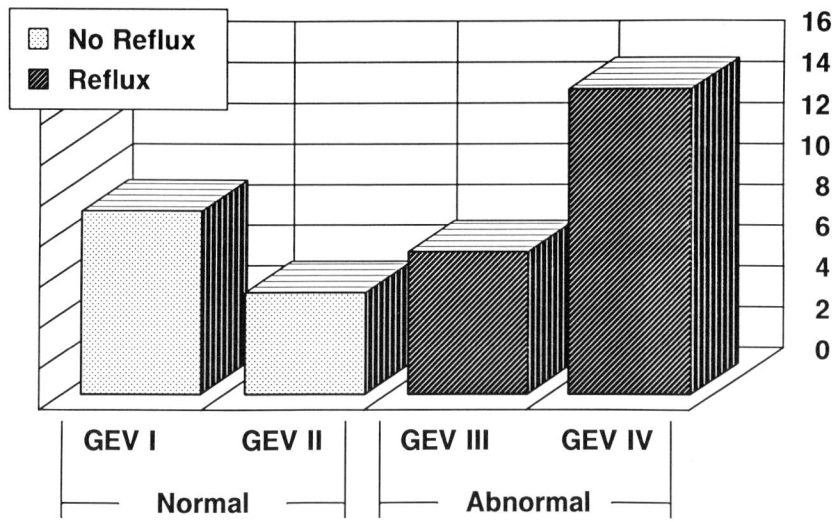

Fig. 1. Grading system of the GEV developed from retroflexed endoscopy in 32 patients with and without GERD.

across the GE junction and the maneuver of depressing the cardia to eliminate the gradient, helps to confirm the importance of the valve in an in situ preparation.

The appearance of the valve through the retroflexed endoscope in 20 normal volunteers without reflux was studied in order to determine how the normal valve appears.

Thirty-two patients, with and without reflux, were examined with a retroflexed endoscope and the valves were graded by a gastroenterologist blinded to the clinical status of the patient. From this study, a grading system of the valve was developed (Fig. 1).

In a separate study of 33 patients seen in the gastric laboratory who had both standard acid reflux test and grading of the GEV, the results were shown in terms of prediction of the clinical status of the patient. The results are shown in Table 1. It is noteworthy that grading of the GEV predicted the clinical picture in 32 of 33

Table 1. This study demonstrates the correlation with clinical status of patients seen in the GI laboratory. Grading of the GEV correlated more closely with clinical picture than measurement of the LESP

Measurement of LESP	Grading of esophageal value
33 patients	
Correlation with clinical picture of GERD	
LESP	Grading of GEV
17 of 33	32 of 33
Endoscopist blinded to clinical picture	

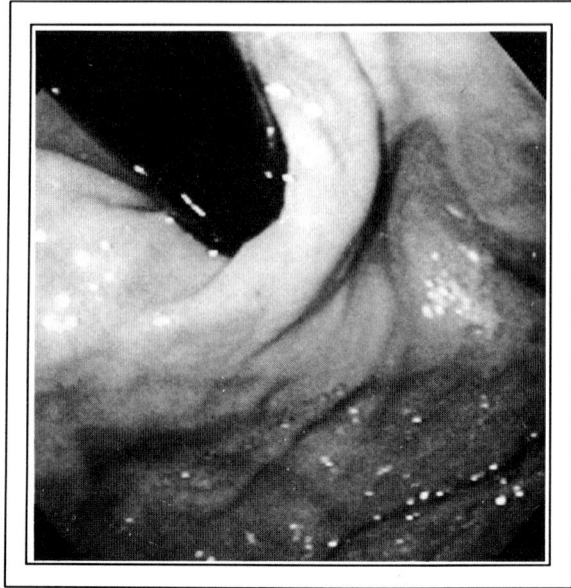
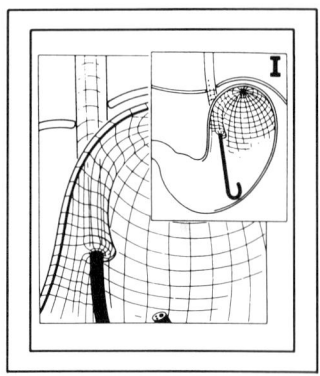

Fig. 2. Grade I valve is a normal valve. It is a musculomucosal fold that adheres to the retroflexed endoscope through all phases of respiration, opens for swallowing, but closes promptly.

patients; whereas measurement of the LESP correlated with the clinical picture in only 17. This study showed clearly that grading of the GEV more accurately portrays the clinical status than does measurement of the LESP.

The grade I valve is a normal valve (Fig. 2). This consists of a musculomucosal fold adherent to the endoscope through all phases of respiration. It opens for swallowing and belching, and closes promptly. The grade II gastroesophageal valve is only slightly less well defined and shorter. It opens but closes promptly (Fig. 3). The grade III valve opens frequently, remains open for varying periods of time, is poorly defined and often is associated with a hiatal hernia (Fig. 4). The grade IV valve shows no well-defined musculomucosal fold; the esophageal orifice is wide open and it is invariably accompanied by a hiatal hernia (Fig. 5).

It is noteworthy that in 32 patients with or without a history of varying degrees of reflux, the GEV was graded by gastroenterologists blinded to the clinical status of the patient. No patient with grade I or II GEV showed reflux; whereas, all patients with grade III and IV valves showed reflux (Fig. 1).

In a separate study of 33 patients seen in the gastric laboratory who had both a standard acid reflux test and grading of the GEV, the results were shown in terms of prediction of the clinical status of the patient. The results are shown in Table 1. It is noteworthy that grading of the GEV predicted the clinical picture of 32 of the 33 patients whereas measurement of the LESP correlated with the clinical picture in only 17.

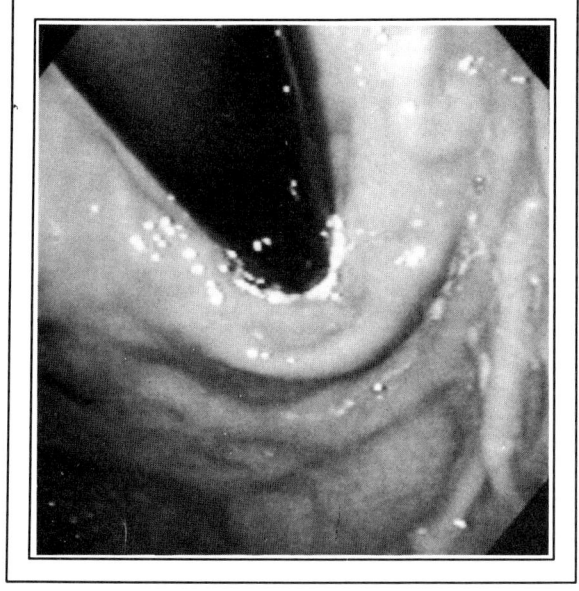
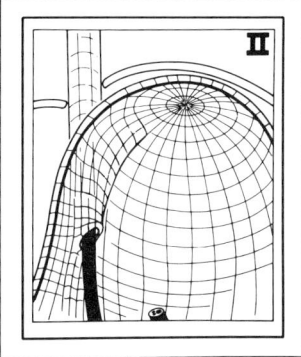

Fig. 3. Grade II GE valve, slightly less well-defined, but one which still opens for swallowing, closes promptly and does not allow reflux.

These studies show clearly that the GEV is an important component of the gastroesophageal barrier. The role of surgery, therefore, is to re-establish a normal grade I, 180° valve in a patient who has lost the valve and is therefore suffering from reflux.

In addition to recreating the valve, calibrating of the LES is important and can be done with intraoperative measurement of the sphincter pressure. The relationship of the LES to the valve is shown in Fig. 6. This computer generated view shows that the sphincter resides inside the valve and aids the valve in discriminating between gas, liquids and solids, and does the discriminatory work while the valve does the heavy work, in terms of preventing reflux. Increased intragastric pressure serves to close the valve against the lesser curve.

Posterior fixation of the GEJ is essential. This is lost when the patient develops a hiatal hernia and the GEJ ascends into the posterior mediastinum. The esophagus can no longer generate propulsive waves that are necessary for esophageal clearance since the esophagus no longer has a fulcrum or point of fixation from which to work. It should be recalled that the entire GI tract, including the hollow as well as solid viscera in humans and most vertebrate animals, is suspended by the dorsal mesentery to the posterior body wall. The esophagus is no exception to this rule. Extensive cadaver dissections demonstrate that the esophagus is primarily fixed posteriorly by a dense plate of fibroareolar tissue extending from the median arcuate ligament all the way to the aortic arch. The posterior attachment of the GE junction by the dorsal

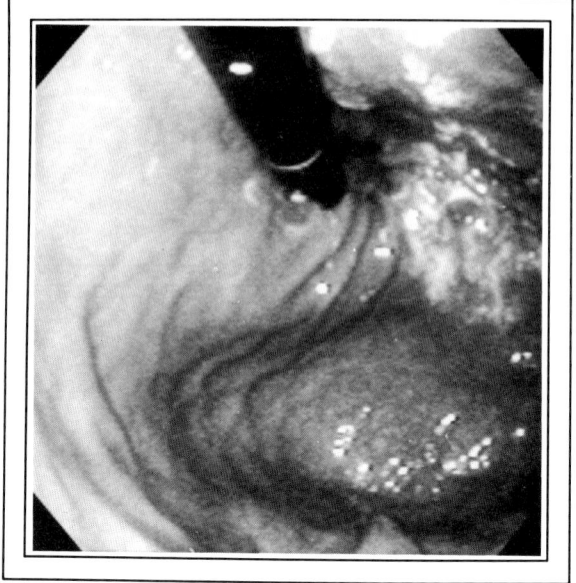
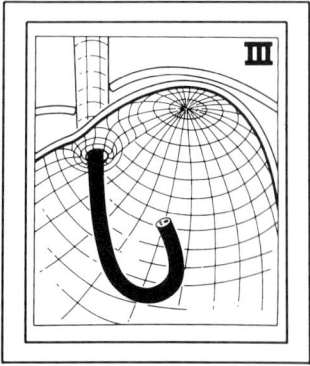

Fig. 4. The grade III valve opens frequently, closes poorly, is poorly defined and may be associated with a hiatal hernia.

mesentery to the preaortic fascia is key to the integrity of the entire barrier to reflux. It has been demonstrated in the cadaver that, with division of the posterior attachment the GEJ slides into the chest and the effect of the GEV is lost. This is also demonstrated with the retroflexed endoscope in the human. As the GE junction ascends into the posterior mediastinum, the valve is lost and the sphincter is distracted. Reattachment of the GE junction is therefore important for restoration of esophageal function.

Closure of the enlarged diaphragmatic opening is important to prevent recurrence of hiatal hernia. The diaphragm should be closed loosely about the esophagus so that at least one finger can be placed alongside the esophagus with a nasogastric tube in the lumen. Fixation of the cardia to the rim of the diaphragm is also important to accentuate the valve and to close the opening into the posterior mediastinum to prevent herniation of the cardia into the posterior mediastinum. To summarize, the goals of surgery are:
— Restoration of the GEV.
— Calibration of the LES to the proper range.
— Posterior fixation of the GE junction to restore esophageal peristalsis and clearance.
— Reduction of the hiatal hernia.
— Closure of the diaphragm.

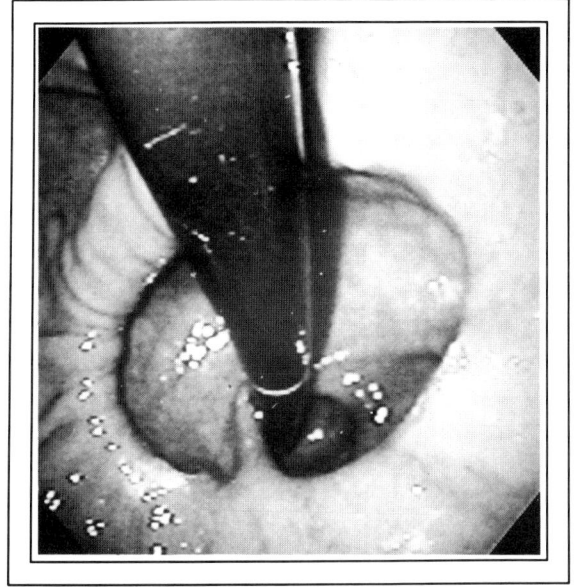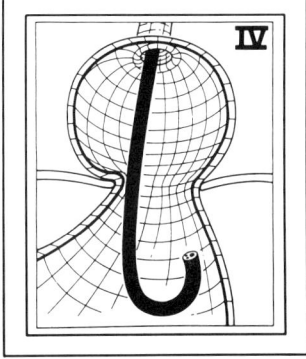

Fig. 5. In patients with a grade IV valve, there is no definable mucosal fold and the esophagus remains open the majority of the time viewed, and a hiatal hernia is invariably present.

Technique

The conventional open technique is accomplished through an upper abdominal midline incision. The abdomen is thoroughly explored. The pylorus, in particular, is examined carefully for any evidence of pyloric stenosis which might impede gastric emptying. The triangular ligament of the left lobe of the liver is divided so that the left lobe can be retracted to the patient's right. This exposes the esophageal hiatus with its covering phrenoesophageal membrane. An upper hand retractor with two blades is placed to facilitate exposure of the upper abdomen. The phrenoesophageal membrane is then divided on the diaphragm (Fig. 7), keeping as much of the fibroareolar tissue that makes up the phrenoesophageal bundles as possible with the GE junction. It is these bundles that normally hold the GE junction in place in the diaphragm and these bundles will be used to anchor the GE junction to the preaortic fascia. The lesser omentum is divided and the esophageal hiatus is exposed. The esophagus is gently diverted to the patient's left and the attachment of the cardia to the diaphragm is divided. The repair can be accomplished without dividing the short gastric vessels. Only rarely do we need to divide a short gastric vessel. This dissection must be done with care so as not to damage the spleen. Capsular tears of the spleen may be repaired by cautery or by suturing and applying Avitene. Division of the phrenogastric and superior portions of the gastrosplenic ligament mobilizes the

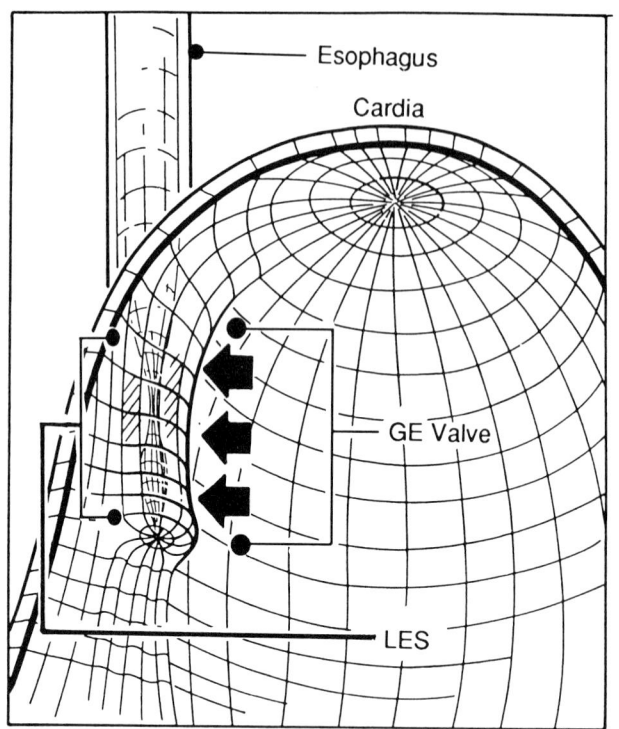

Fig. 6. The relationship of the LES to the valve is shown. This computer-generated view shows the relationship of the sphincter and the GEV. The sphincter resides inside the valve and aids the valve in discriminating between gas, liquid and solids, and aids in the prevention of reflux. The arrows are pressure vectors demonstrating that increased intragastric pressure closes the valve.

upper part of the gastric fundus. The fundus can then be rotated so that the posterior part of the stomach can be visualized. This allows the GE junction to be retracted down and the hiatal hernia reduced. The bundles of tissue that constitute the anterior and posterior attachments of the GE junction to the diaphragm, the anterior and posterior phrenoesophageal bundles, can then be displayed. By retracting these caudally, an intra-abdominal segment of esophagus becomes visible. The anterior and posterior vagus nerves are visualized and kept in view so as not to be damaged.

Attention is again turned to the pylorus. If the pylorus is scarred because the patient has had a duodenal ulcer or if there is a pyloric diaphragm obstructing the outlet of the stomach, a pyloromyotomy or pyloroplasty is planned. These findings should be interpreted in light of the patient's history. If the patient has a history of duodenal ulcer, not only should a pyloroplasty or pyloromyotomy be planned, but a vagotomy to decrease the gastric acid should be added. These findings should be anticipated by careful preoperative workup. Preoperative endoscopy should rule out pyloric stenosis or duodenal ulcer. Only if the duodenum is markedly scarred or if there is active ulceration should pyloroplasty and vagotomy be performed. We generally employ a highly selective vagotomy and Jaboulay pyloroplasty. If the pylorus is simply scarred and there is no active ulceration, the pylorus may be dilated

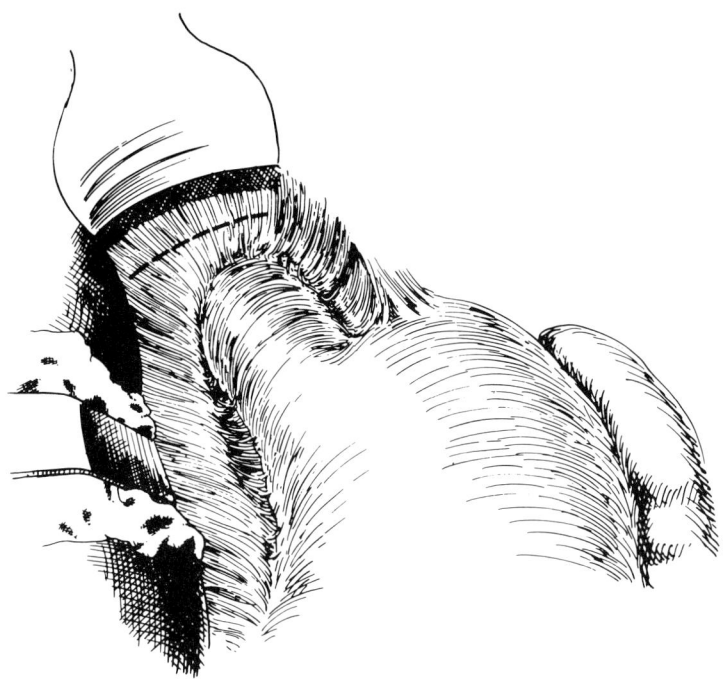

Fig. 7. The phrenoesophageal membrane is divided on the diaphragm in order to retain the fibroareolar tissue on the stomach to be used in the repair.

and a pyloromyotomy performed. It is imperative to relieve any gastric outlet obstruction to obtain a good result from an antireflux procedure. On the other hand, to add a vagotomy to a routine hiatal hernia repair is unwise. In our experience, this has led to complications of vagotomy without benefit to the patient.

Retracting the stomach to the patient's left exposes the preaortic fascia. The aorta and celiac axis are easily felt. The median arcuate ligament (MAL) lies immediately above the celiac trunk. It can be exposed by careful blunt dissection at this point over the midpoint of the aorta. The celiac artery usually arises cephalad to the median arcuate ligament. When the free edge of the MAL has been exposed, the celiac artery can be compressed into the aorta and the fibroareolar tissue overlying the artery can be carefully divided. An instrument such as a Goodell dilator is then passed beneath the median arcuate ligament. If the instrument is in the correct plane, it should simply float beneath the preaortic fascia. If the instrument meets an obstruction, there may be a branch of the celiac artery in the midline. The branch may be damaged if force is used on insertion.

Dissection of the celiac axis has been the deterrent to performing this operation in the opinion of other surgeons. If it is difficult to locate the MAL and if the surgeon is not familiar with vascular surgery and is uncomfortable dissecting out the celiac axis, a safer alternative procedure is recommended.

By retracting the esophagus to the patient's left, the surgeon can expose the

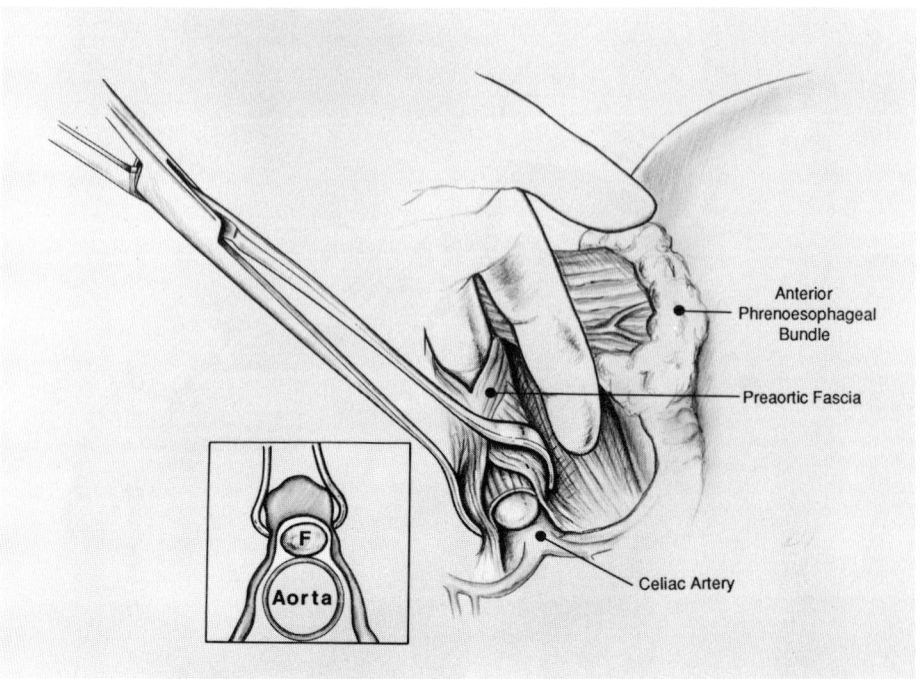

Fig. 8. The fibroareolar tissue in the esophageal hiatus is divided and a finger is passed down posterior to the preaortic fascia. Sutures may then be placed in the preaortic fascia without dissecting out the median arcuate ligament. The preaortic fascia is lifted off the aorta with a Babcock of stay suture.

esophageal hiatus. The fibroareolar tissue overlying the aorta and the esophageal hiatus can be simply divided by sharp dissection, thereby exposing the aorta. A finger is then passed gently beneath the preaortic fascia, down to the celiac artery and the preaortic fascia can be lifted off the aorta. The fascia can be grasped with a Babcock clamp and sutures simply placed through the preaortic fascia. This is a much simpler and safer approach than dissecting out the celiac artery. This technique was described by Vansant (Fig. 8) and is used quite frequently. In passing the finger behind the fascia, care must be taken not to damage short branches that pass from the aorta to the crura. By staying in the midline, these branches are avoided. We find that this approach is preferable and we now rarely dissect out the median arcuate ligament.

The crura of the esophageal hiatus are loosely approximated behind the esophagus with nonabsorbable sutures. The crura are closed so that a finger can be placed alongside the esophagus, making certain the closure is not too tight.

The stomach is then rotated to expose the anterior and posterior phrenoesophageal bundles. The bundles are grasped with Babcock clamps well above the left gastric artery, taking care not to traumatize the vagal nerves. Strong, nonabsorbable sutures are used for the repair. Sutures are taken through the anterior and posterior phrenoesophageal bundles. These are then passed through the preaortic fascia which is lifted well off the aorta with a Babcock clamp. Usually five sutures are placed in the anterior and posterior phrenoesophageal bundles and carried through the preaortic

664

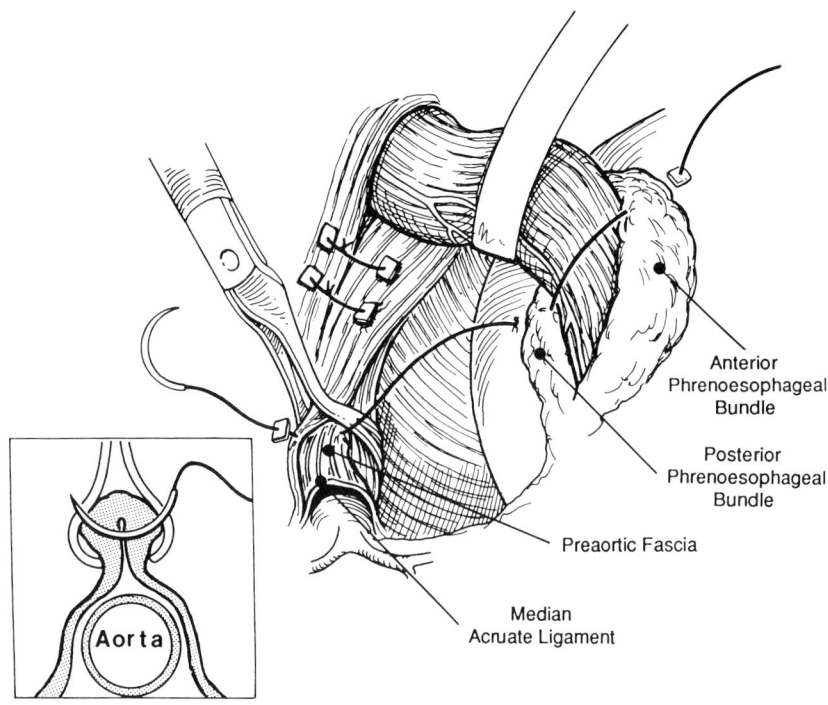

Fig. 9. The hiatus is closed loosely about the esophagus and sutures are commenced in the anterior and posterior phrenoesophageal bundles and carried through the preaortic fascia. The median arcuate ligament is not dissected out. Four such sutures are placed and the top suture is tied with a single throw and a knot to allow for pressure measurements and alteration of the sutures according to the pressure obtained.

fascia (Fig. 9). These sutures are placed with the vagus nerves in full view, in order not to damage them. A single knot is then placed in the top three sutures which are then clamped with long hemostats. Measurement of the barrier pressure is then obtained by passing the side hole of the modified nasogastric tube attached to a monitor through the GE junction. If the pressure is above 40 mmHg, the sutures are loosened. If it is below 25 mmHg, the sutures are tightened, depending on the problem at hand. After the proper pressure is obtained, all five sutures are tied and a final pressure measurement is taken. The barrier is usually 3–4 cm long. Additional cardiodiaphragmatic sutures are taken. The final appearance of the repair is shown in Fig. 10. In addition to restoring the sphincter, the GEV is accentuated and can be readily palpated through the wall of the stomach. The valve measures from 3–4 cm along the lesser curve and is important in the prevention of reflux. In patients who have had previous operations with scarring and destruction of the GEJ, the valve may be destroyed or inadequate. In these cases, a gastrostomy is performed, and the valve is secured with sutures in the anterior and posterior edges of the valve, thereby lengthening the valve to 3–4 cm. Attempts to calibrate the cardia with a bougie are unsatisfactory. It is impossible to determine whether the wrap around the bougie is too tight or too loose.

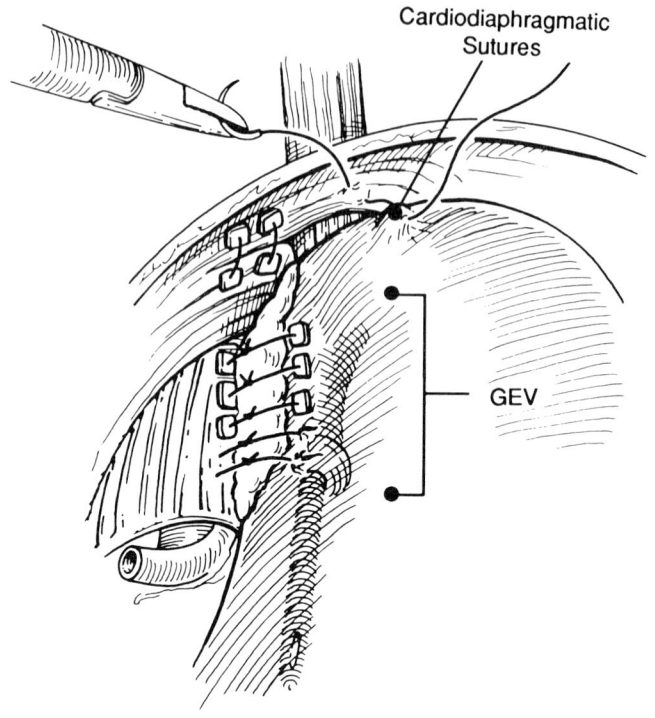

Fig. 10. The final appearance of the repair is shown. All 4–5 sutures are tied, anchoring the GE junction to the preaortic fascia. If the procedure is done open, the GEV can be palpated. If it is done closed, endoscopy is done to check the valve. Cardiodiaphragmatic sutures are placed in to prevent herniation back into the posterior mediastinum.

Intraoperative manometry

In 1977 the authors' group first reported the use of a simplified method of measuring the pressure in the antireflux barrier during operation to give the surgeon an objective determination of the pressure that has been created. This measurement is obtained by simply modifying the nasogastric tube which is routinely used in these patients. The tip of the smaller silastic sump portion of the tube is sealed at the end and a 1 mm side hole is cut 18 cm from the tip of the tube (Fig. 11). This small silastic tube is attached to a strain gauge and to a manometer that produces a digital reading. If this manometer is not available, the pressure tube can simply be attached to the arterial line that the anesthesiologist has available. The tube is constantly perfused at a slow rate (0.7 ml/min). This apparatus is identical to the one that has been used in the gastric lab for over a decade and has been thoroughly standardized and used in over 19,000 patients at the institution. The side hole is passed across the GEJ at operation and a baseline pressure is obtained prior to repair. Most often there is no pressure whatever in the GE junction. As the side hole passes through the junction, both a

666

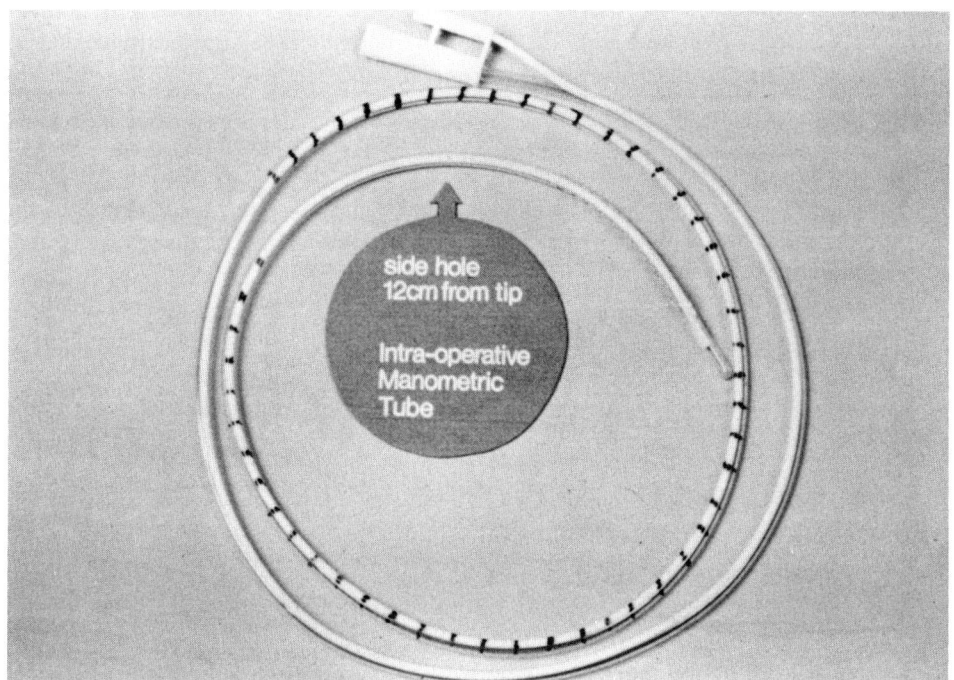

Fig. 11. Modified nasogastric tube with a side hole which can be passed back and forth across the lower esophageal sphincter during surgery to determine the appropriate barrier pressure.

tracing and a digital readout are obtained. After the repair, if the pressure is over 40 mmHg, the sutures which have been placed are loosened. If the pressure is less than 20 mmHg, the sutures are tightened. This process is continued until a pressure of somewhere between 25 and 35 mmHg is obtained. The side hole must be pulled at a steady rate through the barrier. If it is pulled through too rapidly, a peak pressure will be missed.

In the repair of recurrent hernias, there is no doubt that intraoperative pressure measurement could avoid some of the disastrous complications of the Nissen procedure which occur when the wrap is either too loose or too tight. Further efforts to simplify intraoperative manometrics and to make the technique more readily available are underway. The present technique is safe and simple and requires only a few minutes to obtain valuable information. It is in the authors' opinion that in a major antireflux operation, so dependent upon the construction of an adequate barrier, intraoperative assessment of the barrier should become a standard part of any technique that is used.

It is important to point out that the Hill repair is not a fundoplication. The phrenoesophageal bundles are imbricated together and there is no wrap of stomach around the lower esophagus. Very often this operation is erroneously described as partial fundoplication or a wrap. There is no intention upon the part of the authors of this procedure to do a blind wrap around of the stomach, but rather a careful calibration of the antireflux barrier, restoration of the GEV and posterior fixation of the GEJ. There is no wrap to slip. The basic differences between the gastroesophageal restoration repair and the Nissen repair are as follows:

- The Hill procedure depends upon augmentation of the intrinsic pressure and its special features. By placing tension on the collarsling musculature, the repair automatically restores the GEV which has been shown to be important in the prevention of reflux. The Nissen repair, on the other hand, depends upon extrinsic pressure of a wrap around the lower esophagus with indirect pressure on the lower esophagus.
- The Hill procedure anchors the GEJ posteriorly to its normal primary attachment, the preaortic fascia. The Nissen repair is allowed to float freely and the GEJ is not anchored. The unanchored esophagus has no fulcrum from which to operate and almost always develops a dysmotility since the esophagus cannot generate propulsive waves.
- In the Hill procedure, no sutures into the esophagus are used because the esophagus has no serosa and no strength. The Nissen procedure employs esophageal sutures to hold the wrap in place. The weakness of these sutures accounts for the frequency of the slipped Nissen. If these sutures are taken deeply, there is a risk of fistula formation from the esophagus.
- In the Hill procedure, intraoperative pressure measurement is used to calibrate the barrier created at operation, giving an objective assessment of the competence of the reflux barrier. This should be used in all repairs, whether it is the Hill, the Belsey or the Nissen. In the Nissen procedure, the surgeon either relies on a bougie or a finger placed up into the esophageal lumen. A number of patients have been seen in whom a large bougie was used only to find that as soon as the bougie was removed the wrap, which was made too tight, simply closed down or the wrap that was made loosely remains open after removal of the bougie.

Results

Several reviews of our own series, and those reported by others, have shown good results for follow-up extending to 8 years. To determine how these early results stand the test of time, the authors conducted a long-term follow-up study. In this recent report of patients undergoing the Hill procedure with reconstruction of the GE junction and restoration of the flap valve for primary GE reflux, 447 patients were reviewed from the time of their initial operation to follow-up assessment. These assessments were conducted after 5 to 10 years and 15 to 20 years. All operations were performed during a 5-year period between 1968 and 1973 by the same surgeon. The mean follow-up was 17.5 years.

All patients (240 men and 207 women; mean age 54.3 years; range 18 to 79 years) had suffered from primary symptoms of GE reflux of heartburn and regurgitation prior to surgery. Twenty-nine of these patients also had significant dysphagia.

Patients rated the results of their operations on a scale ranging from excellent to poor. The proportion of patients subjectively rating their operative results as good to excellent, increased from 82% during the 1977—1978 evaluation period to 88.5% during the 1987—1988 evaluation period. Of the total number of patients assessed, 95% rated their results as excellent to good with only 5.5% rating their outcome as fair. Eight patients in this series rated their surgical outcome as poor. Only three patients from the original operative series of 447 patients were found to have required reoperation for recurrent symptoms during the follow-up period. Therefore, the anatomical recurrence rate is less than 1%. It was gratifying to find that there were none of the severe complications such as esophageal fistula, thoracic incarceration, obstruction and severe gas bloat, that have been reported with other types of antireflux repairs.

This study clearly shows that a carefully done Hill repair with reconstruction of the GE junction and restoration of the flap valve has proved to be safe and reliable, providing a definitive antireflux repair which stands the test of time. The addition of intraoperative manometry has resulted in an even more precise operation, thus even better long-term results are predicted for the future. A complete follow-up, multi-center study is in progress.

Reproducibility

For an operation to be of value, it should be reproducible with good results in other hands. The Hill repair has been performed and reported by a number of surgeons around the world: Csendes and Larrain in Chile, Hermreck and Coates in the United States, along with Thomas, Vansant, Warshaw, Ottinger, Mercer of Canada and Russell of Australia, to name a few. Csendes and Larrain achieved a 93% good results and no radiologic recurrence in 29 patients followed up to 16 months. Mercer has performed the Hill procedure in 110 patients with 95% good results. Vansant et al. have reported treating up to 400 patients with around 90% good results. A multi-institution study is underway which will include around 2,500 patients and the analysis thus far appears to yield a 90% good result over the long term without the complications reported with the Nissen procedure.

Summary and Conclusion

In summary, the Hill procedure includes reconstruction of the normal gastro-esophageal junction and restoration of the gastroesophageal valve. This restores the esophagus to its normal point of attachment or fulcrum, allowing it to generate forceful peristaltic waves to propel food aborally into the stomach. In short, the esophageal motility is restored. The sphincter is calibrated, and the pressure measured so that a range of pressure is created that is high enough to prevent reflux but not so high as to create dysphagia. The gastroesophageal valve is restored and the diaphragm is closed loosely about the esophagus. With careful selection of patients and careful performance of the procedure, good results can be obtained over the long term.

References

1. Allison PR, Johnstone AS. The oesophagus lined with gastric mucous membrane. Thorax 1953;8:87—101.
2. Barrett NR. The lower esophagus lined by columnar epithelium. Surgery 1957;41:881—894.
3. Brand DL, Eastwood IR, Martin D et al. Esophageal symptoms, manometry, and histology before and after antireflux surgery: a long-term follow-up study. Gastroenterology 1979;76:1393—1401.
4. Cameron AJ, Ott BJ, Payne WS. The incidence of adenocarcinoma in columnar-lined (Barrett's) esophagus. N Engl J Med 1985;313:857—859.
5. Fyke RE, Code CF, Schleggel JF. The GE sphincter in healthy human beings. Gastroenterologia 1956;86:135—150.
6. Hameeteman W, Tytgat GNJ, Houthoff HF et al. Barrett's esophagus: development of dysplasia and adenocarcinoma. Gastroenterology 1989;96:1249—1256.
7. Hamilton SR, Smith RRL, Cameron JL. Prevalence and characteristics of Barrett's esophagus in patients with adenocarcinoma of the esophagus or esophagogastric junction. Hum Pathol 1988;19:942—948.
8. Havelund T, Laursen LS, Skoubo-Kristensen E et al. Omeprazole and ranitidine in treatment of reflux oesophagitis: double-blind comparative trial. Br Med 1988;296:89—92.
9. Hill LD. Intraoperative measurement of lower esophageal sphincter pressure. J Thorac Cardiovasc Surg 1978;75:378—382.
10. Hill LD, Chapman KW, Morgan EH. Objective evaluation of surgery for hiatus hernia and esophagitis J Thorac Cardiovasc Surg 1961;41:60.
11. Hill LD, Gelfand M, Bauermeister D. Simplified management of reflux esophagitis with stricture. Ann Surg 1970;172: 639—651.
12. Hill LD, Morgan EH, Kellogg HB. Experimentation as an aid in management of esophageal disorders. Am J Surg 1961; 102:240—253.
13. Klinkenberg-Knol EC, Jansen JMB, Festen HPM et al. Double-blind multicenter comparison of omeprazole and ranitidine in the treatment of reflux oesophagitis. Lancet 1987;349—351.
14. Leonardi HK, Crozier RE, Ellis FH. Reoperation for complications of the Nissen fundoplication. J Thorac Cardiovasc Surg 1981;81:50—56.
15. Little AG, Ferguson MK, Skinner DB. Reoperation for failed antireflux operations. Surgery 1986;91:511—517.
16. Mittal RK, Dudley F, Rochester DF, McCallum RW. Sphincteric action of the diaphragm during a relaxed lower esophageal sphincter in humans. J Am Physiol Soc 1989:G 139.
17. Morgan EH, Hill LD, Siemsen JK et al. Studies of intraluminal esophageal and gastric pressure and pH. Bull Mason Clin 1960;14:53—89.
18. Negre JB. Postfundoplication symptoms. Do they restrict the success of Nissen fundoplication? Ann Surg 1983;198:698—700.
19. Nissen R. Eine einfache Operation zur beeinflussung der Refluxösophagitis Schweiz Med Wochenschr 1956;86:590.
20. Ovaska J, Miettinen M, Kivilaakso E. Adenocarcinoma arising in Barrett's esophagus. Dig Dis Sci 1989;34:1139—1336.
21. Patterson DJ, Graham DY, Smith IL et al. Natural history of benign esophageal stricture treated by dilatation. Gastroenterology 1983;85:346— 350.
22. Rabinovitch PS, Reid BJ, Haggitt RC et al. Progression to cancer in Barrett's esophagus is associated with genomic instability. Lab Invest 1988;60:65—71.
23. Reid BJ, Haggitt RC, Rubin CE, Rabinovitch PS. Barrett's esophagus. Correlation between flow cytometry and histology in detection of patients at risk for adenocarcinoma. Gastroenterology 1987;93:1—11.
24. Reid BJ et al. Endoscopic biopsy can detect high-grade dysplasia or early adenocarcinoma in Barrett's esophagus without grossly recognizable neoplastic lesions. Gastroenterology 1988;94:81—90.
25. Rossetti M, Hell K. Fundoplication for the treatment of gastroesophageal reflux in hiatal hernia. World J Surg 1977;I:439—444.
26. Russell COH. Control of reflux. In: Hill LD, Kozarek RA, McCallum RW, Mercer CD (eds) The Esophagus: Medical and Surgical Management. Philadelphia: WB Saunders, 1988;45—46.
27. Skinner DB, Walther BC, Riddell RH et al. Barrett's esophagus. Comparison of benign and malignant cases. Ann Surg 1983;198:554—565.
28. Thor K, Silander T. Long-term randomized prospective trial of the Nissen procedure vs. a modified Toupet technique. Ann Surg 1989;210:719—724.
29. Watson A. The role of antireflux surgery combined with fiberoptic endoscopic dilatation in peptic esophageal stricture. Am J Surg 1984;148:346—349.

Selected references

Hill LD, Aye RW, Ramel S. Antireflux surgery: a surgeon's look. Gastroenterol Clin North Am 1990; 19:745–775. This publication is an excellent review of the present status of antireflux surgery.

Larrain A, Pope CE. Respiratory complications of gastroesophageal reflux. In: The Esophagus: Medical and Surgical Management. Hill LD, Kozarek RA, McCallum RW, Mercer CD (eds). Philadelphia: WB Saunders, 1988, pp 70–77. It has become recognized that respiratory complications account for a large portion of the gastroesophageal reflux problem. This is a very important review of that complication of reflux.

Low DE, Anderson RP, Ilves R et al. Fifteen- to twenty-year results after the Hill antireflux operation. J Thorac Cardiovasc Surg 1989;98:444–450. This study represents the longest follow-up of antireflux surgery to be published. There was a mean follow-up of 17.5 years and the results are excellent considering the fact that these patients were among the early patients done with this technique and were low on the learning curve and done prior to the availability of new technology, including measurement of sphincter pressures.

Low DE, Mercer CD, James EC, Hill LD. Post-Nissen syndrome. Surg Gynecol Obstet 1988;167:1–5. This review represents the largest series of post-Nissen problems from any institution in the world. It represents an excellent survey of the serious problems that are being seen all too frequently with the Nissen procedure.

Mercer CD, Hill LD. Surgical management of peptic esophageal stricture. J Thorac Cardiovasc Surg 1986; 91:371–378. This important article demonstrates clearly that a simplified antireflux procedure will correct most patients with peptic esophageal stricture. Resection is reserved only for those patients who have a destroyed esophagus.

Reid BJ, Haggitt RC, Rubin CE. Barrett's esophagus and esophageal adenocarcinoma. In: The Esophagus: Medical and Surgical Management. Hill LD, Kozarek RA, McCallum RW, Mercer CD (eds). Philadelphia: WB Saunders, 1988;157–166. The Reid, Haggitt, and Rubin group has the largest collection of biopsies in Barrett's esophagus in the world. From this experience they are able to show that there is a direct relationship between Barrett's esophagus and adenocarcinoma.

Thor K, Hill LD, Mercer CD, Kozarek RA. Reappraisal of the flap valve mechanism: A study of a new valvuloplasty procedure in cadavers. Acta Chir Scand 1987;153:25–28. This paper represents publication of the cadaver work done to illustrate the importance of the gastroesophageal valve which is the main component of the antireflux barrier. The valve, when visualized with the retroflexed endoscope, gives a better assessment of the clinical picture than measurement of the sphincter pressure.

Belsey operation

 ## Is Belsey's operation preferable if there is a disorder of esophageal motility?

T. Lerut (Leuven)

Motor disturbances of the esophagus are generally classified into two groups:
1. Primary motor disorders
— achalasia;
— vigorous achalasia;
— diffuse esophageal spasm (DES) (cork-screw esophagus);
— painful esophageal peristalsis (nut-cracker esophagus);
— transitional forms and nonspecific disorders.
2. Secondary motor disorders secondary to gastroesophageal reflux (GER).
In the first group, the best known indication for surgery is achalasia and, to a lesser extent, vigorous achalasia and diffuse spasm.

The first question to be answered is whether or not an antireflux operation is necessary when performing surgery for primary motor disorders: this is extremely difficult to answer since data from literature, usually dealing with retrospective studies mostly on achalasia, are very conflicting. It seems, however, that over the years the trend to add an antireflux procedure after a myotomy is growing [1]. It appears from the available data that indeed the incidence of GER is significantly lower when an antireflux procedure was performed (Table 1). As far as the problems of DES are concerned, some groups [2] are performing a myotomy across the gastroesophageal junction only when the lower esophageal sphincter (LES) is hypertensive, in which case an antireflux procedure is recommended. Others usually

Table 1. Gastroesophageal reflux following esophageal myotomy for achalasia

Study (without antireflux procedure)	Number of patients	Number with postoperative reflux	Study (with antireflux procedure)	Number of patients	Number with postoperative reflux
Ellis 1964 [14]	113	4	Okike 1979	16	1
Okike 1979 [15]	456	14	Pai 1984	17	2
Pai 1984 [16]	16	0	Belsey 1966	62	0
Ferguson 1960 [17]	44	4	Peyton 1979 [20]	8	2
Belsey 1966 [18]	64	10	Bjorck 1982	11	0
Jara 1979 [19]	121	63			
Bjorck 1982 [21]	41	8			
Total	855	103 (12%)	Total	114	5 (4%)

find a myotomy over the LES necessary to reduce outflow obstruction and consequently add an antireflux procedure [1].

The second question is whether to perform a total or partial fundoplication.

Again, there are few scientific data to answer this question. It is however generally accepted that the use of an antireflux procedure after a myotomy introduces the potential to recreate the problem the surgeon is trying to solve, namely outflow obstruction hindering esophageal emptying, as the powerless myotomized esophagus may show difficulty in pushing a swallowed bolus across a recreated high pressure zone. This is reported to be the main cause of recurrent dysphagia together with an incomplete myotomy. Stipa [3] observed 11.5% recurrent dysphagia after myotomy plus Nissen for achalasia. To overcome this problem, Del Genio [4] uses preoperative manometric calibration of the Nissen fundoplication, resulting in a transitory dysphagia in only four out of 54 patients operated for achalasia, and no patients had pathologic reflux. Duranceau has been performing a short (2 cm) Nissen fundoplication in addition to the myotomy on a number of patients who were followed up for many years. In a first report with a follow-up of 1 to 2 years, there was no recurrent dysphagia [5]. However, in two subsequent publications [6,7], reflecting the results at a much longer follow-up, respectively 50% and 75% of his patients showed recurrent symptoms (Table 2). These recurrent symptoms came along with a progressive increase in diameter of the distal esophagus on barium swallow, and a worsening of stasis on radionuclide transit studies. Duranceau's work shows the importance of a very extended long-term follow-up before making any conclusion. Most authors, however, advocate the use of a partial fundoplication, with a low incidence of recurrent dysphagia [8–11].

The third and final question then is whether a Belsey Mark IV should to be performed when dealing with motor disturbances of the esophagus. This question of course deals completely with the approach for the myotomy. A Belsey Mark IV can only be performed through a thoracic approach. The choice of the approach is highly dependent on the surgeon's personal preferences as, again, no scientific evidence supports either the abdominal or thoracic approach. The rationale for an abdominal approach is its supposedly less traumatic aspect with lower morbidity. The abdominal

674

Table 2. Partial or total fundoplication?

Partial fundoplication and recurrent dysphagia

	Type of fundoplication	Number of patients	Dysphagia
Perrault 1991 [8]	Belsey	14	0
Little 1988 [9]	Belsey	38	0
Csendes 1988 [10]	Dor	100	1

Total fundoplication (Nissen) and recurrent symptoms

Stipa [3]	:	11.5% recurrent dysphagia.
Del Genio [4] :	Intraoperative manometry and calibration (n = 54)
	Four transient dysphagia - no reflux.
Duranceau	:	Myotomy and short Nissen (2 cm).
[5]	1981: Follow up: 1–2 years (n = 12)
	0% recurrent dysphagia.
[6]	1988: Follow up: 6–8 years (n = 15)
	50% recurrent symptoms.
[7]	1992: Follow up: 6–10 years (n = 17)
	75% recurrent symptoms.

approach theoretically allows a longer downward extension of the myotomy, reducing the risks of recurrent dysphagia. In this setup, a partial fundoplication of the Dor type is often recommended.

The thoracic approach has the advantage that it allows a longer cephalad extension of the myotomy. Some groups prefer to perform systematically a long myotomy, as in many patients the motor disturbance is rather a mixture of different disorders, and abnormal motility in the esophageal body can interfere with bolus transit [9]. The thoracic approach is also preferred in obese patients or in patients who have had previous abdominal surgery. In these cases the modified Belsey Mark IV, in which two rows of two mattress sutures are placed on each side of the myotomy, is the operation of choice. From our own experience, we have analyzed the data of a group of 11 patients, who were followed up for at least 5 years postoperatively, and who underwent a long myotomy for achalasia combined with a modified Belsey Mark IV antireflux procedure. Until today, no patient has had recurrent dysphagia or important regurgitation while one patient had a poor result due to severe gastroesophageal reflux.

Finally, in patients with motor disturbances secondary to reflux, as for most patients with indications for antireflux surgery, we prefer a Belsey Mark IV since from our experience with this operation, patients are enjoying better eating and drinking than after a Nissen operation, with the same percentage of reflux control [11]. Moreover, evidence is growing that, in patients with severe motor disturbances of the esophageal body secondary to GER, antireflux is not resulting in recovery of normal motility [12]. Persisting motor disturbances after a total Nissen-type fundoplication eventually may result in increasing difficulties to propel the food bolus across the fundoplication. It is not unlikely to assume that, in the long-term follow-up, these motor disturbances may even become worse, resulting in late dysphagia [13].

Conclusion

A scientifically based response to the question whether a Belsey Mark IV procedure is the preferred antireflux procedure in patients suffering from esophageal motor disturbances is difficult. The reason for this is the lack of prospective and randomized studies, resulting in a great deal of controversial aspects to this kind of surgery. However, it seems that there is a growing consensus to systematically add a fundoplication in patients who undergo a myotomy for a primary motor disorder. Most authors today advocate a partial type of fundoplication. When a thoracic approach is used, the modified Belsey Mark IV should be the preferred antireflux procedure. In patients with secondary motor disorders related to gastroesophageal reflux, we also prefer the classic Belsey Mark IV antireflux procedure.

References

1. DeMeester TR, Stein HJ. Surgery of esophageal motor disorders. In: Castell DO (ed) The Esophagus. Boston: Little Brown, 1992;401–439.
2. Jamieson GG. Is there a risk of late esophageal obstruction when myotomy is not extended into the oesophagogastric junction? In: OESO, Giuli R, McCallum RW, Skinner DB (eds) Primary Motility Disorders of the Esophagus. Paris: John Libbey Eurotext, 1991;722–723.
3. Stipa S, Iascone C, Moraldi A. Esophagomyotomy with antireflux procedures for achalasia of the oesophagus clinical comparison of Nissen fundoplication and Belsey MIV. In: Siewert JR, Holscher AR (eds) Diseases of the Esophagus. Berlin: Springer Verlag, 1988;966–969.
4. Del Genio A, Di Martino N, Fei L, Maffetone V, Ambrosio A. L'esame manometrico intraoperativo dell'esophago serve a migliorare l'interventi e quindi anche la prognosi dei pazienti? Acta Chir Ital 1986;42:762–769.
5. Duranceau A, Lafontaine ER, Vallières B. Effects of total fundoplication on function of the esophagus of myotomy for achalasia. Am J Surg 1982;143:22–28.
6. Duranceau A, Cardin JL, Taillefer R. Long-term effects of total fundoplicaiton on the myotomised esophagus. In: Siewert JR, Hölscher AH (eds) Diseases of the Esophagus. Berlin: Springer Verlag, 1988;1206–1209.
7. Topart P, Deschamps C, Taillefer R, Duranceau A. Long-term effect of total fundoplication on the myotomised esophagus. Ann Thorac Surg 1992;54;1046–1052.
8. Perrault L, Beauchamp G, Bastien E, Laurendeau F, Jobin G, Archambault A. Surgical treatment of achalasia in a general hospital. Can J Surg 1991;34:487–490.
9. Little AG, Soriano A, Ferguson MK, Winans CS, Skinner DB. Surgical treatment of achalasia: results with esophagomyotomy and Belsey repair. Ann Thorac Surg 1988;45:489–494.
10. Csendes A, Braghetto I, Mascaro J, Henriquez A. Late subjective and objective evaluation of the results of esophagomyotomy in 100 patients with achalasia of the esophagus. Surgery 1988;104:469–475.
11. Lerut T, Coosemans W, Christiaens R, Gruwez JA. The Belsey Mark IV antireflux procedure: indications and long-term results. Acta Gastroenterol Belg 1990;53:585–590.
12. Lundell LR, Myers JC, Jamieson GG. The influence of preoperative oesophageal motor dysfunction on the long-term outcome of antireflux surgery. Gullet 1993;3:50–55.
13. Luostarinen M. Nissen fundoplication for reflux esophagitis: long-term clinical and endoscopic results in 109 of 127 consecutive patients. Ann Surg 1993;217:329–337.
14. Ellis FH, Crozier RE, Watkins E. Operation for esophagal achalasia: results of esophagomytomy without an antireflux operation. J Thorac Cardiovasc Surg 1984;88:344–351.
15. Okike N, Payne WS, Neufeld DM et al. Esophagomyotomy versus forceful dilatation for achalasia of the esophagus: results in 899 patients. Ann Thorac Surg 1979;28:119–125.
16. Pai GP, Ellison RG, Rubin JW et al. Two decades of experience with modified Heller's myotomy for achalasia. Ann Thorac Surg 1984;38:201–206.
17. Ferguson TB, Burfor TH. An evaluation of the modified Heller operation in the treatment of achalasia of the esophagus. Ann Surg 1960;152:1–15.
18. Belsey R. Functional disease of the esophagus. J Thorac Cardiovasc Surg 1966;62:164–188.
19. Jara FM, Toledo-Pereyra LH, Leweis JW, Malligan DJ. Long-term results of esophagomyotomy for achalasia of esophagus. Arch Surg 1979;114:935–936.
20. Peyton MD, Greenfield LD, Elkins RC. Combined myotomy and hiatal herniorraphy: a new approach to achalasia. Am J Surg 1974; 128:786–790.
21. Bjorck S, Dernevik L, Gatzinsky P, Sanberg N. Oesophagocardiomyotmy and antireflux procedures. Acta Chir Scand 1982;148:525–529.

Collis operation

What are the respective indications for:
— the Collis-Belsey procedure?
— the Collis-Nissen procedure?

H.C. Urschel (Dallas)

The original indication for the Collis-Belsey operation was for a stricture of the lower esophagus [1]. To avoid resection, the stricture was dilated and, to lengthen the esophagus for an adequate fundoplication procedure, the Collis maneuver was used on the lesser curvature of the stomach [2—4]. It lengthened the esophagus with a gastric tube so that, which ever fundoplication procedure (Belsey or Nissen) was employed, there was no tension. The new cardia was well in the abdomen, allowing positive pressure of the abdomen on the long intra-abdominal tube [5—7]. Subsequently, the indications have included people requiring repair for significant gastroesophageal reflux not treatable by medical means with a short esophagus, Barrett's esophagus, pulmonary aspiration, as well as complications such as obesity and recurrent hiatal hernia with gastroesophageal reflux [8—12].

The final indication is for the standard patient with gastroesophageal reflux (with or without hiatal hernia), whose symptoms of gastroesophageal reflux cannot be controlled by medical means. The reason for extending the procedure to this group is that there was a known recurrence rate between 10 and 15% for the "Belsey" procedure, even in the uncomplicated cases where there was no evidence of pulmonary complications, a short esophagus or stricture, and no evidence of a recurrent hiatal hernia or gastroesophageal reflux [13—18]. Due to the safety of the procedure (no leaks in the past) and the theoretical advantages of a longer esophagus and a fundoplication likely to be performed without any tension, we felt that this procedure should be applied to every surgical patient with the hope that it would lower the recurrence rate. The Collis-Belsey procedure reduced the recurrence to only 6% over a period of 15 years [9].

All of the indications for the Collis-Belsey procedure would pertain for the Collis-Nissen operation. The main difference is that the Collis-Nissen is an easier reconstruction from the intra-abdominal approach. When the intra-abdominal route is mandated by such problems as gallstones, gastric surgery etc., this is the easier procedure. It also may be employed where the surgeon is not confident or qualified to perform thoracic surgery. The Belsey procedure is difficult to perform through the abdomen. The Collis-Nissen can be used easily in the chest if it is preferred by the surgeon. The advantages and indications for the Collis-Nissen operation are the same as listed above for the Collis-Belsey procedure.

References

1. Pearson FG, Langer B, Henderson RD. Gastroplasty and Belsey hiatal hernia repair. J Thorac Cardiovasc Surg 1971;61:50.
2. Collis JL. An operation for hiatus hernia with short esophagus. Thorax 1957;12:181.
3. Collis JL. An operation for hiatus hernia with short esophagus. J Thorac Cardiovasc Surg 1957;34:768.
4. Collis JL. Gastroplasty. Thorax 1961;16:197.
5. Hiebert CA, Belsey RH. Incompetence of the gastric cardia with radiologic evidence of hiatal hernia. J Thorac Cardiovasc Surg 1961;42:352.
6. Hill LD. Intraoperative measurement of lower esophageal sphincter pressure. J Thorac Cardiovasc Surg 1978;75:378.
7. Skinner DB, Belsey RH, Hendrix TR, Zuidema GD. Surgical management of esophageal reflux and hiatal hernia. In: Gastroesophageal Reflux and Hiatal Hernia. Boston: Little, Brown and Company, 1972.
8. Urschel HC Jr, Paulson DL. Gastroesophageal reflux and hiatal hernia. J Thorac Cardiovasc Surg 1967;53:21.
9. Urschel HC Jr, Razzuk MA. Recommendation of "Collis-Belsey" fundoplication for uncomplicated hiatal hernia and gastro-esophageal reflux. Ann Thorac Surg 1979;27:564.
10. Pearson FG, Henderson RD. Long-term follow-up of peptic strictures managed by dilatation, modified Collis gastroplasty and Belsey hiatus hernia repair. Surgery 1976;80:396–404.
11. Urschel HC Jr, Razzuk MA, Wood RE, Galbraith NF, Paulson DL. An improved surgical technique for the complicated hiatal hernia with gastroesophageal reflux. Ann Thorac Surg 1973;15:443.
12. Wood RE, Campbell D, Razzuk MA et al. Surgical advantages of selective unilateral ventilation. Ann Thorac Surg 1972;14:173.
13. Skinner DB, Belsey RHR, Russell PS. Gastroesophageal reflux and hiatal hernia. J Thorac Cardiovasc Surg 1967;53:33.
14. Orringer MB, Skinner DB, Belsey RH. Long-term results of the Mark IV operation for hiatal hernia and analysis of recurrence and the treatment. J Thorac Cardiovasc Surg 1972;63:25.
15. Orringer MB, Sloan H. Complications and failings of the combined Collis-Belsey operation. J Thorac Cardiovasc Surg 1977;74:726–735.
16. Orringer MB, Sloan H. Combined Collis-Nissen reconstruction of the esophagogastric junction. Ann Thorac Surg 1978;25:16–21.
17. Henderson RD. Personal communication, 1972.
18. Henderson RD. Reflux control following gastroplasty. Ann Thorac Surg 1977;24:206.

What are the comparative results of the Collis-Nissen procedure,
— with gastric section
— without gastric section?

A.G. Little (Las Vegas)

The Collis gastroplasty is a technique designed to functionally lengthen the esophagus by adding a tube of stomach with the exact dimensions as the esophagus. This operation is illustrated in Fig. 1. Collis initially proposed this operation as a primary and stand-alone procedure for reflux, particularly in the presence of a reflux stricture. Over time, ingenious surgeons have learned to combine the benefits of the gastric lengthening operation with the standard techniques of Belsey and Nissen for reflux control. In essence, this entails a thoracotomy with lengthening of the esophagus using the Collis technique when the surgeon feels that because of inflammation, there will be difficulty in reducing a completed standard antireflux procedure within the abdomen. The Collis is designed to relieve vertical tension and seems particularly appropriate for use in patients with severe and/or long-standing esophagitis or a fibrous reflux stricture. The severely inflamed esophagus can be stretched below the

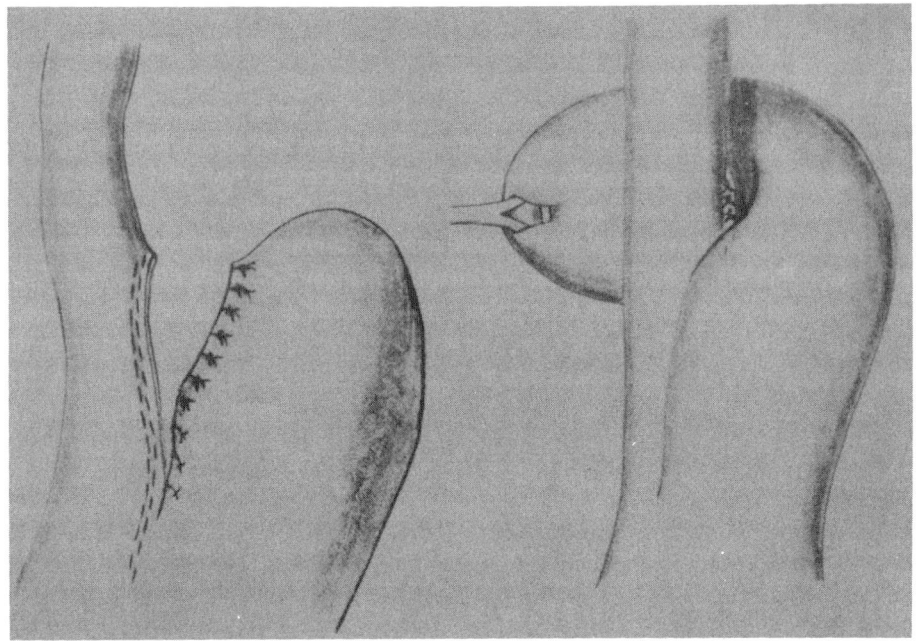

Fig. 1. The Collis procedure is performed via a left thoracotomy. After mobilization of the esophagus and gastric fundus, a GIA stapler is placed against a Maloney bougie passed through the esophagus and held against the lesser curve. After firing the stapler, the appearance is as shown on the left. Subsequently, the fundus can be wrapped around the "neo-esophagus" to construct a Nissen fundoplication as shown in the right-hand drawing.

diaphragm after an antireflux operation, but this vertical tension will subsequently tend to distract and disrupt the fundoplication, causing it to lose its efficiency. The Collis procedure helps prevent this development. After construction of the gastroplasty or neo-esophagus tube, either a Belsey Mark IV procedure or a Nissen fundoplication is performed, in the standard fashion, with the fundoplication being based upon the neo-esophagus of gastric mucosa.

Sufficient experience has been gained to show that the results of this approach to antireflux surgery are entirely satisfactory [1]. Unfortunately, a prospective randomized comparison of antireflux procedure with and without a Collis procedure has not been performed, so the exact indications for use of the Collis lengthening procedure are undefined.

A complication of the Collis procedure is a leak from the gastric suture line. This is presumably more likely to happen when previous antireflux or other gastroesophageal surgery has taken place, as multiple dissections interfere with the blood supply to this area. In addition, leaks were more common with hand-sewn gastric closure than are seen with current stapling techniques. With use of a GIA type stapler, the leak incidence is quite low. Nonetheless, to completely avoid this risk, an alternative approach has been suggested which involves stapling the gastroplasty tube but not actually cutting it to separate it from the fundus [2]. Although there has been less reported experience with this technique, it appears that results are similar to the so-called cut Collis gastroplasty experience. I have not had any personal experience with this technique. I do feel that the chance of leak using a GIA stapler and oversewing the staple line is so low that I would prefer to have the fundic mobility produced by cutting the gastroplasty rather than to leave it stapled and uncut. However, there is no reason to think that the uncut gastroplasty cannot be successful and this does not seem to be an issue on the cutting edge of surgery at this time.

References

1. Stirling MC, Orringer MB. Continued assessment of the combined Collis-Nissen operation. Ann Thorac Surg 1989;47:224–230.
2. Demos NJ. Stapled, uncut gastroplasty for hiatal hernia: twelve-year follow-up. Ann Thorac Surg 1984;38:393–399.

What are the advantages of the Collis-Nissen procedure in cases of stricture?

M.B. Orringer (Ann Arbor)

Esophageal reflux strictures are the end result of inflammation caused by reflux from the stomach of both acid and alkaline secretions, through an incompetent lower esophageal sphincter mechanism. The erosion of esophageal squamous epithelium by refluxed acid and bile is associated with acute submucosal inflammation which may extend into the esophageal muscular layers and adjacent periesophageal tissues. Healing of this process results in varying degrees of fibrosis. Repetition of this acute inflammation followed by healing produces progressive mural fibrosis which begins in the esophageal submucosa and may extend panmurally and involve adjacent tissues. As fibrous deposition continues and contraction of collagen fibers within the stricture occurs, circumferential narrowing of the lumen of the esophagus as well as varying degrees of esophageal shortening follow.

Esophageal reflux strictures occur clinically in three general varieties. The most common type is short (1–2 cm in length) and is localized to the esophagogastric junction, typically just proximal to a sliding hiatal hernia. The second more extensive reflux stricture involves the distal half or third of the esophagus for 3 to 5 cm or more in length. This type of stricture is typically seen after prolonged nasogastric intubation, especially in a critically ill patient who is supine for many days and at times after severe protracted vomiting, as in hyperemesis gravidarum or gastric outlet obstruction. The third type of reflux stricture occurs in the mid or upper thoracic esophagus, at the squamocolumnar epithelial junction in patients with Barrett's esophagus (columnar epithelium-lined lower esophagus). Regardless of the type of reflux stricture, it should be realized that a reflux stricture, no matter how "mild" the narrowing, represents an *advanced* stage of esophagitis for which aggressive institution of appropriate therapy is mandatory.

When confronted with an esophageal stricture, the surgeon must answer two basic questions: is the stricture benign or malignant, and if benign, can the stricture be dilated? Both of these questions are answered by esophagoscopy, which is mandatory in the evaluation of every esophageal stricture. The technique of endoscopic assessment of reflux strictures is beyond the scope of this discussion, but is of essential importance in the evaluation of these patients. The stricture should be both biopsied and brushed for cytologic assessment to rule out the presence of carcinoma. The "severity" of a reflux stricture cannot be predicted from its radiographic appearance. In assessing the severity of the stenosis, the surgeon is interested in knowing the degree of resistance encountered as an esophageal dilator is passed through it. This is a reflection of the degree of fibrosis associated with the stricture and has direct correlation with the clinical outcome of operations designed to treat the problem. Esophageal strictures are, therefore, graded in accordance with the degree of resistance encountered as the dilator is passed: 1) mild: no resistance; 2) moderate: requiring some force to dilate; and 3) severe: requiring very forceful dilation. As a general rule, strictures which can be dilated by passage of a bougie orally to the range of a 40 French size, can be further dilated intraoperatively to the 50–60 French range and will, therefore, be amenable to treatment with a concomitant antireflux procedure. Using currently available technology, particularly the Savary dilating system, at least 95% of all esophageal reflux strictures are dilatable. Since 25% of patients with reflux strictures complain only of dysphagia and have little if any symptoms of gastroesophageal reflux, they may respond extremely well to a periodic esophageal dilation 1 to 3 times a year and institution of aggressive antireflux medical therapy. In the remainder of patients with reflux strictures, persistent ulcerative esophagitis or refractory reflux symptoms warrant surgical intervention.

As one considers the available surgical options in the treatment of the patient with an esophageal reflux stricture, it is clear from reported series that the long-term success of a standard antireflux procedure (e.g., the Hill, Belsey, or Nissen operation) in controlling gastroesophageal reflux is influenced by the degree of esophagitis present at the time of operation. The presence of a stricture clearly increases the risk of recurrent herniation and/or reflux after any of these operations [6,7]. This is not particularly surprising, since the intramural inflammation and esophageal shortening associated with a reflux stricture prevent the *tension free* reduction of the prerequisite 3 to 5 cm segment of distal esophagus below the diaphragm. Since each of the standard antireflux operations seeks to achieve an intra-abdominal location of the esophagogastric junction and utilizes sutures into the distal esophageal or periesophageal tissues, the long-term success of these antireflux operations must be jeopardized in the presence of mural inflammation and esophageal shortening. For these factors require that sutures be taken into inflamed tissues and also that the esophagogastric junction be brought below the diaphragm under tension. While distal esophagectomy and reconstruction with either a jejunal or short segment colonic interposition provide good relief of dysphagia and reflux symptoms in patients with peptic strictures, these are sizeable and technically demanding operations which may be avoided by utilization of more conservative nonresective techniques.

Pearson and associates in 1971 reported success using the Collis gastroplasty operation in combination with the Belsey Mark IV hiatal hernia repair, in patients with severe reflux strictures and secondary esophageal shortening [1]. After intraoperative dilation of the stricture and construction of the gastroplasty tube over a large (56 or 58 French) intraesophageal dilator, Pearson advocated a standard Belsey repair around the "new" distal esophagus, i.e., the gastroplasty tube. This combined Collis-Belsey operation was conceptually sound as it lengthened the functional distal esophageal tube, thereby eliminating the need to "drag" the old esophagogastric junction beneath the diaphragm under tension, and the gastroplasty tube provided a resilient healthy stomach wall rather than the inflamed esophagus around which to suture the fundoplication. Pearson reported excellent relief of both dysphagia and reflux symptoms following dilation of peptic strictures and the Collis-Belsey operation in 25 of 33 patients so treated and followed for 5–12 years [2]. These results, however, were not duplicated by other investigators, and in an attempt to improve reflux control after performance of the Collis gastroplasty, Henderson [3] and Orringer and Sloan [4] began to advocate use of a 360° Nissen-type fundoplication.

Operative technique

The combined Collis-Nissen operation is performed through a left 6th interspace posterolateral thoracotomy. The costal margin is not divided and a diaphragmatic counter-incision is not utilized, unless adhesions from prior operations prevent mobilization of the cardia and upper stomach through the diaphragmatic hiatus. As in the routine Belsey Mark IV procedure, the gastric fundus is mobilized through the diaphragmatic hiatus after incising the phrenoesophageal attachments. Division and ligation of an average of six high short gastric vessels is carried out. Once complete mobilization of the cardia from all diaphragmatic hiatal attachments has been achieved, the esophageal stricture is supported by the surgeon's hand as progressively larger Maloney tapered esophageal dilators are passed by the anesthetist through the patient's mouth and are guided across the esophagogastric junction by the surgeon. Once the stricture has been dilated, the gastroplasty tube is constructed over a 54 French dilator in women or a 56 French dilator in men. The dilator is displaced against the lesser curvature of the stomach, and as the fundus is retracted in the opposite direction, the GIA surgical stapler is applied to the stomach adjacent and parallel to the dilator (Fig. 1). Use of the GIA stapler eliminates the need for a manually sewn gastric suture-line, simplifies construction of the gastroplasty tube and prevents gastrointestinal contamination of the field. Once the knife assembly is advanced, a 5-cm gastric tube extension of the esophagus is thereby created. It is occasionally necessary to partially apply the stapler a second time to gain an additional 2 to 3 cm of "esophageal" length if there is a great deal of esophageal

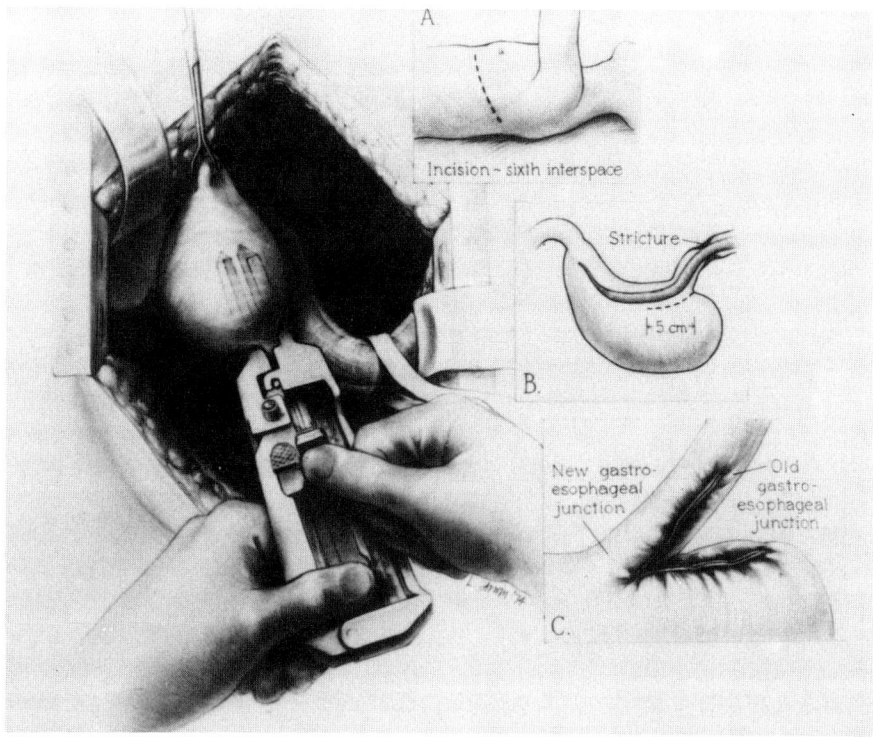

Fig. 1. Construction of the Collis gastroplasty tube utilizing the GIA surgical stapler. (A) Six left intercostal space posterolateral thoracotomy used. (B) 54 or 56 French Maloney dilator passed through the esophageal stricture and displaced against the lesser curvature of the stomach. Dotted line indicates subsequent placement of the surgical stapler. Main illustration showing knife assembly of the stapler being advanced. (C) Appearance of the neo-esophagus after removal of the surgical stapler. (Reproduced with permission of the CV Mosby Company from Orringer MB and Sloan H. J Thorac Cardiovasc Surg 1974;68:298–302 [8]).

shortening and fibrosis. In more than 97% of patients, however, one application of the GIA stapler is sufficient. The stapled suture-line is oversewn with running 4-0 polypropylene suture. An average of three to five #1 posterior crural sutures are placed but left untied for the present.

With the intraesophageal dilator still in place, the gastric fundus is passed posterior to the gastroplasty tube and is positioned for the fundoplication (Fig. 2). The fundoplication is constructed with four interrupted 2-0 silk sutures, each suture passing through the gastric fundus then the gastroplasty tube and then through the fundus again, beginning at the new esophagogastric junction and proceeding proximally (Fig. 3). The four sutures are placed 1 cm apart and as they are tied, a 3-cm long fundoplication around the gastroplasty tube is thereby achieved. The silk suture-line is then oversewn with a running 4-0 polypropylene Lembert stitch through the seromuscular layers on either side as a prophylactic measure against subsequent leak from the fundoplication sutures. The esophageal dilator is then removed, the

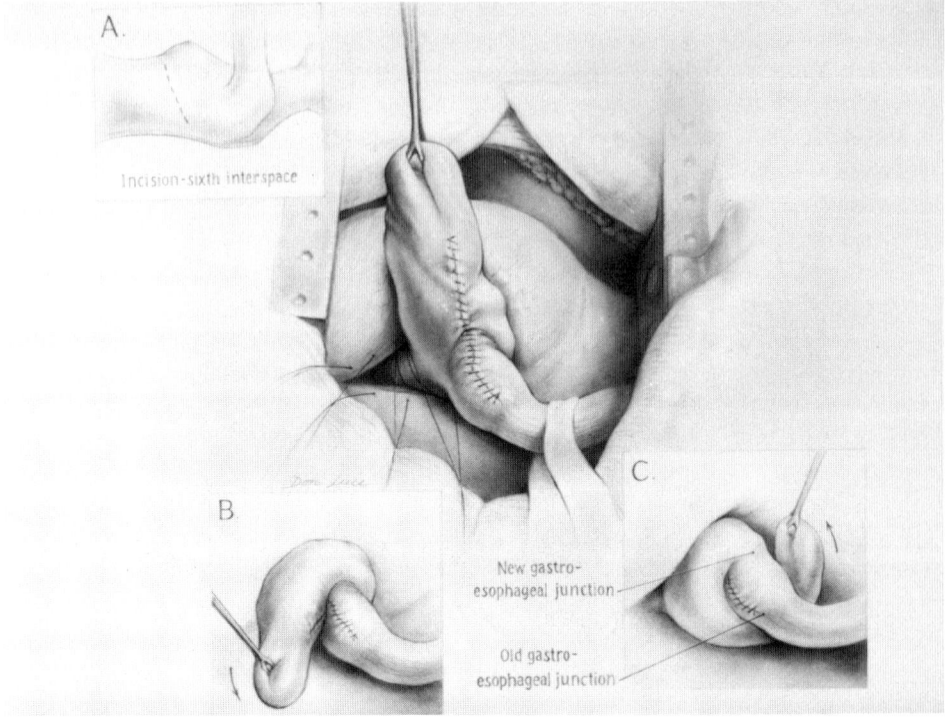

Fig. 2. Main drawing shows the elongated narrowed gastric fundus resulting after construction of the gastroplasty tube. Inset A shows the left 6th intercostal space thoracotomy used. Insets B & C show placement of the gastric fundus around the gastroplasty tube in preparation for construction of the fundoplication. The posterior crural sutures (main illustration) are left untied for the time being (reproduced with permission of Elsevier from Orringer MB and Sloan H. Ann Thorac Surg 1978;25:16–21 [11]).

fundoplication is reduced beneath the diaphragm, and the posterior crural sutures are tied until the diaphragmatic hiatus admits one finger loosely alongside the esophagus. At the conclusion of the operation, the distal esophagus rests loosely and without tension in the posterior mediastinum. Silver clip markers placed intraoperatively, two at the new esophagogastric junction (the apex of the gastroplasty tube) and two at the edges of the diaphragmatic hiatus, serve to identify the length of intra-abdominal segment of the functional neo-esophagus that is encircled by the gastric wrap.

Results

Sixty-four patients (average age 51 years) with esophageal reflux strictures have been treated by the author with intraoperative dilation and a combined Collis-Nissen procedure as described above [5]. There was one postoperative death (1.6% mortality) from a pulmonary embolus 2 weeks after operation. Esophageal leaks occurred in two

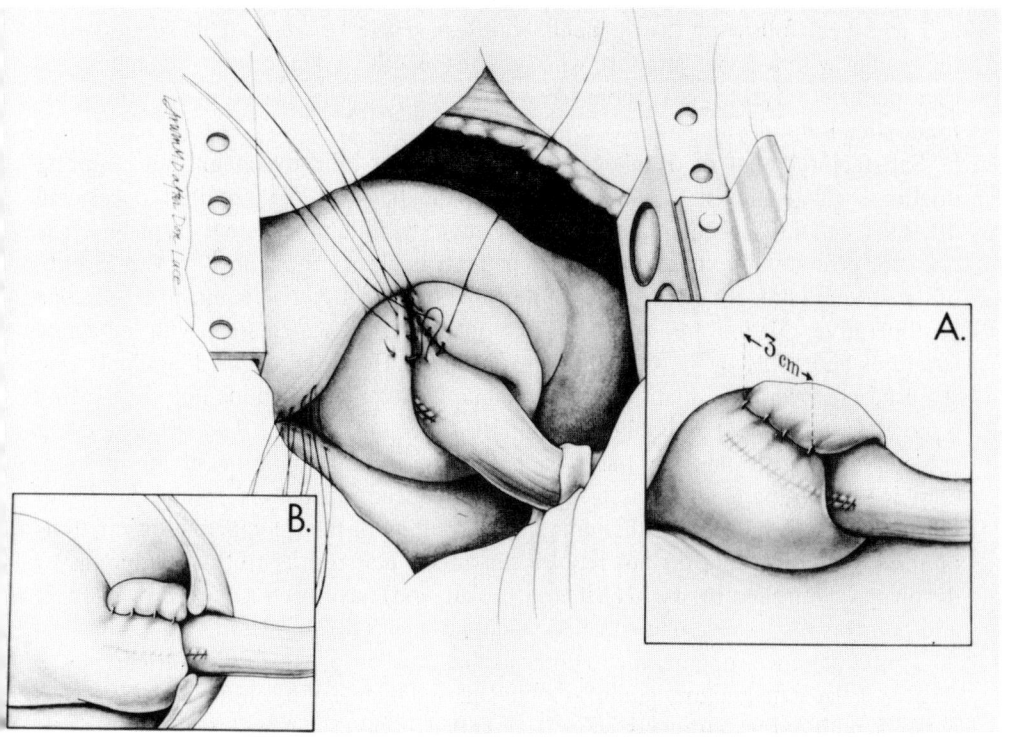

Fig. 3. Construction of 3-cm long fundoplication. Beginning at the distal end of the gastroplasty tube, i.e., the new esophagogastric junction, four seromuscular 2-0 silk sutures are placed 1 cm apart (main illustration) to achieve a 3-cm long fundoplication around the gastroplasty tube. Inset A shows the 3-cm long fundoplication. Inset B shows the fundoplication reduced beneath the diaphragm. The posterior crural sutures are then tied (reproduced with permission from Elsevier from Stirling MC, Orringer MB. Ann Thorac Surg 1988;45:148−155 [5]).

patients (3%) and both healed after drainage. The strictures were graded at the time of dilation as mild (easily dilated) in 37, moderate (requiring some force to dilate) in 17 and severe (requiring very forceful dilation) in 10. Four patients were lost to follow-up. Fifty-nine patients were followed for an average of 43 months. At the time of most recent follow-up, reflux symptoms were eliminated or mild in 88% of the patients, 8% required an antireflux medical regimen to control their reflux symptoms and 3% had poorly controlled reflux symptoms. Objective follow-up of these patients has been obtained by routine use of postoperative esophageal manometry and standard acid reflux testing with the intraesophageal pH electrode. Good reflux control was evident in 94% of 50 patients studied 1-year postoperatively but in only 66% of 29 patients studied 2 to 5 years postoperatively. However, seven of these 10 patients with abnormal reflux detected by the pH electrode did not have significant reflux symptoms. Distal high pressure zone pressure and length increased considerably after the Collis-Nissen operation and this increase was maintained over time. Patients judged to have severe strictures on the basis of the amount of force required to dilate them were significantly ($p < 0.05$) more prone to objective reflux recurrence at 2 to 5-year follow-up than patients with less severe strictures. This suggests that the patient with a severe stricture who requires repetitive dilations postoperatively to treat persistent dysphagia is more likely to develop at least partial disruption of the fundoplication.

Satisfactory relief of dysphagia (no dysphagia or mild dysphagia not requiring dilation) was achieved in 81% of these patients; 7 (12%) required occasional dilations; and 4 (7%) required regular dilations to treat their persistent dysphagia. The need for postoperative dilation in these patients is clearly influenced by the severity of the stricture preoperatively, 50% of those with mild strictures requiring at least one postoperative dilation for dysphagia, compared to 73% of those with moderate strictures and 100% of those with severe strictures. However, of the 38 patients who required postoperative dilation for dysphagia, 27 required dilations only in the first 6 months after surgery and only 11 continued to require dilations. Overall, evaluating subjective clinical status of these patients, intraoperative dilation of the stricture combined with the Collis-Nissen repair has produced satisfactory results in 77% of our patients who have had either complete resolution of their preoperative symptoms or mild symptoms that do not require treatment. Fair results (reflux symptoms or dysphagia controlled by medical therapy or dilation) have been achieved in 9 (15%) and poor results (severe uncontrolled symptoms) in 5 (8%).

This experience supports the hypothesis that most esophageal reflux strictures will resolve if the inflammatory stimulus which caused them can be eliminated. However, patients with reflux strictures who have failed previous antireflux operations are significantly less likely to have a satisfactory result than those who have had no previous operation. Intraoperative dilation and a combined Collis-Nissen operation is indicated in most patients with esophageal reflux strictures [9,10]. Resection is needed for those few who cannot be dilated adequately or when the esophagus is disrupted during attempted dilation. Patients with associated esophageal pathology such as megaesophagus, severe dysplasia in Barrett's epithelium, or caustic strictures also require resection. Since 50% of our patients with strictures and a history of previous antireflux surgery had unsuccessful results with the Collis-Nissen procedure, we now recommend resection in this group, with preference to a total thoracic esophagectomy and cervical esophagogastric anastomosis. Since patients with severe strictures are significantly less likely to have good objective long-term reflux control and also show a tendency to poor subjective results, we believe that the patient with a tough, "hard" stricture from panmural fibrosis is also better treated by resection.

The evolution of the surgical management of gastroesophageal reflux and its complications continues from the Belsey Mark IV repair to the Collis-Belsey procedure and now the Collis-Nissen operation. Meticulous follow-up and analysis of long-term subjective and objective results continue to permit further refinements in the indications for the various surgical options available to the patient with a reflux stricture.

References

1. Pearson FG, Langer B, Henderson RD. Gastroplasty and Belsey hiatal hernia repair. J Thorac Cardiovasc Surg 1971; 61:50—63.
2. Pearson FG. Surgical management of acquired short esophagus with dilatable peptic stricture. World J Surg 1977;1: 463—473.
3. Henderson RD. Reflux control after gastroplasty. Ann Thorac Surg 1977;24:206—214.
4. Orringer MB, Sloan H. Complications and failings of the combined Collis-Belsey operation. J Thorac Cardiovasc Surg 1977;74:726—735.
5. Stirling MC, Orringer MB. The combined Collis-Nissen operation for esophageal reflux strictures. Ann Thorac Surg 1988;45:148—155.
6. Donnelly RJ, Deverall PB, Watson DA. Hiatus hernia with and without stricture: experience with the Belsey Mark IV repair. Ann Thorac Surg 1973;16:301.
7. Orringer MB, Skinner DB, Belsey RHR. Long-term results of the Mark IV operation for hiatal hernia and analyses of recurrences and their treatment. J Thorac Cardiovasc Surg 1972;63:25.
8. Orringer MB, Sloan H. An improved technique for combined Collis-Belsey approach to dilatable esophageal strictures. J Thorac Cardiovasc Surg 1974;68:298—302.
9. Orringer MB, Orringer JS. The combined Collis-Nissen operation: early assessment of reflux control. Ann Thorac Surg 1982;33:534—539.
10. Henderson RD, Maryatt GV. Total fundoplication gastroplasty (Nissen gastroplasty): five-year review. Ann Thorac Surg 1985;39:74—79.
11. Orringer MB, Sloan H. Combined Collis-Nissen reconstruction of the esophagogastric junction. Ann Thorac Surg 1978;25:16—21.

What is the risk of dehiscence of the suture of the neo-esophageal tube?

J. Testart (Rouen)

Every digestive suture, either hand sewn or stapled, has a risk of leaking. In the Collis operation, there are two suture lines: one on the neo-esophageal tube, the other on the neofundus. This last one is below the diaphragm and lying on the serous of other parts of the stomach since it is used in the construction of a gastric cuff (Collis-Nissen) or a gastric valve (Collis-Belsey). This suture is not at risk of stretching and then leaking.

Conversely, the neo-esophageal suture is subject to many hazards:
1. Mechanical
— transverse stretching when the upper part of the stomach is calibrated on a bougie in order to have the stapler well in place;
— longitudinal stretching when the neocardia is pulled down;
— it is above the diaphragm, and therefore subjected to negative pressure;
— it has no covering in the left pleural cavity;
— its lower part is against the diaphragmatic hiatal edge, which can injure it at each breath;

2. Biological
— due to inflammation at the mucosal junction;
— moreover, ischemia that could occur when the neo-esophageal tube is long and when it has been isolated from its meso (upper part of the minor omentum along the lesser curvature of the stomach), where vessels and nerve branches of the Latarjet nerves arrive together. The separation of this upper part of the lesser curvature from the stomach could be deliberate in order to quell the acid secretion in the tube, it could also be inadvert, as could be the case in difficult dissections of a reoperation.

It seems that the authors advocating a peeling of the lesser curvature of the neo-esophagus do not exceed 4 cm when shaping the neo-esophageal tube [1]. These same authors have stretched out the indications of Collis operation to uncomplicated gastroesophageal reflux with a normal length esophagus. However, when an 8-cm neo-esophageal tube is needed, in order to place the neocardia below the diaphragm, i.e., when the cardia is truly irreducible, then the peeling seems to be too hazardous for the vasculature of the tube.

There is indeed a large difference among the rates of leakage on the suture line of a Collis operation depending on the pathological circumstances.

In large series the rate of leakage is either zero (in more than 600 operations [2] or more than 300 operations [3]), or very low (in 320 cases, two leaks and five perforations [4]; in 424 cases, six leaks [1]). Even in these large series it seems that leaking affected only brachyesophagus; for instance, in Orringer's series, the two leaks occurred in his 64 cases of brachyesophagus [5].

In the literature the only author who, as we did, restricted the indications of Collis operation to the true brachyesophagus had two leaks in 58 cases [6]. We performed 59 Collis operations in 13 years with four leaks (two deaths) [7]. Causal circumstances and previous history are summarized in Table 1. The diagnosis of leakage was suspected at day 2 in two cases and day 4 in two cases because of hyperthermia (four cases) or of digestive fluid in a drain (two cases), and it was asserted with X-ray opacification (four cases). One patient (case 2) died before reaching the operating room from a pneumothorax after venous puncture at the neck. The three other patients were operated immediately using the same approach as before: in three cases, the disruption was located at the upper extremity of the staple line. In one case, the leak was at the junction of the two applications of the stapler. In these three reoperations a continuous hand suture was made covering the staple line. One patient (Number 1) died on day 6 from staphylococcal septicemia. The two other patients healed and left on day 20 and day 60 but suffered from sequelae.

Case 3 had occasional dysphagia during the first 3 postoperative years and after 12 years follow-up, occasional pyrosis still persisted once or twice a week. On X-rays, the neo-esophageal tube seemed too wide, and a gastroesophageal reflux could be instigated. Red congo did not turn dark in the neo-esophageal tube.

Case 4 complained of occasional dysphagia and epigastric fullness, but never suffered pyrosis again. All pH-metries were normal and the red congo test was unacid. There was no esophagitis, however, on endoscopy as on X-ray, the tube appeared with a zigzag shape. Manometry evidenced insufficient relaxation of the

688

Table 1. Leaks on the suture line of Collis' operation: etiology

History	Associated procedure	Approach	Suture
Case 1 (female: 69 years) — oily-thorax-collapsotherapy for tuberculosis — gastroenteral anastomosis — antireflux operation (Lortat-Jacob) — Redo antireflux operation (Nissen)	Pleural peeling	Left thoracotomy	GIA (8 cm) 2 staplers
Case 2 (male: 75 years) — Pneumothorax (collapsotherapy for tuberculosis)	Truncal vagotomy pyloroplasty-Bougie No. 38	Middle line abdominal	TA 55 (5 cm)
Case 3 (female: 56 years)		Middle line abdominal	TA 90 (8 cm)
Case 4 (female: 64 years)	Resection of a giant epiphrenic diverticula	Left thoracotomy	GIA (8 cm) 2 staplers

lower esophageal sphincter (LES) after swallowing. Increasing dysphagia and dyspnae were explained by the fact that the early Belsey valve had progressively become a true paraesophageal hernia, due to disruption of the suture on the phrenotomy made at the time of the Collis operation. Reoperation was conducted after 10 years through the same approach (left thoracotomy). Complete dissection was made, a Nissen fundoplication was performed around the neo-esophageal tube, and the diaphragm was sewn with nonresorbable thread.

After the reoperation, the absence of gastroesophageal reflux was demonstrated from pH-metry, endoscopy and radiography. The red congo test was negative, and manometry again showed the insufficient relaxation of the LES.

A risk of disruption seems to exist when Collis operation has been made for truly irreducible cardia, that bears a high risk of lethality. How can this risk be reduced?
— Routinely checking the tightness of the suture by insufflation at end of operation appeared to us to give insufficient warrant;
— we preserved the vessels along the upper part of the lesser curvature, and none of the leaks that we observed could be related to ischemia;
— in our cases, the staple line was covered with a hand made suture, and we detected no leak;
— we have no experience of biological glue.

References

1. Pearson FG, Cooper JD, Patterson GA, Ramirez J, Todd TR. Gastroplasty and fundoplication for complex reflux problems. Ann Surg 1987;206:473—481.

2. Henderson RD. The advantage of Collis-Nissen procedure via an abdominal or thoracic approach. In: Giuli R, McCallum RW (eds) Benign Lesions of the Esophagus and Cancer. Berlin: Springer Verlag, 1988;471—474.
3. Payne WS. Why have so many antireflux procedures been devised? Can specific factors be defined in order to properly choose the procedure to offer? In: Giuli R, McCallum RW (eds) Benign Lesions of the Esophagus and Cancer, Berlin: Springer Verlag, 1988;523—525.
4. Orringer MB. Results of Collis-Nissen operation. In: Giuli R, McCallum RW (eds) Benign Lesions of the Esophagus and Cancer. Berlin: Springer Verlag, 1988;474—479.
5. Stirling MC, Orringer MB. Collis-Nissen operation for esophageal reflux strictures. Ann Thorac Surg 1988;45:148—155.
6. Beauchamp G. The Collis-Nissen procedure. In: Giuli R, McCallum RW (eds) Benign Lesions of the Esophagus and Cancer. Berlin: Springer Verlag, 1988;463—466.
7. Testart J, Peillon C. Les complications de l'opération de Collis. Lyon Chir 1992;88/2 bis:193—195.

What are the undesirable effects of Collis operation?

R.J. Ginsberg (New York)

In 1957, Collis first described the results of an operation for hiatus hernia with short esophagus [1,2]. This esophageal lengthening procedure utilized a short segment of the proximal cardia along the lesser curvature of the stomach fashioned into a tube, thereby creating a "neo-esophagus" and lengthening the gullet by 3—5 cm. This was combined with an anterior crural repair. In 1971, Pearson described the use of a partial fundoplication (Belsey Mark IV) combined with the Collis "gastroplasty" for the treatment of an acquired short esophagus [3—5]. Henderson and Orringer advocated the use of a total fundoplication with the Collis gastroplasty, following failures of reflux control with the Pearson modification [6—15]. Langer and Bingham were the first to describe the "uncut" gastroplasty more recently popularized by Evangelist, Demos and Payne. A variant is now utilized in barosurgery as the "vertical banded" gastroplasty [16—20]. These procedures may be accomplished with a thoracic, abdominal or thoraco-abdominal approach, all equally effective.

Physiology of the gastroplasty tube

Pearson, Henderson and Ellis have reported on the physiology of the gastroplasty tube [21—23]. The tube itself is aperistaltic with a minor effect on the high pressure zone. The intra-abdominal position, adds only minimally to high the pressure zone but does not prevent reflux. The addition of a partial fundoplication increases the high pressure zone and a total fundoplication strengthens it even more [24].

690

Early undesirable effects

The early undesirable effects of gastroplasty creation involves mainly technical mishaps. These include: postoperative gastroplasty leaks, gastroplasty necrosis, early dysphagia and early recurrent reflux. In addition, complications related to all antireflux procedures may occur following creation of the gastroplasty and antireflux repair. These will not be discussed, but may occur with increased frequency, since the indications for adding a gastroplasty often include the most difficult cases (e.g., severe structure, redo surgery).

Postoperative leaks

The incidence of postoperative leaks following gastroplasty is about 1%. Most gastroplasties are created using mechanical staplers. Failure of the stapler may occur. For this reason, most authors oversew the staple line with a continuous absorbable suture. Inadvertent necrosis of the wall of the proximal esophagus by the "heel" of the stapler can occur and be obviated by initiating the oversewing just proximal to the staple line on the esophagus. Similarly, leaks can occur along the suture line of the newly created fundus or at the angle between the gastroplasty tube and fundus.

Gastroplasty necrosis

This is an extremely rare event and has been reported only occasionally. Theoretically, this is more apt to occur when gastroplasty is utilized following subtotal gastrectomy with division of the main left gastric artery. Despite this potential complication, it is a very rare event.

Postoperative dysphagia

Postoperative dysphagia can occur from complications related to the antireflux procedure but can also result from a poorly created gastroplasty tube. Most authors advocate utilizing a 50–60 French bougie in creating a sufficient sized tube in order to prevent this problem. The original description by Collis, however, utilizes as narrow a tube as a number 32 French and other authors utilize a variety of diameters as low as 40 French. The creation of a gastroplasty distal to a myotomized esophagus has resulted in significant postoperative dysphagia and reflux and is now not recommended by most authors.

Early reflux

Technical failure of the antireflux procedure is the usual cause of early reflux.

Late complications

The late complications following gastroplasty include: recurrent reflux, diverticula formation within the gastroplasty, gastroplasty-fundic fistulae and the potential of adenocarcinoma developing in the gastroplasty tube. As well, a myriad of late complications related to the associated antireflux operation can occur, but will not be discussed.

Recurrent reflux

Collis described a significant incidence of recurrent reflux, suggesting the need for a more adequate added antireflux procedure. Both Henderson and Orringer described significant reflux (15–20%) occurring after partial fundoplication following gastroplasty. They have, therefore, advocated total fundoplication gastroplasty. Too long a total fundoplication results in prolonged dysphagia and most authors now recommend a total fundoplication of no more than 1.5 cm, applied either to the gastroplasty tube or to the distal esophagus. On the other hand, Pearson has not noted this problem and continues to use a Belsey Mark IV fundoplication. He attributes some of the reflux occurring to be due to a patulous, wide distal tube.

Dysphagia

The incidence of persisting mild or moderate dysphagia occurs in 10–15% of gastroplasty operations. This is increased in dysmotility states (e.g., scleroderma) or reconstruction following previously failed antireflux procedures and is seen more frequently with total fundoplication, with too narrow a gastroplasty tube, or with ill-constructed antireflux procedures.

Gastroplasty diverticula

An ill-constructed gastroplasty, especially one with too wide a tube or too tight a hiatal closure or antireflux wrap, can result in dilatation and diverticula formation in the proximal portion of the gastroplasty. This is obviated if the antireflux procedure is performed on the distal esophagus rather than only on the distal gastroplasty.

Development of carcinoma

Scattered reports have suggested that there may be an increased incidence of adenocarcinoma developing in the distal esophagus or within the gastroplasty tube. However, the extremely small numbers so far reported suggest that there is no greater an incidence than that seen after other antireflux procedures and frequently may be related to "missed" early carcinoma at the time of operation or persisting to dysplastic change of the lower esophageal mucosa after gastroplasty formation.

Complications of "uncut" gastroplasty

The original series of Langer utilized interrupted silk sutures to develop an uncut gastroplasty and resulted in a modest number of late gastro-gastric fistulae with resultant recurrent reflux. The technique of Henderson, reapplying the fundic closure against the gastroplasty closure has resulted in similar fistulae. If the fundic closure and gastroplasty closure are not opposed, the incidence of gastro-gastric fistulae appears lessened. It appears that the uncut gastroplasty, even with the use of stapling devices will inevitably lead to the occasional gastro-gastric fistulae because of staple failure with recurrent uncontrollable reflux as the resultant complication.

Summary

Despite these early and late problems that may develop following gastroplasty creation, the gastroplasty tube, designed by Collis to lengthen the esophagus in dealing with the acquired short esophagus combined with an antireflux procedure has proven to be an excellent approach to these difficult lower esophageal problems with extremely low morbidity. It has been mainly applied in treating patients with a high risk of recurrence following standard antireflux procedures. These include: the acquired short esophagus and peptic stricture, massive obesity, recurrent reflux after antireflux repair and combined type I and type II hiatal hernias. Care should be taken in employing this technique in patients with severe motility disorders, and it appears to be contraindicated following myotomy of the lower esophageal sphincter. Despite the occasional problems related to gastroplasty malfunction, the procedure has stood the test of time and is associated with few technical problems.

References

1. Collis JL. An operation for hiatus hernia with short esophagus. J Thorac Surg 1957;14:768–778.
2. Collis JL. Gastroplasty. Thorax 1961;16:197–206.
3. Pearson FG, Langer B, Henderson RD. Gastroplasty and Belsey hiatus hernia repair. J Thorac Cardiovasc Surg 1971;61: 50–63.
4. Pearson FG, Henderson RD. Long-term follow-up of peptic strictures managed by dilatation, modified Collis gastroplasty and Belsey hiatus hernia repair. Surgery 1976;80:396–404.
5. Pearson FG, Cooper JD, Nelems JM. Gastroplasty and fundoplication in the management of complex reflux problems. J Thorac Cardiovasc Surg 1978;76:665–672.
6. Henderson RD, Marryatt G. Recurrent hiatus hernia: management by thoracoabdominal total fundoplication gastroplasty. Can J Surg 1981;24:151–157.
7. Henderson RD. Reflux control following gastroplasty. Ann Thorac Surg 1977;24:206–214.
8. Henderson RD, Marryatt G. Total fundolication gastroplasty (Nissen gastroplasty): five-year review. Ann Thorac Surg 1985;39:74–79.
9. Henderson RD, Marryatt G. Recurrent hiatal hernia: management by thoracoabdominal total fundoplication gastroplasty. Can J Surg 1981;24:151–154.
10. Henderson RD, Marryatt G. Total fundoplication gastroplasty: long-term follow-up in 500 patients. J Thorac Cardiovasc Surg 1983;85:81–87.
11. Henderson RD. Dysphagia complicating hiatal repair. J Thorac Cardiovasc Surg 1984;88:922–928.
12. Henderson RD. Surgical management of the failed gastroplasty. J Thorac Cardiovasc Surg 1986;91:46–52.
13. Orringer MB, Sloan H. Complications and failings of the combined Collis Belsey operation. J Thorac Cardiovasc Surg 1977;74:726–735.
14. Orringer MB, Sloan H. Combined Collis-Nissen reconstruction of the esophagogastric junction. Ann Thorac Surg 1978;25: 16–21.
15. Stirling MC, Orringer MB. Continued assessment of the combined Collis-Nissen operation. Ann Thorac Surg 1989;47: 224–230.
16. Langer B. Modified gastroplasty: a simple operation for reflux esophagitis with moderate degrees of shortening. Can J Surg 1973;16:1–8.

17. Bingham JAW. Evolution and early results of constructing an antireflux valve in the stomach. Proc R Soc Med 1974; 67:4–8.
18. Bingham JAW. Hiatus hernia repair combined with the construction of an antireflux valve in the stomach. Br J Surg 1977; 64:460–465.
19. Evangelist FA, Taylor FH, Alford JD. The modified Collis-Nissen operation for control of gastroesophageal reflux. Ann Thorac Surg 1978;26:107–111.
20. Demos NJ. A simplified improved technique for the Collis gastroplasty for dilatable esophageal strictures. Surg Gynecol Obstet 1976;142:591–594.
21. Pearson FG, Henderson RD. Experimental and clinical studies of gastroplasty in the management of acquired short esophagus. Surg Gynecol Obstet 1973;136:737.
22. Henderson RD, Bosszko A, Gashe F et al. Esophageal replacement by a gastric tube: an experimental study of the properties of the gastric tube. Br J Surg 1974;61:533.
23. Ellis FH, Leonardi HK, Dabuzhsky L, Crozier RE. Surgery for short esophagus with structure: an experimental and clinical manometric study. Ann Surg 1978;188:341–350.
24. Tomas-Ridocci M, Paris F, Antoli CC et al. Total fundoplication with or without gastroplasty for gastroesophageal reflux: comparative study. Ann Thorac Surg 1985;39:308–311.

How to interpret the persistence of esophageal acidity after Collis operation?

J. Testart (Rouen)

The detection of esophageal acidity, whatever the chosen pH-metric procedure, is usually considered as the mark of gastroesophageal reflux (GER). This was also the case in the papers relating acid pH-metry after Collis operation:
— 11% in a series of 242 Collis operations [1];
— 23% of 10 Collis-Belsey [2] and 3% of 31 Collis-Nissen [2].
Orringer [1] had noticed that among his 27 patients with postoperative esophageal acidity, 10 had no symptoms that could refer to GER.

This question was also addressed [3] in our prospective study that included pH-metry with a standard meal [4], and showed:
— considerable variations of the score in some patients;
— acidity, although the antireflux valve appeared hyperefficient, both on X-rays and physiological exploration.

Such findings justified the search for an acid secretion in the nco-csophageal tube. We used mucous coloration with red congo under esophagoscopy. This marker turns dark blue at pH 3. Twelve patients were examined. In six, red congo did not change color, and these patients had neither pyrosis, nor esophagitis at esophagoscopy, nor acidity at pH-metry; however, three had dysphagia (one had a zigzag-shaped neo-esophageal tube, one a narrow tube with insufficient relaxation of the inferior esophageal sphincter, and the third had only insufficient relaxation, with 30% of

694

esophageal nonpropulsive contractions). Three patients had dyspepsia with postprandial feeling of fullness and delay of gastric evacuation.

In the six other patients, red congo turned dark, either along the whole neo-esophageal tube or only on its lower part (for instance 2 or 3 cm on a 7 cm long tube). Two patients had no pyrosis, no esophagitis, normal esophageal contractions, but partial relaxation of the inferior esophageal sphincter, and pH-metry showed fluctuating scores. The four other patients still suffered pyrosis, with esophagitis at esophagoscopy and acid scores at pH-metry. However, on X-rays GER was not demonstrable in two of these patients: one had undergone 3 years before Collis operation a resection of an epiphrenic diverticula with myotomy; the other had an important kyphoscoliosis. In both, esophageal dyskinesia was shown at physiological explorations.

In addition to these 12 patients, 34 others underwent a postoperative pH-metry with standard meal. A pathological acid score (above 90) was found in 13 patients. Eleven of them had one or two other pH-metry examinations, with at least one of them being normal. The pH probe was most often set blindly, occasionally after measurement of the range of the Z line. The acid pH-metric scores coincided with cases in which the pH probe was set on the gastric mucosa of the neo-esophageal tube.

Therefore, the presence of acid in the esophagus after Collis operation could be explained as linked with:
— either failure to cure GER;
— or acid secretion in the gastric mucosa of the neo-esophageal tube, with stasis of acid due to insufficient esophageal clearance.

In our four failed cases, we found two to be related to each of these causes.

References

1. Orringer MB. Results of Collis-Nissen operation. In: Giuli R, McCallum RW (eds) Benign Lesions of the Esophagus and Cancer. Berlin: Springer Verlag, 1988;474—478.
2. Paris F, Ridocci MT, Mora F, Benages A. Comparison of Collis-Nissen and Collis-Belsey procedures. In: Giuli R, McCallum RW (eds) Benign Lesions of the Esophagus and Cancer. Berlin: Springer Verlag, 1988;482—486.
3. Testart J, Kartheuser A, Peillon C, Galmiche JP, Denis P. L'opération de Collis pour brachy oesophage. Gastroenterol Clin Biol 1991;15:512—518.
4. Galmiche JP, Guillard JF, Denis P. Etude du pH oesophagien en période post prandiale chez le sujet normal et au cours du syndrome de reflux gastro-oesophagien. Gastroenterol Clin Biol 1990;4:531—539.

Failures after Collis operation

How to evaluate persistent reflux?

N.J. Demos (New York)

The incidence of significant recurrent gastroesophageal reflux, on long-term follow-up after various types of hiatal hernioplasties varies from 10 to 18 to 20% [1—3].

The common denominator of recurrent reflux is usually some type of anatomic or physiologic recurrence. Therefore, clinical evaluation of the patient's symptoms is in order. Heartburn, epigastric pain at times radiating to the back, neck or shoulders, especially after eating or in the recumbent position, are highly suggestive of reflux.

Information regarding the previous antireflux operation or operations is usually unobtainable or unreliable. Therefore, other methods have to be used to assess and properly diagnose the presence and the extent of reflux.

A therapeutic trial of antacids, diet and acid suppression for several weeks is carried out. Esophagram, endoscopy, manometry, acid clearing study and 24-h pH testing are usually performed on a selective basis.

Esophagram might or might not reveal reflux or recurrent hiatal hernia. One of the 145 patients studied showed definite anatomic recurrence on esophagram 4.5 years after repair. He also had a mild stricture, which was easily dilated. Generally speaking, endoscopy may show esophagitis, ulcer or stricture.

Lacking the above evidence of gastroesophageal reflux, one has to rely on physiological testing to provide evidence of reflux explaining the symptoms.

A manometric recording of low resting pressure in the lower esophageal sphincter means partial or complete recurrence of the hiatal hernia. Dysmotility in the body of the esophagus, which is a new development or a recurrence of preoperative findings, suggests some type of failure of the antireflux procedure. Recurrence of symptoms has been found to have a defective acid clearance alone in 13% or combined with sphincteric failure in 61% of recurrent reflux cases in Little's series [4].

Twenty-four-hour pH studies are rather diagnostic of the presence and magnitude of reflux. Two of our patients (total of 145) had enough symptoms to justify 24-h pH testing. The computer scores were 55 and 125, the normal reference range being 0–20. They were both managed well with intermittent antacid therapy.

In 52 of our patients, who were either tested routinely or because of vague upper abdominal symptoms, the 24-h test was normal. The patients with vague upper abdominal symptoms usually proved to have either duodenal ulcer or moderate or severe gastritis, frequently associated with the presence of *Helicobacter pylori*.

The management of recurrent reflux or other complications is covered well in the work of Little et al. [4].

References

1. Ellis FH Jr, El-Kurd MF, Gibb SP. The effect of fundoplication on the lower esophageal sphincter. Surg Gynecol Obstet 1976;143:1–5.
2. Belsey RHR. Mark IV repair of hiatal hernia by the transthoracic approach. World J Surg 1977;1:475–481.
3. Hill LD. Progress in the surgical management of hiatus hernia. World J Surg 1977;1:425–436.
4. Little AG, Ferguson MK, Skinner DB. Reoperation for failed antireflux operations. J Thorac Cardiovasc Surg 1986;91:511–517.

Does deterioration of manometric findings often occur?

M.B. Orringer (Ann Arbor)

The Collis gastroplasty, in combination with the Belsey hiatal hernia repair, was initially advocated as a means of reducing the incidence of recurrent gastroesophageal reflux in patients with reflux strictures known to predispose them to recurrence after a standard Belsey Mark IV repair. Adding length to the functional distal esophagus eliminated tension on the repair, and the gastroplasty tube provided more resilient uninflamed tissue to which the stomach could be sewn in performing the Belsey fundoplication. This operative approach was undertaken with a commitment to careful preoperative evaluation and postoperative follow-up using esophageal manometry and intraesophageal acid reflux testing, in order to provide an objective assessment of reflux control. Of 83 patients undergoing the combined Collis-Belsey operation, 77 had postoperative esophageal manometry and acid reflux testing [1]. Seventy had postoperative esophageal function tests within 1 to 6 months of operation, 37 between 12 and 17 months, eight between 18 and 23 months and 13 between 24 and 33 months after operation. The average follow-up was 13 months when these data were reviewed. From a subjective standpoint, among these 77 patients, 38% had an excellent result (completely asymptomatic), 43% a good result (no reflux symptoms, but mild nonspecific complaints such as incisional pain or occasional abdominal discomfort), 8% had a fair result (mild reflux symptoms but greatly improved over preoperative status); and 11% a poor result (moderate to severe symptoms of reflux). From an objective standpoint, of the 75 patients undergoing preoperative manometry and acid reflux testing, 50% had no demonstrable distal esophageal high pressure zone, and moderate to severe gastroesophageal reflux was documented with the intra-esophageal pH electrode in 87%. All but three of the 70 patients who had post-operative esophageal function tests within the first 6 months after operation had a definite high pressure zone. The average mean and peak pressures in the HPZ nearly doubled from preoperative values, from 2.61 to 4.96 mmHg and from 5.60 to 10.60 mmHg, respectively. The average length of the HPZ increased from 1.63 preopera-tively to 3 cm at 6 months postoperatively. At the time of their first acid reflux test within 6 months of operation, 83% had no or insignificant reflux, whereas moderate to severe reflux was detected in 17%. Over the ensuing period of follow-up, 11 additional patients developed moderate to severe reflux on standard pH reflux testing, so that all told, 23 of 77 patients, or 30% of the group, had moderate to severe reflux on obstructive pH reflux testing. Eight of these patients, however, had no subjective symptoms of reflux, and clinically were rated as having good or excellent reflux control.

We concluded that in many patients, the elongated gastric fundus remaining after construction of the gastroplasty tube is not sufficiently wide to allow the 240° Belsey fundoplication originally described and was responsible for failure to control gastroesophageal reflux in an appreciable number of these patients. This was the basis for our recommendation that, after construction of the gastroplasty tube, the gastric fundus be used as a 360° Nissen-type fundoplication to better control reflux.

In 1989, we reported the results of the combined Collis-Nissen operation in 353 patients [2]. The average length of follow-up for 261 patients (74%) followed at least 12 months was 43.8 months. Fifty-eight percent were followed at least 36 months; 41%, 48 months; and 29%, 60 months or longer. Subjectively, in these 261 patients, reflux was eliminated in 75%, was mild in 11%, moderate in 9%, and severe in 5%. Seventeen percent required either periodic or regular esophageal dilations for dysphagia. Objectively intraesophageal pH reflux testing showed good reflux control in 91% and poor reflux control in 9%. Ten percent of the patients had required reoperation for recurrent reflux or dysphagia. The combined Collis-Nissen operation resulted in an increase in the distal high pressure zone pressure from an average preoperative value of 4 mmHg to a postoperative value of approximately 10 mmHg. Similarly, high pressure zone length increased after operation from 3.5 to 4.3 cm compared with an average preoperative length of 1.7 cm. Both distal esophageal high pressure zone pressure and length remained constant in long-term follow-up. It is emphasized that, when performing the combined Collis-Nissen operation, the gastroplasty tube should be constructed over either a 54 French dilator in women or a 56 French dilator in men and the length of the fundoplication should be limited to 3 cm to minimize the postoperative dysphagia from too long a wrap. Incorporation of a Collis gastroplasty with a fundoplication of any type to control gastroesophageal reflux after performance of an esophagomyotomy should *not* be carried out. The resulting distal high pressure zone pressure is too great for the myotomized esophagus to overcome and postoperative dysphagia is a major cause for an unsatisfactory postoperative result.

References

1. Orringer MB, Sloan H. Complications and failings of the combined Collis-Belsey operation. J Thorac Cardiovasc Surg 1977; 74:726–735.
2. Stirling MC, Orringer MB. Continued assessment of the combined Collis-Nissen operation. Ann Thorac Surg 1989;47: 224–230.

Is the diameter and the angle of the tube important?

D.B. Skinner (New York)

The Collis gastroplasty procedure, when coupled with a partial or total fundoplication, can be an effective solution to controlling reflux in complicated patients. However, the operation is technically demanding because of the exposure required, the variability of the angle of entry of the esophagus into the stomach, the potential problems created by making a tube of varying diameter and the fact that the tube is nonperistaltic and can cause dysphagia if too long a segment is used.

The gastroplasty segment should be created over a large bougie (preferably 60 French) which must be applied closely along the lesser curvature aspect of the upper stomach adjacent to the cardia. The segment should not be constructed longer than 5 cm. Care must be taken that the tube is of uniform diameter without a narrowing or a dilatation near the distal end as it enters the stomach. The Law of Laplace applies. If the junction of the tube with the residual stomach is narrower than the proximal tube, a partial obstruction with proximal dilatation will occur. Follow-up of more than 20 years of a gastric tube interposition patient demonstrates that remarkable proximal dilatation can occur in a gastric tube if its point of entry into the stomach is too narrow.

On the other hand, if the distal end of the tube is of greater diameter, an inverted funnel effect occurs, which makes control of reflux less effective. This undoubtedly accounts for some of the variability in reports describing the effectiveness of the gastroplasty in controlling gastroesophageal reflux.

A third technical problem may result in reoperative cases in which the blood supply to the cardia has been previously disturbed. If the left gastric and/or short gastric vessels are interrupted and the tube is of too narrow a diameter, the tube may become ischemic and even perforate.

Other techniques

What can be expected from posterior fundoplasty in treatment of gastroesophageal reflux?

V. Guarner (Mexico City)

The Nissen fundoplication has a high rate of undesirable side effects. In 1969, after a long experimental evaluation [1] we introduced another antireflux procedure that we conventionally called: the posterior fundoplasty, which is essentially a modification of the Nissen procedure but not a hemifundoplication [2].

As was demonstrated for the first time in 1975 [3], the side effects with this late procedure were, from the beginning, considerably less frequent than with the Nissen.

In 1980, a comparative study was published [4] with a 10-year follow-up of 135 patients, who had been operated on using the posterior fundoplasty method, compared with 40 patients who were operated on employing Nissen fundoplication. The 10-year evaluation was done clinically, with endoscopy, radiology and manometric studies in both groups.

Technique

Either a right transverse or a vertical midline incision is performed. The left lobe of the liver is retracted without sectioning the left triangular ligament. The spleen is protected with a large sponge, previously rolled. Both crura of the diaphragm are dissected and closed behind the esophagus.

The upper part of the anterior wall of the fundus, in the area in which there are

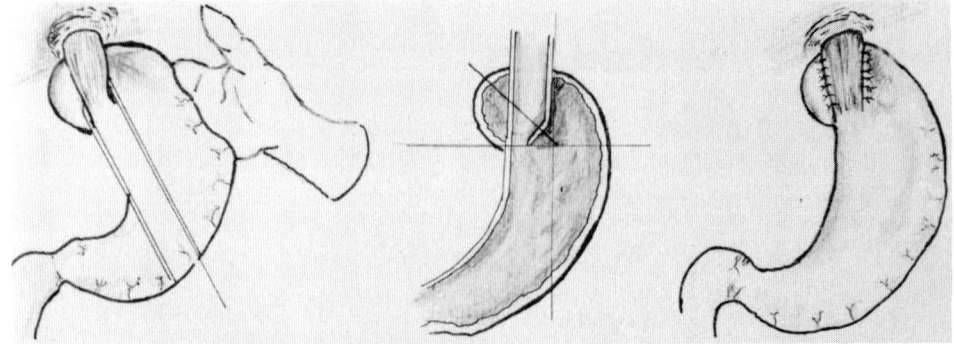

Fig. 1. Left: the right hand passes the anterior wall of the fundus to the right side of the esophagus; middle: the fundus does not wrap around the esophagus, but forms a 110° angle with the wall of the esophagus; right: the esophagus is sutured to the anterior wall. (Reprint from Surg Gynecol Obstet 1990;170:451–452. ©1990, by The Franklin H. Martin Foundation.)

no vasa brevia (so the omentum does not need to be transected), is passed behind the esophagus to its right side, forming more or less a 110° angle between the esophagus and the fundus, as seen in Fig. 1. This angle does not refer to the degree in which the stomach wraps around the esophagus, as it is often misinterpreted. The clue to the operation (and the reason for insisting on the technique) is the amount of fundus that is passed to the right side of the esophagus. It is precisely the internal part of this portion of the fundus which is attached with interrupted stitches of three or four zero silk to the esophagus (Fig. 1).

The difference between our technique and the Toupet [5] is that, in the latter procedure, the operation is done with both the anterior and the posterior walls of the fundus.

Table 1.

Clinical evaluation	Preoperative		Postoperative	
	Posterior fundoplasty	Nissen	Posterior fundoplasty	Nissen
Substernal burning	135	40	7 (5.1%)	2 (5%)
Regurgitation	135	40	7 (5.1%)	2 (5%)
Dysphagia	9	0	0	5 (12.5%)

Table 2.

Postoperative clinical evaluation	Fundoplication	Posterior fundoplasty
Vomiting block	24/40 (60%)	3/135 (2.2%)
Difficulties in belching	14/40 (35%)	4/135 (2.9%)

704

Discussion

This operation accomplishes three purposes. First, it elongates the abdominal esophagus even more than does the Nissen procedure and as it has been demonstrated by many authors, this is an important point. Secondly, it forms a fold or a type of valve on the left side of the esophagus, which prevents gastric content to reach the esophagus. Thirdly, it also creates, as other procedures, a posterior bag with the stomach in which the gastric acid finds an easier access.

In 1980, we published a 10-year comparative evaluation between 135 cases operated with posterior fundoplasty and 40 patients with classical Nissen fundoplication. Both procedures had the same effectiveness in the control of gastroesophageal reflux, however, dysphagia was lower with our procedure (2.9 vs. 12.5%), inability to vomit 2.2 vs. 60%, difficulties in belching, 2.9 vs. 35% (Tables 1 and 2; Fig. 2).

Sliding of the fundoplication that occurred in one patient, and produced occlusion of the esophagogastric junction, was not seen after fundoplasty, because in this technique the fundus is fixed all its way to the abdominal esophagus. By the same fact, the length of the lower sphincter is manometrically longer with posterior fundoplasty compared to the Nissen (Fig. 3).

From 1966 until 1992, we have operated on more than 1,500 patients with the technique of posterior fundoplasty. The evaluation of long-term results are 90% excellent, with the same low average of side effects.

FREQUENCY (%)

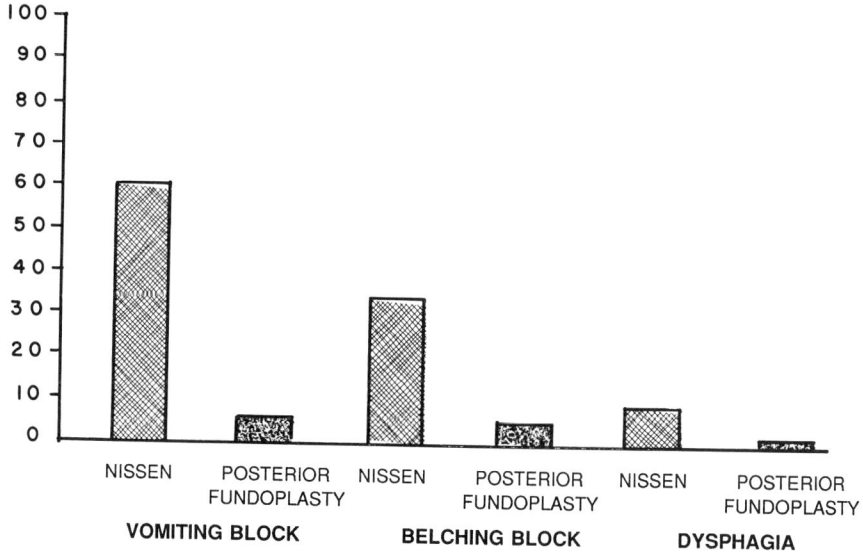

Fig. 2.

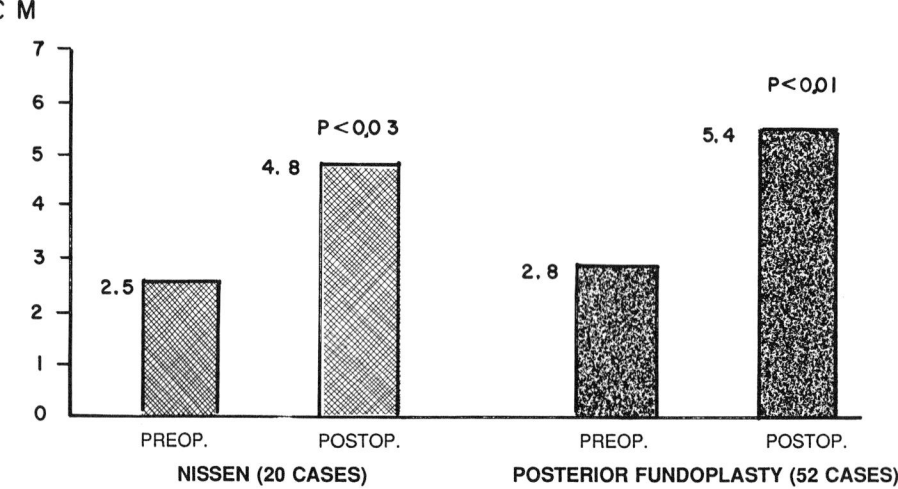

Fig. 3. Length of the lower esophageal sphincter before and after surgical treatment.

References

1. Guarner V, Ramirez DJ, Martinez Toro N. Valoración experimental y clinica de un nuevo procedimiento antireflujo en la union esofago gástrica. Gaceta Med Mex 1969;99:541—551.
2. Skinner DB. In: Atlas of Esophageal Surgery. New York: Churchill Livingstone, 1991.
3. Guarner V. A new antireflux procedure in the esophagogastric junction. Arch Surg 1975;110:101—106.
4. Guarner V, Martinez Toro N, Gaviño J. Ten-year evaluation of the posterior fundoplasty in the treatment of esophagogastric reflux. Am J Surg 1980;139:200—203.
5. Guarner V. The posterior fundoplasty in the treatment of gastroesophageal reflux. Surg Gynecol Obstet 1990;170:451—452.

Should a gastrolysis be done at the fundus to construct an antireflux valve?

P. Thomas, T. Lonjon, R. Giudicelli, P. Fuentes (Marseilles)

A variety of transabdominal surgical techniques can be used to manage reflux esophagitis. The choice depends on whether plication involves all or part of the circumference of the esophagus, and on whether the posterior and/or anterior side of the fundus is used. Several techniques, not requiring mobilization of the fundus, have been proposed. A number of anatomical factors and surgical requirements contribute to the effectiveness of this surgery.

Anatomical relations and surgical requirements

Three contiguous structures are mainly responsible for maintaining the gastroesophageal junction: the meso-esophagus which connects the front and sides of the esophagus to the preaortic layer and to the diaphragm, the left gastric artery and the gastrophrenic ligament which attaches the fundus to the left diaphragmatic dome.

While the meso-esophagus must be dissected in order to lengthen the abdominal esophagus, the extent of dissection of the esocardiofundic area depends on the plication technique. All antireflux procedures, except the anterior hemifundoplication technique as described by Dor, require transection of the gastrophrenic ligament. This minimum mobilization is prerequisite, although not necessarily adequate for fundoplication using the posterior side of the fundus (Nissen, Toupet), and provides the space necessary for passage of the valve behind the esophagus, even when it is composed of the anterior side of the fundus (Nissen-Rossetti, modified Toupet). Release of the posterior side can be done either from top to bottom and left to right after division of the anterior leaf of the gastrophrenic ligament at the top of the fundus [1], or from bottom to top and vertically after opening the gastrocolic ligament and exposing the posterior side of the fundus via the omental bursa [2].

In addition to these basic technical factors, certain unfavorable anatomic features may exist. The configuration of the upper part of the stomach can vary with regard to several factors including height of fundus, angle of His, surface of bare area of stomach and distance apex hiatus to the first superior short gastric artery [3]. Morphologic conditions such as obesity and kyphosis also influence the extent of mobilization on the gastrosplenic ligament. In some cases it may be necessary to section the first short vessels.

Incidence on results

The main peroperative complication of antireflux surgery for esophagitis is spleen damage. Splenectomy is necessary in about 3.5% of cases regardless of the technique used [4]. Section of the short gastric vessels during mobilization of the fundus appears to be a risk factor for this complication [4]. However, even when fundoplication is performed without mobilization (e.g., using the anterior side of the fundus), the splenectomy rate remains around 1.5% [1]. Moreover, consideration of the splenectomy rate alone overlooks minor injuries in which conservative surgery or using fibrin glue was possible. A short distance between the hiatus and the superior short gastric arteries is predisposing anatomical factor for spleen damage [3]. In these patients, mobilization should be limited in order to avoid tension on the gastrosplenic ligament.

The incidence of gastroesophageal injury is lower, i.e., 0.4% in the multicentric AFC study [4]. The fact that the main theoretical cause of this type of lesion is excessive tension supports the argument in favor of extensive mobilization of the fundus, especially when posterior gastropexy is associated with fundoplication. However, it should be emphasized that the reduction of the blood supply to the upper portion of the stomach that results from extensive mobilization can facilitate gastroesophageal lesions. In practice poor surgical technique, i.e., stitches too deep and too tight is the main cause [5]. This complication has rarely been reported by surgeons with long experience in transabdominal antireflux surgery.

The incidence of gas bloat syndrome varies depending on the procedure used. The main causes are injury of the pneumogastric nerves and especially excessive tightness of the gastroesophageal junction [4]. Routine performance of extensive mobilization of the fundus can result in a bulky plication, while inadequate mobilization contributes to excessive tightness.

The main problem is postoperative failure. Immediate failure is due to poor surgical technique resulting in a loose gastroesophageal junction [6]. Long-term recurrence results from loss of functional integrity [5]. In addition to aging of tissue and weight gain, the primary cause of stretching is excessive plication [7]. Thus an adequate, flexible plication is the best guarantee of long-term results. Depending on the anatomical relations, extensive mobilization of the fundus may be necessary to reach this objective.

Is mobilization of the fundus a prerequisite?

The antireflux procedure that we prefer is posterior hemifundoplication. As previously reported, satisfactory results have been achieved with no reflux detectable by pH-metry at 1 year in 91.3% of cases [6]. Plication is always made mainly using the anterior side of the fundus. A review of our recent experience indicates that the need for extensive mobilization, including the short vessels, depends on the anatomical configuration: out of 138 patients who underwent antireflux surgery between 1987 and 1992, mobilization was unnecessary in 75 cases (54.3%), while dividing of the short vessels was required in 61 patients (44.2%). In the remaining two patients (1.5%), more extensive mobilization was required. Morbidity was low and was not correlated with the extent of mobilization of the fundus. No splenectomies were performed and no esophageal injuries occurred. Postfundoplication syndrome was observed in four patients (2.9%): two without and two with mobilization of the fundus.

The essential condition for effective antireflux surgery is the availability of sufficient fundus for plication with minimum tension. In order to fulfill this condition, the extent of resection of the esocardiofundic area must be adapted not only to the plication procedure used but also to anatomical features that can vary greatly from one patient to another.

References

1. Boutelier Ph, Jonsell G. An alternative fundoplicature maneuver for gastroesophageal reflux. Am J Surg 1982;143:260–264.
2. Barbin JY, Barbin JG, Chaillou Ph. Le procédé de Toupet. In: Giuli R (ed) OESO Lésions Bénignes de l'Oesophage et Cancer: Réponses à 210 Questions. New York, Berlin, Heidelberg: Springer Verlag, 1988;459–470.
3. Wald H, Polk HJ. Anatomical variations in hiatal and upper gastric areas and their relationship to difficulties experienced in operations for reflux esophagitis. Ann Surg 1983;197:389–392.

4. Boutelier Ph, Chipponi J. In: Le Traitement Chirurgical du Reflux Gastro-oesophagien de l'Adulte. Paris: Masson, 1989; 93–139.
5. Leonardi HK, Ellis FH. Reoperative surgery for gastroesophageal reflux. In: Jamieson GG (ed) Surgery of the Esophagus. London: Churchill Livingstone, 1988;411–414.
6. Fuentes P, Dupin B, Giudicelli R, Reboud E. Posterior hemifundoplication for gastroesophageal reflux. In: Siewert JR, Hölscher AH (eds) Diseases of the Esophagus. New York, Berlin, Heidelberg: Springer Verlag, 1987;1233–1235.
7. Payne WS, Trastek VF, Pairolero PC. Reflux esophagitis. Surg Clin North Am 1987;67:443–454.

What can be achieved with the Toupet procedure?

Ph. Boutelier (Paris)

The purpose of surgical treatment for gastroesophageal reflux is to re-establish normal physiology of the esogastric function: 1) to permit the passing of food; 2) to prevent gastroesophageal reflux; and 3) to permit incidental occurence of eructations and vomiting. This is, therefore, a matter of functional surgery.

Manometric studies have shown that two factors are essential for cardial continency: LES tonicity and length of the abdominal esophagus. LES tonicity is sensibly higher than gastric pressure when relaxed, preventing in this way gastric content to reflux into the esophagus. This tonicity depends on several hormonal and nervous factors.

The existence of an adequate length of the abdominal esophagus allows the LES to undergo intra-abdominal pressure variations and also to resist to abdominal hyperpressures, since the difference between stomach and LES pressure remains the same.

Principles of Toupet procedure

The Toupet procedure realizes a partial retroesophageal fundoplicature which is fixed to the folds of the diaphragm (Fig. 1). I personally advise to make an esophageal insert of a constant length of 4 cm, with a surrounding wrap ranging from 200° to 270°, depending on the tone of the LES. Therefore, this procedure allows reconstitution of an adequate length of the abdominal esophagus, which is the first aim of antireflux surgical treatment. Then it creates close anatomical connections between the abdominal esophagus and fundus, thus allowing transmission of gastric hyperpressures towards the LES. In addition, this operation accentuates the angle of His or the flap valve mechanism, which can be seen clearly when viewed postoperatively from an endoscope. Finally, the retroesophageal fundus is securely fixed over its

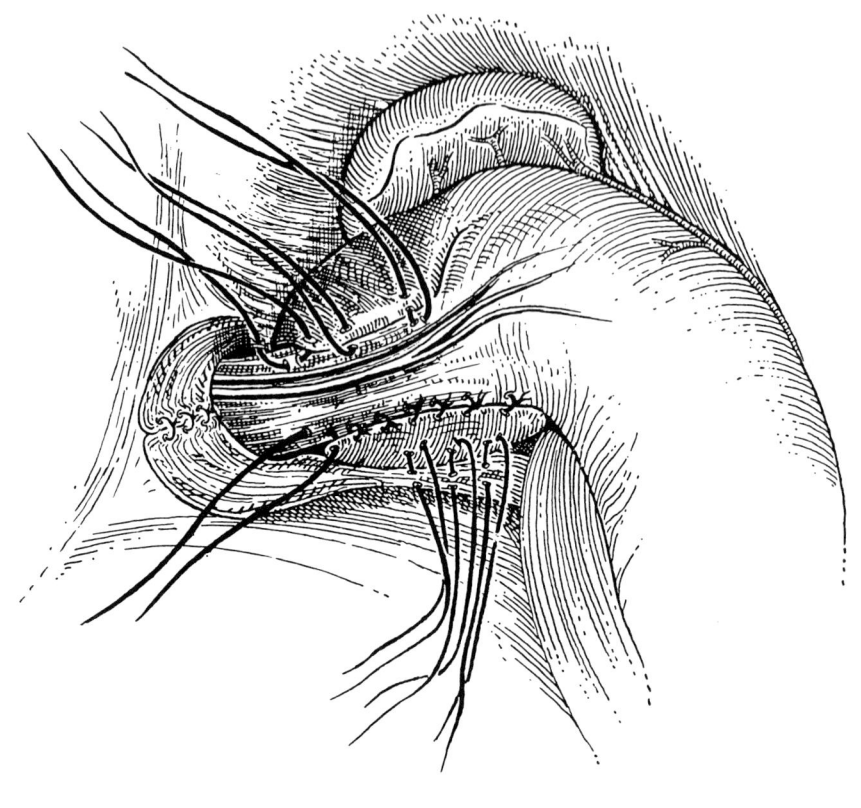

Fig. 1.

entire length by several stitches to the folds of the diaphragm, to prevent the assembly either from passing into the thorax, or going flat and shifting under the diaphragm.

Results

I have obtained good results regularly with this procedure [1], with a recurrence rate of less than 10% and with no gas bloat syndrome in patients with Nissen fundoplication. More recently [2], 100 patients operated upon according to the modified Toupet procedure have been investigated with a minimum of 3 years follow-up. All patients have been followed up both preoperatively and postoperatively with X-ray, manometry, Bernstein tests, pH measurement and endoscopy with biopsies. Good or excellent results have been obtained in over 90% with a recurrence rate of 7%, no operative deaths, and one splenectomy. Then, the same authors have realized a long-term randomized prospective trial of Nissen procedure vs. modified Toupet technique [3]. All patients were followed up on a long-term basis for 5 years with a standard questionnaire, endoscopy and manometry. Ninety-five percent of the patients in the modified Toupet group had good or excellent results vs. 67% for the Nissen group.

However, both procedures are effective in curtailing esophagitis with an improvement of the endoscopic grading by 91% in the Nissen group and 69% in the group undergoing the modified Toupet procedure. A significant improvement in symptoms (acid regurgitation, hearthbrun, retrosternal pain) was noted in both groups, except for dysphagia in the Nissen group. Three patients with a Nissen fundoplication had a slipped Nissen requiring reoperation, and two suffered from gas bloat syndrome. These specific complications of the Nissen procedure were not found in the modified Toupet group.

Discussion

One criticism may be said about this operation which fails to calibrate the cardia. This point is probably essential in cases where the major mechanism of the gastroesophageal reflux (GER) consists of spontaneous relaxations of the cardia [4], thus probably explaining some failures of this procedure. For this reason, when a pathological gastroesophageal reflux coexists with a LES subnormal tone, I have

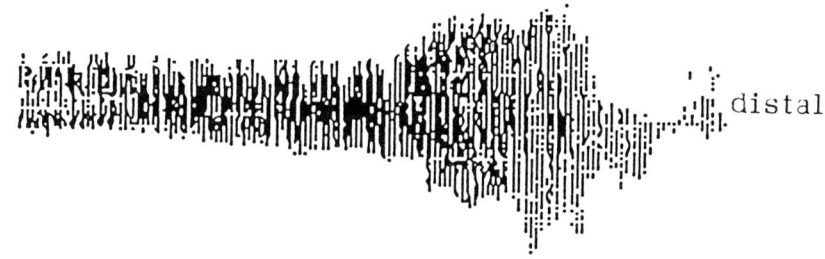

distal

Narrowing of cardia + TOUPET

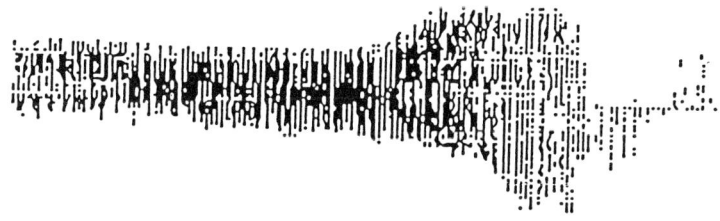

NORMAL LES – Manometric study

Fig. 2.

suggested [5] to combine the modified Toupet procedure with narrowing of the cardia by means of a peritoneal scrap. Postoperative studies with computerized manometry show pictures similar to those of a normal sphincter (Fig. 2).

References

1. Boutelier Ph, Jonsell G. An alternative fundoplicative maneuver for gastroesophageal reflux. Am J Surg 1982;143:260–264.
2. Thor K. The modified Toupet procedure. In: Hill LD (ed) The Esophagus Medical and Surgical Management. W.B Saunders Company 1988;135–138.
3. Thor K, Silander T. A long-term randomized prospective trial of the Nissen procedure vs. a modified Toupet technique. Ann Surg 1989;210(6):719–724.
4. Dodds WJ, Dent J, Hogan WJ et al. Mechanisms of gastroesophageal reflux in patients with reflux esophagitis. N Eng J Med 1982;307:1547–1552.
5. Boutelier Ph. Une nouvelle méthode de cure de reflux gastro-oesophagien: la fundoplicature rétro-oesophagienne associée au cravatage péritonéal du cardia. Chirurgie 1990;116:597–601.

The Rampal procedure

J.B. Flament, L. Poloma, H. Plet, J.P. Palot, J.F. Delattre, C. Avisse (Reims)

Treatment of gastroesophageal reflux (GER) has long been associated with hiatal hernia repair; this view is no longer valid for surgical indications. On one hand, the frequency of hiatal hernia is increasing with aging of the population, and an operation may be considered only when reflux is complicated with esophagitis. On the other hand, routine endoscopic examinations showed that reflux esophagitis could exist without any evidence of hiatal hernia.

Appreciation of the role of the lower esophageal sphincter (LES) in the prevention of acid reflux has led to the creation of procedures designed to reinforce the LES and to restore its normal competence. It is important to create an artificial valve at the gastroesophageal (GE) junction, preferably behind the esophagus, lengthening the subdiaphragmatic esophagus and maintaining the sphincteric mechanism in the positive pressure environment of the abdominal cavity [1]. The narrowing of the hiatus itself is no longer considered essential, even though it may be a useful additional procedure. The principle should help to improve results in the current 15% of failures reported in surgical literature. This value corresponds with the results obtained using the Lortat-Jacob procedure. Over a long period these results were thought satisfactory; failures were not as severe as those associated with Nissen fundoplication. However, a better procedure could be sought after.

This report describes our experience with 282 operations combining a partial fundoplication with a cardiopexy using the ligamentum teres (Fig. 1). The technique

712

was inspired by the work of Pedinielli [2] and Rampal [3], and is similar to the procedure used by Marchal [4] and Narbona [5].

Methods

During a 10-year period, from January 1983 to December 1992, 317 consecutive patients were operated on for gastroesophageal reflux. Of these, 282 underwent circular cardiopexy with the round ligament and a posterior semifundoplication.

There were 112 female and 180 male patients. The mean age was slightly higher in females (58.6 to 47.9 years), with a range of 25—85 years.

Nine patients (3%) were operated on for recurrent reflux esophagitis 2 to 6 years after an earlier operation. The other 273 (97%) had a primary repair: 135 (49.8%) were suffering from an isolated GER uncontrolled by medical therapy; in 138 (50.5%) patients, GER was associated with another digestive disease (64 gallstones, 29 duodenal ulcers, 1 colonic cancer etc.); reflux was the main complaint in 52 of these 138 patients (37%). In all cases GER was clinically evident and had been documented by endoscopic and/or manometric studies. We have never done a preventive repair of an uncomplicated hiatal hernia in the course of a supramesocolic operation.

Eighty-eight percent of the patients were evaluated with fiberoptic endoscopy. Esophagitis was evaluated in four grades according to DeMeester's scale: grade 0 = no esophagitis (64 patients); grade I = erythematous mucosa (58 patients); grade II =

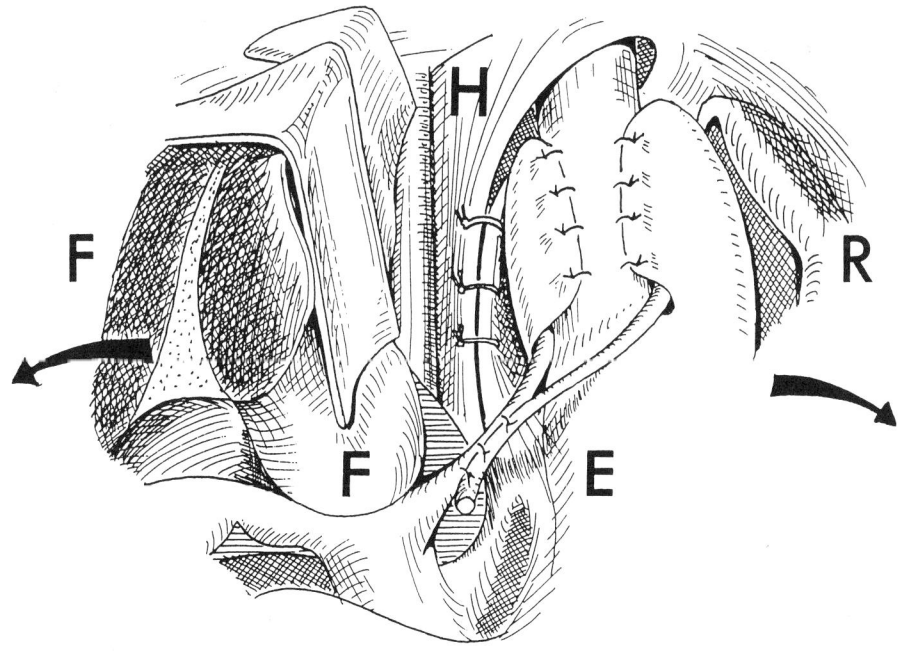

Fig. 1. The assembly.

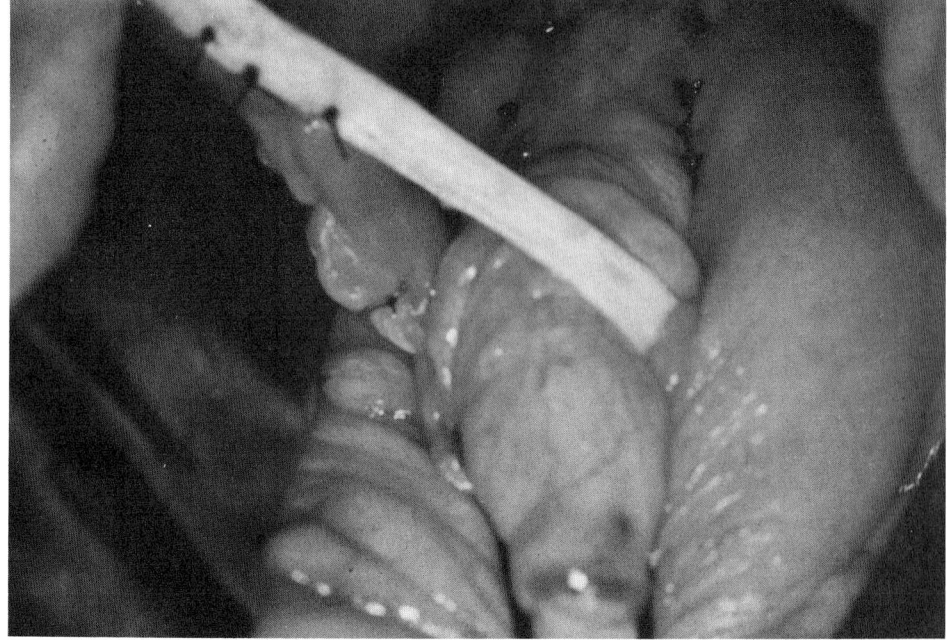

Fig. 2. Surgical view: round ligament extended by a cutaneous strip.

presence of erosions and pseudomembranous mucosa (70 patients); grade III = ulceration or stenosis (64 patients). Of the 283 patients, 134 patients had grades II and III (69.8%).

Upper gastrointestinal (GI) X-ray examination was carried out in 149 patients. Fourteen were normal, 93 had reflux and hiatal hernia, 23 had reflux without hernia and 32 had hernia without reflux. A manometric study was performed in 166 patients and postprandial 3-h pH-monitoring in 170 patients.

Three major points are included in our procedure: approximation of the crura of the diaphragm, cardiopexy with the ligamentum teres and posterior semifundoplication.

All operations were performed transabdominally, 131 through an upper midline incision, 151 through an upper transverse incision, depending on the morphology of the patient. The standard procedure contains five steps.

The first step is dissection and freeing of the ligamentum teres from its umbilical insertion up to the bottom of the fissure for the ligamentum teres on the inferior surface of the liver.

The second step is exposure of the hiatus. We use a self-retaining Olivier's retractor to elevate the thoracic wall; the left triangular ligament is divided and the left lobe of the liver retracted. The vestibule of the lesser sac is then divided, and the anterior and posterior nerves of Latarget are retracted medially along the lesser curvature of the stomach; these nerves must be carefully protected. Division of the upper part of the gastrohepatic ligament provides an excellent exposure of the right crus of the diaphragm. The esophagus is then mobilized after division of the peritoneal reflection and of the phrenoesophageal membrane. The distal esophagus is dissected until a long intra-abdominal segment is obtained. In 28 patients (10%) this necessitated a bilateral truncal vagotomy. The esophagus and the anterior vagus nerve are encircled with a tape and the posterior vagus nerve is usually left off the tape posteriorly. Dissection of the gastrophrenic ligament and division of one or two short gastric vessels provide a wide exposure of the left crus.

The third step is approximation of the crura of the diaphragm posteriorly to the esophagus with three or four nonabsorbable sutures. These sutures must be tied with a tension that causes tissue approximation but avoids any laceration of the muscles. The esophageal hiatus, now narrowed, is displaced forward and upward and the surgeon must be able to insert the index finger next to the esophagus.

The fourth step is mooring of the GE junction. The ligamentum teres is pulled behind and around the esophagus from the right to the left and then fixed to itself by two or three nonabsorbable stitches that form a loop. The loop must not be too tight and must accept a fingertip.

The final step is the creation of a semifundoplication including an anterior and a posterior fundic fold. The fundus is pulled behind the esophagus with a clamp and then sutured on its right border with a vertical row of five or six nonabsorbable sutures. An anterior valve is obtained similarly and fixed by a second row of stitches placed either right or left to the anterior vagus nerve.

Variations included a ligament that was too short, and was reinforced by a skin strip in 28 cases, no hiatus closure in 31 patients, and in 19 patients the ligamentum teres was fixed to the anterior abdominal wall (Fig. 2).

Other associated procedures in 133 patients included operation on biliary tract in 64 cases, treatment of a duodenal ulcer in 29 cases (25 parietal cell vagotomies and four bilateral truncal vagotomies) and right hemicolectomy for cancer in one patient.

Our patients were clinically evaluated at 3 weeks, 6 months and from then on annually. Three-week postoperative controls also included 191 upper GI X-ray examinations, 161 fiberoptic endoscopies, 120 manometric studies, and 132 three-hour pH-monitorings.

Results

There were 10 minor splenic tears without consequence. Five splenic injuries required subsequent splenectomy (1.7%), and there was one subphrenic abscess. In two patients, dissection of the esophagus produced an esophageal tear that was closed and buttressed by the fundoplication without consequence. Eleven wound infections (3.9%) were responsible for one immediate postoperative evisceration (successfully treated with an absorbable prosthesis) and for 12 delayed incisional hernias (4.2%).

There were two postoperative deaths (0.7%): a 70-year-old patient died suddenly after an operation that included cholecystectomy and external biliary drainage for angiocholitis. A pulmonary embolus was confirmed by postmortem examination. Another patient died from myocardial infarction.

The symptoms of GER immediately disappeared in all cases. Seventy-four patients (25%) suffered from a transient dysphagia, relieved in all cases within 3 weeks to 6 months. Only one patient reported painful belching, that disappeared after 8 months. No other side effects were reported. Endoscopic examination was performed in 161 patients. X-ray examination was performed in 188 patients with satisfactory results in 180 cases (96%). Evidence of esophageal dilatation was present in 25 patients, but only five suffered from dysphagia. Manometric functional studies were carried out in 146 patients, showing restoration of a competent LES in all cases; the average lower esophageal sphincter pressure (LESP) was 12.05 ± 6.95 cm preoperatively and 23.9 ± 12.9 cm postoperatively. This difference is highly significant ($p < 0.001$). In 27 patients, manometric studies revealed motility disorders in the distal esophagus: their interpretation is unclear, but these disorders were accompanied in 10 cases with transient dysphagia. Absence of reflux, in 95% of the 139 patients examined postoperatively, was verified by pH monitoring.

Two patients died 3 months and 8 months after surgery from concomitant disease. Seven have been lost for follow-up. The other 271 patients underwent postoperative clinical evaluation (follow-up = 100%). The mean follow-up period was 38 months, with a range of 1–8 years.

On subjective clinical evaluation, 264 out of 271 patients (97%) were satisfied with the results of the operation. Recurrent symptoms were present in five cases. Four of these were 60 year-old patients whose reflux was controlled by medical therapy, and one patient was a 45 year-old woman operated on for recurrent reflux presenting intermittent regurgitations but normal endoscopic findings. Asymptomatic reflux was evidenced by upper GI X-ray examination in only one female patient in whom endoscopic and manometric controls were normal. In two other cases a persistent reflux was demonstrated by pH monitoring without any clinical and endoscopic symptoms.

Discussion

Pedinielli [2] was the first to propose a procedure of cardiopexy slinging the GE junction and called it "technique du collet". He used a strip of skin cut from the abdominal wall at the beginning of the operation. He slung it around the distal esophagus and sutured it to itself. He then attached it tensely to the anterior abdominal wall. The first published results were satisfactory, but questions remained concerning the evolution of the cutaneous strip in the absence of any blood supply.

Rampal et al. [3] in France and Narbona in Spain in 1972 [5], proposed using the ligamentum teres to perform a cardiopexy, a principle directly inspired by Pedinielli's "snare". The advantages were evident: a) blood supply for the ligamentum teres is provided by a little artery branching from the hepatic artery, thus preventing long-term resorption; b) the ligament connects the GE junction to the left lobe of the liver, acting as a "floating anchor" through its movements accompanying respiration; and c) the system thus obtained is most likely to maintain the angle of His, as it pulls the GE junction forward, downward, toward the right. Narbona [5] considered that this

716

procedure could not prevent reflux in itself, and had to be associated with closure of the hiatus and anterior gastropexy.

In 1967 Marchal [4] adopted Rampal's technique with a few modifications, insisting on the restoration of the angle of His by creating a close anatomic contact between the fundus and distal esophagus. The good results obtained from this procedure stem from an understanding of a number of basic theoretical criteria. Sliding hiatal hernia is an acquired disease linked with the failure of the posterior attachments of the GE junction and preceded by shortening of the abdominal portion of esophagus. In most cases, the hernia is accompanied by pathologic reflux due to deterioration of gastroesophageal sphincteric competence. The goal of surgery is to reduce the hernia and to prevent the reflux. Thus, ideal treatment should be conducted along two different concepts, and the operation should include two main steps.

The first is a "plastic" step, corresponding to the creation of an artificial valve. The simplest procedure is to restore the angle of His by suturing the fundus to the distal esophagus. Lortat-Jacob demonstrated its importance [6]. Creation of a zone of hyperpressure by partial (Toupet) or total (Nissen) wrapping of the distal esophagus with the gastric fundus is probably the best way to prevent reflux. Variations of intragastric or intra-abdominal pressure are immediately transmitted to the distal esophageal sphincter, preventing reflux. Adlay showed that a 270° semifundoplication was sufficient and avoided the side effects of the Nissen fundoplication [7]. This high pressure zone exists in normal subjects and corresponds to the diaphragmatic canal limited by the two muscular bundles of the hiatus. Its role in improving the LES has been clearly demonstrated by Delattre [1].

The second step is a "pexic" one, aimed at anchoring the GE junction inside the abdominal cavity. This step ensures a lengthening of the subdiaphragmatic esophagus that favors the transmission of the variations of intra-abdominal pressure. Fixation of the valve to the posterior parietal structures, either the median arcuate ligament as advocated by Hill, or the crura of the diaphragm as recommended by Toupet [8], seems a rigid system.

On the contrary, the attachment of the GE junction by the ligamentum teres provides a flexible system and concomitant mobility with the liver. This may represent a self-adapting and self-regulating system. Contractions of the diaphragm that increase intra-abdominal pressure and provoke reflux when the esophageal hiatus is enlarged, pull the liver and subsequently the insertion of the ligamentum teres in a downward direction. The more powerful the contraction of the diaphragm, the more powerful the traction on the ligament. This procedure reproduces the normal anatomic and physiologic conditions of cardiac competence.

Summary

For the past 10 years, we have used a procedure combining hiatus closure, cardiopexy with the ligamentum teres and a 270° semifundoplication. The procedure is easy to perform, benign and reliable. The results obtained with this technique are slightly superior to those obtained in other series [9], both subjectively and objectively.

Postprandial pH monitoring evidences the absence of postoperative reflux in all cases. Healing of reflux esophagitis can be verified by endoscopy in 100% of cases. Manometric measurements indicate effective restoration of LESP. These results remain stable with time, and there are no uncomfortable side effects.

References

1. Delattre JF, Palot JP, Ducasse A, Flament JB, Hureau J. The crura of the diaphragm and diaphragmatic passage. Applications to gastroesophageal reflux, its investigation and treatment. Anat Clin 1985;7:271–283.
2. Pedinielli L. Traitement chirurgical de la hernie hiatale par la "technique du collet". Ann Chir 1964;18:1461–1474.
3. Rampal M, Perillat Ph, Rougaud R. Notes préliminaires sur une nouvelle technique de cure chirurgicale des hernies hiatales: la cardiopexie par le ligament rond. Marseille Chir 1964;16:488.
4. Marchal G, Balmes M, Bousquet M, Olivier G, Dayan L. Traitement des hernies hiatales par la technique de Rampal. Montpellier Chir 1967;479–482.
5. Narbona B, Olavarrieta L, Lloris JM, de Lera F, Calvo MA. Le traitement du reflux gastro-oesophagien par pexie avec le ligament rond. A propos de 100 opérés suivis entre 16 et 23 années. Chirurgie 1990;116:201–210
6. Lortat-Jacob JL, Dromer M, Lebas P et al. A propos de 221 interventions pour hernie par l'hiatus oesophagien chez l'adulte. Etude d'une statistique hospitalière intégrale. Ann Chir 1962;16:985–990.
7. Adlay ES, Goldsmith HS. Efficacy of fundoplication in preventing gastric reflux. Am J Surg 1973;126:322–324.
8. Toupet A. Technique d'oesophago-gastroplastie avec phrénogastropexie appliquée à la cure radicale des hernies hiatales et comme complément de l'opération de Heller dans les cardiospasmes. Mem Acad Chir 1963;102:700.
9. Boutelier Ph, Chipponi J. Le traitement chirurgical du reflux gastro-oesophagien de l'adulte. Rapport présenté au 91ème Congrès Français de Chirurgie, 1989, Masson.

What procedures are unsuitable for laparoscopy?

F. Dubois (Paris)

This question is multifaceted and has no simple answer. Firstly, the following main principles must be applied:
- the indications for surgical treatment of reflux are governed by the same rules, whether the operation is to be carried out conventionally or by endoscopy; the fact that endoscopic surgery may be more readily accepted by the patient in no way extends the indications;
- clearly, endoscopic surgery should only be considered by those who are skilled in the procedures involved, and who possess all the necessary equipment;
- the type of surgical intervention carried out must be that which is considered to be the most effective, i.e., it is important not to make do with an incomplete or unsatisfactory surgical procedure, simply because it is easy or because it is the only surgical option available by the endoscopic route.

Beyond these essential rules it is much harder to make any firm recommendations, especially as the technique is a recent one which is still under development and its approaches tend to change as experience is gained. For example, from 1989 to 1993 the transition has been made from simpler to more complicated interventions (i.e., Dor anterior valve, followed by Nissen and finally Toupet, which requires greater skill for the sutures).

It appears that all techniques for the surgical treatment of gastroesophageal reflux (GER) have been or could be carried out endoscopically, whether they involve formation of a valve, fixing of the cardia, or both of these procedures. Even if, due to lack of equipment, an operation such as Collis procedure for lengthening the esophagus is not feasible by endoscopy, it can be carried out by thoracoscopy.

Other contraindications, although still major at present, may become relative in the future and in some instances have already been removed:
— the dangers of pneumoperitoneum in patients with emphysematous bullae can be reduced by the suspension technique;
— reintervention for recurrence after surgical treatment of reflux: a few patients have been reoperated endoscopically with varying degrees of difficulty;
— reflux after gastric or esophageal resection: it is possible to imagine carrying out a duodenal diversion by endoscopy and this may well have already been done;
— undilatable esophageal constriction requiring esophageal resection: resections have already been carried out endoscopically and thoracoscopically;
— patients having undergone multiple operations at the supramesocolic level where dissection could be hazardous, or even patients with portal hypertension or severe periesophagitis;
— when there is a very large left liver lobe, it is very difficult to reach an underlying hiatus, and it is necessary to move the lobe in order to reach the hiatus from above. Perhaps one day that route may be used endoscopically.

In theory, therefore, there are no absolute contraindications for the endoscopic treatment of GER. It is only a matter of situations and procedures of varying and increasing difficulty, which the surgeon must take into account when considering the indications and the routes by which to tackle the problem.

Surgical treatment of established alkaline esophagitis

S. Correnti, G. Antonini, A. Mariotti, A. Liverani, G. Caprarola, U. Mercati (Perugia)

Gastroesophageal reflux (GER) disease accounts for approximately 75% of esophageal pathology [1]. Recently, surgeons have been paying much more attention to duodenogastroesophageal reflux (DGER), the identification of which has been given a substantial boost through the "combined" 24-h esophageal and gastric pH monitoring. DGER can be quantified with prolonged gastric pH monitoring, and appears to be related to increased esophageal exposure to alkalinity pH > 7, recorded on esophageal pH monitoring. The disease is insidious. In most instances in fact, the acid gastric environment neutralizes the alkaline reflux; in this situation reflux of gastric juice into the esophagus cannot be detected by pH monitoring and misinterpretations of the results may occur with a "mixed" or "neutral" reflux. ^{99}Tc scintigraphy does not guarantee better results, due to the frequency of false positives (18%) [2]. These shifty peculiarities may be dangerous because acid/alkaline esophageal reflux seems to be more severe than acid reflux.

The potential detrimental effect of duodenal contents on esophageal mucosa has been shown in animal models and humans [3,4]. It has a large role in the development of complications of GER (esophagitis, strictures, Barrett's esophagus), their prevalence being significantly higher in patients with acid/alkaline reflux as compared with those having only acid reflux (86 vs. 51%) [1]. Ingredients in the refluxed juice (gastric acid, pepsin, activated pancreatic enzymes and bile acids) have been implicated as factors predisposing to the development of complications. However, considerable differences of opinion still exist in regard to the relative importance of each of these factors. Trypsin, in physiologic concentrations, seems to be the major injurious agent in an alkaline refluxate [1,4].

Minimal work has been done to investigate the factors involved in the development of esophageal adenocarcinoma. Since adenocarcinoma occurs in patients with Barrett's esophagus, all of whom have severe gastroesophageal reflux, it is likely that the components of the refluxate are involved in the carcinogenic process. Adenocarcinoma was seen only in the esophagus of rats exposed to the combination of a duodenal juice and nitrosamines, while the esophageal tumors produced by nitrosamines alone were pure squamous carcinoma. The presence of bile, pancreatic juice or some other constituent of duodenal juice accelerates the production of esophageal carcinoma and alters the differentiation to produce adenocarcinoma [5]. These experiments complement the animal studies [4], who found a greater destruction of the rat esophageal mucosa after exposure to duodenal juice than to gastric juice. These observations implicate duodenal juice as an important carcinogen or cocarcinogen in the development of adenocarcinoma of the esophagus.

Enterogastric alkaline reflux gastritis and esophagitis are rare, but may exist [1,6,7], in people who have never been operated on previously. Particularly, an increased duodenogastric reflux has been demonstrated in patients with gallstones. Recently, the percentage of patients with cholecystectomy having abnormal pH profiles before operation has been quantified as 30% [8—10]. It is of interest that another recent report demonstrated that no patient without detectable amounts of biliary acids (BA) in the gastric juice before cholecystectomy showed the presence of BA after the operation [7].

DGER is best known after previous foregut surgery (cholecystectomy, vagotomy and pyloroplasty, Billroth II gastric resection, pancreatic resection, etc.) accounting for more than 70% of patients with increased esophageal alkaline exposure

[1,2,11,12]. There is no doubt that, in the case of patients with previous upper gastrointestinal or bilio-pancreatic surgery, complaining of severe and specific symptoms (epigastric pain, nausea, biliary vomiting), DGER must be suspected and investigated . The most common and simple surgical procedure which predisposes to DGER is cholecystectomy [6,8].

The underlying mechanisms would be the higher amounts of bile in the duodenal lumen due to the lack of storage in the gallbladder with a continuous bile flow independent of the meals and a dysfunction of the antroduodenal motor unit with an abnormal function of the pyloric channel [7]. Bile, in an acid medium, is injurious to the gastric mucosa [13], slows gastric emptying [11,12] and becomes a true risk factor of further severe GER.

This could explain why, even if the majority of patients who undergo cholecystec-tomy are satisfied and have no further symptoms, a significant minority, between 20 and 50%, have persistent or new symptoms that, in only rare cases (5.4%), can be explained by retained stones in the bile duct [8]. Several of the so-called postchole-cystectomy syndromes could be attributed to an increase in duodenogastric reflux.

Among 1,237 upper endoscopies using the "combined" pH monitoring test, from the beginning of 1992 up until now, we identified 68 patients with noncomplicated GER and who had never previously undergone surgery. Twenty-seven (39.7%) had acid alkaline reflux and four had gallstones.

Hiatal hernia and low pressure of the distal esophageal sphincter (DESP) have been proved by manometry in five and 18 alkaline refluxers respectively. All the patients with gallstones had low DESP. Grade I esophagitis was present in 17 cases, grade II in nine, and grade III in one. Three of the patients with biliary stones had grade I esophagitis, while one had grade II (Fig. 1).

Table 1 shows the distribution of the alkaline refluxers among 93 patients previously operated on either by us or elsewhere and revisited during the subsequent 16 months.

The relationship between the type of surgery, the LES function and the grade of esophagitis is reported in Table 2. It is worth noting that esophagitis in patients who had previous surgery is worse than in subjects who had never been operated on. It is also of interest that a Roux-en-Y duodenal diversion (DD) was performed by us to correct a B II gastric resection with symptoms of reflux. One year later, the patient

Table 1. Alkaline reflux in patients already operated on

Type of surgery	Number of patients	Alkaline refluxers	Gastric refluxers	DGER
Cholecystectomy	45	8	4	4
Cholecystectomy + B I	1	1	1	0
Cholecystectomy + B II	4	4	2	2
B I	8	8	5	3
B II	34	34	25	9
Roux-en-Y[a]	1	1	1	1
Total	93	56	38	19

[a]Performed 1 year ago after gastric B II resection.

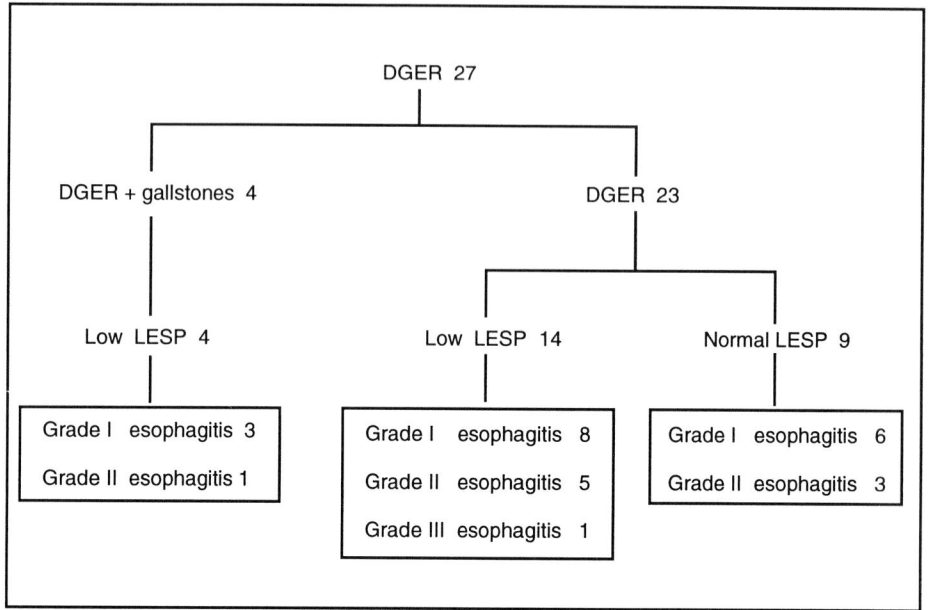

Fig. 1. Acid/alkaline reflux in patients never operated on (27); refluxers (total) = 68; acid GER = 41.

complained of reflux symptoms again, with low LESP. Medical treatment was unsuccessful and surgery was performed. It was impossible to carry out a correct Nissen because of the small gastric stump. All the patients with an entire stomach had acid/alkaline reflux. The total percentage of refluxers with low LESP (20/46 = 43.5%) was higher in patients who had never been operated upon (18/27) than in patients who had undergone previous surgery (2/19).

Up to now, we have 12 patients who have never been operated on (Table 3), and four with previous cholecystectomy (Table 4), grade I esophagitis and normal or low LESP, under medical treatment; their clinical and endoscopical state was balanced but the follow-up is too short as of yet (1—4 months).

One patient with gallstones, low LESP and grade I esophagitis underwent only a cholecystectomy performed by a fellow surgeon: the biliary symptoms disappeared but the outcome is unsatisfactory due to a persistent and worsened reflux.

The remaining patients belonging to the group of "never operated on cases" underwent a 360° Nissen repair (Table 3). A follow-up of 1—8 months is insufficient but, for now, all the subjects with a Nissen antireflux repair (AR) have a "good" Visick clinical grading and satisfactory endoscopical results.

Table 4 summarizes our approach in the case of patients having had previous surgery. The DD with a Roux-en-Y loop is our preferred choice. Two patients with previous cholecystectomy and B II gastric resection were treated with a Van Stiegmann-Goff DD [14]. In two other cases with a very low LESP an antireflux repair was necessary. Specific morbidity and mortality were nil.

Bilious vomiting and heartburn disappeared in all the patients reoperated on, but

Table 2. DGER, LESP and esophagitis in patients already operated on

Type of surgery	Low LESP	Esophagitis grade I	Esophagitis grade II	Esophagitis grade III
Cholecystectomy (4)	0	4	0	0
Cholecystectomy and B II (2)	0	0	2	0
B I (3)	0	1	2	0
B II (9)	1	1	7	1
Roux-en-Y (1)	1	0	1	0
Total	2	6	12	1

the follow-up of these cases is also too short in length (1—14 months) to allow any significant conclusion, but nevertheless, we consider the Roux-en-Y DD as a satisfactory procedure. Grade I (excellent) and grade II (good) were the Visick results in all these cases. Episodic vomiting of food has been seen in some patients who had neglected to keep the suggested rules of their diet, namely to eat little but frequently. These data complement the outcome of an other group of Roux-en-Y reconstructions controlled by us in the past for a different reason: it accounts for 26 operations, and the follow-up was longer (1—5 years). Endoscopy and pH-metry showed only one refluxer: this patient is the one included in the present series and who recently underwent a 270° AR. His outcome is going well 2 months after the operation.

The lack of an accuracy rate of our diagnostic possibilities, leads us to believe that the increased esophageal exposure to a pH > 7 recorded on 24-h esophageal pH monitoring represents only "the tip of the iceberg" of an underestimated disease. Moreover, these findings suggest that all patients presenting with biliary symptoms but no documented acute cholecystitis, should undergo full upper gastrointestinal investigations with esophagogastroduodenoscopy, biopsies and "combined" pH monitoring to exclude esophageal pathology. Perhaps, in the future, one should always take this approach, in spite of the consecutive widening costs of gallbladder disease. The "radiologically excluded" gallbladder, that could be in some way

Table 3. DGER treatment (patients never operated on)

Patients never operated on	Medical therapy	Medical therapy and cholecystectomy	AR 360°
Without gallstones			
Normal LES, grade I esophagitis (6)	6		
Normal LES, grade II esophagitis (3)			3
Low LES, grade I esophagitis (8)	6		2
Low LES, grade II esophagitis (5)			5
Low LES, grade III esophagitis (1)			1
With gallstones			
Grade I esophagitis (1)		1	
Grade II esophagitis (3)			3[a]

[a]+ cholecystectomy.

723

Table 4. DGER treatment (patients already operated on)

Patients already operated on	Medical therapy	AR 270°	DD
Cholecystectomy (normal LES, grade I esophagitis) (4)	4		
Cholecystectomy + B II (normal LES, grade II esophagitis) (2)			2[a]
B I (normal LES, grade I esophagitis = 1, grade II = 2) (3)			3[b]
B II (9) — low LES, grade I esophagitis = 1 — normal LES grade I esophagitis = 1, grade II esophagitis = 7		1	8[b]
Roux-en-Y (low LES, grade I esophagitis) (1)		1	

[a]Van Stiegmann-Goff; [b]Roux-en-Y.

understood as a cholecystectomy, belongs to this group. The so-called "functional" diseases of acalculous gallbladder, the aspecific symptoms of which are often not improved by simple cholecystectomy, can also be added to the biliary causes of suspected DGER. Often, this last group of patients do not benefit by simple cholecystectomy; on the contrary, their preoperative symptoms can even be worsened.

We had 56.5% of alkaline refluxers with normal LESP. Of course, this is not new: in fact, almost half of the subjects with increased esophageal exposure to gastric juice did not have LES incompetence [2,8]. It is well known that there are many other factors leading to reflux (progressive gastric dilatation, increased gastric pressure, persistent gastric reservoir, gastric hypersecretion of acid etc.). Nevertheless, this remark introduces us to an important concept, namely to be mistaken for a normal LES function; therefore, to delay the admission of patients with DGER into a program of therapy with strict follow-up may be extremely dangerous. Perhaps, even the physiological episodes of reflux may become malignant if the esophageal mucosa is repeatedly washed by duodenal content.

Since our review in 1989 [15], some changes in identification and nosology of the disease arose and convinced us that a strong therapeutical protocol should be started immediately in case of DGER.

Without taking into consideration the complicated alkaline esophagitis (i.e., stenosis, Barrett's, etc.), where a prompt resective surgery is mandatory, there is general agreement to state that, unfortunately, medical treatment is rarely of benefit in noncomplicated biliary GER. Acid reduction by pharmacological agents seems unlikely to alter the injurious effects of duodenal juice. Like others, we have not as yet found the new prokinetic agent cisapride to be of significant benefit in treating patients with bilious vomiting [5,8].

Most of the patients with gastric biliary lake but no injured esophagus are clinically silent [11]: to take the bile away from the esophagus seems to be the sole effective treatment to reach this goal, as well as to prevent benign or malignant complications. At the present time, however, there are no reports convincing us of the need of immediate routine surgery. Therefore, in the absence of any other medical option, making, at least in selected cases, a controlled pharmacological attempt seems to be ethical. Moreover, H_2-blockers and antacids may abolish the acid component of the "mixed" refluxate that is the most frequent one at least among patients never operated upon. Reflux of acid juice contaminated with duodenal contents seems to be the most important determinant for the development of mucosal injury in patients with GER [1].

The degree of the esophagitis, the function of the LES and the presence of worsening factors, such as gallstones or cholecystectomy, may act like modulators of the medical strategy.

Patients without previous surgery and complaining of grade I esophagitis, with normal LESP and no gallstones, may be primarily treated with diet, inhibitors of gastric secretion, upper digestive tract prokinetic agents, biliary acids antagonists etc. Of course, a strict follow-up is needed, and worsening of the esophagitis and/or of the LES and/or of the esophageal body function under treatment indicates that a prompt admission of the patient to surgery is necessary.

Much more care is needed in cases of esophagitis grade II or III, which are more frequent in subjects already operated on. In these instances prompt surgery should be mandatory.

When surgery is indicated, two options exist: antireflux repair (AR) and duodenal diversion (DD).

Patients never operated on and without gallstones may primarily benefit by a 360° Nissen fundoplication, particularly if a mechanically defective sphincter exists. The Nissen repair, in our opinion, is the best choice among AR, as long as it is done before loss of esophageal contractility. We also performed this AR in cases of normal LES function with grade II esophagitis and without other evident causes of reflux. At the present time, manometry is not a physiological investigation and false negative results may appear. Medical therapy and strict endoscopic follow-up are mandatory to control the remaining alkaline gastritis which is, however, a slower and easier process to control. Biliary diversion procedures can be reserved for later use if gastric signs and symptoms persist.

The most difficult problem solving of the debate on surgery of DGER in patients without previous surgery occurs when reflux is combined with gallstones. First, biliary symptoms may oblige one to perform surgery quickly, then, cholecystectomy perpetuates and worsens the pre-existent reflux and therefore, the alkaline gastritis. Most of the patients with preoperatively detected biliary acids in the stomach show an important increase after cholecystectomy [7], and in these cases, the increased gastric stasis could neutralize the antireflux effect of the Nissen repair. Therefore, in theory, a DD, combined or not with AR (as in case of normal LESP, and also considering that basal esophageal sphincter pressure does not show a significant reduction following cholecystectomy [9]), could be a more correct choice. On the other hand, a "classic" DD (Roux-en-Y and two-thirds gastric resection) seems to be excessive. Moreover, reports stating only less than 50% of satisfactory results after cholecystectomy and Roux-en-Y DD [12] increase doubts. One reason for such an outcome may be that in some cases the gastric stasis caused by biliary reflux persists also in the gastric stump, particularly if it is too large. The addition of a truncal vagotomy at the time of the DD could further worsen the gastric emptying. Pylorus-preserving procedures such as described by DeMeester ("duodenal switch") [16], could be more appropriate in this type of patient. The procedure, which does not imply vagotomy, may be difficult if duodenal anomalies exist, but has the advantage of preserving the stomach and the pyloric function. The questions remain as to whether the short remaining duodenum is able to "inhibit" the gastric acid secretion, and if the gastric emptying can be restored. We never experienced this procedure.

Concerning major surgery, B II gastric resection was the most frequent cause of postoperative DGER among revisited patients, however, there are many other surgical procedures of the upper digestive tract leading to alkaline reflux [15]. Some of these are performed in people with benign pathology, and thus a long life expectancy. In these cases, particularly, prevention of reflux is the first step of the therapy. For example, truncal vagotomy with pyloroplasty should be avoided and replaced by parietal cell vagotomy without drainage. The procedure is also effective for the treatment of perforated duodenal ulcer, when added to suture. B II gastric resection should be routinely replaced by a Roux-en-Y gastric resection.

However, when the correction of previous surgery is necessary, in our opinion, the "classic" Roux-en-Y DD (large gastric resection, two-thirds, large gastrojejunal anastomosis, Roux-en-Y reconstruction with a loop not less than 50–60 cm in length) remains the treatment of choice.

The protective effect of Roux-en-Y diversion of the duodenal contents downstream has been shown since 1964 [17], and the procedure remains the most common reconstruction for bilious vomiting following previous surgery [12]. In several instances, when an abnormal function of the LES exists, the Roux-en-Y DD alone may, however, be sufficient. Two basic technical concepts should always be observed in order to reach the goal of a satisfactory function of the procedure. First, there is general agreement that the most important reason for failure of bile diversion operations is that the length of the efferent loop is insufficient to prevent reflux of bile and duodenal contents into the gastric remnant [11–13]. Secondly, although there is no common agreement on size of gastric resection, our experience is that the smaller the gastric stump, the better its emptying is. A too wide gastric remnant could be one of the reasons why some authors [12], having performed a simple antrectomy, then report an unsatisfactory outcome in 53% of their patients after a Roux-en-Y DD, persistent upper abdominal pain and vomiting of food being the main symptoms. It should be kept in mind, however, that changes in gastric motility and stasis in the gastric remnant may be permanent in some subjects, leading to definitively delayed gastric emptying. This could also explain why the worst results have been seen in patients with truncal vagotomy before revision.

In our experience, no patients required surgical treatment for stomal ulcer, so we would disagree that Roux-en-Y DD is ulcerogenic.

Malabsorption is reported to be not significantly different from that reported following B II gastrectomy [12]. There is no agreement on the need for truncal vagotomy but, in the past, this procedure gave rise to considerable problems such as diarrhea in addition to the stasis of the gastric remnant, and we preferred to disregard it. In theory, truncal vagotomy could be mandatory to abolish the acid component of mixed refluxate, that is frequently observed after small gastric resections as is antrectomy. In our opinion, the complications of this added procedure outweighs its advantages, and its effects may be equalled by prolonged H_2-blockers administration.

The problem of patients already operated on and having abnormal LES function is also of importance: in the case of a previous simple antrectomy, the gastric stump is usually wide enough to perform a correct Nissen repair. On the other hand, in the case of a correct B II resection or a "classic" Roux-en-Y DD (as after vagotomy and drainage or cholecystectomy), the gastric stump could be too small for a 360° antireflux procedure; its excessive mobilization seems risky for the vascular supply to the remaining stomach, and only one short vessel can be cut with safety. The anatomical conditions only allow the construction of a 270° AR. We adopted this surgical technique in a Roux-en-Y refluxer, and the clinical outcome was very satisfying 2 months later.

The Roux-en-Y DD can also be used in cases of patients with subtotal esophagectomy and intrathoracic gastric transplant [15]. In our experience, among 82 patients controlled after resection for esophageal cancer, alkaline reflux accounted for 29.4% of them, despite an isoperistaltic gastric tube routinely performed, with satisfactory emptying steadily demonstrated (^{99}Tc scintigraphy). Unfortunately, we usually observe stage II B or stage III tumors of the esophagus, developed in weakened patients with a short life expectancy. In these cases, medical therapy seems the best option, and dilatations of eventual stenoses of the esophagogastric anastomosis are preferred over surgery, with good results. On the other hand, DD could be performed in refluxers previously operated on for a benign esophageal disease.

Finally, we would like to stress the good outcome which followed our two Van Stiegmann-Goff procedures. The operation is easy and fast to perform after a B II gastric resection. Perhaps, if more controlled studies can prove its effectiveness, the technique could be recommended as the treatment of choice in these instances.

References

1. Stein HJ, Barlow AP, DeMeester TR, Hinder RA. Complications of gastroesophageal reflux disease. Ann Surg 1992; 216(1):35–43.
2. Stein HJ, Smyrk TC, DeMeester TR, Rouse J, Hinder RA. Clinical value of endoscopy and histology in the diagnosis of duodenogastric reflux disease. Surgery 1992;112(4):796–804.
3. Pellegrini CA, DeMeester TR, Wernly JA et al. Alkaline gastroesophageal reflux. Am J Surg 1978;135:177–184.
4. Kivilaakso E, Fromm D, Silen W. Effect of bile salts and related compounds on isolated esophageal mucosa. Surgery 1980;87:280–285.
5. Attwood SEA, Smyrk TC, DeMeester TR, Mirvish SS, Stein HJ, Hinder RA. Duodenoesophageal reflux and the development of esophageal carcinoma in rats. Surgery 1992;111(5):503–510.
6. Walsh TN, Jazrawi S, Byrne PJ, Hennessy TPJ. Cholecystectomy and gastroesophageal reflux. Br J Surg 1991;78:753 (abstract).
7. Cabrol J, Navarro X, Simo-Deo J, Segura R. Evaluation of duodenogastric reflux in gallstone disease before and after simple cholecystectomy. Am J Surg 1990;160:283–286.
8. Jazrawi S, Walsh TN, Byrne PJ, Hill AD, Li H, Lawlor P, Hennessy TPJ. Cholecystectomy and oesophageal reflux: a perspective evaluation. Br J Surg 1993;80:50–53.
9. Svensson JO, Gelin J, Svanvik J. Gallstones, cholecystectomy and duodenogastric reflux of bile acid. Scand J Gastroenterol 1986;21:181–187.
10. Cranford CA, Kennedy NSJ, Sutton D, Cuschieri A. The relationship between enterogastric reflux of bile and gallbladder function. Am J Gastroenterol 1987;82:972.

11. Alexander-Williams J. Alkaline reflux gastritis: a myth or a disease. Am J Surg 1982;143:17—21.
12. Ferguson GH, MacLennan I, Taylor TV, Torrance HB. Outcome of revisional gastric surgery using a Roux-en-Y biliary diversion. Br J Surg 1990;77:551—554.
13. Gowen GF. Spontaneous enterogastric reflux gastritis and esophagitis. Ann Surg 1985;201(2):170—175.
14. Van Stiegmann G, Goff UJS. An alternative to Roux-en-Y for treatment of reflux gastritis. Surg Gynecol Obstet 1988; 166:69—70.
15. Castrini G, Correnti S. The alkaline esophagitis: an up-date. Dis Eso 1989;II(2):81—90.
16. DeMeester TR, Fuchs KH, Ball CS, Albertucci M, Smyrk TC, Marcus JN. Experimental and clinical results with proximal end to end duodenojejunostomy for pathologic duodenogastric reflux. Ann Surg 1987;206:414—426.
17. Lawson HH. Effect of duodenal content on the gastric mucosa under experimental conditions. Lancet 1964;469—471.

What are the overall results of surgical treatment of GER?

B. Zilberstein, I. Cecconello, A. Nasi, H.W. Pinoti (São Paulo)

When the clinical treatment for reflux esophagitis (RE) fails and the inflammation of the esophageal mucosa persists, or continues to increase, enhancing symptomatology and/or complications like hemorrhage, stenosis, ulcer, or Barrett's mucosa, surgical treatment is indicated [1]. Such an approach is also recommended in patients with simultaneous surgical diseases, abdominal or incisional hernias, complicated peptic ulcer, cholecystitis, the latter coinciding in 15 to 30% with hiatal hernia. Surgery is also indicated in RE caused by previous interventions on the esophagogastric junction (Table 1).

The principles on which the surgical treatment of RE is based are the following:
— restoration of the abdominal portion of the esophagus;
— restoration of His angle;
— reinforcement of the physiological action of "lower esophageal sphincter" (LES).

Table 1. Indications for surgical treatment of reflux esophagitis

1° Complicated esophagitis	3° Simultaneous surgical diseases
— hemorrhage	— cholelithiasis
— ulcer	— peptic Ulcer
— Barrett's mucosa	4° EGJ abnormalities
— cancer	5° Failure of medical treatment
2° Respiratory effects	6° Postoperative esophagitis
— laryngotracheitis	7° Special professional activities
— bronchial asthma	
— acute or recurrent pneumonitis	

These objectives are reached by reducing the hiatal hernia (when present) by reduction or adjustment of the hiatal ring and by fundoplication.

The fundoplications usually allow an increase of the LES pressure being the main factor for the success of the surgical approach. According to DeMeester total or partial fundoplication increases the LES pressure levels by 10 to 20 mmHg [2].

This result is due to mechanical and or functional effects. The mechanical effect occurs as a consequence of the increase in the intragastric pressure or volume which enhances the compression of the esophagus by the stomach. Experimental studies have demonstrated that the tension of the gastric wall interferes with the LES function. Fundoplication changes the direction of strength vectors caused by gastric distension, transferring them no longer to the cardia orifice, but to the distal esophagus wrapped by the stomach.

The functional effect is related to the anatomical arrangement of the muscular fibers of the gastric fundus which continue to be active, and keep their tonus even when they surround the esophagus after fundoplication [3].

Surgical treatment

The most common surgical techniques differ as to the approach and the performance of the wrap.

The approach may be by left thoracotomy [4] or by median abdominal incision. The fundoplication may be total [5] or partial [6,7]. From the practical standpoint, the aim is to create a valvular antireflux mechanism. In those cases in which the esophageal wall is seriously compromised by the esophagitis, Nissen's procedure should be considered owing to the risk of tearing of the sutures. In this technique all the esophageal circumference is surrounded by the stomach. In patients with stenosing esophagitis, dilation of the narrowed portion has to be carried out when needed with probes of progressively increasing diameter before the creation of the valve. In order

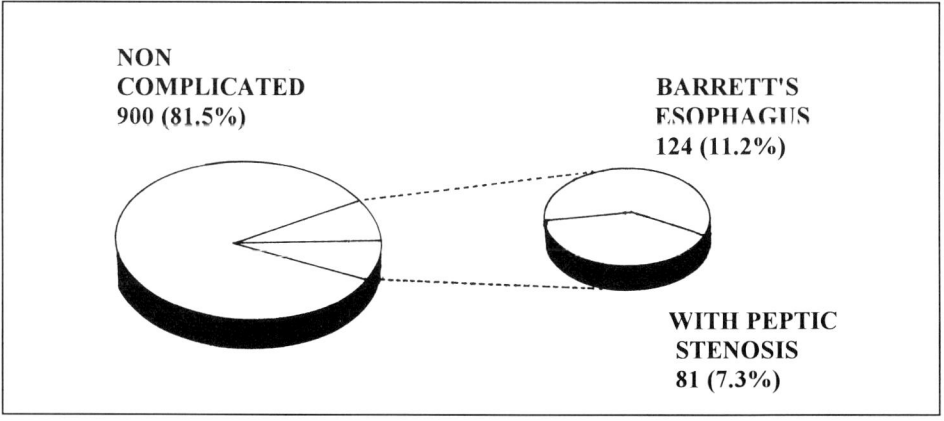

NON
COMPLICATED
900 (81.5%)

BARRETT'S
ESOPHAGUS
124 (11.2%)

WITH PEPTIC
STENOSIS
81 (7.3%)

Fig. 1. Surgical treatment of reflux esophagitis (1105 cases).

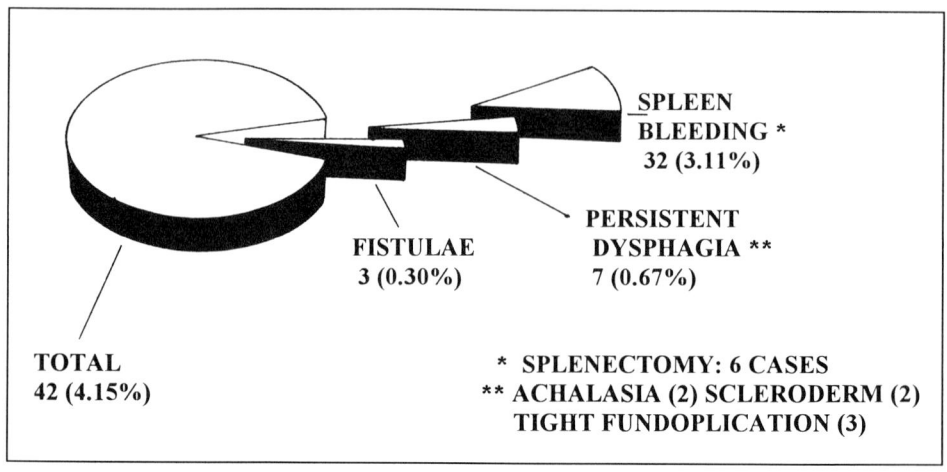

Fig. 2. Reflux esophagitis: complications of abdominal fundoplication (900 cases).

to achieve this goal, it is often necessary to divide the median part of the diaphragm up to the xiphoid process, to allow an ample exposure of the mediastinum [8–11]. In cases where it is not possible to reach a satisfactory intraoperative patency at the level of the stenosis, it is suggested to keep a gastrostomy for further retrograde dilation attempts.

Results

Since 1967, surgical treatment of RE was performed in 1105 cases (Fig. 1). In 900 patients a partial fundoplication was performed. Main complications and mortality are reported in Fig. 2 and Table 2. Late follow-up of 270 patients showed 95% good results following surgical treatment (Fig. 3).

Table 2. Partial abdominal fundoplication of reflux esophagitis

Bronchopneumonia	1
Acute myocardial infarction	1
Pulmonary thromboembolism	1
Stroke	1
Peritonitis	1
Total	5 (0.55%)

Discussion

A review of the international literature on surgical management of RE is shown in Tables 3 and 4.

730

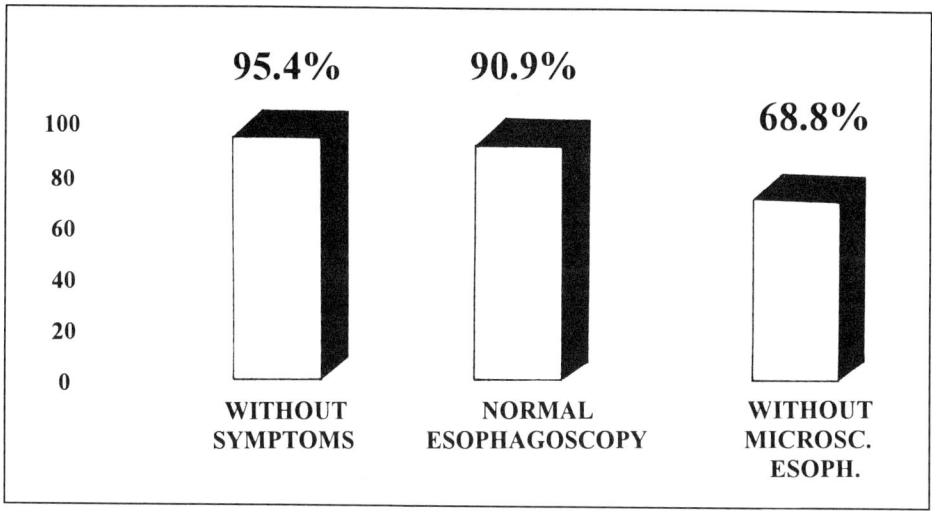

Fig. 3. Reflux esophagitis: partial abdominal fundoplication (5 years follow-up).

A prospective study published by Beauchamp et al. in 1989 with 3 years follow-up is shown in Table 5 [12].

Walker et al. published in 1989 a very elegant study showing that no great difference could be demonstrated between the two main techniques (Table 6) [13].

Table 3. Reflux esophagitis: surgical treatment by fundoplication

	Number	Good results (%)	Recurrent esophagitis (%)	Complications (%)	Mortality (%)
Partial abdominal fundoplication	2001	91	8.6	7.7	0.7
Total abdominal fundoplication (Nissen)	3226	92	9.8	7.9	1.2

Table 4. Reflux esophagitis: surgical treatment from international literature

	Number	Mortality (%)	Good result (%)	RR[a] (%)
Belsey	1656	0.2	83.0	—
	783	0.9	87.6	—
	1512	—	85.0	—
Partial	826	0.1	95.0	—
	1524	1.1	85.0	8.5
Nissen	3260	0.5	92.0	—
	2196	0.7	87.4	—
	1967	—	92.5	—
	1141	1.0	87.0	7.0

[a]RR = reflux recurrence.

731

Table 5. Post floppy-Nissen symptoms: 50 cases; 3-year follow-up

	Incidence (%)	Symptoms (%)
Change ingest. habits	56	0
Meteorism	38	26
Gastric fullness	38	28
Eructation difficulty	22	14
Vomiting difficulty	36	24
Sup. abdom. pain	32	4
Diarrhea	20	4
Persistent diarrhea	16	4

Table 6. Randomized prospective study Lind × Nissen (Visick, endoscopy, manometry, pH 24-h/3-year): 52 cases

Lind = Nissen (p < 0.001)
 — improvement of symptoms
 — immediate and late dysphagia
 — pH 24-h
 — endoscopy
>Nissen
 — late difficulty for eructation

Conclusions

Today, near at the end of the 20th century, surgery has a very precise role in the management of esophageal reflux disease, being the definitive solution of complicated RE. Surgical techniques are definitely efficient. What must be still analyzed and compared is the introduction of minimal invasive techniques such as videolaparoscopic procedures. In our surgical unit, 26 laparoscopic Lind procedures have already been performed with no mortality and very good immediate recuperation.

In spite of immediate good results, these data need to have a long follow-up, and prospective studies are mandatory. Minimal invasive surgery will be the future perspective of curative treatment for esophageal reflux.

References

1. Jamieson GG, Duranceau AC. The development of surgery for gastroesophageal reflux disease. In: Jamieson GG (ed) Surgery of the Esophagus. Edinburgh: Churchill Livingstone, 1988;233—245.
2. DeMeester TR, Fuchs KM. Comparison of operations for uncomplicated reflux disease. In: Jamieson GG (ed) Surgery of the Esophagus. Edinburgh: Churchill Livingstone, 1988;299—308.
3. Liebermann-Meffert D. Architeture of the musculature of the gastroesophageal junction and the fundus. Chir Gastroenterol 1975;9:425—429.
4. Belsey RHR. Mark IV repair of hiatal hernia by the transthoracic approach. World J Surg 1977;1:475—481.
5. Nissen R. Gastropexy and "fundoplication" in surgical treatment of hiatal hernia. Am J Dig Dis 1961;6(10):954—961.
6. Lind JF, Burns CM. MacDougall JT. "Physiological" repair for hiatus hernia — manometric study. Arch Surg 1965;91: 233—237.

7. Toupet A. Technique d'oesophago-gastroplastie avec phréno-gastropexie appliquée dans la cure radicale des hernies hiatales et comme complément de l'opération de Heller dans le cardiospasme. Mem Acad Chir (Paris) 1963;102:700.
8. Pinotti HW, Cecconello I, Pollara WM, Zilberstein B, Carvajal I, Raia AA. Perspectivas quirúrgicas del acceso transdiafragmático al esófago torácico. Rev Esp Enf Apar Dig 1982;62:100.
9. Pinotti HW, Pollara WM, Zilberstein B, Cecconello I, Raia AA. Esofagite de refluxo com estenose. Conduta terapêutica e resultados. Rev Col Bras Cir 1983;10:10—14.
10. Pinotti HW, Pollara WM, Oliveira MA, Zilberstein B, Cecconello I. Esophageal hiatus reoperations. Guidelines for surgical management. Arq Bras Cir Dig. 1986;1:24.
11. Siewert R. Surgical therapy of peptic stenoses. In: Stipa S, Belsey RHR, Moraldi A (eds) Medical and Surgical Problems of the Esophagus. Serono Symposium 43: Academic Press, 1981;146—154.
12. Beauchamp et al. Abstracts of the International Congress on Esophageal Diseases, Chicago, 1989.
13. Walker et al. Abstracts of the International Congress on Esophageal Diseases, Chicago, 1989.

Newborn and children

 ## How to separate the spitters from the serious refluxers in infants?

S.G. Jolley (Las Vegas)

The task of separating the normal "spitting" infant from the infant with serious disease from emesis is not as straightforward as one might presume. Regurgitation of feedings may be effortless or with effort. The material regurgitated may have bile or be nonbilious. Several causes for "excessive" emesis can be found in infants, but the main goal of diagnosis is to exclude obstruction in the alimentary tract as the cause for emesis. Forceful emesis and emesis with bile are more likely to be indicative of alimentary tract obstruction (e.g., pyloric stenosis, intestinal malrotation, intussusception) than is effortless emesis without bile. Since the diagnostic features of alimentary tract obstruction in infants are well described in pediatric surgical texts, this article will focus primarily on excessive emesis in infants which is nonbilious and effortless.

Historically, the barium meal has been used as an initial test for the evaluation of infants with nonbilious, effortless emesis [1,2]. The study is most suited to exclude the presence of anatomical abnormalities which may produce obstruction in the foregut, or may be associated with emesis (e.g., hiatal hernia). Since reflux of barium from the stomach into the esophagus occurs in normal infants [3] and may be absent in infants with serious disease from emesis [3,4], the presence of reflux during the barium meal is not a reliable method for separating infants with disease from the normal "spitty" infant. A radionuclide esophagram [5] is easier to quantitate, but no more accurate than the barium meal for identifying infants with disease from emesis.

Manometric measurements of the esophagus and stomach also have been employed to identify infants with disease resulting from emesis as a consequence of a defective gastroesophageal junction (gastroesophageal reflux disease (GERD)) [6]. Intuition would suggest that infants with a defective gastroesophageal junction causing disease should have a decreased lower esophageal sphincter pressure (LESP). In fact, it is not that simple. Infants with GERD can have a decreased, normal or increased LESP [6]. The dynamic function of the LES is more important than static measurements and shows inappropriate relaxations of the LES or a persistent decreased basal LESP as associated with a defective gastroesophageal junction in infants with GERD [7]. Therefore, a single static measurement of LESP cannot reliably identify the presence or absence of a defective gastroesophageal junction in infants. Prolonged manometric studies in infants are just evolving and will require a critical analysis of data from normal infants to establish a standard reference.

Endoscopy has been used to identify esophageal mucosal abnormalities as an indicator of disease from excessive emesis in infants. The presence of mucosal ulceration, stricture, extreme friability or Barrett's epithelium are clearly evidence of mucosal injury, probably from GERD. However, most infants with GERD do not have these signs of advanced mucosal injury. Furthermore, less obvious findings of mucosal injury on microscopic examination of the esophageal biopsy in infants

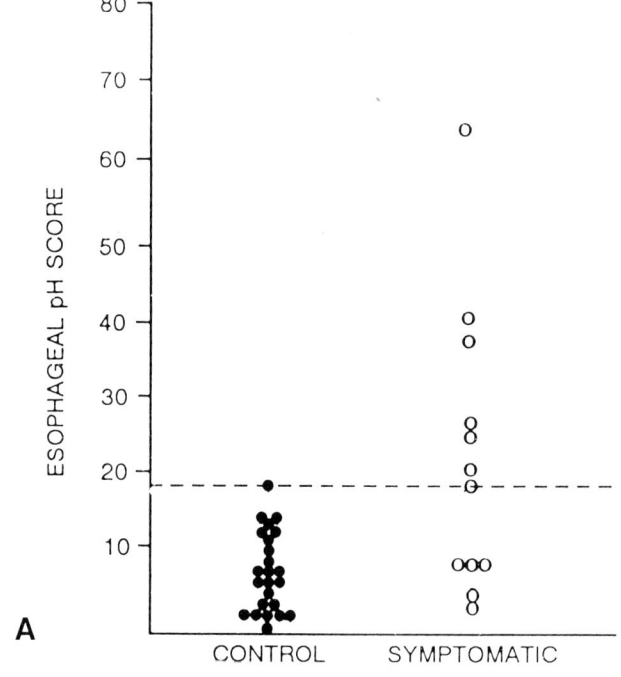

Fig. 1. A comparison of normal infants and children (control, n = 24) and symptomatic infants and children (symptomatic, n = 12) with well documented gastroesophageal reflux disease having 24-h esophageal pH monitoring perfomed and analyzed by a) the Johnson-DeMeester score; b) the percentage of total time that the esophageal pH < 4; and c) the author's method using an esophageal pH score calculated from recording intervals after the first 2 h postcibal. The dotted lines represent the upper limit of normal for the children studied [13].

736

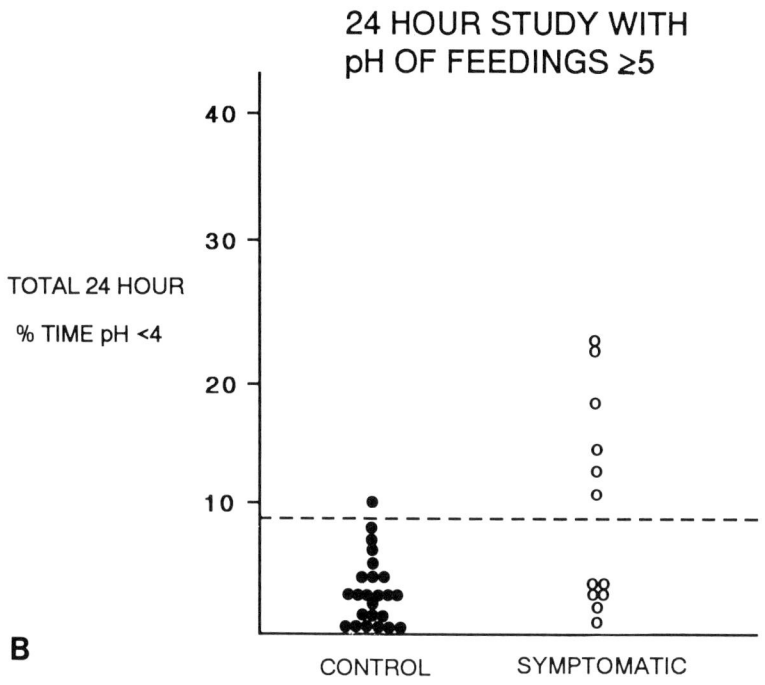

24 HOUR STUDY WITH
pH OF FEEDINGS ≥5

TOTAL 24 HOUR

% TIME pH <4

B

CONTROL   SYMPTOMATIC

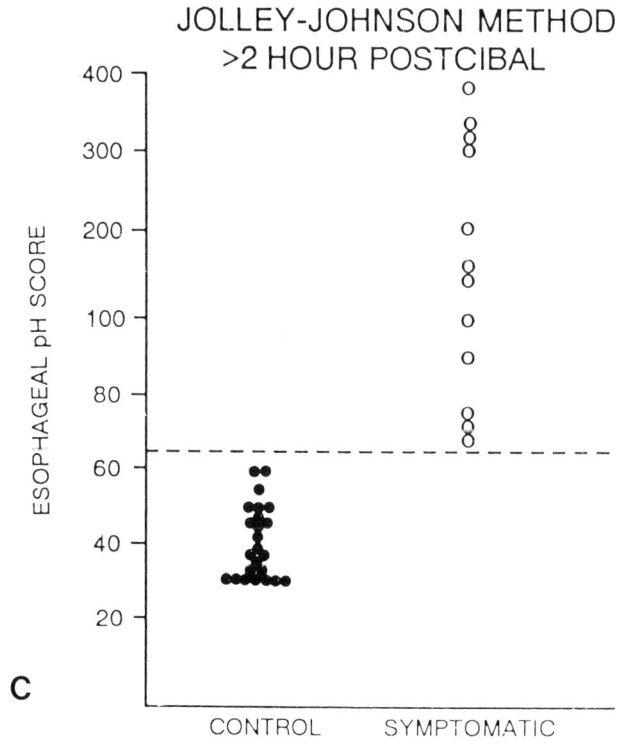

JOLLEY-JOHNSON METHOD
>2 HOUR POSTCIBAL

ESOPHAGEAL pH SCORE

C

CONTROL   SYMPTOMATIC

[8–10] may result from any mechanism (including alimentary tract obstruction) whereby excessive gastric contents are regurgitated into the esophagus and GERD is not present.

Due to the dissatisfaction with the barium meal, manometric methods and endoscopy (in other than severe forms of GERD) to identify disease from excessive emesis, extended esophageal pH monitoring became popular in the 1970s. The methodology utilized by Johnson and DeMeester in adults [11] has been tried in infants and children [12] but has been less successful in identifying infants with GERD than the success reported for adult studies [13]. In 1977, the author attempted to apply the method of Johnson and DeMeester to a group of normal infants and children [13,14]. Unfortunately, the method of Johnson and DeMeester produced a 50% false-negative rate in infants with documented GERD (Fig. 1a). When the percentage of total time esophageal pH < 4, the most commonly reported parameter to indicate GERD, was used, the false-negative rate was 50% and the false-positive rate was 33% (Fig. 1b).

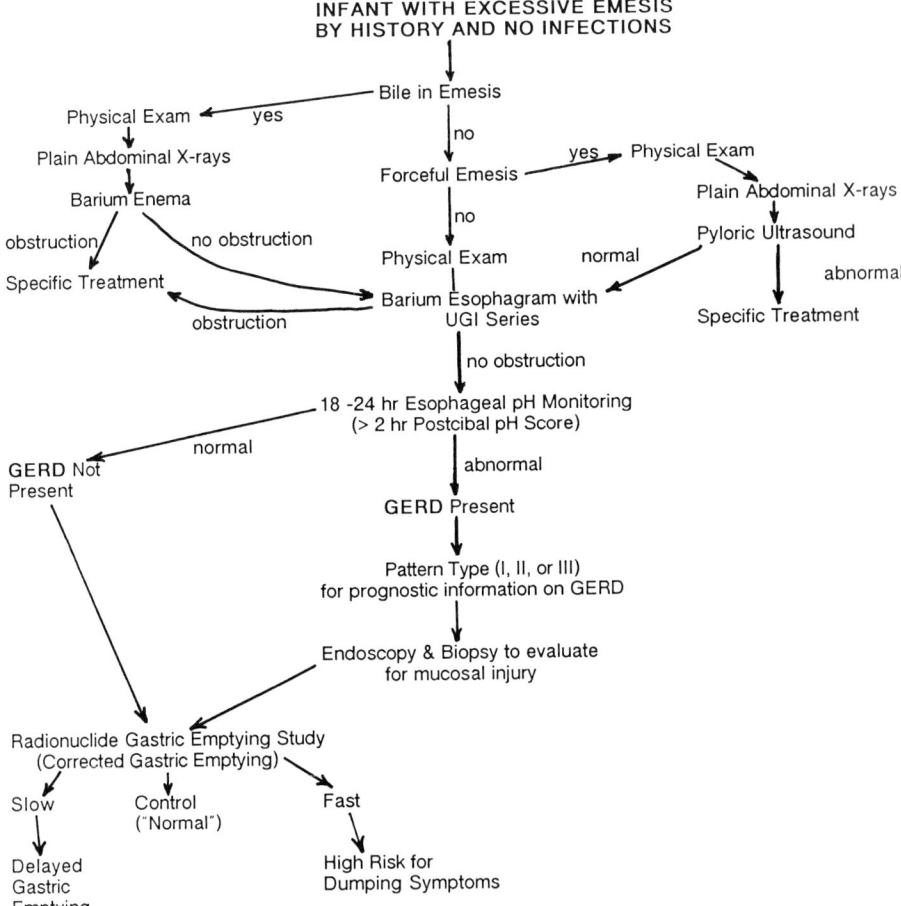

Fig. 2. An algorithm used by the author to separate infant spitters from infants with disease caused by excessive emesis.

738

The reasons behind the low accuracy with the Johnson-DeMeester scoring method, or the use of the percentage of total time with esophageal pH < 4 in infants, were due to these methods of analysis ignoring the basic stimuli for acid reflux episodes in normal children, such as feedings and the state of wakefulness [14,15]. Another method for esophageal pH record analysis devised by the author accounted for both feeding and wakefulness periods separately, thereby resulting in an esophageal pH score which more reliably identifies infants and children with GERD (Fig. 1c). The false-negative rate with the author's method is less than 5%. Although GERD in infants occurs in various patterns (type I, II and III) [16], the method for deriving the pattern type cannot replace the esophageal pH score for identifying GERD in infants. The reflux patterns in infants serve to characterize the GERD rather than to confirm its existence.

The infants with disease resulting from excessive emesis may have gastric emptying abnormalities in addition to GERD, or as the sole cause for the emesis. A radionuclide gastric emptying study with a clear liquid, and mathematically corrected for delay caused by postcibal gastroesophageal reflux episodes, can identify infants with abnormal effective gastric emptying [17]. The corrected gastric emptying may be slow, normal or rapid. A slow corrected gastric emptying is seen in 25% of symptomatic infants with GERD and in 29% without GERD. The slow corrected gastric emptying is a separate cause of disease from excessive emesis in infants. Rapid corrected gastric emptying usually causes dumping symptoms which occasionally are associated with excessive emesis and no GERD in infants [17].

The author's preferred method for identifying infants with disease from excessive emesis is shown in Fig. 2. As mentioned previously, the main goal is to exclude anatomical obstruction. Once that has been accomplished, 18–24-h esophageal pH monitoring and radionuclide gastric emptying studies are important in the symptomat-

Table 1. The combination of findings from esophageal pH monitoring and gastric emptying studies in infants with excessive emesis by history and no indication of alimentary tract obstruction by physical examination and radiographic studies

Esophageal pH score	Pattern type	Corrected gastric emptying	Incidence (%)	Interpretation
Abnormal	I	Slow	14	GERD unlikely to resolve & delayed gastric emptying
	I	Control	17	GERD unlikely to resolve
	I	Fast	24	GERD unlikely to resolve and rapid gastric emptying
	II	Slow	7	GERD likely to resolve & delayed gastric emptying
	II	Control	5	GERD likely to resolve
	II	Fast	11	GERD likely to resolve and rapid gastric emptying
	III	Slow	1	GERD unlikely to resolve & delayed gastric emptying
	III	Control	3	GERD unlikely to resolve
	III	Fast	5	GERD unlikely to resolve and rapid gastric emptying
Normal	Normal	Slow	4	Delayed gastric emptying
	Normal	Control	8	Normal
	Normal	Fast	1	Rapid gastric emptying

ic infant to assess for GERD and abnormalities of effective gastric emptying. Virtually any combination of findings is possible (Table 1), but the abnormalities must be treated separately. Regurgitation of feedings due to poor esophageal emptying has been difficult to quantitate in infants. A delay in esophageal emptying may be suspected by either grossly delayed emptying of barium from the esophagus during a barium meal [18], or the prolonged clearance of apple juice feedings from the esophagus during extended esophageal pH monitoring [19].

In summary, the author's method for performing extended esophageal pH monitoring is the most accurate method currently available to identify infants who have GERD as a cause for excessive emesis. A corrected gastric emptying value from liquid radionuclide gastric emptying studies also allows the clinician to identify infants with excessive emesis secondary to gastric emptying abnormalities, regardless of whether or not GERD is also present.

References

1. Carre IJ, Astley R. The fate of the partial thoracic stomach (hiatus hernia) in children. Arch Dis Child 1960;35:484–486.
2. McCauley RGK, Darling DB, Leonidas JC et al. Gastroesophageal reflux in infants and children: a useful classification and reliable physiologic technique for its demonstration. Am J Roentgenol 1978;130:47–50.
3. Cleveland RH, Kushner DC, Schwartz AN. Gastroesophageal reflux in children: results of a standardized fluoroscopic approach. Am J Roentgenol 1983;141:53–56.
4. Jolley SG, Leonard JC, Tunell WP et al. A comparison of barium and radionuclide esophagography with extended esophageal pH monitoring for the diagnosis of gastroesophageal reflux in children. Clin Res 1985;33:35A.
5. Rudd TG, Christie DL. Demonstration of gastroesophageal reflux in children by radionuclide gastroesophagography. Radiology 1979;131:483–486.
6. Herbst JJ, Book LS, Johnson DG et al. The lower esophageal sphincter in gastroesophageal reflux in children. J Clin Gastroenterol 1979;1:119–123.
7. Werlin SL, Dodds WJ, Hogan WJ et al. Mechanisms of gastroesophageal reflux in children. J Pediatr 1980;97:244–249.
8. Ismail-Beigi F, Horton PF, Pope CE. Histological consequences of gastroesophageal reflux in man. Gastroenterology 1970;58:163–174.
9. Leape LL, Bhan I, Ramenofsky ML. Esophageal biopsy in the diagnosis of reflux esophagitis. J Pediatr Surg 1981;16:379–384.
10. Benjamin B, Pohl D, Bale PM. Endoscopy and biopsy in gastroesophageal reflux in infants and children. Ann Otol 1980;89:443–445.
11. Johnson LF, DeMeester TR. Twenty-four-hour pH monitoring of the distal esophagus: a quantitative measure of gastroesophageal reflux. Am J Gastroenterol 1974;62:325–332.
12. Hill JL, Pellegrini CA, Burrington JD et al. Technique and experience with 24-h esophageal pH monitoring in children. J Pediatr Surg 1977;12:877–887.
13. Jolley SG. Current surgical considerations in gastroesophageal reflux disease in infancy and childhood. Surg Clin North Am 1992;72:1365–1391.
14. Jolley SG, Johnson DG, Herbst JJ et al. An assessment of gastroesophageal reflux in children by extended pH monitoring of the distal esophagus. Surgery 1978;84:16–23.
15. Jolley SG, Herbst JJ, Johnson DG et al. Postcibal gastroesophageal reflux in children. J Pediatr Surg 1981;16:487–490.
16. Jolley SG, Herbst JJ, Johnson DG et al. Patterns of postcibal gastroesophageal reflux in symptomatic infants. Am J Surg 1979;138:946–950.
17. Jolley SG, Leonard JC, Tunell WP. Gastric emptying in children with gastroesophageal reflux. An estimate of effective gastric emptying. J Pediatr Surg 1987;22:923–926.
18. Jolley SG, Herbst JJ, Johnson DG et al. The questionable effect of position on children with gastroesophageal reflux. Clin Res 1980;28:96A.
19. Jolley SG. The role of achalasia in infancy. In: Giuli R, McCallum RW, Skinner DB (eds) Primary Motility Disorders of the Esophagus. Montrouge: John Libbey Eurotext, 1991;985–987.

What are the boundaries between physiologic and pathologic reflux in relation to age in infancy?

S.R. Orenstein (Pittsburgh)

To determine the boundaries between physiologic and pathologic reflux requires a definition of "physiologic" or "normal". Several meanings of this term are possible. The first is purely quantitative, a proportion (for example, 95%) of all individuals are considered to fall within this definition of normal and the "tail(s)" of the distribution are considered abnormal. The other meaning is a qualitative one, which connotes that no harm results.

It is evident that reflux which is quantitatively normal may be qualitatively abnormal: if, for example, the refluxate is aspirated, or if the refluxate triggers harmful bronchospasm. Similarly, reflux which is abnormal in a strictly quantitative sense may, nevertheless, produce no harmful effects and thus be considered qualitatively physiologic. This paper will address both meanings, and explore whether there are age-related boundaries between physiologic and pathologic reflux.

Reflux quantification

Methods of quantifying reflux in children range from the very nontechnical (simple observation for regurgitation), to very technical (barium fluoroscopy, gastroesophageal scintigraphy and pH probe).

Observation for regurgitation was earliest method of documenting reflux and still has a role in identifying reflux in infants, although it is clear that such regurgitant reflux represents at most only "the tip of the iceberg" of reflux episodes and that regurgitant reflux may even result from different mechanisms than nonregurgitant reflux [1]. Data from our Infant Gastroesophageal Reflux Questionnaire (©Susan Orenstein, 1992) indicate that parents report that about 70% of infants referred for evaluation for reflux disease (and a similar proportion of them who are subsequently shown to have reflux disease) will have regurgitation as "a problem" [2], in contrast to about 20% of infants seen in a well baby clinic (unpublished data). Specifically, the parents of the infants with reflux report that about 80% of them regurgitate at least once a day and at least 5 ml per episode, whereas only 40% of nonreferred, well infants do so. It can be seen that there is both significantly more regurgitation in infants with reflux disease and a great deal of overlap between them and normal infants. After a year of age, regurgitation is infrequent in children with reflux disease as well as in normals.

Fluoroscopic barium gastroesophagography has been used for several decades to document the occurrence of gastroesophageal reflux episodes. Without using provocative maneuvers, fluoroscopy demonstrates reflux episodes more often and higher in the esophagus in children with reflux disease than in those without symptoms of reflux disease, although, again, there is overlap between normals and reflux patients. The reflux episodes also decrease in frequency and height in the esophagus during aging in normals. A retrospective study of 470 children delineated the upper range of normal for the number of episodes seen in 5 min of fluoroscopy: younger than 6 weeks, three episodes; 7 weeks–1 year, two episodes; 1–6 years, one episode; and over 6 years, less than one episode [3]. This study also crudely quantified the volume of refluxate, by distinguishing reflux that reached the level of the clavicles from reflux that did not. Of the reflux episodes in each age group of asymptomatic children, the proportion which reached the clavicles decreased with age: 86% of episodes in normal infants younger than 6 weeks old reached the clavicles, whereas only 20% of the episodes in the normal teenagers did.

Scintigraphic gastroesophagography was introduced for evaluation of reflux less than 2 decades ago [4,5]. Scintigraphic monitoring, like fluoroscopic monitoring, documents reflux in the postprandial period. In contrast to fluoroscopy, however, the monitoring can be done during an entire postprandial hour without prohibitive radiation exposure and the "meal" is a physiological meal, rather than barium. Theoretically, one could quantify frequency, actual volume and duration of reflux episodes, but I am aware of no published data quantifying reflux scintigraphically in relation to age in normal children. One could roughly estimate the normal limits of scintigraphic reflux in relation to age from pH probe-measured postprandial reflux following an acid meal [6], but 24-h pH probe values for asymptomatic normal infants and children are only known using milk formula feedings [7,8], which hide postprandial reflux from detection by the pH probe.

The pH probe misses postprandial reflux when nonacid meals are fed, but this method has allowed the detection of reflux frequency, duration and acidity throughout prolonged periods of monitoring, typically recording throughout a 24-h period. Using this method, investigators have characterized the range of normal for total duration of esophageal acidification ($pH < 4$) and for frequency of acid reflux episodes related to age during infancy, childhood and adulthood (Fig. 1) [7,8,10]. The total daily duration of esophageal acidification is a product of the frequency of episodes and their (mean) duration. Two other measures related to total esophageal acid exposure which are often scored on pH probes are the number of episodes longer than 5 min and the duration of the longest episode. Finally, the pH probe's ability to quantify the degree of acidity and the capabilities of computerized scoring systems have led investigators to measure the "area under the curve", a product of the degree of acidity and the duration of exposure [11–14].

Predicting qualitative abnormalities

Only the pH probe measures have been evaluated in detail for their ability to predict qualitative abnormalities (disease) due to gastroesophageal reflux. Several scores have been published which have been mathematically derived to select those patients with reflux disease [15,16], but these derived scores have the disadvantage of obscuring the primary data [17,18]. In contrast, several different simpler scores have been

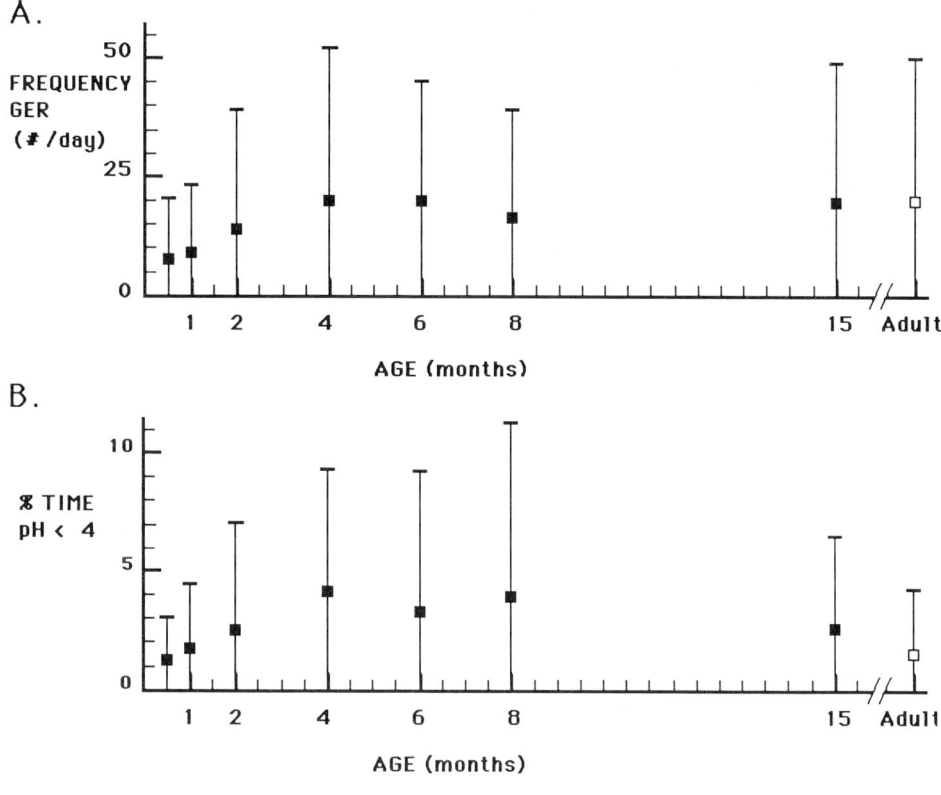

Fig. 1. Physiologic reflux: range of normal values (mean ± 2SD) in children of various ages (n = 285) and in adults (n = 15). Top panel depicts frequency of reflux episodes; bottom panel depicts total duration of esophageal acidification throughout the day, during normal activities and diet [8,10]. Figure previously published [9].

shown to correlate with different manifestations of reflux disease.

Thus the *reflux index* (the percentage of the day with esophageal pH < 4) is greater in those with esophagitis than in those without esophagitis. In both children [19] and adults [20], all controls without esophagitis have a reflux index below 10%, whereas one half to two-thirds of those with esophagitis have a reflux index greater than 10%; this cutoff does not appear to vary much with age. Another study in adults found by Receiver-Operating-Characteristic analysis that the optimal cutoff was slightly lower, 7% with a sensitivity and specificity of 89 and 93%, although half of the "patients" were endoscopically normal (histology was not reported) [21].

The *area under pH 4 curve* (AUC), which correlates with the reflux index [11,14], is also greater in patients with esophagitis than in those without. Extrapolating from data presented graphically [14], it seems that one can calculate that a cutoff value of 20 min-units-below-four (e.g., 20 min of pH 3, or 10 min of pH 2) per hour of monitoring is a good predictor of histologic esophagitis. I have calculated its sensitivity as 93%, its specificity as 88%, its positive predictive value as 84% and its negative predictive value as 95% for the children presented. Other investigators have identified a corresponding value of 32 per day (i.e., 1.3 per hour) to predict reflux disease in general [12]. The 15-fold difference may reflect the insensitivity of esophageal histology from grasp biopsies for identifying children with problematic reflux and the nonspecificity of a reflux index of 4%, the gold standards used by the two groups of investigators. There are no data, however, to assess whether this cutoff value varies with age. For both the AUC and the reflux index, one might expect that the lifetime duration of acid exposure might play a role in the genesis of esophagitis; thus it may be that esophagitis in very young children requires a greater degree or duration of daily acid exposure, because of the necessarily limited lifetime duration of exposure.

The *mean duration of reflux during sleep* is a score which has been correlated with respiratory complications of reflux by several investigators [22–24]. A value of about 4 min has been found to be a useful threshold; again, this value has not been evaluated in relationship to age.

Conclusion

Infants manifest more reflux than adults when evaluated by any of several methods, including simple observation for regurgitation, fluoroscopic monitoring and pH probe monitoring. However, pH probe studies of normal infants and adults clearly show that this decrease in acid gastroesophageal reflux during infancy is much less than one might anticipate from the decrease in observable regurgitation during this period of maturation.

The decrease in some manifestations of reflux disease (such as malnutrition or apnea) during development is unlikely to be due to simple reduction in reflux quantity, but rather to be due to other developmental changes (such as suppression of regurgitation or of abnormal respiratory reflexes). Similarly, the increase in other manifestations of reflux disease (such as esophagitis, Barrett's esophagus, or stricture) is likely to be due to a cumulative increase in lifetime esophageal exposure to injurious material.

References

1. Orenstein SR, Deneault LG, Lutz JW, Wessel HB, Dent J. Regurgitant reflux, in contrast to non-regurgitant reflux, is associated with rectus abdominus contraction in infants. Gastroenterology 1991;100:A135.
2. Orenstein SR, Cohn JF, Shalaby TM, Kartan R. Reliability and validity of an infant gastroesophageal reflux questionnaire. Clin Pediatr 1993;32:472–484.
3. Cleveland RH, Kushner DC, Schwartz AN. Gastroesophageal reflux in children: results of a standardized fluoroscopic approach. Am J Roentgenol 1983;141:53–56.
4. Fisher RS, Malmud LS, Roberts GS, Lobis IF. Gastroesophageal (GE) scintiscanning to detect and quantitate GE reflux. Gastroenterology 1976;70:301–308.
5. Heyman S, Kirkpatrick JA, Winter HS, Treves S. An improved radionuclide method for the diagnosis of gastroesophageal reflux and aspiration in children (milk scan). Radiology 1979;131:479–482.
6. Orenstein SR, Klein HA, Rosenthal MS. Scintigraphic images for quantifying pediatric gastroesophageal reflux: a study of simultaneous scintigraphy and pH probe using multiplexed data and acid feedings. J Nucl Med 1993;34:1228–1234.
7. Vandenplas Y, Govaerts H, Helven R, Sacre L. Gastroesophageal reflux, as measured by 24-h pH monitoring, in 509 healthy infants screened for risk of sudden infant death syndrome. Pediatrics 1991;88:834–840.
8. Vandenplas Y, Sacre SL. Continuous 24-h esophageal pH monitoring in 285 asymptomatic infants 0-15 months old. J Pediatr Gastroenterol Nutr 1987;6:220–224.

9. Orenstein SR. Gastroesophageal reflux. In: Stockman J, Winter R (eds) Current Problems in Pediatrics. Chicago: Mosby Year Book Medical Publishers, 1991;193—241.
10. Johnson LF, DeMeester TR. Twenty-four-hour pH monitoring of the distal esophagus: a quantitative measure of gastro-esophageal reflux. Am J Gastroenterol 1974;62:325—332.
11. Stoker D, Williams J, Colin-Jones D. Use of the area under the curve to assess the esophageal pH test. Gastroenterology 1991;100(5,Pt2):A169.
12. Tovar J, Izquierdo M, Eizaguirre I. The area under pH curve: a single-figure parameter representative of esophageal acid exposure. J Pediatr Surg 1991;26:163—167.
13. Izquierdo M, Tovar J, Eizaguirre I. L'exposition acide oesophagienne en un seul chiffre: la surface sous la courbe de pH. Chir Pediatr 1989;30:1—5.
14. Vandenplas Y, Franckx GA, Pipeleers MM, Derde MP, Sacre SL. Area under pH 4: advantages of a new parameter in the interpretation of esophageal pH monitoring data in infants. J Pediatr Gastroenterol Nutr 1989;9:34—39.
15. Jolley SG, Johnson DG, Herbst JJ, Pena A, Garnier R. An assessment of gastroesophageal reflux in children by extended monitoring of the distal esophagus. Surgery 1978;84:16—23.
16. Euler AR, Byrne WJ. Twenty-four-hour esophageal intraluminal pH probe testing: a comparative analysis. Gastroenterology 1981;80:957—961.
17. Grill BB. Twenty-four-hour esophageal pH monitoring: what's the score? J Pediatr Gastroenterol Nutr 1992;14:249—251.
18. Friesen CA, Hayes R, Hodge C, Roberts CC. Comparison of methods of assessing 24-h intraesophageal pH recordings in children. J Pediatr Gastroenterol Nutr 1992;14:252—255.
19. Baer M, Maki M, Nurminen J, Turjanmaa V, Pukander J, Vesikari T. Esophagitis and findings of long-term esophageal pH recording in children with repeated lower respiratory tract symptoms. J Pediatr Gastroenterol Nutr 1986;5:187—190.
20. Schlesinger PK, Donahue PE, Schmid B, Layden T. Limitations of 24-h intraesophageal pH monitoring in the hospital setting. Gastroenterology 1985;89:797—804.
21. Schindlbeck NE, Heinrich CH, Konig A, Dendorfer A, Pace F, Muller-Lissner SA. Optimal thresholds, sensitivity, and specificity of long-term pH-metry for the detection of gastroesophageal reflux disease. Gastroenterology 1987;93:85—90.
22. Johnson DG, Jolley SG, Herbst JJ, Cordell LJ. Surgical selection of infants with gastroesophageal reflux. J Pediatr Surg 1981;16(4, suppl 1):587—594.
23. Halpern LM, Jolley SG, Tunell WP, Johnson DG, Sterling CE. The mean duration of gastroesophageal reflux during sleep as an indicator of respiratory symptoms from gastroesophageal reflux in children. J Pediatr Surg 1991;26:686—690.
24. Eizaguirre I, Tovar JA. Predicting preoperatively the outcome of respiratory symptoms of gastroesophageal reflux. J Pediatr Surg 1992;27:848—851.

G.H. Willital (Münster)

What are the diagnostic procedures for gastroesophageal reflux in children?

The diagnostic procedure to be undertaken in children suspected of gastroesophageal reflux (GER) is a program of several points (Tables 1—3):

a. Family history: the most striking general symptoms in newborns and babies with GER are microaspirations with pulmonary distress syndrome at different intervals of time. Main clinical signs are recurrent atelectasis, recurrent pneumonia, and recurrent respiratory distress syndrome. One has to keep in mind that the lower esophageal sphincter (LES) has to undergo a maturation which takes between 1 and 1.5 years. This means that children may have, within this interval of time, a physiological reflux.

Table 1. Normal values for 24-h monitoring of intraesophageal pH in children

Parameter	pH < 4 (% of time)	Reflux episodes (longest <12 min)
Overall	<3.4%	#/d + 4(#>5'/day) < 50
Fasting	<2.2%	1/h
2-h postprandial	<10%	< 5/h

Table 2. Classification of endoscopic findings in esophagitis according to Savary and Miller

Stage	Endoscopic findings
0	Symptoms of reflux without epithelial defects
I	Few erosions
II	Confluent but not circular erosions
III	Circular erosions or ulcers
IV	Peptic stricture

b. Measurement of pH, performed as a 24-h pH-metry in order to determine: length of reflux periods, frequency of reflux periods, deepest pH value during reflux episodes.

c. Manometry studies: these manometry studies are performed with double or triple tip catheter in order to record the pressure inside the abdomen, at the level of the LES and in the lower part of the esophagus. This enables the determination of the resting pressure inside the LES (between 15—25 mmHg in babies, toddlers and children). Furthermore, pressure upon the abdomen, and consecutively pressure inside the stomach, will not be registered in cases of a competent LES to the lower distal esophagus. This also can be registered by esophageal manometric studies.

d. Endoscopic investigations: they enable to determine whether alterations of the distal part of the esophagus can be recognized (edema, erosions, ulcers, scar formations, stenosis, classification of Savary and Miller). Furthermore, endoscopic investigations enable the determination of whether the esophagogastric junction is open or can be opened by air insufflation: if the sphincter is competent, air insufflation will cause no visible, spontaneous opening of the LES.

e. Scintigraphic investigations: they enable to determine scintigraphically the passage and the motility of the esophagus as well as the function of the LES and the function of the pylorus. One has to keep in mind that pylorus spasms are combined with a GER in about 15—18% of the cases.

Table 3. Normal values for manometry of the lower esophageal sphincter (LES) in children

Parameters	Normal	Pathological
Pressure LES	10—20 mmHg	< 6 mmHg
Abdominal length LES	2—4 cm	< 1 cm
Total length LES	2.5—6 cm	< 2 cm

What is the indication for surgery in GER in children?

There is a physiological reflux in newborns and babies within the first year of life with an incompetent LES, reaching its normal activity within the 12 to 18 months after birth. The indication for reflux operation in children depends very much upon histology, pH-metry, endoscopy and esophageal manometry, especially if the reflux endoscopically demonstrates signs to be classified in the group of Savary and Miller type III and IV (i.e., alterations, bleeding, scar formations and stenosis), and is independent from age. In all other cases reflux below the age of 1—1.5 years should be treated conservatively.

In children not older than 1.5 to 2 years, if reflux occurs clinically and if manometric, endoscopic, and pH investigations demonstrate GER clearly, indication for surgery is also mandatory.

Which is the adequate operative procedure to treat GER in children?

There are four main surgical steps to be observed:
a. Intraoperative endoscopy of the esophagus, in order to determine the esophago-gastric junction, is important to perform the retroesophageal hiatus plasty at the right level; this means not too low and not too high with regard to the gastroesophageal junction. The other point is that the endoscope lying inside the esophagus should be just the right size, in order to create the pathway through the diaphragm in an adequate diameter, not too wide and not too narrow. Therefore, intraoperative endoscopy is a very helpful method to perform the retroesophageal hiatus plasty adequately. The surgeon himself can see the light of the intraesophageal endoscope, so that this procedure can be performed with extreme precision by diaphanoscopy .
b. Fixation of the hiatus muscle to the esophagus at the right level, to be determined by intraoperative endoscopy.
c. Fixation of the fundus to the abdominal esophagus in order to create the angulation of His.
d. Fixation of the fundus of the stomach to the diaphragm in order to avoid recurrencies.

When does the maturation process really occur?

S.R. Orenstein (Pittsburgh)

The question of when maturation occurs with regard to reflux in infants may be approached from several directions. Symptomatic clinical maturation can be examined, or the maturation of mechanisms underlying reflux can be evaluated.

Symptoms of reflux: changes during development

As noted in the section on physiologic vs. pathologic reflux, infants manifest more reflux than adults when evaluated by any of several methods, including simple observation for regurgitation, fluoroscopic monitoring and pH probe monitoring. However, pH probe studies of normal infants and adults clearly show that this decrease in acid gastroesophageal reflux during infancy is much less than one might anticipate from the decrease in observable regurgitation during this period of maturation.

Infants are usually not symptomatic with reflux disease at birth, but develop symptoms during the first month or two of life [1]. The symptoms tend to peak by 4–6 months and usually decline thereafter, disappearing between 8 and 18 months of age [2]. Symptoms persistent beyond 24 months are far less likely to resolve. In this respect, they are similar to symptoms in older children and adults [3].

Mechanisms of reflux: changes during development

Mechanisms contributing to the occurrence of reflux episodes include: 1) hypotonia of the lower esophageal sphincter (LES); 2) transient relaxations of the LES; and 3) increases in intragastric pressure or volume, the latter often due to delayed gastric emptying [4–6]. Factors contributing to the damage done by reflux episodes include: 1) impaired esophageal clearance and neutralization; and 2) increased noxiousness of gastric contents. The presence of other abnormalities, such as a propensity to laryngospasm, aspiration, or bronchospasm, may make reflux more likely to produce disease; these abnormalities, too, may change during development.

The LES tone (and length) has been found to increase during the first months of life in normals [7], although others have found a higher tone in infants than in older children [8].

Esophagitis probably lowers LES tone in both infants and adults. The frequency of transient LES relaxations in adults is debated, ranging up to seven per hour in normals [9–13]; the frequency in infants has not been completely described. We have identified transient increases in intra-abdominal pressure as probable precipitants of regurgitant reflux [14] and similar findings have been reported in rare adults with regurgitation, but the frequency of those events and their modification during development are unknown.

The average esophageal clearance time in normal infants and adults can be calculated from data from several authors [15—18]. The data suggest that the average reflux episode is 2 to 3 min in normal infants and perhaps minimally less in the adult, although differences in techniques may explain these small differences. Similarly, normal infants have peristaltic amplitudes which should produce effective esophageal clearance [19,20]. Decreased peristaltic amplitude and impaired clearance are present in adults and infants with reflux disease, and are probably secondary phenomena like LES hypotonia, due to esophagitis [17,19,20]. The noxious gastric contents probably actually increases during development, as gastric, biliary and pancreatic secretion mature and as the frequency of neutral liquid meals decreases.

There are probably *not* important maturational changes between young infancy and adulthood in most of the above-noted reflux mechanisms.

The most important maturational change is the marked decrease in regurgitant reflux during the first 12 months — the cause for this change is unknown and requires further study. Since nonregurgitant acid reflux does not change much during development, the other mechanisms for reflux probably do not change much either. Auxiliary mechanisms, however, may be important. These include the unclear developmental phenomena which allow apnea to occur as a response to reflux or to other stresses prior to about 6 months of age. Other manifestations of reflux disease, particularly esophagitis and its sequelae (Barrett's esophagus and stricture), actually increase during maturation, but this increase is due to the cumulative total duration of esophageal exposure to refluxate rather than to a maturational change in reflux mechanisms.

References

1. Orenstein SR, Cohn JF, Shalaby TM, Kartan R. Reliability and validity of an infant gastroesophageal reflux questionnaire. Clin Pediatr 1993;32(8):472—484.
2. Carre IJ. The natural history of the partial thoracic stomach (hiatus hernia) in chlidren. Arch Dis Child 1959;34:344—353.
3. Treem W, Davis P, Hyams J. Gastroesophageal reflux in the older child: presentation, response to treatment and long-term follow-up. Clin Pediatr 1991;30(7):435—440.
4. Cucchiara C, Staiano A, DiLorenzo C, DeLuca G, dellaRocca A, Auricchio S. Pathophysiology of gastroesophageal reflux and distal esophageal motility in children with gastroesophageal reflux disease. J Pediatr Gastroenterol Nutr 1988;7(6): 830—836.
5. Werlin SL, Dodds WJ, Hogan WJ, Arndorfer RC. Mechanisms of gastroesophageal reflux in children. J Pediatr 1980;97(2): 244—249.
6. Hillemeier AC, Lange R, McCallum RW, Seashore J, Gryboski J. Delayed gastric emptying in infants with gastro esophageal reflux. J Pediatr 1981;98(2):190—193.
7. Boix-Ochoa J, Canals J. Maturation of the lower esophagus. J Pediatr Surg 1976;11(5):748—756.
8. Moroz S, Espinoza J, Cumming W et al. Lower esophageal sphincter function in children with and without gastroesophageal reflux. Gastroenterology 1976;71(2):236—241.
9. Mittal RK, McCallum RW. Characteristics of transient lower esophageal sphincter relaxation in humans. Am J Physiol 1987;252(Gastrointest Liver Physiol 15):G636—G641.
10. Mittal RK, Stewart W, Schirmer B. Effect of a catheter in the pharynx on the frequency of transient lower esophageal sphincter relaxations. Gastroenterology 1992;103(4);1236—1240.
11. Holloway RH, Kocyan P, Dent J. Provocation of transient lower esophageal sphincter relaxations by meals in patients with symptomatic gastroesophageal reflux. Dig Dis Sci 1991;36(8):1034—1039.
12. Freidin N, Ren J, Sluss J, McCallum RW. The effect of large meal on the frequency and quality of transient LES relaxations (TLESR). Gastroenterology 1989;96(5,Pt2):A159.
13. Freidin N, Fisher M, Boyd D, Taylor W, Sluss J, McCallum RW, Mittal RK. Pattern of sleep and acid reflux in normal subjects and gastroesophageal reflux patients. Gastroenterology 1989;96(5):A158.

14. Orenstein SR, Deneault LG, Lutz JW, Wessel HB, Dent J. Regurgitant reflux, in contrast to non-regurgitant reflux, is associated with rectus abdominus contraction in infants. Gastroenterology 1991;100:A135.

15. Johnson LF, DeMeester TR. Twenty-four-hour pH monitoring of the distal esophagus: a quantitative measure of gastroesophageal reflux. Am J Gastroenterol 1974;62;325—332.

16. Orenstein SR. Gastroesophageal reflux. In: Stockman J, Winter R (eds) Current Problems in Pediatrics. Chicago: Mosby Year Book Medical Publishers, 1991:193—241.

17. Sondheimer JM. Clearance of spontaneous gastroesophageal reflux in awake and sleeping infants. Gastroenterology 1989;97(4):821—826.

18. Vandenplas Y, Sacre SL. Continuous 24-h esophageal pH monitoring in 285 asymptomatic infants 0—15 months old. J Pediatr Gastroenterol Nutr 1987;6(2):220—224.

19. Hillemeier AC, Grill BB, McCallum RW, Gryboski J. Esophageal and gastric motor abnormalities in gastroesophageal reflux during infancy. Gastroenterology 1983;84(4):741—746.

20. Kahrilas PJ, Dodds WJ, Hogan WJ. Effect of peristaltic dysfunction on esophageal volume clearance. Gastroenterology 1988;94(1):73—80.

In infancy, the symptoms may take special forms

M. Bellaiche, M.A. Maspoli, A.L. Lapeyraque, N. Boige,
P. Foucaud (Versailles)

There is considerable variation in the reported incidence of gastroesophageal reflux (GER) in infants. One of the reasons for this may be that the clinical picture is polymorphic. Although upper gastrointestinal symptoms are an essential part of the diagnostic picture for GER, there are also more atypical manifestations. Certain pulmonary and ENT disorders, certain serious infantile diseases and even sudden deaths may be attributable to GER that has eluded diagnosis. GER can be identified under these clinical situations by 24-h pH monitoring, although nothing can be said about the cause-effect relation. The etiopathogenesis of these disorders is often multifactorial and only the correction of these extra-alimentary manifestations after antireflux treatment can give an indication of the true role of GER.

GER and respiratory disorders in the infant

Physiopathology

a. *Induction of respiratory diseases by GER.* Two mechanisms have been schematically proposed to account for the pulmonary complications of GER: bronchial aspiration of gastrointestinal fluid and reflex bronchoconstriction [1].

Bronchial inhalation of gastric juice causes pulmonary disease. Its toxic effects can cause bronchoconstriction [2], surfactant destruction with atelectasis and an increase in total pulmonary resistance [3]. In some cases the clinical picture is very suggestive of an aspiratory mechanism. An acid taste in the mouth, confirmed by pH measurement, prior to the onset of cough or an asthma attack [4] is one example here. The combination of difficulty in swallowing and global loss of sphincter tone, in children with encephalopathy presenting lung disease associated with repeated swallowing, is another example.

Direct diagnostic methods based on tracheal intubation or bronchoscopy have been envisaged: detection in the airways of macrophages infiltrated with lipid droplets [5], lactose [6] or intragastrically administered dyes. However, these procedures are too invasive and not sufficiently specific. In addition, the intubation itself can influence the results. Radiological investigations can also assist the diagnosis, as when a bronchographic image is obtained after esophagogastroduodenal examination after administration of barium or pulmonary contamination after esophageal technetium scintigraphy. Unfortunately the sensitivity of these investigations is still insufficient, especially for the detection of repeated microaspiration [3]. Therefore, objective demonstration is not always possible and the diagnosis must be supported by the history and compatible radiological data [7,8].

Reflex bronchospasm was first evoked in adults with a combination of asthma and GER [9]. It is in fact known that intraesophageal infusion of acid causes bronchospasm and potentiates the effect of the cholinergics [10]. A pediatric population with this same disease combination was investigated by Davis et al. [11]. The authors found that intraesophageal instillation of decinormal hydrochloric acid only causes bronchospasm in children with esophagitis and not in asthmatic subjects with uncomplicated GER. The damaging effects of esophagitis on the afferent nerve impulses may account for the increased sensitivity to variations of pH [12]. Animal studies indicate that the vagus nerve plays a part in this reflex bronchoconstriction [9] and this would explain the efficacy of atropine here. This mechanism should therefore be suspected, especially in asthmatics with nocturnal symptoms that are resistant to treatment with the usual bronchodilators.

b. *GER induced by respiratory disease*. Chronic respiratory disease causes symptoms and requires treatment which themselves can render the patient susceptible to GER. The excessive abdominal pressure created by forced expiration during wheezing and cough potentiate GER. This has been observed especially in patients with cystic fibrosis, asthma, bronchopulmonary dysplasia and infective lung disease. Negative intrathoracic pressure secondary to stridor or hiccup may have the same consequences on GER. Breathing exercises involving forced expiratory and postural maneuvers also facilitate the disorder [13].

The pressure of the lower esophageal sphincter (LES) may be reduced in subjects with respiratory disease, either because of the thoracic distension, or as a result of treatment with drugs such as the β adrenoceptor stimulants, the anticholinergics, or theophylline (which also increases gastric acidity) [14]. By combined evaluation of GER by pH monitoring and determination of respiratory function, Berquist et al. [15] confirmed that episodes of GER accompany bronchodilator therapy, but also showed that there are no spirometric repercussions.

GER and chronic respiratory disease present the risk of mutual exacerbation. However, Hampton et al. [16] found no significant correlation between the severity of GER and the change in respiratory function in 38 children suffering from chronic respiratory disease. The authors suggested that there may be individual susceptibility.

Epidemiology

In large-scale, multicenter pediatric studies, the incidence of respiratory disorders seen in conjunction with GER fluctuates between 15 and 45% [3,17–20]. It is very important to take into account the general condition of the patients when interpreting these figures. As was already seen, chronic respiratory disease can cause secondary GER. Analysis of six cumulative pediatric populations showed a 56% incidence of GER confirmed by 24-h pH monitoring. Cystic fibrosis [21] and asthma [22] are at the forefront here and are diseases in which antireflex treatment is often an integral part of the therapeutic scheme.

Patients with fixed or progressive encephalopathy are also very prone to the pulmonary complications of GER because of global hypotonia, disorders of swallowing, restraining devices, scoliosis and the need for physiotherapy. Deforming diseases can also be associated with reflux: operated atresia of the esophagus where there is major impairment of motility, and to a lesser degree, gastroschisis or omphalocele, cleft lip/palate and Pierre-Robin syndrome [3,8,20]. Short bowel syndrome, because of the impaired motility and the frequent dependence on gastrostomy feeding, is also a predisposing condition [23]. Age seems to play a part as witnessed by the variability of the percentage of respiratory disease in GER as a function of the mean age of the population considered. Ghisolfi et al. [19] found only 1% respiratory complications in babies under 3 months, compared with 20% in infants and 33% in children.

Clinical characteristics

The respiratory symptoms secondary to GER are very heterogeneous: bronchitis, with or without an asthma-like component, cough, wheezing, lung disease. A number of characteristics of these episodes suggest that GER might be responsible. GER should be checked for if the respiratory symptoms are recurrent, exacerbated in the supine position with a predominance of cough at night, especially 1 to 3 hours after going to bed [24,25], if the disorders are not seasonal in character [20] and if they affect the middle lobe in particular [3,17,20]. The existence of other potential complications of GER such as apnea, faintness or repeated episodes of ENT disease tends to support the diagnosis, as does the existence of patent gastrointestinal symptoms, especially if these predominate at night [20].

Paraclinical characteristics

It is much easier to demonstrate the existence of GER in a patient exhibiting respiratory symptoms than to confirm the cause-effect relation between these disorders. The supplementary investigations carried out for these respiratory conditions can give useful pointers here, however.

A high level of reflux of barium or disorders of swallowing during radiological examination of the esophagus, stomach and duodenum following administration of barium, can be indicative of aspiration. However, the observation period is too short and the main value of these examinations is that it allows visualization of the anatomy of the upper gastrointestinal tract [3]. Twenty-four hour pH monitoring is the investigation of choice for confirmation of GER [3,19,20,26]. Respiratory symptoms coinciding with a fall in pH or increased esophageal acidity at night are useful indicators. However, in the experience of the French-speaking pediatric nutrition and gastroenterology group, it would seem that the traces examined show a greater tendency to reveal very short-lived and repetitive acid refluxes predominating during the day without GER at night (unpublished data). Although esophageal scintigraphy, by revealing pulmonary contamination, is of theoretical interest, in practice its sensitivity is not greater than 25% [3,19,20,27]. Manometric analysis has shown a reduction in the pressure of the LES in several studies [28–30]. The results concerning the pressure of the upper esophageal sphincter are more questionable, however: Cargill et al. [28] and Gerhardt et al. [31] observed hypotonia of the upper esophageal sphincter whereas Sondheimer et al. [8] did not. The value of esophago-gastric endoscopy resides in its ability to detect esophagitis which is recognized as a potential inducer of bronchospasm [12].

Treatment

A number of factors must be taken into consideration when deciding on the therapeutic strategy for this type of reflux. The ventral tilting position can render respiratory physiotherapy difficult. A compromise is therefore necessary. Most authors contraindicate the use of bethanechol because of its potential bronchospastic properties [32,33]. Treatment of the esophagitis must be optimal as this condition tends to maintain the disease. In patients receiving theophylline, it is advisable to use H_2-receptor antagonists other than cimetidine. The course is usually favorable except in certain cases (bronchodysplasia, encephalopathy, esophageal atresia and gastrostomy feeding) where surgical treatment is often required [3,18,20].

GER and "near miss" sudden infant death syndrome

Episodes of suffocation, apnea or fainting can be life-threatening or may be premonitory signs of sudden death (main cause of death in children under 1 year of age). Investigations for etiological factors have emphasized the important role of GER [3,20,34,35].

Physiopathology

Several studies have shown that there is a correlation between the fall in intraesophageal pH and apnea [9,36,37]. Bradycardiac apnea was found to be induced by instillation of decinormal hydrochloric acid in five infants admitted to hospital after a "near miss" sudden death syndrome [3]. This was not caused by instillation of milk. The monitoring of pH visualized this phenomenon during acid reflux occurring at the same time as apnea in 40 to 100% of cases investigated for serious fainting and GER [38]. Furthermore, this sudden fall in esophageal pH was found to precede a fall in transcutaneous oxygen pressure in half of the premature babies investigated by Pasquis et al. [39]. Menon et al. [40] observed brief or even prolonged apnea associated with postprandial reflux in infants. However, this chronological relationship between GER and apnea was not seen in polygraphic studies [3,27,41] performed with infants who had been saved from sudden death.

The apnea can be accompanied by laryngospasm and bradycardia. The mechanism appears to be a vagal reflex triggered by esophageal and/or laryngeal chemoreceptors. This vagal hyperreflexia has been demonstrated by decelerations in ECG traces obtained with Holter ECG monitoring equipment and studies of the oculocardiac reflex in certain "near miss" infants [42,43]. In this population, GER was found in 18 to 30% of cases [27,34,44]. This vagal dystonia is very probably related to a process of deficient maturation [34,35]. This is supported by the fact that anatomopathological and functional studies of the brain stem [45,46] have revealed immaturity of the autonomic nervous system. A common embryological origin for the triggering of fainting, apnea and GER has even been suggested in the Pierre-Robin syndrome. At the esophageal level, the vagal hyperreflexia also manifests by incomplete achalasia of the LES [34,35]. This has been observed in 75% of "near miss" infants with vagal hyperreflexia compared with 30% of infants without this condition [47].

Anatomopathological study

Systematic postmortem examinations have allowed considerable advances to be made in the understanding of the etiopathogenesis of sudden infant death, which is nowadays less and less inexplicable. The presence of esophagitis in 20 to 40% of cases [48,49] demonstrates the importance of the reflux factor in these infants.

Clinical studies

The initial demonstrations of GER in infants who had suffered respiratory arrest [36,37] were very encouraging. However, although the link between these two disorders is not in doubt, subsequent studies failed to confirm that all cases of "near miss" sudden infant death are the same. Near misses tend to exhibit polymorphic symptoms of necessarily fairly short duration. The episodes described comprise cyanosis and/or pallor, hypotonia, loss of contact, suffocation, apnea or cardiorespiratory arrest which responds to resuscitation. These episodes can be prolonged and life-threatening. A history of regurgitation or vomiting argues in favor of the link with GER. However, this parameter is lacking in sensitivity [3,27]. In practice, a history of this type was only found in one-third of cases on average in the various published studies [35,49–52]. Symptoms of esophagitis, the triggering of the disorder on a change of posture and repeated respiratory symptoms are also factors to be checked for.

The incidence of GER among near miss infants ranges from 10 to 100% according to the study considered [35,49–52]. However, these figures are invalidated by recruitment biases and the methods of investigation used, and the true incidence is probably between 10 and 20% [3,20,27].

The diurnal character of near miss sudden infant death can perhaps assist in determining its etiology. The GER diagnosed in near miss infants by polygraphic investigations was found to occur in the waking period in 60 to 75% of cases [52–54]. In the cases where GER developed at night, however, Jeffrey et al. [54] have found that it occurs most frequently during REM sleep.

The efficacy of antireflux treatment is the most convincing argument here. The disappearance of the near miss episodes during treatment demonstrates the responsibility of the GER [34,35,37,49]. If medical treatment is not sufficient to improve the clinical picture and to normalize esophageal pH, the infant may require surgical treatment [3,20,27].

Paraclinical studies

In all cases of near miss sudden infant death syndrome, an exhaustive investigation is required to check for pre-existing neurological, metabolic, cardiac or ENT disease. A systematic investigation for GER must also be carried out. Barium meal, scintigraphic and endoscopic investigations have the same value as in patients with respiratory disorders associated with GER. The monitoring of pH can be combined with permanent ECG monitoring using a Holter apparatus or, better still, integrated into a single polygraphic trace. In addition to its diagnostic value, it helps to guide patient management. In practice, optimal antireflux treatment is based on the results obtained for control pH measurements. Esophageal manometry designed to check for incomplete achalasia will give useful information concerning the state of esophageal immaturity [47]. In addition, a greatly diminished lower esophageal sphincter pressure (LESP) is the best indication for the use of urecholine.

Treatment

Hygienic-dietetic treatment of reflux (ventral tilting at 30°, thickening and fractionating of meals, early diversification of diet, large cot, absence of passive smoking) is initially sufficient. However, recent studies [55] have reported a reduced incidence of sudden infant death syndrome in the Netherlands following a government advisory circular recommending that all infants should always be placed in lateral decubitus in their cots. Initially pronate ventral decubitus appears to be a risk factor, especially because of the stifling and hyperthermia that it can generate.

Drug therapy is often required, mainly with cisapride and bethanechol. The presence of vagal hypertonia in addition to the GER complicates management. Prescription of an atropine-like drug such as diphemanil in theory reduces the lower esophageal sphincter pressure (LESP) and antagonizes the parasympathomimetic motility stimulants used. However, in clinical practice the anticholinergics do not appear to aggravate GER [56] or to reduce LESP in infants receiving antireflux treatment [57].

Where medical treatment fails, surgical treatment should be considered. Cardiorespiratory monitoring at home is sometimes combined with antireflux treatment until the esophagus has matured.

GER and ENT disorders

The physiopathological mechanisms that engender ENT symptoms in GER are the same as those described for the respiratory symptoms. GER also acts to maintain lesions in cases of laryngeal surgery or acquired stenosis in intubated children. In these cases antireflux treatment can reduce the morbidity caused by inflammation and edema that obstructs the upper airways.

ENT symptoms can develop at several levels. GER should be checked for in subjects with a chronic, dry, barking cough occurring mainly at night, once the possibility of malformation, allergy or a foreign body have been eliminated. Recurrent acute laryngitis, as observed in the adult [58], occurring without fever or nasopharyngitis and without any seasonal factor, is more frequently a sign of GER than of allergy or adenoiditis. This diagnosis is supported if laryngoscopy reveals erythema of the posterior rim [59].

Pharyngeal symptoms resulting from GER often take the form of acute or repeated pharyngitis or pharyngeal paraesthesia in older children [60]. Posterior pharyngeal or retrocricoid granulations surrounded by erythema are often visible. By extrapolation, the GER could favor the development of otitis or nasopharyngitis. However, this is very difficult to demonstrate, especially in these multifactorial disorders. In order to corroborate these pediatric clinical findings, a 2-channel esophageal and oro/hypopharyngeal pH monitoring technique was used in a recent study [61] to demonstrate the pathogenic role of GER in a population of 21 children suffering from recurrent otitis and pharyngitis, by comparison with a control group. A significant difference was observed for both the esophageal trace and the pharyngeal trace, thus confirming the presence of gastric fluid in the ENT sphere in these children. The role of GER in this type of condition will be best established, however, by analysis of the symptoms, 24-h pH monitoring and the success of antireflux therapy.

References

1. Barish CF, Wu WC, Castell DO. Respiratory complications of gastroesophageal reflux. Arch Intern Med 1985;145;1882–1888.
2. Mendelson CL. The aspiration of stomach contents into the lungs during obstetric anesthesia. Ann J Obstet Gynecol 1946;52:191–205.
3. Orenstein SR, Orenstein DM. Gastroesophageal reflux and respiratory disease in children. J Pediatr 1988;112:847–858.
4. Pellegrini CA, DeMeester TR, Johnson LF et al. Gastroesophageal reflux and pulmonary aspiration: incidence, functional abnormality, and results of surgical therapy. Surgery 1979;86:110–119.
5. Nussbaum E, Maggi JC, Galant SP. Association of lipid-laden alveolar macrophages and gastroesophageal reflux in children. Pediatr Res 1986;20:475A.

6. Hopper AO, Kwong LK, Stevenson DK et al. Detection of gastric contents in tracheal fluid of infants by lactose assay. J Pediatr 1983;102:415–418.

7. Darling DB, McCauley RGK, Leonidas JC et al. Gastroesophageal reflux in infants and children: correlation of radiological severity and pulmonary pathology. Radiology 1978;127:735–740.

8. Sondheimer JM, Morris BA. Gastroesophageal reflux among severely retarded children. J Pediatr 1979;94:710–714.

9. Mansfield LE, Hameister HH, Spaulding HS et al. The role of the vagus nerve in airway narrowing caused by intraesophageal hydrochloric acid provocation and esophageal distention. Ann Allergy 1981;47:431–434.

10. Herve P, Denjean A, Jian R et al. Intraesophageal perfusion of acid increases the bronchomotor response to methacholine and to isocapnic hyperventilation in asthmatic subjects. Am Rev Respir Dis 1986;134:986–989.

11. Davis RS, Larsen GL, Grunstein MM. Respiratory response to intraesophageal acid infusion in asthmatic children during sleep. J Allergy Clin Immunol 1983;72:393–398.

12. Baer M, Maki M, Nurminen J et al. Esophagitis and findings of long-term oesophageal pH recording in children with repeated lower respiratory tract symptoms. J Pediatr Gastroenterol Nutr 1986;5:187–190.

13. Vandenplas Y, Dierics A, Becker U et al. Esophageal pH monitoring data during chest physiotherapy. J Pediatr Gastroenterol Nutr 1989;9:250–254.

14. Christensen J. Effects of drugs on esophageal motility. Arch Intern Med 1976;136:532–537.

15. Berquist WE, Rachelefsky GS, Kadden M et al. Gastroesophageal reflux associated to recurrent pneumonia and chronic asthma in children. Pediatrics 1981;68:29–35.

16. Hampton FJ, MacFadyen UM, Beardsmore CS et al. Gastroesophageal reflux and respiratory function in infants with respiratory symptoms. Arch Dis Child 1991;66:848–853.

17. Baculard A, Maufroy C, Grimfeld A et al. Etude critique du rôle du reflux gastro-oesophagien dans les bronchopneumopathies de l'enfant de plus de 3 ans. A propos de 500 observations. Ann Ped 1981;28:393–401.

18. Carre IJ. Pulmonary infections in children with a partial thoracic stomach (hiatus hernia). Arch Dis Child 1960;35:481–487.

19. Ghisolfi J, Baculard A, Olives JP et al. Manifestations cliniques et évolution du reflux gastro oesophagien de l'enfant. XXVI Congrès de Pédiatrie, Toulouse, June 30–July 2, 1981;33–47.

20. Hermier M, Descos B. Reflux gastro-oesophagien et manifestations respiratoires. Pédiatrie 1983;38:125–135.

21. Cucchiara S, Santamaria F, Andreotti M et al. Mechanism of gastroesophageal reflux in cystic fibrosis. Arch Dis Child 1991;66:617–622.

22. Scheinman P, Le Bourgeois M, Deblic J et al. Reflux gastro-oesophagien et asthme de l'enfant. Rev F Allerg 1987;27:71–76.

23. Brand J, Brodsky, Hurt H. No evidence of aspiration in intubated infants fed by orogastric or oroduodenal routes. Pediatr Res 1986;20:405A.

24. Euler AR, Byrne WJ, Ament ME et al. Recurrent pulmonary disease in children: a complication of gastroesophageal reflux. Pediatrics 1979;63:47–51.

25. Jolley SG, Herbst JJ, Johnson DG et al. Esophageal pH monitoring during sleep identifies children with respiratory symptoms from gastroesophageal reflux. Gastroenterology 1981;80:1501–1506.

26. Euler AR, Byrne WJ. Twenty-four hour esophageal intraluminal pH probe testing: a comparative analysis. Gastroenterology 1981;80:957–961.

27. Foucaud P, Navarro J. Explorations gastro-oesophagiennes au cours des malaises graves du nourrisson. In: Dehan M, Gilly R (eds) Mort Subite du Nourrisson. Paris: Doins éditeurs, 1989;253–268.

28. Cargill G, Goutet JM, Vargas J et al. Analyse manométrique du reflux gastro-oesophagien du nourrisson et de l'enfant. Pediatrie (Lyon) 1982;37:311 (abstract).

29. Cucchiara S, Tussi F, Minella et al. Pathophysiologic mechanism of gastroesophageal reflux (GER) in patients with GER disease complicated by respiratory symptoms. XXVI Annual Meeting of the European Society for Pediatric Gastroenterology and Nutrition (ESPGAN), Göteborg; 28–30 June 1993.

30. Goutet JM, Cargill G, Vargas J et al. Intérêt de l'étude manométrique de l'oesophage dans le reflux gastro-oesophagien de l'enfant. Arch Fr Pediatr 1981;38:897.

31. Gerhardt D, Schuck T, Bordeaux R et al. Human upper esophageal sphincter response to volume osmotic and acid stimuli. Gastroenterology 1978;75:268 274.

32. Euler AR. Use of betanechol for the treatment of gastroesophageal reflux. J Pediatr 1980;96:321–324.

33. Sondheimer JM, Mintz HL, Michaels M. Betanechol treatment of gastroesophageal reflux in infants: effect on continuous esophageal pH records. J Pediatr 1984;104:128–131.

34. Benhamou Ph, Dupont C. Lien entre reflux gastro-oesophagien et malaise grave du nourrisson. Press Med 1992;21:1673–1676

35. Foucaud P, Cargill G, Navarro J. Malaises du nourrisson et reflux gastro-oesophagien. In: Journées Parisiennes de Pédiatrie 1985. Paris: Flammarion Médecine-Sciences, 1985;191–197.

36. Herbst JJ, Book LS, Bray PF. Gastroesophageal reflux in the "near miss" sudden infant death syndrome. J Pediatr 1978;92:93–95.

37. Leape LL, Holder TM, Franklin JD et al. Respiratory arrest in infants secondary to gastroesophageal reflux. Pediatrics 1977;60:924–928.

38. Chakraborry T, Ogilvie A, Heading R et al. Abnormal cardiovascular reflexes in patients with gastroesophageal reflux. Gut 1989;30:46–49.

39. Pasquis P, Tardif C, Nouvet G. Reflux gastro-oesophagien et affections respiratoires. Bull Eur Physiopathol Respir

1983;19:645—658.

40. Menon AP, Schefft GL, Thach BT. Apnea associated with regurgitation in infants. J Pediatr 1985;106:625—629.
41. Southall DP, Richards J, Brown DJ et al. Twenty-four-hour tape recording of ECG and respiration in the newborn infant with finding related to sudden death and unexplained brain damage in infancy. Arch Dis Child 1980;55:7—16.
42. Kahn A, Riazi J, Blum D. Oculocardiac reflex in near miss for sudden infant death syndrome. Pediatrics 1983; 71:49—52.
43. Lucet V, Toumieux MC, Pajot N et al. Hypertonie vagale paroxystique du nourrisson. Arch Fr Pediatr 1984;41:527—531.
44. Weereman G, Bochner A, Van Lailliem et al. Gastroesophageal reflux in infants with a history of near miss sudden infant death. J Pediatr Gastroenterol Nutr 1991;12:313—323.
45. Pettigrew AG, Rahilly PM. Brainstorm auditory evoked response in infants at risk of sudden infant death. Early Hum Dev 1985; 11:99—111.
46. Quattrochi JJ, McBride PT, Yates AJ. Brain stem immaturity in sudden infant death syndrome: a quantitative rapid Golgi study of dendritic spines in 95 infants. Brain Res 1985;28:39—46.
47. Foucaud P, Boige N, Cargill G et al. Esophageal achalasia and dysautonomia in childhood. XXIst Annual Meeting of the European Society for Pediatric Gastroenterology and Nutrition (ESPGAN). Copenhagen; 19—21 May 1988.
48. Dehan M, Imbert MC, Gautier JP et al. Etude clinique et anatomo-pathologique de 59 cas de mort subite du nourrisson. Arch Fr Pediatr 1988;45:541—548.
49. Herbst JJ, Myers WF. Gastroesophageal reflux in children. Adv Pediatr 1981;28:159—186.
50. Newman M, Russe L, Glasman M. Patterns of gastroesophageal reflux on patients with apparent life-threatening events. J Pediatr Gastroenterol Nutr 1989;8:157—160.
51. Rosen CL, Forst JD, Harrisson JM. Infant apnea polygraphic studies and follow-up monitoring. Pediatrics 1983;71:731—736.
52. Spitzer AR, Boyle JT, Tuchman DN et al. Awake apnea associated with gastroesophageal reflux: a specific clinical syndrome. J Pediatr 1984;104:200—205.
53. Ariagno RL, Guilleminault C, Baldwin R et al. Movement and gastroesophageal reflux in awake term infants with "near miss" SIDS, unrelated to apnea. J Pediatr 1982;100:894—897.
54. Jeffery HE, Reid I, Rahilly P et al. Gastroesophageal reflux in "near miss" sudden infant death infants in active but not quiet sleep. Sleep Res 1980;3:393—339.
55. Engelberts, De Jonge. Choice of sleeping position for infants: possible association with cot death. Arch Dis Child 1990;65:462—467.
56. Lamireau E, Barbier J, Demarquez J. Les anticholinergiques n'aggravent pas le reflux gastro-oesophagien. Groupe Francophone de Gastroentérologie et Nutrition Pédiatriques, Genève 1990 (abstract).
57. Benzakour A, Munck A, Boige N et al. Pression du sphincter inférieur de l'oesophage lors de l'association diphemanil, traitement antireflux au cours des malaises graves du nourrisson. Groupe Francophone de Gastroentérologie et Nutrition Pédiatriques, Tunis 1991 (abstract).
58. Jacob P. Proximal oesophageal pH-metry in patient with "reflux laryngitis" Gastroenterology 1991;100:305—310.
59. Andrieux J, Dehesdind, Le Luyer B et al. Rôle du reflux gastro-oesophagien au cours des dyspnées laryngées aiguës récidivantes de l'enfant. Ann Otol Chir Cervicofac 1984;101:141—149.
60. Contencin P, Viaia P, Narcy P. Etude des variations du pH rhinopharyngé dans les rhinopharyngites de l'enfant. Press Med 1991;33:1595—1598.
61. Contencin P, Adjoua P, Viaia P et al. La pH-métrie couplée, oesophagienne et oro/hypopharyngée, de longue durée dans les formes ORL de reflux gastro-oesophagien de l'enfant. Ann Otolaryngol 1992;109:129—133.

Are the histologic changes associated with reflux different in adults and children?

D.A. Antonioli (Boston)

The histologic changes associated with gastroesophageal reflux (GER) are basically similar in children and adults. In well-oriented esophageal mucosal biopsy specimens taken 2 cm or more above the gastroesophageal junction, a basal zone occupying more than 20% of the thickness of the squamous epithelium and stromal papillae extending more than two-thirds of the distance through the epithelium are excellent markers of GER. However, since most esophageal mucosal biopsies in the pediatric population are obtained using grasp biopsy forceps that result in small, poorly-oriented specimens, basal zone hyperplasia and papillary lengthening cannot be evaluated. Thus, as in adults, detection of intraepithelial inflammation becomes a major component in evaluating GER-related esophagitis in children [1].

Intraepithelial neutrophils are uncommon but are a good indicator of GER, being most often noted in patients with esophageal erosions or ulcers. Intraepithelial eosinophils are more frequent than neutrophils in GER-related injury and they are often the sole marker of injury in children. Even a small number of eosinophils in a specimen taken 2–3 cm above the gastroesophageal junction correlates with GER. Although intraepithelial eosinophils are a very specific indicator of acid reflux, they are not a highly sensitive one [2]. Intraepithelial lymphocytes may be increased in childhood GER [1,3]. Other, nonspecific markers of mucosal injury may be noted; these include increased mitoses in the epithelium, spongiosis and balloon-cell change (swelling) of keratinocytes [4]. Vascular congestion in papillae is a nonspecific response to endoscope trauma.

Like adults, children may develop Barrett's esophagus (BE) as a complication of severe GER. The precise incidence and prevalence of BE in the pediatric population are difficult to determine, because clinical studies in this age group are few in number and typically retrospective in nature. Within these limitations, however, BE has been diagnosed between infancy and age 19 years in 10 to 13% of children with severe GER and/or histologically proven esophagitis [5,6]. These percentages are similar to those for adults with severe GER; also like adults, BE in children has a marked male predominance [6,7].

Barrett's esophagus may be overrepresented in certain subsets of pediatric patients. For example, there may be an excess of BE in children (and adults) who have had an esophageal atresia or tracheoesophageal fistula surgically repaired. These congenital lesions are associated with esophageal dysmotility, resulting in poor esophageal acid clearance and a high prevalence of esophagitis [8]. Likewise, young people who are severely developmentally disabled are numerous in studies of BE in childhood [9], forming up to 40–70% of the BE patients in some series [6,7,10]. Severe GER is common in these patients; however, since they often cannot articulate their symptoms, the diagnosis of esophagitis is often delayed, thus allowing time for BE to develop [10]. The recognition of BE is important in children because of its malignant potential. Although they are rare, 10 cases of adenocarcinoma arising in BE before the age of 25 years have been reported [11].

The histologic features of BE in children are, in many respects, similar to those in adults. Fundic, junctional and specialized columnar epithelium may all be found, with the specialized epithelium typically at the upper end and the fundic and junctional types at the distal end of the BE segment [5–7,9,10]. As in adults, the fundic and junctional variants usually have an atrophic appearance, unlike that of normal stomach [5].

The major histologic difference between pediatric and adult BE is that specialized columnar epithelium is less frequent in children. Whereas specialized columnar epithelium can be identified in over 90% of adults with BE, it has been detected in only 15 to 50% of children with BE [5–7]. Its presence appears to be age related, in that specialized columnar epithelium increases in prevalence in older, as compared to younger, cohorts of children with BE [6].

The relative paucity of specialized epithelium in younger children may make the diagnosis of BE problematic; caution should be exercised if only fundic or junctional tissue is obtained in biopsy specimens, since they may represent normal proximal stomach or gastric mucosa in a hiatal hernia [12]. Multiple biopsies and careful endoscopic measurements of the length of columnar mucosa may aid in determining if BE is present. Alcian blue staining (at pH 2.5) of biopsy specimens may be helpful in detecting otherwise inapparent goblet cells [12].

References

1. Dahms BB, Rothstein FC. Mucosal biopsy of the esophagus in children. In: Rosenberg HS, Bernstein J (eds) Respiratory and Alimentary Tract Diseases (Perspectives in Pediatric Pathology, vol. II). Basel: Karger, 1987;97–123.
2. Winter HS, Madara JL, Stafford RJ et al. Intraepithelial eosinophils: a new diagnostic criterion for reflux esophagitis. Gastroenterology 1982;83:818–823.
3. Groben PA, Siegal GP, Shub MD et al. Gastrointestinal reflux and esophagitis in infants and children. In: Rosenberg HS, Bernstein J (eds) Respiratory and Alimentary Tract Diseases (Perspectives in Pediatric Pathology, vol II). Basel: Karger, 1987;124–151.
4. Jessurun J, Yardley JH, Giardiello FM, Hamilton SR. Intracytoplasmic plasma proteins in distended esophageal squamous cells (balloon cells). Mod Pathol 1988;1:175–181.
5. Dahms BB, Rothstein FC. Barrett's esophagus in children: a consequence of chronic gastroesophageal reflux. Gastroenterology 1984;86:318–323.
6. Qualman SJ, Murray RD, McClung J, Lucas J. Intestinal metaplasia is age-related in Barrett's esophagus. Arch Pathol Lab Med 1990;114:1236–1240.
7. Hassall E, Weinstein WM, Ament ME. Barrett's esophagus in childhood. Gastroenterology 1985;89:1131–1137.
8. Biller JA, Allen JL, Schuster SR, Treves ST, Winter HS. Long-term evaluation of esophageal and pulmonary function in patients with repaired esophageal atresia and tracheoesophageal fistula. Dig Dis Sci 1987;32:985–990.
9. Roberts IM, Curtis RL, Madara JL. Gastroesophageal reflux and Barrett's esophagus in developmentally disabled patients. Am J Gastroenterol 1986;81:519–523.
10. Snyder JD, Goldman H. Barrett's esophagus in children and young adults: frequent association with mental retardation. Dig Dis Sci 1990;35:1185–1189.
11. Hassall E, Dimmick JE, Magee JF. Adenocarcinoma in childhood Barrett's esophagus: case documentation and the need for surveillance in children. Am J Gastroenterol 1993;88:282–288.
12. Hassall E. Barrett's esophagus: congenital or acquired? Am J Gastroenterol 1993;88:819–824.

What is the contribution of scintigraphy in gastroesophageal reflux in children

C. Maurage, F. Baulieu, N. Faure, K. Dieckmann,
J.C. Rolland (Tours)

Supplementary investigations for gastroesophageal reflux in children

The physician who looks after a child with suspected gastroesophageal reflux (GER) must answer various questions:
— Is there genuine and abnormal GER?
— What is the cause (or mechanism)?
— How often, how much, how long and how acid is the reflux into the esophagus?
— Is there any esophagitis?
— Is there any aspiration into the bronchi/lungs?
— Finally, did the GER disappear after treatment?
Each of the various investigations available to supplement the clinical findings offers a different contribution to these questions.

Barium transit through the esophagus, stomach and duodenum

This remains the most readily available and easiest investigation to establish the existence of reflux, and in particular it is the only one for proper examination of the anatomy of the region of the esophagus/cardia. Nevertheless, there are various problems with clinically-doubtful cases. These include difficulties in standardizing the investigation (volume, positions, etc.) and difficulties in interpretation, and, in particular, some lack of sensitivity in both confirmation of intermittent reflux (not occurring at the time of the investigation) as well as in the detection of esophagitis. Exposure to irradiation depends largely on the equipment and on the number of films taken. The cost (Z120), which is not negligible, is often ignored.

Esophagoscopy

The main and specific purpose of this is to visualize any esophagitis and to confirm it by histology of a biopsy (an invasive procedure which is reasonably well tolerated). A general anaesthetic is sometimes required. Cost: K50.

Esophageal manometry

This more recent and less widespread investigation is a technique for examining normal esophageal function and the various mechanisms involved in its abnormalities rather than a method for diagnosing reflux. (It only detects pressure changes and cannot, strictly speaking, confirm reflux). Cost: K20.

Measurement of pH in the esophagus

This is carried out continuously with miniature electrodes over 12 or 24 h; it is very reliable, sensitive and safe.

The disadvantages are the length of recording, the unpleasantness of having tubes in place and, in small children, the difficulty of establishing an intrabuccal reference electrode.

It is an excellent method for detecting very small or late reflux and for defining the rate, amount and duration of reflux, but it is only a test of acid reflux at a restricted level in the esophagus (the site of the lower end of the catheter). The cost varies with technique and duration (in the clinic: K40).

Scintigraphy

This is less-widely used for the diagnosis of GER in children.

The inherent qualities of a radioisotope test (sensitivity, scanty irradiation which is not influenced by the number of films or the length of the investigation, the ability to carry out kinetic and quantitative analyses) make it a priori very suitable for the study of GER and for looking for possible inhalation into the lungs.

We thought it would be helpful to draw up a protocol and to carry out the test in children. As a result, we have learned something of the practical problems involved in its performance and interpretation, and we can discuss its place among other available methods on the basis of personal experience.

The technique involves labeling a meal with 0.5 mCi of ^{99m}Tc colloidal sulfide. An aliquot of the meal is mixed with colloidal technetium. The rest is taken without any radioactive product and has the effect of washing residual activity out of the esophagus. Subsequently, recording is continued for 1 h with 60 images being taken at intervals of 1 min. Later images are taken from several directions (anterior, posterior, right and left lateral) 4 and 24 h after the meal. The recordings from an investigation can then be used for kinetic and quantitative studies (activity curves over the course of time in selected areas of interest − quantification).

In children with reflux confirmed by barium studies or pH measurement the images on scintigraphy, and the activity curves show one, two or more bouts of reflux. Sometimes a focus can be seen outside the esophagus which gives rise to a suspicion of aspiration into the lungs.

Discussion

Arrangement of this protocol and the results of two recent studies in children with respiratory symptoms have allowed the advantages and disadvantages of this technique to be confirmed and defined, as well as uncovered certain problems with interpretation.

Advantages

Some of the advantages are linked to the protocol employed. There is little inconvenience for the child who does not have to undergo anesthesia, premedication, additional fasting, passage of tubes or intravenous injection. The product is given with a normal meal and the test is carried out in as physiological manner as possible.

Irradiation is scanty. The dose of 500 μCi delivers a mean 100 mrads to the whole body which is clearly less than a series of X-rays during a barium investigation.

There are other advantages associated with isotope technology:

— *Sensitivity.* One of the aims of this study was to measure this and define its limits. However, it is already clear from the nature of the findings that very small refluxes of the isotope can be detected but this raises the problem of their pathological significance.
— Measurement of activity at intervals of time and in predefined areas enables an objective study of the rate, amount and duration of reflux (esophageal clearance) and gastric emptying. These last two parameters appear to be particularly closely-associated with the pathological nature of the reflux. This ability to quantify the results also means that comparative tests could be envisaged, especially of the effects of different symptomatic and curative forms of treatment.
— Finally, scintigraphy has the specific advantage of allowing detection of aspiration of fluid from the stomach into the bronchi and lungs. The significance of such reflux aspirations in the pathogenesis of certain asthma-like syndromes and repeated bronchopneumonias in infants and children is now well understood.

Disadvantages

As shown previously these are scanty for the child; however, they are important to the medical team, though they are not unique to scintigraphy. The disadvantages are the problems involved in transporting the child to the department where examinations are to be carried out, and in accompanying the child during the examinations (4–5 h). The cost, Z150 + ERA154, is relatively high but should be kept in proportion (by comparison with barium studies).

Problems of interpretation

Two problems have arisen: the first one is a product of the sensitivity of the technique and takes the form of how much significance to attach, particularly in very young infants, to scanty, small, short bouts of reflux which occur close to meals. Continuous pH measurement poses problems of the same nature but it does not record reflux which is buffered by a meal.

Because it allows precise, objective and comparable measurements to be taken, it is reasonable to suppose that scintigraphy can make a major contribution to this study and to decisions whether or not GER in children are abnormal.

The other problem is particularly important because it concerns confirmation of aspiration into the lungs which is the specific advantage of scintigraphy over other investigations. When faced with a focus of activity high-up and close to the side of the esophagus, it is sometimes difficult to distinguish between aspiration into the chest and intrabuccal reflux. This difficulty is obviously greater as the dimension becomes smaller in younger children. The solution certainly lies in meticulous pin-pointing of the levels and by careful observation of the child with particular attention to changes in the position of its head and any regurgitation which takes place during the investigation.

At this point in our study, we formed an opinion that scintigraphy with technetium sulfide is as interesting as there was reason to suppose in the investigation of GER in children. This study has been continued in a more systematic manner mainly to define the links between respiratory disease and GER [4].

This investigation, therefore, is of interest:
— in clinical circumstances which suggest reflux where barium studies, which are less sensitive, are negative, and facilities for pH measurement are not available;
— when it is desirable to identify the timing, rate, amount and duration of an established GER and its relationship with gastric emptying regardless of the pH;
— as a sensitive supplementary criterion for assessment of a child's response to treatment for GER which is not unpleasant for the child;
— finally, and for this purpose, there is no substitute for scintigraphy for recognition of reflux aspiration, particularly when looking for the etiology of asthma-like dyspnea and recurrent bronchopneumonia in children. The timing should, of course, be chosen on the basis of the clinical circumstances and the results of the more usual investigations (biochemical, radiological, immunological) which are often requested in this context.

Conclusion

Scintigraphy with technetium sulfide has a role in the investigation of GER and its complications in children. In the light of its inherent qualities, it may well be that further study of this method of investigation will improve our understanding of the physiopathology of GER in children and of the extent of its involvement in complex disease processes.

References

1. Berquist WE, Rachelefsky GS, Kadden M, Siegel SC, Katz RM, Fonkalsrud EW, Ament ME. Gastro-oesophageal reflux-associated recurrent pneumonia and chronic asthma in children. Pediatrics 1981;68:29—35.
2. Boonyaprapa S, Alderson O, Garfinkel DJ, Chipps BE, Wagner N. Detection of pulmonary aspiration in infants and children with respiratory disease: concise communication. J Nucl Med 1980;21:314—318.

3. De Blic J, Revillon Y, Scheinman P. Relations entre reflux gastro-oesophagien et pathologie respiratoire chronique. Rev Intern. Ped. 1992;221:6–14.
4. Maurage C, Caurier B, Bergeat MA, Robert M, Rolland JC. Reflux gastro-oesophagien de l'enfant et manifestations respiratoires. A propos de 70 observations. Revue Med de Tours 1987;2:325–329.

Are reflux-related strictures in children different from those in adults?

N. Meadows (London)

Over the last 5 years, the presence of stricture formation in the esophagus attributable solely to reflux esophagitis has declined in children. This is undoubtedly due to the more aggressive therapeutic approach and the increased application of endoscopy and pH study in the management of gastroesophageal reflux in infancy. Indeed a 20-year study from Navarro in France has identified the incidence of stricture formation in 89 patients of 232 infants diagnosed as having reflux [1].

Any consideration of esophageal stricture in children has to take into account the contribution of other congenital defects that may be present (Table 1). These are all associated with reflux, but in addition may have combined esophageal dysmotility. The best examples of such associations would be Down's Syndrome, Hirschprung's and tracheoesophageal fistulae and atresias. In these situations, delayed acid clearance resulting from both reflux and disordered motility predispose the child more readily to stricture formation.

In adults the situation is slightly clearer, with a higher number of reflux patients progressing to stricture formation (approximately 10%). Of perhaps more significance is that 25% of the patients are entirely asymptomatic [2]. Recently, much interest has arisen in the association of Barrett's epithelium and strictures. It has been estimated that approximately 60–80% of strictures show evidence of Barrett's changes, the stricture occurring at the squamo-columnar junction. Certainly this association is increased in the presence of strictures found in patients with hiatus hernia [3].

Table 1.

Associations with congenital stenosis	Acquired strictures
Tracheoesophageal fistula	Caustic ingestion
Duodenal atresia	Peptic esophagitis
Anorectal anomalies	Severe infections
Cardiac anomalies	Epidermolysis Bullosa
Down's syndrome	

Table 2. Esophageal stricture Queen Elizabeth Hospital (5-year experience)

4 caustic ingestion
3 tracheoesophageal atresia
2 gastroesophageal reflux

In children it is now believed that the association between Barrett's epithelium and stricture formation is equally strong. Initially it was felt that Barrett's epithelium may represent a congenital change, but it is now clear that this is not the case and does indeed represent change associated with reflux. However, care must be taken in the diagnosis and several of the early studies in which Barrett's epithelium was described may represent single gastric metaplasia. The site from which the biopsy was taken has also to be considered, particularly in the case of hiatus hernia, as exemplified in the recent review of the available pediatric studies by Hassall [4,5].

So what are the major differences between adult strictures and those in children? This is probably best illustrated from experience of esophageal strictures obtained at the Queen Elizabeth Hospital for Children in London. In a 5-year period, we have seen a total of 10 children with esophageal strictures. Four of these were associated with caustic ingestion and were in no way related to gastroesophageal reflux. Of the remainder, five were associated with tracheoesophageal atresia or fistula and in four of these gastroesophageal reflux was thought to play an important contributory role. The remaining two patients had pure gastroesophageal reflux-related strictures, both associated with Barrett's epithelium. This change was also present in three of the patients with tracheoesophageal atresia. The most significant finding was that both patients with gastroesophageal strictures were severely cerebrally palsied.

In conclusion, in children, pure reflux strictures are much more likely to be associated with disorders where esophageal dysmotility is also present. The more aggressive diagnostic work-up and management of reflux has resulted in a reduced risk in children with simple reflux. However, in children with handicap, because of the often silent nature of their reflux, consideration of surgical correction has been suggested as an early therapeutic option. The role of treatment in Barrett's epithelium changes remains a matter for debate, although it is the feeling of many clinicians that consideration should be given to early surgery to prevent complications in childhood, particularly stricture formation.

References

1. Navarro J, Cargill G, Foucaud P. Gastro-oesophageal reflux in pediatric gastroentorology. In: Navarro J, Schmitz J (eds) Gastro-oesophageal Reflux in Paediatric Gastroenterology. Oxford: Oxford Medical Publications, 1992;105–123.
2. Katzka DA. Barrett's oesophagus: introduction and management. Gastroenterol Clin North Am 1989;18:339–357.
3. Cameron AJ, Zinsmeister AR, Ballard DJ, Carry JA. Prevalence of columnar-lined (Barrett's) oesophagus. Gastroenterology 1990;99:918–922.
4. Hassall E, Weinstein WM, Ament ME. Barrett's oesophagus in childhood. Gastroenterology 1985;89:1331–1337.
5. Hassall E. New definitions and approaches in children. J Ped Gastroenterol Nutr 1993;16:345–364.

For how long should medical treatment be continued?

S.R. Orenstein (Pittsburgh)

The simple answer to the question posed in the title is: "until it is cured or requires surgery".

Ascertaining the success of medical treatment, or deciding that it has failed and requires surgery, are, however, rather complex issues. The complexity arises, first, from ambiguity regarding what constitutes optimal medical therapy (which components of conservative therapy are included? Should both a prokinetic and an acid suppressor be used? Should a proton pump inhibitor be used in children?). Second, the complexity results from different responses to therapy by the various manifestations of reflux. Third, the complexity is caused by the need to use invasive testing to evaluate persistence of disease. Fourth, the complexity results from maturational issues — different responses in infants and in older children.

In this discussion, I will not deal with the components of medical therapy, but my personal biases are that "conservative therapy" (advice regarding positioning and feeding) is a very helpful underpinning for reflux therapy, particularly in infants; that a prokinetic agent should usually be used for reflux disease, with an H_2 blocker added in those patients with esophagitis; that H_2-blocker therapy may be optimized with higher than previously used doses [1]; and that proton pump therapy in children should be reserved for intractable symptoms and used on a temporary basis, often prior to a decision for surgery. I will evaluate the evidence regarding both the success and failure of medical therapy for reflux disease in children, attempting to address the various symptomatic presentations individually and to identify when invasive testing is needed. Due to the different natural history of reflux disease in infants and in older children, these two developmental groups will be discussed separately.

Infants

Success of medical therapy — discontinuing therapy

How one determines the success of medical therapy for reflux disease in infants varies with the presenting manifestations of the reflux. In infants with *regurgitation and failure to thrive*, controlling regurgitation enough to allow adequate weight gain is the measure of treatment success and persistence of adequate weight gain when therapy is withdrawn indicates "cure" of the problem. Data are limited, but clinical experience suggests that this problem usually resolves between 8 and 12 months, the period when regurgitation frequency is markedly reduced in normal infants.

In contrast to the nutritional consequences of regurgitation, which can be monitored noninvasively when therapy is withdrawn, esophagitis due to reflux cannot be observed directly. Discontinuing therapy therefore requires: 1) assumptions that esophagitis resolves in concert with observable signs (such as crying or regurgitation); or 2) assumptions that the timing of its persistent resolution can be predicted by pharmacologic studies (largely in adults); or 3) invasive evaluation. Thus one should treat esophagitis for at least 2 or 3 months and until the observable signs have resolved, or until invasive evaluation (esophageal histology) demonstrates resolution.

Apnea, one of the most threatening symptoms of reflux, is essentially confined to infancy. The decision that therapy of the reflux has been successful and can be terminated is undertaken in a more conservative manner than such a decision to terminate therapy for other manifestations of reflux in infants, because of the importance of *assuring that apnea will not recur when therapy is discontinued*. A decision to terminate therapy in infants with reflux-associated apnea utilizes knowledge of the maturational time course of infantile apnea of any cause, as well as the knowledge of the particular infant's symptoms since initiation of antireflux therapy. A conservative plan is to continue therapy until the infant is older than 6 months and no apnea has occurred for 2 months. Evidence that other signs of reflux are eliminated is also supportive. Infants who have been monitored should not have both the pharmacologic therapy for reflux and the monitor discontinued simultaneously.

Infants with other respiratory manifestations definitely attributable to reflux often require fundoplication for adequate control. However, many such infants deserve a trial of aggressive medical therapy before consigning them to surgery, to allow those who are able to avoid surgery to do so. If medical therapy does result in complete resolution of the respiratory symptoms for a period of time, it is reasonable to attempt to discontinue pharmacologic therapy, but to keep surgical therapy in reserve for those who are unable to remain off therapy.

Failure of medical therapy — advancing to surgical therapy

Surgical therapy is warranted in three general situations. These are, in decreasing order of necessity: 1) symptom hazard: when the danger of persistent reflux is so great that primary fundoplication is preferable to relying on imperfect medical therapy; 2) symptom intractability: when medical therapy fails to resolve serious symptoms; or 3) medication dependence: when medical therapy resolves serious symptoms, but is unable to be withdrawn without resumption of the symptoms. Because the natural history of infantile reflux disease is to resolve in the first year or so of life, surgery should be postponed until after that time, if possible.

Symptom hazard has often been cited as a reason for primary surgical therapy for reflux-associated apnea in infants [2], but pediatric gastroenterologists have managed large numbers of such infants without surgery and without adverse outcome [3]. Many infants who have experienced a cyanotic episode or ALTE, apparently due to reflux, can have their risk for subsequent such episodes markedly reduced by very careful nursing practices (e.g., cautious feeding, diligent burping and prone positioning) as well as by pharmacologic intervention. Nonetheless, occasional infants with recurrent severe reflux-associated apneic episodes may demonstrate the

768

intractability which would prompt surgical intervention. The utility of cardiorespiratory monitoring in the meantime is ambiguous, although often used, in this situation as in many others; the awake, obstructive, postprandial apnea associated with reflux is particularly unlikely to be detected early by such monitoring.

Two other situations in which symptom hazard may prompt primary fundoplication are Barrett's esophagus and reflux stricture; since both of them are uncommon in infants, they will be considered in the section on older children.

Symptom intractability should not be used as the sole justification for surgery until comprehensive medical therapy (a prokinetic agent, an acid-lowering agent in adequate doses and aggressive conservative management) has been used for at least several months, or if persistent symptoms produce unacceptable hazard. Esophagitis does not resolve in most patients with less than 2 or 3 months of therapy, and related respiratory symptoms may take at least that long [4]. Even esophagitis which has been documented to persist for 12 months or more of treatment in infancy may resolve as the infant becomes a toddler (author's personal experience). A coexisting large hiatal hernia [5,6] or other anatomic defect may prompt earlier surgery including fundoplication. Infants who are particularly likely to manifest symptom intractability during medical therapy of reflux are infants with chronic respiratory disease [7,8] such as bronchopulmonary dysplasia or cystic fibrosis, infants with neurologic disease, infants with other congenital anomalies [7,9] and infants who require gastrostomy feedings [10]. One may reasonably decide after several months of therapy in these patients that the disease is intractable, particularly if the symptoms are producing chronic morbidity. Several groups have attempted to determine whether medical intractability could be predicted by a pH probe study, thus justifying primary surgical therapy. These surgeons have retrospectively identified several parameters of 24-h pH probe monitoring which have "predicted the need for surgery": frequency greater than 34 [11] or ~45 [12] reflux episodes per day, daily reflux duration greater than 27% of the monitored time [13], sleep reflux duration greater than ~4 min/day [14,15] and frequency of prolonged episodes (lasting longer than 5 min) greater than 20 per day [13]. The logic is often circular, however, since the pH probes were considered in the decision for surgery and using the authors' decision that surgery was required as the gold standard is suspect, since some of the authors report a rather large number of patients "requiring" surgery. Other groups studying adults and children have found that the pH probe was a poor predictor of intractability [16–18]. One must conclude, with the group from Salt Lake City, that "the clinical history and the patient's response to medical treatment remain the most important factors in the decision for or against surgery" [15].

Medication dependence generally should not be used as the sole justification for surgery in infants, because of the natural history of infantile reflux to resolve by 2 years of age.

Older children

Success of medical therapy – discontinuing therapy

The natural history of reflux disease in older children is similar to that in adults; unlike most infants, many older children will not achieve persistent resolution of reflux-associated symptoms. However, since some reflux disease does resolve after a course of therapy, even in older children, most reflux disease is initially treated for at least 6–12 weeks, based on the usual course of healing of esophagitis. When such therapy is used empirically. it should not be continued longer than the 6–12 weeks (if the symptoms persist during 3 months of therapy, or return after its discontinuation, endoscopic evaluation is required). If *esophagitis* has been documented prior to starting medical therapy, a longer course of treatment may be used if the symptoms persist and treatment can be discontinued based on symptom resolution.

Symptoms other than esophagitis, such as chronic *respiratory* symptoms (e.g., asthma, recurrent pneumonia, hoarseness), may also be treated with at least 6–12 weeks of therapy; the medications are withdrawn after this period if the symptoms have resolved. Recent evidence in adults suggests that treatment ameliorates the symptoms of esophagitis more rapidly than any associated respiratory symptoms, which may take months to respond and which may require high-dose proton pump therapy [4]. If the symptoms recur when medication is withdrawn, more protracted medical therapy may be required, or surgery may be considered.

Failure of medical therapy – advancing (retreating?) to surgical therapy

Recent work in adults has suggested that primary surgical therapy could be a therapeutic option for severe or complicated esophagitis, with greater efficacy than medical therapy persisting for up to 2 years [19–21]. Analysis has suggested that such an approach is of more benefit to younger adults than to older ones [20] and an age threshold in the sixth decade has been identified. Extrapolating such data, it is possible to conclude that primary surgical therapy might be of even more benefit in older children, particularly since relatively long-term function has been documented for fundoplication [22–25], modulating earlier concerns regarding the stability of fundoplication. The development of laparoscopic techniques may further support early fundoplication for children. Modulating such a conclusion is the possibility that ongoing research will provide new medications which are more effective, safe and economical than those now available, and will allow our pediatric patients to avoid the surgeon's knife.

Symptom hazard can be cited as justification for primary surgical intervention in children with *Barrett's specialized epithelium* [26] and in children with *strictures* [27–29]. Although some experts argue that adults with these findings might be managed without surgery, the anticipated long duration of disease, the concerns about lifetime proton pump use in young children and the probable additional need for preventing duodenogastroesophageal reflux in these settings argue for primary surgery for children with these presentations.

Symptom intractability during therapy is readily justified as a reason for fundoplication in the older child. Children particularly likely to require surgery for this reason are those with chronic or recurrent respiratory symptoms, neurologic disease and provocative anatomic abnormalities such as esophageal atresia or a large hiatal hernia [7,30—33]. Some might even recommend primary fundoplication prior to medical therapy in such children, but primary aggressive medical therapy has several advantages. First, it should help the surgeon by decreasing esophageal inflammation in those patients who will eventually come to surgery. Second, it may allow a few patients to avoid surgery if their symptoms resolve completely and do not recur. Third, intractability of symptoms during aggressive medical therapy should raise concerns that the diagnosis of a reflux-associated symptom might have been incorrect.

For the reasons noted above in support of primary surgical therapy, *medication dependence* may be used more often than in the past to justify surgery in older children. If anticipated requirement for medical therapy in a child is lifelong, the relative efficacy and safety of fundoplication make it a very reasonable alternative. Medication dependence is best used to justify surgery in a child who is at least 18 to 24 months old, who has been treated for at least 3 months and who has been demonstrated to relapse after withdrawal of medication at least once, and preferably twice. Such an irreversible decision should be made in consultation with a family well-informed as to the relative risks and benefits.

References

1. Lambert J, Mobassaleh M, Grand R. Efficacy of cimetidine for gastric acid suppression in pediatric patients. J Pediatr 1992;120:474—478.
2. Jolley SG, Halpern L, Tunell WP, Johnson D, Sterling C. The risk of sudden infant death from gastroesophageal reflux. J Pediatr Surg 1991;26:691—696.
3. Farrell MK, Wolske S, Brocker D. Is surgery required for the infant with gastroesophageal reflux (GER) and apnea? A prospective study. Pediatr Res 1983;17:187A.
4. Kamel P, Kahrilas P, Hanson D, McMahan J, Brenic S. Prospective trial of omeprazole in the treatment of "reflux laryngitis". Gastroenterology 1992;102:A93.
5. Friedland GW, Sunshine P, Zboralske FF. Hiatal hernia in infants and young children: a 2- to 3-year follow-up study. J Pediatr 1975;87:71—74.
6. Cahill J, Aberdeen E, Waterston D. Results of surgical treatment of esophageal hiatal hernia in infancy and childhood. Surgery 1969;66:597—602.
7. Jolley SG, Herbst JJ, Johnson DG, Matlak ME, Book LS. Surgery in children with gastroesophageal reflux and respiratory symptoms. J Pediatr 1980;96:194—198.
8. Guiffre RM, Rubin S, Mitchell I. Antireflux surgery in infants with bronchopulmonary dysplasia. Am J Dis Child 1987;141:648—651.
9. Parker AF, Christie DL, Cahill JL. Incidence and significance of gastroesophageal reflux following repair of esophageal atresia and tracheoesophageal fistula and the need for anti-reflux procedures. J Pediatr Surg 1979;14:5—8.
10. Jolley SG, Smith E, Tunell WP. Protective antireflux operation with feeding gastrostomy. Ann Surg 1985;201:736—740.
11. Evans DF, Haynes J, Jones JA, Stower MJ, Kapila L. Ambulatory esophageal pH monitoring in children as an indicator for surgery. J Pediatr Surg 1986;21:221—223.
12. Ramenofsky ML, Powell RW, Curreri PW. Gastroesophageal reflux. pH probe-directed therapy. Ann Surg 1986;203:531—536.
13. Da Dalt L, Mazzoleni S, Montini G, Donzelli F, Zacchello F. Diagnostic accuracy of pH monitoring in gastro-oesophageal reflux. Arch Dis Child 1989;64:1421—1426.
14. Eizaguirre I, Tovar JA. Predicting preoperatively the outcome of respiratory symptoms of gastroesophageal reflux. J Pediatr Surg 1992;27:848—851.
15. Johnson DG, Jolley SG, Herbst JJ, Cordell LJ. Surgical selection of infants with gastroesophageal reflux. J Pediatr Surg 1981.

16. Olden K, Triadafilopoulos G. Failure of initial 24-h esophageal pH monitoring to predict refractoriness and intractability in reflux esophagitis. Am J Gastroenterol 1991;86:1142—1146.
17. Boesby S, Wallin L, Myrhoit T, Andersen LI. Twelve-hour overnight oesophageal pH monitoring in patients with reflux symptoms. Gut 1991;32:10—11.
18. Tovar JA, Angulo JA, Gorostiaga L, Arana J. Surgery for gastroesophageal reflux in children with normal pH studies. J Pediatr Surg 1991;26:541—545.
19. Spechler SJ, Group at DoVAGRDS. Comparison of medical and surgical therapy for complicated gastroesophageal reflux disease in veterans. N Engl J Med 1992;326:786—792.
20. Richter JE. Surgery for reflux disease — reflections of a gastroenterologist [editorial]. N Engl J Med 1992;326:825—827.
21. Behar J, Sheahan D, Biancani P, Spiro H, Storer E. Medical and surgical management of reflux esophagitis. N Engl J Med 1975;293:263—268.
22. Vos A, Boerema I. Surgical treatment of gastroesophageal reflux in infants and children: long-term results in 28 cases. J Pediatr Surg 1971;6:101—111.
23. Johansson J, Johansson F, Joelsson B, Floren CH, Walther B. Outcome 5 years after 360° fundoplication for gastro-oesophageal reflux disease. Br J Surg 1993;80:46—49.
24. Martinez de Haro L, Ortiz A, Parrilla P, Garcia Marcilla J, Aguayo J, Morales G. Long-term results of Nissen fundoplication in reflux esophagitis without strictures: clinical, endoscopic and pH-metric evaluation. Dig Dis Sci 1992; 37:523—527.
25. Luostarinen M. Nissen fundoplication for reflux esophagitis: long-term clinical and endoscopic results in 109 of 127 consecutive patients. Ann Surg 1993;217:329—337.
26. Hassall E, Weinstein WM. Partial regression of childhood Barrett's esophagus after fundoplication. Am J Gastroenterol 1992;87:1506—1512.
27. Rode H, Millar AJW, Brown RA, Cywes S. Reflux strictures of the esophagus in children. J Pediatr Surg 1992;27:462—465.
28. Nihoul C, Mitrofanoff P, Lortat—Jacob S. Les sténoses peptiques de l'oesophage chez l'enfant. Ann Pediatr 1979;26:692—698.
29. Larrain A, Csendes A, Pope CE II. Surgical correction of reflux: an effective therapy for esophageal strictures. Gastroenterology 1975;69:578—583.
30. Stringel G, Delgado M, Guertin L, Cook JD, Maravilla A, Worthen H. Gastrostomy and Nissen fundoplication in neurologically impaired children. J Pediatr Surg 1989;24:1044—1048.
31. Stringel G. Gastrostomy with antireflux properties. J Pediatr Surg 1990;25:1019—1021.
32. Wilkinson JD, Dudgeon DL, Sondheimer JM. A comparison of medical and surgical treatment of gastroesophageal reflux in severely retarded children. J Pediatr 1981;99:202—205.
33. Byrne WJ, Euler AR, Ashcraft E, Nash DG, Seibert JJ, Golladay ES. Gastroesophageal reflux in the severely retarded who vomit: criteria for and results of surgical intervention in 22 patients. Surgery 1982;91:95—98.

The cylindric mucosa

# What are the defining indices of the esophagogastric junction and the defining criteria for columnar lined esophagus (CLE)?

H.W. Boyce Jr. (Tampa)

Anatomic features of the normal esophagogastric junction

The esophagus in the average adult passes through the diaphragmatic hiatus at approximately 38 cm and joins the stomach near the squamocolumnar junction at about the 40 cm level. The normal level of the squamocolumnar mucosal junction may vary 1 to 2 cm depending on the body habitus, type of endoscope used and the care with which measurements are made. More accurate distance measurements are made on endoscope withdrawal than during insertion because the instrument is in a more straightened position. If minimal air insufflation of the proximal and mid-esophagus is utilized during endoscopy, the closed lower esophageal sphincter (LES) region may be readily demonstrated. At the point of closure of the proximal end of the sphincter, several (usually four to six) longitudinal symmetrical mucosal folds can be seen to disappear in the center of the closed lumen. This closure produces a rosette appearance with the lumen being precisely centered at the point where these longitudinal folds converge. The tone of the LES relaxes with primary or secondary peristalsis and also opens in response to gentle insufflation. As the closed normal esophageal sphincter is approached with the endoscope it will relax with gentle scope pressure and with passage through the sphincter there is little or no detectable resistance. As the high pressure sphincter zone relaxes, one can identify the squamocolumnar mucosal junction 1 to 2 cm beyond and see into the short tubular cavity of the proximal stomach, the cardia. The proximal end of the LES is most easily demonstrated in patients with achalasia because of the dilation of the body of the esophagus and typical hypertonicity of the closed sphincter [1,2].

The level of the hiatal margin is not as readily demonstrated in normal patients as in those who have a hiatal hernia. However, it is possible in most instances to determine the level with relative precision. As the lumen is gently insufflated with air, the patient is asked either to sniff or inhale rapidly, at which time the diaphragmatic hiatal margin moves inferiorly either quickly or gradually depending upon the breathing maneuver used to demonstrate its location. The wall of the esophagogastric junction is slightly indented as the hiatal margin moves distally with a sniff or deep breath.

The squamous mucosa of the esophagus is pearly pink or pinkish-grey in color and contrasts sharply with the orange-red color of the gastric columnar epithelium. The esophageal mucosa is only slightly transparent and reflects light moderately. The gastric mucosa has a glistening surface because of the presence of mucus, but is more transparent and consequently absorbs a great deal of light. For this reason gastric mucosa requires more light for adequate photography.

The junction of the squamous and columnar epithelium appears after minimum inflation as a slightly irregular or undulating line, the so-called ora serrata or "Z" line. With continued inflation pressure, the irregular junction often becomes straight with only minimal serration. This junction normally is located in the distal half of the LES segment at or just below the esophageal diaphragmatic hiatus. This line of demarcation between the two types of mucosa is readily identifiable in the absence of pathologic changes. If there is uncertainty about the location of this mucosal junction, it can be dramatically demonstrated by application of several milliliters of 50% Lugol's solution through an endoscopic catheter [3]. This will stain the glycogen in the esophageal mucosa in about 30 s. In addition to surface characteristics and color, the normal distal extent of the esophageal squamous epithelium is also clearly demarcated by the level of abrupt disappearance of multiple, linear, frequently branching, small blood vessels just proximal to the upper end of the gastric folds of the cardia at the junction of squamous and columnar epithelium.

After the endoscope is passed into the proximal stomach, a retroversion maneuver should be performed to view the cardia and fundus from below. In the normal setting the insertion tube of the endoscope can be seen coming through a snugly fitting intra-abdominal segment of esophagus. The snug fit in this region is sustained throughout respiration and during moderate insufflation of the stomach, except that transient relaxation in response to primary or secondary peristalsis can be detected. The classic snug appearance of the region is nearly always demonstrated in patients with achalasia because of the increased tone in the LES segment. The angle of His on the greater curvature aspect demarcates the distal end of the sphincter region, also called the submerged or abdominal segment of the esophagus. The normally located squamocolumnar mucosal junction cannot be identified radiographically. However, in patients with herniation of the proximal stomach through the diaphragmatic hiatus, a lower esophageal ring may be demonstrated, the location of which corresponds with the level of the intrathoracically displaced squamocolumnar mucosal junction.

Earlier radiographic and anatomic studies have caused much confusion about this area relative to the structures that are seen in normal patients and in patients with hiatal hernias. In an individual with normal anatomy there are no rings, no asymmetrical bulges, no bulbous contour of the distal esophagus, and no displacement of the squamocolumnar mucosal junction greater than 2 cm cephalad to the diaphragmatic hiatus. These alterations are seen only in patients with a hiatal hernia [1,2].

Several linear gastric folds normally are seen in the cardia, especially when a hiatal hernia is present. These folds normally terminate within 0.5 to 1.0 cm of the normal location of the squamocolumnar mucosal junction. Therefore, this termination point of the folds can be utilized endoscopically and radiographically as a marker for the approximate location of the normal squamocolumnar mucosal junction. The cephalad margins of these longitudinal gastric folds correspond to the level of the esophagogastric muscular junction as well. The proximal margins of these folds provide the best endoscopic landmark for the muscular junction between esophagus and stomach and as a marker for the normal location of the squamocolumnar junction. These relationships to the esophagogastric muscular junction can be demonstrated on surgical and autopsy specimens as well.

In some patients with a hiatal hernia and normal LES tone, the esophageal wall in the region of the esophageal sphincter will be closed snugly around the endoscope. Some relaxation may be apparent in relation to primary and secondary peristalsis or after greater degrees of air insufflation. In patients with reflux esophagitis, especially those with a columnar lined esophagus (CLE) who tend to have the lowest sphincter pressures, there is considerable free space around the endoscope in the region of the LES just proximal to the hernia pouch. Patients with a CLE nearly always have a widely patent sphincter region on antegrade and retrograde endoscopy.

When viewing the region of the squamocolumnar junction by retroversion in patients with hiatal hernia and normal sphincter pressure, the closure of the proximal end of the LES can be observed. The point of maximum closure in these cases appears about 1 cm above the squamocolumnar mucosal junction. This level of closure corresponds with the so-called esophageal A-ring or sphincter contraction ring, both in location and contour seen during radiography and antegrade endoscopy.

With a hiatal hernia of moderate or larger size the retroverted endoscope can be pulled back to the level of the diaphragmatic hiatus, or even a short distance into the hernia pouch, thus affording a close-up examination of the hernia pouch and the squamocolumnar mucosal junction from below.

It is important to observe carefully and record the characteristics of the distal esophagus and proximal stomach in all patients. The location of the diaphragmatic hiatus in relation to the proximal stomach, the level of the squamocolumnar mucosal junction and the proximal extent of the gastric mucosal folds in the hernia pouch are characteristics utilized in the precise endoscopic diagnosis of hiatal hernia and reflux sequelae, including the earliest stages of CLE. The levels of these landmarks should be recorded on every esophagoscopy report.

Endoscopic anatomy of the columnar-lined (Barrett's) esophagus

In the past few years so-called Barrett's or columnar lined esophagus (CLE) has been recognized as more common than previously believed [4–7]. Since metaplastic epithelium in CLE is considered premalignant, its early recognition is imperative. It is possible to recognize minimal degrees of columnar lined esophagus based on an understanding of the normal lumenal topographic relationships discussed above. Short segments of CLE appear to have premalignant potential similar to larger segments extending to the proximal esophagus.

CLE rarely, if ever, occurs without both a markedly hypotensive LES and a hiatal hernia. The recognition of this relationship is important for accurate diagnosis. Mucosal biopsies taken from a hernia pouch have resulted in overdiagnosis and confusion in surveillance reports. These problems result from the failure of the endoscopist to understand normal endoscopic anatomy, especially recognition of small sliding hiatus hernias.

The endoscopic features that aid in the diagnosis of CLE include: the location of the cephalad margin of the linear gastric mucosal folds in the ever-present hiatal hernia pouch, the displacement of the squamocolumnar junction greater than 1.0 cm cephalad from these folds, the level of disappearance of the linear esophageal vessels, the patulous LES region and the absence of a lower esophageal Schatzki or "B" ring [1].

Identification of the squamocolumnar mucosal junction in normal patients and in those with the typical CLE is not usually difficult because of differences in mucosal color and texture. The mucosal color in the columnar lined segment is orange-red to red; the color usually is more reddish than normal gastric mucosa and is distinctly different from the pinkish-grey color of normal esophageal squamous mucosa. It may be impossible to precisely locate the squamocolumnar junction in the presence of severe esophagitis or a stricture. Close-up observation of the texture of metaplastic intestinalized columnar mucosa will reveal a pitted or villoid pattern. Several biopsies from areas of suspected columnar metaplasia usually will provide histologic proof of the diagnosis. The exact location of biopsies and the relation of this site to surrounding landmarks should be recorded when the samples are obtained. Normal squamous esophageal mucosa is characterized by a pink-grey smooth surface and many underlying small vessels oriented parallel to the long axis of the lumen. These small vessels disappear at the site of the normal muscular junction between esophagus and stomach, and are not observed when severe inflammation or neoplasm are present. The level where these vessels disappear is another reasonably accurate endoscopic landmark for the level at which the true esophagogastric muscular junction should lie. When the location of the junction remains uncertain, several milliliters of Lugol's solution can be instilled to stain squamous epithelium a brownish-black [3]. Islands of residual squamous epithelium in the columnar-lined segment also are readily identified by this stain.

The squamocolumnar mucosal junction in CLE can vary widely in location and appearance. It often has an undulating appearance with orange-red, finger-like cephalad extensions of metaplastic epithelium between peninsulas of squamous mucosa, the whole junction appearing asymmetrical and interrupted. There is a common tendency to attribute this appearance to esophagitis with erosion alone, when in some cases the orange-red proximally directed streaks are due to metaplastic columnar epithelium at the site of previous healed linear erosions. Areas of metaplastic columnar epithelium rarely contain adherent surface exudate as is typical for erosions. In some patients, islands of metaplastic columnar epithelium surrounded completely by squamous epithelium may be found proximal to the level of the main squamocolumnar junction.

When the squamocolumnar junction is displaced proximally 2 cm or more above the esophageal hiatus, a hiatal hernia is present and one can readily recognize the gastric folds of the gastric cardia that extend through the hiatus. These normal folds begin at a point 0.5 to 1 cm distal to the normal position of the squamocolumnar junction. Excessive air inflation usually obliterates these folds so that their cephalad margins appear to be more distally located than they really are. Since a measurement of 1 cm above the proximal end of the gastric folds indicates the expected site of a normally positioned squamocolumnar mucosal junction in patients with a hiatal hernia, it is easy to determine whether the junction is displaced more proximally as seen with CLE [1,2].

Others believe that CLE should be diagnosed only when the squamocolumnar mucosal junction is located more than 2 cm [8,9] or 3 cm [10,11] proximal to the cephalad margin of the gastric folds. This diagnosis can only be suspected by endoscopic examination, and biopsy confirmation of the presence of specialized epithelium (intestinal metaplasia) is required. Whether one uses the 1 cm, the 2 cm or the 3 cm distance of squamocolumnar mucosal junction location, biopsy proof of specialized columnar epithelium in this segment is required. It seems that a presumptive endoscopic diagnosis and a nondiagnostic biopsy using the 1 cm distance criterion is better than an unsuspected endoscopic diagnosis using the 2 or 3 cm distance criteria for separation of gastric fold margins from mucosal junction. The latter patient would never have had the potential benefit of surveillance. In general, the agreement between endoscopy and histology for diagnosis of CLE has been good. The sensitivity, specificity and accuracy of endoscopy have been shown to be 89%, 93% and 91% respectively [12].

With the use of these endoscopic definitions and landmarks, minimal degrees of metaplastic epithelial change in the distal esophagus can be suspected and confirmed by biopsy. It is, therefore, not necessary to await development of the classic later stages of CLE with squamocolumnar junction dislocation into midesophagus in order to diagnose this condition. CLE of short length often exists in patients with minimal symptoms and will not be diagnosed in such cases if considered only in relation to severe reflux symptoms, proximal esophageal stricture, an esophageal ulcer or a long segment of columnar-lined esophagus.

The endoscopic landmarks and topography described above should be used to avoid missing the diagnosis of CLE. Overdiagnosis occurs when the mucosa in a hiatal hernia pouch is interpreted as being in the tubular esophagus or the presence of an inlet patch in the cervical esophagus is interpreted as CLE. An adequate number of biopsy specimens (preferably with large forceps) and precise histologic interpretation usually prevents misdiagnosis. Underdiagnosis occurs with failure to recognize short segments of columnar mucosa lining the distal esophagus or failure to recognize the lining of most of the esophagus by columnar epithelium, when there is a markedly dislocated squamocolumnar junction as far proximal as the cervical esophagus. This error is more likely when proximal esophagitis and/or stricture are absent and the endoscopist is careless and fails to examine every millimeter of the esophageal mucosa with care.

References

1. Boyce HW. The esophagogastric junction: 25 years looking and learning. ASGE Distinguished Lectureship, May 1984.
2. Boyce HW. Hiatus hernia and peptic diseases of the esophagus. In: Sivak MV (ed) Gastrointestinal Endoscopy. Philadelphia: WB Saunders, 1987;401—418.
3. Nothmann BJ, Wright JR, Schuster MM. In vivo vital staining as an aid to identification of esophagogastric mucosal junction in man. Am J Dig Dis 1972;17:919—924.
4. Naef AP, Savary M, Ozzello L. Columnar-lined lower esophagus: an acquired lesion with malignant predisposition. Report on 140 cases of Barrett's esophagus with 12 adenocarcinomas. J Thorac Cardiovasc Surg 1975;70:826—835.
5. Sjogren RW Jr, Johnson LF. Barrett's esophagus: a review. Am J Med 1983;74:313—321.
6. Herlihy KJ, Orlando RC, Bryson JC, Bozymski EM, Carney CM, Powell DW. Barrett's esophagus: clinical, endoscopic, histologic, manometric and electrical potential difference characteristics. Gastroenterology 1984;86:436—443.
7. Armstrong D, Blum AL, Savary M. Reflux disease and Barrett's esophagus. Endoscopy 1992;24:9—17.
8. Tytgat GNJ, Hameeteman W, Onstenk R, Schotborg R. The spectrum of columnar-lined esophagus — Barrett's esophagus. Endoscopy 1989;21:177—185.
9. Spechler SJ, Goyal RK. Barrett's esophagus. N Engl J Med 1986;315:362—371.
10. Monnier Ph, Fontolliet Ch, Savary M, Ollyo JB. Barrett's esophagus or columnar epithelium of the lower esophagus. Bailliere's Clin Gastroenterol 1987;1:769—789.
11. Dent J, Bremner CG, Collen MJ, Haggitt RC, Spechler SJ. Barrett's oesophagus. Working Party Reports, World Congresses of Gastroenterology 1990:17—26.
12. Woolf GM, Riddell RH, Irvine EJ, Hunt RH. A study to examine agreement between endoscopy and histology for the diagnosis of columnar-lined (Barrett's) esophagus. Gastrointest Endosc 1989;35:541—544.

Epidemiology

 ## Is it possible to specify the prevalence of CLE in esophagitis?

A.J. Cameron (Rochester)

A review of work relevant to this question is complicated by the lack of uniform definition of terms. The length of esophageal columnar mucosa required to diagnose CLE varies from 2 to 5 cm. The presence of intestinal metaplasia may or may not be a criterion. Reflux esophagitis may be defined by either endoscopic findings or histologic changes. Some series were collected retrospectively, and their data base may be less than ideal. Despite these problems, a reasonable answer to the question can be given.

CLE may occur with or without esophagitis. In CLE patients, esophagitis takes the form of inflammation in the squamous mucosa proximal to the CLE. Table 1 shows the proportion of patients with reflux-related esophageal mucosal abnormality that had CLE in six series. CLE was found in 7 to 33% (mean: 12%) of patients with endoscopic evidence of gastroesophageal reflux disease.

The difficulty in specifying the prevalence of CLE in esophagitis is that esophagitis often resolves when treated, but CLE does not. Although antacids alone are not very effective, clinical trials have shown that treatment of reflux esophagitis with H_2 receptor antagonist drugs for 8 to 12 weeks results in healing of esophagitis in about 50% of cases. Treatment with proton pump inhibitor drugs (such as omeprazole) for a similar period can heal esophagitis in about 90% of cases. By contrast, we have shown that the length of CLE usually remains unchanged over years in patients given antacids and H_2 blockers [1], and treatment with omeprazole

Table 1.

Year of publication	Authors	Patients with esophagitis or CLE	Patients with CLE
1975	Naef et al. [2]	1225	140 (11%)
1979	Burbige and Radigan [3]	41	8 (20%
1984	Starnes et al. [4]	439	40 (9%)
1985	Schnell et al. [5]	163	54 (33%)
1986	Rothery et al. [6]	776	58 (7%)
1987	Winters et al. [7]	56	12 (21%)

or lansoprazole for 1 or 2 years causes little [8] or no regression of CLE [9]. Therefore, the relative numbers of patients with esophagitis and CLE in different series may depend on whether previous treatment has been given.

From the epidemiologic standpoint, more useful information is obtained by prospective studies of consecutive patients with gastroesophageal reflux symptoms. The following series were found:

Schnell et al. [5] performed endoscopy in 428 patients with frequent heartburn and regurgitation. Fifty-four (13%) had CLE and 109 (25%) had erosions or ulcer without CLE. Thus, 33% of patients with mucosal changes had CLE.

Winters et al. [7] endoscoped 97 patients with reflux symptoms (heartburn, regurgitation, dysphagia) occurring every week. Twelve patients had CLE (12%) and 44 (45%) had esophagitis without CLE. Thus, 21% of patients with mucosal changes had CLE.

Mann et al. [10] endoscoped 180 male patients with symptoms of reflux esophagitis. CLE was found in 20 (11%). Of interest, the severity of esophagitis was the same in patients with and without CLE. After 6 months of treatment with antacids, cimetidine, and metoclopramide, esophagitis resolved or was much improved, but no regression of CLE was seen.

In summary, the prevalence of CLE in three series of patients endoscoped for symptoms of gastroesophageal reflux was very similar, 11, 12 and 13%. The prevalence of esophagitis without CLE was higher, 25 to 45%. However, the prevalence of CLE is likely to remain stable, whereas the prevalence of esophagitis depends on whether treatment for reflux has been given.

References

1. Cameron AJ, Lomboy CT. Barrett's esophagus: age, prevalence, and extent of columnar epithelium. Gastroenterology 1992;103:1241–1245.
2. Naef AP, Savary M. Columnar-lined esophagus: an acquired lesion with malignant predisposition. J Thor Cardiovasc Surg 1975;70:826–834.
3. Burbige EJ, Radigan JJ. Characteristics of the columnar-cell lined (Barrett's) esophagus. Gastrointest Endosc 1979;25:133–136.
4. Starnes VA, Adkins RB, Ballinger JF et al. Barrett's esophagus. A surgical entity. Arch Surg 1984;119:563–566.
5. Schnell TG, Sontag SJ, Wannier J et al. Endoscopic screening for Barrett's esophagus, esophageal adenocarcinoma and other mucosal changes in ambulatory subjects with symptomatic gastroesophageal reflux. Gastroenterology 1985;88:1576 (Abstract).

6. Rothery GA, Patterson JE, Stoddard CJ et al. Histological and histochemical changes in the columnar-lined (Barrett's) oesophagus. Gut 1986;27:1062–1068.
7. Winters C, Spurling TJ, Chobanian SJ et al. Barrett's esophagus. A prevalent, occult complication of gastroesophageal reflux disease. Gastroenterology 1987;92:118–124.
8. Gore S, Healey CJ, Sutton R et al. Regression of columnar-lined (Barrett's) oesophagus with continuous omeprazole therapy. Gut 1992;33(suppl):S32 (Abstract).
9. Sampliner RE, Mackel C, Jennings D et al. Effect of 12 months of a proton pump inhibitor (lansoprazole) on Barrett's esophagus – a randomized trial. Gastroenterology 1992;102:A157 (Abstract).
10. Mann NS, Tsai MF, Nair PK. Barrett's esophagus in patients with symptomatic reflux esophagitis. Am J Gastroenterol 1989;84:1494–1496.

What is the cell line giving rise to the columnar mucosa?

P.J. Kahrilas (Chicago)

The most severe histologic consequence of chronic gastroesophageal reflux is Barrett's esophagus. Barrett's mucosa is metaplastic columnar epithelium that has replaced the native squamous epithelium thereby providing greater resistance to the effects of gastroesophageal reflux. Cell types encountered in Barrett's mucosa include constituents of gastric, small intestinal and colonic epithelium (e.g., columnar mucus containing cells that stain with PAS; goblet cells that stain with PAS, Alcian blue and mucicarmine; columnar cells with brush borders and a paucity of mucus vacuoles similar to small intestinal absorptive epithelial cells; Paneth cells; parietal cells; chief cells and endocrine cells) [1]. Barrett's mucosa may exhibit a variety of topographic appearances on endoscopic and pathologic examination. It may appear as a circumferential sheet, islands of columnar mucosa interspersed with squamous mucosa, or finger-like projections coming from the squamocolumnar junction. Furthermore, the architecture of the mucosa can include glands with deep and shallow pits as in gastric mucosa and villous structures resembling small intestinal mucosa. A given patient may exhibit one or more histopathologic appearance in either a mosaic [2] or zonal [3] pattern.

The histopathologic pattern of Barrett's epithelium seen in the vast majority of affected adult patients is a distinctive, specialized columnar epithelium with mucus cells, goblet cells and a villous structure. The columnar cells lack intestinal absorptive capabilities or ultrastructural characteristics of true intestinal cells making them an example of incomplete intestinal metaplasia [4]. Less common histopathologic patterns of Barrett's epithelium include: junctional or cardiac-type Barrett's mucosa with a predominantly foveolar surface pattern containing mucus glands and resembling the epithelium of normal gastric cardia, except that it is atrophic, fundic-type which is the only variety of Barrett's epithelium that contains both parietal and chief cells with sparse and atrophic glands, and an indeterminate category which shows a wide spectrum of histopathologic and mucosal features [1]. These cells may secrete hydrochloric acid and pepsin. The glandular structures of the fundic epithelium, however, are sparse and foreshortened, causing it to appear atrophic compared to the normal gastric mucosa.

The origin and pathogenesis of the columnar epithelium lining the distal esophagus have been disputed since the time of their initial description by Barrett [5,6]. Initially, there was dispute as to whether the columnar mucosa was a congenital remnant as a result of incomplete replacement of the columnar epithelium by squamous epithelium during development, or acquired as a result of chronic gastroesophageal reflux. Although the persistence theory may well apply to inlet patches in the proximal esophagus, the overwhelming bulk of evidence supports the notion that columnar epithelium in the distal esophagus represents an acquired condition. Proposed mechanisms for acquisition of Barrett's epithelium are the upward growth of cardiac or gastric epithelium after destruction of the squamous epithelium [7], proliferation of the superficial cardiac glands of the esophagus [8], and replacement of the squamous epithelium by metaplastic epithelium [9–11].

Supportive evidence for the upward growth of cardiac epithelium in the pathogenesis of Barretts' comes from both dogs, in which the distal esophageal mucosa was denuded and allowed to regenerate in the presence of gastroesophageal reflux [7], and observation of humans after esophagogastrostomy [12]. In both instances, the distal esophageal mucosa sometimes regenerates with a columnar mucosa consistent with an upward growth of the junctional epithelium. However, the migration theory of pathogenesis has been effectively rejected by elegant studies of Gillen et al. [13]. In Gillen's experiments, the distal esophagus was again denuded of mucosa, but in this case a ring of squamous epithelium was left intact between the denuded area and the stomach, thereby making migration impossible. Dogs were then divided into five groups: acid reflux, acid and bile reflux, reflux plus cimetidine, no reflux and control. Only dogs in the acid reflux group and the acid plus bile reflux group developed a columnar epithelium in the upper denuded ring suggesting that acid (but not bile) reflux was a necessary condition for the development of a columnar mucosa and proving that the columnar did not arise by migration from the gastric cardia.

Another line of evidence strongly supporting the contention that Barrett's epithelium arises from a progenitor cell that can differentiate into either squamous or columnar epithelium comes from recent attempt to ablate Barrett's using laser photoablation [14,15]. In this study, ablation of the columnar epithelium was attempted in 10 men by first burning it with an argon laser, and then allowing the epithelium to regenerate during concomitant high dose acid suppressive therapy (omeprazole 40 mg q.i.d.). In 38 of 40 treated areas of columnar epithelium, squamous mucosa was partially or completely restored. The best success was achieved in areas that had a squamous border or, best of all, in columnar islands. Thus, there must be progenitor cells within the metaplastic tissue that can differentiate into squamous epithelium, provided that differentiation occurs in a neutral as opposed to an acid environment. As in other body tissues, Barrett's appears to be a reversible metaplastic change.

References

1. Hamilton SR. Reflux esophagitis and Barrett esophagus. Monogr Pathol 1990;31:11.
2. Thompson JJ, Zinsser KR, Enterline HT. Barrett's metaplasia and adenocarcinoma of the esophagus and gastroesophageal junction. Hum Pathol 1983;14:42–61.
3. Paull A, Trier JS, Dalton MD, Camp RC, Loeb P, Goyal RK. The histologic spectrum of Barrett's esophagus. N Engl J Med 1976;295:476–480.
4. Rothery GA, Patterson JE, Stoddard CL, Day DW. Histologic and histochemical changes in the columnar-lined Barrett's esophagus. Gut 1986;27:1062–1068.
5. Barrett NR. Chronic peptic ulcer of the oesophagus and "oesophagitis". Br J Surg 1950:38:175–182.
6. Barrett NR. The lower esophagus lined by columnar epithelium. Surgery 1957:41:881–894.
7. Bremner CG, Lynch VP, Ellis FH Jr. Barrett's esophagus: congenital or acquired? An experimental study of esophageal mucosal regeneration in the dog. Surgery 1970:68:209–216.
8. Adler RH. The lower esophagus lined by columnar epithelium. Its association with hiatal hernia, ulcer, stricture and tumor. J Thorac Cardiovasc Surg 1963:45:13–34.
9. Hayward J. The lower end of the esophagus. Thorax 1961:16:36–41.
10. Berenson MM, Herbst JJ, Freston JW. Enzyme and ultrastructural characteristics of esophageal columnar epithelium. Am J Dig Dis 1974:19:895–907.
11. Berenson MM, Herbst JJ, Freston JW. Esophageal columnar epithelial β-galactosidase and β-glucuronidase. Gastroenterology 1975:68:1417–1420.
12. Hamilton SR, Yardley JH. Regeneration of cardiac type mucosa and acquisition of Barrett mucosa after esophagogastrostomy. Gastroenterology 1977:72:669–675.
13. Gillen P, Keeling P, Byrne PJ, West AB, Hennessy TPJ. Experimental columnar metaplasia in the canine oesophagus. Br J Surg 1988:75:113–115.
14. Berenson MM, Johnson TD, Markowitz NR, Buchi KM, Samowitz WS. Restoration of squamous mucosa after ablation of Barrett's esophageal epithelium. Gastroenterology 1993;104:1686–1691.
15. Spechler SJ. Laser photoablation of Barrett's epithelium: burning issues about burning tissues. Gastroenterology 1993:104:1855–1858.

What is the prevalence of Barrett's mucosa in children and young adults? Do these groups carry particular risk factors?

E. Hassall (Vancouver)

It has been estimated that the prevalence of Barrett's esophagus (BE) in children is 13% of those with reflux esophagitis [1]. However, in that study, only two of the 13 "children" described (one of the two was 19 years of age) had specialized Barrett's mucosa with goblet cell metaplasia. Based on our experience at BC Children's Hospital over the last 9 years, I estimate the prevalence of bona fide BE to be less than 2% of children presenting with symptoms of gastroesophageal reflux (GER) or reflux esophagitis.

Of the small number of children with BE, those at higher risk for developing BE are children with neurologic impairment [2], or cystic fibrosis (CF) [3]. Both of these conditions predispose to severe, chronic GER, which is often silent. In both conditions, and in children without these conditions who develop BE, hiatal hernia is present in the majority.

Neurologically impaired children may have one or more of many mechanisms which predispose them to pathologic GER, such as esophageal and gastroduodenal dysmotility, delayed gastric emptying, hiatal hernia, kyphoscoliosis, body casts and prolonged recumbency. When reflux does occur, it is often silent, as central nervous system problems such as severe cerebral palsy and/or mental retardation make verbal or motor responses to esophageal symptoms difficult, subtle, nonspecific or absent [4]. Such children may be apparently asymptomatic or present with "feeding problems"/gagging/recurrent cough, which are often attributed to this underlying neurologic problem alone. Thus, chronic GER in these children often goes unrecognized until presenting with a complication. One recent study showed that mental retardation per se was an independent risk factor for the development of Barrett's esophagus in children and young adults [2]. Another study identified BE in seven of 27 institutionalized adults, but found no higher rate in spastic than in ambulatory patients [5]. Neurologic handicap was present in at least three of nine children and young adults under 25 years of age who presented with adenocarcinoma in a Barrett's esophagus [6].

Due to several pathogenetic mechanisms, children with CF also have a marked predilection to develop pathologic GER [7–9]. In one study [10], 26.5% of CF patients older than 5 years of age reported gastrointestinal symptoms suggestive of reflux (heartburn or regurgitation) compared with only 5.6% of their normal siblings. However, intraesophageal pH studies in CF patients detect a much higher prevalence of pathologic GER [7,11,12], i.e., reflux is silent in the majority of CF patients. Reflux may be silent because gastrointestinal (GI) symptoms may be truly absent, or these symptoms might be relatively ignored by CF patients because of their plethora of other problems. Many patients with CF may consider upper GI symptoms (e.g., heartburn, chest pain, occasional vomiting) as "part of CF" and therefore not report them [3]. Reflux may also cause or contribute to pulmonary disease without causing GI symptoms [8,13] and in CF patients this may go unrecognized in many patients because of their pre-existing pulmonary disease.

Only recently has CF been described as a risk factor for BE [3]. With the high prevalence of pathologic reflux in CF patients, it is surprising that BE had not previously been described in CF. Perhaps BE is truly extremely rare in CF because Barrett's specialized metaplasia takes some years to develop in response to chronic, severe GER [14,15] and the life span of CF patients is relatively short. However, BE does occur in children with chronic, severe reflux, and the median life span in CF has doubled from 14 to 28 years between 1969 and 1990 [16], i.e., ample life span for BE to occur and be detected. A more plausible explanation is that cases of BE are being missed in children and young adults with CF. A likely reason for this is reflected in the literature which shows an apparent reluctance to perform detailed endoscopy with documentation of landmarks and multiple esophageal biopsies in patients with CF. In most reports of esophageal disease in CF, the diagnosis of esophagitis has been made by inference without endoscopy [7,17–19], or by naked eye endoscopy without multiple biopsies [17,18,20]. Similar comments regarding reluctance to perform endoscopy with biopsies apply to neurologically handicapped children.

It is well recognized that Barrett's mucosa shows decreased pain sensitivity compared with that of esophageal squamous mucosa, hence the predilection for late presentation of BE, i.e., with complications. In children with CF or neurologic impairment, the silence of the pathologic reflux itself makes these groups doubly at risk for having reflux missed.

While Barrett's esophagus carries its own morbidity and implications, in CF and the neurologically impaired, its additional importance is that it is a marker for particularly severe reflux which may exacerbate the nutritional and pulmonary problems of both these groups of patients.

Children with CF should be closely questioned for the presence of upper GI symptoms. Patients with even apparently mild symptoms should undergo upper GI endoscopy with documentation of landmarks, multiple biopsies and recording of the sites of origin of biopsies relative to the landmarks. Similarly, handicapped children may benefit from sensitive vigilance and earlier diagnostic studies. Both groups stand to benefit from earlier diagnosis of GER and of Barrett's esophagus, since effective medical and surgical treatment of reflux is available [21,22].

Another group of children who may be at risk for development of BE are those with a positive family history of proven BE, based on anecdotal reports of families with BE [15]. However, the magnitude of this risk is as yet not quantifiable, as there are no extensive studies screening the offspring of affected parents.

References

1. Dahms BB, Rothstein FC. Barrett's esophagus in children: a consequence of chronic gastroesophageal reflux. Gastro-enterology 1984;86:318—323.
2. Snyder JD, Goldman H. Barrett's esophagus in children and young adults. Frequent association with mental retardation. Dig Dis Sci 1990;10:1185—1189.
3. Hassall E, Israel DM, Davidson AGF, Wong LTK. Barrett's esophagus in children with cystic fibrosis: not a coincidental association. Am J Gastroenterol 1993;88:1934—1938.
4. Byrne WJ, Campbell M, Ashcroft E et al. A diagnostic approach to vomiting in severely retarded patients. Am J Dis Child 1983;137:259—262.
5. Roberts IM, Curtis RL, Madara JL. Gastroesophageal reflux and Barrett's esophagus in developmentally disabled patients. Am J Gastroenterol 1986;81;519—523.
6. Hassall E, Dimmick JE, Magee JF. Adenocarcinoma in childhood Barrett's esophagus. Case documentation and the need for surveillance in children. Am J Gastroenterol 1993;88:282—288.
7. Cucchiara S, Santamaria F, Andreotti MR et al. Mechanisms of gastroesophageal reflux in cystic fibrosis. Arch Dis Child 1991;66:617—622.
8. Orenstein SR, Orenstein DM. Gastroesophageal reflux and respiratory disease in children. J Pediatr 1988;112:847—858.
9. Vandenplas Y, Diericx A, Blecker U et al. Esophageal pH monitoring data during chest physiotherapy. J Pediatr Gastroenterol Nutr 1991,13.23—26.
10. Scott RB, O'Loughlin EV, Gall DG. Gastroesophageal reflux in patients with cystic fibrosis. J Pediatr 1985;106:223—227.
11. Dab I, Malfroot A. Gastroesophageal reflux: a primary defect in cystic fibrosis? Scand J Gastroenterol 1988;23(suppl 143): 125—131.
12. Malfroot A, Dab I. New insights on gastroesophageal reflux in cystic fibrosis by longitudinal follow-up. Arch Dis Child 1991;66:1339—1345.
13. Boyle JT, Tuchman DN, Altschuler SM et al. Mechanisms for the association of gastroesophageal reflux and bronchospasm. Am Rev Respir Dis 1985:13(suppl):S516—520.
14. Hassall E. Barrett's esophagus: new definitions and approaches in children. J Pediatr Gastroenterol Nutr 1993;16:345—364.
15. Hassall E. Barrett's esophagus: congenital or acquired? Am J Gastroenterol 1993;88:819—824.
16. Fitzsimmons SC. The changing epidemiology of cystic fibrosis. J Pediatr 1993;122:1—9.
17. Vinocur CD, Marmon L, Schidlow DV, Weintraub WH. Gastroesophageal reflux in the infant with cystic fibrosis. Am J Surg 1985;149:182—186.

18. Bendig DW, Wagner ML, Gunyon MH. Complications of gastroesophageal reflux in patients with cystic fibrosis. J Pediatr 1982;100:536–540.
19. Stringer DA, Sprigg A, Juodis E et al. The association of cystic fibrosis, gastroesophageal reflux and reduced pulmonary function. J Can Assoc Radiol 1988;39:100–102.
20. Feigelson J, Girault F, Pecau Y. Gastroesophageal reflux and esophagitis in cystic fibrosis. Acta Paediatr Scand 1987;76:989–990.
21. Hassall E, Weinstein WM. Partial regression of childhood Barrett's esophagus after fundoplication. Am J Gastroenterol 1992;87:1506–1512.
22. Gunasekaran TS, Hassall E. Efficacy and safety of omeprazole for severe gastroesophageal reflux in children. J Pediatr 1993;123:148–154.

Does Barrett's mucosa develop in children not suffering from reflux?

E. Hassall (Vancouver)

In 1976, Borrie and Goldwater proposed a congenital etiology for BE in children and an acquired etiology in adults [1], based on their finding of a bimodal distribution of patients — a group 0–10 years and a group over 40 years of age. However, their youngest patient with columnar mucosa (of unspecified nature) on biopsy was 11 years old, therefore the accuracy of diagnosis and conclusions regarding their under 10-year-olds is questionable.

Since that proposal, other evidence has been cited in support of a congenital etiology. One newborn in an autopsy study [2] was found to have an esophagus "completely lined with columnar epithelium except for two tiny patches of squamous epithelium", however, the type of columnar epithelium was not specified, as in a previous study [3], it was likely ciliated columnar epithelium which had not yet desquamated. There is no evidence it was Barrett's specialized epithelium. Further evidence against a purely congenital etiology is that BE has not been found in any autopsy study of neonates [2–4]. The occurrence of BE in very young children could suggest a congenital cause, however, claims of BE occurring in children under 5 years of age [5–7] are not supported by adequate documentation [8], all cases have been single biopsy diagnoses without specialized epithelium. The mere occurrence of BE in children [5,6,9,10] is not supportive of a purely congenital cause, as in all well-documented childhood cases of BE, chronic severe GE reflux has been present. Similarly, the presence per se of a total columnar-lined esophagus in an adult [11] is not supportive as the patient had a hiatal hernia and longstanding reflux. An interesting report [12] was that of a 14-month-old child with a bleeding, penetrating giant ulcer in the distal esophagus. The ulcer had gastric mucosa at the margins and was surrounded by squamous mucosa. The authors concluded that this was a congenital Barrett's ulcer but specialized mucosa was not present. Rather, it may represent congenital gastric heterotopia of the esophagus, with an unusual course analogous to Meckels diverticulum. Thus, most of the evidence for a purely congenital etiology can be refuted.

That genetic factors may play a role is illustrated by the occurrence of BE in several families [13]. However, GE reflux was present in all cases. Due to these cases, an autosomal dominant inheritance has been proposed, however, it is unclear whether it is Barrett's epithelium or GE reflux that might be inherited [14,15]. In any case, the overwhelming number of patients with BE has no family history of such, therefore it is necessary to consider etiologies other than purely genetic for the majority of cases.

In contrast there is voluminous and compelling evidence to implicate GE reflux as the usual inciting and ongoing injurious factor in the pathogenesis of BE [13,16]. A severe injury and an abnormal chemical environment (continued exposure to refluxate) during repair, might result in BE. That BE is a purely congenital disorder in some patients is unsupported by any evidence, but a congenital component cannot be entirely ruled out. This factor might explain the development of BE in only some persons with reflux.

This question also raises the issue of the development of BE due to other injuries (e.g., following mucositis due to chemotherapy). Barrett's esophagus has been described at autopsy in three children who had received chemotherapy for leukemia [17]. One child had the lower one-third of esophagus occupied by fundic gland mucosa, another had 4 cm of fundic gland mucosa distally, and the third child had 4 cm of mixed fundic and cardiac gland mucosa. In another study of 16 women who underwent chemotherapy for breast cancer [18], nine had the Z-line displaced 4–9 cm proximally, but columnar mucosa was present in biopsies ≥ 4 cm in only six patients. Of these six patients only three had "intestinal type" mucosa, which was not further described.

While the children [17] might not meet current criteria for BE and only three of the adults may have developed BE [18], the concept that some form of columnar metaplasia may develop after chemotherapy is intriguing. It does fit with one hypothesis of pathogenesis of BE, that is, severe mucosal injury (in this case, mucositis) healing abnormally in an injurious milieu, i.e., acid or alkaline reflux. While reflux was not documented in these studies [17,18], it is recognized that cancer patients undergoing chemotherapy often have delayed gastric emptying, nausea, vomiting and esophagitis, i.e., some of these patients may have de novo or transient pathologic reflux due to their cancer or cancer therapy.

However, the implication of these studies that BE often follows cytotoxic therapy, has been challenged by a recent report in which none of 15 women receiving chemotherapy for breast cancer developed BE [19]. In Sartori's study [18], endoscopy had been performed before chemotherapy and 1 month after the completion of 6 months of chemotherapy. In a more recent report [19], follow-up endoscopy was done at a mean of 31 months after completion of chemotherapy. It is possible that columnar metaplasia developed during treatment, then regressed in the 2.5 years after treatment ended.

One may conclude that, at present, there is little evidence to support a solely nonreflux etiology of BE in children.

References

1. Borrie J, Goldwater L. Columnar cell-lined esophagus: assessment of etiology and treatment. A 22-year experience. J Thorac Cardiovasc Surg 1976;71:825−834.
2. Postlethwait RW, Musser AW. Changes in the esophagus in 1,000 autopsy specimens. J Thorac Cardiovasc Surg 1974;31: 285−294.
3. Rector LE, Connerley ML. Aberrant mucosa in the esophagus in infants and in children. Arch Pathol 1941;31:285−294.
4. de la Pava S, Pickren JW, Adler RH. Ectopic gastric mucosa of the esophagus. A study on histogenesis. NY State J Med 1964;65:1831−1835.
5. Dahms BB, Rothstein FC. Barrett's esophagus in children: a consequence of chronic gastroesophageal reflux. Gastroenterology 1984;86:318−323.
6. Cheu HW, Grosfeld JL, Heifetz SA et al. Persistence of Barrett's esophagus in children after antireflux surgery: influence on follow-up care. J Pediatr Surg 1992;27:260−266.
7. Conti Nibali S, Barresi G, Tuccari G et al. Barrett's esophagus in an infant: a long-standing history with final postsurgical regression. J Pediatr Gastroenterol Nutr 1988;7:602−607.
8. Hassall E, Dimmick JE. Absence or regression of Barrett's esophagus. J Pediatr Gastroenterol Nutr 1989;8:544−545.
9. Hassall E, Weinstein WM, Ament ME. Barrett's esophagus in childhood. Gastroenterology 1985;89:1331−1337.
10. Snyder JD, Goldman H. Barrett's esophagus in children and young adults. Frequent association with mental retardation. Dig Dis Sci 1990;10:1185−1189.
11. Haque AK, Merkel M. Total columnar-lined esophagus: a case for congenital origin? Arch Pathol Lab Med 1981;105: 546−548.
12. Heydenrych JJ, Keet AD. Giant lower oesophageal ulcer in a Bushman baby. S Afr Med J 1983;63:331−333.
13. Hassall E. Barrett's esophagus: congenital or acquired? Am J Gastroenterol 1993;88:819−824.
14. Everhart CW, Holtzapple PG, Humphries TJ. Barrett's esophagus: inherited epithelium or inherited reflux? J Clin Gastroenterol 1983;5:357−360.
15. Cameron AJ. Barrett's esophagus and adenocarcinoma: from the family to the gene. Gastroenterology 1992;102:1421−1424.
16. Hamilton SR. Pathogenesis of columnar cell-lined (Barrett's) esophagus. In: Spechler SJ, Goyal RK (eds) Barrett's Esophagus: Pathophysiology, Diagnosis and Management. New York: Elsevier Science, 1985:29−37.
17. Dahms BB, Greco MA, Strandjord SE, Rothstein EC. Barrett's esophagus in three children after antileukemia chemotherapy. Cancer 1987;60:2896−2900.
18. Satori S, Nielsen I, Indelli M et al. Barrett's esophagus after chemotherapy with cyclophosphamide, methotrexate and 5-fluorouracil (CMF): an iatrogenic injury? Ann Int Med 1991;114:210−211.
19. Herrera JL, Uzel C, Martino R et al. Barrett's esophagus: lack of association with adjuvant chemotherapy. Gastrointest Endosc 1992;38:551−553.

What factors suggest a genetic origin for this disorder?

S.J. Sontag (Hines, Illinois)

More than 40 years since Barrett made the original observation of the disease named after him, the etiology of Barrett's esophagus remains an enigma. Based on 22 years of experience, Borrie and Goldwater [1] proposed that Barrett's esophagus in children was congenital and in adults was acquired. They suggested a bimodal distribution consisting of a 0 to 10-year-old group and a group 40 years and older. Unfortunately, the investigators had no patients under the age of 11 to support their proposal.

A number of reports suggest that Barrett's esophagus may be genetic in origin. Gelfand reported Barrett's esophagus in identical female twins in their sixties [2]. Crabb reported Barrett's esophagus in an 80-year-old male, his son and his two daughters [3]. Everhart reported a 40-year-old male and his two teenage sons, all of whom had Barrett's esophagus [4]. Jochem reported Barrett's esophagus in six males over 3 generations in one family [5]. The distribution of Barrett's epithelium in these cases suggests a genetic autosomal dominant inheritance. It has been suggested by several authors that the gastroesophageal (GE) reflux, not the Barrett's epithelium, is the condition that is inherited [6,7].

The belief that gastric columnar epithelium in the tubular esophagus has a congenital (existing at birth) component has been difficult to support. Up until 17 weeks of gestation, the embryological esophagus is lined with ciliated columnar epithelium. At about this time, a small focus of squamous epithelium, which appears in the columnar epithelium at the level of the midesophagus, begins to migrate proximally and distally [8]. By 40 weeks gestation, the original columnar lined esophagus should be completely replaced by squamous epithelium. If Barrett's epithelium were truly congenital, one would expect to find newborn infants and very young children with specialized columnar or gastric epithelium in the distal esophagus. Such findings have not been reported in autopsy studies of neonates [9]. In addition, Barrett's esophagus with specialized columnar epithelium occurs rarely in young children. In six studies of children with Barrett's esophagus, comprising more than 1500 children, specialized columnar epithelium was documented in only 34 — the youngest of which was 5 years old [10–15].

It is likely, therefore, that Barrett's epithelium results from congenital GE reflux. We propose the following sequence of events to explain the development of squamous esophagitis in some individuals and Barrett's epithelium in others and the finding of gastric epithelium in younger children and specialized columnar epithelium in adults. Our hypothesis is as follows: 1) an incompetent antireflux barrier at the GE junction is a congenital condition that occurs as a result of incomplete development due to premature birth; 2) subsequent acid reflux may cause either squamous esophagitis or the development of Barrett's epithelium, depending on how much squamous epithelial replacement of the embryonic columnar epithelium had occurred in utero. If squamous epithelium had not completely replaced the columnar epithelium, then an incomplete squamocolumnar junction will be present along with the congenital GE reflux. In such a case, biopsy of the distal esophagus in the area of columnar epithelium during early childhood may reveal gastric-type of epithelium; 3) as reflux worsens, however, and bile becomes a component of the acid reflux, the pleuripotential cell may differentiate into specialized columnar epithelium. On the other hand, if the squamocolumnar junction has been completed at birth, despite the presence of congenitally-acquired GE reflux, squamous esophagitis will be the result of the chronic acid injury. Such a scenario might explain why junctional and fundic epithelium are found so frequently in younger patients with reflux, whereas specialized columnar epithelium is reserved for older children and adults. It is possible that the change from gastric epithelium to specialized epithelium requires years of reflux in addition to the presence of bile in the refluxate. It is not known why some patients with Barrett's esophagus go on to develop adenocarcinoma while the vast majority do not.

Prevalence of Barrett's in children

A number of authors have attempted to define the prevalence of Barrett's esophagus in the pediatric population [10–15]. Unfortunately, these studies give little insight into the true prevalence of Barrett's esophagus in children. For example, most of the studies were retrospective, the sites of biopsies often were haphazard and not planned and most of the biopsies were taken at least 2 cm proximal to the visual GE junction, which would easily miss all the children with short segment Barrett's. Furthermore, the method used to report the prevalence of Barrett's was incorrect: the ratio of specialized columnar epithelium patients to total columnar epithelium patients was used to report the prevalence of Barrett's, rather than the ratio of specialized columnar patients to the total pediatric population undergoing endoscopy. Thus the prevalence of specialized columnar, which ranges from less than 1.0 to 5%, is based on a total of only 34 children with specialized columnar epithelium. The true number of patients with Barrett's may have been overestimated (due to the use of an inappropriately low total number of patients at risk) or underestimated (due to sampling errors immediately above the gastroesophageal junction). These studies, however, do suggest that specialized columnar epithelium in children is rare.

In conclusion, genetic factors may possibly be involved in some cases of Barrett's esophagus, probably as an autosomal dominant factor, but genetic factors as a major cause of Barrett's cannot be supported or refuted based on the available data. Most of the available data suggest that GE reflux is congenital. Finally, the apparently lower prevalence of Barrett's in children and higher prevalence in adults suggest that Barrett's esophagus is acquired as a result of the congenital GE reflux.

References

1. Borrie J, Goldwater L. Columnar cell-lined esophagus: assessment of etiology and treatment. A 22-year experience. J Thorac Cardiovasc Surg 1976;71:825–834.
2. Gelfand MD. Barrett's esophagus in sexagenarian identical twins. J Clin Gastroenterol 1983;5:251–253.
3. Crabb DW, Berk MA, Hall TR et al. Familial gastroesophageal reflux and development of Barrett's esophagus. Ann Intern Med 1985;103:52–54.
4. Everhart CW, Holtzapple PG, Humphries TJ. Occurrence of Barrett's esophagus in three members of the same family: first report of familial incidence. Gastroenterology 1978;74:1032A.
5. Jochem VJ, Fuerst PA, Fromkes JJ. Familial Barrett's esophagus associated with adenocarcinoma. Gastroenterology 1992;102:1400–1402.
6. Everhart CW, Holtzapple PG, Humphries TJ. Barrett's esophagus: inherited epithelium or inherited reflux? J Clin Gastroenterol 1983;5:357–360.
7. Cameron AJ. Barrett's esophagus and adenocarcinoma: from the family to the gene. Gastroenterology 1992;102:1421–1424.
8. Johns BAE. Developmental changes in the oesophageal epithelium in man. J Anat 1952;86:431–439.
9. Rector LE, Connerley ML. Aberant mucosa in the esophagus in infants and children. Arch Pathol Lab Med 1941;31:285–294.
10. Dahms BB, Rothstein FC. Barrett's esophagus in children: a consequence of chronic gastroesophageal reflux. Gastroenterology 1984;86:318–323.
11. Hassall E, Weinstein WM, Ament ME. Barrett's esophagus in childhood. Gastroenterology 1985;89:1331–1337.

12. Cooper JE, Spitz L, Wilkins BM. Barrett's esophagus in children: a histologic and histochemical study of 11 cases. J Pediatr Surg 1987;22:191—196.
13. Snyder JD, Goldman H. Barrett's esophagus in children and young adults. Frequent association with mental retardation. Dig Dis Sci 1990;10:1185—1189.
14. Qualman SJ, Murray RD, McClung J et al. Intestinal metaplasia is age related in Barrett's esophagus. Arch Pathol Lab Med 1990;114:1236—1240.
15. Cheu HW, Grosfeld JL, Heifetz SA et al. Persistence of Barrett's esophagus in children after antireflux surgery: influence of follow-up care. J Pediatr Surg 1992;27:260—266.

What are the endoscopic criteria for diagnosing columnar metaplasia?

G.N.J. Tytgat (Amsterdam)

A columnar-lined esophagus develops when damaged squamous mucosa in the distal esophagus is replaced by metaplastic columnar mucosa [1]. Usually, gastroesophageal reflux is the factor that injures the squamous mucosa.

Presumably columnar mucosa often develops to its full extent in a short period of time, usually many years before the abnormality is discovered. In all probability the process of columnar metaplasia does not progress substantially in time after the initial injurious episode [2].

Definition of esophageal columnar metaplasia or Barrett's esophagus

Esophageal columnar metaplastic mucosa consists of one or any combination of three types of columnar epithelia: 1) gastric fundic type epithelium, characterized by surface mucus cells and adjacent parietal and chief cells; 2) junctional type epithelium, with mucus secreting cells similar to the normal cardiac epithelium; and 3) specialized columnar epithelium, which is a variant of incomplete intestinal metaplasia [3]. It is the latter specialized epithelium that appears associated with the development of dysplasia and carcinoma. Therefore, there is an increasing trend to consider the presence of specialized epithelium as the sole criterion for the diagnosis of Barrett's esophagus. In practice, only histology allows the identification of

795

specialized metaplasia. Since its distribution may be patchy, it is recommended to take biopsies every 2 cm from all quadrants of the columnar-lined segment.

The columnar mucosa is probably derived from either the esophageal submucosal glands, the gastric cardia or possibly residual pluripotent stem cells located in the basal area of the squamous epithelium.

The definition of esophageal columnar metaplasia, or Barrett's esophagus, is somewhat controversial. The endoscopic diagnosis may be problematic in part because of difficulties in localizing accurately the esophagogastric junction. Theoretically, the squamocolumnar mucosal junction, or Z-line, or *ora serrata*, should coincide with the esophagogastric junction at the lower border of the lower esophageal sphincter. The esophagogastric junction is identified endoscopically as the proximal extent of the gastric folds. However, even in normal individuals, the distal 2—3 cm of the esophagus may be lined, in whole or in part, by columnar epithelium. Therefore, most authors feel that columnar metaplasia should be diagnosed only when the squamocolumnar mucosal junction is situated more than 2—3 cm proximal to the proximal extent of the gastric folds, regardless of the subtype of epithelium which is present [4,5]. Obviously the question should be raised of what constitutes so-called "short segment Barrett's esophagus", consisting of short tongues or patches of columnar mucosa in the very distal segment [4,6]. When such limited columnar epithelium is of the "distinctive", or "specialized", or "intestinal" type, the diagnosis of esophageal columnar metaplasia is also appropriate.

If one uses as definition: the presence of "specialized" columnar epithelium containing goblet cells etc. instead of the definition of the presence of more than 3 cm of columnar epithelium, then the prevalence rates are slightly higher because of the inclusion of patients with short segments of columnar metaplasia.

Columnar metaplasia is easily recognized endoscopically with the salmon pink columnar mucosa contrasting sharply with the paler esophageal squamous epithelium. The upper margin may be accurately defined, and regular or irregular with many tiny islands of remaining squamous mucosa scattered throughout. As the upper margin is often grossly irregular, measurement of its length can be difficult with no generally agreed points of measurement. The proximal margins of the gastric folds provide the only reliable endoscopic landmark for identifying the junction of the muscular wall of the esophagus and the stomach [4,7,8].

The proximal extent of the gastric folds should serve as a fixed reproducible anatomic landmark whose distance from the incisor teeth should not vary from one endoscopy to the next. The squamocolumnar mucosal junction is normally located within 2 cm of the proximal extent of the gastric folds.

Appearance of the displaced squamocolumnar mucosal transitional area

The squamocolumnar mucosal junction is readily seen because of the contrast between the pearly white or pinkish squamous mucosa and the redder columnar mucosa. The mucosal junction may be relatively straight, but more commonly the junction is rather irregular with tongues or fingers or flame-like extensions. Often small patches of squamous mucosa are scattered around the squamocolumnar junction, the so-called "island type" [9,10]. A rather straight line is said to occur more often in congenital metaplasia, whereas the island type is more common in reflux-induced metaplasia.

Endoscopic appearance of the columnar mucosa

To the astute endoscopist it may be readily obvious that the mucosal appearance at the esophagogastric junction differs from the mucosa covering the gastric hiatal hernia. There is a different degree of shininess, and usually a slightly minor degree of pinkish coloration.

Columnar epithelium typically has a velvety surface and a salmon pink appearance. Not uncommonly, tiny remaining patches of squamous mucosa indicate the level of the original squamocolumnar mucosal junction. The metaplastic columnar epithelium is usually readily recognized endoscopically, the salmon-pink velvety-like appearance contrasting with the more pearly whitish squamous mucosa. Occasionally the appearances of the columnar segment may, however, be quite variable. Sometimes the mucosa is completely smooth and glistening. Sometimes there are irregularities in color, with patches of erythema and zones of white scarring. Also punctate erythema and a somewhat reticulated or pitted appearance may be visible, resembling the appearance of the corpus mucosa in the stomach [11,12]. Sometimes the appearance resembles that of atrophic gastritis, the vascular pattern being visible through the transparent mucosal layer. Occasionally there is conspicuous accentuation of the vascular pattern, especially of the level of the original gastroesophageal junction. In other patients the mucosal relief is slightly uneven, finely nodular and almost "mammillary" in appearance.

Ulceration is not uncommon within the columnar-lined segment. Often the ulcers are rather superficial and whitish in appearance. Barrett ulcers may be either single or multiple. Occasionally there is evidence of extensive ulceration. Most often Barrett ulcers are present in the distal part of the columnar segment. Complications of Barrett ulcers are bleeding and, rarely, perforation. Not uncommonly, areas of linear or intertwining lines of scarring are seen within the Barrett segment, presumably representing scarring following prior ulceration.

Concluding remarks

Endoscopy and multiple biopsies are of vital importance in diagnosing esophageal columnar metaplasia. Unequivocal discovery of the proximal extent of the gastric folds and of the displaced squamocolumnar mucosal junction are essential elements for correct diagnosis. Short segment columnar metaplasia requires the histologic demonstration of "specialized" or "intestinal" type columnar epithelium.

References

1. Spechler SJ, Goyal RK. Barrett's esophagus. N Engl J Med 1986;315:362–371.
2. Cameron AJ, Lomboy CT. Barrett's esophagus: age, prevalence and extent of columnar epithelium. Gastroenterology 1992;103:1241–1245.
3. Paull A, Trier JS, Dalton MD, Camp RC, Loeb P, Goyal RK. The histologic spectrum of Barrett's esophagus. N Engl J Med 1976;295:476–480.
4. Tytgat GNJ, Hameeteman W, Onstenk R, Schotborg R. The spectrum of columnar-lined esophagus – Barrett's esophagus. Endoscopy 1989;21:177–185.
5. Dent J, Bremner CG, Collen MJ, Haggitt RC, Spechler SJ. Barrett's oesophagus. J Gastroenterol Hepatol 1991;6:1–22.
6. Schnell TG, Sontag SJ, Chejfer G. Adenocarcinomas arising in tongues or short segments of Barrett's esophagus. Dig Dis Sci 1992;37:137–143.
7. McClave SA, Boyce HW, Gottfried MR. Early diagnosis of columnar-lined esophagus: a new endoscopic diagnostic criterion. Gastrointest Endosc 1987;33:413.
8. Tytgat GNJ. Endoscopic diagnosis of columnar-lined esophagus. Motility 1989;7:14–15.
9. Monnier Ph, Savary M. Contribution of endoscopy to gastro-oesophageal reflux disease. Scand J Gastroenterol 1984;19:26.
10. Monnier Ph, Fontolliet Ch, Savary M, Ollyo JB. Barrett's oesophagus or columnar epithelium of the lower oesophagus. Bailliere's Clin Gastroent 1987;1:769.
11. Robertson CS, Mayberry JF, Nicholson DA et al. Value of endoscopic surveillance in the detection of neoplastic change in Barrett's oesophagus. Br J Surg 1988;75:760–763.
12. Palley SL, Sampliner RE, Garewal HS. Editorial: management of high-grade dysplasia in Barrett's esophagus. J Clin Gastroenterol 1989;11:369–372.

Is any lower esophagus lined by columnar epithelium always Barrett's mucosa?

K.R. Geisinger (Winston-Salem)

According to Rector and Connerley, the earliest description of glandular epithelium in the esophagus was provided by Schmidt in 1805 [1]. The now classic article by the above two authors exhaustively reviewed the literature and reported the findings of their large-scale autopsy investigation of pediatric esophagi [1]. One premise of their study was that the normal esophageal mucosa consisted solely of stratified squamous epithelium and thus glandular elements were considered aberrant; such was the case in nearly 12% of their autopsies. A minority of specimens had residual fetal-type ciliated columnar epithelium in either the upper or lower segments of the organ. However, it never persisted beyond 72 h of life, apparently being exfoliated before or shortly after birth. More commonly and important clinically, gastric-type elements were identified and subdivided into those with and without parietal cells (fundic versus cardiac mucosa). The latter subgroup probably represents the cardiac glands found within the lamina propria throughout the length of the esophagus in a large proportion of normal individuals. Mucosa with parietal cells was never found in a lower segment of an esophagus and probably represented gastric heterotopias or inlet patches [2,3].

The following decade witnessed the publication of a number of important papers including several by Barrett [4,5]. Initially, Barrett believed the columnar epithelium present in the lower segment was gastric in origin and resulted from a congenitally short esophagus [4]. Allison and Johnson, and subsequently Barrett, revised this concept claiming that the distal glandular tissue was gastric mucosa but present within the esophagus; the theory of a congenital origin persisted [5,6].

In 1961, an essay by Hayward significantly altered our thoughts about this [7]: he claimed that the normal gastroesophageal junction was defined grossly and externally by the upward reflection of the peritoneum from the stomach to the diaphragm. The tubular organ proximal to this point was the esophagus. Furthermore, in most individuals, glandular epithelium is present in the distal-most 1 to 2 cm of this tube and thus is a normal component of the esophageal mucosa. He preferred the term junctional (rather than cardiac) epithelium. Hayward also discussed the cephalic extension of this mucin-producing columnar epithelium as a protective metaplastic process secondary to reflux damage to the squamous epithelium [7]. More recently, these concepts have been eloquently reviewed and expanded by several well recognized experts [8–10].

The main point of this is that the lumen of the distal-most esophageal segment is normally lined by glandular epithelium, which histologically and histochemically is indistinguishable from that covering the cardiac region of the stomach. It may be assumed that some individuals uncommonly will have a larger length of such junctional mucosa, and consequently many authors and workers in this field will not endoscopically diagnose Barrett's esophagus, unless columnar epithelium extends more than 3 cm above the gastroesophageal junction [9,10]. In these circumstances, at least in order to diagnose Barrett's esophagus histologically, the intestinal (or specialized) variant of metaplasia needs to be recognized [8–10]. Others would not require the presence of the intestinal form of glandular metaplasia [11].

Two other normal types of glandular tissue in the distal esophagus should be mentioned [10]. First, the lamina propria may contain cardiac type glands beneath the overlying squamous epithelium. These glands transport their secretions to the lumen through the squamous layer via columnar cell-lined ducts. The other consideration is the submucosal glands which produce acidic mucins which are carried to the lumen through squamous-lined ducts. These elements may be found throughout the entire length of the organ.

From a clinical viewpoint, a potentially important and practical consideration consists of the origin of adenocarcinomas occurring in the distal esophagus and the gastroesophageal junction (perijunctional adenocarcinomas). Various authors provide different classification schemes [8,10,11]. In part, this diversity exists due to the heterogeneity in the definition of Barrett's epithelium, as mentioned previously. Other reasons include the necessarily subjective, arbitrary and somewhat artificial subdivisions.

For example, Haggitt and Dean discussed four groups, two of which account for the bulk of all such tumors: those arising on a background of Barrett's esophagus and those originating in the proximal stomach (cardia) with extension into the esophagus [8]. They provided specific criteria for the separation of these two categories. If dysplastic Barrett's epithelium is found in addition to the cancer, then it is considered to have arisen in the pre-existing metaplastic segment (Fig. 1). These authors would also classify a neoplasm as occurring in Barrett's esophagus if benign Barrett's mucosa without dysplasia is present and the majority of the tumor resides in the esophagus [8]. Otherwise, a gastric origin is declared. Haggitt and Dean proposed two other categories [8]. In one of these, adenocarcinomas arise in superficial glands; they required the presence of squamous epithelium between the more proximal cancer and the distal gastroesophageal junction. Finally, a small number of malignancies may be derived from the esophageal submucosal glands; many of these will histologically resemble salivary gland tumors [12]. However, it may be that a larger proportion of these, at least the adenoid cystic type, actually originate from the overlying squamous epithelium [13].

The system proposed by Potet et al. is similar [11]. For the birth of a carcinoma to be considered from Barrett's esophagus, glandular or columnar epithelium (not necessarily of the intestinal type) must be interposed between the proximal tumor and the more distal squamous epithelium or the junction. These authors combined tumors arising in the cardia and the gastroesophageal junction as another distinct category [11]. Their criteria included restriction of the tumor mass to the proximal 5 cm of the stomach, involvement of the junction and no evidence of Barrett's epithelium. With their less stringent definition of Barrett's epithelium, it would seem that a larger proportion of cancers in this region would be classified as esophageal rather than gastric in origin. Their third group were those adenocarcinomas restricted to the lower esophagus without any evidence of an associated glandular metaplasia. To further

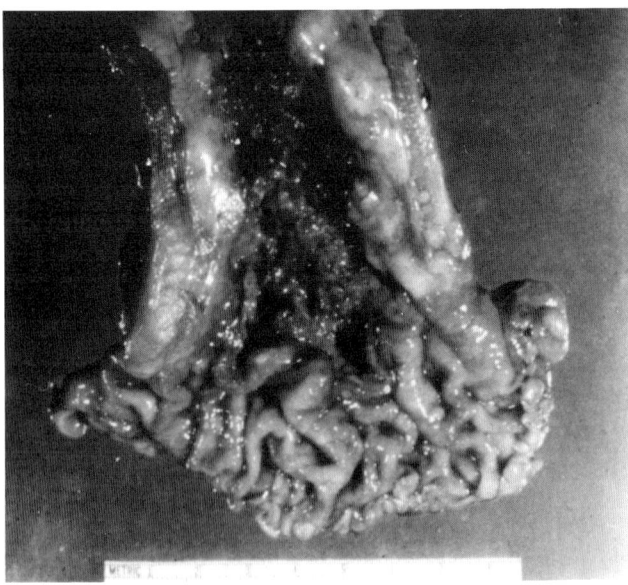

Fig. 1. This Barrett's associated adenocarcinoma has mutilated the mucosa of the distal esophagus and thickened its wall. It appears to terminate rather abruptly at the gastroesophageal junction.

qualify, squamous epithelium had to be situated between the tumor and the cardia. They proposed the possibility of a submucosal glandular origin [11].

The scheme of DeNardi and Riddell included adenocarcinomas arising in Barrett's esophagus, the gastric cardia and the distal 1 to 2 cm of the esophagus (Hayward's junctional mucosa) [10]. Cardial tumors are those located at or below the gastroesophageal junction, with the bulk of the cancer in the cardia. Barrett's carcinomas are those situated primarily within the esophagus and usually associated with glandular metaplasia. Carcinomas originating within junctional epithelium are, in the classification of these others, combined with the cardiac lesions, unless Barrett's metaplasia is demonstrated, in which case they are considered esophageal.

I would like to provide a classification of perijunctional adenocarcinomas (Table 1) which should not be misconstrued as original or novel, but rather a combination of already existing classifications [8,10,11]. The latter, as described above, resemble each other fairly closely, but each differs in some minor way from the others. This scheme is based on a combination of gross anatomic and histogenetic microscopic features. A basic premise is that adenocarcinomas may arise in (or morphologically recapitulate) any glandular epithelium. The gastroesophageal junction is defined externally by the reflection of the gastric peritoneum to the diaphragm. As stated by Haggitt and Dean, however, this region may also be so mishappened by neoplasm that this usual guidepost is destroyed [8]. In this situation, the morphologist may define the origin of a histologic section as from the esophagus if submucosal glands are recognized. Of course, neither of these criteria can be applied frequently or consistently to conventional endoscopically-obtained biopsy specimens (Fig. 2).

Much more important overall is that perijunctional adenocarcinomas are quite similar with regard to their biology and clinical courses, as well as apparently related epidemiologies [14–20]. Any subdivision of neoplasms attains "true weight" only

Table 1. Perijunctional adenocarcinomas

---

1. Tumors of the gastric cardia with proximal extension into the esophagus
   Grossly, the mass occurs predominately distal to the gastroesophageal junction (GEJ), but does not extend into the more distal stomach. Histologically, it may be associated with glandular dysplasia in adjacent gastric epithelium. Typically, Barrett's epithelium will not be seen.
2. Tumors arising in Barrett's metaplasia
   Grossly, the mass occurs predominately in the esophagus. Usually, it is associated with Barrett's epithelium with or without dysplasia distal to the cancer and proximal to the GEJ. If the entire distal esophagus is destroyed by the neoplasm, then Barrett's epithelium must be proximal to the mass.
3. Tumors arising in Hayward's junctional epithelium
   Grossly, the mass occurs predominately in the esophagus, but usually it straddles the junction and mutilates the region so that there is no residual junctional epithelium in which to identify dysplasia.
4. Tumors arising in gastric heterotopia or cardiac glands
   Grossly, the mass occurs predominately in the esophagus. Histologically, squamous epithelium is present between the proximal cancer and the distal GEJ. These tumors might also represent neoplasms of submucosal gland origin without an appearance resembling salivary gland malignancies.
5. Tumors arising in submucosal glands and histologically resembling salivary gland cancers
6. Salivary gland-like tumors arising in squamous epithelium

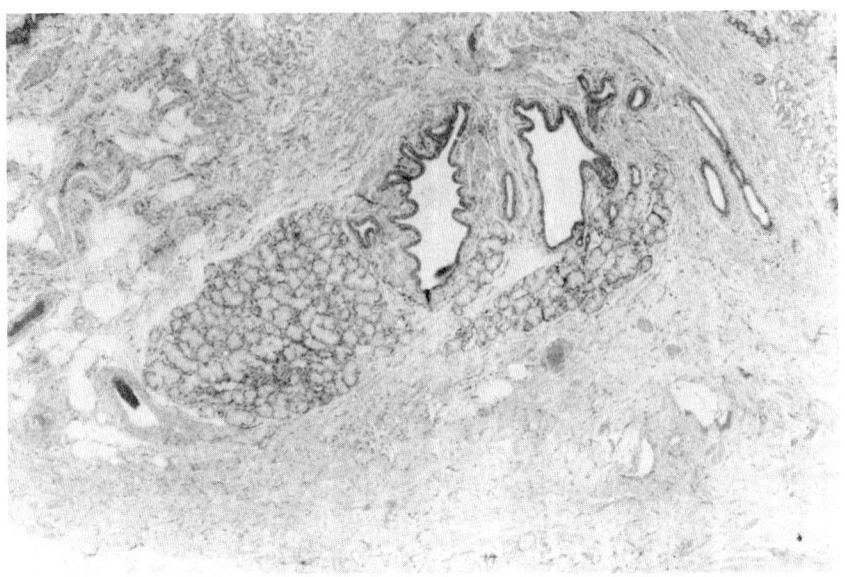

Fig. 2. Submucosal glands and their squamous-lined ducts lie deep to a dysplastic Barrett's epithelium in the right upper corner (× 20).

when it sheds light significantly into different pathways of neoplastic progression or potential etiologies for the various tumors. These are the puzzle pieces that require additional investigation.

References

1. Rector LE, Connerley ML. Aberrant mucosa in the esophagus in infants and children. Arch Pathol 1941;31:285–294.
2. Yarborough CS, McLane RC. Stricture related to an inlet patch of the esophagus. Am J Gastroenterol 1993;88:275–276.
3. Christensen WN, Sternberg SS. Adenocarcinoma of the upper esophagus arising in ectopic gastric mucosa. Two case reports and review of the literature. Am J Surg Pathol 1987;11:397–402.
4. Barrett NR. Chronic peptic ulcer of the oesophagus and "oesophagitis." Br J Surg 1950;38:175–182.
5. Barrett NR. The lower esophagus lined by columnar epithelium. Surgery 1957;41:881–894.
6. Allison PR, Johnstone AS. The oesophagus lined with gastric mucous membrane. Thorax 1953;8:87–101.
7. Hayward J. The lower end of the esophagus. Thorax 1961;16:36–41.
8. Haggitt RC, Dean PJ. Adenocarcinoma in Barrett's epithelium. In: Spechler SJ, Goyal RK (eds) Barrett's Esophagus: Pathophysiology, Diagnosis and Management. New York: Elsevier, 1985;153–166.
9. Reid BJ, Weinstein WM. Barrett's esophagus and adenocarcinoma. Ann Rev Med 1987;38:477–492.
10. DeNardi FG, Riddell RH. The normal esophagus. Am J Surg Pathol 1991;15:296–309.
11. Potet F, Flejou J-F, Gervax H, Paraf F. Adenocarcinoma of the lower esophagus and the esophagogastric junction. Sem Diagn Pathol 1991;8:126–136.
12. Bell-Thompson J, Haggitt RC, Ellis FH Jr. Mucoepidermoid and adenoid cystic carcinomas of the esophagus. J Thorac Cardiovasc Surg 1980;79:438–446.
13. Epstein JI, Sears DL, Tucker RS, Eagan JW Jr. Carcinoma of the esophagus with adenoid cystic differentiation. Cancer 1984;53:1131–1136.
14. Antonioli DA, Goldman H. Changes in the location and type of gastric adenocarcinoma. Cancer 1982;50:775–781.
15. Kalish RJ, Clancy PE, Orringer MB, Appelman HD. Clinical, epidemiologic, and morphologic comparison between adenocarcinomas arising in Barrett's esophageal mucosa and in the gastric cardia. Gastroenterology 1984;86:461–467.
16. Wang HH, Antoniolo DA, Goldman H. Comparative features of esophageal and gastric adenocarcinomas: recent changes in type and frequency. Human Pathol 1986;17:482–487.

17. MacDonald WC, MacDonald JB. Adenocarcinoma of the esophagus and/or gastric cardia. Cancer 1987;60:1094—1098.
18. Hamilton SR, Smith RRL, Cameron AJ. Prevalence and characteristics of Barrett's esophagus in patients with adeno-carcinoma of the esophagus or esophagogastric junction. Human Pathol 1988;19:942—948.
19. Hesketh PJ, Clapp RW, Doos WG, Spechler SJ. The increasing frequency of adenocarcinoma of the esophagus. Cancer 1989;64:526—530.
20. Blot WJ, Devesa SS, Kneller RW, Fraumeni JF Jr. Rising incidence of adenocarcinoma of the esophagus and gastric cardia. J Am Med Assoc 1991;265:1287—1289.

What are the differences in endoscopic appearances of Barrett's mucosa in children and adults?

E. Hassall (Vancouver)

Endoscopic appearance

It has been previously asserted by this author [1] and others [2] that, in children, Barrett's mucosa was not always recognizable endoscopically by a proximally located Z-line with a continuous sleeve of pink mucosa lining the tubular esophagus. It was suggested by the author and others that somehow columnar mucosa was obtained on biopsy from a white-appearing mucosa of the tubular esophagus at endoscopy [1,2]. Having studied more cases in children and adults with much more care, I now believe that this assertion was quite incorrect. I believe that the error was due to our inexperience as pediatricians in accurately documenting esophageal landmarks due to:
— the failure in carefully documenting the color of mucosa from which biopsies came;
— the fact that many of the children were reported on the basis of retrospective review of inadequately detailed endoscopy reports [1,2], and others on the basis of blind suction biopsy [2];
— error in reporting white mucosa present, when this likely represented white exudate rather than truly white esophageal mucosa.
At initial endoscopy of a child with severe reflux esophagitis, the tubular esophagus may appear white in patches or uniformly, due to exudate camouflaging the underlying mucosa and landmarks; this phenomenon was previously described in adults by Burbige and Radigan [3]. Having now carefully studied several children pre- and posttreatment with fundoplication or omeprazole, it has become clear that effective antireflux treatment allows accurate identification of the esophageal landmarks and reveals that the mucosa of the tubular esophagus in BE is always pink or red in children, as it is in adults. In children as in adults, islands of white mucosa, squamous on biopsy, are often present just below the Z-line [4—6]. White squamous

islands are present more numerously and extensively (throughout the body of the Barrett's mucosa) following effective fundoplication, constituting partial regression of Barrett's mucosa, in children [7] as well as in adults [8]. *Thus the endoscopic appearance of BE is the same in children as in adults.*

Histology

Several descriptions have asserted that BE in children is characterized far less often by the presence of specialized columnar metaplasia with goblet cells than by the presence of fundic gland or cardiac gland mucosa [1,2,9–12] and that the "commonest types" of BE in children are fundic gland and cardiac gland metaplasia. This assertion, of course, depends on how BE is defined in children. Many would now diagnose BE only when specialized columnar metaplasia with goblet cells staining positive with Alcian blue at pH 2.5 is present in the tubular esophagus. The reasoning for this is as follows.

There is good reason to have precise and restrictive criteria for the diagnosis of BE in children, as well as in adults. Barrett's esophagus is a premalignant condition in adults [13] and children [14]. A diagnosis of BE, therefore, may have implications for life expectancy, follow-up with surveillance endoscopy and biopsies, life insurance and health insurance. Adenocarcinoma of the esophagus arises virtually always in Barrett's esophagus, short or long segment; strong evidence suggests that it arises only from Barrett's specialized metaplastic epithelium, not from fundic or cardiac mucosa [4,8,13–23]. Therefore, surveillance endoscopy is required only when this type of epithelium is present [8,15–18,22]. For these reasons, there is increasing consensus that the diagnosis of BE be restricted to only those patients who have epithelium which may be premalignant [4,15–18], namely Barrett's specialized epithelium (i.e., with goblet cells positive with Alcian blue stain at pH 2.5). By this approach, BE is unequivocally present, with all its implications, only if specialized mucosa with goblet cells is present for any length in the tubular esophagus. Accurate diagnosis requires endoscopy with careful documentation of the landmarks of diaphragmatic pinchcock, top of gastric folds, lower esophageal sphincter (LES) zone and Z-line [4,25] (Fig. 1). When this is done, hiatal hernia is much less likely to be missed, and misdiagnosis of hiatal hernia as BE is a less frequent occurrence [16,26]. In addition, multiple biopsies with careful documentation of their source in relation to the landmarks are necessary to ensure that the extent and nature of metaplasia are documented [4,15].

With these factors in mind, the major childhood studies of BE in the literature to date are now scrutinized and it becomes apparent that the diagnosis of BE is often questionable. Detailed examination of these studies is constructive as it reveals pitfalls avoidable in future studies. Table 1 summarizes salient features of the largest childhood studies to date [1,2,9–12].

In the study by Dahms and Rothstein [2], the diagnosis was made in five patients on the basis of only a single biopsy 3 or 4 cm above the LES showing fundic mucosa only. Their patients had few biopsies (average 1.3 per patient), many of which were

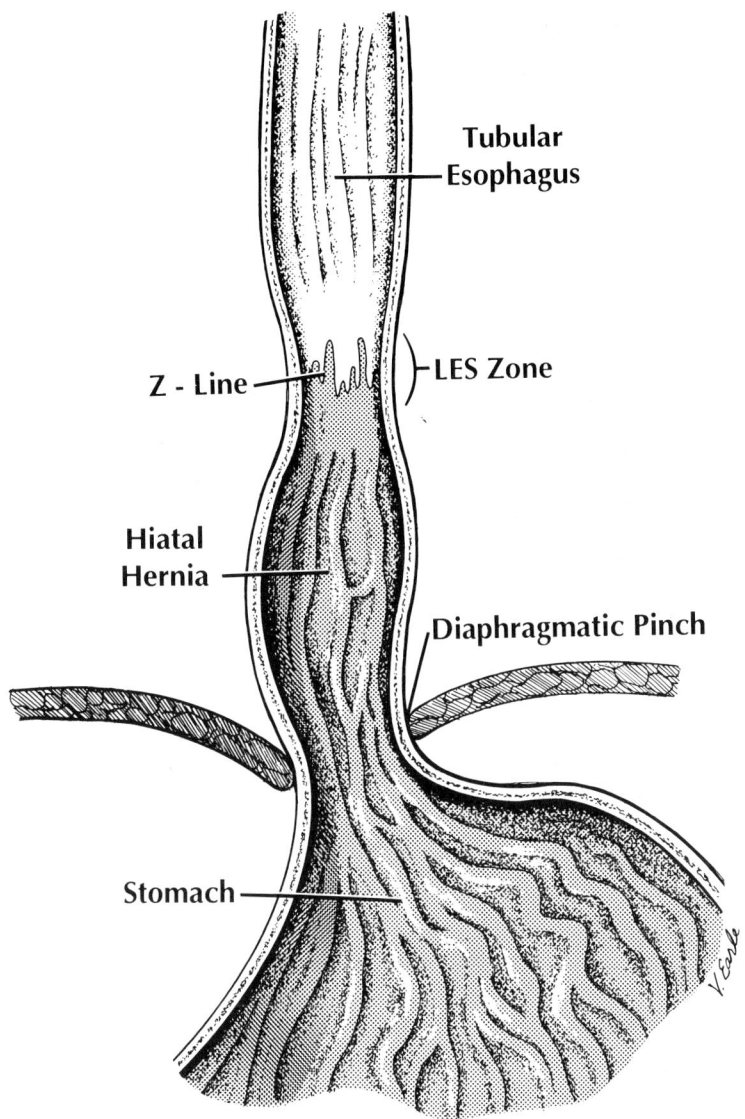

Fig. 1. Diagram showing relationships of the landmarks of the tubular esophagus and stomach when hiatal hernia is present. Barrett's esophagus is not present in this figure [4].

blind suction biopsies and details of careful landmark documentation were not given. That no hiatal hernias were diagnosed and relatively few strictures were present is somewhat out of keeping with other pediatric and adult studies. All patients and biopsy data were retrospectively gathered and, most importantly, specialized mucosa with goblet cells was present in only two patients. It seems likely that many of these patients had hiatal hernias and not BE. Similar observations apply to the study of Cheu et al [12]. Seven of their 16 patients had "small intestinal type epithelium" which was not further defined. This is potentially misleading because normal cardiac

Table 1. Childhood Barrett's studies

Author	No. of pts.	Age range (average)	Sex M:F	Hiatal hernia	Stricture	Mano-metry	pH study	Biopsies in columnar mucosa per patient (average)	Length of Barrett's mucosa (cm) (average)	Number with goblet cell meta-plasia
Hassall [1]	11	6.0–14.0 (9.7)	10:1	6	8	11	9	2–7 (4.6)	4–13 (7)	5
Dahms [2]	13	0.7–19.0 (9.8)	NS	0	5	7	8	1–3 (1.3)	3–8 (4)	2
Cheu [12]	16	1.2–16.0 (10.3)	11:5	NS	NS	NS	NS	NS	NS	7
Cooper [9]	11	1.1–13.3 (5.9)	8:3	11	5	NS	NS	1–3 (1.4)	NS	1
Snyder [10]	10	3.7–27.0 (19)	8:2	NS	1	NS	NS	NS	NS	7
Qualman [11]	28	1.0–23.0 (12.0)	19:9	NS	NS	NS	NS	NS	NS	14

NS = not stated. Adapted from [4].

mucosa can be villiform and resemble small bowel mucosa, in contrast to *Barrett's specialized mucosa* which may or may not be villiform but which contains goblet cells, as its definitive feature.

In another report [27], three children with surgically repaired esophageal atresia were said to have BE based on the presence of fundic or fundic and cardiac mucosa at 3.5 and 10 cm above the LES in one or two biopsies. It is likely that columnar mucosa was present proximally in these patients because the surgeon put it there at the time of anastomosis. Patients with esophageal atresia are at high risk for complications of severe GE reflux and may be, therefore, candidates for the development of BE. However, because of their surgically altered anatomy, the diagnosis of BE in these patients should be made only if landmarks are carefully documented and specialized mucosa is present. None of the patients in that study had specialized mucosa with goblet cells [27].

An interesting report [28] along similar lines described BE occurring in the cervical esophagus 2.2–13.9 years (mean 8.2) after gastric tube replacement of the esophagus. Ten of 14 children had endoscopic changes described as "salmon-red flamelike projections rising from the anastomosis", or "irregular red patches of gastric mucosa surrounded by normal, pale esophageal epithelium". However, these changes were present "just above" the surgical anastomosis and biopsies taken from "just above" the anastomosis showed fundic or junctional mucosa in eight patients. None had specialized mucosa with goblet cells. Not stated were the linear extent of the endoscopic and histologic changes, the number of biopsies, nor details of how the anastomotic landmark was identified with certainty at endoscopy. The description of changes occurring at a neo-anastomotic site is interesting, but the diagnosis of BE is not substantiated. Hopefully, more detailed reports with longer follow-up will become available in these patients; perhaps BE will develop.

Several pitfalls are shown by another case [29] in which BE was diagnosed in an 8-month-old infant on the basis of a single biopsy showing villiform cardiac mucosa without goblet cells but with focal sulfomucin positivity. These cannot be considered adequate grounds for a diagnosis of BE [30]; the biopsy was from a site unclear and mucosa of the normal gastric cardia is often villiform. Thus the diagnosis hinged entirely on focal sulfomucin positivity, which is common both in normal adults [31] and in the fetus [32]. Specialized mucosa with goblet cells was not present to begin with.

In the study by Cooper et al. [9], the presenting symptoms, male predominance, prevalence of hiatal hernias and presence of strictures in 5 of 11 patients are all clinical features suspicious of BE (Table 1). Furthermore the authors took care to document the endoscopic landmark of the LES. Their biopsies were said to be >2 cm above the LES, but actual biopsy sites and lengths of Barrett's mucosa were not given. Most patients were diagnosed on the basis of a single biopsy and only one had specialized mucosa with goblet cells (type I or "complete" metaplasia). This was primarily a study of mucin histochemistry claiming that a further seven patients had specialized mucosa (without goblet cells) on the basis of having type IIA and/or type IIB mucosa (both "incomplete" metaplasia). Type IIA is defined by the presence of neutral mucin and traces of sialated mucin and type IIB by sulfated mucin [31,32]. However, both sialomucins and sulfomucins are also present in cardiac glands of some normal humans [31–33] and some reflux patients without BE [31]. It would be difficult to make a case for BE for the 10 patients without goblet cell metaplasia, because the significance of types IIA and IIB (i.e., without goblet cells) is unknown.

In the study by Hassall et al. [1], the high M:F ratio and prevalence of hiatal hernia and strictures are all consistent with the profiles of BE in adults. However, only five patients had specialized mucosa with goblet cells. Those five had been studied recently, prospectively and with multiple large "jumbo" biopsies. The current proposal to limit the diagnosis of BE to only those with goblet cell metaplasia would exclude six patients with biopsies containing cardiac mucosa as proximal as 10, 6, 5, 8, 15 and 4 cm above the LES. Compared to the patients with specialized mucosa, the slides and endoscopy reports were obtained retrospectively, there were fewer and smaller biopsies and the landmarks had not been documented with the same thoroughness. While one could exclude those whose most proximal biopsies were 4, 5 and 6 cm above the "LES" by suggesting that the landmarks had not been well documented, it is less likely that biopsies 8, 10 and 15 cm above the "LES" containing cardiac mucosa were actually in proximal hiatal hernia. There are two possible explanations for the absence of goblet cell metaplasia in these circumstances:
a. that biopsies were insufficient in number and size and that areas of goblet cell metaplasia were missed (this seems very likely);
b. that even a 10- or 15-cm BE in a child does not contain some goblet cell metaplasia (this seems much less likely).

Qualman [11] has shown that even when goblet cell metaplasia is present in children or young adults, it is quantitatively much less than in older patients. However, it is not clear whether they had adequate tissue samples in the younger children to compare with those taken in older children and adults. In other words, if fewer biopsies were taken from younger children (as has tended to be the case in pediatric studies), perhaps some of their findings could be accounted for by sampling error. A 5-year-old patient in that study is the youngest patient in the literature to have well documented goblet cell metaplasia, suggesting that this type of metaplasia likely takes at least a few years to develop. Whether or not goblet cell metaplasia develops directly from primordial pluripotent cells or via cardiac mucosa is unknown [34,35]. In other words, it is possible, but by no means certain, that cardiac mucosa in the tubular esophagus is a precursor of goblet metaplasia (i.e., BE) in children.

In order not to exclude this possibility, the following is proposed for the diagnosis of BE in children.

1. When specialized mucosa with goblet cell metaplasia is unequivocally demonstrated on multiple biopsies in the tubular esophagus for any length above the LES, BE is present.
2. When only fundic mucosa is present, BE is not present.
3. When only cardiac mucosa (without specialized mucosa/goblet cell metaplasia) is present >3 cm above the LES in a child, that patient should be diagnosed as "possible BE". The diagnosis should be verified within a year with endoscopy and biopsies. Since these patients are not at risk for malignancy, regular surveillance endoscopy is not indicated. However, repeat evaluation with endoscopy and biopsy is advisable 4–5 years later to determine whether goblet cell metaplasia has developed.

By the above proposed criteria, all the childhood studies have overdiagnosed BE and a diagnosis of BE under age 4–6 years should be viewed with particularly critical attention. The most common pitfall has been absence of correlation between biopsies and landmarks. It is probable that BE may also be missed due to absence of recognition of goblet cell metaplasia. This occurs when biopsies are too few, too small and alcian blue stain at pH 2.5 is not used. Careful histologic mapping makes possible accurate diagnosis, evaluation of regression [7] and early detection of dysplasia [14,22,24]. One may conclude that when stringent criteria are used for the diagnosis of BE, *the histologic appearances of BE in children are similar to those in adults.*

References

1. Hassall E, Weinstein WM, Ament ME. Barrett's esophagus in childhood. Gastroenterology 1985;89:1331–1337.
2. Dahms BB, Rothstein FC. Barrett's esophagus in children: a consequence of chronic gastroesophageal reflux. Gastroenterology 1984;86:318–323.
3. Burbige EJ, Radigan JI. Characteristics of the columnar-cell lined (Barrett's) esophagus. Gastrointest Endosc 1979:133–136.
4. Hassall E. Barrett's esophagus: new definitions and approaches in children. J Pediatr Gastroenterol Nutr 1993;16:345–364.
5. Herlihy KJ, Orlando RC, Bryson JC et al. Barrett's eophagus: clinical, endoscopic, histologic, manometric and electrical potential difference characteristics. Gastroenterology 1984;86:436–443.
6. Bozymski EM. Barrett's esophagus: endoscopic characteristics. In: Spechler SJ, Goyal RK (eds) Barrett's Esophagus: Pathophysiology, Diagnosis and Management. New York: Elsevier Science, 1985;113–119.
7. Hassall E, Weinstein WM. Partial regression of childhood Barret's esophagus after fundoplication. Am J Gastroenterol 1992;87:1506–1512.
8. Skinner DB, Walther BC, Riddell RH et al. Barrett's esophagus: comparison of benign and malignant cases. Ann Surg 1983;198:554–566.

9. Cooper JE, Spitz L, Wilkins BM. Barrett's esophagus in children: a histologic and histochemical study of 11 cases. J Pediatr Surg 1987;22:191–196.

10. Snyder JD, Goldman H. Barrett's esophagus in children and young adults. Dig Dis Sci 1990;10:1185–1189.

11. Qualman SJ, Murray RD, McClung J, Lucas J. Intestinal metaplasia is age related in Barrett's esophagus. Arch Pathol Lab Med 1990;114:1236–1240.

12. Cheu HW, Grosfeld JL, Heifetz SA et al. Persistence of Barrett's esophagus in children after antireflux surgery: influence on follow-up care. J Pediatr Surg 1992;27:260–266.

13. Spechler SJ, Goyal RK. Barrett's esophagus. N Engl J Med 1986;315:362–371.

14. Hassall E, Dimmick JE, Magee JF. Adenocarcinoma in childhood Barrett's esophagus. Case documentation and the need for surveillance in children. Am J Gastroenterol 1993;88:282–288.

15. Haggitt RC. Adenocarcinoma in Barrett's esophagus: a new epidemic? Hum Pathol 1992;23:475–476.

16. Reid BJ, Haggitt RC, Rubin CE. Barrett's esophagus and esophageal adenocarcinoma. In: Hill L et al. (eds) The Esophagus: Medical and Surgical Management. Philadelphia: WB Saunders Company 1988:157–166.

17. Schnell TG, Sontag SJ, Chefjec G. Adenocarcinoma arising in tongues or short segments of Barrett's esophagus. Dig Dis Sci 1992;37:137–143.

18. DeMeester TR, Attwood SEA, Smyrk TC et al. Surgical therapy in Barrett's esophagus. Ann Surg 1990;212:528–542.

19. Rubio CA, Aberg B. Barrett's mucosa in conjunction with squamous carcinoma of the esophagus. Cancer 1991;68:583–586.

20. Haggitt RC, Tryzelaar J, Ellis FH, Colcher H. Adenocarcinoma complicating columnar epithelium-lined (Barrett's) esophagus. Am J Clin Pathol 1978;70:1–5.

21. McArdle JE, Lewin KJ, Randall G et al. Distribution of dysplasia and early invasive carcinoma in Barrett's esophagus. Hum Pathol 1992;23:479–482.

22. Reid BJ, Blount PL, Rubin CE et al. Flow cytometric and histologic progression to malignancy in Barrett's esophagus prospective endoscopic surveillance of a cohort. Gastroenterology 1992;102:1212–1219.

23. Thompson JJ, Zinsser KR, Enterline HT. Barrett's metaplasia and adenocarcinoma of the esophagus and gastroesophageal junction. Hum Pathol 1983;14:42–61.

24. Reid BJ, Weinstein WM, Lewin KJ et al. Endoscopic biopsy can detect high-grade dysplasia or early adenocarcinoma in Barrett's esophagus without grossly recognizable neoplastic lesions. Gastroenterology 1988;94:81–90.

25. McClave SA, Boyce HW, Gottfried MR. Early diagnosis of columnar-lined esophagus: a new endoscopic criterion. Gastrointest Endosc 1987;33:413–416.

26. Lewin KJ, Riddell RH, Weinstein WM. In: Gastrointestinal Pathology and its Clinical Implications, vol 1. New York: Igaku-Shoin, 1992;413–422.

27. Rothstein FC, Dahms BB. Barrett's esophagus in children. In: Spechler SJ, Goyal RK (eds) Barrett's Esophagus: Pathophysiology, Diagnosis and Management. New York: Elsevier Science, 1985:129–141.

28. Lindahl H, Rintala R, Sariola H, Ilmo L. Cervical Barrett's esophagus: a common complication of gastric tube reconstruction. J Pediatr Surg 1990;25:446–448.

29. Conti Nibali S, Barresi G, Tuccari G et al. Barrett's esophagus in an infant: a long-standing history with final postsurgical regression. J Pediatr Gastroenterol Nutr 1988;7:602–607.

30. Hassall E, Dimmick JE. Absence of regression of Barrett's esophagus. J Pediatr Gastroenterol Nutr 1989;8:544–545.

31. Peuchmaur M, Potet F, Goldfain D. Mucin histochemistry of the columnar epithelium of the oesophagus (Barrett's oesophagus): a prospective biopsy study. J Clin Path 1984;37:607–610.

32. Filipe I. Mucins in the human gastrointestinal epithelium: a review. Invest Cell Pathol 1979;2:195–216.

33. Ganter P, Marche CL. Histochemie des mucins gastrointestinales de l'homme. Ann Anat Path (Paris) 1970;15:321–346.

34. Cameron AJ, Lomboy CT. Barrett's esophagus: age, prevalence, and extent of columnar epithelium. Gastroenterology 1992;103:1241–1245.

35. Hassall E. Barrett's esophagus: congenital or acquired? Am J Gastroenterol 1993;88:819–824.

809

Is the routine detection of CLE in a general population important?

A.J. Cameron (Rochester)

Most patients with CLE (Barrett's esophagus) have gastroesophageal reflux symptoms such as heartburn and acid regurgitation. Reflux symptoms are similar in patients with or without CLE [1], so that endoscopy with biopsy is required to establish the diagnosis. Treatment of reflux esophagitis is the same whether or not CLE is present. Therefore, detection of CLE is not necessary for management of reflux.

Patients with CLE have an increased risk of esophageal cancer, estimated to be 30 to 125 times greater than the general population incidence. The incidence of adenocarcinoma in CLE is between 1 in 52 and 1 in 441 patient years [2]. Patients with CLE are often advised to have endoscopy at 1- or 2-year intervals for early cancer detection [3–5].

This brings us to the question, "Is the routine detection of CLE in a general population important for cancer detection?" To answer this question, I will especially use our statistics for the population of Olmsted County, Minnesota.

The incidence of adenocarcinoma of the esophagus has risen steadily since 1970 and is now about 1.0 per 100,000 population per year [6]. Adenocarcinoma of the esophagogastric junction is about twice as common, approximately 2.0 per 100,000. In a surgical study [7], macroscopic evidence of CLE was found in 85% of esophageal and 35% of junction adenocarcinomas. The incidence of CLE-related adenocarcinoma is, therefore, about 1.55 cases per 100,000 per year. This is the theoretical maximum yield from any cancer detection program for CLE.

Early cancer detection is unlikely to prevent all cancer deaths. We have observed the development of unresectable carcinoma in a patient undergoing regular surveillance. When a cancer is found, surgical resection may carry a 5% mortality rate and early cases may have an 80% surgical cure rate. This does not take any account of possible lead time bias. A patient with early cancer may die of unrelated illness before the cancer becomes clinically apparent. Patients with adenocarcinoma who are not found in a surveillance program, but who first present with tumor-related symptoms may still sometimes be saved. A 5-year survival of 15 to 22% following surgical resection in such cases is reported [8,9]. Taking into account those deaths that would not be prevented by a CLE surveillance program and those that would not be lost without such a program, we think that a maximally effective program might prevent 1.1 CLE related deaths per 100,000 population per year.

Based on a comparison of clinical and autopsy findings, we have estimated that, for every known patient with CLE, there are 20 more undetected cases in the general population [10]. It is in this large pool of undetected cases that most adenocarcinomas now develop. It would not be easy to find these presently undiagnosed CLE cases as a further examination of data will show.

In Olmsted County, a population-based study of adults aged 30 to 64 showed that heartburn occurred in 13% and acid regurgitation in 6.5% of residents every week [11]. When patients with frequent reflux symptoms were examined by endoscopy, CLE was found in 12 to 13% [1,12]. It should also be noted that up to one-third of patients with adenocarcinoma in CLE do not have a history of preceding reflux symptoms [13].

Let us estimate the effect of a screening program in a population of 100,000. We might exclude the 48% of our population who are less than 30 years old and at low risk for esophageal cancer. For the remaining 52,000 people, we might try to contact and perform endoscopy on the 13% with weekly reflux symptoms (6,760 people). If the population screening was repeated every 5 years, we would initially do 1,352 screening endoscopic examinations per year, somewhat less after the first 5 years. Out of 6,760 examinations, 12.5% or 845 cases of CLE might be found. These 845 cases might be re-examined at 1-year intervals for surveillance. Thus, screening plus surveillance to detect early adenocarcinoma in CLE would require 2,197 endoscopic examinations per year. This program would not detect cases of CLE in people with infrequent or absent reflux symptoms, so let us assume that one-third of CLE cases would be missed. Performance of 2,197 endoscopic examinations per year might prevent, not 1.1, but 0.73 cancer deaths per year in our 100,000 population. If an endoscopy costs $500, it would cost about 1.5 million dollars to prevent one death from CLE-related adenocarcinomas. The number of endoscopic examinations required for this screening and surveillance program would exceed by a factor of 4 the number of examinations currently performed for all other indications combined in the same population; about 500 per year.

An attempt to detect all cases of CLE in the general population over 30 by performing endoscopy on all people aged 30 or older every 5 years would carry an even worse cost/benefit ratio. Performance of 10,400 endoscopic examinations for screening above would cost $5,200,000 per year to save 1.1 deaths per year.

There are two conclusions: first, the routine detection of CLE in a general population by mass screening with endoscopy would not be a cost efficient use of medical resources. Secondly, and directly relevant to clinical practice, endoscopic examination of a patient with reflux symptoms for the sole reason of preventing death from adenocarcinoma at some future date is probably not necessary.

References

1. Winters C, Spurling TJ, Chobanian SJ et al. Barrett's esophagus. A prevalent, occult complication of gastroesophageal reflux disease. Gastroenterology 1987;92:112–124.
2. Williamson WA, Ellis FH, Gibb SP et al. Barrett's esophagus. Prevalence and incidence of adenocarcinoma. Arch Intern Med 1991;151:2212–2216.
3. Spechler SJ. Endoscopic surveillance for patients with Barrett's esophagus: does the cancer risk justify the practice? Ann Int Med 1987;106:902–904.
4. Achkar E, Carey W. The cost of surveillance for adenocarcinoma complicating Barrett's esophagus. Am J Gastroenterol 1988;83:291–294.
5. Atkinson M. Barrett's oesophagus – to screen or not to screen? Gut 1989;30:2–5.
6. Pera M, Cameron AJ, Trastek VF, Carpenter HA, Zinsmeister AR. Increasing incidence of adenocarcinoma of the esophagus and esophagogastric junction. Gastroenterology 1993;104:510– 513.
7. Lomboy CT, Pera M, Cameron AJ, Carpenter HA, Trastek VF. Adenocarcinoma of the esophagus and esophagogastric junction are both associated with Barrett's epithelium. Gastroenterology 1993;102:A373 (Abstract).

8. Skinner DB, Walther BC, Riddell RH et al. Barrett's esophagus. Comparison of benign and malignant cases. Ann Surg 1983;198:554−565.

9. Sanfey H, Hamilton SR, Smith RRI, Cameron JL. Carcinoma arising in Barrett's esophagus. Surg Gynecol Obstet 1985; 161:570−574.

10. Cameron AJ, Lomboy CT. Barrett's esophagus: age, prevalence, and extent of columnar epithelium. Gastroenterology 1992;103:1241−1245.

11. Talley NJ, Zinsmeister AR, Schleck CD, Melton LJ. Dyspepsia and dyspepsia subgroups: a population-based study. Gastroenterology 1992;102:1259−1268.

12. Schnell TG, Sontag SJ, Wannier J et al. Endoscopic screening for Barrett's esophagus, esophageal adenocarcinoma and other mucosal changes in ambulatory subjects with symptomatic gastroesophageal reflux. Gastroenterology 1985;88:1576 (Abstract).

13. Spechler SJ, Goyal RK. Barrett's esophagus. N Engl J Med 1986;315:362−371.

Physiopathology

 Is there evidence of enhanced duodenogastric reflux in Barrett's esophagus?

R.C. Heading (Edinburgh)

The role of refluxed bile acids and other constituents of duodenal luminal fluid in causing esophageal mucosal damage has long been a topic of controversy. Part of the controversy comes about because of methodological difficulties in detecting and quantitating abnormal duodenogastric reflux. It is now certain that some duodenogastric reflux is physiological and occasional measurements may demonstrate quite substantial reflux in apparently healthy subjects. This has made for difficulties in defining the "normal range".

A substantial body of literature nevertheless points to enhanced duodenogastric reflux in patients with esophageal reflux disease, including those with Barrett's esophagus. This is entirely compatible with pathophysiological concepts, if gastro-esophageal reflux disease is regarded primarily as a disorder of upper gastrointestinal motility. It is then understandable that motor dysfunction in the esophagus and its lower sphincter may be accompanied by disordered gastric or pyloroduodenal motor function, but the occurrence of increased duodenogastric reflux in such patients does not prove a causal role for refluxed duodenal content in relation to esophageal mucosal damage.

There is less certainty with respect to the occurrence of enhanced duodenogastric reflux in Barrett's esophagus relative to its occurrence in uncomplicated esophagitis. Recently published data appears to suggest that duodenogastric reflux is little different between them, though some evidence points to significantly increased duodenogastric reflux in complicated Barrett's esophagus (i.e., Barrett's esophagus accompanied by strictures or ulcers) [1,2]. Comparing uncomplicated Barrett's esophagus with uncomplicated reflux esophagitis, however, studies of bile salt concentrations in upper gastrointestinal aspirates and studies based on dual (intragastric and intraesophageal) pH monitoring are in agreement in showing no abnormality specifically associated with Barrett's esophagus [3–5]. Consequently, although duodenogastric reflux appears to be enhanced in such individuals relative to healthy control subjects, there is no sound experimental basis for suggesting duodenogastric reflux has a major role in the causation of Barrett's metaplasia.

References

1. Gillen P, Keeling P, Byrne PJ, Healy M, O'Moore RR, Hennessy TPJ. Implications of duodenogastric reflux in the pathogenesis of Barrett's oesophagus. Br J Surg 1988;75:540–543.
2. Attwood SEA, De Meester TR, Bremner CG, Barlow AP, Hinder RA. Alkaline gastroesophageal reflux: implications in the development of complications in Barrett's columnar-lined lower oesophagus. Surgery 1989;106:764–770.
3. Gillen P, Keeling P, Byrne PJ, Hennessy TPJ. Barrett's oesophagus: pH profile. Br J Surg 1987;74:774–776.
4. Gotley DC, Morgan AP, Gall D, Owen RW, Cooper MJ. Composition of gastro-oesophageal refluxate. Gut 1991;32:1093–1099.
5. Singh S, Bradley LA, Richter JE. "Alkaline" pH environment in controls and patients with gastro-oesophageal reflux disease. Gut 1993;34:309–316.

What is the effect of gastric juice on Barrett's mucosa?

R.M. Bremner, T.R. DeMeester (Los Angeles)

Continued erosion of the lower esophageal mucosa by gastroesophageal reflux can result in replacement of the squamous epithelium with columnar cells. This appears to occur because the columnar cells are more resistant to acid. Evidence of this is seen at endoscopy where erosive esophagitis occurs in the squamous epithelium above a quiescent Barrett's lining. In effect, the columnar change is an attempt to protect the esophagus from further acid injury. Complications such as ulceration, stricture, dysplasia and carcinoma that can occur in the metaplastic Barrett's mucosa are likely, due to the composition of the refluxed material. Reflux of duodenal contents has long been suspected to cause gastric mucosal injury and has been causally implicated in the development of gastric carcinoma [1,2]. There is growing evidence that a similar process is involved in the columnar lined esophagus. Experimental animal models have shown that bile and various enzymes can cause significant esophageal injury. A similar process is thought to occur in humans, although it remains to be shown which specific components of the refluxed juice are important [3,4]. We have recently found that there was a close relationship between esophageal injury and increased esophageal exposure to pH < 2 and to pH > 7, suggesting that alkaline components of refluxed gastric juice contribute to esophageal injury in humans [5]. Many studies have shown that duodenal contents can reflux through the stomach and into the esophagus. Gowen reported on 42 patients with hypochlorhydria who had prominent gastric bile pool on endoscopy and histological evidence of gastritis, as well as esophagitis with heartburn unrelieved by antacids. An increase in gastric bile salts in patients with reflux esophagitis and strictures has also been reported [6,7]. Bremner supported his early hypothesis that bile reflux may be related to Barrett's ulceration by reports of increased bile acids in the stomachs of some Barrett's patients and later, in the gastric juice of Barrett's patients with stricture [8–10]. This was independently supported by Gillen who showed that postprandial gastric bile concentrations in patients with complicated Barrett's was greater than that of patients with uncomplicated Barrett's [11].

Attwood et al. used 24-h pH monitoring to compare patients with uncomplicated to complicated Barrett's disease. They used esophageal exposure to pH > 7 as an indirect indicator of entero-gastroesophageal reflux. They adhered to the use of glass combined electrodes and dilated all patients with strictures prior to pH monitoring. They found a similar acid exposure and a definite increase in the alkaline esophageal exposure in the patients with complicated disease (Fig. 1) [12]. More recently, Stein and colleagues used esophageal aspirate studies to quantitate duodenal contents in the esophagus, and found an increase in bile acids in the esophagus of patients with

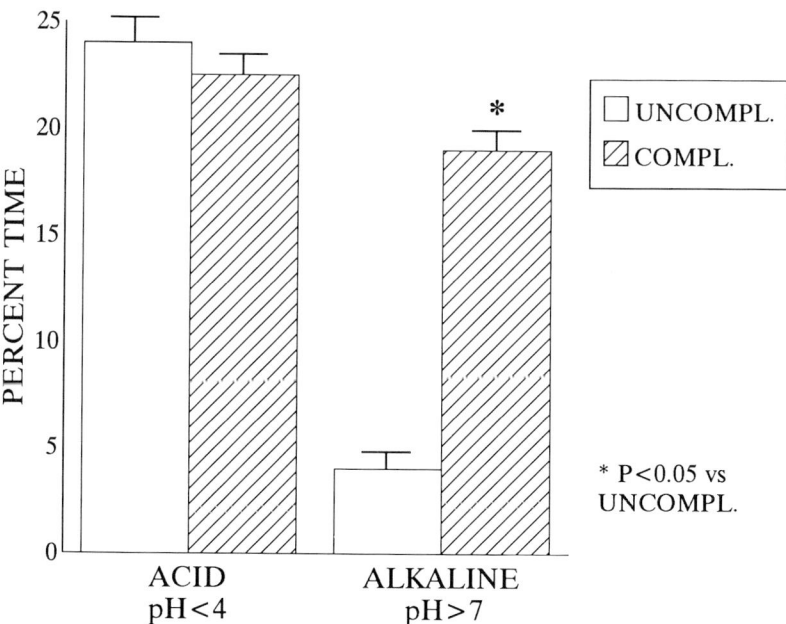

Fig. 1. The 24-h esophageal pH profiles in patients with complicated and uncomplicated Barrett's esophagus.

815

strictures or Barrett's esophagus [13]. They performed simultaneous pH monitoring in these patients and showed a good correlation between bile concentration and pH > 7 supporting the early assumptions of Attwood and DeMeester that pH > 7 is a reflection, albeit the "tip of the iceberg" of the presence of duodenal contents in the esophagus. The use of the recently developed bile spectrophotometric probe, which measures bile more directly, may clarify the controversies in this area [14,15].

There is other evidence that duodenal contents may be causally related to the development of the Barrett's epithelium and to the development of carcinoma in the columnar lined epithelium [16,17]. Clark recently performed an esophagoduodenostomy with gastric preservation in rats and showed that continued exposure of the esophagus to duodenal contents led to the development of columnar lined esophagus, dysplasia and even carcinoma. When a carcinogen was added to the rat model, 50% of the animals developed carcinoma [18].

In conclusion, the colunmar lining of the Barrett's mucosa represents an attempt to protect the esophagus from further acid injury as it is relatively resistant to acid. Contamination of the refluxate with duodenal contents is a plausible explanation for the complications that are seen in this disease. New technology, which will be able to measure bile salts directly promises to provide answers to the relationship of the components of refluxed gastric juice to various forms of esophageal injury.

References

1. Du-Plessis DJ. Pathogenesis of peptic ulceration. Lancet 1965;1:974–978.
2. Yasui A, Hoeft SF, DeMeester TR, Bremner RM, Nimura Y, Hinder RA, Leichman L. An alkaline stomach is common to Barrett's esophagus and gastric carcinoma. Gastroenterology 1992;102(4):A411.
3. Lillemoe KD, Johnson LF, Harmon JW. Taurodeoxycholate modulates the effects of pepsin and trypsin in experimental esophagitis. Surgery 1985;97:662–667.
4. Schweizer EJ, Harmon JW, Bass BL. Bile acid reflux precedes mucosal barrier disruption in the rabbit esophagus. Am J Physiol 1984;247:G280.
5. Bremner RM, Crookes PF, DeMeester TR, Peters JH, Stein HJ. Concentration of refluxed acid and esophageal mucosal injury. Am J Surg 1992;164:522–527.
6. Kay MD, Showalter JP. Pyloric incompetence in patients with symptomatic gastroesophageal reflux. J Lab Clin Med 1974;83:198–206.
7. Gotley DC, Morgan AP, Cooper MJ. Bile acid concentration in the refluxate of patients with reflux oesophagitis. Br J Surg 1988;75:587–590.
8. Bremner CG. The columnar-lined (Barrett's) esophagus. Ann Surg 1977;9:103–123.
9. Bremner CG, Hamilton DG. The columnar-lined (Barrett's) esophagus: surgical techniques. In: Stipa S, Belsey RHR, Moraldi A (eds) Medical and Surgical Problems of the Esophagus, vol 43, 2nd Symposium. Academic Press, 1981; 204–207.
10. Bremner CG, Hamilton DG. Barrett's esophagus: controversial aspects. In: DeMeester TR, Skinner DB (eds) Esophageal Disorders: Pathophysiology and Therapy. New York: Raven Press, 1985;233–239.
11. Gillen P, Keeling P, Byrne PJ, Healy M, O'Moore RR, Hennessy TPJ. Implication of duodenogastric reflux in the pathogenesis of Barrett's oesophagus. Br J Surg 1988;75:540–543.
12. Attwood SEA, DeMeester TR, Bremner CG, Barlow AP, Hinder RA. Alkaline gastroesophageal reflux: implications in the development of complications in Barrett's columnar-lined lower esophagus. Surgery 1989;106:764–770.
13. Stein HJ, Feussner H, Kauer W, DeMeester TR, Siewert JR. "Alkaline" gastroesophageal reflux: assessment by ambulatory esophageal aspiration and pH monitoring. Presented at the Annual Meeting of the Society for Surgeons of the Alimentary Tract. Boston, 1993.
14. Bechi P, Falciai R, Baldini F, Cosi F, Pucciani F, Travaglini F, Boscherini S. Ambulatory assessment of enterogastric reflux and nonacid gastroesophageal reflux by means of a fiber optic sensor. Gastroenterology 1992;102(4):A39.
15. Burdiles P, Hoeft SF, Clark G, Bremner RM, Crookes PF, Dreuw B, DeMeester TR, Peters JH. Evaluation of a fiber-optic sensor for bilirubin. Gastroenterology 1993;103(4):A485.
16. Pera M, Cardesa A, Bombi JA, Ernst H, Pera C, Mohr U. Influence of esophago jejunostomy on the induction of adeno-

carcinomas of the distal esophagus in Sprague-Dawley rats by subcutaneous injection of 2,6-dimethylnitrosomorphine. Cancer Res 1989;46:6803–6808.

17. Attwood SEA, Smyrk TC, DeMeester TR, Mirvisch SS, Stein HJ, Hinder RA. Duodenoesophageal reflux and the development of esophageal adenocarcinoma in rats. Surgery 1992;111:503–510.

18. Clark GWB, Smyrk TC, Mirvish SS, Anselmino M, Yamashita Y, Hinder RA, DeMeester TR, Birt DF. The effect of gastroduodenal juice and dietary fat on the development of Barrett's esophagus and esophageal neoplasia. Ann Surg Oncol (in press).

Is the mucosa in the CLE usually the site of acid hypersecretion?

C.G. Bremner, S.F. Hoeft (Los Angeles)

The columnar lining of a Barrett's esophagus is unstable and is prone to complications, such as stricture (62%), ulceration (20%), bleeding (18%), and adenocarcinoma [1]. Spontaneous esophageal perforation of Barrett's ulcer has also been described [2]. The pathogenesis of these complications has been debated and current evidence suggests that gastroesophageal reflux of duodenal contents may be responsible [3]. One other theory is that acid secretion within the wall of the columnar segment is responsible for the mucosal breakdown [4]. This neo-epithelium is a complicated tissue in which a multitude of cells can be identified. Herschfield [5] first reported on the histological appearance of chief cells with pepsinogen granules and parietal cells which responded to histamine stimulation by the secretion of hydrochloric acid (0.51 meq/h). Mangla et al. [6] performed pepsin and acid secretory studies by balloon isolation of the esophagus and also showed that Barrett's epithelium produced pepsin and acid. The acid output in one case studied was 0.17 meq/h and this increased to 0.34 meq/h after histamine stimulation. Ustach et al. [7] also studied the secretory capability of Barrett's esophagus and found that no acid was present in the unstimulated state, but after histalogical stimulation, 10 ml of secretion containing 5 meq/l of acid was obtained. Gastric parietal cells can also be detected in the columnar lined esophagus by technetium pertechnetate esophageal imaging. The sensitivity of this test for detecting Barrett's epithelium is only 47% and pentagastrin stimulation does not increase the sensitivity [8]. This suggests that the secretory potential of Barrett's epithelium is limited.

Paull et al. [9] defined the three types of columnar epithelium in Barrett's and noted parietal cells in the atrophic gastric fundic type of epithelium. The presence of parietal cells in the columnar lining may not be a consistent finding because no parietal cells were found in studies by Burgess [10] or Pedersen [11]. The specialized epithelium characteristics of Barrett's esophagus are distinguished by its villiform surface, mucous glands and goblet cells, which are always found proximally and the

817

gastric fundic epithelium, which is always the most distal [9]. Patches of heterotopic gastric mucosa in the upper esophagus have also been detected using ^{99m}Tc-pertechnetate scintigraphy [12] and acid production by this epithelium has been demonstrated using red congo staining [13]. The small basal acid output and the minimal response to histamine stimulation from columnar epithelium in the esophagus questions whether this amount of acid secretion in the esophagus is of clinical significance. Moreover, prevention of gastric acid reflux by fundoplication cures ulceration in Barrett's esophagus [14] suggesting that esophageal secretion of acid is clinically insignificant.

Specific endocrine cell populations have also been identified in 62—78% of Barrett's epithelium. Immunohistochemical studies have identified serotonin (82%), somatostatin (54%), secretin (22%), pancreatic polypeptide (17%) and neurotensin-immunoreactive cells [15,16]. Histochemical stains show that the mucous cells contain largely neutral mucins, but sialomucins and sulfomucins were found in 70% of biopsies in one series [17]. These secretions apparently have no effect on acid secretion by parietal cells.

Conclusion

There is therefore no evidence to suggest that hypersecretion of acid in the columnar lined esophagus takes place. Secretory studies from the excluded esophagus report on only small amounts of acid after histamine stimulation. It is, therefore, unlikely that the secretion of acid from parietal cells in the esophagus is of clinical importance. Following antireflux surgery, Barrett's ulcers heal. Pearson [14] treated 10 Barrett's ulcers on medical treatment, and none healed. All of these patients underwent antireflux surgery and complete healing occurred in eight, after a follow-up of 1 to 11 years. Two of the patients developed adenocarcinoma. The small amount of acid secretion from the columnar segment in some patients is, therefore, insufficient to perpetuate esophageal damage.

There is, however, evidence from some studies that a high basal gastric output (greater than 10 meq/h) is present in Barrett's patients who did not respond to ranitidine 150 mg twice daily [18,19]. There is also an increased acid exposure (pH < 4) of the esophagus in Barrett's patients [3] and this is a result of gastroesophageal reflux of gastric contents, and is not related to acid secretion from within the esophagus.

References

1. Bremner CG. The management of columnar-lined oesophagus. In: Jamieson GG (ed) Surgery of the Oesophagus. Edinburgh: Churchill Livingstone, 1988;223—232.
2. Limburg AJ, Hesselink EJ, Kleibeuker JH. Barrett's ulcer: cause of spontaneous oesophageal perforation. Gut 1989; 30(3):404—405.
3. Attwood SEA, DeMeester TR, Bremner CG, Barlow AP, Hinder RA. Alkaline gastroesophageal reflux: implications in the development of complications in Barrett's columnar-lined lower esophagus. Surgery 1989;106:764—770.
4. Barrett NR. Chronic peptic ulcer of the oesophagus and "oesophagitis". Br J Surg 1950;38:175—182.
5. Hershfield NB, Lind JF, Hildes JA, McMorris LS. Secretory function in Barrett's epithelium. Gut 1965;6:535—539.

818

6. Mangla JC, Schenk EA, Desbaillets L, Guarasci G. Kubasik NP, Turner MD. Pepsin secretion, pepsinogen, and gastrin in "Barrett's esophagus". Clinical and morphologic characteristics. Gastroenterology 1976;70:669–676.

7. Ustach TJ, Tobon F, Schuster M. Demonstration of acid secretion from esophageal mucosa in Barrett's ulcer. Gastrointest Endosc 1969;16:98–100.

8. Mangla JC. Acid and pepsin production by Barrett's epithelium: role of radionuclide imaging in diagnosis. In: Spechler SJ, Goyal RK (eds) Barrett's Esophagus: Pathophysiology, Diagnosis and Management. New York: Elsevier, 1985;49–57.

9. Paull A, Trier JS, Dalton MD et al. The histologic spectrum of Barrett's esophagus. N Engl J Med 1976;295:476–480.

10. Burgess JN, Payne WS, Anderson HA et al. Barrett's esophagus; the columnar epithelial-lined lower esophagus. Mayo Clin Proc 1971;46:728–734.

11. Pedersen SA, Hage E, Neilsen PA, Sorensen HR. Barrett's syndrome: morphological and physiological characteristics. Scand J Thorac Cardiovasc Surg 1972;6:191–205.

12. Yegelwel EJ, Bushnell DL, Fisher SG, Keshavarzian A. Technetium pertechnetate esophageal imaging for detection of Barrett's esophagus. Dig Dis Sci 1989;34(7):1075–1078.

13. Hamilton JN, Thune RG, Morrissey JF. Symptomatic ectopic gastric epithelium of the cervical esophagus. Dig Dis Sci 1986;31:337–342.

14. Pearson FG, Cooper JD, Patterson GA, Prakash D. Peptic ulcer in acquired columnar-lined esophagus: results of surgical treatment. Ann Thorac Surg 1987;43:241–244.

15. Ritchie AJ, Johnston C, McGuigan J, Gibbons JRP. Endocrine cells in Barrett's esophagus. Specificity and clinical implications. Gastroenterol 1993;104:178A.

16. Feurle GE, Helmstaedter V, Buehring A, Bettendorf U, Eckardt VF. Distinct immunohistochemical findings in columnar epithelium of esophageal inlet patch and of Barrett's esophagus. Dig Dis Sci 1990;35:86–92.

17. Lee RG. Mucins in Barrett's esophagus: a histochemical study. Am J Clin Pathol 1984;81:500–503.

18. Collen MJ, Lewis JH, Benjamin SB. Gastric acid hypersection in refractory gastroesophageal reflux disease. Gastroenterology 1990;98(3):654–661.

19. Mulholland MN, Reid BJ, Levine OS, Rubin CE. Elevated gastric acid secretion in patients with Barrett's metaplastic epithelium. Dig Dis Sci 1989;34:1329–1334.

What is the pH measurement profile in patients with CLE?

S. Bruley des Varannes, J.P. Galmiche (Nantes),
C. Scarpignato (Parma)

The association between Barrett's esophagus (BE) and gastroesophageal reflux (GER) is well established. Barrett's esophagus is present in 5–20% of patients with chronic symptoms of GER and the role of GER in the pathogenesis of BE is now widely established [1,2].

Several studies have demonstrated abnormal esophageal acid exposure in the distal esophagus (Table 1), which is significantly higher than in patients with erosive esophagitis. In BE patients, esophageal acid exposure is especially high during the upright and supine periods [4,5,11]. This severe reflux is apparently related to the poor tone of the lower esophageal sphincter (LES) frequently observed in these patients [11].

In patients with BE, there are frequent nonspecific esophageal motor abnormalities, especially a lack of motor response to swallowing, intermittent nonpropagated contractions or esophageal contractions with low amplitude.

Table 1. Acid exposure in the distal esophagus in patients with Barrett's esophagus

Authors	Patients	% time pH < 4 (mean or median)	Number of reflux episodes > 5 min in duration
Patel et al. [3]	7	34.5	ND
Iascone et al. [4]	22	28.0	12.5
Gillen et al. [5]	24	32.9	11.0
Schlesinger, Schmid [6]	16	15.0	8.8
Orr et al. [7]	13	19.0	ND
Attwood et al. [8]	23	23.0	ND
Zaninotto et al. [9]	12	28.0	ND
Parrilla et al. [10]	20	26.7	13.8
Bruley des Varannes et al. [11]	18	12.7	8.5

ND: not determined.

These characteristics may account for prolonged acid clearance time, as indicated by a mean duration of acid refluxes significantly longer than in controls, or in patients with reflux symptoms, with or without esophagitis [11]. The number of long-lasting refluxes (>5 min) is also higher. It is still unclear whether these characteristics are secondary or not to mucosal lesions.

Until now, studies have measured acid exposure in the distal esophagus. Recently, we compared acid exposure, not only in the distal esophagus, but also in the mid-esophagus, by using dual 24-h pH monitoring in controls, patients with esophagitis and patients with BE. Electrodes were placed 5 and 10 cm proximal to the LES. The results are summarized in Table 2. Patients with BE not only had more prolonged acid exposure in the distal esophagus, but also more reflux in the midesophagus than patients with reflux esophagitis and no BE.

It has been reported that duodenogastric reflux is higher in patients with BE, especially during the postprandial period [12,13]. Thus, increased gastric bile acid or pancreatic enzyme concentration could potentiate the noxious action of refluxed-action. Moreover, some authors have noted abnormal esophageal exposure above pH 7, suggesting alkaline reflux. However, esophageal pH monitoring does not appear to be a reliable tool for measuring esophageal exposure to bilio-pancreatic components. It has been clearly demonstrated that no correlation exists between pH level and bile acid concentration, at least in gastric juice [14]. Recently, Champion et al., using an esophageal probe directly sensitive to bile acids (absorption spectrophotometry), showed that bile acid exposure was proportionally higher as acid exposure increased [15]. With this technique, both bile acid exposure and acid exposure were higher in patients with BE than in those with esophagitis or controls. These new results do not indicate that duodenogastric reflux is greater in BE, but that volumes of refluxate are higher [15].

It would thus appear that acid reflux parameter values are higher in patients with BE than in those with esophagitis, although some studies show no significant differences in the case of severe esophagitis, suggesting that other factors, in addition to high esophageal acid exposure, may play a role in development of BE.

Table 2. Results of 24-h pH monitoring (median and range) 10 cm proximal to the LES in patients with Barrett's esophagus (BE), patients with gastroesophageal reflux (GER) with and without esophagitis, and healthy volunteers

	Healthy volunteers (n = 9)	GER (n = 14)	BE (n = 17)
% time pH < 4			
— total time	0.5 (0.3–3.2)	2.1[a] (0.0–3.3)	6.6[ab] (0.1–60.2)
— upright	0.3 (0.5–4.8)	2.6 (0.3–12.9)	7.5 (0.3–50.7)
— supine	0.1 (0.0–1.2)	2.1[a] (0.0–11.7)	6.8[a] (0.0–83.8)
Number of reflux episodes			
> 5 min in duration	0.0 (0.0–3.0)	2.0[c] (0.0–6.0)	4[a] (0.0–19.0)
Mean duration (min/reflux)	0.8 (0.4–4.0)	1.3 (0.1–5.5)	3.4[ab] (0.3–28.7)

[a] p < 0.01 vs. healthy volunteers; [b] p < 0.05 vs. GER; [c] p < 0.05 vs. healthy volunteers; Kruskall-Wallis and Mann-Whitney.

References

1. Jutel P, Galmiche JP. Endobrachy esophage. In: Galmiche JP, Colin R (eds) Troubles de la Motricité de l'Oesophage. Reflux gastro-oesophagien. Paris: Doin, 1987;177–191.
2. Winters C, Spurling TJ, Chobanian SJ et al. Barrett's esophagus. A prevalent, occult complication of gastroesophageal reflux disease. Gastroenterology 1987;92:118–124.
3. Patel GK, Clift SA, Read RC. Mechanism of gastroesophageal reflux (GER) in patients with Barrett's esophagus. Gastroenterology 1982;82:1146.
4. Iascone C, DeMeester TR, Little AG, Skinner DB. Barrett's esophagus. Functional assessment, proposed pathogenesis and surgical therapy. Arch Surg 1983;118:543–549.
5. Gillen P, Keeling P, Byrne PJ, Hennesy TPJ. Barrett's esophagus: pH profile. Br J Surg 1987;74:774–776.
6. Schlesinger PK, Schmid B. Esophageal pH profiles fail to identify patients at risk for development of Barrett's esophagus. Gastroenterology 1987;92:1622.
7. Orr WC, Lackey C, Robinson MG, Johnson LF, Welsh JD. Esophageal acid clearance during sleep in patients with Barrett's esophagus. Dig Dis Sci 1988;33:654–659.
8. Attwood SEA, DeMeester TR, Bremner CG, Barlow AP, Hinder RA. Alkaline gastroesophageal reflux: implications in the development of complications in Barrett's columnar-lined lower esophagus. Surgery 1989;106:764–770.
9. Zaninotto G, De Meester TR, Bremner CG, Smyrk TC, Cheng SC. Esophageal function in patients with reflux-induced strictures and its relevance to surgical treatment. Ann Thorac Surg 1989;47:362–370.
10. Parrilla P, Ortiz A, Martinez de Haro LF, Aguayo JL, Ramirez P. Evolution of the magnitude of gastroesophageal reflux in Barrett's oesophagus. Gut 1990;31:964–967.
11. Bruley des Varannes S, Ravenbackht-Charifi M, Cloarec D, Pujol P, Simon J, Galmiche JP. Endobrachyeosophage et reflux gastro-oesophagien acide. Enregistrements pH-métriques étagés et étude manométrique. Gastroenterol Clin Biol 1992;16: 406–412.
12. Gillen P, Keeling P, Byrne PJ, Healy M, O'Moore RR, Hennesy TPJ. Implication of duodenogastric reflux in pathogenesis of Barrett's oesophagus. Br J Surg 1988;75:540–543.
13. Waring JP, Legrand J, Chinichian A, Sanowski RA. Duodenogastric reflux in patients with Barrett's esophagus. Dig Dis Sci 1990;759–762.
14. Hostein J, Bost R, Faure H, Lachet B, Fournet J. Valeur diagnostique de la pH-métrie gastrique au cours du reflux duodénogastrique. Gastroenterol Clin Biol 1987;11:206–211.
15. Champion G, Singh S, Bechi P, Richter JE. Duodenogastric reflux: relationship to esophageal pH and response to omeprazole. Gastroenterology 1993;104:A51.

What is the mean distal sphincteric pressure in patients with CLE?

C. Iascone, A. Moraldi, D. Castiglia (Rome)

Barrett's esophagus (BE), or columnar lined esophagus (CLE), is a condition in which the squamous mucosa that normally lines the distal esophagus is replaced by a columnar epithelium resembling that of the stomach and intestine. Early controversy regarding the pathogenesis of Barrett's epithelium focused on whether the aberrant mucosa was congenital or acquired, as result of chronic gastroesophageal reflux. Reports of families with high prevalence of BE [1], and the finding that the disorder is rare among blacks [2], suggest that genetic factors may be involved in the development of BE. However, although it is not possible to exclude a congenital origin in some patients [3,4], it is generally accepted that BE is a consequence of gastroesophageal reflux in most cases. Bremner et al. [5] found that esophageal mucosal defects in dogs were replaced by columnar epithelium under concomitant histamine stimulated acid reflux. Presently it is reasonable to think that BE occurs in predisposed patients with severe gastroesophageal reflux. In the last few years, several studies focused on esophageal function in patients with CLE. Comparing patients with BE to subjects with esophagitis and to a group of normals, we found that patients with esophagitis had a lower esophageal sphincter pressure (LESP) significantly higher than those with BE and both were significantly lower than that measured in the control subjects. LESP had also a statistically significant linear relationship with the extent of Barrett's mucosa involvement [6]. Most of these findings were confirmed by the following studies, showing that the mean LES pressure of patients with BE was significantly lower than that of normal controls (Table 1) [7–13].

A mechanically defective cardia was found in 90% of 41 patients with BE in one of these reports [8]. Pressure and overall length of LES were significantly decreased in 17 patients with BE, when compared with those of nine healthy volunteers in the study of Bruley des Varannes [7]. Similarly, in all studies but one [9], LES pressure was significantly lower in patients with BE than in patients with non-Barrett esophagitis (Table 2).

Sarr et al. [14] found a LESP <10 mmHg in all patients with BE and in half of the subjects with gastroesophageal reflux symptoms; pressure and length of LES were significantly altered in 17 patients with BE, when compared to 38 patients without

Table 1. BE vs. controls

Author	Year	BE	Controls	LESP BE	LESP controls	p value
Iascone [6]	1983	22	33	4.9 ± 0.8	16.7 ± 1.1	0.001
Herlihy [10]	1984	20	2	14 ± 2	19.0 ± 1	0.05
Parrilla [13]	1990	20	20	10 ± 6.1	17.2 ± 6.5	0.01
Li [11]	1992	9	26	6.8 ± 6.2	18.0 ± 5.6	0.0001

Table 2. BE vs. non-Barrett esophagitis (NBE)

Author	Year	BE	NBE	LESP BE	LESP NBE	p
Iascone [6]	1983	22	31	4.9 ± 0.8	8.7 ± 1.01	0.05
Gillen [9]	1987	24	25	15 (median)	17 (median)	NS
Hann [12]	1989	20	160	11.5 ± 4.4	19.5 ± 5.7	0.005
Parrilla [13]	1990	20	28 (severe)	10 ± 6.1	9.1 ± 4.1	NS
			25 (mild)		14 ± 5.2	0.05

esophagitis and 62 patients with non-Barrett esophagitis [7]. Parrilla [13] found that LES pressure was significantly lower in patients with BE than in patients with mild non-Barrett esophagitis and similar to that of subjects with severe esophagitis. Data obtained from five University Departments in Italy showed a mean LESP in patients with BE ranging from 7.27 to 13.6 mmHg (Table 3).

Table 3. Mean LESP

University	BE	LESP
Rome	7	7.3 ± 5.5
Bologna	21	8.2 ± 4.2
Milan	17	10.3 ± 3.1
Turin	21	10.6 ± 7.15
Genoa	6	12.4 ± 9.3

In 16 patients with limited BE and in 17 patients with extended BE, LES pressure was 9.9 ± 6.3 mmHg and 8.2 ± 4.6, respectively, confirming previous personal observation [6] and results published by Ranson [15] and Herlihy [10], indicating that patients with circumferential-type BE had lower LES pressures than patients with island-type BE. Finally, no different LES pressures have been found in patients with BE or without complications [8,9].

Conclusion

Based on several reports it can be concluded that a defective sphincter has been found in the majority of patients with BE. Also that LES pressure is significantly lower than that of healthy volunteers and that of patients with non-Barrett esophagitis.

Even though complications of BE do not affect the sphincter tone, however, a significant relationship seems to be present between LES pressures and extent of columnar lining.

Acknowledgements

The authors would like to thank the following colleagues and friends for their cooperation in sending their data on Barrett's patients:

- Prof. Giuseppe Gozzetti and Sandro Mattioli, University of Bologna (II Clinica Chirurgica e Terapia Chirurgica).
- Prof. Francesco Mattioli and Nicola Pandolfo, University of Genoa (Clinica Chirurgica Generale).
- Prof. Alberto Peracchia and Luigi Bonavina, University of Milan (Istituto di Chirurgia Generale ed Oncologia Chirurgica).
- Prof. Marcello Dei Poli, University of Turin (Chirurgia Generale).

References

1. Everhart CW Jr, Holtzaapple PG, Humphries EJ. Barrett's esophagus inherited epithelium on inherited reflux? J Clin Gastroenterol 1983;5:357–358.
2. Smith RRL, Hamilton SR, Boitnott JK, Rogers EI. The spectrum of carcinoma arising in Barrett's esophagus: a clinicopathologic study of 26 patients. Am J Surg Pathol 1984;8:563–573.
3. Haque AK, Merkel M. Total columnar-lined esophagus; a case for congenital origin? Arch Pathol Med 1981;105:546.
4. Law SW, Sheeman EE. Benign esophageal stricture and the lower esophagus lined by columnar epithelium; report of 2 cases. Dis Chest 1965;48:214.
5. Bremner CG, Lynch VP, Ellis FH Jr. Barrett's esophagus: congenital or acquired? An experimental study of esophageal mucosal regeneration in the dog. Surgery 1970;68:209–216.
6. Iascone C, DeMeester TR, Little AG, Skinner DB. Barrett's esophagus: functional assessment, proposed pathogenesis, and surgical therapy. Arch Surg 1983;118:543–549.
7. Bruley des Varannes S, Ravenbakht-Charifi M, Cloarec D, Pujol P, Simon J, Galamiche JP. Endobrachyoesophage et reflux gastro-oesophagien acide. Enregistrements pH-métriques étagés et étude manometrique. Gastroenterol Clin Biol 1992;16:406–412.
8. DeMeester TR, Atwood SEA, Smyrk TC, Therkildsen DH, Hinder RA. Surgical therapy in Barrett's esophagus. Ann Surg 1990;212:528–540.
9. Gillen P, Keeling P, Byrne PJ, Hennessy TPJ. Barrett's esophagus: pH profile. Br J Surg 1987;74:774–776.
10. Herlihy KJ, Orlando RC, Bryson JC, Bozymski EM, Carney CN, Powell DW. Barrett's esophagus: clinical, endoscopic, histologic, manometric, and electrical potential difference characteristics. Gastroenterology 1984;86:436–443.
11. Li V, Bost R, Caravel JP, Fournet J, Hostein J. Endobrachyesophage, reflux gastro-oesophagien acide et reflux duodenogastrique en période inter-digestive postprandiale. Gastroenterol Clin Biol 1992;16:978–983.
12. Hann NS, Tsai MF, Nair PK. Barrett's esophagus in patients with symptomatic reflux esophagitis. Am J Gastroenterol 1989;84:1494–1496.
13. Parrilla P, Ortiz A, Martinez de Haro LF, Aguayo JL, Ramirez P. Evalutation of the magnitude of gastroesophageal reflux in Barrett's esophagus. Gut 1990;31:964–967.
14. Sarr GM, Hamilton SR, Marione GC, Cameron JL. Extended and limited types of Barrett's esophagus in the adult. Am J Surg 1985;149:87–91.
15. Ranson JM, Patel GK, Clift FA, Womble SE, Read RC. Barrett's esophagus: its prevalence and association with adenocarcinoma in patients with symptoms of gastroesophageal reflux. Ann Thorac Surg 1982;33:19–27.

824

Does esophageal dysfunction in CLE influence bolus propulsion through the esophagus? Does it differ from that of reflux esophagitis?

H.J. Stein (Munich), *T.R. DeMeester* (Los Angeles)

Esophageal clearance function is a major determinant of esophageal exposure to gastric juice. Factors important in esophageal clearance include esophageal peristalsis, gravity, salivation and anchoring of the distal esophagus in the abdomen. A defect in any one can prolong esophageal exposure to refluxed gastric content and contribute to the development of mucosal injury. Of the factors mentioned, effective esophageal peristalsis is the most important determinant of esophageal clearance function [1]. In addition, disordered esophageal peristalsis may also hamper propulsion of a swallowed bolus from the negative intrathoracic pressure environment to positive intra-abdominal pressure environment, and thus cause dysphagia [2].

Using simultaneous manometric and video-fluoroscopic recording of barium swallows, Kahrilas and co-workers have shown that propulsion of a bolus and clearance of refluxed gastric contents depends on peristaltic contractions of sufficient amplitude [3]. In their study nonperistaltic contractions (i.e., simultaneous, interrupted and isolated contractions) and peristaltic contractions of insufficient amplitude resulted in splitting of a swallowed barium suspension and retention of contrast medium in the esophageal body. The minimal contraction amplitude required to occlude the esophageal lumen and propel a liquid bolus was about 30 mmHg in the distal esophagus [3]. This indicates that esophageal clearance function can be assessed by manometry of the esophageal body.

Detailed functional studies of the esophageal body using standard manometry show that the mean amplitude of contractions in the distal half of the esophagus, following 10 wet swallows, is decreased in patients with Barrett's esophagus, as compared to patients with gastroesophageal reflux disease and esophagitis (Fig. 1) [4,5]. A decreased esophageal contraction amplitude in patients with Barrett's esophagus during the upright, supine and meal periods can also be documented with the new technique of ambulatory 24-h esophageal motility monitoring [6]. Ambulatory motility monitoring also shows that, compared to patients with esophagitis, patients with Barrett's esophagus also have an increased frequency of isolated contractions and contractions with an amplitude below 30 mmHg (Fig. 2), resulting in a markedly increased prevalence of contractions that are ineffective for bolus propulsion and clearance of refluxed gastric juice [5]. Combined ambulatory esophageal manometry and pH monitoring confirms that a compromised clearance function results in a prolonged duration of reflux episodes, particularly during the night when the subject is in the supine position and gravity does not aid in clearance of the refluxate [5]. This explains the increased frequency of prolonged reflux episodes in patients with Barrett's esophagus as compared to patients with gastroesophageal reflux and esophagitis (Fig. 3).

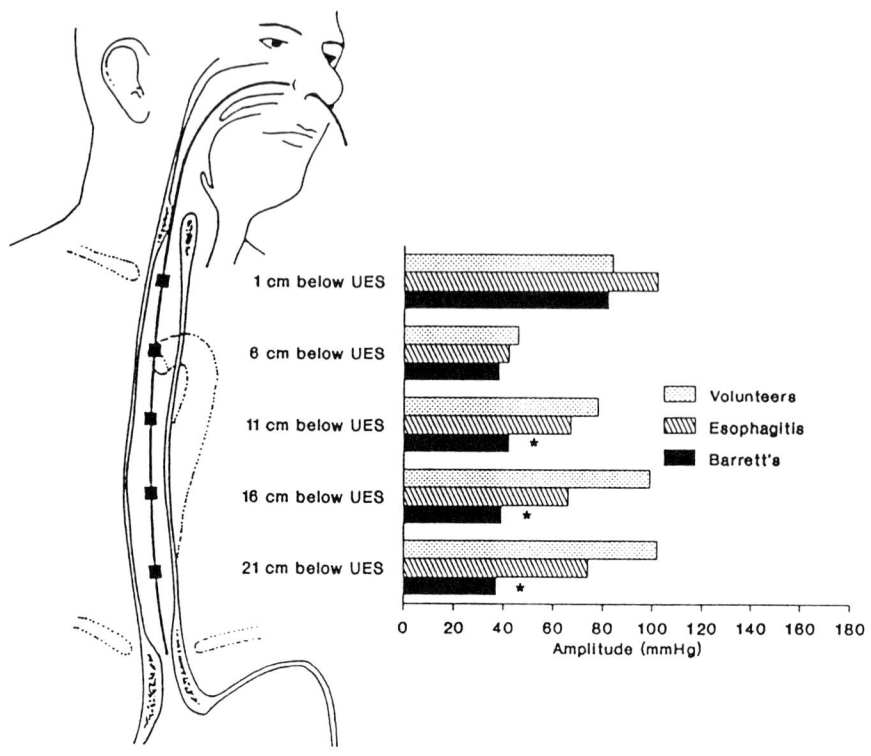

Fig. 1. Mean of amplitude of esophageal contractions following 10 wet swallows measured 1, 6, 11, 16, and 21 cm below the upper esophageal sphincter (UES) in normal volunteers, patients with esophagitis and patients with Barrett's esophagus. *: p < 0.01 vs. esophagitis and normal volunteers. From [5], with permission.

These observations have two important implications regarding surgical therapy in patients with Barrett's esophagus. First, the loss of peristaltic function in Barrett's esophagus appears to be, at least in part, secondary to persistent reflux across a mechanically defective lower esophageal sphincter (LES). Since the loss of clearance function further prolongs esophageal exposure to gastric juice, a vicious cycle is initiated. Even with complete suppression of reflux by an antireflux procedure or proton pump inhibitors, esophageal contractility may not recover once fibrosis of the esophageal wall has developed and the mean amplitude of contractions has deteriorated below 30 mmHg [6,7]. Consequently, a correction of the underlying defect, i.e., the mechanically defective LES, should be encouraged early in the course of the disease. Secondly, once esophageal peristalsis has deteriorated, an antireflux repair with little outflow obstruction, i.e., a partial fundoplication, should be considered to avoid induction or accentuation of postoperative dysphagia.

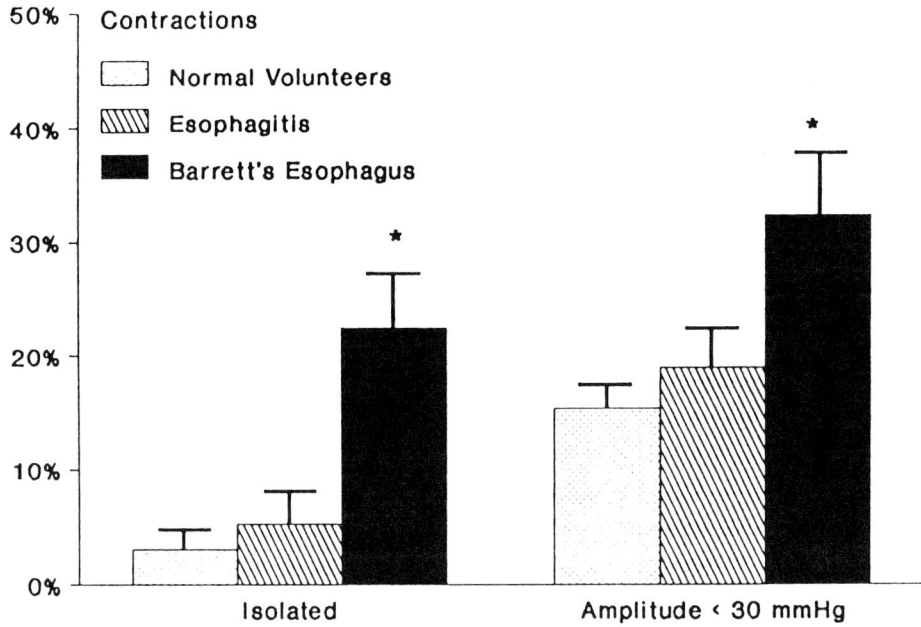

Fig. 2. Mean frequency of isolated and low amplitude contractions (<30 mmHg) on ambulatory 24-h esophageal motility monitoring in normal volunteers, patients with esophagitis and patients with Barrett's esophagus. *: p < 0.01 vs. esophagitis and normal volunteers.

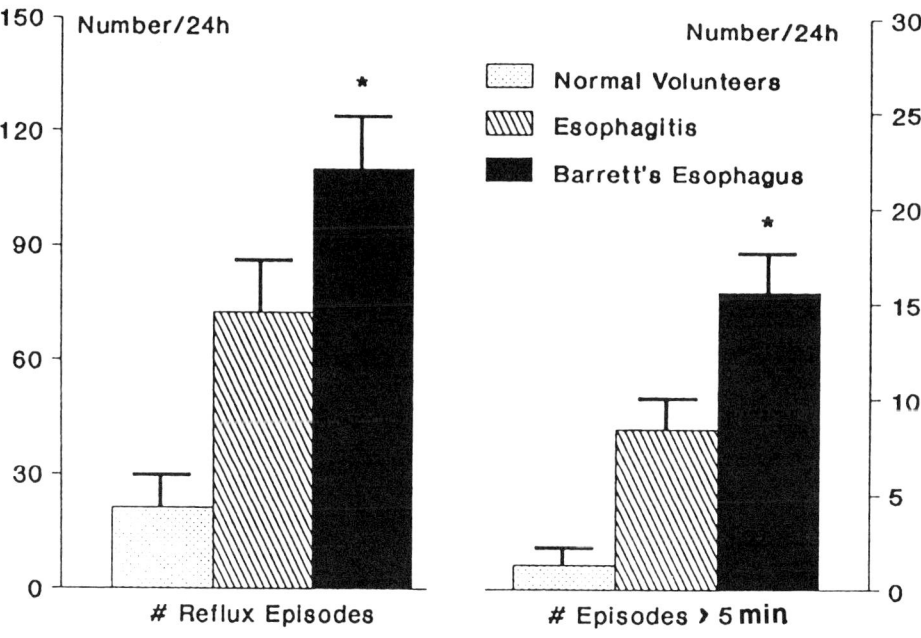

Fig. 3. Frequency of reflux episodes and reflux episodes lasting longer than 5 min (pH < 4) on ambulatory 24-h esophageal pH monitoring in normal volunteers, patients with esophagitis and patients with Barrett's esophagus. *: p < 0.01 vs. esophagitis and normal volunteers. From [5] with permission.

References

1. Helm JF, Dodds WJ, Riedel DR, Teeter BC, Hogan WJ et al. Determinants of esophageal acid clearance in normal subjects. Gastroenterology 1983;85:607–612.
2. Singh S, Stein HJ, DeMeester TR, Hinder RA. Nonobstructive dysphagia in gastroesophageal reflux disease – a study with combined ambulatory pH and motility monitoring. Am J Gastroenterol 1992;87:562–567.
3. Kahrilas PJ, Dodds, WJ, Hogan WJ. Effect of peristaltic dysfunction on esophageal volume clearance. Gastroenterology 1988;94:73–80.
4. Iascone C, DeMeester TR, Little AG, Skinner DB. Barrett's esophagus: functional assessment, proposed pathogenesis, and surgical therapy. Arch Surg 1983;118:543–549.
5. Stein HJ, Hoeft SF, DeMeester TR. Functional foregut abnormalities in Barrett's esophagus. J Thorac Cardiovasc Surg 1993;105:107–111.
6. Stein HJ, Eypasch EP, DeMeester TR. Circadian esophageal motor function in patients with gastroesophageal reflux disease. Surgery 1990;108:769–777.
7. Stein HJ, Bremner RM, Jamieson J, DeMeester TR. Effect of Nissen fundoplication on esophageal motor function. Arch Surg 1992;127:788–791.

 O. Ekberg (Malmö)

The intestinal metaplasia seen in Barrett's esophagus is confined only to the mucosa. It may involve the muscularis mucosa but never reaches into the muscularis propria [1]. Therefore, the mucosal metaplasia does not per se influence esophageal motility. However, Barrett's esophagus is regularly seen together with reflux esophagitis, which might be severe. Areas of squamous epithelium between mucosal metaplasia is therefore regularly, to a more or less advanced degree, altered by reflux esophagitis. Such esophagitis may reach into the muscularis propria, and thereby have an influence on the motility of the esophagus. However, superficial esophagitis, e.g., grade I, is also regularly seen together with abnormal motility, which for instance can be registered during barium swallow and/or manometry. Such dysmotility can be either hypomotility with defective propulsion in the esophagus or hypermotility seen as nonpropulsive vigorous contractions. The mucosal metaplasia as well as esophageal dysmotility are both likely to be secondary to gastroesophageal reflux disease.

Patients with Barrett's esophagus actually have been shown to regularly suffer from severe mechanical dysfunction, both in terms of lower esophageal sphincter dysfunction and also defective clearance of reflux material (both acid and alkaline, from the esophagus) [2].

It has been shown that the mean amplitude and the propagation rate of the contractile waves in the distal third of the esophageal body in Barrett's esophagus is similar to those found in mild and severe reflux esophagitis [3]. The proportion of abnormal waves are, however, significantly higher in the Barrett's group than in patients with severe esophagitis. In patients with Barrett's esophagus, the manometric esophageal pattern is not different from that found in patients with reflux esophagitis

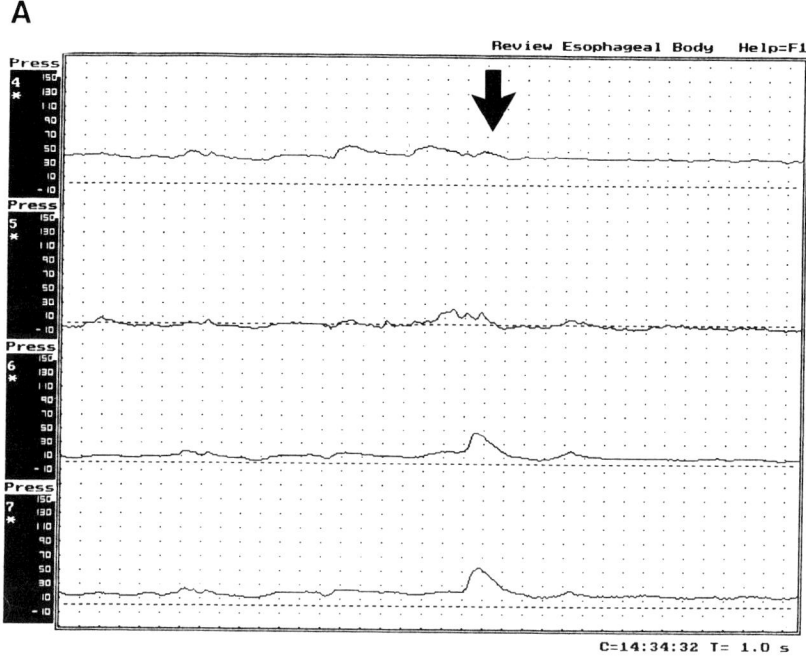

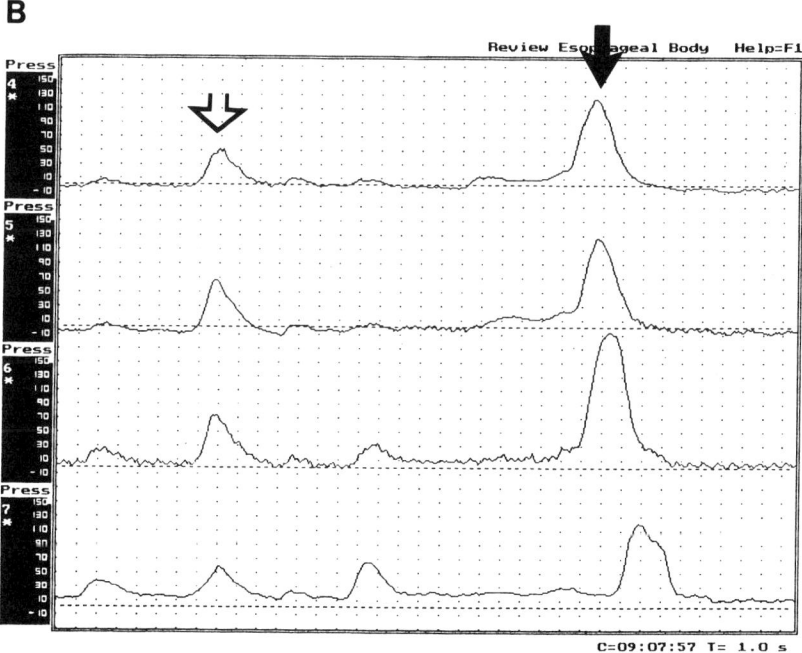

Fig. 1. Esophageal manometry from mid and distal esophagus before (A) and after (B) fundoplication in a patient with Barrett's esophagus and reflux esophagitis. In (A) there are very weak and simultaneous contractions (arrows) in the distal esophagus and absence of peristalsis in mid esophagus. After surgery (B) peristalsis returned to almost normal (arrow). However, still some simultaneous contractions (open arrow) were registered.

(Fig. 1). The amplitude of esophageal contractions in patients with Barrett's esophagus is proximally normal but regularly markedly reduced in the distal three fifth [4]. There is also a high prevalence of simultaneous, dropped and/or interruptive waves. Such peristaltic abnormalities are found in up to 83% of patients with Barrett's esophagus [3]. The presence of nonpropulsive contractions and pharyngeal swallow not being followed by esophageal peristalsis is not specific for Barrett's esophagus. However, Barrett's esophagus is regularly seen with severe esophagitis and the degree of reflux esophagitis does correlate with motor abnormalities of the esophagus.

References

1. Gottfried MR, McClave SA, Boyce HW. Incomplete intestinal metaplasia in the diagnosis of columnar-lined esophagus (Barrett's esophagus). Am J Clin Pathol 1989;92:741–746.
2. Stein HJ, Barlow AP, DeMeester TR, Hinder RA. Complications of gastroesophageal reflux disease. Role of the lower esophageal sphincter. Esophageal acid and acid/alkaline exposure, and duodenogastric reflux. Ann Surg 1992;216:35–43.
3. Parrilla P, Ortiz A, Martinez de Haro LF, Aguayo JL, Ramirez P. Evaluation of the magnitude of gastro-oesophageal reflux in Barrett's oesophagus. Gut 1990; 31:964–969.
4. DeMeester TR, Attwood SEA, Smyrk TC, Therkildsen DH, Hinder RA. Surgical therapy for Barrett's esophagus. Ann Surg 1990;212:528–540.

Do the etiologic factors in disorders of esophageal motility suggest that regression is no longer possible?

T.R. DeMeester (Los Angeles)

Esophageal motility in patients with Barrett's esophagus are similar to those in patients with less complicated reflux disease, with the exception that contraction amplitude is lower [1]. Consequently, their response to therapy is likely to be similar.

We have studied the effect of Nissen fundoplication on the compromised esophageal body function in patients with gastroesophageal reflux disease (GERD). In the first study, stationary manometry of the distal esophageal body was performed in 50 normal volunteers and compared with that in 40 patients with increased esophageal acid exposure, before and 11 to 68 months (median: 30 months) after successful reflux control and healing of acute mucosal injury with Nissen fundoplication [2].

Prior to the operation, patients had a lower mean amplitude of contractions, higher prevalence of low amplitude and interrupted and simultaneous contractions in the distal esophagus compared with normal volunteers. Nissen fundoplication restored the lower esophageal sphincter to normal, increased contraction amplitude and reduced the prevalence of low-amplitude contractions but did not improve contraction amplitude in patients with a mean amplitude below 35 mmHg (Fig. 1).

The prevalence of interrupted and simultaneous contractions in the distal esophagus was significantly increased in patients with GERD compared with the normal volunteers ($p < 0.001$). Nissen fundoplication had no effect on the prevalence of these contraction abnormalities.

In the second study, the outcome of Nissen fundoplication in patients with a nonspecific motility abnormality was compared to the outcome in patients with normal motility [3]. One hundred consecutive patients undergoing primary Nissen fundoplication were evaluated before and a median of 50 months following operation, with emphasis on the presence of a preoperative motility disorder and its relationship to preoperative symptoms and outcomes after surgery. Compared with patients who had normal motility, patients with a nonspecific motility abnormality had a greater prevalence and severity of heartburn and regurgitation before operation. These patients also had a greater esophageal exposure to gastric juice on pH monitoring due to poorer esophageal clearance function. The prevalence and severity of preoperative dysphagia was not related to the presence of a motility disorder. An overall 93% actuarial success rate was achieved in the relief of heartburn and regurgitation over a 96-month period. This success rate was similar in patients with or without a motility abnormality (Fig. 2). Dysphagia was rarely caused or made more severe by the procedure; if present before surgery, it was relieved in most patients. The prevalence of persistent postoperative dysphagia was similar in patients with normal

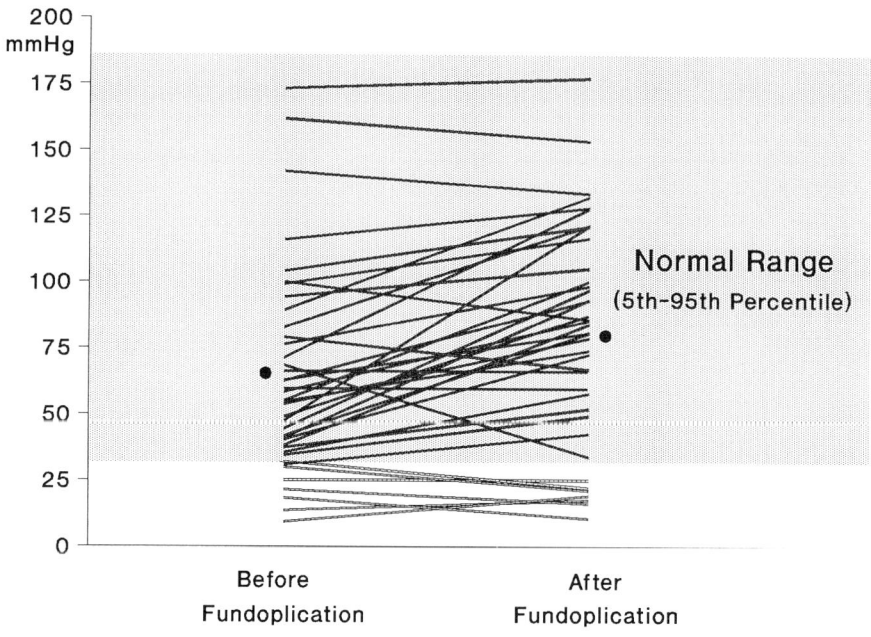

Fig. 1. Mean amplitude of contractions of the lower esophagus of patients before and after Nissen fundoplication. No improvement was noted in patients who had a preoperative mean contraction amplitude in the distal esophagus below 35 mmHg; ● = group mean before and after fundoplication ($p < 0.05$).

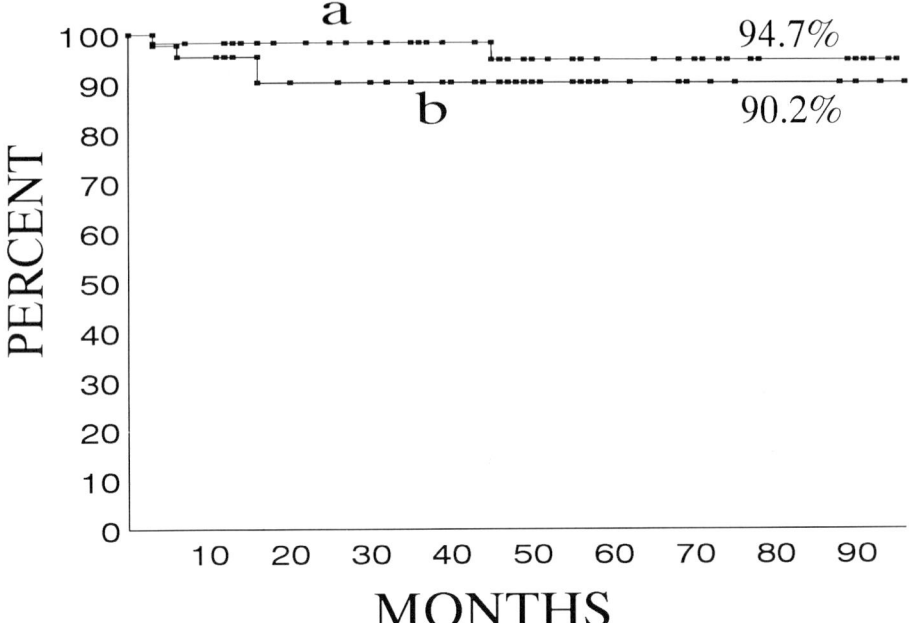

Fig. 2. The actuarial success of Nissen fundoplication in controlling symptoms of: a) heartburn and regurgitation for patients with normal motility (n = 56); and b) abnormal motility (n = 44). There was no difference in the ability to relieve these symptoms based on the presence of normal or abnormal esophageal motility prior to surgery. (Mantel-Cox, χ^2 = 1.29, p = NS).

or abnormal motility. The success of the Nissen fundoplication is not affected by the presence of a nonspecific motility disorder.

On the basis of these studies performed in patients with less complicated GERD, it can be concluded that motility abnormalities in patients with Barrett's esophagus are unlikely to regress, even if all gastroesophageal reflux were prevented. The presence of a motility abnormality is unlikely to affect the outcome of a Nissen fundoplication, unless the amplitude of esophageal contractions are below the fifth percentile of normal.

References

1. Stein HJ, Hoeft SF, DeMeester TR. Functional foregut abnormalities in Barrett's esophagus. J Thorac Cardiovasc Surg 1993;105(1):107–111.
2. Stein HJ, Bremner RM, Jamieson J, DeMeester TR. Effect of Nissen fundoplication on esophageal motor function. Arch Surg 1992;127(7):788–791.
3. Bremner RM, DeMeester TR, Crookes PF, Costantini M, Hoeft SF, Peters JH, Hagen J. The effect of symptoms and nonspecific motility abnormalities on surgical therapy for gastroesophageal reflux disease. J Thorac Cardiovasc Surg (in press).

What are the possible reasons for the differing results of tests of gastric emptying?

G.G. Jamieson (Adelaide)

We now have relatively sophisticated means by which we can measure gastric emptying in patients. As a result, it might be thought that tests of gastric emptying would be relatively standardized, enabling us to draw useful comparisons between different groups who are having their gastric emptying measured. Unfortunately, nothing could be further from the truth. Looking at the example of patients with gastroesophageal reflux disease (GERD) who have had their gastric emptying studied, quite varying results can be found. Some investigators have found delayed gastric emptying of both solids and liquids, and believe it is an important component of the pathogenesis of the disorder. Some investigators have found delay in gastric emptying but believe it is an epiphenomenon and not related to the pathogenesis of the disorder. Furthermore, some have found delayed solid emptying only, some delayed solid and liquid emptying, some delayed liquid emptying only, and yet other investigators have found no delay in emptying at all [1—6]. How can we explain these discrepancies?

The first problem is that there is no internationally agreed way of classifying patients with GERD. This means that the patient groups being studied may not be comparable, and this may account for some of the differences which are found. Nevertheless, it is hard to see this as a major factor since nearly all investigators tend to be looking at patients towards the severe end of the reflux spectrum.

To begin to understand the situation, I think we need to understand the mechanisms of gastric emptying and its control. Liquids tend to empty from the stomach in an exponential fashion with the rate of emptying, appearing to be under both caloric control and osmotic control. As the liquid becomes stronger in osmotic terms, then the slower the emptying of it becomes. Thus, if we drink isotonic saline or water we get rapid emptying of the liquid from the stomach. This is controlled mainly by the passage of propagated waves passing along the stomach to the duodenum with the pylorus playing little, if any, role. However, if one drinks 5, 10 or 20% dextrose in water, one gets progressive slowing of gastric emptying. A similar effect is seen if one increases the lipid concentration in the solution or if one increases the osmolarity of the saline from one normal to two normal to three normal. This slowing of emptying is due to a diminution of propagated pressure waves in the stomach and an increase in pyloric closure, with both of these effects tending to keep fluid in the stomach.

The situation with solids differs. Solids are received into the reservoir area of the stomach (the fundus and body) and then transferred to the antrum where grinding of food begins. It seems that the stomach has to grind the solids to sizes of less than 1 mm^3 before the particles begin to empty. In effect, the stomach has to turn the solid into a liquid suspension before the solids begin to empty. Quite clearly, the transference of food from the reservoir of the stomach to the grinding portion of the stomach takes time and so does the grinding of the particles down to less than 1 mm^3. Until this transference and grinding of the solid has taken place, no emptying of it occurs. This no emptying phase is usually called the lag phase of solid emptying. If the food is unable to be ground down, it is called indigestible and it will remain in the stomach until phase three contractions occur during fasting. These are known as the housekeeper waves of the stomach and these waves sweep any remaining contents of the stomach through into the duodenum. Furthermore, the caloric content of the solid food is important as the stomach appears to empty itself at a relatively standard rate of 1 kcal/min. This means that denser foods, such as fat, tend to be emptied more slowly than equivalent amounts of less dense foods such as carbohydrate.

When one looks at tests of gastric emptying, many differences can be seen. Firstly, some investigators have concentrated on liquid emptying only and furthermore, different groups have used different liquids. For instance a 10% dextrose drink (e.g., Coca Cola) will empty differently from a milk shake.

Secondly, a lot of investigators have used what they describe as a mixed meal, that is, a mixture of liquids, and solids and the results produced by such a meal depend greatly on what is being mixed. If the solid is represented by preground gruel, then the gastric emptying test is really measuring caloric rich liquid emptying. If oatmeal is being used, then some grinding will have to occur and gastric emptying will take longer. Scrambled eggs as the solid component of a meal has become popular because of its ease of preparation, and it is clear that this will be much more easily ground down than hamburger beef which is another popular meal used in solid gastric emptying.

Thus meals which are either liquid, or easily rendered to liquid, test predominantly relatively simple gastric and pyloric motor function. Meals which have a greater solid component also test the transfer of food from the proximal to the distal stomach and some degree of grinding, while meals which are less readily digestible may be testing predominantly the grinding function of the distal stomach. Furthermore, depending on the content of the meal, one meal may be testing duodenal feedback mechanisms to a greater degree than another (the fact that the amount of acid produced in response to the meal may also influence the rate of gastric emptying has been left out altogether).

It should also be pointed out that just about all investigators, except our own group, have looked only at emptying from the total stomach. Thus it is quite possible that a patient may have normal total emptying measured and yet have grossly delayed proximal to distal emptying, counter-balanced by accelerated distal emptying and such a situation could be a potent cause of GERD.

We have used a dual isotope method to examine solid (hamburger) and liquid (dextrose solution) gastric emptying in patients with GERD, and found that 60% of patients had delay in either solid or liquid emptying or both [4]. Furthermore, it was shown that the major cause of delayed emptying relates to delayed transfer of food from the proximal to the distal stomach [3]. As we have also demonstrated structural abnormalities in the muscle of the proximal stomach, this is strong evidence for the presence of a neural disorder. This suggests that the abnormality precedes and may play a pathogenetic role in the cause of abnormal reflux [7].

We have recently completed a study in 19 patients with reflux disease and found that delayed solid emptying from the proximal stomach is significantly correlated with the number of postprandial sphincter relaxations and reflux episodes. This adds further weight to the thesis that delayed gastric emptying is a pathogenetic mechanism inducing GERD.

In summary, unless one uses patients with broadly similar degrees of GERD and identical test meals of solids and liquids given under similar test conditions, then gastric emptying tests are going to vary greatly when compared between different groups of investigators.

References

1. Dubois A. Clinical relevance of gastroduodenal dysfunction in reflux esophagitis. J Clin Gastroenterol 1986;8:17–25.
2. Horowitz M, Akkermans LMA. Scintigraphic measurement of gastric emptying. In: Read NW (ed) Gastrointestinal Motility: Which Test?, Chapter 8. London: Wrightson Biomedical Publishing Ltd, 1989.
3. Jamieson GG, Myers J, Collins P, Dehn T, Maddern G, Horowitz M. Which region of the stomach is responsible for delay in gastric emptying of solids in patients with gastroesophageal reflux disease (GERD) in diseases of the esophagus. In: Little AG, Ferguson MK, Skinner DB (eds) Diseases of the Esophagus, vol 2. New York: Mount Kisco, 1990;121–126.
4. Maddern GJ, Chatterton BE, Collins PJ, Horowitz M, Shearman DJC, Jamieson GG. Solid and liquid gastric emptying in patients with gastro-oesophageal reflux. Br J Surg 1985;72:344–347.
5. McCallum RW, Berkowitz DM, Lerner E. Gastric emptying in patients with gastroesophageal reflux. Gastroenterology 1981;80:285–291.
6. Schwizer W, Hinder RA, DeMeester TR. Does delayed gastric emptying contribute to gastroesophageal reflux disease. Am J Surg 1989;157:74–81.
7. Wattchow DJ, Furness J, Jamieson GG, Maddern GJM. The distribution of peptide containing nerve fibres in the gastric musculature of patients with gastroesophageal reflux disease. Ann Surg 1992;216:153–160.

Should the use of pharmacologic agents promoting gastric emptying be reconsidered?

R.W. McCallum (Charlottesville)

Gastroesophageal reflux (GER) occurs more often in the postprandial than in the fasting state. One reason is that the volume of contents present in the stomach determines the frequency of reflux. In fact, the volume of fluid in the stomach required to produce a GER episode has been used as an index of lower esophageal sphincter (LES) strength. In the postprandial state, the volume of fluid present in the stomach depends on the following factors: volume of food and saliva ingested; volume of gastric secretions; duodenogastric reflux; and gastric emptying.

GER is more common after a large meal. Gastric acid secretion in patients with reflux esophagitis has been studied. GER patients as a group have normal acid secretory parameters, although up to 5% may be hypersecretors [1]. There is an increased incidence of GER in patients with Zollinger-Ellison syndrome [2], and this is attributed to an overwhelming effect of hypersecretion of acid. Pyloric incompetence facilitating duodenogastric reflux was proposed as an important contributing factor in a number of ways a large volume of refluxed material would increase the gastric volume and may even slow the gastric emptying rate; bile acid may induce antral gastritis and therefore cause antral hypomotility, and bile acids and other alkaline secretions may reflux into the esophagus, damaging the esophageal mucosa directly.

It has been reported that patients with GER disease have higher concentrations of bile acids in the stomach and therefore larger volumes of duodenogastric reflux [3]. However, recent studies using radionuclide methods have shown that duodenogastric reflux is a physiologic phenomenon; concentrations of bile acids in the gastric juice of patients with erosive esophagitis are similar to those of normal subjects [4]. Therefore, the significance of duodenogastric reflux remains controversial. However, recent strokes in patients with GER and more severe disease, such as structure and/or Barrett's esophagus, suggest more bile present in the fluid refluxing into the esophagus in these subjects of patients.

Gastric retention, with accumulation of acid and gastric contents, may be postulated as a contributory factor in the production of GER. McCallum and colleagues [5,6] reported delayed gastric emptying of solids in a significant number

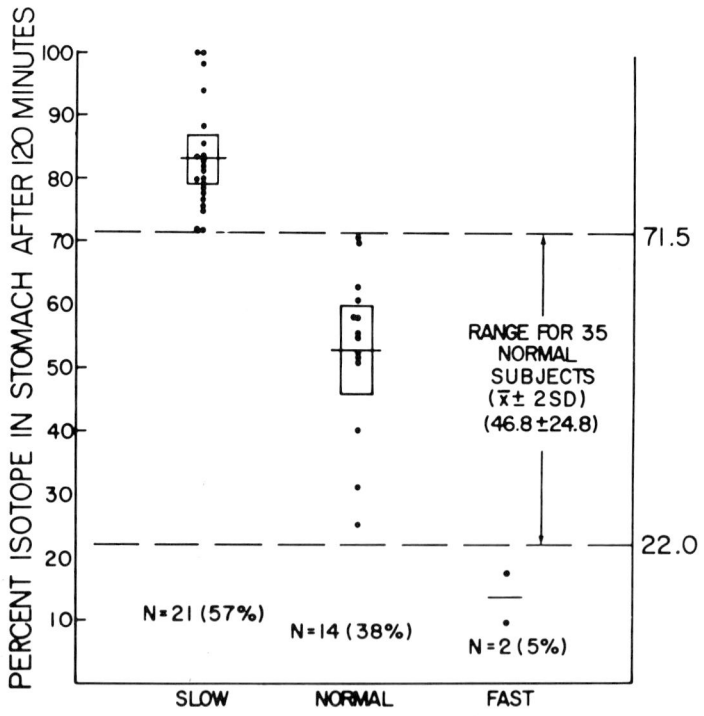

Fig. 1. Gastric emptying G-E reflux patients (n = 37, with 95% confidence limits).

836

of patients with GER (Fig. 1). Behar and Ramsey [7] found that there was an abnormality in the gastric antral motility, but that liquid emptying was normal.

An antireflux operation, fundoplication, is often successful in patients with reflux esophagitis. When gastric emptying studies are performed, surgical failures appear to correlate with slower solid emptying [8,9], whereas increased liquid emptying occurs more often. This latter phenomenon is probably attributable to impaired receptive relaxation related to surgical trauma or entrapment of the vagus nerve. The author has also observed that a population of postfundoplication patients presenting with increasing symptoms of GER (and therefore termed "relative" or "absolute failure") had an accompanying delay in gastric emptying. This delay may have been present in this patient group from the onset; thus there would be no reason to suppose that a fundoplication would have any real effect on improving the rate of solid gastric emptying in these patients. Interestingly, the literature indicates that symptoms tend to recur over a period of 3 to 5 years, such that after 5 years there is significant development of reflux as documented by esophageal pH studies. It may indicate that the continued delay in gastric emptying in some patients slowly weakens the efficacy of the antireflux procedure.

Fink and colleagues [1] have reported that the slow gastric emptying of solids in patients with GER can be correlated with the degree and severity of antral gastritis. Presumably this antral gastritis continues after surgery. The cause of the gastritis is not clear. Is it possible that gastric stasis itself could promote gastritis, or could gastritis induce a smooth muscle impairment? In the latter case, the cause of the gastritis could be bile reflux, which raises questions about the competence of the pylorus and the status of duodenal motility in GER.

Therapeutic role of gastric prokinetic agents in gastroesophageal reflux

The study of gastrointestinal motility has been advanced by the development of such diagnostic techniques as the use of perfused catheter and microtransducer recordings, measurement of myoelectric activity and radionuclide methodology. These techniques have provided a new understanding of gastrointestinal pathophysiology, and thus offer a rational basis for pharmacotherapy for gastrointestinal motility studies. The term "applied pharmacology" of the gut reflects the promise of new "prokinetic" agents, which have stimulated a renewed interest in defining disease mechanisms involving abnormalities in smooth muscle. These prokinetic agents, which also have important therapeutic benefits in disorders of gastrointestinal smooth muscle, are discussed in this review.

"Kinetic," as defined in the Dorland Medical Dictionary, means "pertaining to or producing motion". "Prokinetic" implies favoring "forward motion". This review concentrates on metoclopramide and domperidone, which is still experimental in the USA and the newer agent cisapride, which has just become available in the USA and approved by the FDA for treatment of GERD patients who have nocturnal heartburn as part of their presentation.

Prokinetic agents

The use of prokinetic agents, which increase the LES tone and stimulate gastric emptying, is appealing in the management of GER because it addresses the chronic underlying factors that contribute to the condition. The amount of gastric contents available for reflux into the esophagus and the interrelationship of delayed gastric emptying to GER has been summarized (Fig. 2).

Bethanechol

Bethanechol was the first smooth muscle stimulant to be used to treat patients with GER. The agent increases LES pressure and esophageal clearance but it does not augment gastric emptying. It has a negative effect, in that it stimulates gastric acid secretion and also decreases the velocity of esophageal peristalsis.

The studies on the use of the bethanechol in GER have produced conflicting results. In endoscopically controlled studies it appears to be as effective as cimetidine [10]. In another report bethanechol and antacids were compared with placebo and antacids and there were no differences. Another study demonstrated complete healing of esophagitis in 45% of bethanechol-treated patients compared with 13.5% healing in an antacid-placebo group [11].

Bethanechol at a dose of 25 mg, 4 times a day, is often not well tolerated. Side effects including abdominal cramps, diarrhea, urinary frequency and blurred vision have limited its acceptance as a treatment for GER.

Metoclopramide

Metoclopramide, a procainamide derivative, stimulates gastrointestinal (GI) smooth muscle [12]. It increases LES pressure and the amplitude of esophageal contractions as well [1]. It also accelerates gastric emptying in retention states and improves small

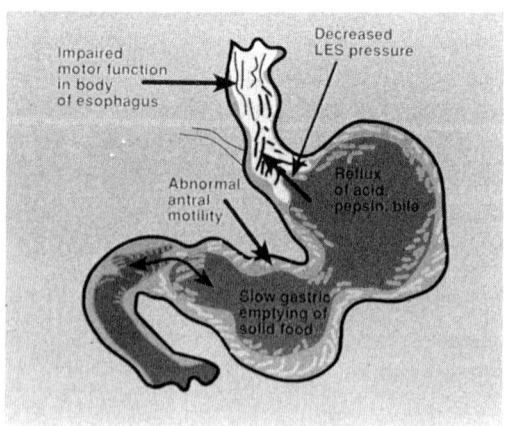

Fig. 2. Etiology of reflux (adapted from McCallum and Champion).

bowel transit. The exact mechanism that produces these effects on GI smooth muscle has not been precisely defined, but it is partially explained through dopamine antagonism. Although dopamine is regarded as an inhibitory neurotransmitter, the actual existence of dopaminergic neurons in the GI tract has not been clearly established in humans. Metoclopramide also augments acetylcholine release from postganglionic cholinergic nerve terminals and sensitizes muscarinic receptors of GI smooth muscle. It may have a direct stimulating effect on smooth muscle, as suggested by its effect on opossum LES, which is not abolished by tetrodotoxin or atropine [13].

Metoclopramide has the ability to not only stimulate the GI smooth muscle but to co-ordinate gastric, pyloric and duodenal motor activity, resulting in net aboral movement. This property is incompletely understood, but crucial to the class of prokinetic agents. It differentiates its action from the nonspecific cholinergic effect of bethanechol on gastric emptying [14].

Studies showed that metoclopramide, both parenterally and orally, increased the rate of gastric emptying in GER patients in whom emptying was delayed [15]. On the other hand, bethanechol did not produce a significant improvement in gastric retention. In the same patients with symptomatic reflux and low LES pressure, 20 mg of metoclopramide produced a greater increase in sphincter pressure than 25 mg of bethanechol, whereas responses to 10 mg of metoclopramide and 25 mg of bethanechol were similar. Metoclopramide does not increase gastric acid secretion or stimulate endogenous gastrin release, thus presenting a theoretical advantage over bethanechol.

Metoclopramide also significantly enhanced gastric emptying in the subgroups of GER patients with slow as well as normal emptying rates [16]. The improvement in the group of esophagitis patients with normal emptying was greater than that reported by Metzger and colleagues [17] in normal volunteers using the same test meal. This result was obtained in a larger population and, although significant, the mean decrement of 10.8%, 90 min after the meal, was only half the improvement achieved with metoclopramide in the slow emptying reflux patients (20.3%). For a given patient, this improved emptying rate (although still in the normal range) may be clinically important by reducing the residual gastric volume available to reflux, particularly when combined with the purported reduction in the duodenogastric reflux attributed to metoclopramide. These effects, augmented by the accompanying increase in LES pressure, may reduce GER.

A double-blind study showed that metoclopramide significantly reduced day and night time heartburn and regurgitation, as well as decreasing the need for antacid use [18]. In addition, the magnitude of increase in LES pressure after metoclopramide did not predict symptomatic response, indicating that the clinical response to this prokinetic compound is more related to enhanced gastric emptying and decreased duodenogastric reflux, thus facilitating acid removal from the region of the proximal stomach and the gastroesophageal junction.

In a follow-up study, metoclopramide significantly improved symptoms in a double-blind trial and this symptom improvement was correlated more with increasing gastric emptying and LES pressure than any other parameter [19].

Guslandi and colleagues [20] randomly treated 45 patients with symptomatic GER and confirmed histologic esophagitis with either metoclopramide (10 mg, 3 times a day) or ranitidine (150 mg twice a day). During the 6-week trial, both drugs were effective in producing symptomatic and endoscopic improvement. More recently, metoclopramide with cimetidine was shown to provide symptom relief in patients not already adequately improved by cimetidine alone [21].

The recommended dose of metoclopramide is 10 mg before meals and at bedtime. On a physiologic basis it can be recommended that, for long-term maintenance therapy, a larger single dose of 20 mg, either at bedtime or before a large (evening) meal or a known provocative event, should be considered.

The limiting factor with metoclopramide is the high incidence of side effects, which occur in approximately 20% of patients at a dose of 10 mg, 4 times a day. The most troublesome side effects appear to be restlessness, agitation, somnolence and extrapyramidal symptoms related to intracerebral dopamine antagonism [22].

Domperidone

Domperidone is a peripheral dopamine antagonist, which, unlike metoclopramide, does not readily enter the central nervous system. It thus has none of the side effects that restrict the use of metoclopramide.

Results of pharmacologic studies on the effects of domperidone on esophageal motility have proved inconsistent. Studies by Brock-Utne and colleagues [23] and Weihrauch and co-workers [24] using domperidone intravenously, found increased LES pressure following administration, but other studies have not [25]. Likewise, trials using oral domperidone have produced variable results [23–25]. In addition, pH monitoring [26] found no difference between domperidone and placebo.

Domperidone's prokinetic effect on the stomach and its ability to improve gastric emptying, thereby reducing gastric volume and possibly helping to prevent reflux, have been well documented [27–31]. Therapeutic trials of domperidone in treating GER, however, have also produced equivocal results and overall have been negative in well-controlled double-blind studies [32].

Goethals [33] in a double-blind crossover study comparing domperidone with placebo, found domperidone to be superior in alleviating heartburn and regurgitation. Similarly, Valenzuela [25] found domperidone significantly more effective than placebo in relieving regurgitation but did not significantly improve heartburn or endoscopic healing.

In a study comparing domperidone and ranitidine alone and in combination, both agents were equally effective in reducing symptoms and promoting healing of esophagitis, but the combination therapy was not significantly superior to either drug alone [34].

Conversely, in another study comparing domperidone with placebo as add-on therapy to a standard antacid regimen, concomitant domperidone administration did not significantly affect LES pressure, the number of reflux episodes (as recorded by pH meter), or heartburn [26]. However, the domperidone-treated group did show a significant decrease in antacid use over baseline.

These studies suggest that the primary effect that domperidone may have in patients with reflux esophagitis may be due to improved gastric emptying, with movement of gastric contents, acid and pepsin away from the lower esophageal sphincter rather than improved esophageal motility. This is consistent with domperidone's dopamine-antagonist activity on D_2 receptors in the stomach.

The recommended dose of domperidone is 10 mg to 20 mg before meals and at bedtime. The overall incidence of side effects with domperidone is less than 7%. Headaches and endocrinologic problems related to the hyperprolactinemia (e.g., breast enlargement, nipple tenderness, galactorrhea and amenorrhea), which occur with all dopamine antagonists, appear to be the most troublesome. A dose of 20 mg, 4 times a day, has proved to be effective therapy in a large number of patients with GER in European and other studies and doses of 20 or 30 mg before large meals, or on an intermittent basis, could be an approach for long-term maintenance therapy.

Cisapride

Cisapride (Propulsid) is unique among prokinetic agents because it does not have an antidopaminergic action. Instead, it exerts its effect by increasing the availability of acetylcholine from postganglionic nerve endings of the myenteric plexus, leading to improved propulsive motor activity of the esophagus, stomach, small bowel and large bowel. It has no known direct antiemetic properties. Its full pharmacology profile and effects in GER have been extensively reviewed recently [35].

Cisapride appears to exert its beneficial effects in patients with GER by stimulating esophageal peristalsis, increasing LES tone (Fig. 3), and stimulating gastric emptying (Fig. 4).

These effects have been investigated both in normal subjects and in patients with

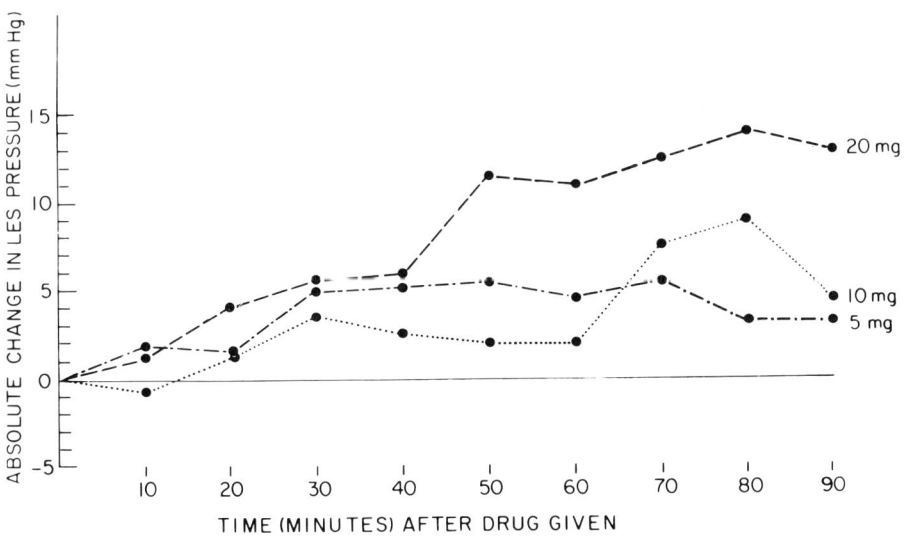

Fig. 3. Summary of dose-response effects of cisapride on LES pressure in men (n = 8).

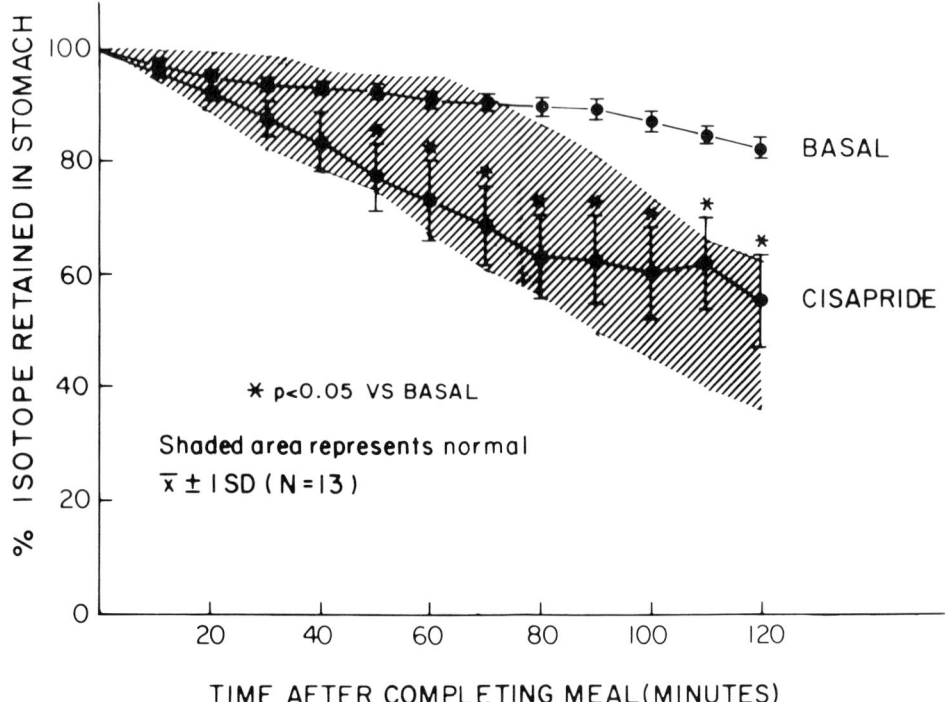

Fig. 4. Summary of effects of 10 mg i.v. cisapride on gastric emptying of a solid meal (n = 19).

GER in short-term studies. In healthy volunteers, cisapride increased the LES tone following intravenous and oral administration [36–38]. In GER patients who had an abnormally low LES pressure (<10 mmHg), cisapride raised the amplitude of esophageal peristaltic contractions and normalized the LES [36].

This effect was confirmed in a study by Collins and Love [39] in which cisapride, 10 mg, 3 times a day, was administered over a 1-month period to patients with symptoms and endoscopic evidence of GER. In this study, radionuclide esophageal transit times were not significantly altered by cisapride. However, duration of GER, especially at night, was significantly reduced after treatment with cisapride when compared with placebo (p = 0.007).

Conversely, Holloway and colleagues [40] studied 16 patients in a randomized double-blind, placebo-controlled crossover trial to evaluate postprandial reflux. Esophageal manometry and pH were monitored after loading a dose of cisapride, 10 mg, 3 times a day, for 3 days. The investigators found no significant effect on the rate of reflux, duration of esophageal acid exposure, mechanism of LES incompetence, esophageal peristalsis, or basal LES pressure.

Comparison of cisapride with placebo

To assess cisapride's efficacy in healing and symptomatic relief, several double-blind randomized trials have been conducted in which the agent was administered in parallel with placebo to patients with grades 0 to III esophagitis (Savary Miller classification). Mucosal damage was confirmed by endoscopy at the commencement of the trials and attempts were made to eliminate placebo responders during an initial period of 1 to 2 weeks [41,42].

Cisapride was more effective than placebo in symptomatic and objective improvement in patients with endoscopically proved reflux esophagitis. Thus, as assessed objectively and subjectively, these European studies show that cisapride therapy seems to be superior to placebo in patients with reflux esophagitis. Two multicenter double-blind studies in the U.S. have demonstrated significant reductions in nocturnal heartburn during treatment with cisapride. The study population in both trials had moderated to severe heartburn for more than 3 months and at least grade I esophagitis documented on endoscopy. A 2-week placebo run-in period enabled exclusion of placebo responders before randomization to placebo or active treatment. Antacid use was permitted on a p.r.n. basis during both trial periods.

In the earlier trial, 147 reflux patients with day *or* night heartburn (35% of whom had esophageal ulceration) were randomly assigned to treatment with placebo or cisapride 10 mg q.i.d. for 8 weeks. Cisapride 10 mg q.i.d. significantly ($p < 0.01$ vs. placebo) improved nocturnal heartburn throughout the trial. In addition, antacid consumption declined significantly ($p = 0.04$) with cisapride, but not with placebo.

The effectiveness of cisapride in treating patients with nocturnal heartburn was confirmed in a dose-response trial. A total of 177 patients with daytime *and* nocturnal heartburn were randomized to treatment with placebo, cisapride 10 mg q.i.d., or cisapride 20 mg q.i.d. for 12 weeks. At 4 weeks, cisapride 10 mg q.i.d. was significantly ($p < 0.05$) more effective than placebo in reducing night time heartburn, with symptomatic improvement with cisapride 10 mg q.i.d. continuing to be superior to placebo at 8 and 12 weeks (Fig. 5). Treatment with the 20 mg q.i.d. cisapride resulted in significantly ($p < 0.05$) greater improvement in night time heartburn at all times evaluated (Fig. 5). Average daily antacid use was also significantly ($p < 0.05$ vs. placebo) reduced at 4 weeks with cisapride 10 mg q.i.d. and at all evaluations with cisapride 20 mg q.i.d. (Fig. 5). Side effects reported in each treatment group were similar and there were no serious adverse reactions.

The effectiveness of cisapride 10 mg q.i.d. in reducing night time heartburn has also been shown in non-U.S. clinical trials involving 366 patients in all.

Comparison of cisapride with other drugs in combination therapy

Cisapride has been compared with ranitidine and metoclopramide in clinical studies. In combination therapy the use of cisapride, with or without cimetidine, has also been studied.

Cisapride administered in a dose of 10 mg, 4 times a day tended to affect healing in a higher percentage of patients than ranitidine, 150 mg twice a day, after 6 to 12 weeks of treatment, but the differences were not significant [43]. Similar results were obtained in a study by Manousos and colleagues [44].

Galmiche and colleagues compared the efficacy of cisapride, 10 mg, 4 times a day and cimetidine with placebo and cimetidine in the treatment of 47 patients with

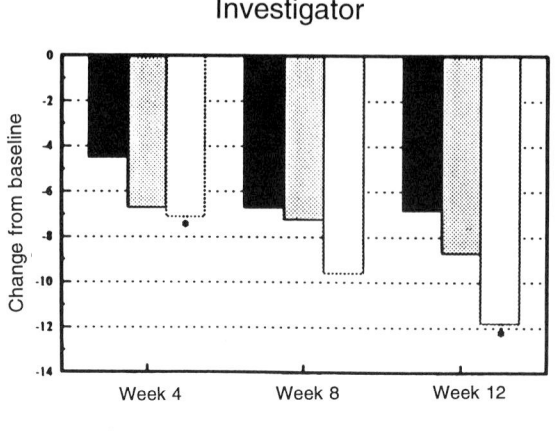

Investigator

* p < 0.05 vs. placebo using ANCOVA

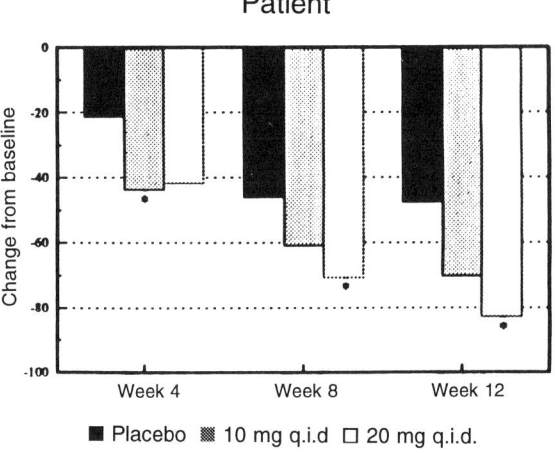

Patient

■ Placebo ▨ 10 mg q.i.d □ 20 mg q.i.d.

Fig. 5. Total symptoms.

erosive or ulcerative esophagitis (Savary Miller grades II and III) [45]. The percentage of patients with good or excellent response, in terms of healing rates, was significantly higher ($p < 0.025$) in the cisapride-cimetidine group compared with the placebo-cimetidine group.

Further studies are required regarding the role of cisapride, either as an alternative to H_2-receptor antagonists or in combination with a proton pump blocker. In this latter case the dose of the proton pump agent could be decreased, while cisapride is used to address bile and pancreatic reflux, which could be occurring in patients with esophageal stricture or Barrett's esophagus.

Long-term therapy

GERD is a chronic lifelong disease in 90% of patients encountered initially as "acute" GERD. Therefore, long-term therapy is needed in order to address symptomatic recurrences. Cisapride is the only prokinetic agent that has proven effective in the maintenance treatment of esophagitis. Three placebo-controlled multicenter studies have confirmed the efficacy of cisapride in delaying the relapse of GERD, prolonging the duration of endoscopic and symptomatic remission at recommended chronic long-term doses ranging from 20 mg b.i.d. to even 20 mg t.i.d. [46—48]. The effects are most pronounced in patients with recurrent mild to moderate esophagitis, as defined by the initial degree of esophageal mucosal injury. Clinical response in these trials to cisapride was less pronounced on patients with aggressive GERD who required proton-pump inhibitors to achieve symptom control and/or induce healing. However, even in this severe subset of patients, the duration of remission was doubled compared to placebo. A clear message from these and other studies in Europe ranging from 6 months 5.5 years in over 1,000 patients [49] is that cisapride is an amazingly safe and well-tolerated agent. Apart from transient loosening of stools, borborygmi or abdominal pain, which may occur at the initiation of therapy, rare headaches have also been reported. No significant changes in biochemical or hematological variables have been observed.

Conclusion

Etiologically, GER disease can be regarded as a motility disorder and gastric acid secretion is normal in nearly all patients. Although blocking acid is effective in the treatment of GER disease, it does not overcome or address the underlying pathologic factors that facilitate acid to reflux into the esophagus. Prokinetic agents address the upper gastrointestinal motility disturbances contributing to GER disease, and thus have an important role in the acute and long-term medical management of this entity.

References

1. Fink SM, Barwick K, DeLuca V et al. The association of histologic gastritis with gastroesophageal reflux and delayed gastric emptying. J Clin Gastroenterol 1984;6:301—305.
2. McCallum RW, Walsh JH. Relationship between lower esophageal sphincter pressure and serum gastrin concentration in Zollinger-Ellison syndrome and other clinical settings. Gastroenterology 1979;76:76—81.
3. Kaye MD, Showalter JP. Pyloric incompetence in patients with symptomatic gastroesophageal reflux. J Lab Clin Med 1974;83:198—206.
4. Kean FB, Dimagno EP, Malagelada JR. Duodenogastric reflux in humans: Its relationship to fasting antroduodenal motility and gastric, pancreatic and biliary secretion. Gastroenterology 1981;81:726—731.
5. McCallum RW, Berkowitz DM, Lerner E. Gastric emptying in patients with gastroesophageal reflux. Gastroenterology 1981;80:285—291.
6. McCallum RW, Mensh R, Lange R. Definition of gastric emptying abnormalities present in gastroesophageal reflux patients. In: Weinbeck M (ed) Motility of the Digestive Tract. New York: Raven, 1982;355—356.
7. Blackwell JN, Heading RC, Fettes MR. Effects of domperidone on lower esophageal sphincter pressure and gastroesophageal reflux in patients with peptic esophagitis. R Soc Med Int Cong Symp Series 1981;36:57—65.
8. Brandsborg O, Brandsborg M, Loygreen NA et al. Influence of parietal cell vagotomy and selective gastric vagotomy on gastric emptying rate and serum gastrin concentrations. Gastroenterology 1977;72:212—214.
9. Maddern GJ, Jamieson GG, Chatterton BE et al. Is there an association between failed antireflux procedures and delayed gastric emptying? Ann Surg 1985;202:162—165.
10. Thanik KD, Chey WY, Shah AN et al. Bethanechol or cimetidine in the treatment of symptomatic reflux esophagitis. Arch Intern Med 1982;142:1479—1481.

11. Saco LS, Orlando RC, Levison SL et al. Double-blind controlled trial of bethanechol and antacid versus placebo and antacid in the treatment of erosive esophagitis. Gastroenterology 1982;82:1369–1372.

12. Eisner M. Gastrointestinal effects of metoclopramide in man: in vivo experiments with human smooth muscle preparation. Br Med J 1968;4:679–680.

13. Cohen S, DiMarino AJ. Mechanism of action of metoclopramide on opossum lower esophageal sphincter muscle. Gastroenterology 1976;71:996–998.

14. McCallum RW, Kline MM, Curry N et al. Comparative effects of metoclopramide and bethanechol on lower esophageal sphincter pressure in reflux patients. Gastroenterology 1975;68:1114–1118.

15. McCallum RW, Fink SM, Lerner E et al. Effects of metoclopramide and bethanechol on delayed gastric emptying present in gastroesophageal reflux patients. Gastroenterology 1983;84:1573–1577.

16. Fink SM, Lange RC, McCallum RW. Effect of metoclopramide on normal and delayed gastric emptying in gastroesophageal reflux patients. Dig Dis Sci 1983;28:1057–1061.

17. Metzger WH, Cano R. Sturdevant RAL. Sturdevant RAL: effects of metoclopramide in chronic gastric retention after gastric surgery. Gastroenterology 1976;71:30–32.

18. McCallum RW, Ippolitti AF, Cooney C et al. A controlled trial of metoclopramide in symptomatic gastroesophageal reflux. N Engl J Med 1977;296:354–357.

19. McCallum RW, Fink SM, Winnan GR et al. Metoclopramide in gastroesophageal reflux disease: rationale for its use and results of a double-blind trial. Am J Gastroenterol 1984;79:165–172.

20. Guslandi M, Testoni PA, Passaretti S et al. Ranitidine vs. metoclopramide in the medical treatment of reflux esophagitis. Hepatogastroenterology 1983;30:96–98.

21. Lieberman DA, Keefe EB. Double-blind controlled trial of metoclopramide and cimetidine vs. cimetidine in the treatment of severe reflux esophagitis [abstract]. Gastroenterology 1985;88:1476.

22. Albibi R, McCallum RW. Metoclopramide: pharmacology and clinical applications. Ann Intern Med 1983;98:86–95.

23. Brock-Utne JG, Downing JW, Dimpoulos GE et al. Effect of domperidone on lower esophageal sphincter tone in late pregnancy. Anesthesiology 1980;52:321–323.

24. Weihrauch TR, Forster CRF, Krieglstein J. Evaluation of the effect of domperidone on human esophageal and gastroduodenal motility by intraluminal manometry. Postgrad Med J 1979;55:7–10.

25. Valenzuela JE. Effects of domperidone on the symptoms of reflux esophagitis. R Soc Med Int Cong Symp Series 1981;36:51–56.

26. Blackwell JN, Heading RC, Fettes MR. Effects of domperidone on lower esophageal sphincter pressure and gastroesophageal reflux in patients with peptic esophagitis. R Soc Med Int Cong Symp Series 1981;36:57–65.

27. Baeyens R, Reyntjens A, Van de Velde E. Effects of domperidone (R33,812) on the motor function of the stomach and small intestine. Arzneim Forsch 1978;28:682–686.

28. Champion MC, Gulenchyn KY, O'Leary T et al. Domperidone improves symptoms and solid phase gastric emptying in diabetic gastroparesis [abstract]. Am J Gastroenterol 1987;82:213.

29. Corinaldesi R, Stanghellini V, Zarabini GE et al. The affect of domperidone on the gastric emptying of solid and liquid phases of a mixed meal in patients with dyspepsia. Curr Ther Res 1983;34:982–986.

30. Del Genio A, Di Martino N, Piccolo S et al. The effect of domperidone on gastric emptying in reflux esophagitis: a radioisotopic study. J Nucl Med Allied Sci 1984;28:251–256.

31. Horowitz M, Maddern GJ, Chatterton BE et al. Acute and chronic effects of domperidone on gastric emptying in diabetic autonomic neuropathy. Dig Dis Sci 1985;30:1–9.

32. Champion MC. Domperidone: minireview. Gen Pharmacol 1988;19:499–505.

33. Goethals C. Domperidone in the treatment of postprandial symptoms suggestive of gastroesophageal reflux. Curr Ther Res 1979;26:876–880.

34. Masci E, Testoni PA, Passaretti S et al. A comparison of ranitidine, domperidone maleate and ranitidine + domperidone maleate in the short-term treatment of reflux esophagitis. Drugs Exp Clin Res 1985;10:1–6.

35. McCallum RW, Prakash C, Campoli-Richards DM et al. Cisapride: a review. Drugs 1988;36:652–681.

36. Janssens J, Ceccatelli P, Vantrappen G. Cisapride restores the decreased lower esophageal sphincter pressure in reflux patients. Digestion 1986;34:139.

37. Weinbeck M, Cuder-Wiessinger E, Berges W. Cisapride acts as a motor stimulator in the human esophagus. Gastroenterology 1984;86:1298.

38. Weiser HF, Holscher A, Zimmerman T. Effect of cisapride and metoclopramide on the lower esophageal motility pressure: a pressure and pH study. Digestion 1986;34:142.

39. Collins BJ, Love AHG. The effect of chronic oral administration of cisapride on the 16-h pH profile, oesophageal transit and gastric emptying of patients with evidence of gastro-oesophageal reflux: a placebo-controlled trial [abstract]. Digestion 1986;34:142 (Abstract).

40. Holloway RH, Dent J, Downton J et al. Effect of cisapride on postprandial gastroesophageal reflux. Digestion 1986;34:141.

41. Lepourtre L, Bollen J, Vandewalle N et al. Therapeutic side effects of cisapride in reflux oesophagitis: a double-blind, placebo-controlled study. In: Progress in the Treatment of Gastrointestinal Motility Orders. Amsterdam: Excerpta Medica, 1988;63–65.

42. Van Outrye M, Vanderlinden I, Dedullen G et al. Dose-response study with cisapride in gastroesophageal reflux disease. Curr Ther Res 1988;43:408–415.

43. Janisch HD, Huttermann W, Bouzo MH. Cisapride vs. ranitidine in the treatment of reflux esophagitis. Hepatogastro-

enterology (in press).

44. Manousos ON, Mandidis A, Michailidis D. Treatment of reflux symptoms in esophagitis patients: comparative trial of cisapride and metoclopramide. Curr Ther Res 1987;42:807—813.
45. Galmiche JP, Vitaux J, Brandstaetter G et al. Benefit of adding cisapride to cimetidine in the treatment of severe reflux esophagitis [abstract]. Gastroenterology 1987;92:1400.
46. Toussaint J, Gossium A, Deruyttere M et al. Healing and prevention of reflux esophagitis by cisapride. Gut 1991;32:1280—1285.
47. Tytgat GNJ, Anker Hansen OJ, Carling Z et al. Effect of cisapride on relapse of reflux esophagitis, healed with an antisecretory drug. Scand J Gastroenterol 1992;27:175—183.
48. Blum AL, Adams B, Borzo M et al. Effect of cisapride on relapse of esophagitis. A multinational, placebo-controlled trial in patients healed with an antisecretory drug. Dig Dis Sci 1993;38:551—560.
49. Verlinden M. An evaluation of adverse experiences, intercurrent conditions and clinical laboratory data based on 4 clinical trials, in 1046 patients evaluating the effectiveness of cisapride for the prevention of recurrence of reflux esophagitis. Janssen Researth Foundation, December 1990. (Data on file).

Can the development of Barrett's mucosa be found after esophagogastrostomy?

P.H. Cugnenc, Ph. Wind, M. Bouchoucha, J.Ph. Barbier
(Paris)

Replacement of the squamous epithelium, which normally lines the esophagus with a glandular mucosa [1] (Barret's mucosa), is one of the complications of gastroesophageal reflux (GER). Carrying out an esophagogastrostomy sets up the conditions for the onset of esophageal reflux. These conditions are identical to those reproduced experimentally by Bremner et al. in dogs [2]. The two traditional operations which involve esophagogastrostomy are esophagectomy with excision of the upper pole of the stomach and extensive resection of the esophagus with esophagogastroplasty.

Esophagogastrectomy with excision of the upper pole of the stomach involves excision of a limited amount of the esophagus together with gastrectomy of the upper part of the stomach and esophagogastric anastomosis. Such operations are rarely performed nowadays precisely because of the major risk of GER. Hamilton et al. [3] carried out a retrospective study of 17 patients who had undergone gastrectomy involving the upper pole and partial excision of the esophagus with esophagogastric anastomosis. After a period of 18 ± 14 months (range 2 to 43 months) Barrett mucosa covered the region of the anastomosis in seven of these patients. In three patients Barrett mucosa was found in the lower esophagus after a delay of 100 ± 22 months (range 76 to 114 months). Seven had normal mucosa in the esophagus and at the anastomosis. Severe symptoms of GER and bile reflux were found only in those with Barrett's esophagus. In addition, pyloroplasty had often been carried out more frequently in this group.

Extensive resection of the esophagus with esophagogastroplasty and esophagogastric anastomosis is usually carried out for malignant disease in adults and for nonmalignant disease (atresia) in children. Using an endoscope, Lindahl et al. [4] examined the remaining esophagus in 14 children who had undergone extensive resection of the esophagus with esophagogastroplasty (mainly for esophageal atresia) for the past 2 years. When endoscopy was performed (a mean 8.2 years, range 2.2 to 13.9 years, after operation) 10 of these patients had glandular metaplasia in the remaining esophagus.

In adults, Naef et al. [5] described a patient who developed Barrett's esophagus 13 years after extensive resection of the esophagus with esophagogastroplasty for stenosis caused by chemical burns. We have an experience of a group of 65 esophagectomies for cancer carried out consecutively between 1986 and 1992 with esophagogastroplasty and esophagogastric anastomosis in the neck. Thirty of these patients were included in a study which involved endoscopy with esophageal and gastric biopsies, 24-h pH measurement in the gastric transplant and manometry carried out 3 months after operation and then every year [6]. No Barrett's esophagus was found after 3 to 47 months. Esophagitis was found 3 times macroscopically and 15 times histologically. Lesions of gastritis were found in the gastric transplant on histology only on three occasions. The mean pH was 4.3 ± 1.0 and the percentage of times on which it was lower than 4 was 42.6 ± 10.9. The only conclusion to be drawn from these findings is that acidity continues in the gastric transplant in spite of vagotomy and the extent of the resection. The amount of acid could not be calculated because the volume of gastric secretion was not measured. This test was not carried out in the remaining segment of the esophagus.

When conditions for GER are created experimentally, Barrett's esophagus is possible after esophagogastrostomy and the mechanism is probably the same as when it is a complication of traditional GER. There is probably a long delay before its onset. This last finding explains the rarity with which glandular metaplasia of the remaining esophagus is found in adults after extensive esophagectomy and esophagogastroplasty for cancer. Lindahl et al. [4] urge the prevention of this complication in children by systematic treatment for GER. Although no cancer has been reported in Barrett's esophagus following esophagogastrostomy, the risk certainly appears to be the same as in other forms of Barrett's esophagus, and endoscopic monitoring is essential.

References

1. Spechler S, Goyal R. Barrett's esophagus. N Eng J Med 1966;315:362–371.
2. Bremner C, Lynch V, Ellis P Jr. Barrett's esophagus: congenital or acquired? An experimental study of esophageal mucosal regeneration in the dog. Surgery 1970;68:209–216.
3. Hamilton S, Yardley J. Regeneration of cardiac type mucosa and acquisition for Barrett mucosa after esophagogastrostomy. Gastroenterology 1977;72:669–675.
4. Linahl H, Rintala R, Sariola H, Louhimou L. Cervical Barrett's esophagus: a common complication of gastric tube reconstruction. J Pediatr Surg 1990;25:446–448.
5. Naef P, Savary M, Ozzelo L. Columnar-lined lower esophagus: an acquired lesion with malignant predisposition. Report of 140 cases of Barrett's esophagus with adenocarcinomas. J Thorac Cardiovasc Surg 1975:70:826–835.
6. Bouchoucha M, Cugnenc PH, Drévillon C, Faye A, Boboc B, Arhan P, Barbier JPh. Functional evaluation of gastric transplants used in esopohageal reconstruction. Dysphagia 1969;4:53–57.

Mucosa and radiology

 Is the radiologic appearance of Barrett's esophagus distinguishable from that of severe reflux esophagitis?
— What value should be given to reticular mucosal pattern?

M.S. Levine (Philadelphia)

Barrett's esophagus is an acquired condition in which there is progressive columnar metaplasia of the distal esophagus due to long-standing gastroesophageal reflux and reflux esophagitis. Current data suggest that Barrett's esophagus is a much more common condition than has previously been recognized. In various studies, the prevalence of Barrett's esophagus in patients with reflux esophagitis has ranged from 8 to 20%, with an overall prevalence of about 10%. These figures may be skewed in favor of Barrett's esophagus, because patients with reflux symptoms who undergo endoscopy are more likely to have significant reflux disease. Nevertheless, Barrett's esophagus is being diagnosed with greater frequency as the number of patients who undergo endoscopy increases.

Many authors believe that barium studies have a limited role in evaluating patients with possible Barrett's esophagus, and that endoscopy and biopsy are required for diagnosing this condition. However, recent data suggest that double contrast esophagography is a useful screening examination in patients with reflux symptoms to determine the relative need for endoscopy and biopsy in these patients.

Radiographic aspects

The classic radiologic features of Barrett's esophagus consist of a high esophageal stricture or ulcer, often associated with a hiatal hernia or gastroesophageal reflux [2,7]. The unusual location of these strictures and ulcers can be attributed to the fact that they often occur in the proximal zone of columnar metaplasia near the squamocolumnar junction. The strictures may appear as ring-like constrictions (Fig. 1) or, less commonly, as smooth, tapered areas of narrowing (Fig. 2) in the midesophagus. Barrett's ulcers typically appear as relatively deep ulcer craters within the columnar mucosa at a considerable distance from the gastroesophageal junction. Other patients may have both a stricture and an ulcer in the midesophagus (Fig. 3). Since these findings are unusual in uncomplicated reflux esophagitis, the presence of a high esophageal stricture or ulcer, particularly if associated with a hiatal hernia or gastroesophageal reflux, should be strongly suggestive of Barrett's esophagus. However, studies have found that strictures are actually more common in the distal esophagus and that most cases do not fit the classic description of a high stricture or ulcer [1,6,8]. Thus, esophagography is an inadequate screening examination for Barrett's esophagus when the diagnosis is made only in patients who have the classic radiologic features of this condition.

A reticular mucosal pattern has also been described as a relatively specific sign of Barrett's esophagus, particularly if located adjacent to a stricture [6]. This delicate reticular pattern is characterized radiographically by innumerable tiny, barium-filled grooves or crevices on the esophageal mucosa, often resembling the areae gastricae pattern found on double contrast studies of the stomach (Fig. 4). In most cases, there is an adjacent stricture in the middle, or less commonly, distal third of the esophagus, with the reticular pattern extending distally a short but variable distance from the stricture. Occasionally, however, a reticular or villous pattern of the mucosa may be observed as the only morphologic abnormality in Barrett's esophagus without evidence of strictures [5]. Whether or not a stricture is present, this distinctive reticular pattern should be highly suggestive of Barrett's esophagus and endoscopy and biopsy should be performed for a definitive diagnosis. Nevertheless, this finding has been observed in only 5 to 30% of patients with Barrett's esophagus and its specificity has also been questioned [1–3,6,9]. Thus, most cases of Barrett's esophagus will be missed on double contrast esophagography if a reticular mucosal pattern is used as the primary radiologic criterion for diagnosing this condition.

Since Barrett's esophagus develops as the sequelae of long-standing reflux esophagitis, it is not surprising that these patients often have radiologic evidence of hiatal hernias, gastroesophageal reflux, reflux esophagitis, and peptic strictures (Fig. 5) [1–3,6–9]. However, these findings often occur in patients with uncomplicated reflux disease. As a result, inclusion of these findings as criteria for Barrett's esophagus increases the sensitivity of the radiologic examination but decreases its specificity, so that many patients would be referred unnecessarily for endoscopy and biopsy [3]. Thus, radiographic findings that are relatively specific for Barrett's esophagus are not sensitive and those findings that are sensitive are not specific. Many investigators therefore believe that esophagography has limited value

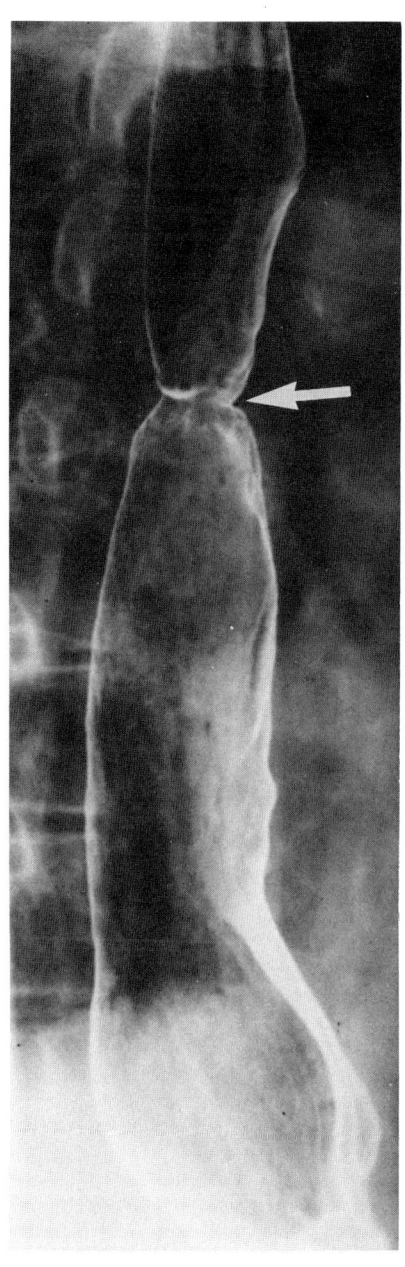

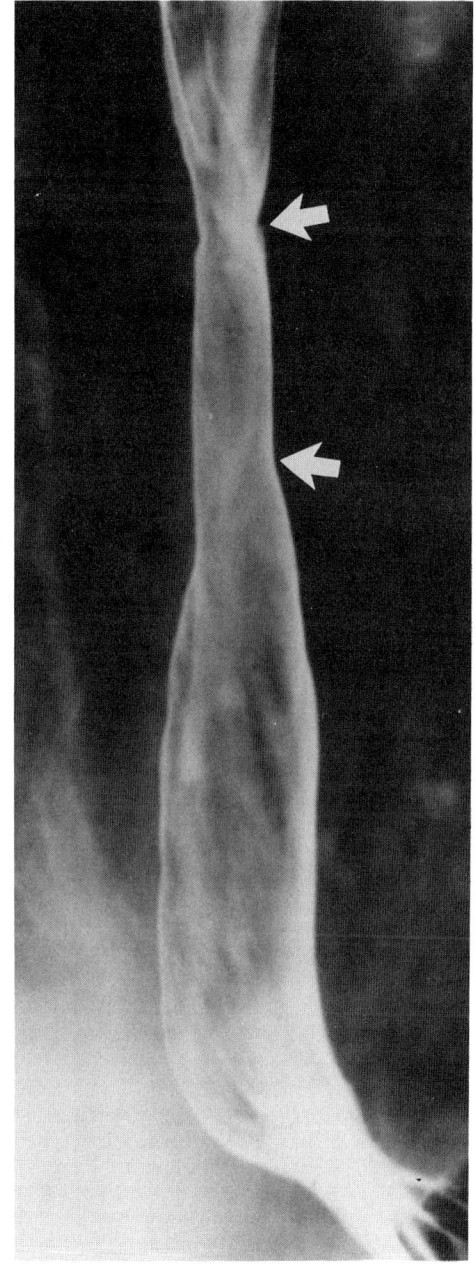

Fig. 1. Barrett's esophagus with a midesophageal stricture. A focal ring-like constriction (arrow) is seen in the midesophagus. In the presence of a hiatal hernia and gastroesophageal reflux, a high stricture should be virtually diagnostic of Barrett's esophagus.

Fig. 2. Barrett's esophagus with a midesophageal stricture. A relatively smooth, tapered area of narrowing (arrows) is present in the midesophagus.

as a screening examination for Barrett's esophagus and that endoscopy and biopsy are required to diagnose this condition.

Recently, however, Gilchrist et al. performed a blinded, retrospective study of 200

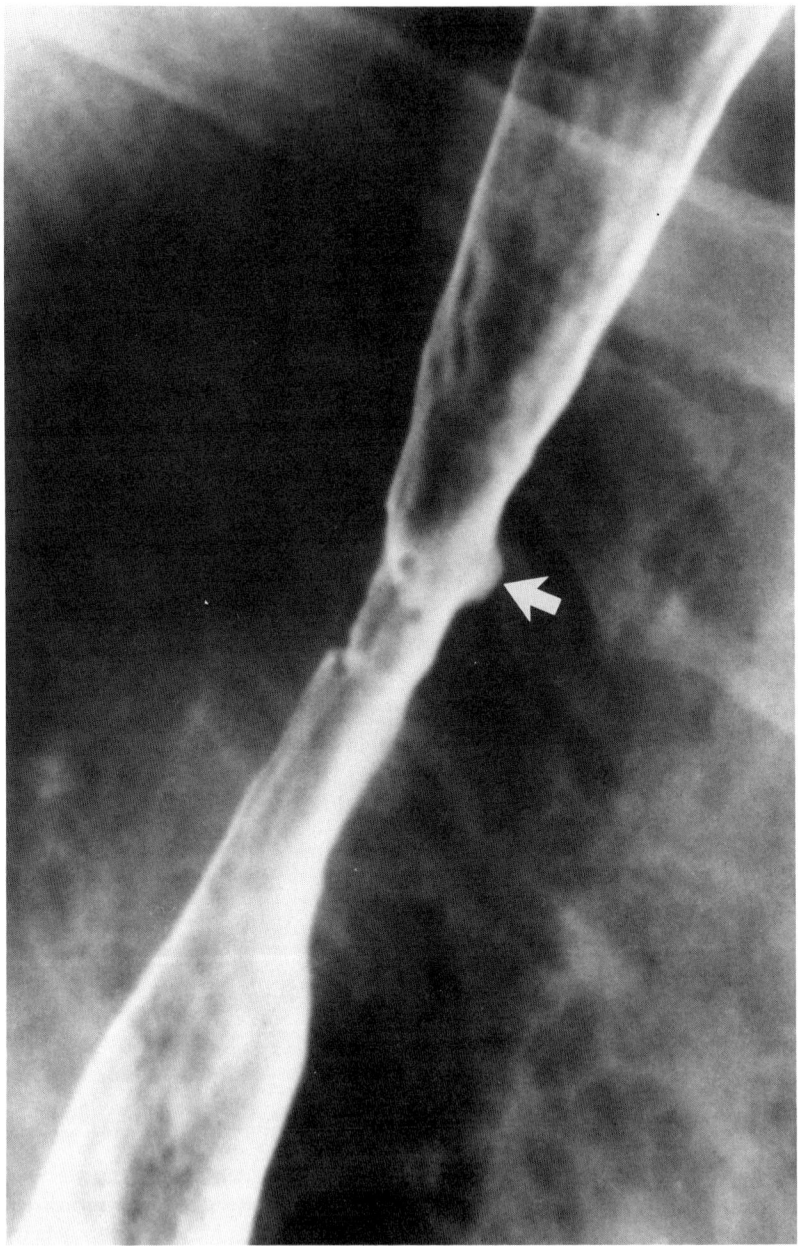

Fig. 3. Barrett's esophagus with a midesophageal stricture and ulcer. A concentric area of narrowing is seen in the midesophagus, with a discrete ulcer (arrow) in the region of the stricture.

patients who had both double contrast esophagrams and endoscopy because of severe reflux symptoms [4]. The patients were classified into high-, moderate- and low-risk

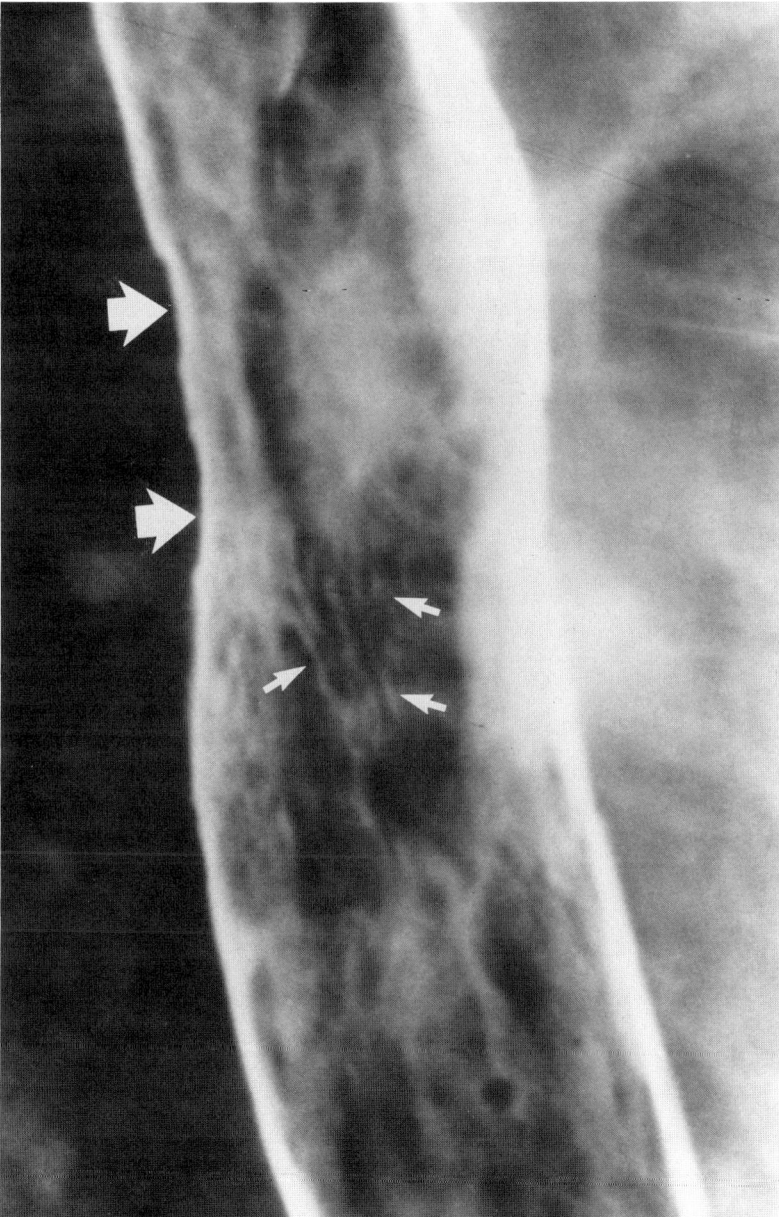

Fig. 4. Barrett's esophagus with a reticular mucosal pattern. There is the earliest stage of a stricture in the midesophagus with slight flattening of one wall (large arrows). A lacy reticular pattern (small arrows) is seen extending distally from the region of the stricture. This reticular pattern is a relatively specific radiologic criterion for Barrett's esophagus, particularly if located adjacent to the distal aspect of a high stricture.

groups for Barrett's esophagus on the basis of the radiographic findings. Patients were classified at high risk for Barrett's esophagus if the radiographs revealed a high stricture or ulcer or a reticular pattern; at moderate risk, if the radiographs revealed a distal peptic stricture and/or reflux esophagitis (because previous studies have shown that about 40% of patients with peptic strictures and 10% with reflux esophagitis have Barrett's esophagus); and at low risk, if none of these findings were present. When these radiologic criteria were used, 10 patients (5%) were thought to be at high risk, 73 (37%) at moderate risk and 117 (58%) at low risk for Barrett's esophagus. Endoscopic correlation revealed biopsy-proven Barrett's mucosa in nine of 10 patients (90%) at high risk, 12 of 73 patients (16%) at moderate risk and only one of 117 patients (<1%) at low risk for Barrett's esophagus. Although the overall

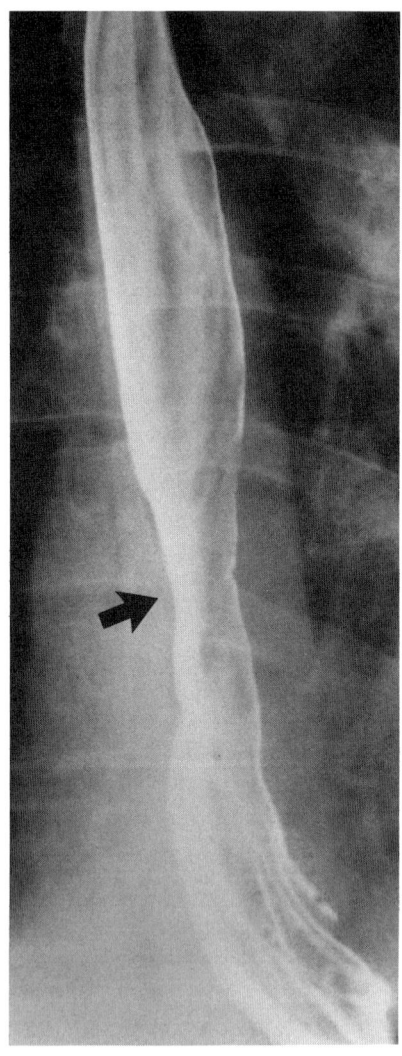

Fig. 5. Barrett's esophagus with a distal stricture. There is a smooth, tapered area of narrowing (arrow) in the distal esophagus above a hiatal hernia. An ordinary peptic stricture without Barrett's esophagus could produce identical radiographic findings.

854

sensitivity in diagnosing reflux esophagitis was only 53%, most cases of reflux esophagitis missed radiographically were mild and only one of those patients had Barrett's esophagus. The data suggest that esophagitis severe enough to cause Barrett's esophagus can almost always be detected on technically adequate double contrast examinations. This observation has important implications for the management of these patients, since unnecessary endoscopy can be avoided when there is no radiologic evidence of esophagitis or stricture formation.

On the basis of the study by Gilchrist et al., it seems reasonable to classify patients into high-, moderate- and low-risk groups for Barrett's esophagus based on the findings of double contrast esophagography [4]. Patients who are at high risk for Barrett's esophagus because of a high stricture or ulcer or a reticular mucosal pattern should undergo early endoscopy and biopsy for a definitive diagnosis. A larger group of patients are at moderate risk for Barrett's esophagus because of reflux esophagitis or peptic strictures, so clinical judgement should be used regarding the decision to perform endoscopy in this group based on the severity of reflux symptoms, age and overall health of the patient. However, the majority of patients have no radiologic evidence of esophagitis or strictures and the risk of Barrett's esophagus is so low in this group that endoscopy does not appear to be warranted. Patients who have a normal double contrast esophagram can therefore be treated empirically for their reflux symptoms without need for endoscopic intervention.

Thus, double contrast esophagography is a useful screening examination for Barrett's esophagus in patients with reflux symptoms, as it allows these individuals to be separated into high-, moderate- and low-risk groups for Barrett's esophagus, to determine the relative need for endoscopy and biopsy in these patients.

References

1. Agha FP. Radiologic diagnosis of Barrett's esophagus: critical analysis of 65 cases. Gastrointest Radiol 1986;11:123−130.
2. Chen YM, Gelfand DW, Ott DJ et al. Barrett's esophagus as an extension of severe esophagitis: analysis of radiologic signs in 29 cases. Am J Radiol 1985;145:275−281.
3. Chernin MM, Amberg JR, Kogan FJ et al. Efficacy of radiologic studies in the detection of Barrett's esophagus. Am J Radiol 1986;147:257−260.
4. Gilchrist AM, Levine MS, Carr RF et al. Barrett's esophagus: diagnosis by double-contrast esophagography. Am J Radiol 1988;150:97−102.
5. Glick SN, Teplick SK, Amenta PS et al. The radiologic diagnosis of Barrett's esophagus: importance of mucosal surface abnormalities on air-contrast barium studies. Am J Radiol 1991;157:951−954.
6. Levine MS, Kressel HY, Caroline DF et al. Barrett's esophagus: reticular pattern of the mucosa. Radiology 1983;147:663−667.
7. Robbins AH, Hermos JA, Schimmel EM et al. The columnar-lined esophagus: analysis of 26 cases. Radiology 1977;123:1−7.
8. Robbins AH, Vincent ME, Saini M et al. Revised radiologic concepts of the Barrett's esophagus. Gastrointest Radiol 1978;3:377−381.
9. Shapir J, DuBrow R, Frank P. Barrett's oesophagus: analysis of 19 cases. Br J Radiol 1985;58:491−493.

How useful is a reticular mucosal pattern as a specific indicator of Barrett's mucosa?

O. Ekberg (Malmö)

The classic radiologic features of Barrett's esophagus consist of a high esophageal stricture or ulcer, often associated with a sliding hernia and gastroesophageal reflux [1] (Fig. 1). A reticular mucosal pattern has also been described as a relatively specific sign of Barrett's esophagus on double contrast esophagography, particularly if located adjacent to a stricture [1]. However, such a reticular mucosal pattern can only be identified in 5—30% of patients with Barrett's esophagus proved endoscopically [2—4].

The radiographic appearance of the reticular pattern is that of delicate, tiny barium filled groves or crevices on the mucosal surface of the esophagus (Fig. 2). Such a reticular pattern may somewhat resemble "ariae gastricae" that can be demonstrated on double contrast examination of the stomach. When such a reticular pattern is present together with a proximally located stricture and/or a relatively deep ulcer crater, this constellation of signs is relatively specific to Barrett's esophagus (Fig. 1).

Differential diagnosis in patients with this reticular pattern include drug-induced esophagitis which, however, is usually located in the mid upper esophagus [5]. Primary or metastatic tumors can never be excluded in these patients and therefore, the reticular pattern, per se, is an indication for further endoscopic workup. When pronounced (Fig. 2), the reticular pattern may simulate varices, which are, however, usually located in the distal esophagus. This part of the esophagus is usually spared in Barrett's esophagus. However, downhill esophageal varices due to superior vena cava obstruction is located in the same area as the reticular pattern due to Barrett's esophagus [6].

A nodular appearance of esophageal mucosa can also be due to glycogenic acanthosis [7]. The nodules in glycogenic acanthosis are usually spread apart and the streaks of barium between the nodules are therefore less well defined.

A superficial "varicoid" carcinoma may mimic the appearance of Barrett's esophagus when the latter is pronounced [8]. Therefore, endoscopy is always indicated for biopsy and confirmation.

Thus, the radiographic finding of a reticular pattern is relatively specific to Barrett's esophagus when present together with a stricture or local ulcer. However, in other settings the reticular pattern is not sensitive.

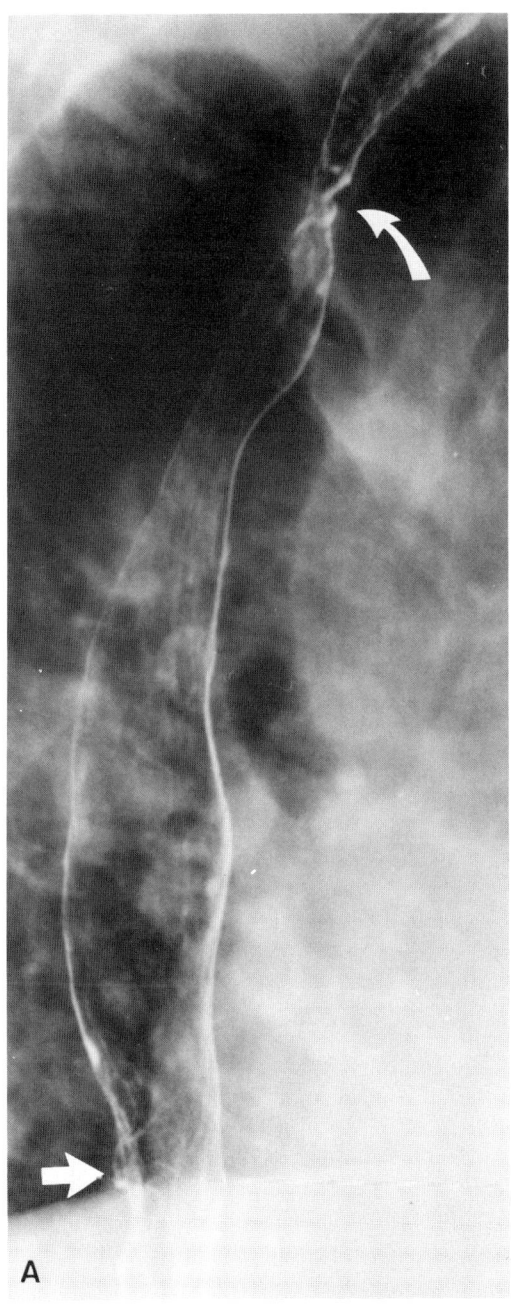

A

Fig. 1. Forty-five-year-old male with a 15-year history of solid bolus dysphagia. Double contrast esophagography was performed. A) Overview; B) (*following page*) detail of proximal stenosis; C) detail of distal ulcer and reticular pattern. A proximal stenosis of the esophagus with somewhat irregular contours was revealed (bent arrow). In the distal esophagus there was a 2 by 3 cm area (small arrow) of reticular pattern surrounding a relatively deep ulcer crater (arrow). The proximal stricture could not be dilated. Endoscopy, therefore, had to be performed during laparotomy via the stomach in retrograde

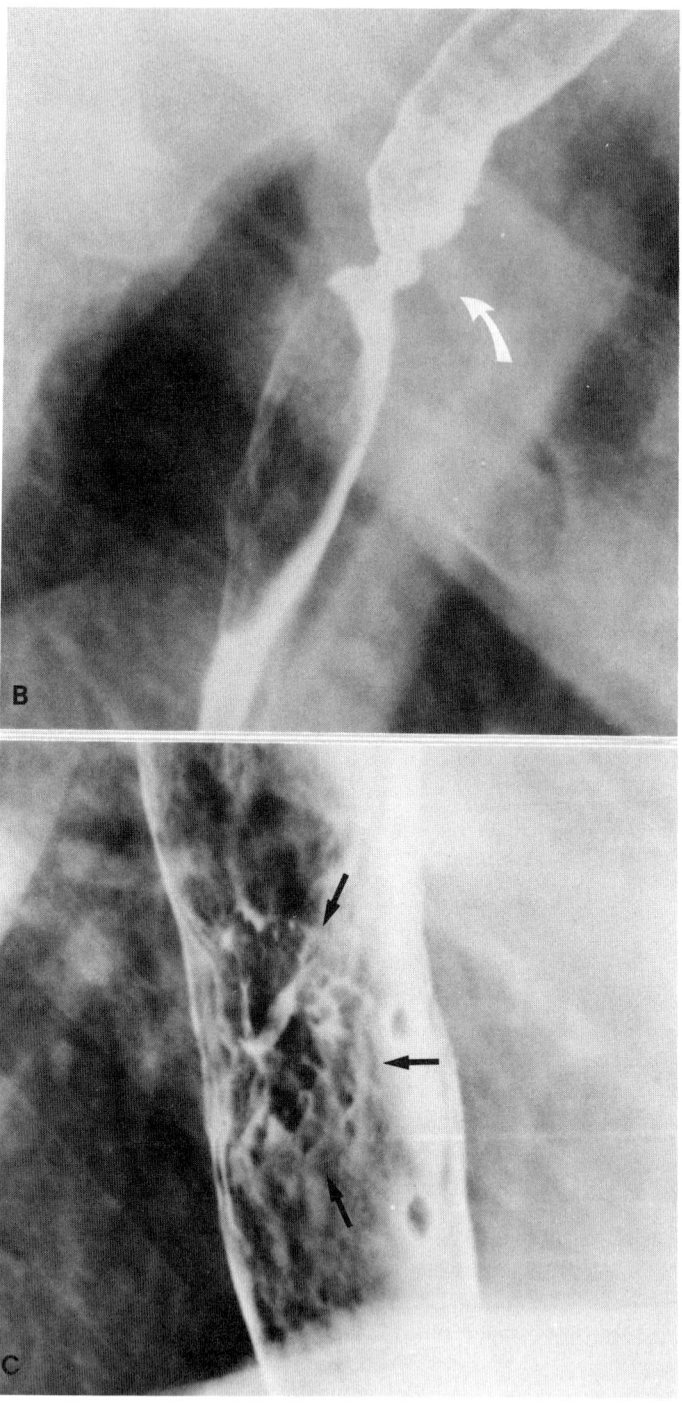

(Fig. 1 B,C, continued) direction. This showed typical Barrett's mucosa and an ulcer. Histology verified the diagnosis. In this patient the localized ulcer with upheaped edges suggested malignancy and the reticular pattern submucosal spread. Resection of the esophagus was performed and no carcinoma was present.

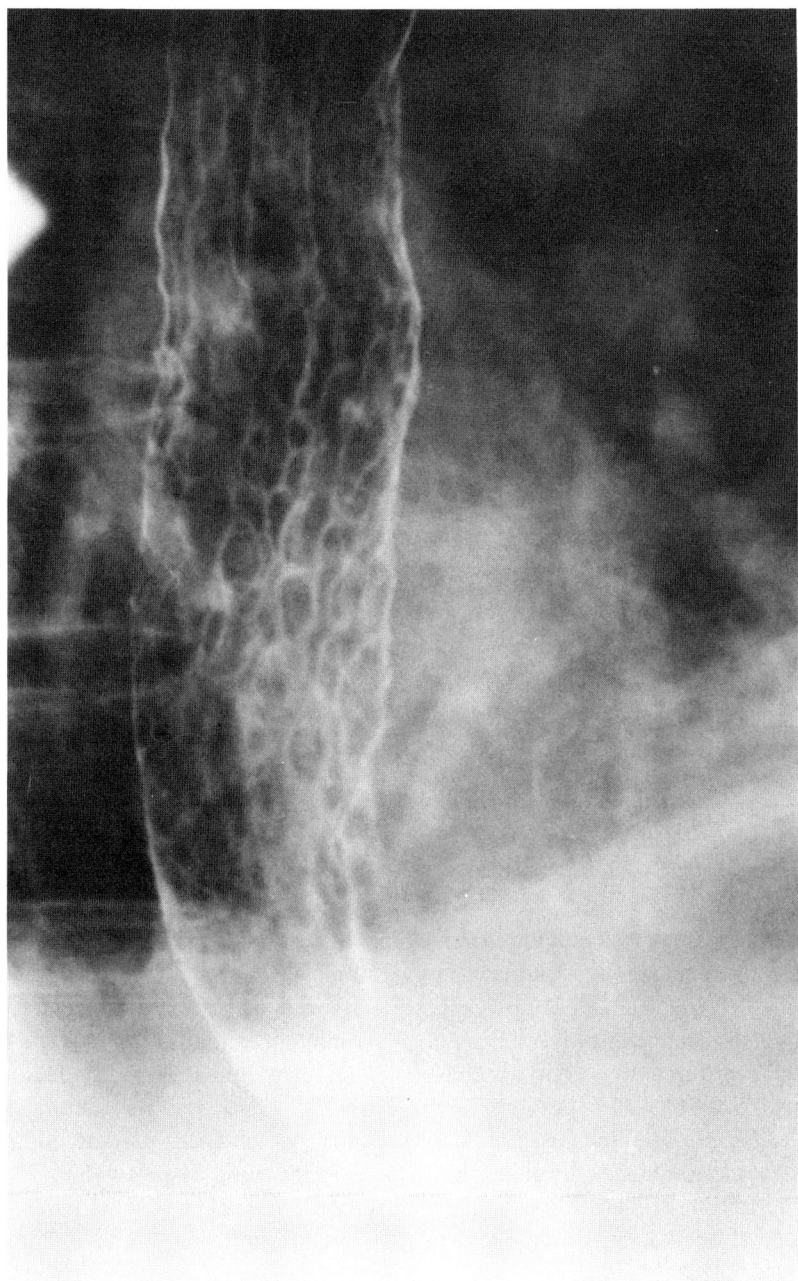

Fig. 2. Sixty-year-old female with ovarial carcinoma who presented with difficulties swallowing. Double contrast esophagography showed a pronounced reticular pattern with multiple barium-filled groves and inbetween demarcated areas of smooth featureless areas of intact or nodular mucosa. Although the reticular pattern was fairly characteristic there was no other lesion in the esophagus, particularly no stricture. Differential diagnosis in this patient therefore included varices, although the most distal part of the esophagus was spared. Another differential was superficial metastasis of the patient's ovarial carcinoma. Endoscopy and histology showed mild intestinal metaplasia.

References

1. Levine MS. Reflux esophagitis. In: Radiology of the Esophagus. Philadelphia: WB Saunders Company, 1989;39–44.
2. Chen YM, Gelfand DW, Ott DJ, Wu WC. Barrett's esophagus as an extension of severe esophagitis: analysis of radiologic signs in 29 cases. Am J Radiol 1985;145:275–281.
3. Levine MS, Kressel HY, Caroline DF, Laufer I, Herlinger H, Thompson JI. Barrett's esophagus: reticular pattern of the mucosa. Radiology 1983;147:663–667.
4. Gilchrist AM, Levine MS, Carr RF, Saul SH, Katzka DA, Herlinger H, Laufer I. Barrett's esophagus: diagnosis by double-contrast esophagography. Am J Radiol 1988;150:97–102.
5. Teplick JG, Teplick SK, Ominsky SH, Haskin ME. Esophagitis caused by oral medication. Radiology 1980;134:23–25.
6. Levine MS. Varices. In: Radiology of the Esophagus. Philadelphia: WB Saunders Company, 1989;200–202.
7. Laufer I. Double-contrast gastrointestinal radiology. In: Double Contrast Gastrointestinal Radiology. Philadelphia: WB Saunders Company, 1979;126.
8. Glick SN, Teplick SK, Goldstein J, Stead JA, Zitomer N. Am J Radiol 1982;139:683–688.

In radionuclide scans of Barrett's esophagus, what is the involvement of mucoid and parietal cells in pertechnetate excretion?

Tapin K. Chaudhuri, Tuhin K. Chaudhuri (Hampton),
S. Fink (San Antonio)

Barrett's esophagus is a condition in which the squamous mucosa of the lower esophagus is replaced by columnar epithelium [1]. The significance of Barrett's epithelium lies in the incidence of cancer [2] associated with the finding. It appears that patients with aneuploidy (abnormal DNA content within cells) or evidence of increased proliferative activity within cells, as determined by flow cytometry, predisposes to neoplastic progression in Barrett's esophagus [3]. Estimates vary widely [4,5], but the increased risk is sufficiently validated so that endoscopic surveillance is now under consideration and its value being assessed [6,7].

The definition of Barrett's esophagus specifies a lower esophageal location, but it is noteworthy that heterotopic gastric mucosa may also be found in the upper esophagus [8]. Patients with proximal heterotopic gastric mucosa show a basic fundic-type or antral-type gastric mucosa with few variations and no intestinal metaplasia. In this series of 61 patients, five demonstrated Barrett's columnar epithelium in the distal esophagus, this was cardiac-type columnar mucosa with variable intestinal metaplasia in this area [8,9]. Heterotopic gastric mucosa in the upper esophagus is best explained by a congenital theory of origin: it does not correlate with reflux esophagitis and clinical complications, or even symptoms alone, are extremely rare.

Radionuclide scanning

Diagnosis and surveillance of Barrett's esophagus is accomplished primarily by endoscopic means, but radionuclide scintigraphy may be used to diagnose Barrett's esophagus. Since 1973 the selective concentration of ^{99m}Tc-pertechnetate in gastric mucosa has been used to diagnose Barrett's esophagus [10,11] and this technique allows for simple, reproducible studies as these patients are followed clinically.

Clinical experience suggests that this technique has a high specificity; in one study, seven patients with esophagitis serving as controls all had negative scans [12]. Sensitivity, however, was low, with only eight of 17 patients (47%) with Barrett's esophagus giving positive images. Imaging was more frequently positive in those patients with more extensive disease. Sensitivity in detecting Barrett's esophagus was not enhanced by pentagastrin.

The technique [13] of scintiscanning Barrett's esophagus is as follows: after intravenous injection of 5 to 10 mCi of ^{99m}Tc-pertechnetate, imaging is performed over the thorax with the patient standing. The patient is instructed not to swallow saliva, which can create false-positive results [13]. Images are obtained at 20 to 30 and 40 to 60 min postinjection. Normal results are characterized by an absence of tracer accumulation at the lower end of the esophagus; abnormal results are characterized by uptake of the isotope in this area. Figure 1 shows a positive scintiscan for BE.

If a false-positive result for Barrett's esophagus is seen secondary to swallowed saliva, the simplest way to make the differential diagnosis is to have the patient drink a glass of water and to repeat the imaging. The activity due to true Barrett's esophagus will not be washed away by water, but the false-positive activity secondary to swallowed saliva will be eliminated [13].

Animal studies suggest that cimetidine retards the excretion of pertechnetate from the mucus cells and might thereby improve the sensitivity of pertechnetate imaging [14]. Unfortunately, a vast majority of the patients in one study, in which the sensitivity of scanning for Barrett's esophagus was only 47%, were taking cimetidine or ranitidine at the time of the examination. Experiments comparing scan appearance in Barrett's patients with and without simultaneous intravenous cimetidine have not yet been carried out.

Initial studies suggested that radioactive technetium (^{99m}Tc04) is secreted by the gastric parietal cells [15], but later evidence from several directions indicates that the mucus cells are mainly responsible. Berquist [10,11] pointed out that ^{99m}Tc-per-technetate is taken up and concentrated throughout the normal stomach, which is consistent with the distribution of the mucus-secreting gastric cells. Autoradiographic studies on animals [16–18]) show heavy uptake in the gastric mucous lining and little or no uptake in the parietal and chief cells. Human studies confirm that parietal cells do not secrete ^{99m}Tc, in patients with pernicious anemia and histamine-fast achlorhydria concentrate ^{99m}Tc-pertechnetate in their stomachs [19] . Also, it has been suggested that a ^{99m}Tc-abdomen scan could help to locate gastric mucosa in a retained antral cuff [20] . This area is devoid of parietal cells, but does contain gastric mucus secreting cells.

Barrett's Esoph.

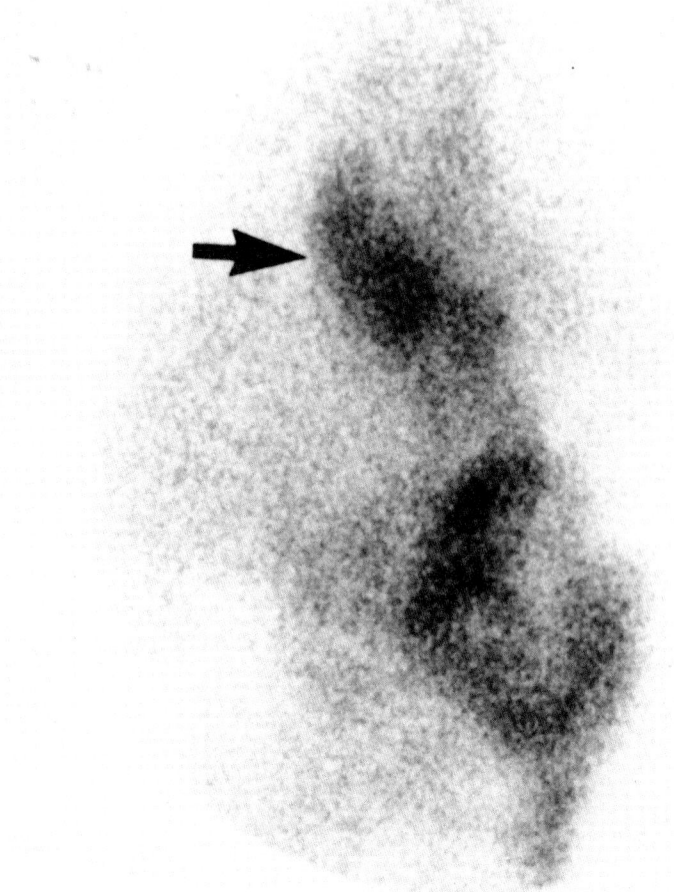

Fig. 1. Positive scintiscan for Barrett's esophagus. (Reproduced with permission of the publisher and author [13]).

Conclusion

It is now generally accepted that ^{99m}Tc-pertechnetate uptake in Barrett's esophagus is mediated by gastric mucus secreting cells, and not parietal or chief cells.

References

1. Spechler SJ, Goyal RK. Barrett's esophagus. N Engl J Med 1986;315:362—371.
2. Hassall E, Dimmick JE, Magee JF. Adenocarcinoma in childhood Barrett's esophagus: case documentation and the need for surveillance in children. Am J Gastroenterol 1993;88:282—288.
3. Fennerty MB, Sampliner RE. Flow cytometry in Barrett's esophagus: when all is said and done, more is said than done! Am J Gastroenterol 1993;88:319—320.
4. Cameron AJ, Ott DJ, Payne WS. The incidence of adenocarcinoma in columnar-lined (Barrett's) esophagus. N Engl J Med 1985;313:857—859.
5. Hameeteman W, Tytgat GNJ, Houthoff HJ, Van den Tweel GJ. Barrett's esophagus: development of dysplasia and adeno-carcinoma. Gastroenterology 1989;96:1249— 1256.
6. Lee FL, Isaacs PE. Barrett's ulcer: response to standard dose ranitidine, high dose ranitidine and omeprazole. Am J Gastroenterol 1988;83:914—916.
7. Spechler SJ. Endoscopic surveillance for patients with Barrett's esophagus: does the cancer risk justify the practice? Ann Intern Med 1987;106:902—904.
8. Borhan-Manesh F, Farnum JB. Incidence of heterotopic gastric mucosa in the upper esophagus. Gut 1991;32:968—972.
9. Cox AJ, McClave SA. Incidence of heterotopic gastric mucosa in the upper esophagus (review of article by Borham-Manesh). Gastrointest Endosc 1992;38:108—109.
10. Berquist TH, Nolan NG, Stephens DH. Diagnosis of Barrett's esophagus by pertechnetate scanning. Mayo Clin Proc 1973;48:276—279.
11. Berquist TH, Nolan NG, Stephens DH et al. Radiosotope scintigraphy in diagnosis of Barrett's esophagus. Am J Radiol 1975;123:401—411.
12. Yegelwel EJ, Bushnell DL, Fisher SG, Keshavarzian A. Technetium pertechnetate esophageal imaging for detection of Barrett's esophagus. Dig Dis Sci 1989;34:1075—1078.
13. Chaudhuri TK, Fink S, Bird JA. Radionuclide study of esophageal disorders: current clinical status and future directions. Appl Radiol 1988;17:70—77.
14. Sagar IV, Piccone JM. The effect of cimetidine on blood clearance, gastric uptake and secretion of ^{99m}Tc-pertechnetate in dogs. Radiology 1981;139:729—731.
15. Meier-Ruge W, Fridrich R. Die Verteilung von Tecnetium 99m und Jod-131 in der Magenschleimhaut. Histochemie 1969;19:147—154.
16. Chaudhuri TK, Polak JJ. Autoradiographic studies of distribution in the stomach of ^{99m}Tc-pertechnetate. J Nuc Med 1976;17:559.
17. Chaudhuri TK, Polak JJ. Autoradiographic studies of distribution in the stomach of ^{99}Tc-pertechnetate. Radiology 1977;123:223—224.
18. Chaudhuri TK, Polak JJ. Some differences in the cellular distribution of ^{131}I and ^{99m}Tc in animal stomachs. Clin Res 1979;27:264A.
19. Chaudhuri TK. Can ^{99m}Tc-pertechectate be used to assess the secretion of gastric acid in pernicious anemia? J Nucl Med 1977;18:121—122.
20. Chaudhuri TK, Chaudhuri TK, Shirazi SS, Condon RE. Radioisotope scan — a possible aid in differentiating retained gastric antrum from Zollinger-Ellison syndrome in patients with recurrent peptic ulcer. Gastroenterology 1973;65:697—698.

What are the differences in radiographic findings between children and adults?

M.Y.M. Chen, D.J. Ott, S.T. Auringer (Winston-Salem)

Barrett's esophagus in childhood is a complication of longstanding gastroesophageal reflux (GER) disease. Common clinical presentations, reflecting underlying reflux esophagitis, include vomiting, chest or abdominal pain, dysphagia and heartburn. Risk factors for pediatric Barrett's esophagus include chronic GER, psychomotor-retardation-cerebral palsy, repaired esophageal atresia, or esophageal replacement (gastric tube) surgery, connective tissue diseases and other entities associated with GER.

The true prevalence of Barrett's esophagus in children is unknown. In two series of pediatric patients, 2.5–13% of their population followed for GER had Barrett's esophagus [1,2], in comparison to a 3% prevalence of Barrett's esophagus in adults examined endoscopically [3]. Barrett's esophagus has been found in infants as young as 3 weeks old, suggesting that the metaplastic process may begin in the perinatal or even antenatal period [4].

Radiologic signs of Barrett's esophagus not seen in children

As infants and young children poorly tolerate a double contrast examination, most radiologic findings of pediatric Barrett's esophagus are observed on a single-contrast full-column barium esophagram. Therefore, most signs of Barrett's esophagus, such as the granular and reticular mucosal patterns shown by double-contrast examinations in adults, are not seen in children (Table 1).

Radiologic signs seen in both children and adults

Hiatal hernia has a high prevalence (75–94%) but low specificity in adults with Barrett's esophagus, but it is much less common (13%) in children with this condition

Table 1. The prevalence of radiographic signs in children and adults with Barrett's esophagus

	Adults % [3,11]	Children (%) [4–7]
Reflux	45–63	31/45 (69)
Hiatal hernia	75–94	6/45 (13)
Thickened folds	28–86	uncertain
Granular pattern	67	–
Reticular pattern	3–30	–
Ulcer	69	10/45 (22)
Stricture	71	22/45 (49)
Pseudodiverticula	21	1/45 (2)
Distal dilatation	34–66	uncertain

(Fig. 1) [4—7]. The youngest child with Barrett's esophagus, in association with hiatal hernia, was presented in this report.

Cycles of ulceration and healing may induce stricture formation at or below the migrated squamocolumnar junction (Fig. 2 and 3). The prevalence of strictures is

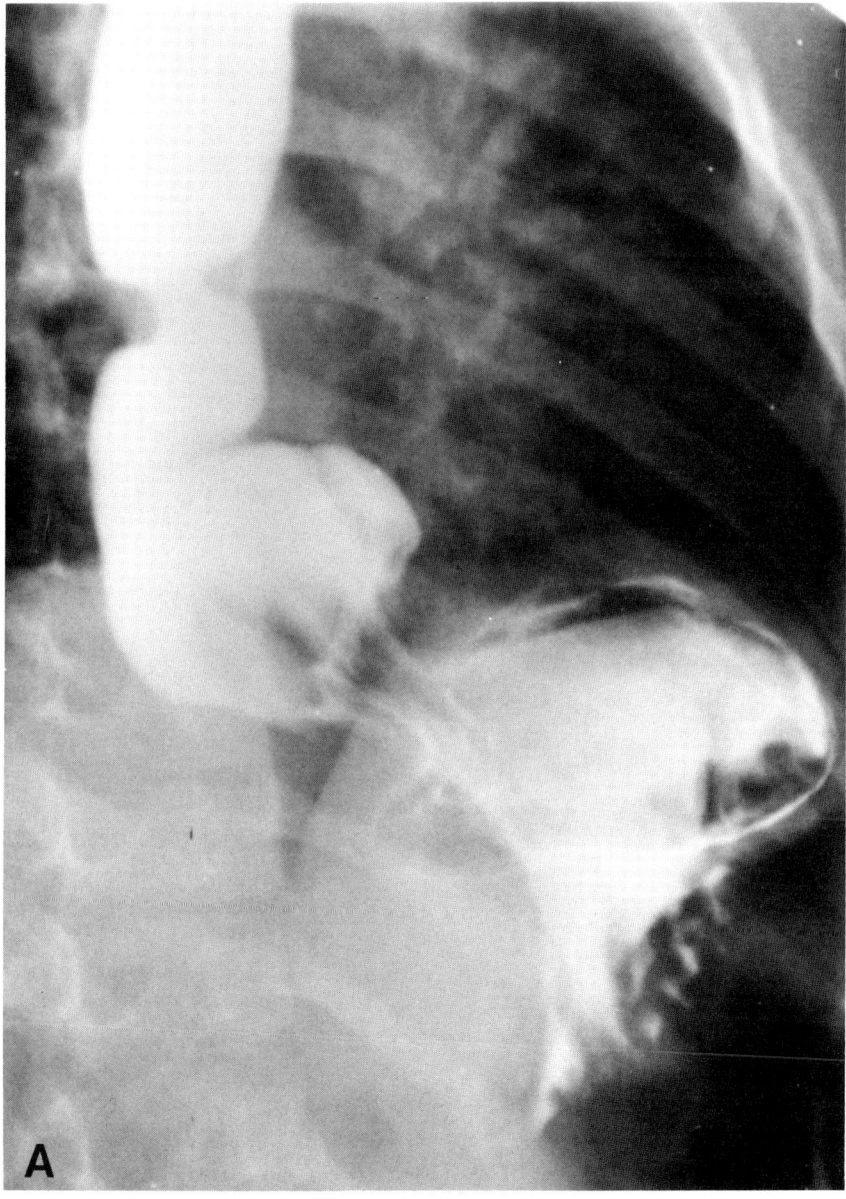

Fig. 1A. A large hiatal hernia shown in a 5-year-old boy with Barrett's esophagus.

lower (49%) in children with Barrett's esophagus than in adults (71%). This lower prevalence of strictures in children is assumed to be related to the longer time required to produce a stricture, and the fact that adults with Barrett's esophagus usually have a longer history of GER. Also, some midesophageal strictures in

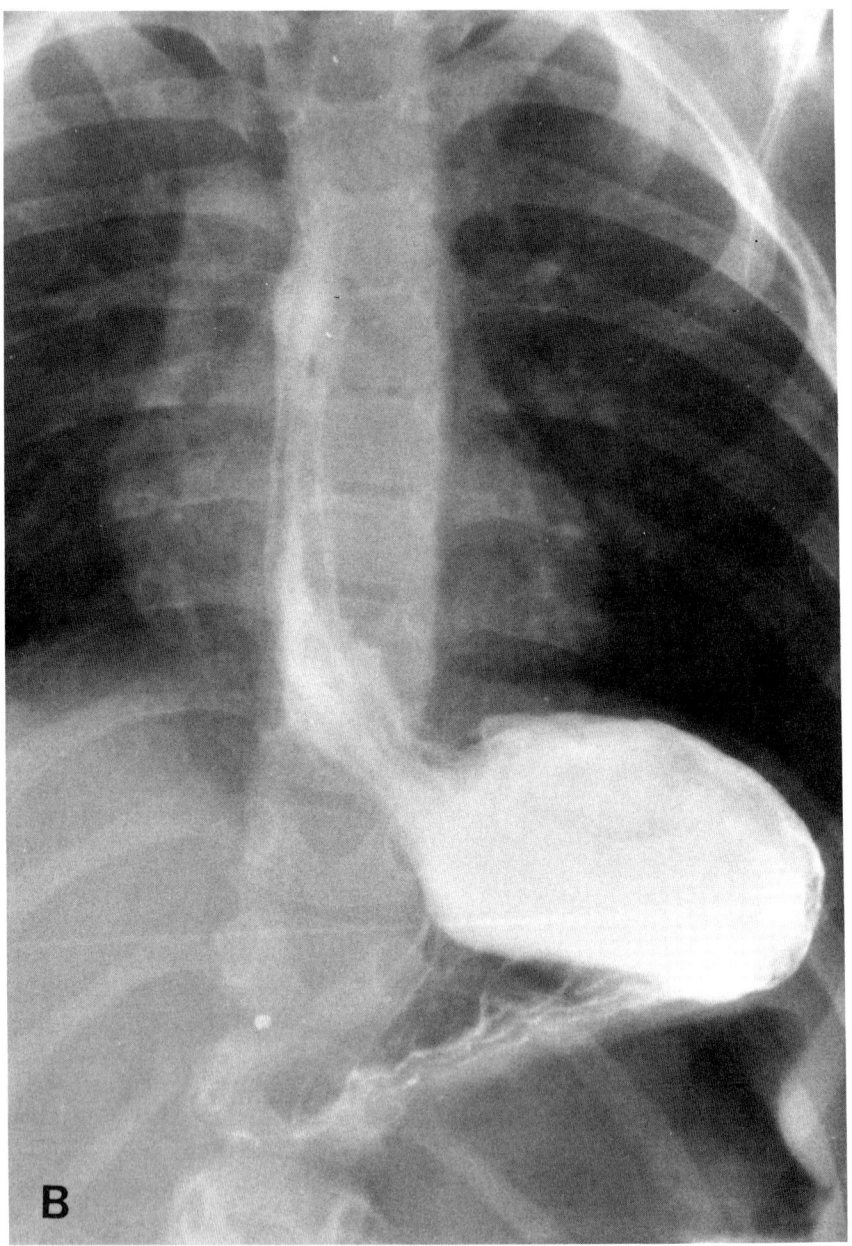

Fig. 1B. Gastroesophageal reflux shown in a 5-year-old boy with Barrett's esophagus.

children may have other causes, such as repaired esophageal atresia and congenital tracheobronchial remnants (Fig. 2) [5].

Deep esophageal ulcers are characteristically located at the squamocolumnar transition zone or below the level of stricture in patients with Barrett's esophagus.

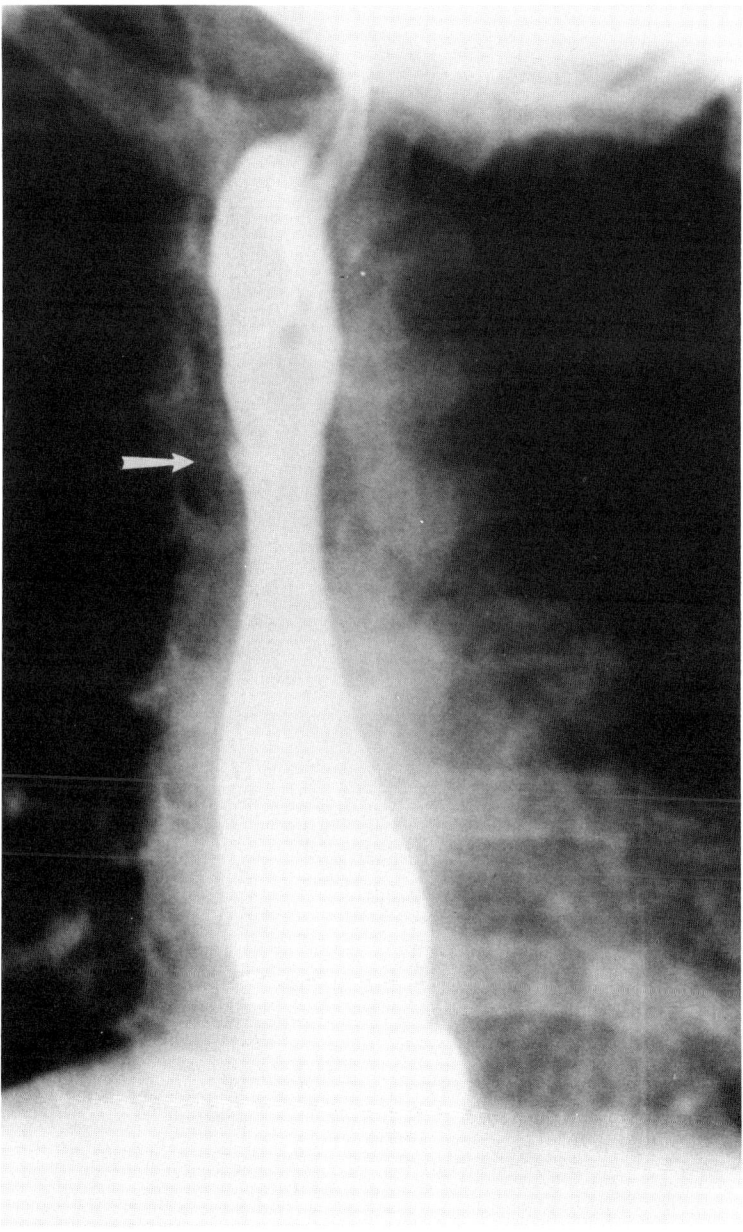

Fig. 2. A midesophageal stricture and ulcer (arrow) present in the area of repaired esophageal atresia and columnar epithelium were found distal from the stricture [5] (used with permission).

Ulcerations are more commonly detected by means of endoscopy than by radiographic examinations. In one study [1], endoscopy showed that 10 of 13 children with Barrett's esophagus had esophagitis with ulcers and exudates, but only four of these ulcers were seen by radiography.

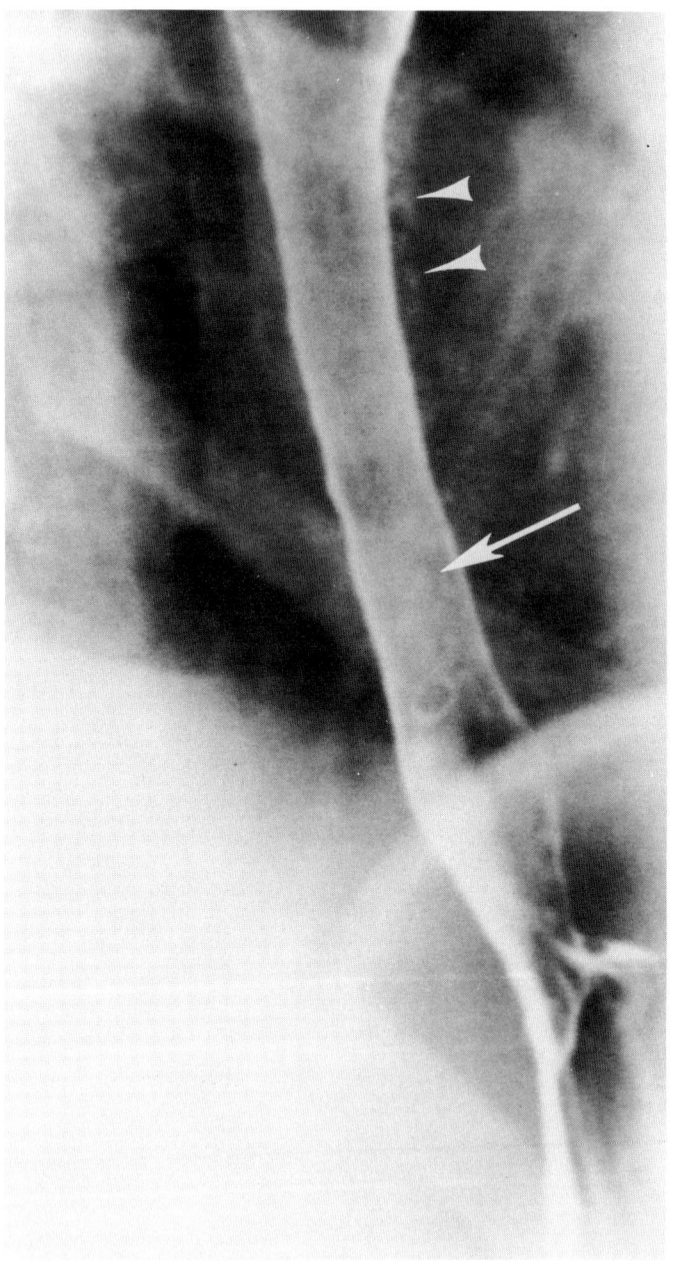

Fig. 3. Distal stricture, ulcers (arrow) and intramural diverticula (arrow heads) shown in a 6 year-old-boy with Barrett's esophagus [5] (used with permission).

Gastroesophageal reflux is observed fluoroscopically in about one-half of adults with Barrett's esophagus (Fig. 1); however, reflux is a more common finding (69%) in children with Barrett's esophagus. Many children with an underlying disease, such as psychomotor retardation, asthma, or familial dysautonomia are predisposed to GER. Pseudodiverticula have been reported in one child (Fig. 3) [5].

Esophageal strictures and signs of reflux esophagitis are suggestive of Barrett's esophagus, however, in one study [5], three of 13 patients (23%) with Barrett's esophagus appeared normal radiographically. A final diagnosis of Barrett's esophagus is based on biopsy because pinkish columnar epithelium is difficult to differentiate from inflamed squamous epithelium at endoscopy in children.

Malignant transformation

The prevalence of adenocarcinoma resulting from Barrett's esophagus averages 10% in adults [3]. The prevalence of adenocarcinoma in children with Barrett's esophagus is uncertain, but there have been four cases of esophageal adenocarcinoma reported in children with Barrett's esophagus [8–10]. The radiographic appearances of esophageal adenocarcinoma in children are nonspecific strictures or mass effects. Most children with Barrett's esophagus have the junctional or fundic type of Barrett's epithelium [1], however, the intestinal variant of Barrett's mucosa (15–45%), which is most common in adults, is responsible for malignant changes [5,6].

References

1. Dahms BB, Rothstein FC. Barrett's esophagus in children: a consequence of chronic gastroesophageal reflux. Gastroenterology 1984;86:318–323.
2. Snyder JD, Goldman H. Barrett's esophagus in children and young adults. Dig Dis Sci 1990;35:1185–1189.
3. Chen MYM, Gelfand DW, Ott DJ, Wu WC. Barrett's esophagus: the radiologist's role. Appl Radiol 1992;21:30–33.
4. Robins DB, Zaino RJ, Ballantine TVN. Barrett's esophagus in a newborn. Pediatr Pathol 1991;11:663–667.
5. Yulish BS, Rothstein FC, Halpin TC Jr. Radiographic findings in children and young adults with Barrett's esophagus. Am J Radiol 1987;148:353–357.
6. Hassall E, Weinstein WM, Ament ME. Barrett's esophagus in childhood. Gastroenterology 1985;89:1331–1337.
7. Herlihy KJ, Orlando RC, Bryson JC, Bozymski EM, Carney CN, Powell DW. Barrett's esophagus: clinical, endoscopic, histologic, manometric, and electrical potential difference characteristics. Gastroenterology 1984; 86:436–443.
8. Hassall E, Dimmick JE, Magee JF. Adenocarcinoma in childhood Barrett's esophagus: case documentation and the need for surveillance in children. Am J Gastroenterol 1993;88:282–288.
9. Hoeffel JC, Nihoul C, Schmitt M. Esophageal adenocarcinoma after gastroesophageal reflux in children. J Pediatr 1989;115:259 261.
10. Elliott MJ, Ashcroft T. Primary adenocarcinoma of the gastro-oesophageal junction in childhood. Scand J Thor Cardiovasc Surg 1983;17:65–66.
11. Chen YM, Gelfand DW, Ott DJ, Wu WC. Barrett esophagus as an extension of severe esophagitis: analysis of radiologic signs in 29 cases. Am J Radiol 1985;145:275–281.

Mucosa and histology

Are parietal and chief cells present in Barrett's esophagus, and are such cells functional?

D.A. Antonioli (Boston)

Parietal and chief cells are found in two of the three types of Barrett's epithelium: the fundic type and the junctional type. They are more numerous in the fundic type mucosa, which resembles normal gastric corpus-fundic mucosa to some degree. However, the fundic type mucosa in Barrett's esophagus is typically atrophic appearing, with glands decreased in number and size compared to the normal stomach. In addition, the glands tend to be separated from one another by fibrous tissue and strands of smooth muscle extending upwards from the muscularis mucosae [1,2]. In fact, if the histology has the appearance of normal gastric fundus, the specimen has most likely been inadvertently obtained from the proximal stomach or gastric mucosa within a hiatal hernia. The junctional type mucosa may contain a few parietal cells among the cellular elements of its mucous glands. Both fundic and junctional mucosa tend to be concentrated at the distal end of the Barrett's esophagus segment [1], but they may be found along its entire length [3]. Also, both types are much less common than specialized columnar epithelium.

Thus, although both parietal and chief cells can be identified in Barrett's esophagus, they are much less numerous than their counterparts in the stomach. Studies of their functional significance have been infrequent. However, Mangla did demonstrate increased acid and pepsin secretion within the esophagus in Barrett's esophagus patients with fundic-type mucosa. The quantities produced were small and the author did not feel that they contributed to the propagation of esophagitis [4]. At present, therefore, intraesophageal production of acid and pepsin does not appear to be a significant factor in the pathogenesis of esophagitis.

References

1. Paull A, Trier JS, Dalton MD et al. The histologic spectrum of Barrett's esophagus. N Engl J Med 1976;295:476–489.
2. Meuwissen SG, Bosma A, van Donk E et al. Immunohistochemical localization of pepsinogen A and C containing cells in Barrett's oesophagus. Virchows Arch (A) 1988;413:13–16.
3. Rothery GA, Patterson JE, Stoddard CL, Day DW. Histological and histochemical changes in the columnar-lined (Barrett's) oesophagus. Gut 1986;27:1062–1068.
4. Mangla JC. Acid and pepsin production by Barrett's epithelium: role of radionuclide imaging in diagnosis. In: Spechler SJ, Goyal RK (eds) Barrett's Esophagus: Pathophysiology, Diagnosis and Management. New York: Elsevier, 1985;49–57.

Does such a finding explain that Barrett's ulcers do not respond to conservative medical regimen?

G. Delpre (Petah Tikva),
A. Neeman, A. Leiser, U. Kadish (Tel-Aviv)

Although the concept of columnar lined esophagus (CLE) has existed for many years, it was first formalized by Norman R. Barrett in 1950 [1] and hence bears his name under the label of Barrett's esophagus (BE). When Barrett expressed his opinion that this portion belonged to the gastric area, he set off the first part of what has turned out to be a continuing controversy. In 1953 Allison and Johnstone [2] as well as Lortat-Jacob and Robert [3] stated that this portion was in fact esophagus lined with gastric mucosa. The initial controversy ended with the recognition by Barrett himself [4] that the intermediate columnar-lined segment is the esophagus. Another point of controversy has been the origin of BE, whether congenital [1] or acquired [2]. While continuing to advocate a congenital origin, Barrett later recognized the contributory role of reflux [4]. Further studies strongly support the concept that Barrett's metaplasia is acquired from long-standing reflux of gastric acid or bile-containing small bowel contents [5]. A third point of controversy has also arisen concerning the direction of differentiation [6]. In accordance with their biopsy findings, Paull and co-workers [7] have suggested that the metaplasia occurs in three zones – the most proximal being the specialized columnar epithelium (SCE) with a villiform surface; the next the "junctional" zone with cardiac glands, resembling the gastric cardia; the third and most distal zone (when present) resembled atrophic gastric fundus. Ulcerations, when observed, were at the junction of the squamous and columnar epithelium. These findings contrast with those of Thomson et al. [6], who studied the entire segments of eight specimens of BE. They found the following: a) with the exception of a slight tendency for gastric fundic epithelium to occur distally, no zonation was observed; b) ulcerations and residual squamous islands were always present when the whole segment was studied.

Yet another controversial issue concerns the absence, presence or relative quantity of parietal cells, to be found only in the gastric fundic type of epithelium [6]. In their early study, Allison and Johnstone and other authors were unable to demonstrate parietal cells in the specimens investigated [2,8,9]. Trier [10] and Berenson [11], in nine patients with complicated BE, stated that no parietal cells were present on the basis of light and ultramicroscopic studies. Other authors [6,12–15], however, clearly identified parietal cells in CLE. The controversy which naturally follows concerns the absence or presence of chief cells in the fundic-type epithelium [6]. Some authors [10–12] reported having found none, whereas others [13–15] emphasized this finding as well as that of parietal cells. Parietal cells are defined as pyramidal or triangular cells with fine granular cytoplasm, whereas chief cells are irregular polygonal vacuolated cells. In both cells the nucleus is located near the basement membrane [6,15] (Fig. 1). It should be noted that much of the controversy revolving around the identification of parietal and chief cells stems from the fact that conclusions have been drawn from biopsy specimens and this involves sampling errors [6].

Yet another point of disagreement relates to the stated belief of Barrett himself in his later writings [4] that the abnormal mucosa was incapable of secreting neither acid nor pepsin. Jones and Gummer [16] identified parietal cells in the CLE but produced

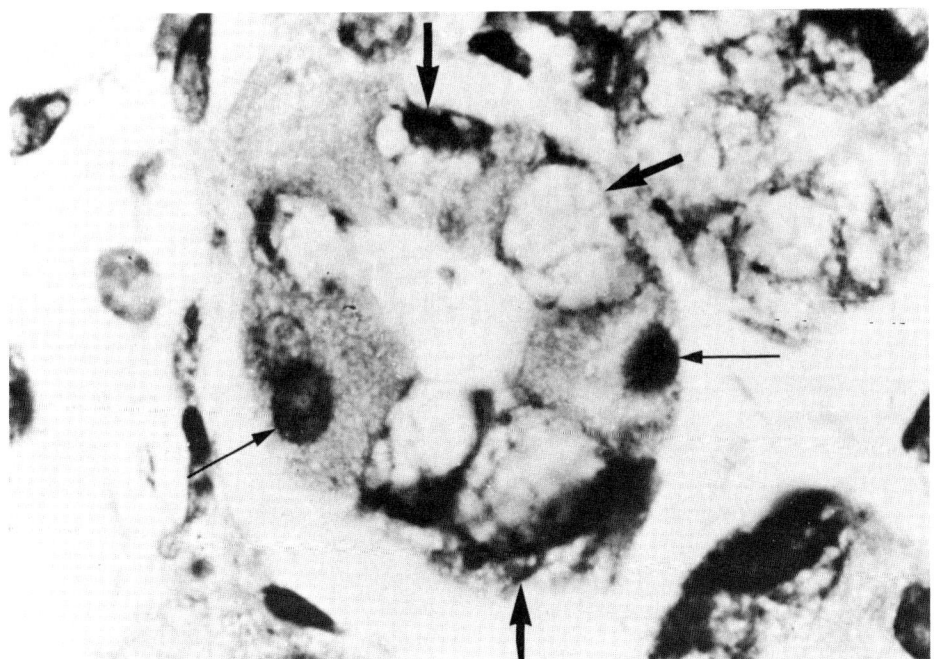

Fig. 1. Deep mucosal glands lined by irregular polygonal vacuolated chief cells (large arrows) and by pyramidal or triangular parietal cells with fine granular cytoplasm (fine arrows) [15] (reprinted with permission of publisher).

873

no evidence that acid was actually secreted. However, there are several studies [13–15,17] in which separate aspirates were obtained from the esophagus and stomach before and after histalog stimulation (Table 1). Special measures taken during the procedure prevented reflux of gastric contents to the esophagus and expectoration of saliva into the samples collected. 1) Using these techniques it was possible to prove local autonomous acid secretion. After histamine stimulation, 10 ml of secretion containing 5 mEq/l of acid was obtained from the esophagus, as compared to 30 ml containing 40 mEq/l acid obtained from the stomach [17]; 2) the apparent discordance in some of the results [15] indicates that the inflammation, frequently present and leading to atrophy, is associated with a loss of specialized cell function such as the production of acid or pepsin [6]; 3) the presence of esophageal acid secretion in the absence of parietal cells further supports the inadequacy of sampling [15]; 4) the demonstration of *pepsinogens* [13–15,18], of *cathepsin* [15,18] and of *autonomous pepsin secretion* [15] in the BE is of great interest.

Pepsin is a potent proteolytic enzyme synthesized, stored and secreted in the chief cells as its active precursor form, pepsinogen [19]. Pepsinogens 1 through 5 (Pepsinogen I) originate solely in chief and mucus neck cells in the fundus and body of the stomach, whereas the more slowly migrating pepsinogens 6 and 7 (Pepsinogen II) are found in the antrum and duodenum [15,19], as is another slow moving protease (SMP), immunologically distinct from Pepsinogens I and II, which is a cathepsin (acid protease resistant to alkalinization) [15].

In a patient with ulcerated stricture situated in the upper esophagus [13], esophageal biopsies revealed parietal and secretory cells filled with pepsinogen granules. In another patient [14], agar gel electrophoresis zymogram of biopsies, taken below an ulcer in the upper esophagus, showed slow- and fast-moving proteolytic components in a pattern akin to that of the fundus. Pepsinogens were not found in squamous epithelium, or in five normal midesophagus controls. In another study [15] of four patients, pepsin production was ascertained by chemical studies in two and by agar gel electrophoresis in three. In all four, the mucosa was shown to contain pepsinogens and/or cathepsin, the latter alone in a small amount (one case) or combined and present in notable amounts (two cases with ulcer and stricture in the upper esophagus). In a group of 22 noncomplicated BE patients Meuwissen et al.

Table 1. Data of samples collected from esophageal secretions, before and after histalog stimulation in Barrett's esophagus

Patients N/Author	1-h basal				1-h stimulation			
	Pepsin (U/h)	Acid			Pepsin (U/h)	Acid		
		pH	Volume (ml)	Conc./total acid output		pH	Volume (ml)	Conc./total acid output
(1) Hershfield	—	4.33	44	0.79 mEq/h	—	3.88	15	0.51 mEq/h
(1) Ustach	—	—	0	0.00 mEq/l	—	—	10	5.0 mEq/l
(1) Mangla	78.765	1.6	43	0.17 mEq/h	40.243	1.0	49	0.34 mEq/h
(2) Mangla	19.456	2.45	17	0.02 mEq/h	4.076	2.75	35	0.015 mEq/h

[18], using electrophoretic analysis of biopsy specimens, demonstrated the *ubiquity* and also *heterogeneity* of the isozymogen patterns in BE (also known for its histological pleomorphism [6,7,18]). All the precursors were found in most of the biopsies of Barrett's epithelium, although at a lower concentration than in the adjacent gastric fundus. The permanence of the secretory process of pepsinogens and cathepsin in BE is attested to by the fact that even after fundoplication, there were no significant changes in zymograms in patients followed for up to 3 years [15].

No less controversial is the opening question as to the role of parietal and chief cells in influencing the response of Barrett's ulcer to conventional medical regimens. In the attempt to clarify this question, the discussion will be divided into two parts: 1) parietal; and 2) chief cells i.e., 1) acid; and 2) pepsin secretion. The above considerations as well as conclusions summarized elsewhere will constitute the basis for this.

Parietal cells — acid secretion

The local autonomous acid secretion depends on the type of Barrett's epithelium (fundic type) and on the parietal cells present. Their number and function are readily reduced (metaplastic inflammatory condition), which can explain: 1) the low values of acid in samples from esophagus as compared with those from the stomach [13,17]; 2) individual differences (Table 1); 3) sampling errors and discordant results [6,15]. The added insult of local esophageal acid secretion, if present, may have only a minimal additive effect, if at all, on the following main pathogenetic mechanisms: elevated gastric acid secretion, defective esophageal clearance, reduced esophageal acid sensitivity [5]. From this viewpoint, the effectiveness of conventional medical regimens is almost independent of the finding of parietal cells and their direct acid secretion.

Chief cells — pepsin secretion

Chief cells are inconstantly present and only in fundic-type epithelium, but the ability of Barrett's epithelium to secrete pepsinogens and/or cathepsin appears to be unrelated to the type of epithelium or the presence of chief cells [15,18]. It is possible that cathepsin is more frequently found in BE complicated in its upper part [14,15]. It is known that the activity of this slowest moving band is not affected by sequential acidification and alkalinization [15,20]. In fact, it is the plurality of pathophysiologic mechanisms which causes the columnar mucosa to lose its ability to resist damage [5]. The factors implied may be interrelated. For instance, in the first step, an acid esophageal environment will potentiate the proteolytic enzymes produced in situ or brought in with the refluxates (pepsinogens, trypsin) together with the bile acids. In the second step, postprandial bile acids in the esophagus causes increased alkaline exposure and additional reflux of duodenal juice. Finally, H_2-receptor antagonists may be harmful since an alkaline environment activates the pancreaticoduodenal enzymes but does not inactivate the cathepsin [15,20].

In summary, it has been shown elsewhere that the wide range of therapeutic alternatives for Barrett's ulcers is related to the varying aspects of BE and ulcerations and their pathogenetic mechanisms. In some, a Barrett's ulcer will initially respond to conservative treatment, provided that high doses of H_2-receptor antagonists are given for long enough periods. In others, acid-pump blockers are usually effective for both initial and maintenance therapy. The finding of parietal and chief cells and the role they may play is discussed. The influence of parietal cells and of acid esophageal secretion in the vicinity of a Barrett's ulcer is questionable in comparison with the other existing mechanisms. On the other hand, the ability of Barrett's epithelium to secrete proteolytic enzymes (gastric proteases), even in the absence of the chief cells, may in part constitute a complicating factor in regard to the conventional medical regimens used in Barrett's ulcers.

References

1. Barrett NR. Chronic peptic ulcer of the esophagus and esophagitis. Br J Surg 1950;38:175–182.
2. Allison PR, Johnstone AS. The esophagus lined with gastric mucosa membrane. Thorax 1953;8:87–101.
3. Lortat-Jacob JL, Robert F. Les malpositions cardiotuberositaires. Arch Hal App Dig 1953;42:750–760.
4. Barrett NR. The lower esophagus lined by columnar epithelium. Surgery 1957;41:881–894.
5. Scarpignato C, Franze A. Columnar-lined (Barrett's) esophagus. Curr Opin Gastroenterol 1990;6:580–585.
6. Thompson JJ, Zinsser KR, Enterline HT. Barrett's metaplasia and adenocarcinoma of the esophagus and gastroesophageal junction. Hum Pathol 1983;14:42–61.
7. Paull AP, Trier JS, Dalton MD, Camp RC, Loeb P, Goyal RK. The histologic spectrum of Barrett's esophagus. N Engl J Med 1976;295:476–480.
8. Adler RM. The esophagus with columnar epithelium: its clinical significance. Geriatrics 1965;20:109–115.
9. Delpre G, Kadish U, Glantz I, Avidor I. Prolonged cimetidine therapy in ulcerated Barrett's columnar-lined esophagus. Am J Gastroenterol 1984;79:8–11.
10. Trier JS. Morphology of the epithelium of the distal esophagus in patients with midesophageal peptic strictures. Gastroenterology 1970;58:444–461.
11. Berenson MH, Herbst JJ, Freston JU. Enzyme and ultra-structural characteristics of esophageal columnar epithelium. Dig Dis Sci 1974;19:895–907.
12. Burgess JN, Payne WS, Andersen HA, Weiland LH, Carlson HC. Barrett's esophagus — the columnar epithelial-lined lower esophagus. Mayo Clin Proc 1971;46:728–734.
13. Hershfield NB, Lind JF, Hildes JA, McMorris LS. Secretory function of Barrett's epithelium. Gut 1985;6:535–539.
14. Mangla JC, Kim Y, Guarasci G, Schenk EA. Pepsinogens in epithelium of Barrett's esophagus. Gastroenterology 1973;65:949–955.
15. Mangla JC, Schenk EA, Desbaillets L, Guarasci G, Kubasit NP, Turner MD. Pepsin secretion, pepsinogen, and gastrin in "Barrett's esophagus". Gastroenterology 1976;70:669–676.
16. Jones FA, Gummer JWP. Clinical gastroenterology. In: Clinical Gastroenterology. Springfield, Illinois: Charles C. Thomas, 1960;317.
17. Ustach TJ, Tobon F, Schuster MM. Demonstration of acid secretion from esophageal mucosa in Barrett's ulcer. Gastrointest Endosc 1988;16:98–100.
18. Westerveld BD, Pals G, Bosma A, Defize J, Pronk JC, Frahts RR, Eriksson AW, Meuwissen SG. Gastric proteases in Barrett's esophagus. Gastroenterology 1987;93:774–778.
19. Basson MD, Modlin IM. Pepsinogen: prolate ellipsoid or unrecognized pathogen? J Clin Gastroenterol 1987;9:475–479.
20. Samloff IM. Slow movement protease and the seven pepsinogens: electrophoretic demonstration of the existence of eight proteolytic fractions in human gastric mucosa. Gastroenterology 1969;57:659–669.

Are there histologic differences between Barrett's mucosa of long segment (over 3 cm above the LES) and short segment (3 cm or less above the LES)?

S.R. Hamilton (Baltimore)

Barrett's esophagus can be defined pathogenetically by columnar epithelial replacement of previously squamous epithelium-lined esophageal mucosa, usually due to chronic gastroesophageal reflux. Clinical and pathological definition, however, is difficult in some patients because the segment of Barrett's mucosa is short, anatomic landmarks are uncertain and a hiatal hernia may be present. Nonetheless, it is clear in specimens from esophagectomy, endoscopy with confirming biopsies, and autopsy that short segments of Barrett's esophagus, less than 3 cm in length, are relatively frequent in adults. These short segments of Barrett's mucosa often do not involve the entire circumference of the esophagus, but rather appear as fingers or tongues extending above the remainder of the squamocolumnar junction. When the entire circumference is involved uniformly, distinguishing short-segment Barrett's esophagus from gastric cardia, intestinalized gastric cardia, and hiatal hernia is made difficult.

The histopathologic differences between long and short segments of Barrett's esophagus can be considered for two characteristics: the types of columnar-lined mucosa present and the occurrence of dysplasia (intraepithelial neoplasia) and adenocarcinoma. The spectrum of histopathology in Barrett's mucosa can be classified as distinctive-type (specialized columnar), cardiac-type (junctional) and fundic-type. Histopathologic examination of short segment cases shows that any or all of these mucosal types can be identified. The mucosal types are often in a mosaic pattern in short-segment Barrett's esophagus, as is the case in long segments. There is a tendency for cardiac type mucosa to be predominant in the lowermost portions of the Barrett-lined segment. Development of incomplete intestinalization over time in cardiac-type Barrett's mucosa may explain the pathogenesis of distinctive-type mucosa [1,2].

The occurrence of dysplasia and adenocarcinoma in short-segment Barrett's esophagus is well documented [3,4] but the frequency is not well defined. As described above, diagnosis of short-segment Barrett's esophagus can be difficult. Based on evident cases, the occurrence of carcinoma has been reported to be rare in short segments [5,6]. This finding may be related to the small surface area of Barrett's mucosa at risk, as compared to patients with long-segment Barrett's esophagus. However, in patients with symptomatic adenocarcinoma of the esophago-gastric junction region, the precursor short-segment Barrett's esophagus may be overgrown by the tumor and made unidentifiable. Thus, neoplastic complications in short-segment cases could be more frequent than is appreciated at present. Long-term follow-up in cohorts of patients with short-segment Barrett's esophagus would be needed to establish the frequency.

In conclusion, short-segment Barrett's esophagus is quantitatively, but not qualitatively, different from long-segment disease. The relationship of length to development of neoplasia is not yet defined precisely, but columnar epithelial dysplasia and adenocarcinoma clearly can develop in short segments. As a consequence, evaluation by multiple endoscopic biopsies and brush cytology of short-segment, as well as long-segment, cases at the time of initial presentation is prudent. The value of surveillance in patients with short-segment Barrett's esophagus is uncertain.

References

1. Hamilton SR, Yardley JH. Regeneration of cardiac type mucosa and acquisition of Barrett's mucosa after esophagogastrectomy. Gastroenterology 1977;72:669–675.
2. Qualman SJ, Murray RD, McClung HJ, Lucas J. Intestinal metaplasia is age-related in Barrett's esophagus. Arch Pathol Lab Med 1990;114:1236–1240.
3. Hamilton SR, Smith RRL, Cameron JL. Prevalence and characteristics of Barrett's esophagus in patients with adenocarcinona of the esophagus or esophagogastric junction. Hum Pathol 1988;19:942–948.
4. Schnell TG, Sontag SJ, Chejfec G. Adenocarcinomas arising in tongues of short segments of Barrett's esophagus. Dig Dis Sci 1992;37:133–143.
5. Ransom JM, Patel GK, Cliff SA et al. Extended and limited types of Barrett's esophagus in the adult. Ann Thorac Surg 1982;33:19–27.
6. Iftikhar SY, James PD, Steele RJC, Hardcastle JD, Atkinson M. Length of Barrett's esophagus – an important factor in the development of dysplasia and adenocarcinomas. Gut 1992;33:1155–1158.

Is the presence of specialized epithelium necessary for the diagnosis of Barrett's esophagus?

H.D. Appelman (Ann Arbor)

The characteristic, specialized or distinctive epithelium covering the esophagus in classical Barrett's mucosa has tall, apical-mucin-containing, columnar cells resembling gastric surface cells, interspersed among which are intestinal-type goblet cells. This type of epithelium has been designated as incomplete intestinal metaplasia, incomplete, because only the goblet cells are intestinal cells, the columnar cells are not. Furthermore, in classic Barrett's mucosa, this epithelium covers villiform projections and dips into the mucosa as crypt-like tubules. When this mucosa is present in a biopsy, the histologic diagnosis of Barrett's mucosa is obvious. However, a few biopsy diagnostic problems surface from time to time. For instance, sometimes this specialized or distinctive mucosa is not present, but the biopsy contains gastric-type mucosa with either cardiac or fundic glands at the base and gastric-type pits on the surface. The question always arises as to whether it is possible to diagnose Barrett's esophagus from such mucosae. The situation is complicated by the facts that virtually every patient with Barrett's mucosa has a hiatal hernia and that the exact location of the lower esophageal sphincter is sometimes not clear endoscopically. Therefore, biopsies of what the endoscopist thinks is the lower esophagus may, in fact, be from the hiatal hernia. As a result, biopsies, supposedly from distal esophagus, which contain only normal gastric components are always suspect as being from the hiatal hernia and not from a Barrett's mucosa.

In our institution, the unequivocal histologic diagnosis of Barrett's is reserved for those biopsies containing the distinctive epithelium with incomplete intestinal metaplasia and/or for those mucosae for which there is absolutely no doubt that the biopsies came from the tubular esophagus, even if only relatively normal gastric type epithelium is present. One way of proving the latter to be truly Barrett's is to see a mucous gland in the underlying submucosa or its duct penetrating the columnar mucosa. Furthermore, in children, particularly those 5 years of age and younger, Barrett's mucosa rarely has the distinctive or specialized epithelium, so we have to accept Barrett's in very young children with only normal gastric mucosal elements [1].

It has been my experience, and that of others, that any Barrett's mucosa is a disorganized distorted mucosa. Even when Barrett's esophagus contains only normal gastric elements, the mucosa is architecturally different from normal gastric mucosa [2,3]. Usually the glandular component is too small, or it is uneven with patches of normal glands alternating with patches of atrophy, and the pits are too long and often distorted as well, with branched, dilated and serrated forms. This type of disorganized gastric type mucosa is probably diagnosable as Barrett's, but it is always comforting for the pathologist to know that such mucosa comes from the tubular esophagus and from nowhere else.

References

1. Qualman SJ, Murray RD, McClung J, Lucas J. Intestinal metaplasia is age-related in Barrett's esophagus. Arc Pathol Lab Med 1990;114:1236–1240.
2. Geboes K, Geboes KP, Ectors N. The histologic classification of Barrett's esophagus. Acta Endoscopica 1992;22:485–495.
3. Hamilton SR. Reflux esophagitis and Barrett's esophagus. In: Goldman H, Appelman HD, Kaufman N (eds) Gastrointestinal Pathology. Baltimore: Williams & Wilkins, 1990:33–39.

Apart from the specialized mucosal type, how can Barrett's mucosa be distinguished from the normal cardia mucosa?

H.D. Appelman (Ann Arbor)

Barrett's mucosa has a number of different, nondysplastic epithelial components. The most common and diagnostically useful is the specialized with incomplete intestinal metaplasia. Possibly equally common are clusters of small glands at the base of the mucosa which contain neutral mucin, so that they are cytologically identical to gastric cardiac glands. The superficial mucosa overlying these glands may have the specialized features, but on occasions, it has only neutral mucus-containing epithelium, identical to gastric surface epithelium. This has been called the "junctional" type of Barrett's mucosa. Separating junctional Barrett's epithelium from gastric cardia may be difficult. This is especially a problem in very young children who commonly do not have the specialized Barrett's epithelium. There are a few tricks or hints that allow the distinction to be made.

First, knowing from the endoscopic report that the site of the biopsy is, without any doubt, within the tubular esophagus indicates that the mucosa is Barrett's. This is not always as clear-cut as one would like. Second, finding an acid mucin-producing submucosal gland beneath the epithelium or a gland duct penetrating the epithelium, indicates that the biopsy came from the esophagus and not from the stomach and confirms the diagnosis of Barrett's. Third, in Barrett's mucosa, even in the absence of the specialized epithelium, the surface is likely to have a villiform configuration and the cardiac-type glands are likely to be fewer, less clustered and more separated than in normal cardiac mucosa. Experienced gastrointestinal pathologists are more likely to be capable of recognizing these subtle distinctions.

If all of these options fail, then the mucosa will look so much like cardiac mucosa that there will be absolutely no way to tell whether it is Barrett's or cardiac. On very rare occasions, we cannot tell.

Are all different types of Barrett's epithelium originally present, or do they appear only after some period of evolution?

D. Parekh, G.W.B. Clark, T.R. DeMeester (Los Angeles)

The most severe histological consequence of chronic gastroesophageal reflux is Barrett's esophagus. Barrett's mucosa is a metaplastic columnar epithelium that replaces the normal squamous epithelium in the esophagus. A wide variety of cell types and histological patterns are encountered in Barrett's mucosa. A distinctive specialized columnar epithelium (SCE) is diagnostic of this condition [1,2]. SCE is characterized by columnar cells, goblet cells and a villous like structure. The columnar cells lack absorptive capabilities or ultrastructure characteristics of true intestinal cells making them thus, an example of incomplete intestinal metaplasia [1]. The other two types of histopathological patterns described in Barrett's epithelium include junctional or cardiac type Barrett's mucosa with a predominantly foveolar surface containing mucous glands and resembling gastric cardia type mucosa and fundic type which is the only variety of Barrett's epithelium that contains both parietal and chief cells with atrophic fundic glands [1–3]. The glandular structures of the fundic type epithelium appear sparse and shortened causing it to appear atrophic compared to normal gastric mucosa [1–3].

It is now well established that Barrett's mucosa is a premalignant lesion and relative to the general population the risk of a patient with Barrett's esophagus developing an esophageal cancer is increased 30–50-fold [1,3]. The development of adenocarcinoma in Barrett's esophagus is preceded by areas of underlying dysplasia, thereby providing evidence in support of the dysplasia-carcinoma sequence in this lesion [4]. The specialized columnar epithelium in Barrett's mucosa has a special significance in this condition: when adenocarcinoma of the esophagus develops in Barrett's mucosa, it virtually always arises in a short or long segment of specialized metaplastic columnar epithelium and not from fundic or cardiac type epithelium [3].

A commonly used definition of Barrett's esophagus has been the presence of columnar epithelium extending more than 3 cm above the normal cardioesophageal junction [1]. This is due to an imprecise relationship between lower esophageal sphincter (LES) and the squamocolumnar junction i.e., there may be a 2–3 cm disassociation between the Z-line and manometrically-defined LES in normal adults. Accurate diagnosis of Barrett's esophagus requires endoscopy with careful documentation of landmarks of the diaphragm (crural impression), gastroesophageal junction and Z-line. In patients with hiatal hernia this is particularly important; otherwise an excess amount of cardiac type Barrett's esophagus may be diagnosed if the biopsies have been obtained from the hiatal hernia. It is because of this difficulty that the prevalence of different types of mucosa in Barrett's esophagus have been controversial.

Paull and colleagues [2] studied 11 patients with Barrett's esophagus by taking multiple biopsies from the esophagus in relation to the distance from the LES as defined by manometric techniques. These workers found that in some patients a zonal distribution of the different types of mucosa was found. Nine of the 11 patients had specialized columnar epithelium, and in five of the nine patients in whom the specialized epithelium was present, either gastric fundic type epithelium with parietal and chief cells or junctional type epithelium (without parietal cells) was interposed between the specialized columnar epithelium and the lower esophageal sphincter zone. The gastric fundic type epithelium extended over at least 2–10 cm above the lower esophageal sphincter in three of these patients, and in the two patients with junctional epithelium this extended for at least 1–4 cm above the lower esophageal sphincter. These workers did not find gastric fundic or junctional type epithelium proximal to specialized columnar epithelium. Furthermore, junctional type epithelium, when present, was interposed between gastric fundic type and specialized columnar epithelium in this study. This study has provided the strongest basis for a zonal distribution of the three types of epithelium in Barrett's esophagus (Fig. 1).

The findings from this study suggested that development of the different epithelial types in Barrett's esophagus is sequential with specialized type Barrett's mucosa being preceded by the other two types of mucosa. Failure to detect the other two types of mucosa consistently in all patients with Barrett's esophagus represents a regression of junctional and fundic type mucosa.

The findings of zonation of the three different types of epithelium in Barrett's esophagus have not been reproduced by other investigators. Thompson and colleagues [3] found in a detailed study of Barrett's mucosa from resected segments for adenocarcinoma of the esophagus that the different cell and epithelial types were randomly and not zonally distributed. Chief and parietal cells were found in four of eight cases, in all cases these cell types (representative of fundic mucosa) were found distally in the metaplastic mucosa, however, in two cases they were found in the middle of and in one case they were found proximal to the distribution of SCE. Fundic glands had a similar distribution as chief and parietal cells with a slight tendency towards distal location, but were randomly distributed throughout the Barrett's mucosa.

Gottfried and colleagues [5] in a study of 17 patients with Barrett's mucosa found that junctional mucosa coexisted, randomly with SCE in five patients, SCE only was present in eight, junctional mucosa only in one, fundic in one and zonation in two patients.

A definition of at least 3 cm of columnar segment has been used to make a diagnosis of Barrett's esophagus since the distal esophagus may be lined by cardiac type columnar metaplasia for a distance of up to 2 cm in normal subjects. Little attention, however, has been directed towards the type of columnar lining in the short segments of metaplastic mucosa. Adenocarcinoma may arise from a short segment of SCE; furthermore, short segment of SCE may be the only histological type of columnar mucosa in Barrett's esophagus [5,6]. This has led to renewed interest in determining the pathophysiology of short segment Barrett's with SCE. In a group of 51 patients with Barrett's metaplasia with SCE, there were 20 patients in whom the length of the SCE was <3 cm as measured endoscopically, and in 31 patients SCE was >3 cm [6].

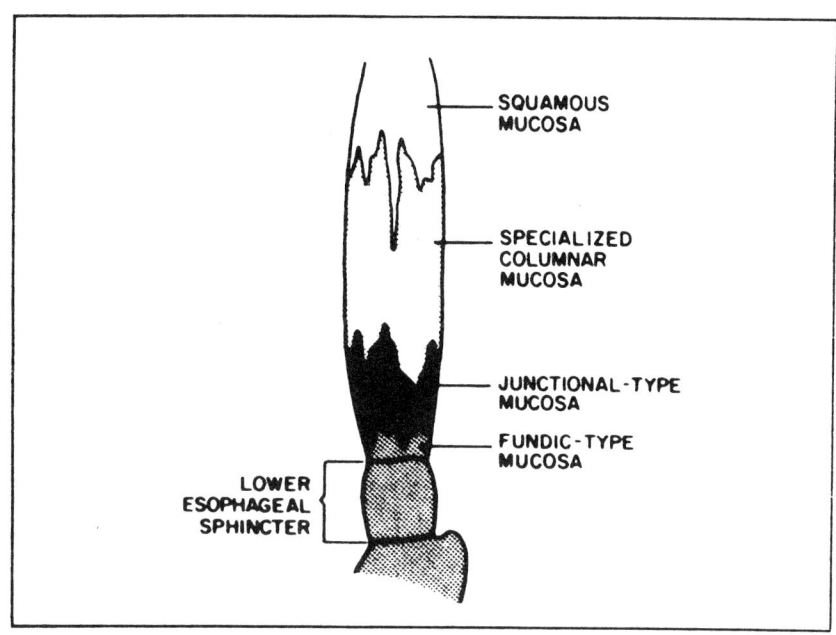

Fig. 1. Zonal distribution of the three types of epithelia in Barrett's esophagus (reproduced with permission from Spechler et al. [1]).

These patients are referred to as short segment Barrett's and extended Barrett's, respectively. Table 1 compares our manometric and pH findings in these two groups of patients. Patients with short segment Barrett's have a high prevalence of mechanically defective LES with abnormal acid exposure on esophageal pH testing. Similar pathophysiologic abnormalities were identified in patients with more extensive Barrett's metaplasia. Furthermore, patients with short segment Barrett's metaplasia had poor esophageal body motility in the distal four-fifths of the esophagus, despite the fact that the length of the Barrett's was restricted to less than 3 cm. Our study shows that the extent of the pathophysiological abnormalities in patients with short segment Barrett's are similar to those seen in patients with gastroesophageal reflux disease (GERD) with esophagitis. This together with a gradation of increase in abnormality of esophageal function as one goes from GERD with no esophagitis to

Table 1. Pathophysiologic abnormalities in short and long segment Barrett's esophagus. Data shown as percentage of patients with abnormal findings

	GERD with esophagitis (%)	Short segment Barrett's (%)	Long segment Barrett's (%)
Number of patients	51	20	31
Defective LES	74	65	87
Abnormal acid exposure	100	83	100
Hiatal hernia	43.5	55	76.9
Complications	0	40	63
Dysplasia	0	20	21

extended Barrett's suggests that short segment Barrett's occurs at an earlier stage of disease compared to patients with extended Barrett's esophagus [6].

Few authors have documented progression of the length of Barrett's over time. Cameron and Lomboy [7] in a study of 374 patients with columnar epithelium 3 or more cm in length found that the mean length of columnar epithelium did not increase on follow-up in 21 patients who were followed up for a mean of 7.3 years (mean initial length was 8.29 ± 0.85 cm; mean final length, 8.33 ± 0.077 cm). These investigators suggested that the data were consistent with the rapid evolution of Barrett's esophagus to its full length, with little subsequent change. In this small series, patients with short segment Barrett's were not studied. It is obvious that further work is necessary on the progression of Barrett's esophagus.

Esophageal adenocarcinoma is the fastest rising cancer in the United States, and the incidence for adenocarcinoma of the gastric cardia is increasing in a parallel fashion. Adenocarcinomas of the esophagus are associated with Barrett's esophagus in more than 75% of cases. In 25% of patients in this study early adenocarcinomas arose from short segment Barrett's mucosa. High-grade dysplasia was present in all of the tumors suggesting that Barrett's metaplasia was the source of these tumors. Our study suggests that specialized intestinal epithelium metaplasia, when present even in a single biopsy, is sufficient to make the diagnosis of Barrett's esophagus [6]. A short segment Barrett's with specialized intestinal metaplasia has the same prognosis as a long segment, and these patients should be carefully followed up for development of adenocarcinomas.

In a further study, we biopsied the distal esophagus and the gastric cardia (after retroflexing the endoscope) in 87 consecutive patients with symptoms of gastro-esophageal reflux undergoing routine endoscopic examination. In five patients unsuspected CLE was identified histologically and was located in the gastric cardia. One of the five patients had high grade dysplasia. Four of the five patients had evidence on manometry and on pH monitoring of severe gastroesophageal reflux. This study clearly shows that CLE may occur as the initial microscopic change in patients with Barrett's esophagus [8].

In conclusion, earlier studies which demonstrated that different types of epithelium in Barrett's mucosa were zonally distributed suggested that these epithelial subtypes develop in a sequential fashion. It is probable that in a few patients there is zonation of the different epithelial types in Barrett's mucosa. On the other hand, the finding of zonation has not been reproducible in all patients. While further work is necessary in this area, the body of evidence available today suggests that the different types of Barrett's epithelium may appear randomly and not necessarily in a sequential fashion. To a certain extent this is a moot argument, because it is the type of epithelium present that is of significance rather than its topological distribution. The presence of even a few millimeter segments of SCE is ominous since these patients are pre-disposed to development of adenocarcinoma of the esophagus or the gastroesophageal junction. The 3-cm rule, based largely on distribution of cardiac mucosa, is therefore not applicable to development of SCE in Barrett's mucosa. Furthermore, our studies suggest that SCE may be a very early finding of Barrett's esophagus to the extent where this epithelial type may be present only at the gastric cardia.

References

1. Spechler SJ, Goyal RK. Medical progress in Barrett's esophagus. N Engl J Med 1986;315:362–371.
2. Paull A, Trier JS, Dalton MD, Camp RC, Loeb P, Goyal RK. The histologic spectrum of Barrett's esophagus. N Engl J Med 1976;295:476–480.
3. Thompson JJ, Zinsser KR, Enterline HT. Barrett's metaplasia and adenocarcinoma of the esophagus and gastroesophageal junction. Hum Pathol 1983;14:42–60.
4. Levine DS, Haggitt RC, Blount PL, Rabinovitch PS, Rusch VW, Reid BJ. An endoscopic biopsy protocol can differentiate high-grade dysplasia from early adenocarcinoma in Barrett's esophagus. Gastroenterology 1993; 105:40–50.
5. Gottfried MR, McClave SA, Boyce HW. Incomplete intestinal metaplasia in the diagnosis of columnar-lined esophagus (Barrett's esophagus). Am J Clin Pathol 1989;42:741–746.
6. Clark GWB, Peters JH, Ireland AP, Hoeft SF, Smyrk TC, DeMeester TR, Bremner CG. Short segments of Barrett's esophagus are associated with gastroesophageal reflux disease and are premalignant (unpublished data).
7. Cameron AJ, Lomboy CT. Barrett's esophagus: age, prevalence and extent of columnar epithelium. Gastroenterology 1992;103:1241–1245.
8. Clark GWB, Ireland AP, Chandrasoma P, DeMeester TR, Peters JH, Bremner CG. Inflammation and metaplasia in the transitional epithelium of the gastroesophageal junction: a new marker for gastroesophageal reflux disease. Gastroenterology (in press).

Does Barrett's mucosa have the same histologic features in adults and children?

D.A. Antonioli (Boston)

The histologic changes associated with gastroesophageal reflux (GER) are basically similar in children and adults. In well-oriented esophageal mucosal biopsy specimens, taken 2 cm or more above the gastroesophageal junction, a basal zone occupying more than 20% of the thickness of the squamous epithelium, and stromal papillae extending more than two-thirds of the distance through the epithelium are excellent markers of GER. However, since most esophageal mucosal biopsies in the pediatric population are obtained using grasp biopsy forceps that result in small, poorly-oriented specimens, basal zone hyperplasia and papillary lengthening cannot be evaluated. Thus, as in adults, detection of intraepithelial inflammation becomes a major component in evaluating GER-related esophagitis in children [1].

Intraepithelial neutrophils are uncommon but are a good indicator of GER, being most often noted in patients with esophageal erosions or ulcers. Intraepithelial eosinophils are more frequent than neutrophils in GER-related injury, and they are often the sole marker of injury in children. Even a small number of eosinophils in a specimen taken 2–3 cm above the gastroesophageal junction correlates with GER. Although intraepithelial eosinophils are a very specific indicator of acid reflux, they are not a highly sensitive one [2]. Intraepithelial lymphocytes may be increased in childhood GER [1,3].

Other nonspecific markers of mucosal injury may be noted: these include increased mitoses in the epithelium, spongiosis and balloon-cell change (swelling) of keratinocytes [4]. Vascular congestion in papillae is a nonspecific response to endoscope trauma.

Like adults, children may develop Barrett's esophagus (BE) as a complication of severe GER. The precise incidence and prevalence of BE in the pediatric population are difficult to determine, because clinical studies on this age group are few in number and typically retrospective in nature. Within these limitations, however, BE has been diagnosed between infancy and age 19 years in 10 to 13% of children with severe GER and/or histologically-proven esophagitis [5,6]. These percentages are similar to those for adults with severe GER; also like adults, BE in children has a marked male predominance [6,7].

Barrett's esophagus may be over-represented in certain subsets of pediatric patients. For example, there may be an excess of BE in children (and adults) who have had an esophageal atresia or tracheoesophageal fistula surgically repaired. These congenital lesions are associated with esophageal dysmotility, resulting in poor esophageal acid clearance and a high prevalence of esophagitis [8]. Likewise, young people who are severely developmentally disabled are numerous in studies of BE in childhood [9], forming up to 40 to 70% of the BE patients in some series [6,7,10]. Severe GER is common in these patients, however, since they often cannot articulate their symptoms, the diagnosis of esophagitis is often delayed, thus allowing time for BE to develop [10]. The recognition of BE is important in children because of its malignant potential. Although they are rare, 10 cases of adenocarcinoma arising in BE before the age of 25 years have been reported [11].

The histologic features of BE in children are, in many respects, similar to those in adults. Fundic, junctional and specialized columnar epithelium may all be found, with the specialized epithelium typically at the upper end and the fundic and junctional types at the distal end of the BE segment [5–7,9,10]. As in adults, the fundic and junctional variants usually have an atrophic appearance, unlike that of normal stomach [5].

The major histologic difference between pediatric and adult BE is that specialized columnar epithelium is less frequent in children. Whereas specialized columnar epithelium can be identified in over 90% of adults with BE, it has been detected in only 15 to 50% of children with BE [5–7]. Its presence appears to be age-related, in that specialized columnar epithelium increases in prevalence in older, as compared to younger, cohorts of children with BE [6].

The relative paucity of specialized epithelium in younger children may make the diagnosis of BE problematic; caution should be exercised if only fundic or junctional tissue is obtained in biopsy specimens, since they may represent normal proximal stomach or gastric mucosa in a hiatal hernial [12]. Multiple biopsies and careful endoscopic measurements of the length of columnar mucosa may aid in determining if BE is present. Alcian blue staining (at pH 2.5) of biopsy specimens may be helpful in detecting otherwise inapparent goblet cells [12].

References

1. Dahms BB, Rothstein FC. Mucosal biopsy of the esophagus in children. In: Rosenberg HS, Bernstein J (eds) Respiratory and Alimentary Tract Diseases (Perspectives in Pediatric Pathology, vol 11). Basel: Karger, 1987;97–123.
2. Winter HS, Madara JL, Stafford RJ et al. Intraepithelial eosinophils: a new diagnostic criterion for reflux esophagitis. Gastroenterology 1982;83:818–823.
3. Groben PA, Siegal GP, Shub MD et al. Gastrointestinal reflux and esophagitis in infants and children. In: Rosenberg HS, Bernstein J (eds) Respiratory and Alimentary Tract Diseases (Perspectives in Pediatric Pathology, vol 11). Basal: Karger, 1987;124–151.
4. Jessurun J, Yardley JH, Giardiello FM, Hamilton SR. Intracytoplasmic plasma proteins in distended esophageal squamous cells (balloon cells). Mod Pathol 1988;1:175–181.
5. Dahms BB, Rothstein FC. Barrett's esophagus in children: a consequence of chronic gastroesophageal reflux. Gastroenterology 1984;86:318–323.
6. Qualman SJ, Murray RD, McClung J, Lucas J. Intestinal metaplasia is age-related in Barrett's esophagus. Arch Pathol Lab Med 1990;114:1236–1240.
7. Hassall E, Weinstein WM, Ament ME. Barrett's esophagus in childhood. Gastroenterology 1985;89:1131–1137.
8. Biller JA, Allen JL, Schuster SR, Treves ST, Winter HS. Long-term evaluation of esophageal and pulmonary function in patients with repaired esophageal atresia and tracheoesophageal fistula. Dig Dis Sci 1987;32:985–990.
9. Roberts IM, Curtis RL, Madara JL. Gastroesophageal reflux and Barrett's esophagus in developmentally disabled patients. Am J Gastroenterol 1986;81:519–523.
10. Snyder JD, Goldman H. Barrett's esophagus in children and young adults: frequent association with mental retardation. Dig Dis Sci 1990;35:1185–1189.
11. Hassall E, Dimmick JE, Magee JF. Adenocarcinoma in childhood Barrett's esophagus: case documentation and the need for surveillance in children. Am J Gastroenterol 1993;88:282–288.
12. Hassall E. Barrett's esophagus: congenital or acquired? Am J Gastroenterol 1993;88:819–824.

Which epithelial differentiations predispose to dysplasia and carcinoma?

F. Potet (Paris)

Barrett's esophagus is defined as a columnar epithelium lining a variable length of the lower esophagus. This term is used when the columnar epithelium extends to at least 3 cm. In our experience, the prevalence is 6% in gastroesophageal reflux disease. The severity of this pathology is due to the frequent development of adenocarcinoma in this type of mucosa [1]. Barrett's mucosa could be considered as a "precancerous condition".

Barrett's mucosa consists of one or a combination of three types of columnar epithelium [2]: 1) the junctional type epithelium resembles normal cardiac epithelium, with the surface and pits lined by typical mucus secreting cells; 2) the gastric fundic type epithelium resembles the epithelium found in the gastric body, but is slightly atrophic; 3) the specialized type epithelium appears to be a particular variant of incomplete intestinal metaplasia (IM): the surface is almost villous and lined by columnar and goblet cells. The columnar cells usually resemble gastric mucus-secreting pit cells rather than intestinal absorptive cells, interspersed with sparse goblet cells; deep in the mucosa are some clear mucus-secreting glands.

The poor prognosis of Barrett's adenocarcinoma incites to an early detection of carcinoma in patients followed by endoscopic biopsy surveillance program, and mainly in patients with a diagnosis of high grade dysplasia [3]. This high grade dysplasia (HGD) pattern is mainly observed in the specialized type of Barrett's esophagus. Most authors agree with the sequence: "Specialized IM mucosa — dysplastic mucosa (low grade and high grade) — adenocarcinoma" [4,5]. Dysplasia in Barrett's mucosa arises most often in specialized mucosa [2,4,5]. Dysplasia is always observed around Barrett's adenocarcinoma. In our experience of 67 Barrett's adenocarcinomas, in all cases specialized mucosa was observed surrounding the cancer. This type of mucosa was dysplastic in 76% of cases. Dysplasia was low grade type in 30% and high grade in 70% of cases.

The existence of this sequence dysplasia-carcinoma incites to the early detection of carcinoma in patients with IM and dysplasia. In some studies [4,6], the surveillance of patients with HGD allows diagnosis of many superficial Barrett's carcinoma. Our hypothesis is that the diagnosis of dysplasia in Barrett's mucosa is the key to the early diagnosis of Barrett's carcinoma.

According to Riddell et al. [7], dysplasia is defined as an unequivocal neoplastic alteration in colonic mucosa. They propose a classification of dysplasia in Barrett's mucosa similar to that in colonic inflammatory diseases. This classification consists of three groups: negative for dysplasia, indefinite for dysplasia and positive for dysplasia, low grade and high grade. This classification may be difficult to apply [8], particularly in intermediate grade (indefinite and low grade); change due to inflammation or regeneration may be difficult to distinguish from low grade dysplasia. On the other hand, it may be difficult to distinguish HGD from invasive adenocarcinoma; the histological abnormalities described to diagnose HGD are rather severe and the diagnosis with carcinoma mainly consists of the absence of extension to the lamina propria. This is why it is necessary to have numerous sections to eliminate adenocarcinoma. In questionable cases, it is recommended to repeat biopsies from the abnormal area, the dysplastic lesions being often observed surrounding invasive carcinoma.

On the whole, is it important to keep a close watch on these patients? Most of the patients with Barrett's esophagus will never develop carcinoma. Specialized mucosa seems to be the mandatory passage from Barrett's mucosa to carcinoma. Carcinoma develops almost always in dysplastic mucosa. The diagnosis of dysplasia in specialized mucosa seems to be the check point of the surveillance of these patients.

Concerning the surveillance of Barrett's esophagus, Reid et al. [6] recommend for all patients with Barrett's esophagus an initial endoscopy with systematic sampling. The biopsy specimens should be obtained at a maximum of 2 cm intervals. If the biopsy specimens do not show any specialized mucosa, the interval between endoscopies could be as long as 2 years. If biopsies show IM specialized mucosa, endoscopy is recommended at 1-year intervals. If dysplasia is diagnosed, Reid et al. recommend re-endoscopy with multiple biopsies to rule out a coexisting adenocarcinoma. If no carcinoma is found at this second endoscopy, they suggest to repeat endoscopy and biopsies every 6 months. They conclude that surveillance of Barrett's esophagus is necessary and useful in detecting adenocarcinoma before the invasive stage.

References

1. Potet F, Flejou JF, Gervaz E, Paraf F. Adenocarcinoma of the lower esophagus and the esophagogastric junction. Sem Diagn Path 1991;8:126−136.
2. Potet F, Duchatelle V. Barrett's oesophagus. In: Williams GT (ed) Current Topics in Gastrointestinal Pathology, vol 81. Berlin: Springer Verlag, 1990;43−60.
3. De Baecque C, Potet F, Molas G, Flejou JF, Barbier P, Martignon C. Superficial adenocarcinoma of the oesophagus arising in Barrett's mucosa with dysplasia: a clinico-pathological study of 12 patients. Histopathology 1990;16:213−220.
4. Hameeteman W, Tytgat GNJ, Houthoff HJ, Van den Tweel GJ. Barrett's esophagus: development of dysplasia and adeno-carcinoma. Gastroenterology 1989;96:1249−1256.
5. Miros M, Kerlin P, Walker N. Only patients with dysplasia progress to adenocarcinoma in Barrett's oesophagus. Gut 1991;32:1441−1446.
6. Reid BJ, Weinstein VM, Lewin KJ, Haggitt RC, VanDeventer G, Den Besten L, Rubin CE. Endoscopic biopsy can detect high-grade dysplasia or early adenocarinoma in Barrett's esophagus without grossly recognizable neoplastic lesions. Gastroenterology 1988;94:81−90.
7. Riddell RH, Goldman H, Ransohoff DF et al. Dysplasia in inflammatory bowel disease: standardized classification with provisional clinical applications. Hum Pathol 1983;14:931−966.
8. Potet F, Barge J. La dysplasie dans le tube digestif. Ann Pathol 1991;11(3):153−161.

Does columnar metaplasia ever derive from a proliferation of the submucosal glands or their ducts, after chronic reflux has destroyed the squamous mucosa?

P. Keeling (Dublin)

Barrett's esophagus is a condition in which, in a variable segment of the esophagus, the normal squamous epithelium becomes replaced by columnar epithelium. The development of a columnar-lined esophagus is believed to be secondary to gastro-esophageal reflux [1]. Both clinical and experimental studies support a causal relationship between acid reflux and columnar-lined esophagus [2−6]. Prolonged intraesophageal pH recordings have established that the patterns of acid reflux in Barrett's esophagus display a markedly increased number of acid events and more prolonged clearance times of acid, when compared with patients presenting with esophagitis without the presence of columnar epithelium [7−8].

Endoscopic studies have shown that the upper limit of columnar epithelium may extend proximally at successive examinations, in the presence of continuing reflux [2,3], thereby suggesting that a process of "creeping substitution" of gastric columnar epithelium may be responsible for the pathogenesis of this condition. However,

Barrett's epithelium may include a variety of epithelial types and histological appearances [9] and may present as islands of columnar epithelium remote from the gastric cardia [10]. These findings cannot be explained on the basis of proximal migration of cardiac epithelium alone. Controversy surrounds the pathophysiology of this condition, and neither the cell of origin nor the method of replacement of squamous epithelium by columnar epithelium has been established.

The influence of luminal contents on the regenerating esophageal mucosa is also uncertain and a hypothesis exists that alteration of luminal reflux contents may alter the morphology of the epithelium.

The demonstration by Gillen et al. [11] of regenerating columnar epithelium originating from cells lining esophageal gland ducts suggests that this is the cell of origin of this epithelium. Esophageal gland ducts in both the dog and man may possess a squamocuboidal junction at varying levels within the duct lining. Reflux-induced mucosal injury may then expose cuboidal cells and possibly stem cells to luminal reflux. It has been postulated that stem cells in the esophagus possess multipotentiality for cell differentiation, and that this would account for the variety of cell types and histological appearances seen in Barrett's epithelium in man. This variety of histological appearances is unlikely to be accounted for by proximal migration of cardiac epithelium alone.

References

1. Hamilton SR. Pathogenesis of columnar cell-lined (Barrett's) esophagus. In: Spechler SJ, Goyal RK (eds) Barrett's Esophagus: Pathophysiology, Diagnosis and Management. New York: Elsevier Science, 1985;29–37.
2. Goldman MC, Beckman RC. Barrett syndrome; case report and discussion about concepts of pathogenesis. Gastroenterology 1960;39:104–110.
3. Mossberg SM. The columnar-lined esophagus (Barrett syndrome) an acquired condition? Gastroenterology 1966;50:671–676.
4. Halvorsen JF, Semb BKH. The Barrett syndrome (the columnar-lined lower oesophagus): an acquired condition secondary to reflux oesophagitis, a case report with discussion of pathogenesis. Acta Chir Scand 1975;141:683–687.
5. Hamilton SR, Yardley JH. Regeneration of cardiac type mucosa and acquisition of Barrett's mucosa after oesophagogastrostomy. Gastroenterology 1977;72:669–675.
6. Bremner CG, Lynch VP, Ellis FH Jr. Barrett's esophagus congenital or acquired?: an experimental study of esophageal mucosal regeneration in the dog. Surgery 1970;68:209–216.
7. Iascone C, DeMeester TR, Little AG, Skinner DB. Barrett's esophagus, functional assessment, proposed pathogenesis and surgical therapy. Arch Surg 1983;118:543–549.
8. Flook D, Stoddard CJ. Gastro-oesophageal reflux (GOR) in patients with oesophagitis or a columnar lined (Barrett's) oesophagus. Gut 1983;24:A1007 (abstract).
9. Thompson JJ, Zinsser KR, Enterline HT. Barrett's metaplasia and adenocarcinoma of the oesophagus and gastro-oesophageal junction. Hum Pathol 1983;14:42–61.
10. Savary M, Monnier P. Diagnosis, pathophysiology and adenocarcinogenesis of Barrett's esophagus. In: DeMeester TR, Skinner DB (eds) Esophageal Disorders: Pathophysiology and Therapy. New York: Raven Press, 1985;101–108.
11. Gillen P, Keeling P, Byrne PJ, West AB, Hennessy TPJ. Experimental columnar metaplasia in the canine oesophagus. Br J Surg 1988;75:113–115.

Can Barrett's mucosa develop following an injury other than reflux, such as irradiation or chemotherapy?

W.V. Bogomoletz (Reims)

Barrett's esophagus (BE) is defined as the replacement of squamous epithelium lining the lower esophagus by gastric-like metaplastic columnar epithelium. In humans, compelling evidence indicates that BE is an acquired disorder resulting from prolonged gastroesophageal reflux (GER) [1,2]. In addition to acid reflux, hereditary factors may contribute to the pathogenesis of BE, as suggested by several case reports of familial association [3]. Moreover, it is not possible to entirely exclude a congenital origin of BE in some patients.

The development of BE has also been described in two unusual situations, both apparently unrelated to GER:

1. BE has been reported following total gastrectomy [4,5]. Some factors other than acid reflux from the stomach must presumably operate in such a surgically created environment. Bile, intestinal or pancreatic secretion could certainly be involved. The possibility of gastric metaplasia in the duodenum contributing acid secretion to "alkaline reflux" in the vicinity of the anastomosis could even be entertained.

2. The possible development of BE following a "toxic" injury to the esophageal mucosa in some patients treated with chemotherapy has been suggested by some workers [6], but refuted by others [7]. This remains a controversial and unresolved issue so far, and further prospective studies are needed to confirm or dismiss this possibility.

In the upper esophagus, the situation is somewhat complicated by the so-called "heterotopic gastric mucosa" (HGM) or "inlet patch". Although the traditionally held view of the congenital nature of HGM has been recently reaffirmed [8], the possibility of HGM being related to acquired inflammation secondary to reflux cannot be entirely dismissed [9]. Development of BE has not been described in radiation-induced esophagitis so far [10].

References

1. Spechler SJ, Goyal RK. Barrett's esophagus. N Engl J Med 1986;315:362–371.
2. Potet F, Duchatelle V. Barrett's oesophagus. In: Williams GT (ed) Current Topics in Gastrointestinal Pathology, vol 81. Berlin: Springer-Verlag, 1990;43–60.
3. Jochem VJ, Fuerst PA, Fromkes JJ. Familial Barrett's esophagus associated with adenocarcinoma. Gastroenterology 1992;102:1400–1402.
4. Hamilton SR, Yardley JH. Regeneration of cardia type mucosa and acquisition of Barrett's mucosa after esophagogastrostomy. Gastroenterology 1977;72:669–675.
5. Meyer W, Vollmar F, Bär W. Barrett's esophagus following total gastrectomy: a contribution to its pathogenesis. Endoscopy 1979;11:121–126.
6. Sartori S, Nielsen I, Indelli M, Trevisani M, Pazzi P, Grandi E. Barrett's esophagus after chemotherapy with cyclophosphamide, methotrexate and 5-fluorouracil (CMF): an iatrogenic injury? Ann Intern Med 1991;114:210–211.

7. Herrera JL, Uzel C, Martino R, Cooke C, DiPalma JA. Barrett's esophagus: lack of association with adjuvant chemotherapy for localized breast carcinoma. Gastrointest Endosc 1992;38:551–553.
8. Borhan-Manesh F, Farmin JB. Incidence of heterotopic gastric mucosa in the upper esophagus. Gut 1991;32:968–972.
9. Bogomoletz WV, Geboes K, Feydy P, Nasca S, Ectors N, Rigaud C. Mucin histochemistry of heterotopic gastric mucosa of the upper esophagus in adults: possible pathogenic implications. Hum Pathol 1988;19:1301– 1306.
10. Fajardo LF. Radiation-induced pathology of the alimentary tract. In: Whitehead R (ed) Gastrointestinal and Oesophageal Pathology. Edinburgh: Churchill Livingstone, 1989;377–383.

Are Barrett's mucosa and the neoplastic colonic mucosa evidence of a diffuse gastrointestinal inflammatory reaction?

A. Keshavarzian, S.J. Sontag (Hines)

We previously reported in a series of 65 patients with well-documented Barrett's esophagus that benign colon adenomas were present in about 30% of the patients and malignant colonic tumors were present in 15% of the patients. After adjusting for several types of statistical biases and deleting patients from the analysis who had already had colonic surgery before the diagnosis of Barrett's was made, we found that 5.5% of the remaining 55 patients had malignant colonic tumors and 29% had benign adenomas [1]. We had no appropriate control group. Since the true prevalence rate of colon cancer and benign colonic adenomas in the general population is not known, we could conclude only that a 5.5% prevalence rate of colon cancer appeared to be very high for the general population.

Since that publication, four other studies in patients with Barrett's esophagus have been published [2–5]. One of the studies [3] reported a 9% prevalence rate of colon cancer (three of 32 patients) and a 25% prevalence rate of benign adenomas (eight of 32 patients). In the remaining three studies [2,4,5], no cancers were found in a total of 97 patients.

First assumption

Without knowing for certain whether the presence of Barrett's esophagus truly correlates with the presence of benign and malignant colonic neoplasms, let us assume that Barrett's metaplastic mucosa and the colonic neoplastic mucosa respond similarly to several stimuli.

The first question asked is, "why would Barrett's esophagus and colonic neoplasia occur together?" One possible explanation is that certain dietary factors that affect bile composition may be associated in some way with both conditions. Elements in the bile have been implicated as colonic mucosal tumor promoters. The same elements that affect the colon may also be involved in mucosal changes in the esophagus, especially since bile is often present in the esophagus in individuals with gastroesophageal reflux (GER). In other words, a tumor promoter or carcinogen in the bile could potentially affect any segment of the gut in which it makes contact. Individuals with GER therefore would likely be exposed to biliary elements that are travelling up to the distal esophagus as well as down to the colon. One might argue that prolonged reflux of acid promotes the gastric junctional type of columnar epithelium in the esophagus, while reflux of bile promotes the specialized intestinal type.

A reasonable sequence of events might begin with "acid" reflux causing gastric-type Barrett's and progress to "acid and bile" reflux, causing goblet cell metaplasia with specialized columnar-type Barrett's. The scenario could end with subsequent malignant transformation as a result of the tumor-promoting elements in the bile.

Possible mechanisms

It is well known that acid is the most important factor in the development of esophagitis. The exact mechanism by which acid causes the inflammatory reaction and subsequent mucosal damage is not known. Reactive oxygen metabolites (ROM), produced by epithelial cells, phagocytic cells and neutrophils, can cause tissue injury both in peptic disorders such as gastric and duodenal ulcer and inflammatory disorders such as ulcerative colitis and Crohn's disease [6—8]. Recent studies have documented the production of ROM by the inflamed esophageal mucosa as well as by Barrett's mucosa, with or without inflammation [9], indicating that the presence of inflammation is not necessary for ROM production. Indeed, the uninvolved rectal mucosa of patients with colonic neoplasia produces ROM [10].

In the last decade, ROM as a factor in human diseases has gained considerable attention [11—13]. In rats and in humans, studies show that ROM are an important factor in increased colonic cell proliferation [14—17]. Since colon cancer is the final phase of the increased colonic cell proliferation sequence (normal mucosa → proliferative mucosa → adenomatous polyp → carcinoma), the cancer may result from ROM control of mutagenesis and carcinogenesis [18]. In this regard, the entire gastrointestinal tract, especially the esophagus and colon, may be under the powerful influence of the dreadful "secret and invisible" ROM.

Several studies have shown that the technique of chemiluminescence is an accurate method to estimate ROM production [19,20]. The technique measures light production as a cellular by-product of oxidative metabolism and has been utilized to demonstrate the involvement of ROM in various diseases [14]. We used chemiluminescence to estimate ROM levels in different areas of the gut during health and disease [9,10,21,22]. The analysis consisted of noninflamed and inflamed esophageal squamous mucosa, noninflamed and inflamed Barrett's epithelium, Barrett's epithelium with and without low grade/high grade dysplasia, Barrett's epithelium with adenocarcinoma, gastric mucosa, normal colonic mucosa, uninvolved and involved

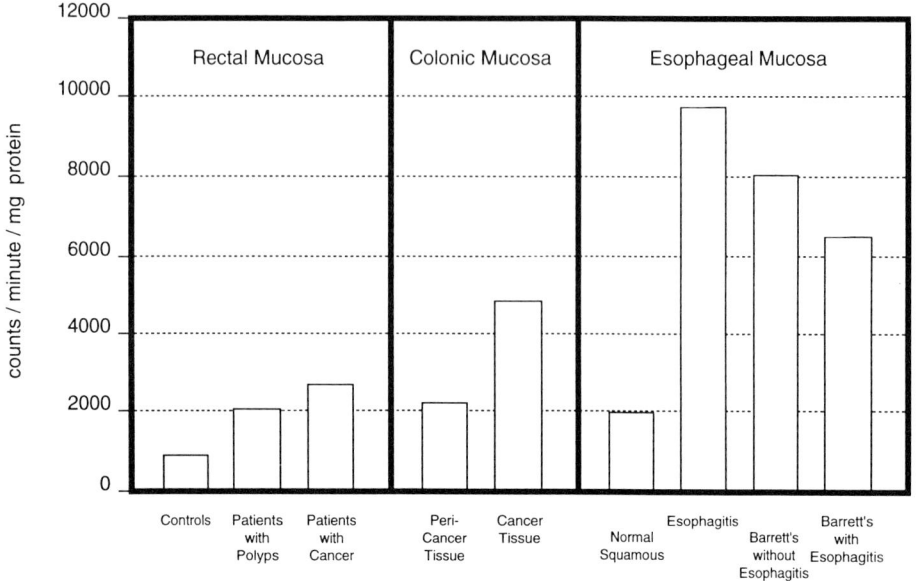

Fig. 1. Production of reactive oxygen metabolites (ROM) measured by chemiluminescence.

rectal and colonic mucosa harboring benign and malignant neoplasms, postsurgical colonic mucosa and rectal mucosa of inflammatory bowel disease and Crohn's colitis.

Figure 1 demonstrates that ROM is present in both normal and diseased tissues. The first column has three bars: the first bar shows that the rectum of normal healthy controls with no polyps or cancer has a level of ROM of about 800 counts/min/mg protein; the second bar shows that the uninvolved rectal mucosa of patients who had had previous polypectomies for benign adenomas produces twice as many ROM; the third bar shows that the uninvolved rectal mucosa of patients with previous cancer produces almost 3 times as many ROM, despite the fact that the benign adenomas and the malignant cancers had been removed. These data suggest that the rectal mucosa of patients who have had previous neoplasia continues to produce significantly higher levels of ROM than normal healthy mucosa.

The second column with two bars shows the very high levels of ROM produced by both the pericancer tissue and the malignant tissue itself. As would be expected, the uninvolved mucosa surrounding the cancer tissue produces similar quantities of ROM as the uninvolved rectal mucosa of patients with previous cancer (column 1, bar 3).

The last column has four bars demonstrating the ROM production of different disease states of the esophageal mucosa. The mucosa of patients with esophagitis, with Barrett's and no esophagitis and with Barrett's with esophagitis produces up to 4 times as many ROM as the normal squamous mucosa of healthy control patients. The high production of ROM seen in the diseased esophageal mucosa is present with or without inflammation.

We have tried to show that the esophageal and colonic mucosa produce ROM

894

regardless of the presence of tumor and regardless of the presence of inflammatory activity. From these data it appears that the gut mucosa (at least the esophagus and colon) respond in similar fashion to certain stimuli in the production of inflammatory mediators such as ROM.

References

1. Sontag SJ, Schnell TG, Chejfec G et al. Barrett's oesophagus and colonic tumors. Lancet 1985;1:946–948.
2. Tripp MR, Sampliner RE, Kogan FJ et al. Colorectal neoplasms and Barrett's esophagus. Am J Gastroenterol 1986;81:1063–1064.
3. Robertson DA, Ayres AC, Smith CC. Screening for colonic cancer in patients with Barrett's oesophagus. Br Med J 1989;298:650.
4. Rothstein RI, Smith RE, Power GC. Barrett's esophagus and colonic neoplasia. Gastroenterology 1991;100(5):A150 (Abstract).
5. Post AB, Achkar E, Carey WD. Prevalence of colonic neoplasia in patients with Barrett's esophagus. Am J Gastroenterol 1993;88(6):877–880.
6. Babbs CFC. Free radicals and the etiology of colon cancer. Free Radic Biol Med 1990;8:191–200.
7. Parks D, Buckley G, Granger N. Role of oxygen-derived free radicals in digestive tract disease. Surgery 1983;94:415–422.
8. Terpstra OT, Blankenstein M, Dees J. Abnormal pattern of cell proliferation in the entire colonic mucosa of patients with colon adenoma or cancer. Gastroenterology 1987;92:704–748.
9. Olyaee M, Sontag S, Schnell T, Salman W, Liao Y, Mobarhan S, Frommel T, Fields JZ, Keshavarzian A. Mucosal reactive oxygen metabolites production in esophagitis and Barrett's esophagus. Gastroenterology 1993;104:A164.
10. Keshavarzian A, Olyaee M, Sontag S, Mobarhan S. Increased levels of luminol-enhanced chemiluminescence by rectal mucosa of patients with colonic neoplasia: a possible marker for colonic neoplasia. Nutr Cancer 1993;19(2):201–206.
11. Buckley GB. The role of oxygen free radicals in human disease processes. Surgery 1983;94:407–411.
12. McCord JM, Fridovich I. The biology and pathology of oxygen radicals. Ann Intern Med 1978;89:121–127.
13. Fantone JC, Ward PA. Role of oxygen-derived free radicals and metabolites in leukocyte-dependent inflammatory reactions. Am J Pathol 1982;107:397–418.
14. Paganelli GM. Rectal cell proliferation and colorectal cancer risk level in patients with nonfamilial adenomatous polyps of the large bowel. Cancer 1991;68:2451–2454.
15. Keshavarzian A, Morgan G, Sedghi S, Gordon JH, Doria M. Role of reactive metabolites in experimental colitis. Gut 1990;31:786–790.
16. Keshavarzian A, Haydek J, Zabihi R, Doria M, D'Astice M, Sorenson Jr. Agents capable of eliminating reactive oxygen species. Catalase, WR-2721, or Cu(II)2(3),5-DIPS)4 decrease experimental colitis. Dig Dis Sci 1992;37(12):1866–1873.
17. Keshavarzian A, Zapeda D, List T, Mobarhan S. High levels of reactive oxygen metabolites in colon cancer tissue: analysis by chemiluminescence probe. Nutr Cancer 1992;17(3):243–249.
18. Moody CS, Hassan HM. Mutagenicity of oxygen-free radicals. Proc Natl Acad Sci USA 1982;79:2855–2859.
19. Boveris A, Cadenas E, Reiter R, Fillipowski M, Nakase Y et al. Organ chemiluminescence: noninvasive assay for oxidative radical reactions. Proc Natl Acad Sci USA 1980;77:347–351.
20. Boveris A, Cadenas E, Chance B. Ultraweak chemiluminescence: a sensitive assay for oxidative radical reactions. Fed Proc 1980;40:195–198.
21. Grande A, Keshavarzian A, Olyaee M, Papa V, Durkin M, Sontag S, Frommel T, Mobarhan S. Increased reactive oxygen metabolites (ROM) and arachidonic acid (AA) levels in rectal mucosa of subjects with colonic neoplasia. 57th Annual Scientific Meeting ACG, October 26–28, 1992.
22. Keshavarzian A, Sedghi S, Kanofsky J, List T, Robinson C, Ibrahim C, Winship D. Excessive production of reactive oxygen metabolites by inflamed colon: analysis by chemiluminescence probe. Gastroenterology 1992;103:177–185.

Does *Helicobacter pylori* colonize the gastric metaplasia of CLE and induce additional disease in that site?

P. Vincent (Lille)

It is now accepted that *Helicobacter pylori* is the causal agent of type B gastritis and an etiological agent in the pathogenesis of most peptic ulcers. An association between *H. pylori* infection and gastric precancerous lesions has also been established and *H. pylori* infection might occupy a key position in the sequence of events leading to gastric cancer.

Little is known about the potential pathogenesis of *H. pylori* in the esophagus where the bacteria is not usually found. However, since *H. pylori* can only colonize the gastric mucosa specifically, one can wonder whether it can colonize the gastric metaplastic area of Barrett's esophagus and promote additional pathology. A review shows that the relationship between *H. pylori* and esophageal pathology is inconstant and suggests that the bacteria might be only a contaminant. Clinical relevance of *H. pylori* in the esophagus remains to be demonstrated.

Helicobacter pylori and pathogenicity

Microbiology

Since *H. pylori* (originally called *Campylobacter pyloridis* and then changed to *Campylobacter pylori*) was first isolated in 1983 [1], efforts have been focused on isolating gastric bacteria and studying their potential pathogenesis. Several species of mucus-associated bacteria have been discovered. They are curved, spiral, microaerophilic, asacharolytic and non-spore-forming Gram-negative rods. Although they look like campylobacteria, significant morphologic, structural, biochemical and genomic features indicated that they should be placed in a new genus now named *Helicobacter* [2]. In humans, *H. pylori* is found commonly in gastric biopsies from symptomatic patients undergoing upper gastrointestinal endoscopy. Many studies have demonstrated that *H. pylori* can also frequently be found in asymptomatic, otherwise healthy, persons. All such infected persons have histologic gastritis. *H. pylori* is arguably the commonest chronic bacterial infection in man. In industrialized countries, prevalence of infection rises with age and in low social classes. Approximately 50% of adults are colonized by the age of 60. In developing countries, 80–90% rates are commonly found, even in children [3]. The lack of a plausible environmental reservoir, the extensive prevalence of infection in humans and the clustering of cases in families and cohabiting persons suggest that humans might be the unique reservoir of *H. pylori* and that person-to-person contacts might be the major way of spread. However, whether the origin of contamination is fecal or oral is still questioned [4].

Colonization of mucosa

All evidence to date is consistent with the hypothesis that *H. pylori* is the human associated *Helicobacter* species [5]. It has evolved with its human host and has acquired properties to withstand the hostile gastric environment. So it is well suited for survival in its ecological niche of antral mucus [6]. Urease production is the major factor of adaptation. This enzyme is essential for initial colonization. Unlike other urease enzymes, the gastric *H. pylori* urease retains significant activity at low pH. Neutralization of local gastric acidity by ammonia (which is the end product of the breakdown of mucosal urea) protects the bacteria against prolonged acidity. Thus, as the organism enters the stomach it is protected long enough to allow penetration of mucus. Motility, due to the flagellae and the spiral shape of the bacteria, is another adaptation factor. It allows the organism to move quickly from the gastric lumen into the viscous environment of gastric mucus [7]. It has been shown that nonmotile variants of *H. pylori* cannot colonize gnotobiotic piglets [8]. Microaerophily is another factor of adaptation, since the atmosphere in the mucus overlaying the gastric cells is microaerobic. Growth of *H. pylori* is possible down to 5% oxygen concentration. Once *H. pylori* has penetrated the mucus layer, adhesion allows the bacterium to settle in intercellular spaces. *H. pylori* has some lectin-like proteins, and gastric type epithelial cells owns a glycerolipid which is a specific receptor for *H. pylori* adhesins [9]. Consequently, natural barriers to microbial colonization of the stomach are inefficient against *H. pylori*. It can colonize all sites where mucus and gastric-type epithelial cells are present, whether normally present in the stomach or metaplastic. This specificity is high and *H. pylori* cannot colonize squamous epithelial cells of the esophagus or absorptive-type duodenal epithelial cells, even when these are metaplastic in the stomach [10].

Induced lesions

H. pylori infection is specifically associated with the presence of type B gastritis but not with type A gastritis (autoimmune gastritis), bile reflux or secondary gastritis. Thus when *H. pylori* is present, gastric inflammation is not the cause of bacterial colonization but its consequence. Several bacterial factors are implied in *H. pylori* induced lesions. Ammonia, produced close to the cell surface by urease activity, has a cytotoxic action on epithelial cells [11]. *H. pylori* produces a phospholipase C [12], which is basically a hemolytic enzyme. Cell alterations can occur equally due to a cytotoxin which is found for many strains, especially in patients with peptic ulcer [13]. Other effects found in *H. pylori* epithelium colonization are modifications in the mucus environment. The presence of the organism decreases the mucus hydrophobicity and reduces the mucus gel thickness. Although the mucus synthesis is not modified, *H. pylori* adherence pedestals obstruct mucin exoxytosis. *H. pylori* secretes a chemotactic factor for neutrophils and monocytes. There is then a lymphocyte activation and a cytokine release. A local secretory immunoglobulin-A response occurs. IgA can overlay bacterial cells [14], but is inefficient to fetter the bacterium and any bacterial toxin. The presence of endotoxins and other bacterial products in the gastric tissue promotes complement activation resulting in a vigorous local and systemic immune response. However, phagocytosis of *H. pylori* by polymorpho-nuclear cells is unusual due to an environment hostile to phagocytic cells. The host's response to infection fails to eradicate bacteria and a chronic infiltration of inflammatory cells occurs, with a persistent systemic humoral immune response to the organism.

Pathology

The role of *H. pylori* in nonulcer dyspepsia is still questioned. However, it is now evident that the type B form of atrophic gastritis (symptomatic or not) is a sequel to long-standing chronic *H. pylori* infection in the mucosa. An increasing prevalence of glandular atrophy with age has been shown, implying a transition from nonatrophic to atrophic gastritis, according to the duration of inflammation [15].

Into the duodenum, where gastric metaplasia occurs in case of increased acid production, *H. pylori* colonizes metaplastic mucus-secreting mucosa. This duodenal colonization leads to active duodenitis (which, strictly from an histological point of view, is "gastritis" in the duodenum), glandular atrophy and ultimately ulceration of metaplasia. It has been widely shown that eradication of *H. pylori* was necessary to allow duodenal ulcers to heal with lower relapse rates.

The key position of *H. pylori* infection in the sequence of events leading to gastric cancer is now in question [16], since cohort follow-up studies support a dynamic progression through chronic atrophic gastritis, intestinal metaplasia to dysplasia and gastric cancer [17]. *H. pylori* infection seems to be associated to a decrease of gastric ascorbic acid [18] whose protective role is known (by preventing the formation of carcinogenetic nitrosamines) [19].

H. pylori and esophagus

Role in gastroesophageal reflux

The relationship between gastric *H. pylori* infection and gastroesophageal reflux (GER) has been studied. In children, the bacteria was found in a minority with reflux (3/80) without relation to macroscopic esophagitis (1/26). Authors concluded that *H. pylori* is unlikely to have an etiologic role in reflux esophagitis [20]. In adults, a paper reported seven cases of gastric infection among 21 patients with reflux [21], which is not a higher prevalence rate than expected in general population of the same range of age in industrialized countries. In this study, the presence of infection seemed to correlate with the grade of esophagitis (according to Savary and Miller's classification). However, the authors discussed neither the small size of their sample nor the possible confounding role of age.

In Barrett's esophagus, the role of *H. pylori* gastric infection has not yet been demonstrated. In the same paper, infection rate was about the same in Barrett's esophagus and esophagitis alone (4/11 vs. 2/6). Another study reported similar frequency of gastric infection in patients with Barrett's esophagus and in age- and sex-matched controls: 10/26 vs. 11/26 [22].

Colonization of esophageal mucosa

The colonization of normal esophagus by *H. pylori* from the gastric area of infection has never been reported. Animal experimentation found no case of implantation of the bacteria in esophagus of gnotobiotic piglets [23]. Among seven gastric infected patients [21] and 25 [22], *H. pylori* was never found in esophageal biopsy specimens. In dyspeptic patients undergoing esogastroduodenoscopy with endoscopic abnormality or histological inflammation of upper gastrointestinal tract, *H. pylori* was cultured in 8/30 cases from the esophagus [24]. However, the bacteria could not be seen in the mucosa at this site by light microscopy or electron microscopy. Authors concluded that isolated *H. pylori* was either a commensal or a contaminant probably originating from the stomach.

H. pylori which specifically colonizes acid secreting gastric epithelium can only settle into Barrett's esophagus where columnar epithelium lines the esophagus, instead of the usual stratified squamous epithelium. Although no *H. pylori* was found by Giemsa staining in esophageal biopsies from 34 patients in the Barrett's esophagus [25] and was not cultured from the esophagus of 11 patients [21], colonization of acid secreting gastric epithelium in the esophageal tissue has been reported a great number of times [22,24,26–33]. In all cases, *H. pylori* was found to be colonizing only the gastric-type tissue in the esophagus. The prevalence of colonized Barrett's esophagus was variable: with the exception of 12 Yemeni patients with Barrett's esophagus, all (100%) colonized [33], the prevalence rate in western countries ranged from 15 to 52% in five series of seven to 100 patients with Barrett's esophagus [22,24,28,29,32]. The absence of Barrett's esophagus colonization without gastric infection demonstrates that esophageal *H. pylori* comes from the stomach. However, as shown in several series, less than half of antral *H. pylori* infection extends to the columnar epithelium of Barrett's esophagus. These findings suggest a difference in mucosal reactivity of columnar epithelium between esophagus and stomach towards *H. pylori* invasion. This might be due to a distinct immunologic reactivity or to a protection by a relatively high acid output, as seen in the gastric corpus. Furthermore, junctional-type epithelium (the type most closely resembling antral mucosa) is found in only about 25% of Barrett's esophagus [25,34]. Thus, it is possible that the metaplastic epithelium of Barrett's esophagus lacks in some cases the prerequisite receptor for attachment of the bacteria.

Esophagitis

Since it can cause inflammation of gastric tissue in the stomach, *H. pylori* has been assumed to have the same effect on gastric tissue in esophagus and thus to contribute to the overrated risk of ulceration and adenocarcinoma in Barrett's esophagus [35—37]. It has been reported a coincidence between the presence of *H. pylori* with areas of esophagitis in a 14-year-old child [27] and an association with acute inflammation of the esophageal columnar mucosa, as compared with Barrett's mucosa from patients with gastric but not esophageal colonization: 4/4 vs. 1/6 [22]. However, further studies show that the relationship is inconstant. Acute esophageal inflammation (polymorphonuclear leukocytes infiltration) was found in only one case among 23 patients with *H. pylori* infection in Barrett's epithelium [29] and in eight cases among 19 [32]. On the other hand, polymorphonuclear cells have been found even when *H. pylori* infection of esophageal columnar epithelium was absent: among 20 patients with endoscopic and histological Barrett's inflammation, 15 had no *H. pylori* infection [24]. Among 81 Barrett's esophagus without *H. pylori* infection, 27 had an active inflammation [32].

Other infections of esophageal columnar epithelium have been described. *Candida* and moniliasis for instance, were found in association with 6/25 (24%) of cases of Barrett's esophagus (vs. 19% of *H. pylori* infection) [28]. Candidiasis is generally regarded as an opportunistic infection in peptic ulcer and it is possible that the presence of esophagitis lesions promotes colonization by *H. pylori* as well as *Candida*. Such contaminant organisms might have no etiologic role in esophageal inflammation.

Ulcer and adenocarcinoma

Ulceration and adenocarcinoma are well known complications associated with Barrett's esophagitis [38] and the possible role of *H. pylori* has been studied. Barrett's esophagus ulceration has been found no more frequently in *H. pylori* infected patients than in noninfected patients: 4/10 vs. 5/16 [22]. In another study, among 25 Barrett's esophagus ulceration, only six patients (24%) were *H. pylori* infected (vs. 17% in nonulcerated cases, the difference was not significant) [28]. These two studies reported that about half *H. pylori* infected patients had no ulceration of their Barrett's mucosa (6/10 and 6/12, respectively).

Association of *H. pylori* with carcinoma of Barrett's esophagus has been rarely documented. Among 30 patients with esophageal columnar epithelium, from which 27% were *H. pylori* infected, one patient had a carcinoma but was not *H. pylori* infected [24]. In 12 cases of *H. pylori* infected Barrett's esophagus, the gastric-type mucosa showed no evidence of dysplasia in any cases but intestinal metaplasia was present in three patients [33]. Among 64 cases of Barrett's esophagus, from which 19% were *H. pylori* infected, one patient had a dysplasia but was not infected.

Conclusion

H. pylori, which may be isolated from gastric juice in infected subjects, can be transmitted by means of GER of contaminated gastric juice to acid secreting gastric-type epithelium of esophagus. The potential analogy to duodenal ulcer of patients

900

with *H. pylori* infected Barrett's esophagus remains evocative. However, the relationship between colonization and esophagitis, ulceration or adenocarcinoma of Barrett's esophagus is inconstant. *H. pylori*, which is not of relevance in GER and not an acquisition of Barrett's esophagus, does not seem to contribute to the natural history of this affection. It is possible that, through migrating from the stomach to the lower third of the esophagus, *H. pylori* undergoes environmental alteration. Observations do not support the hypothesis that *H. pylori* causes inflammatory, ulcerative or precancerous lesions of Barrett's esophagus. Whether or not colonization of esophageal gastric-type epithelium is more than an overinfection of pre-existent lesions by a transient contaminant, remains to be proved.

References

1. Warren JR, Marshall BJ. Unidentified curved bacilli on gastric epithelium in active chronic gastritis. Lancet 1983;2: 1273–1275.
2. Goodwin CS, Armstrong JA, Chilvers T, Peters M, Collins M, Sly L, McConnell W, Harper WES. Transfer of *Campylobacter pylori* and *Campylobacter mustelae* to *Helicobacter* gen. nov. as *Helicobacter pylori* comb. nov. and *Helicobacter mustelae* comb. nov., respectively. Int J Syst Bacteriol 1989;39:397–405.
3. Taylor DN, Blaser MJ. The epidemiology of *Helicobacter pylori* infection. Epidemiol Rev 1991;13:42–59.
4. Vincent P. Epidémiologie de l'infection à *Helicobacter pylori*: quand et comment risque-t-on de s'infecter? La lettre de l'infectiologue 1993;8:184–189.
5. Lee A, Hazell SL. *Campylobacter pylori* in health and disease: an ecological perspective. Microbial Ecol Health Dis 1988;1:1–16.
6. Lee A. Infection causes of gastroduodenal inflammation in humans. Eur J Gastroenterol Hepatol 1992;4:51–57.
7. Hazell SL, Lee A, Brady L, Hennessy W. *Campylobacter pyloridis* and gastritis: association with intercellular spaces and adaptation to an environment of mucus as important factors in colonization of the gastric epithelium. J Infect Dis 1986;153: 658–663.
8. Eaton KA, Morgan DR, Krakowka S. *Campylobacter pylori* virulence factors in gnotobiotic piglets. Infect Immun 1989;57: 1119–1125.
9. Lingwood CA, Pellizani A, Law H, Sherman P, Drumm B. Gastric glycerolipid as a receptor for *Campylobacter pylori*. Lancet 1989;2:238–241.
10. Buck GE, Gourley WK, Lee WK, Subramanyam K, Latimer JM, Di Nuzzo AR. Relation of *Campylobacter pyloridis* to gastritis and peptic ulcer. J Infect Dis 1986;153:664–669.
11. Megraud F, Neman-Simha, Brugmann D. Further evidence of the toxic effect of ammoniac produced by *Helicobacter pylori* urease on human epithelial cells. Infect Immun 1992;60:1858.
12. Daw MA, Keane CT, O'Moore R, O'Morain C. Phospholipase C activity: new pathogenicity marker for *Helicobacter pylori*. Ital J Gastroenterol 1991;23(S2):37–38.
13. Figura N, Guglielmetti P, Rossolini A. Cytotoxin production by *Campylobacter pylori* strains isolated from patients with peptic ulcers and from patients with chronic gastritis only. J Clin Microbiol 1989;27:225–226.
14. Wyatt JI, Rathbone BJ, Heatley RV. Local immune response to gastric *Campylobacter* in nonulcer dyspepsia. J Clin Pathol 1986;39:863–870.
15. Correa P. Precursors of gastric and esophageal cancer. Cancer 1982;50:2554–2565.
16. Forman D. *Helicobacter pylori* infection and gastric carcinogenesis. Eur J Gastroenterol Hepatol 1992;4:531–535.
17. Correa P, Haenzel W, Cuello C, Zavala D, Fontham E, Zarama G. Gastric precancerous process in a high risk population: cohort follow-up study. Cancer Res 1990;50:4737–4740.
18. Sobala GM, Schorah CJ, Shires S, Axon ATR. Impairment of gastric ascorbic acid concentration by acute *Helicobacter pylori* infection. Gut 1990;31:A1180.
19. Mirvish SS. The etiology of gastric cancer intragastric nitrosamide formation other theories. J Natl Cancer Inst 1983;71:631–647.
20. Stewart RJ, Boston VE, Dodge JA, Emmerson AM. *Campylobacter pylori* and reflux oesophagitis. Acta Paediatr Scand 1990;79:107.
21. Francoual S, Lamy Ph, Le Quintrec Y, Luboinski J, Petit JC. *Helicobacter pylori*: has it a part in the lesion of the gastroesophageal reflux? J Infect Dis 1990;161:626–633.
22. Paull G, Yardley JH. Gastric and esophageal *Campylobacter pylori* in patients with Barrett's esophagus. Gastroenterology 1988;95:216–218.
23. Lambert J, Borromeo M, Pinkard K, Turner H, Chapman C, Smith M. Colonization of gnotobiotic piglets with *Campylo-*

bacter pyloridis — an animal model? J Infect Dis 1987;155:1344.

24. Walker SJ, Birch PJ, Stewart M, Stoddard CJ, Hart CA, Day DW. Patterns of colonisation of *Campylobacter pylori* in the oesophagus, stomach and duodenum. Gut 1989;30:1334—1338.

25. Houck JA, Lucas JG. Absence of *Campylobacter*-like organisms in Barrett's esophagus. Arch Pathol Lab Med 1989;113: 470—472.

26. Goodwin CS, Blincow ED, Warren JR. Evaluation of cultural techniques for isolating *Campylobacter pyloridis* from endoscopic biopsies of gastric mucosa. J Clin Pathol 1985;38:1127—1131.

27. Mitchell HM, Bohane TD, Berkowicz J, Hazell SL, Lee A. Antibody to *Campylobacter pylori* in families of index children with gastrointestinal illness due to *C. pylori*. Lancet 1987;2:681—682.

28. Kalogeropoulos NK, Whitehead R. *Campylobacter*-like organisms and candida in peptic ulcers and similar lesions of the upper gastrointestinal tract: a study of 247 cases. J Clin Pathol 1988;41:1093— 1098.

29. Talley NJ, Cameron AJ, Shorter RG, Zinsmeister AR, Phillips SF. *Campylobacter pylori* and Barrett's esophagus. Mayo Clin Proc 1988;63:1176—1180.

30. Flejou JF, Potet F, Molas G et al. *Campylobacter*-like organisms in heterotopic gastric mucosa of the upper oesophagus. J Clin Pathol 1990;43:961—968.

31. Lapertosa G. *Helicobacter pylori* in Barrett's oesophagus. Histopathology 1991;18:568—570.

32. Gospe (Precancerous lesions of the esophagus task force). Analysis of the clinical and biological features of the Barrett's esophagus and risk for developing an esophageal adenocarcinoma in patients with this metaplastic condition: a multicentric study. Acta Endoscopica 1987;17:189—194.

33. Guneid AEL, Sherif AMEL, Murray-Lyon IM, Zureikat N, Shousha S. Effect of chewing Qat on mucosal histology and prevalence of *Helicobacter pylori* in the oesophagus, stomach and duodenum of Yemeni patients. Histopathology 1991;19: 437—443.

34. Paull A, Trier JS, Dalton MD, Camp RC, Loeb P, Goyal RK. The histologic spectrum of Barrett's oesophagus. N Engl J Med 1976;295:476—480.

35. Van der Veen AH, Dees J, Blankenstein M. Adenocarcinoma in Barrett's esophagus in patients: an overrated risk. Gut 1989;30:14—18.

36. Muñoz N, Crespi M, Grassi A, Qing WG, Qiong S, Cai LZ. Precursor lesions of oesophageal cancer in high-risk populations in Iran and China. Lancet 1982;1:876—879.

37. Hameeteman W, Tytgat GNJ, Houthoff HJ, Van den Tweel JG. Barrett's esophagus: development of dysplasia and adenocarcinoma. Gastroenterology 1989;96:1249—1256.

38. Sjogren RW, Johnson L. Barrett's esophagus: a review. Am J Med 1983;74:313—321.

Is the incidence of complications of CLE significantly higher in cases of alkaline reflux than in cases of acid reflux?

R.A. Hinder (Omaha)

The basal pressure in the lower esophageal sphincter (LES) is below normal in most patients with Barrett's esophagus and the mean LES pressure tends to be lower than in patients who have esophagitis without Barrett's epithelium. A decrease in the amplitude of contractions in the distal esophagus has also been reported in Barrett's patients. The prolonged exposure to refluxed material is probably the result of both extreme weakness of the LES resting pressure, which predisposes to frequent episodes of reflux, and from the poor contraction of the distal esophagus, which delays esophageal clearance of the refluxate. Indeed, prolonged esophageal acid exposure and poor esophageal acid clearance have been documented in patients with Barrett's esophagus. When Barrett's patients with and without the complications of stricture, ulceration and carcinoma were compared, those with complications were found to have a higher percent time in which esophageal pH > 7 [1,2]. These patients also had a higher incidence of positive gastric pH scores for alkaline reflux and positive ^{99m}Tc-labeled hepatoiminodiacetic acid scans to test for duodenogastric reflux (DGR). Increased DGR has also been reported in patients with Barrett's. DGR would allow the reflux of bile and pancreatic enzymes into the esophagus. Combined esophageal and gastric pH monitoring has shown that esophageal exposure to pH > 7 was increased in gastroesophageal reflux disease (GERD) patients with duodenogastric reflux (DGR) and that DGR was more frequent in GERD patients with a stricture or Barrett's esophagus. It was also shown that Barrett's patients have more pure alkaline reflux, i.e., gastric pH between 4 and 7 with esophageal pH > 7 than other patients with esophagitis. All of these findings suggest that the development of complications of Barrett's esophagus is the result of the damaging effect of refluxed duodenal juice [3].

References

1. Attwood SEA, DeMeester TR, Bremner CG, Barlow AP, Hinder RA. Alkaline gastroesophageal reflux: implications in the development of complications in Barrett's columnar-lined lower esophagus. Surgery 1989;106:764–770.
2. DeMeester TR, Attwood SEA, Smyrk TC, Therkildsen DH, Hinder RA. Surgical therapy in Barrett's esophagus. Ann Surg 1990;212:528–542.
3. Attwood SEA, Smyrk TC, DeMeester TR, Mirvish SS, Stein HJ, Hinder RA. Duodenoesophageal reflux and the development of esophageal adenocarcinoma in rats. Surgery 1992;111:503–510.

What are the characteristic features of stricture in Barrett's mucosa?

K. Moghissi (Hull)

In his original article on the lower esophagus lined by columnar epithelium, Barrett [1] refers to three types of complications associated with this condition, namely adenocarcinoma, ulcer and stricture. Judging by the number of publications and review articles [2–7], adenocarcinoma has received its fair share of attention. The ulcer was the lesion which initially drew Barrett's [8] attention to the very existence of the columnar epithelial lined esophagus (CLE) and was responsible for stimulating other workers such as Allison [9] and Lortat-Jacob [10] to study independently the CLE.

Compared with adenocarcinoma, the stricture in Barrett's esophagus has received little exposure, possibly because its anatomo-pathological characteristics and its therapeutic significance have not been fully appreciated.

In this article, the task is to elaborate on the characteristics of stricture in CLE (Barrett's stricture) and to provide a definition which encapsulates these characteristics. To do so, I have resorted two sources: 1) historical, based on literature search and publications relevant to Barrett's stricture — prominent amongst these are the original works of Barrett [1,8], Allison [9,11] and Lortat-Jacob [10]; and 2) personal experience and research based on a number of prospective clinico-pathological studies.

Historical sources

Barrett [1] stated that, "stricture demonstrated at or above the aortic arch is almost certainly situated above an esophagus lined with columnar epithelium". Allison did a special study of CLE and later drew attention to the stricture in such an esophagus [11]. He suggested that in consequence of an incompetent cardia and gastroesophageal reflux (GER) followed by esophagitis, there develops a stenotic lesion at the squamo-columnar mucosal junction of CLE. He also clearly differentiated between those strictures which are associated with hiatal hernia, in which the stricture initiates at the squamo-columnar epithelium of the esophagogastric junction, and other strictures which develop at the squamo-columnar mucosal junction of an esophagus lined by columnar epithelium (i.e., Barrett's esophagus), which is some 5 cm above the esophagogastric junction.

Lortat-Jacob [10] in his article on *"endobrachy-oesophage"* gives an account of the clinical and radiological features of strictures. He also reports on anatomo-pathological aspects of the resected specimen of such cases, indicating that stenotic lesion is at the squamo-columnar junction of the esophagus, which in the case of *endobrachy-oesophage* is 5—6 cm above the "cardia".

Since any discussion on Barrett's esophagus and its complications is intricately involved with the description of the lower esophagus and definition of the gastro-esophageal junction, it is relevant to elaborate on the anatomy of the lower esophagus in the region of the esophageal hiatus of the diaphragm, and to expand on the anatomo-pathological changes which occur in this area as a result of GER. The work of Hayward [12—14] is particularly pertinent to this discussion, and accords with our own anatomo-pathological study [7,15—19]; these works indicate that the lower esophagus in the region of the hiatus comprises:
— a thoracic part which is situated above the hiatus, and its mucosa covered with squamous epithelium;
— an abdominal part which is below the hiatus, 2—3 cm in length, with its mucosa lined by junctional columnar epithelium.

In the region of the hiatus, the phreno-esophageal ligament (PEL) is attached to the esophagus and represents a recognizable landmark between the thoracic and abdominal portion of the esophagus. It also indicates an approximate site of the squamo-columnar mucosal junction of the esophagus. Hayward [12—14] rightly suggests that the anatomical gastroesophageal junction is where the esophageal tube (abdominal esophagus) ends and the gastric "bag" begins. Here the peritoneum drapes the stomach and, at the esophagogastric junction, reflects to become the parietal peritoneum. Hayward [12—14] refers to the "surgical" junction where the PEL is attached to the esophagus. It therefore follows that: 1) the PEL and peritoneal reflexion are at or around the esophageal hiatus of the diaphragm (Fig. 1) and that in sliding hiatal hernia both structures ascend upwards into the chest; 2) in the cases of long-standing hernia with associated GER, there develops a pan esophagitis with pathological changes affecting all coats of the esophagus. In the lumen this leads to stricture formation and in the esophageal walls to periesophagitis and periesophageal fibrosis. In severe cases the mediastinal pleura and longitudinal esophageal muscles

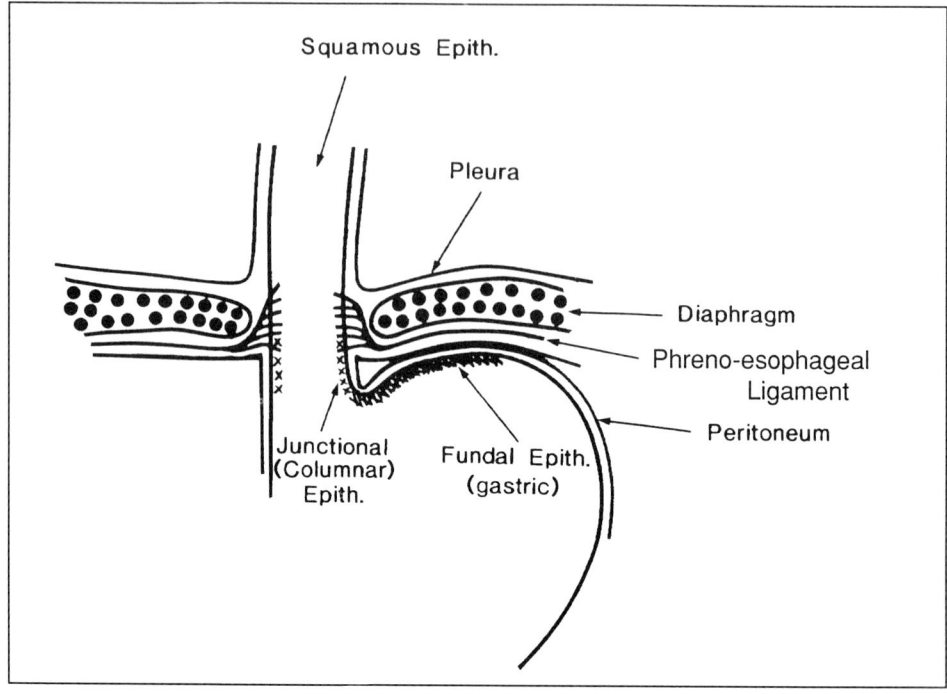

Fig. 1. Anatomy of the lower esophagus in the region of the hiatus.

become incorporated in the fibrous scarring and shortening ensues. In this situation the anatomical esophagogastric junction becomes fixed well above the hiatus and the herniated pouch of the stomach may become tubular in configuration and be dragged upwards (Fig. 2). The degree of shortening can be assessed by the distance between the site of attachment of the phreno-esophageal ligament to the esophagus and the esophageal hiatus of the diaphragm (alternatively, shortening may be assessed by the distance between the lower esophageal sphincter, determined by manometry, and the hiatus). It also follows that, even when the stomach becomes tubular in shape and indistinguishable from the esophagus, the PEL will still mark the boundary of the esophagus and stomach because the tubular structure above (proximal) is the thoracic esophagus, but the structure below is the stomach, and the abdominal esophagus, in these cases, is short and is not its usual 2–3 cm in length.

It should now be clear that in a reflux stricture associated with hiatal hernia, the stenosis is at the squamo-columnar junction of the thoracic-abdominal portion of the esophagus, which in the case of shortening is practically situated between the esophagus and the stomach and, externally, at the approximate level of the insertion of the PEL to the esophagus. In these cases the PEL itself is at some distance upwards from the hiatus in the thorax, depending on the degree of shortening.

In a Barrett's stricture, the stenotic lesion, though usually at the squamo-columnar epithelial junction, is not level with the insertion of the PEL to the esophagus. The ligament is in fact at its usual anatomical site at or near the esophageal hiatus

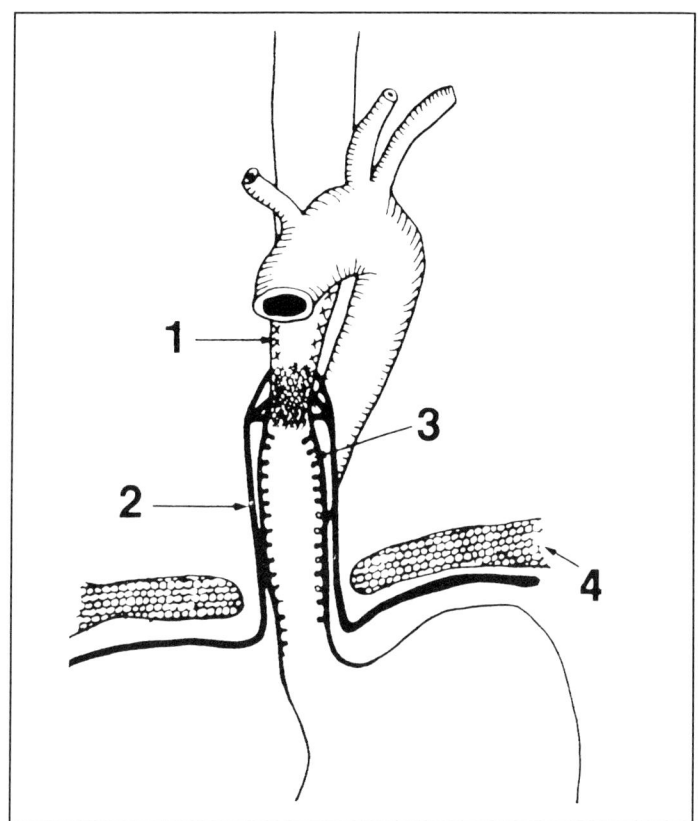

Fig. 2. Anatomy of the esophagogastric junction and phreno-esophageal ligament in high stricture associated with hiatal hernia and acquired short esophagus; 1) squamous epithelium (above the stricture); 2) phreno-esophageal ligament, note its attachment drawn upwards; 3) tubular herniated stomach lined by columnar gastric mucosa; 4) diaphragm.

(Fig. 3). The corollary of this is that in Barrett's stricture the stenosis is, in fact, in the tubular esophagus high above the anatomical gastroesophageal junction, which is not displaced upwards since there is no acquired shortening but "luminal shortening" (*endobrachy-oesophage* of Lortat-Jacob).

Personal experience and research

In the course of a 20-year period (1970–1990) we have undertaken a number of prospective studies covering some 500 patients with esophageal strictures undergoing transthoracic operations, often involving thoraco-phrenotomy [9,15,18]. The protocol of these studies comprised: 1) preoperative, clinical, radiological and endoscopic investigations with biopsy examination above, at and after dilatation below the stricture; 2) intraoperative observations which included:

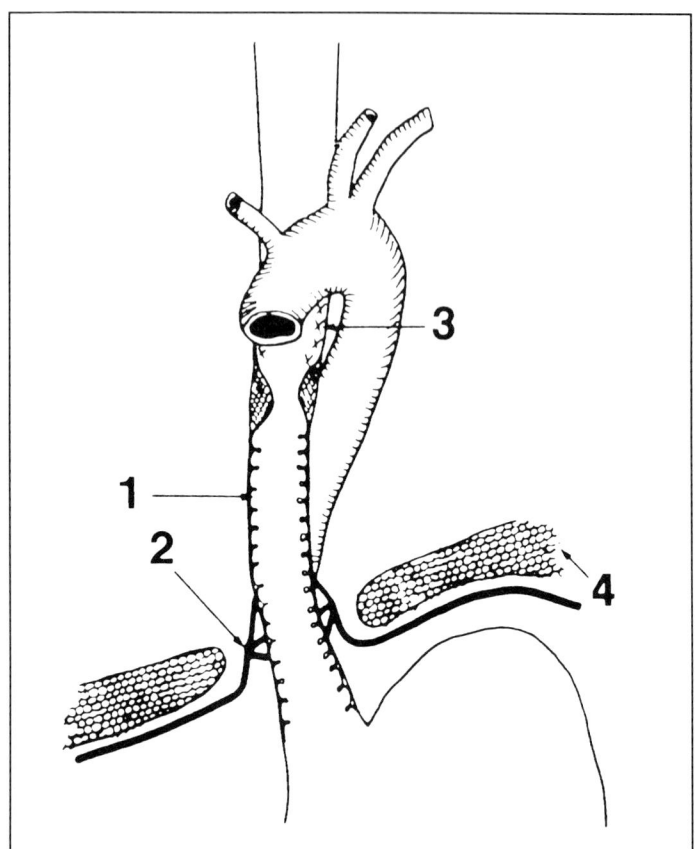

Fig. 3. Anatomy of the lower esophagus in Barrett's stricture; 1) columnar epithelial lined esophagus below the stricture; 2) phreno-esophageal ligament; 3) squamous epithelium above the stricture; 4) diaphragm.

- surgical anatomy and the pathological features of the esophagus and the esophageal hiatus of the diaphragm;
- recording of hernia and shortening of the esophagus;
- the PEL, the site of its attachment to the esophagus, its relationship to the esophageal hiatus of the diaphragm and the esophageal stricture;
- postoperative and histopathological examination of the resected specimen (if resection had been undertaken), with particular reference to the anatomical relationship between the stricture and the PEL and the histology of the mucosal covering.

Data from these investigations have allowed for a complete clinico-pathological diagnosis of cases. Most specifically, it enabled us to distinguish all strictures which developed in CLE and focus attention on the particular features of these cases. Based on these studies and a review of the relevant literature, it is possible to stipulate the following characteristics of strictures in CLE.

Stricture

The stricture is situated high in the esophagus at or near the level of the arch of the aorta (as Barrett suggested) (Figs. 3 and 4A). It is usually mild in consistency and yielding to bouginage.

Mucosa

Mucosa above the stricture is usually squamous and often a mix of columnar and squamous. Below the stricture, the mucosa is always columnar for a length of at least 5 cm of the thoracic esophagus (Fig. 4B–D). Relationship: beside being situated high in the esophagus, the stricture is at least 3 cm above the insertion of PEL to the esophagus and 5 cm above the anatomical gastroesophageal junction and the esophageal hiatus of the diaphragm.

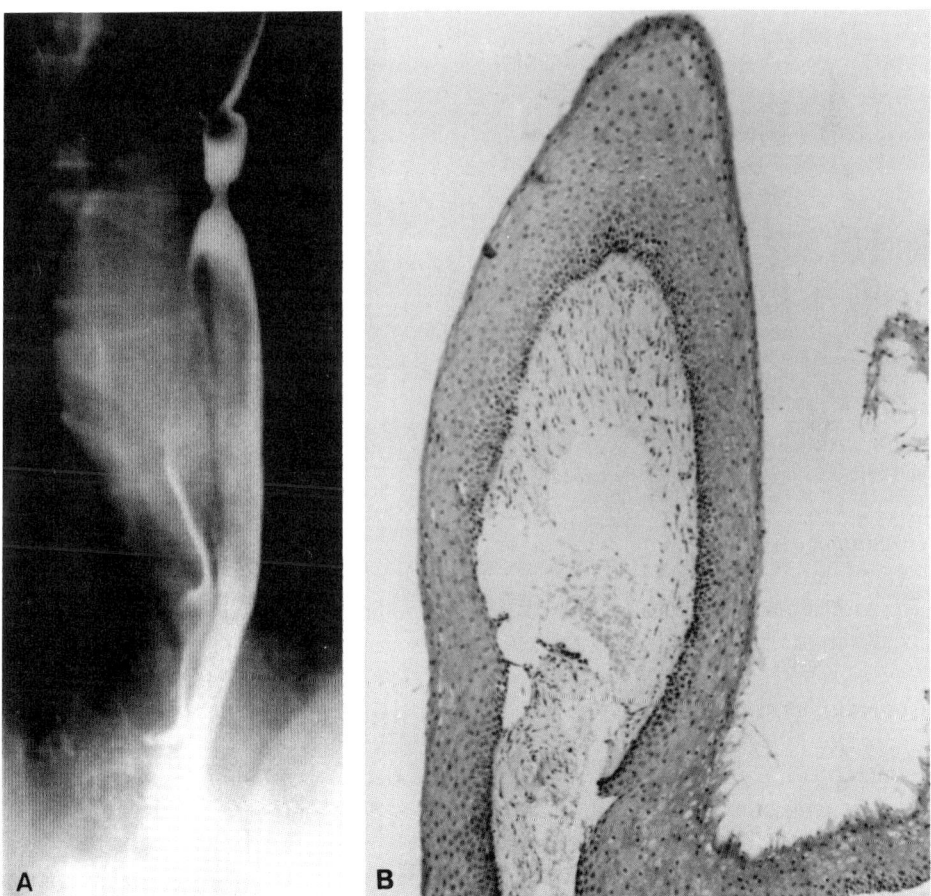

Fig. 4. A) Barium contrast of the esophagus in a typical Barrett's stricture. B) Photo micrograph of an esophageal biopsy above the stricture showing squamous epithelial mucosa.

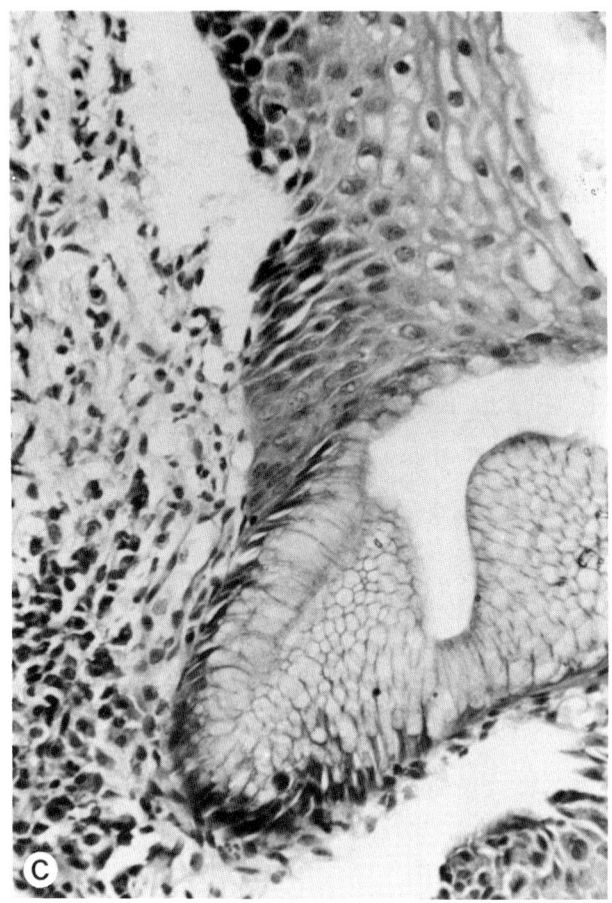

Fig. 4C. Photo micrograph of an esophageal biopsy at the level of the stricture showing mixed squamous and columnar epithelium and inflammatory changes.

Esophageal wall

The esophageal wall is usually unaffected by pathological processes or only affected locally in the area of the stricture with some scarring. PEL is not displaced upward.

Clinical features

Symptomatology in patients with Barrett's stricture is not different from that in patients with other types of esophageal stricture. Predominant amongst symptoms is dysphagia; commonly, patients do suffer from heartburn and dyspepsia prior to development of dysphagia. Unlike cases of reflux stricture associated with hiatal hernia, there is a male sex predominance (in our patients male to female ratio was 3.5:1, whereas in other reflux stricture cases the ratio was 0.6:1). The patients with Barrett's stricture are generally young; a number of them are children and young adults.

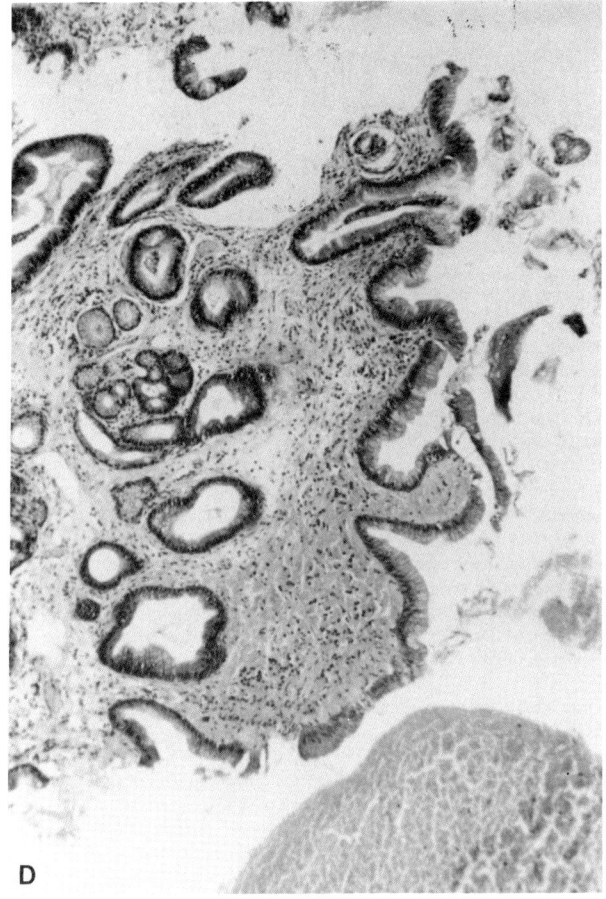

Fig. 4D. Photo micrograph of the oesophageal biopsy below the stricture showing columnar epithelium in Barrett's oesophagus.

Incidence

Barrett's stricture is uncommon when one considers its incidence in esophageal strictures as a whole. In a series of 424 reflux strictures of the esophagus with/without sliding hiatal hernia, 18 (4.2%) we found Barrett's strictures. However, stricture is the most common of the complications of CLE. In our series out of 44 cases of CLE with complications, 18 (nearly 41%) had stricture which is similar to other large series [20,21]. The following definition incorporates the above characteristics of Barrett's stricture: Barrett's stricture is referred to as a stenotic lesion at the squamocolumnar epithelial junction of an esophagus whose lower 5 cm above the gastroesophageal junction (3 cm above the phreno-esophageal ligament) are covered by columnar cell mucosa.

Acknowledgements

I wish to acknowledge with thanks the help and advice given to me by Dr Philip Bury, Consultant Pathologist at Castle Hill Hospital, Cottingham.

References

1. Barrett NR. The lower oesophagus lined by columnar epithelium. Surgery 1957;41:881–894.
2. Naef AP, Ozzello L. Columnar-lined lower oesophagus an acquired lesion with malignant predisposition. J Thorac Cardiovasc Surg 1957;70(5);826–835.
3. Sjogren RW Jr, Johnson LF. Barrett's oesophagus, a review. Am J Med 1983;74:313–321.
4. Skinner DB, Walther BC, Riddell RH, Schmidt H, Iascone C, DeMeester TR. Barrett's oesophagus comparison of benign and malignant cases. Ann Surg 1983;198:544–566.
5. Ribet M, Mensier E, Pruvot FR. Barrett's oesophagus and adenocarcinoma. Eur J Cardiothorac Surg 1987;1:29–32.
6. Streitz JM, Ellis FH, Gibb SP, Balogh K, Watkins E. Adenocarcinoma in Barrett's oesophagus, a clinicopathological study of 65 cases. Ann Surg 1991;213:122–125.
7. Moghissi K, Sharpe DAC, Pender D. Adenocarcinoma and Barrett's oesophagus. Eur J Cardiothorac Surg 1993;7:126–132.
8. Barrett NR. Chronic peptic ulcer of the oesophagus and oesophagitis. Br J Surg 1950;38:175–182.
9. Allison PR, Johnstone AS. The oesophagus lined with gastric mucous membrane. Thorax 1953;8:87–101.
10. Lortat-Jacob JL. Endobrachy oesophage. Ann Chir 1957;11:1247–1254.
11. Allison PR. Peptic oesophagitis and oesophageal stricture. Lancet 1970;11:199–201.
12. Hayward J. The lower end of the oesophagus. Thorax 1961;16:36–41.
13. Hayward J. The phreno-esophageal ligament in hiatal hernia repair. Thorax 1961;16:41–45.
14. Hayward J. The treatment of fibrous stricture of the oesophagus associated with hiatal hernia. Thorax 1961;16:45–55.
15. Moghissi K. Conservative surgery in reflux stricture of the oesophagus associated with hiatal hernia. Br J Surg 1979;66:221–225.
16. Moghissi K. Stenoses hautes de l'oesophage thoracique et leur traitement chirurgical. Chirurgie 1980;106:711–718.
17. Moghissi K, Goebells P. Relevance of anatomopathology of high oesophageal strictures to the design of surgical treatment. Eur J Cardiothorac Surg 1990;4:91–96.
18. Moghissi K. Intra-thoracic fundoplication for reflux stricture associated with short oesophagus. Thorax 1983;38:36–40.
19. Moghissi K, Pender D. Management of proximal oesophageal strictures. Eur J Cardiothorac Surg 1989;3:93–98.
20. Starnes VA, Adkins RB, Ballinger JF, Shayers JL. Barrett's oesophagus: a surgical entity. Arch Surg 1984;119(5):503–567.
21. Bremner CG. In: DeMeester TR, Matthews HR (eds) International Trends in General Thoracic Surgery — Benign Oesophageal Disease. St. Louis, Washington DC, Toronto: The CV Mosby Company, 1987;234.

What is termed a Savary's ulcer?
How does the evolution of a typical Barrett's ulcer differ from that of a Savary's ulcer?

E. Brossard, J.B. Ollyo, C. Fontolliet, M. Savary, Ph. Monnier (Lausanne)

In subjects with Barrett's esophagus, esophageal ulcers are situated either within the metaplastic columnar mucosa in the lower part of the esophagus (Barrett's ulcer), or

912

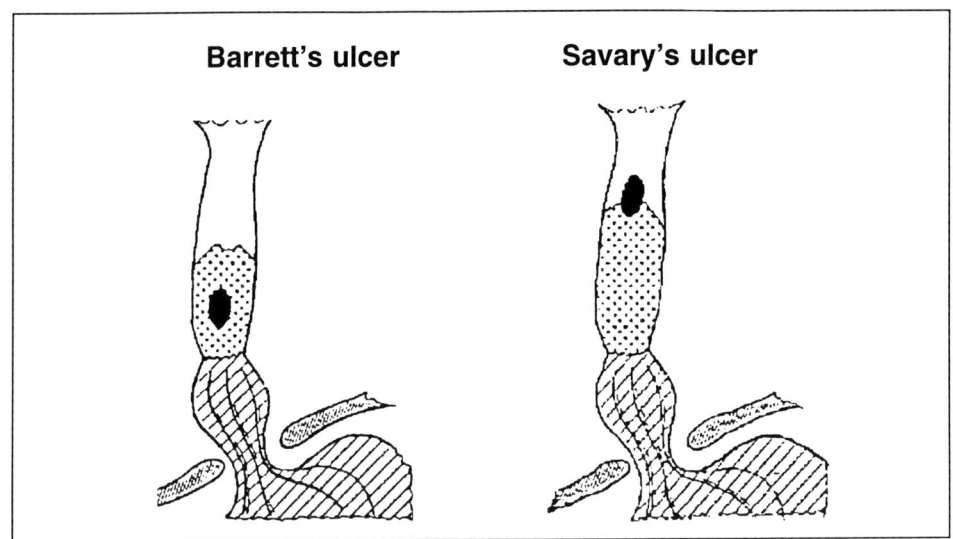

Fig. 1. Barrett's and Savary's ulcers.

higher up in the malpighian region (Savary's ulcer) [1,2] (Fig. 1). Some authors have suggested that Barrett's ulcer is caused by a local secretion of acid by the heterotopic columnar epithelium in the lower part of the esophagus [3]. This etiopathogenesis of Barrett's ulcer is now strongly contested. In 1966, Savary described a junctional peptic ulcer localized on the squamous cell lining, at the upper pole of Barrett's mucosa. This ulcer, known as Savary's ulcer by his students, is thought to be caused by pathological gastroesophageal reflux (GER). Endoscopically, it is characterized by an oval shaped loss of substance, orientated longitudinally, with sharp edges and a crater, whose depth depends on the age of the lesion. This definition excludes superficial ulceration or erosion and all lesions involving diffuse loss of substance over the whole circumference of the esophagus.

Patients and Method

In order to define the differences between Barrett's ulcer and Savary's ulcer, we examined the endoscopic case records of the Centre Hospitalier Universitaire Vaudois in Lausanne over a period of 27 years (from 1963 to 1990). During this period, 44,203 esophagoscopies were carried out. Barrett's esophagus was found in 448 cases. Barrett's ulcer was diagnosed in 50 cases, and Savary's ulcer in 37 cases. Savary's ulcer and Barrett's ulcer were both present in five cases. The prevalence of ulcers in patients with Barrett's esophagus was 20.5%. No significant difference was observed between patients with Savary's ulcer and those with Barrett's ulcer with regard to mean age. In contrast, there was a clear predominance of males among the patients with Barrett's ulcer, and a predominance of females among those with Savary's ulcer (Table 1).

913

Table 1.

	Barrett's ulcer (n = 50)	Savary's ulcer (n = 37)
Age (years)		
— mean	67	63.7
— range	3—85	33—85
Sex		
— Male	72%	43%
— Female	38%	57%

Results

Three quarters of the patients with Savary's or Barrett's ulcer had characteristic and chronic ($\geq$ 5 years) symptoms of GER. Evident gastrointestinal bleeding or anemia of spoliative type was observed in 40% of patients with Savary's ulcer and 72% of patients with Barrett's ulcer. Among the endoscopic characteristics of these two types of ulcer associated with Barrett's esophagus, there was no significant difference with regard to size, and length of Barrett's esophagus and the frequency of concomitant erosive esophagitis. Savary's ulcer differed from Barrett's ulcer by the fact that it was frequently associated with peptic stenosis (Table 2). Biopsies of the rims of Barrett's ulcer revealed a squamous epithelium in 20% of cases. Two patients developed a Barrett's ulcer at a site where 17 and 105 months earlier there had been a large islet of epidermoid mucosa. In 14 cases, repeated endoscopic examinations made it possible to follow the progress of erosive and ulcerative esophagitis of the squamous mucosa into an ulcer surrounded by a columnar mucosa (Barrett's ulcer). These observations argue in favor of a peptic origin of Barrett's ulcer through pathological GER. The vast majority of these ulcers associated with Barrett's esophagus were medically treated, mainly because of the advanced age of the patients. Among the patients who were followed up, the majority of ulcers were healed through medical treatment. There was, however, a significant recurrence rate of ulcers or esophagitis in patients with Savary's ulcer (Table 3). Ninety percent of the 18 patients who underwent antireflux surgery and long-term follow-up were healed. Surgery is consequently the treatment of choice for Savary's and Barrett's ulcers.

Table 2. Endoscopic characteristics

	Barrett's ulcer (n = 50)	Savary's ulcer (n = 37)
Size (cm)	0.5- 5	0.5—2
Length of Barrett's esophagus (cm)		
— mean	7	4.5
— range	3—13	3—10
Erosive esophagitis	34 (68%)	27 (73%)
Peptic stenosis	16 (32%)	25 (67%)

914

Table 3. Medical treatment

	Barrett's ulcer (32/50)	Savary's ulcer (23/37)
Patients followed up	18	15
Follow-up (months)		
— mean	37	52
— range	6–69	6–107
Healed	15 (83%)	14 (93%)
Recurrence of ulcer or esophagitis	5 (28%)	7 (46%)

Discussion

In our opinion, Barrett's ulcer and Savary's ulcer are a complication of GER [4]. In practice, the patient's history almost always reveals typical symptoms of GER. The fact that an acid-secreting mucosa is rarely found in biopsy material collected from areas close to the Barrett's ulcer and that these ulcers commonly heal after antireflux surgery, also argues in favor of a peptic origin of ulcers associated with Barrett's esophagus [5].

In addition, endoscopy has shown that Savary's ulcer, like Barrett's ulcer, is usually associated with other classical lesions of GER (junctional peptic stenosis and/or erosion) [6].

Conclusion

Gastroesophageal reflux can cause two types of ulcers in patients with Barrett's esophagus. Savary's ulcer differs from Barrett's ulcer in its location at the squamo-columnar junction, and by the fact that it is associated with peptic stenosis in 60% of cases. It predominates in elderly women and rarely bleeds. Savary's ulcer frequently recurs after medical treatment, and the treatment of choice is antireflux surgery.

References

1. Ollyo JB, Monnier Ph, Fontolliet Ch, Birchler R, Fasel J, Lévi F, Gonvers JJ. L'ulcère de Savary: une nouvelle complication du reflux gastro-oesophagien. Schweiz Med Wochenschr 1988;118(21):823–827.
2. Barrett NR. Chronic peptic ulcer of the oesophagus and oesophagitis. Br J Surg 1950;38:175–182.
3. Ustach TJ, Tobon F, Schuster MM. Demonstration of acid secretion from oesophageal mucosa in Barrett's ulcer. Gatrointest Endosc 1988;16:98–100.
4. Ollyo JB, Fontolliet Ch, Monnier Ph, Bauerfeind P, Ciluffo T, Gonvers JJ, Savary M. Hétérogénéité pathogénique des ulcères de Barrett. Schweiz Med Wochenschr 1989;119(21):747–751.
5. Ollyo JB, Fontolliet Ch, Wellinger J, Brossard E, Lévi F, Monnier Ph. Peptic ulcers of the esophagus are not a complication of Barrett's epithelium. Acta Endoscopica 1991;21:681–692.
6. Adler RM. The lower esophagus lined columnar epithelium. J Thorac Cardiovasc Surg 1963;45:13–34.

Is *Helicobacter pylori* involved in the pathogenesis of the Barrett type ulcer?

E. Brossard (Lausanne)

Columnar metaplasia of the esophagus is only considered to be pathological if it spreads beyond the upper pole of the lower esophageal sphincter. There are several morphological forms: patch, tongue, or sheath (in which case the condition is known as Barrett's esophagus) [1].

The histology of this disorder is the subject of debate. In 1976, Paull et al. [2] described three types of columnar epithelium: an epithelium of fundic type, an epithelium of cardiac type and an epithelium of specialized type, arranged in layers with the specialized epithelium always situated most proximally. Thompson et al. [3] described a metaplastic epithelium consisting of an intimate mixture of various glands and cells forming a mucosa having an uneven surface and exhibiting a variable degree of atrophy, arranged as a mosaic over the whole area of Barrett's esophagus. However, only the mucosa of specialized type is a precursor for adenocarcinoma.

Two types of ulcer are associated with Barrett's esophagus: Barrett's ulcer situated in the metaplastic columnar mucosa, and Savary's ulcer situated at the squamo-columnar junction. If Savary's ulcer, which is almost always associated with erosive peptic lesions or peptic stenosis, is unquestionably caused by gastroesophageal reflux (GER), the pathogenesis of Barrett's ulcer is still the subject of debate [4–6]. Some authors believe that Barrett's ulcer is a direct complication of Barrett's esophagus, resulting from local acid secretion, or an indirect complication, arising from colonization of the mucosa by *Helicobacter pylori*, or that it develops in a specialized columnar mucosa that is less resistant to reflux. However, others believe that Barrett's ulcer, like Savary's ulcer, is a complication of GER disease. It may develop in a patch of squamous cell mucosa that is progressively circumscribed by the process of columnar cicatrization. It may also develop directly in a columnar mucosa that has been rendered more fragile than normal by *H. pylori* or by the presence of a less resistant specialized epithelium, or it may result from alkaline reflux which is more toxic than acid reflux.

H. pylori, discovered in 1982 by Marshall and Warren [7], is a helical Gram-negative bacillus found in mucosae of gastric type. It is recognized as the agent responsible for type B gastritis and seems to play a role in the pathogenesis of stomach cancer [8,9]. Its role in the pathogenesis of peptic esophageal disorders is more debatable however [10–16].

Materials and Method

To examine the role of *H. pylori* in the pathogenesis of "peptic" ulceration of the esophagus, we compared biopsy specimens obtained from 30 patients with Barrett's ulcer with those obtained from 25 subjects with Savary's ulcer. The group of patients with Barrett's ulcer consisted of 23 men and seven women between 33 and 85 years of age (mean age = 65 years). The group with Savary's ulcer consisted of eight men, 15 women and two children between 3 and 85 years of age (mean age = 59 years). A rigid tube endoscopic examination of the esophagus was carried out on all these patients. One or several biopsy specimens (1—31) were collected from the region of Barrett's esophagus. These specimens were fixed with buffered formol, embedded in paraffin, cut into 5μ sections and stained with hematoxylin-eosin by the usual techniques. *H. pylori* was tested for by staining the histological sections with acridine orange and examining them at a magnification of 400× under a fluorescence micro-scope. As this was a retrospective study, no esophageal cultures were made. The type of mucosa present in Barrett's esophagus was determined. None of these patients underwent gastric biopsy.

Our results are given in Table 1. *H. pylori*, which was only present in mucosa of columnar type, was found in 16% of patients with Barrett's ulcer and 24% of patients with Savary's ulcer. There was no significant difference between these two groups. Six of the 30 patients with Barrett's ulcer and four of the 25 with Savary's ulcer had an acid-secreting mucosa around the ulcer. Sixty per cent of the patients with Barrett's ulcer had a mucosa of specialized type, that is less resistant to reflux. This type of mucosa was found in 36% of the patients with Savary's ulcer. In eight of the 30 patients with Barrett's ulcer the mucosa lining the rim of the ulcers was unaltered.

Discussion

The reported prevalence of esophageal *H. pylori*, which in the majority of cases is found to be localized in the columnar mucosa, varies considerably (Table 2). Our own results indicate a low prevalence of 16 to 24%, the bacteria always being found in the columnar mucosa. Some authors believe that the presence of these bacteria in the esophagus results from contamination by the gastric contents during endoscopy [17]. This cannot be the case in our study as no gastric specimens were collected. Others have demonstrated a relationship, which they attribute to GER, between *Helicobacter* induced antral gastritis and the presence of *H. pylori* in the esophagus [18,19]. The presence of a hiatus hernia, a factor that predisposes to GER, does not,

Table 1. Presence of *H. pylori*

	Barrett's ulcer (n = 30)	Savary's ulcer (n = 25)
Men/women/children	23/7/0	8/15/2
Age range (mean age)	33—85 years (65)	3—85 years (59)
Number of biopsies (range)	7 (1—31)	4 (1—10)
Mucosa of cardiac type	25 (85%)	23 (92%)
Mucosa of fundic type	6 (20%)	4 (16%)
Mucosa of specialized type	18 (60%)	9 (36%)
Presence of *H. pylori*	5 (16%)	6 (24%)

Table 2. Prevalence of H. pylori

Author	No. of patients examined	No. of patients with *Helicobacter*	%
Paull and Yardley [22]	26	4	15.3
Karogelopolous et al. [14]	64	12	19
Talley et al. [15]	23	12	52
Houck et al. [21]	38	0	0
Walker et al. [16]	7	2	29
Hazell et al. [20]	20	3	15
Ferreres et al. [11]	70	31	44.3
Agnholt et al. [10]	11	1	9
Author's personal study	55	11	20

however, appear to be an extra risk factor. In our study there was no difference between the group of patients with Savary's ulcer, unquestionably related to reflux, and the group with Barrett's ulcer, whose etiopathogenesis is less clear. No antral biopsy specimens are available for these patients.

In this study *H. pylori* was identified by histology alone. Although this is a sensitive method when carried out by an experienced specialist, it is not infallible [12,13]. Gastric colonization by *H. pylori* has been described as focal and inconsistent. It is thus reasonable to believe that the same will be true for the esophagus, which would also account for the diversity of published results.

H. pylori has rarely been found in the stomach in a metaplastic mucosa [11]. In our patients, *H. pylori* was found in all types of columnar mucosa. It was not more prevalent, however, in Savary's ulcers which exhibited a specialized mucosa in 36% of cases, than in Barrett's ulcer where a specialized mucosa was found in 60% of cases.

Conclusion

We do not believe that *H. pylori* plays a major part in the natural history of Barrett's esophagus. Our study demonstrated that the colonization of Barrett's esophagus by *H. pylori* is exceptional, and equivalent in patients with Barrett's or Savary's ulcer. Consequently it may be said that this infective agent does not appear to be involved in the pathogenesis of ulceration associated with Barrett's esophagus, whether or not secondary to GER.

References

1. Monnier P, Fontolliet C, Savary M, Ollyo JB. Barrett's oesophagus or columnar epithelium of the lower oesophagus. Clin Gastroenterol 1987;1:769–789.
2. Paull A. Trier JS, Dalton MD, Camp RC, Loeb P, Goyal RK. The histologic spectrum of Barrett's esophagus. N Engl J Med 1976;295:476–480.
3. Thompson JJ, Zinsser KR, Enterline HT. Barrett's metaplasia and adenocarcinoma of the esophagus and gastroesophageal junction. Hum Pathol 1983;14:42–61.

4. Ollyo JB, Monnier P, Fontolliet C, Wellinger J, Levi F, Gonvers JJ. Les ulcères "peptiques" de l'oesophage: ulcère de Wolf, ulcère de Barrett, ulcère de Savary. A Propos de 208 observations. Med Hyg 1988;46:2571−2577.
5. Ollyo JB, Monnier P, Fontolliet C, Birchler R, Fasel J, Levi F, Gonvers JJ. L'ulcère de Savary: une nouvelle complication du reflux gastro-oesophagien? Schweiz Med Wschr 1988;118:823−827.
6. Ollyo JB, Fontolliet C, Wellinger J, Brossard E, Levi F, Monnier P. Les ulcères "peptiques" de l'oesophage ne sont pas une complication de l'épithélium de Barrett. Acta Endoscopica 1991;21:681−692.
7. Warren JR. Unidentified curved bacilli on active chronic gastritis. Lancet 1983;2:1273−1275.
8. Marshall BJ, Warren JR. Unidentified curved bacilli in the stomach of patients with gastritis and peptic ulceration. Lancet 1984;1:1311−1314.
9. Watt JI, Dyxon MF. *Campyobacter*-associated chronic gastritis. Pathol Ann 1990;25(pt1):75−98.
10. Agnholt J, Fallingborg J, Muller-Petersen J, Lomborg S, Christensen L, Sondergaard G, Teglbjaerg PS, Rasmussen SN. The occurrence of *Helicobacter pylori* in the oesophagus. Eur J Gastroenterol Hepatol 1991;3:685−689.
11. Ferreres JC, Fernandez F, Vives AR, Gonzalez-Rodilla I, Ursua I, Ramos R, Val-Bernal JF. *Helicobacter pylori* in Barrett's esophagus. Histol Histopath 1991;6:403−408.
12. Goodwin CS, Blincow ED, Warren JR, Waters TE, Sanderson CR, Easton L. Evaluation of cultural techniques for isolating *Campylobacter pyloridis* from endoscopic biopsies of gastric mucosa. J Clin Pathol 1985;38:1127−1131.
13. Hazell SL, Hennessy WB, Borody TJ, Carrich J, Ralston M, Brady L, Lee A. *Campylobacter pyloridis* gastritis II; distribution of bacteria and associated inflammation in the gastroduodenal environment. Am J Gastroenterol 1987;82: 297−301.
14. Kalogeropoulos NK, Whitehead R. *Campylobacter*-like organisms and *Candida* in peptic ulcers and similar lesions of the upper gastrointestinal tract: a study of 247 cases. J Clin Pathol 1988;41:1093−1098.
15. Talley NJ, Cameron AJ, Shorter RJ, Zinsmeister AR, Phillps SF. *Campylobacter pylori* and Barrett's esophagus. Mayo Clin Proc 1988;63:1176−1180.
16. Walker SJ, Birch PJ, Stewart M, Stoddart CJ, Hart CA, Day DW. Patterns of colonisation of *Campylobacter pylori* in the esophagus, stomach and duodenum. Gut 1989;30:1334−1338.
17. Gruppo operativo per lo studio delle precancerosi esofagee (GOSPE). *Helicobacter pylori* in Barrett's oesophagus. Histopatholology 1991;18:568−570.
18. Cooper BT, Gearty JC. *Helicobacter pylori* in Barrett's oesophagus. Gullet 1991;1:173−176.
19. Loffeld RJ, Ten Tije BJ, Arends JW. Prevalence and significance of *Helicobacter pylori* in patients with Barrett's esophagus. Am J Gastroenterol 1992;87:1598−1600.
20. Hazell SL, Carrich J, Lee A. *Campylobacter pylori* can infect the oesophagus when gastric tissue is present. Gastroenterology 1988;94:178 (abstract).
21. Houck JA, Lucas JG. Absence of *Campylobacter*-like organisms in Barrett's esophagus. Arch Pathol Lab Med 1989;113: 470−472.
22. Paull G, Yardley JH. Gastric and esophageal *Campylobacter pylori* in patients with Barrett's esophagus. Gastroenterology 1988;95:216−218.

Treatments

What are the effects of PPIs on the extent of CLE?

M.A. Bigard (Nancy)

The very fact of trying to answer this question first forces one to examine the reasons which are likely to urge the therapist to try to obtain a regression of the metaplastic columnar epithelium. His main hope is probably to erase or minimize the precancerous nature of this acquired abnormality. However, such hope may turn out to prove of no avail because of certain elements in the natural history of Barrett's esophagus (BE).

In Cameron's and Lomboy's study [1], amongst 51,311 patients who had had an esogastric endoscopy, 377 had a BE of more than 3 cm in length. This study showed that the average age for the diagnosis of a BE without a neoplasm was 63 years, whereas the average age of the adenocarcinoma diagnosis which developed on BE was 64 years. The study of the prevalence in the different age groups suggested that BE appeared at about the age of 40, that is to say more than 20 years its diagnosis or before the development of an adenocarcinoma. Besides, it is likely that BE does not gradually ascend from the cardia but rather that the metaplastic columnar mucosa may replace the squamous mucosa very quickly after the latter has sloughed and been expelled as a cast. These data point out that at the moment of the diagnosis, the evolution of the disease has already been very long and that it is perhaps more important to detect a dysplasia, or to have cellular or biochemical markers which could be predictive of degeneration to develop. This would enable one to detect the high risk patients and to treat them surgically in time. Moreover, the regeneration of the squamous epithelium may be falsely reassuring because it may cover up persistent columnar islets whose evolution remains unknown [2].

The efficiency of the treatment with H_2-receptor antagonists or antacids on the regression of BE was not demonstrated [3]. The efficiency of surgical treatment on this BE regression has been a controversial matter. The studies with positive results relied on serial blind biopsies performed with a hydraulic probe, once one knew there was a lengthening of the esophagus after repositioning the cardia [4]. The study by Perniceni et al. had, however, showed the possibility of regression of BE in one case out of 21 patients treated with total duodenal diversion [5]. Such a regression appears to be uncommon in the different studies, beginning late after the operation (24 months later in the case by Perniceni et al.) and the first stages of the regression being characterized by the reappearance of squamous islands within BE itself.

Gastroesophageal reflux (GER) is widely admitted as playing a role in BE, and it has been demonstrated that acid reflux was more important and came up higher in reflux with BE than without BE [6].

The proton pump inhibitors (PPI) represent the most powerful therapeutic class as far as healing of peptic esophagitis, symptomatic action and long-term healing are concerned [7]. The PPIs are particularly effective in curing esophagitis possibly linked with BE and in the healing of Barrett's ulcers [7].

Several publications examined omeprazole (the first PPI on the market), and its effect on the length of BE in a small number of cases.

A preliminary remark concerning the analysis of these studies should be made as to the difficulty of the reproductibility of measurements of the exact extension of BE and even the very existence of a BE. The usual way of defining it is a 3 cm high columnar epithelium above the endoscopic location of the muscular cardia, theoretically corresponding to the lower esophageal sphincter (LES). This is how 146 patients were assessed by endoscopies with biopsies and manometries in a therapeutic test on patients suffering from complicated GER [8]. Tests were performed at entry and after their 6-week treatment. The manometric location of the LES differed by 3 cm (37 cm by endoscopy, 40 cm by manometry). The endoscopic location of the most proximal level of columnar epithelium differed from the histologic location by 2 cm (31.4 cm vs. 33.1). Important variations of the endoscopic determination of the sphincter and of the squamocolumnar junction during the two endoscopies were frequent (12 patients out of 88 had a change of the squamocolumnar junction of 4 cm or more). The authors concluded that these significant differences could cause substantial confusion in the measurements of the extension of BE.

What are the results of the studies on the effects of the PPIs on the extension of BE? Deviere et al. [9] described the favorable effect of omeprazole treatment on three patients given 60 mg daily. This is how they observed the total disappearance of the columnar mucosa of 16 cm in height after an 18-month treatment in one case, and the regression of 4 cm in length in two cases after 9- and 3-month treatment respectively. The rapidity and the importance of the regression contrast with the results previously obtained with surgery, including the duodenal diversion used by Perniceni et al. [5], which had, however, achieved total abolition of acid reflux and biliopancreatic reflux.

With Salis et al. [10], five patients received 40 mg of omeprazole daily. After 17.6 months, they observed a partial histologic regression for one patient after a 3-month treatment and for a second patient after a 9-month treatment.

Gore et al. [11] studied 12 patients with BE treated with 40 mg of omeprazole daily for 2 years. During 6 months before treatment, there tended to be a small but insignificant increase in the length of BE (6.4 ± 2.6 vs. 7.5 ± 3.4 cm). Under treatment, there was a statistically significant reduction in the length of BE (6.2 ± 2.7 cm at 6 months, 5.6 ± 2.5 cm at 1 year, 4.5 ± 2.6 cm at 2 years). After 2 years of treatment, there had been a complete regression of BE, as defined initially by an extent of more than 3 cm of columnar mucosa above the muscular cardia, in 3 patients. After 2 years of treatment, 11 patients had macroscopic squamous islets in BE.

Thirty-six patients with at least 3 cm of BE were randomized in a study by Sampliner et al. [12]. With a three to one ratio, they either received 60 mg of lansoprazole or a placebo every day for 12 months. The patients were given endoscopic control every 3 months. Four out of nine patients in the placebo group were dropped from the study because the treatment was inefficient on the reflux symptoms. For the lansoprazole-treated patients, the average length of BE was 6.7 cm at the beginning of the study and 6.6 cm after 12 months. In only one patient were major squamous islets in BE. The authors' conclusion was that the treatment is efficient in relieving the symptoms of GER disease, but that there is no significant change in the length of BE after a 1-year treatment.

In their study, Galmiche et al. [13] included 26 patients with a BE of at least 3 cm, their esophagitis lesions being healed after a 2-month omeprazole treatment and presenting no severe dysplasia. The patients received 20 mg of omeprazole each day and benefited from an endoscopic control every 6 months for 2 years. Three patients were excluded from the study because of a high grade dysplasia developing during the 1st year and two were lost track of. The authors observed a slow but significant reduction in BE length (6.0 ± 2.3 cm at entry, 4.0 ± 2.4 cm after 2 years). Out of eight patients followed up for a 2-year period, three had major squamous islets and two had a BE regression with a columnar mucosa of less than 3 cm.

Francis et al. [14] prospectively studied the effect of omeprazole on the length of BE, utilizing an ink tattoo for a fixed reference point. Twelve patients were given 40 mg of omeprazole a day. The junction of the columnar and squamous mucosa had been marked with an india ink tattoo via sclerotherapy needle. The patients returned after 3 and 9 months of treatment for repeat endoscopic evaluation. Measurements were confirmed by two separate operators and serial biopsies were performed. The authors concluded to no extension in the measured length of BE. Indeed, in the group of 12 patients who were checked after 3 months, the length of BE was altered from 6.75 to 6.23 cm. In the group of seven patients checked at 9 months, the length of BE was altered from 7.28 to 7.0 cm.

The results of these various studies do not tally even if, in all likelihood, in certain cases a prolonged PPI treatment causes a regression on the length of BE and/or the appearance of squamous islets within BE. At the moment, it is impossible to fully predict the evolution of BE and whether or not the response will be complete [15].

The efficiency of PPIs on the reflux symptoms in patients with BE does not mean that one should do without endoscopic checks aimed at detecting the appearance of dysplasia. The treatment that will probably be advocated in the future is the association of the endoscopic destruction of BE with a PPI treatment to prevent the columnar mucosa from reappearing. An experimental study on six dogs showed that this was a feasible therapeutic sequence [16]. Half of the circumference of a BE of stable length was destroyed on a patient who was taking high doses of omeprazole. There was a re-epithelialization with a normal squamous mucosa [17].

Laukka et al. [18] treated 14 patients (11 men, three women, their average age being 61) with a 3 cm BE. The destruction of BE was obtained by dynamic phototherapy and the patients then received 20 mg of omeprazole daily for 6 months. There was an endoscopic check between 4.5 and 10.5 weeks after treatment on four patients. The length of BE had decreased in all patients — decreasing from 7 to 6 cm, 10 to 9 cm, 10 to 5 cm and 9 to 8 cm, respectively. There were squamous islands in the residual BE mucosa. The dysplasia remained unchanged in the residual BE. The authors concluded that, by way of dynamic phototherapy followed by antisecretory treatment, there is a possibility of obtaining a BE regression with reappearance of a normal squamous mucosa.

All of these tests are preliminary work, and one should bear in mind that endoscopic treatment may involve complications when assessing the possible benefits of this "aggressive" attitude.

References

1. Cameron AJ, Lomboy CT. Barrett's esophagus: age, prevalence and extent of columnar epithelium. Gastroenterology 1992;103:1241—1245.
2. Riddell RH. Dysplasia and regression in Barrett's epithelium. In: Spechler SJ, Goyal RK (eds) Barrett's Esophagus: Pathophysiology, Diagnosis and Management. New York: Elsevier, 1985;143—152.
3. Jutel P, Galmiche JP. Endobrachyoesophage. In: Galmiche JP, Colin R (eds) Troubles de la Motricité de l'Oesophage. Reflux Gastro-oesophagien. Paris: Doin, 1987;177—191.
4. Galmiche JP. Endobrachyoesophage: la régression est-elle possible? La surveillance est-elle justifiée? Gastroenterol Clin Biol 1988;12:705—708.
5. Perniceni T, Leymarios J, Molas G et al. L'endobrachyoesophage régresse-t-il après diversion duodénale totale? Gastroenterol Clin Biol 1988;12:709—712.
6. Bruley des Varannes S, Ravenbakht-Charifi M, Cloarec D, Pujol P, Simon J, Galmiche JP. Endobrachyoesophage et reflux gastro-oesophagien acide. Enregistrements pH-métriques étagés et étude manométrique. Gastroenterol Clin Biol 1992;16: 406—412.
7. Bardhan KD. Omeprazole in the treatment of gastroesophageal diseases. In: Scarpignato C (ed) Advances in Drug Therapy of Gastroesophageal Reflux Disease. Front Gastrointest Res. Basel: Karger, 1992:246—306.
8. Kim SL, Waring JP, Spechler SJ, Sampliner RE, Doos WG, Krol WF, Williford WO. Accuracy of esophageal measurements in Barrett's esophagus. Gastroenterology 1993;104:A117 (abstract).
9. Deviere J, Buset M, Dumonceau JM, Rickaert F, Cremer M. Regression of Barrett's epithelium with omeprazole. N Engl J Med 1989;320:1497—1498 (letter).
10. Salis GB, Milano C, Chiocca JC, Luis A, Mazure PA, Alvarez F, Garcia A, Stupnik S. Hell J. Esophagus lined by columnar epithelium. Its treatment with omeprazole. Gastroenterology 1992;5:308 (abstract).
11. Gore S, Healey CJ, Sutton R, Sheperd NA, Wilkinson SP. Regression of columnar lined (Barrett's) oesophagus with continuous omeprazole therapy. Gastroenterology 1992;102:A75 (abstract).
12. Sampliner RE, Mackel C, Jennings D, Greski-Rose P. Effect of 12 months of a proton pump inhibitor (lansoprazole) on Barrett's esophagus. A randomized trial. Gastroenterology 1992;102:A157 (abstract).
13. Galmiche JP, Dumas R, Boyer J, Goldfain D, Bury A, Robaszkiewicz M, Cadiot G, Diebold MD. Effet de l'oméprazole à long terme sur l'extension de l'endobrachyoesophage. Gastroenterol Clin Biol 1993;17:A43 (abstract).

14. Francis J, Schaffer R, Kadakia S, Carrougher J. Effect of omeprazole on Barrett's epithelium at 3 and 9 months of therapy. Gastroenterology 1993;104:A80(abstract).

15. Lundell L. Acid suppression in the long-term treatment of peptic stricture and Barrett's oesophagus. Digestion 1992; 51(suppl 1):49–58.

16. Fink MA, Martin CJ, Ewing HP, Thompson ME, Machet D, Rode J. Reversal of experimental Barrett's esophagus by endoscopic laser ablation and reduction of acid reflux. Gastroenterology 1992;102:A924 (abstract).

17. Sampliner RE, Hixson LJ, Fennerty MB, Garewal HS. Regression of Barrett's oesophagus by laser ablation in an anacid environment. Dig Dis Sci 1993;38:365–368.

18. Laukka MA, Wang KK, Cameron AJ, Alexander GL. The use of photodynamic therapy in the treatment of Barrett's esophagus: preliminary results. Gastrointest Endosc 1993;39:291 (abstract).

May CLE progress even during treatment?

J.B. Ollyo, E. Brossard, Ch. Fontolliet, Ph. Monnier, M. Savary (Lausanne)

Barrett's esophagus has been assumed to be an abnormal mode of healing erosive or ulcerative reflux esophagitis. Presuming that erosive or ulcerative reflux esophagitis can relapse to the same grade, or progress to a more severe grade after an inefficient gastroesophageal reflux treatment [1], it is conceivable that some Barrett's esophagus may progress [2], and therefore Cameron's study [3], which supports the contrary, does not apply to all BE.

Patients and Methods

Between January 1, 1963 and December 31, 1992, 428 Barrett's esophagus without adenocarcinoma were diagnosed at the University Hospital of Lausanne. One hundred and forty-five out of 428 adults (33.8%) with Barrett's esophagus (columnar epithelium extending at least 3 cm up the gastric mucosa) were followed up endoscopically and biopsied 1 year or more after the initial diagnosis. Twenty-five out of 145 adults with Barrett's esophagus were excluded from this retrospective study due to an imprecise pre- and/or posttherapeutic protocol. Each patient underwent at least two endoscopic examinations (mean: 5, range: 2–28). Required for inclusion in this study were Barrett's esophagus progression or regression of at least 2 cm, in order to avoid possible errors of estimation between different endoscopists. Regression in the form of squamous epithelium islands amongst Barrett's esophagus and progression in form of isolated columnar epithelium tongues located above Barrett's esophagus were excluded.

Table 1. Natural history of Barrett's esophagus (BE) (Lausanne 1963–1992)

	Regression (7.5%)	Stabilization (68.3%)	Progression (24.2%)
Patients (M/F)	9 (6/3)	82 (56/26)	29 (18/11)
Mean age (range); (years)	53.8 (40–71)	62.2 (20–85)	64.5 (45–87)
Endoscopic follow-up mean (range); (months)	64 (12–156)	61 (12–294)	59 (12–132)
Initial length BE mean (range); (cm)	5.9 (3.5–11)	5.7 (3–15)	5.6 (3–15)
Final length BE mean (range); (cm)	2.1 (0–8)	5.7 (3–15)	9.2 (5–20)

Results

Among 120 Barrett's esophagus, a progression in 29 cases was observed (24.2%) (Table 1). The average Barrett's esophagus length at initial endoscopy was 5.6 cm. The average Barrett's esophagus length observed during the last endoscopy performed between 12 and 132 months (mean: 59) after the initial diagnosis was 9.2 cm. The minimal Barrett's esophagus length was 2 cm and the maximal was 6 cm (mean: 3.6 cm). The only factor which appeared to us to enhance the progression of BE seems to be the patient's age at the moment of the diagnosis (64.5 years of age for progressing and 53.8 years of age for regressing Barrett's esophagus). In our study the consumption of alcohol, tobacco, NSAI, acetylsalicylic acid, the duration of gastroesophageal reflux symptomatology as well as the severity of reflux esophagitis at the moment of the diagnosis do not seem to be implicated in the progression or regression of Barrett's esophagus. Eight out of the 29 patients underwent an ineffective antireflux operation; 21 received medical treatment discontinuously (omeprazole n = 5, H_2-receptor antagonists n = 10, antacids or sucralfate n = 6).

Discussion

Our study proves that a significant percentage of Barrett's esophagus (24.2%) may progress if pathological gastroesophageal reflux is not completely eliminated by the only current effective treatment, namely a successful antireflux operation. Among all influencing factors studied, age at the moment of diagnosis seems to be the most significant.

In our series, we found, like Cameron [3], no evidence of Barrett's esophagus progression in a majority of cases (68.3%) were found. In the remaining cases of Barrett's esophagus (7.5%), we observed regression or disparition due to an efficient treatment of gastroesophageal reflux.

Conclusions

This study demonstrates that Barrett's esophagus, as the reflux esophagitis that preceded [1], may have three evolutive profiles: 1) regression or disparition; 2) stabilization; or 3) extension in height.

References

1. Ollyo JB, Monnier P, Fontolliet C, Savary M. The natural history, prevalence and incidence of reflux oesophagitis. Gullet 1993;3(suppl):3−10.
2. Ollyo JB, Gonvers JJ, Froehlich F, Restellini A, Monnier P, Fontolliet C, Savary M. L'endobrachy-oesophage régresse-t-il après traitement efficace du reflux gastro-oesophagien? Schweiz Med Wochenschr 1990;120:716−720.
3. Cameron AJ, Lomboy CT. Barrett's esophagus: age, prevalence and extent of columnar epithelium. Gastroenterology 1992;103:1241−1245.

Is maintenance of multitherapy mandatory to prevent recurrences?

G. Delpre, U. Kadish (Petah Tikva, Tel Aviv)

The fact that gastroesophageal reflux disease (GERD) has a multifactorial basis explains the proliferation of therapies and why responses to treatments vary so greatly, aside from the element of individual differences from patient to patient.

Peptic complications of gastroesophageal reflux (GER) are strictures, ulcers and Barrett's esophagus (BE). The latter is a condition in which the normal stratified mucosa of the esophagus is replaced by columnar lined epithelium (CLE) and convincing evidence suggests that the development of Barrett's epithelium is mainly a consequence of GER [1]. From this viewpoint BE may be considered to be the end stage of reflux esophagitis rather than a separate disease [2], while strictures and ulcers, also frequent in BE, are the extreme manifestations of this advanced stage. Thus treatment for CLE is in fact the management of a severe chronic reflux esophagitis [3] which must take into consideration aspects of GERD as well as BE. The aim should be to relieve any symptoms present, to heal the inflammation and related damage with short-term therapy and to prevent complications, such as strictures or ulcers through long-term maintenance therapy [4]. However, in attempts to "tailor" therapeutic strategies for each of these steps, one must constantly ask oneself: if what is effective for GER is effective for BE and if what is optimal for GER is optimal for BE.

In the first category of patients with reflux esophagitis, efficient long-term management will include the following: a) lifestyle changes; b) avoidance of abrupt discontinuation of treatment since most patients rapidly become "relapsers", and a slow tapering off of the prescribed drug; c) attainment of optimal acid suppression

— with suboptimal doses, asymptomatic lesions may progress until there are irreversible motility changes [5]. In the second category of patients with erosive esophagitis (implying a more severe GERD) "full-ulcer doses" of H_2-receptor antagonists (H_2-RA) are often required twice daily and for long periods [6]. In a long-term study covering up to 42 months, Lieberman [7] found that some of the patients required both H_2-RA and the prescription of bedtime metoclopramide.

In the third category of patients with complicated GERD and BE (uncomplicated and complicated), the prescription of long-term combined drug therapy is not new (Table 1).

In 1977 short-term "pharmacotherapy" was given by Thompson and Barr [8] in a 70-year-old man with one or two deep Barrett's ulcers. When treated with either carbenoxolone alone (150 mg/day) or cimetidine alone (1,200 mg/day) ulcers showed healing, but upon discontinuation of medication they promptly relapsed. Combining the two drugs (carbenoxolone at the dose of 150 mg and cimetidine at the dose of 1,500 mg) gave a successful result. Wesdorp et al. [9] found a combination of very high doses of cimetidine (1,600 mg/day) with antacids to be beneficial in nine BE patients, two of them with Barrett's ulcers. In another study, Humphries [10] reported having given both cimetidine (1,200 mg/day) and bethanechol (100 mg/day) in six severely symptomatic BE patients, two of whom presented with strictures. Healing was maintained during a mean follow-up of 1 year and there was no recurrence of strictures after initial dilatation. Attempts to decrease the cimetidine were promptly followed by recurrence. In the patient reported by Delpre et al. [11], after initial healing of a strictured esophagus with four esophageal ulcers (Fig. 1), cimetidine was tapered to 400 mg/day with the addition of antacids and metoclopramide 30 mg/day. This "triple" therapy initially was unsuccessful, but when the dose of cimetidine was

Table 1. Multitherapy for maintenance in Barrett's esophagus

| | Evaluable patients | | Therapy | | | |
	BE (n) Complicated (n)		Drugs Nb	Regimen (mg/day)	Duration	Effect (Beneficial)
Thompson	BE (1) ULC (1)		2	CIM (1500) CAR (150)	NS	+
Wesdorp	BE (9) ULC (2) STR (1)		2	CIM (1600) ANT (300)[a]	2 years	+
Humphries	BE (6) STR (2)		2	CIM (1200) BET (100)	1 year	+[b]
Delpre	BE (1) ULC (4) STR (1)		3	CIM (600) MET (30) ANT (NS)	>1 year	+[b]
Spechler	BE (58) DYS (9) OTHERS (NS)		1—4	ANT (450)[a] RAN (300) MET (40) SUC (3000)	1—2 years	+[c]
Patel	BE (3) ULC (1) DYS (3)		4	CIM (1200—1600) BET (100) ALG (NS) ANT (NS)	>18 months	+[d]

Abbreviations: ANT: antacids; BET: Bethanechol; CAR: carbenoxolone; CIM: cimetidine; ALG: alginates; MET: metoclopramide; RAN: ranitidine; SUC: sucralfate; NS: not stated; BE: Barrett's esophagus; STR: stricture; ULC: ulcer; DYS: dysplasia; [a]Antacid neutralizing capacity in mmol/day (approximate value); [b]failure after minimal reduction in CIM; [c]better effect after surgery; [d]regression of BE and dysplasia.

928

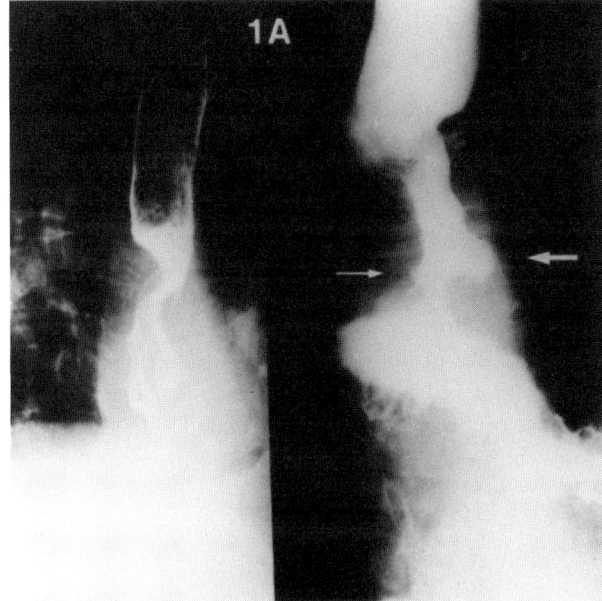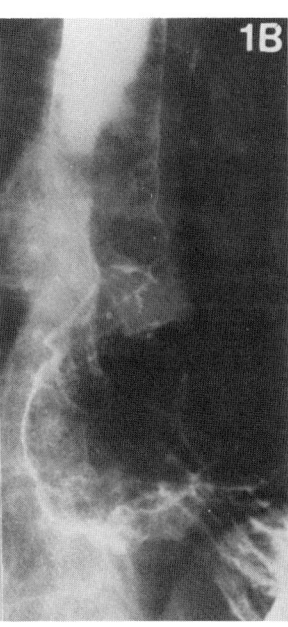

Fig. 1. A) Strictured lower esophagus with proximal overhanging edges and nearby two shallow ulcers (each 1.5 × 1.5 cm). Seen just above the entrance to a diaphragmatic hernia are a third excavated ulcer about 2.0 × 2.5 cm deep (large arrow) and, opposite, a fourth smaller ulcer (fine arrow); B) double contrast view: the esophagus appears to be normal except for a slight mucosal retraction. From [11] (with permission).

increased to 600 mg daily it was found to be beneficial during the follow-up period of more than a year.

The significant effectiveness of "prolonged multipharmacotherapy" has recently been formally evaluated by Spechler and his research group [12] in a long-term (1—2 years) randomized trial. Up to four medications were given, in a stepwise fashion, in accordance with the symptoms and their response to: 1) antacids (12 tablets/day); 2) ranitidine (300 mg/day); 3) metoclopramide (40 mg/day); and 4) sucralfate (3 g/day). Finally, in the three BE patients (one with esophageal ulcer) treated by Patel et al. [13] for over 18 months with a quadruple ("aggressive") continuous therapy — 1) cimetidine (1,200–1,600 mg/day); 2) bethanechol (100 mg/day); 3) alginates; 4) antacids — regression of Barrett's epithelium and even resolution of dysplastic changes were observed, results not described in previous studies [8—12].

Thus, what is the role of maintenance multitherapy in preventing recurrences? Most patients with reflux esophagitis relapse within 1 year, and mild to moderate acid suppression is inadequate in preventing recurrence [4]. Only sustained profound daily acid inhibition can maintain patients with initially "refractory" erosive esophagitis [14]. Management of BE is the life-long management of severe chronic reflux, although no available medical treatment can reverse a defective sphincter [3]. Nevertheless, maintenance multitherapy offers a means for treating simultaneously different pathogenic deficits; the antireflux mechanism of one medication complements the action of the others. Provided that each drug, such as a prokinetic agent, a mucosa-coating drug and an H_2-RA, is given at the optimal dose, it may be postulated that a maximal synergistic effect with possible potentiation will be attained.

In summary, the prophylactic value of maintenance multitherapy, which is supported by our and other previous reports, depends on more specifically adapted responses to the mechanisms involved (i.e., elevated gastric acid secretion, reduced esophageal sensitivity, motility disorders, increased alkaline exposure, reflux of bile and enzymes, etc. [3]), with possible pharmacological potentialization. Multiple maintenance therapy, which is mandatory to prevent recurrence, also provides additional options: 1) its use on a long-term basis instead of the powerful proton pump acid suppression inhibitor; 2) its use in poor-risk patients requiring antireflux surgery or alternatively until inflammatory (dysplastic?) changes clear up; 3) its use to decrease the incidence of high-dose related side effects associated with single drug therapy. The importance of careful follow-up is obvious.

References

1. Spechler SJ, Goyal RK. Barrett's esophagus. N Engl J Med 1986;315:362—371.
2. Iascone C, DeMeester TR, Little AG, Skinner DB. Barrett's esophagus: functional assessment, proposed pathogenesis and surgical therapy. Arch Surg 1983;118:543—549.
3. Scarpignato C, Franze A. Columnar-lined (Barrett's) esophagus. Curr Opin Gastroenterol 1990;6:580—585.
4. Tytgat GNJ, Bianchi Porro G, Feussner H, Pace F, Richter JE, Siewert JR. Long-term strategy for the treatment of gastro-oesophageal reflux disease. Gastroenterol Int 1991;4:21—32.
5. Armstrong D, Nicolet M, Monnier Ph, Chapuis G, Savary M, Blum AL. Maintenance therapy: is there still a place for antireflux surgery? World J Surg 1992;16:300—307.
6. Fennerty MB, Sampliner RE. Medical therapy for gastroesophageal reflux disease. Arch Int Med 1991;151:2365—2366.
7. Lieberman DA. Medical therapy for chronic reflux esophagitis. Long-term follow-up. Arch Int Med 1967;147:1717—1720.
8. Thompson WG, Barr R. Pharmacotherapy of an ulcer in Barrett's esophagus: carbenoxolone and cimetidine. Gastroenterology 1977;73:808—810.
9. Wesdorp IC, Bartelsman J, Schipper ME, Tytgat GNJ. Effect of long-term treatment with cimetidine and antacids in Barrett's esophagus. Gut 1981;22:724—727.
10. Humphries TJ. Long-term treatment and endoscopic follow-up of patients with Barrett's esophagus. Gastrointest Endosc 1982;28:134 (abstract).
11. Delpre G, Kadish U, Glantz I, Avidor I. Prolonged cimetidine therapy in ulcerated Barrett's columnar-lined esophagus. Am J Gastroenterol 1984;79:8—11.
12. Spechler SJ. Comparison of medical and surgical therapy for complicated gastroesophageal reflux disease in veterans. N Engl J Med 1992;326:786—792.
13. Patel GK, Clift SA, Schaeffer RA, Read RC, Texter EC. Resolution of severe dysplasia (Ca in situ) changes with regression of columnar epithelium in Barrett's esophagus on medical treatment. Gastroenterology 1982;82:1147 (abstract).
14. Bardhan KD, Morris P, Thompson M, Dhande DS, Hinchliffe RF, Jones RB, Daly MJ, Carroll NJ. Omeprazole in the treatment of erosive oesophagitis refractory to high dose cimetidine and ranitidine. Gut 1990;31:745—749.

May Barrett's ulcers respond to a conservative medical treatment, as do esophageal ulcers in squamous epithelium?

G. Delpre, A. Leiser, A. Neeman, U. Kadish
(Petah Tikva, Tel Aviv)

When Norman R. Barrett in 1950 described the finding of columnar-lined esophagus (CLE), he expressed the opinion that this portion was part of the gastric area [1]. In 1953, Allison and Johnstone [2] stated that this portion was in fact esophagus lined with gastric mucosa, a condition termed in the same year by Lortat-Jacob and Robert [3] as "endobrachyesophagus", as opposed to "true brachyesophagus" (also called "short congenital esophagus"). In a subsequent report Barrett agreed that the intermediate columnar-lined segment appeared to be esophagus [4]. In fact, the subject of Barrett's initial communication was "the peptic ulcer of the esophagus". In his paper Barrett differentiated two types of esophageal ulcers: those associated with reflux esophagitis and those arising in what he thought was an intrathoracic stomach, behaving much like true gastric ulcers. Once more, Allison and Johnstone [2] correctly characterized the ulcers occurring in the CLE as well-circumscribed penetrating ulcers lying within the columnar segment, labeling them "Barrett's ulcers". They noted that these ulcers are prone to bleed, perforate and cause strictures but could also be healed by "....complete rest, medical treatment, and possible jejunostomy...."

Peptic complications of gastroesophageal reflux (GER) are strictures, ulcers and the development of Barrett's esophagus (BE) [5]. From this viewpoint, Barrett's epithelium and Barrett's ulcers are the extreme manifestations of an advanced stage of gastroesophageal reflux disease (GERD) [6] and at first glance the treatment of either would seem to be the treatment of both. For a better understanding of the therapeutic problems involved, we need to keep in mind a number of aspects of peptic ulcers and Barrett's ulcers.

Peptic ulcerations: Although it is generally accepted that a well-defined ulcer of the esophagus will occur only in BE, large well-documented ulcers have been demonstrated in squamous epithelium in patients with reflux esophagitis, but without BE [7]. According to the endoscopic classification system of Hetzel [8], three types of ulcers of increasing severity may be observed: 1) superficial, located in the last 5 cm of the squamous mucosa and involving less than 10% (grade 2); 2) superficial, located in the last 5 cm of the squamous mucosa and involving up to 50% (grade 3); or 3) deep, located anywhere in the squamous esophagus (grade 4). Wolf et al. [9] have described a particular ulcer situated at the squamocolumnar junction, the "junctional peptic ulcer" or "marginal esophagogastric ulceration". This frequently found Wolf's or Savary's ulcer [10,11] stands in opposition to the classic Barrett's ulcer (Figs. 1—3).

Barrett's ulcer is typically deep and solitary, lying in the posterior wall of the CLE

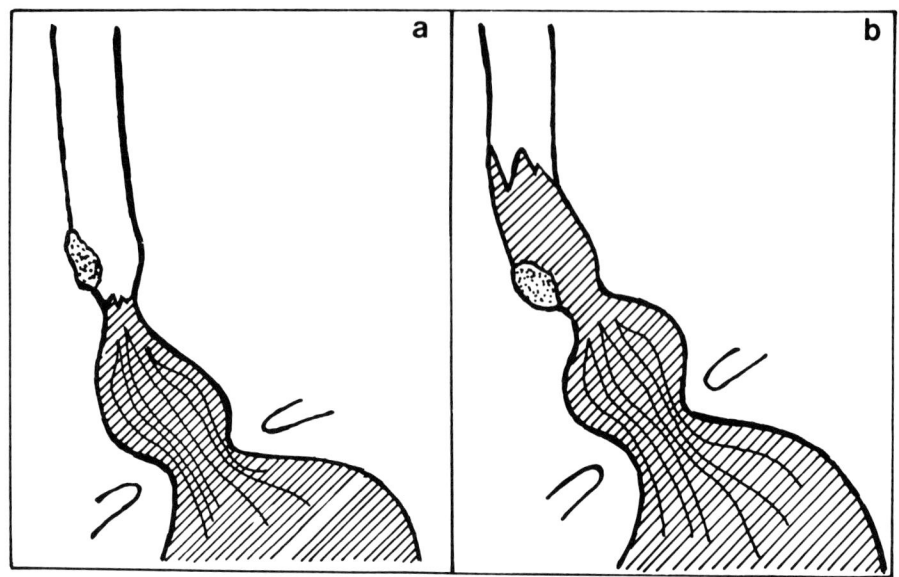

Fig. 1. a) Junctional peptic ulcer (Wolf or Savary); b) Barrett's ulcer. (Adapted from [10].)

[10,11]. However, from the literature it would appear that Barrett's ulcers are very heterogeneous in nature. First, they exhibit a wide spectrum of morphologic appearances. Most often lying in the distal CLE, they may be single, double ("kissing") or multiple; superficial, deep or excavated; small, extensive or very large [5,12–14]. Secondly, they have the same great variability of histological patterns found in the epithelium of Barrett, and beyond the three histological subtypes [15] there may be a mosaic of cells, glands and architectural types with varying degrees of inflammation and ulceration [16]. Moreover, Barrett's ulcers may occasionally

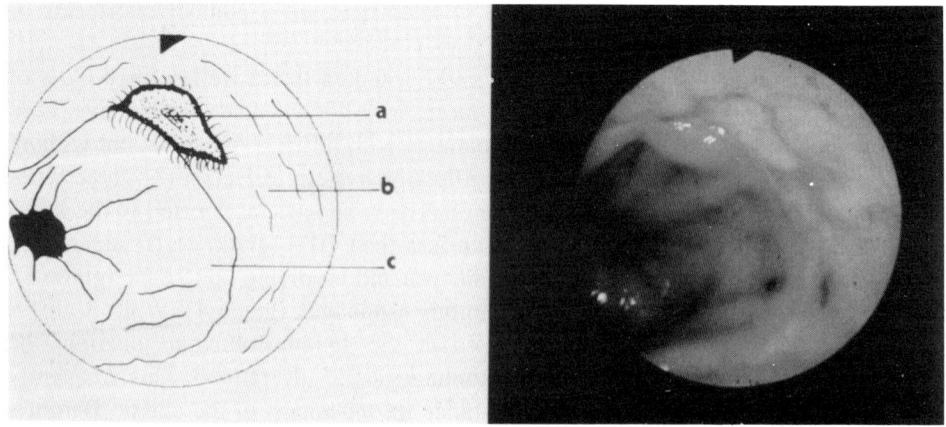

Fig. 2. Junctional ulcer (a) situated at the junction of esophageal (b) and gastric (c) mucosa. (From [11] with permission.)

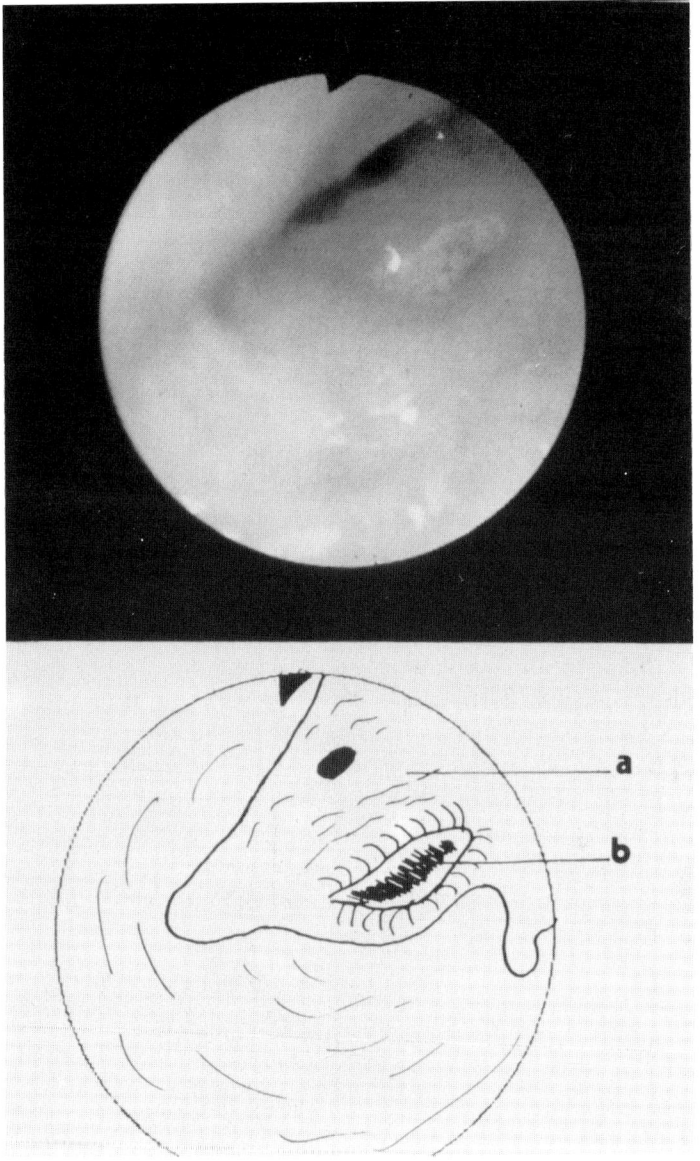

Fig. 3. Within the columnar mucosa (a) — Barrett's ulcer (b). (From [11], with permission.)

develop in residual isolated squamous islands within the CLE [12]. Thirdly, when parietal and chief cells have been present in the vicinity of Barrett's ulcers [16], acid-pepsin secretion has been locally demonstrated [17,18]. Fourthly, a combination of Barrett's and Savary's ulcers is possible [19] (Fig. 4).

When confronted with a proved benign esophageal ulcer (peptic or Barrett's) our aim must be the attainment of effective treatment (in addition to the classic dietary

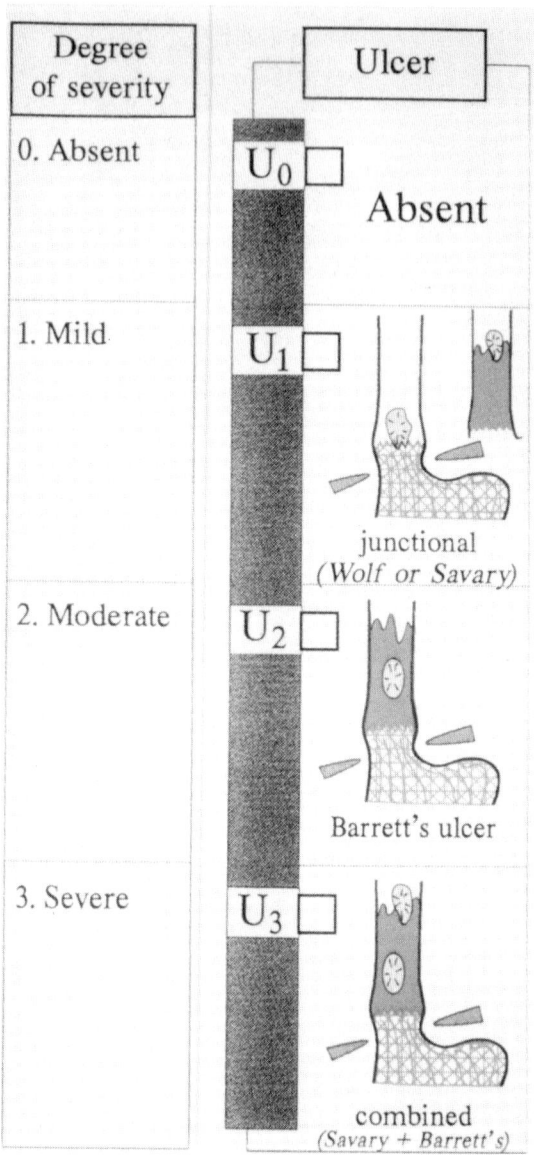

Degree of severity	Ulcer
0. Absent	U_0 ☐ Absent
1. Mild	U_1 ☐ junctional (*Wolf or Savary*)
2. Moderate	U_2 ☐ Barrett's ulcer
3. Severe	U_3 ☐ combined (*Savary + Barrett's*)

Fig. 4. Esophageal ulcers according to the MUSE system of classification. (Adapted from [19], with permission).

and antireflux measures), which will first of all heal the lesion ("acute" therapy) and then prevent its recurrence ("maintenance" therapy). With peptic ulcerations the more severe the ulcer, the greater the need for acid suppression. For grades 2 and 3 superficial ulcers [8] standard therapy may be effective, although in recalcitrant cases additional therapy will be required [20]. For deep ulcers (grade 4) [8] high doses (quadrupled) of H_2 receptor antagonists (H_2RA) may be sufficient [21]. However, there is evidence that superior results may be obtained with acid-pump blockers given at all stages of the disease [19—23]. Barrett's ulcers have a well-deserved reputation for being resistant to healing and prone to complications [12,14]. There are, however, scattered reports in the literature indicating that Barrett's ulcers can be treated successfully by standard conservative regimens, at least in the initial stage, as can esophageal ulcers of low-grade severity in the squamous epithelium. Even in these cases, higher doses over a prolonged period are frequently necessary. In five patients with Barrett's ulcers 1—2 cm in size, 2 months of intensive antacid therapy failed to achieve healing of the ulcers, responding only to high doses of cimetidine (1,200 mg/day) given alone for 1—2 months, and in one patient for 4 months [24]. In one of our patients [13], 4 ulcers (including an excavated ulcer) healed within 3 months on 1,000 mg cimetidine daily. In a patient with a deep ulcer 3 cm in size, ranitidine at the dose of 300 mg/day (in combination with alginates) proved effective within 2 months [25]. Complete healing occurred in 23 out of 27 patients (85%), with ulcers ranging from 0.5 to 3 cm in size, during periods of 2 to 14 months (media. · 4 months). These patients received a combination of antacids and high doses of H_2KA [12]. In one study [26], eight out of 12 patients with Barrett's ulcers showed healing in response to 1,200—1,600 mg cimetidine daily given for a mean time of 8.7 m..'hs (range 2—35 months), and eight out of nine Barrett's ulceration patients showed healing over a mean period of 3.5 months (3—6 months) in response to 300 mg ranitidine daily. Lee and Isaacs [27] reported that 17 out of 28 patients (60%) who received 300 mg/day of ranitidine showed healing of esophageal ulcerations within a treatment period of 2—13 months (mean: 6 months); with 600 mg/day the healing rate was six out of nine within a period of 2—3 months. Edge [28] reported that esophageal ulcerations healed in 18 out of 24 patients given 120 mg famotidine daily. Obviously, the therapeutic strategies remain controversial, although the use of proton-pump inhibitors appears to have opened a new era [12,19,21,22]. Lee and Isaacs [27] reported that two out of three patients with ulcers, which had proved resistant to high doses of ranitidine, showed healing after 4 weeks of omeprazole at the dose of 40 mg/day; in the third patient the ulcer, which was more superficial, persisted after 8 weeks of treatment. Hameeteman and Tytgat [29] reported rapid healing in response to omeprazole 40 mg/day in three patients who proved resistant to very high doses of cimetidine (1,600 mg for 8 months) and, in one, ranitidine (600 mg for 4 months).

Thus there is a great variation in means and responses. Some patients respond to standard medication almost as those with ulcers of the squamous epithelium [13,24—26]. In some, conventional doses of ranitidine will eventually achieve healing, but slowly [27]. In a notable proportion of patients [26—29] only powerful acid-reducing regimens are effective. Very rare cases require surgery [12]. The explanation for this diversity lies in the heterogeneity of the Barrett's ulcer and the multifac-toriality of the Barrett's esophagus, as well as some pharmacologic and epidemiologic factors (Table 1). Regarding the pleomorphism of Barrett's ulcers, however, size in itself is not a determinant factor in its healing as opposed to its penetration beyond the mucosal layer [12,13,18,19,24—27]. One of the seven patients described by Allison and Johnstone in 1953 [2] had a 5 × 7 mm ulcer which perforated!

Variability in histological pattern [5,15,16], together with the action of noxious

Table 1. Factors which may influence the therapeutic response of Barrett's ulcer(s) to conservative medical treatment

Abnormality	Determinant	Consequences
Barrett's ulcer pleomorphism	Number, location, size, bleeding, superficial, deep, excavated	Degree of penetration is a major factor
Histological pattern found in vicinity	1. Specialized (Intestinal) type 2. Islands of squamous epithelium 3. Fundic (Gastric) type	1. Less resistant 2. Easily erodes 3. Local acid-pepsin secretion
Physiopathologic abnormalities both in: uncomplicated and in: Barrett's ulcer	1. Elevated gastric acid secretion 2. Reduced esophageal sensitivity 3. LES failure and motility disorders 4. Low salivary epidermal growth factor 5. Duodenogastric reflux 6. Esophageal postprandial bile acids content	1. Acid esophageal environment 2. Poor recognition 3. Defective esophageal clearance 4. Poor healing esophageal damage 5. Increased alkaline exposure 6. Acid suppression alone questionable
Pharmacologic or etiologic aspects	1. Abnormal cimetidine pharmacokinetics 2. Intake of NSAID 3. Elderly patients	1. Possible cimetidine resistance 2. Superimposed esophageal lesions 3. Greater susceptibility

stimuli [6], may explain at least three mechanisms for ulcer induction and unequal response to treatment (Table 1). The plurality of pathophysiologic mechanisms accounts for the circumstances in which the columnar mucosa loses its ability to resist damage [6,30]. Factors implied may be interrelated. Acid esophageal environment will potentiate proteolytic enzymes (trypsin) and bile acids. Higher postprandial bile acid content in the esophagus causes increased alkaline exposure and more reflux of duodenal juice. In the latter situation, H_2RA may be harmful since in an alkaline environment they will activate the pancreaticoduodenal enzymes [6]. The impact of pharmacologic and etiologic factors must be considered in assessing therapy requirements for Barrett's ulcers in contrast to those for peptic ulcers — these include the abnormal pharmacokinetics of cimetidine in BE [31], the older age of patients with Barrett's ulcers [6], and the use of NSAID's, especially in this older group of patients [32].

Summary

Barrett's ulcers will initially respond to conservative treatment as do esophageal ulcers of low to moderate severity in squamous epithelium, provided that higher doses of H_2RA are given for longer periods. For those that are resistant to this regimen acid-pump blockers are usually effective, as they are for severe peptic ulcers in squamous epithelium. Surgery is rarely necessary. The wide range of therapeutic alternatives for Barrett's ulcers is related to the varying aspects of BE and Barrett's ulcerations.

References

1. Barrett NR. Chronic peptic ulcer of the esophagus and esophagitis. Br J Surg 1950;38:175—182.
2. Allison PR, Johnstone AS. The esophagus lined with gastric mucosa membrane. Thorax 1953;8:87—101.
3. Lortat-Jacob JL, Robert F. Les malpositions cardio tuberositaires. Arch Mal App Dig 1953;42:750—760.
4. Barrett NR. The lower esophagus lined by columnar epithelium. Surgery 1957;41:881—894.
5. Spechler JS, Goyal RK. Barrett's esophagus. N Engl J Med 1986;315:362—371.
6. Scarpignato C, Franze A. Columnar-lined (Barrett's) esophagus. Curr Opin Gastroenterol 1990;6:580—585.
7. Robbins AH, Hermos JA, Schimmel EM, Friedlander DM, Messian RA. The columnar-lined esophagus — analysis of 26 cases. Radiology 1977;123:1—7.
8. Hetzel DJ, Dent J, Reed WD et al. Healing and relapse of severe peptic esophagitis after treatment with omeprazole. Gastroenterology 1988;15:903—912.
9. Wolf BS, Marshak RH, Som HL, Winkelstein A. Peptic esophagitis, peptic ulcer of the esophagus and marginal esophagogastric ulceration. Gastroenterology 1955;29:744—748.
10. Savary M, Miller G. The esophagus. Handbook and Atlas of Endoscopy. Solothurn (Switzerland): Verlag Gassman, 1978.
11. Zeitoun P. Endoscopie et biopsies au cours des oesophagites par reflux. Gastroentérologie 1988;2:11—17.
12. Williamson WA, Ellis FH Jr, Gibb SP, Aretz HT. Barrett's ulcer, a surgical disease? J Thorac Cardiovasc Surg 1992; 103:2—7.
13. Delpre G, Kadish U, Glantz I, Avidor I. Prolonged cimetidine therapy in ulcerated Barrett's columnar-lined esophagus. Am J Gastroenterol 1984;79:8—11.
14. Tytgat GNJ, Hameeteman W, Onstenk R, Schotborg R. The spectrum of columnar-lined esophagus — Barrett's esophagus. Endoscopy 1989;21:177—185.
15. Paull AP, Trier JS, Dalton MD, Camp RC, Loeb P, Goyal RK. The histologic spectrum of Barrett's esophagus. N Engl J Med 1976;295:476—480.
16. Thomson JJ, Zinsser KR, Enterline HT. Barrett's metaplasia and adenocarcinoma of the esophagus and gastroesophageal junction. Hum Pathol 1983;14:42—61.
17. Hershfield NB, Lind JF, Hildes JA, McMorris LS. Secretory function of Barrett's epithelium. Gut 1985;6:535—539.
18. Ustach TJ, Tobon F, Schuster MM. Demonstration of acid secretion from esophageal mucosa in Barrett's ulcer. Gastrointest Endosc 1969;88:98—100.
19. Armstrong B, Nicolet M, Monnier Ph, Chapuis G, Savary M, Blum AL. Maintenance therapy: is there still a place for antireflux surgery? World J Surg 1992;16:300—307.
20. Tytgat GNJ, Bianchi Porro G, Feussner H, Pace F, Richter JE, Siewert JR. Long-term strategy for the treatment of gastroesophageal reflux disease. Gastroenterol Int 1991;4:21—32.
21. Bell NJV, Hunt RH. Role of gastric acid suppression in the treatment of gastroesophageal reflux disease. Gut 1992;33: 118—124.
22. Zeitoun P. Comparison of omeprazole with ranitidine in the treatment of reflux esophagitis. Scand J Gastroenterol 1989; 24(suppl 166):83—87.
23. Hetzel DJ. Controlled clinical trials of omeprazole in the long-term management of reflux disease. Digestion 1992; 51(suppl 1):35—42.
24. Kuthari T, Mangla JC, Kalra TMS. Barrett's ulcer and treatment with cimetidine. Arch Int Med 1980;140:475—477.
25. Andersson R, Löwgren B. Ranitidine therapy of Barrett's ulcer. Acta Chir Scand 1986;152:629—631.
26. Cooper BT, Barbezat GO. Treatment of Barrett's esophagus with H_2 blockers. J Clin Gastroenterol 1987;9:139—141.
27. Lee FI, Isaacs PE. Barrett's ulcer: response to standard dose ranitidine, high dose ranitidine and omeprazole. Am J Gastroenterol 1988,83.914 916.
28. Edge DP. High dose famotidine in ranitidine resistant severe esophagitis: a pilot study. NZ J Med 1990,103:150—152.
29. Hameeteman W, Tytgat GNJ. Healing of chronic Barrett's ulcers with omeprazole. Am J Gastroenterol 1986;81:764—766.
30. Gray MR, Donnelly RJ, Kingsnorth AN. Role of salivary epidermal growth factor in the pathogenesis of Barrett's columnar-lined esophagus. Br J Surg 1991;78:1461—1466.
31. Johnson DA, Kandasamy A, Ezra D, Peck C, Dubois A. Cimetidine pharmacokinetics and pharmacodynamics in Barrett's esophagus. Gastroenterology 1987;92:1456 (abstract).
32. Cooper BT, Barbezat GO. Barrett's esophagus: a clinical study of 52 patients. Q J Med 1987;62:97—108.

Are the early good results of Collis operation in Barrett's esophagus lasting despite the persistence of acid secretion in the gastric tube?

J. Testart (Rouen)

In this article, "good results" will only be considered in terms of esophagitis and gastroesophageal reflux.

Theoretically, the surgical antireflux device which acts as a barrier against gastric acid passage into the esophagus should be placed at the esophagus and gastric mucosae junction level. In fact, the acid-exposed mucosa must be separated from the acid-secreting mucosa. Collis himself, aware of leaving gastric mucosa above the neocardia, believed that this mucosa was not acid-secreting [1]. He drew this presumption from a) the reference to the "Magenstrasse" "devoid of peptic cells and relatively innocuous"; and b) the analogy to those patients "often referred to as having gastric-lined esophagus and in whom symptoms are often slight" (*sic*) [1].

The metaplastic mucosa of endobrachyesophagus has, indeed, no or very little acid or peptic secretions [2], but the mucosa of a neoesophageal tube is different; it does not come from a progressive replacement. It is most often a junctional-type epithelium that fortunately has no parietal or chief cells. Weakness of acid secretions has been noted in the proximal pouch of gastric bipartition made for morbid obesity [3]. However, when the neoesophageal tube is 8 cm long, its lower part could have fundic-type epithelium with glands containing parietal and chief cells. Then it is similar to the long gastric tubes constructed along the greater curvature to replace a resected esophagus. In these tubes, despite resection of the lesser curvature and vagotomy, a near to normal acid secretion has been noticed [4], although other authors have observed weak or no acidity (4 out of 10 cases [5] and 4 out of 12 cases [6]).

In order to lower the acid secretion in the neoesophageal tube, must its nerves be cut? A (truncal) vagotomy has already been proposed by Petrovsky [7] when he described his valvular gastroplication, which is a Nissen fundoplication made around the cardial part of the stomach stretched out into the shape of a tube.

In order to restrict the denervation to the neoesophageal tube, a supraselective vagotomy of the upper part of the lesser curvature can be made. However, vessels are cut at the same time as the nervous branches and ischemia of the tube could therefore occur, particularly if it is long. The authors performing such denervation made tubes that did not exceed 4 cm [8]. This length seems to us insufficient for truly irreducible cardia, and we are not completely convinced by the findings of a case report of complete supraselective vagotomy associated with Collis operation [9].

We have restricted the use of Collis operation to brachyesophagus, which led to us cutting a 6 to 8 cm length tube.

Using mucosal colouring with red congo, we observed acid secretion in the tube in half of the patients [10]. This acid secretion could be observed only on the lower part of the neoesophageal tube, e.g., in one case the endoscopist specified that the mucosa of the endobrachyesophagus did not turn red congo dark, whereas below the gastric mucosa did.

In our prospective study of 32 patients with more than 4 years follow-up, 29 had early good results for esophagitis and reflux and 27 maintained these results 4 years later. We had two late failures, one patient with esophagitis during irradiation for a bronchopulmonary carcinoma, and another one at the time of decompensation of her asthma. Two of these 32 patients, as well as a third patient operated upon just 4 years ago, have had a positive red congo test, and nevertheless good early and late results.

When a neoesophageal tube produces an acid secretion, it is probably small in quantity and easily swept down into the stomach with saliva swallowing, provided there are no motor disturbances. If this requirement is fulfilled, the early good results should abide.

References

1. Adler HR. Collis gastroplasty origin and evolution. Ann Thorac Surg 1990;50:839–842.
2. Gillen P, Hennessy TPJ. Barrett's oesophagus. In: Hennessy TPJ, Cuschieri A, Bennett JR (eds) Reflux Oesophagitis. London: Butterworths, 1989;87–112.
3. Simonowitz DA, Dellinger EP, Stothert JC. Gastroplasty in patients with symptoms of reflux esophagitis. Surg Gynecol Obstet 1982;154:235–237.
4. Domergue J, Veyrac M, Huin-Yan S, Rouanet P, Collet H, Michel H, Pujol H. 24-h pH monitoring for gastroesophageal reflux and gastric function after intrathoracic gastroplasty after esophagectomy. Surg Gynecol Obstet 1990;171:108–110.
5. Pouget X, Valleix D, Descottes B, Caix M. Devenir sécrétoire des gastroplasties tubulées isopéristaltiques. Sem Hop Paris 1988;64:1023–1027.
6. Bouchoucha M, Cugnenc Ph, Faye A, Drevillon C, Arhan P, Barbier JPh. Evaluation fonctionnelle des transplants gastriques utilisés pour reconstruction oesophagienne. Gastroenterol Clin Biol 1989;13.
7. Petrovsky BV, Kanshin NN. The problem of the surgical treatment of sliding hiatus hernias and a shortened esophagus. In: Nyhus LM, Hankins HN (eds) Hernia. Philadelphia: J.B. Lippincott, 1964;513–521.
8. Pearson FG, Cooper JD, Patterson GA, Ramirez J, Todd TR. Gastroplasty and fundoplication for complex reflux problems. Ann Surg 1987;206:473–481.
9. Landreneau RJ, Marshall JB, McClelland RN, Curtis JJ, Johnson JA, Hazelrigg SR. New surgical approach to complicated gastroesophageal reflux disease transthoracic parietal cell vagotomy. Ann Thorac Surg 1991;51:128–130.
10. Testart J, Kartheuser A, Peillon C, Galmiche JP, Denis P. L'opération de Collis pour brachy-oesophage (49 patients). Gastroenterol Clin Biol 1991;15:512–518.

What are the results of long-term follow up of Barrett's esophagus after surgical treatment?

H.W. Pinotti, I. Cecconello, A. Nasi, B. Zilberstein
(São Paulo)

Among 1,105 cases of reflux esophagitis managed surgically in our department during the last 20 years, 124 patients (11.2%) presented with Barrett's esophagus. One hundred of these were treated conservatively by fundoplication. There were 68 males and 32 females in the series, with ages ranging from 9 to 47 years (mean 48.8).

Operative technique

Lind's technique [1] of partial abdominal fundoplication together with approximation of the diaphragmatic pillars was the procedure most utilized. Nissen's technique [2] was employed when the esophageal wall was friable due to severe inflammation. Intraoperative dilatations with Savary bougies of progressive diameters were also realized in severe cases of stenosis, which do not allow passage of the endoscope. Since most esophageal stenoses are intrathoracic, the intraoperative dilatation proceeds as follows:

a) median phrenotomy from the hiatus to the xiphoid appendix to approach the mediastinal esophagus [3];

b) dissection and isolation of the esophagus as far as above the stenosed area;

c) oral introduction of the bougies with the surgeon's help, who guides the dilatation under direct vision and by palpation. If dilatation can be performed with bougies of over 10 mm, it is considered sufficient and discontinued;

d) partial or total fundoplication as already mentioned; and

e) closure of the phrenotomy and approximation of the diaphragmatic pillars, leaving a hiatal opening of one finger.

Table 1. One hundred cases of Barrett's esophagus[a]; management by fundoplication

Procedure	No. of cases
Nissen fundoplication	3
Partial fundoplication	72
Partial fundoplication + intraoperative dilatation	25

[a]Fifty-six cases with peptic stricture.

The procedures employed in these patients are listed in Table 1. Intraoperative and immediate postoperative complications included: laceration of the esophagus during dilatation (five cases); injury to the spleen (three cases); pulmonary atelectasis (one case); and evisceration (one case).

All cases of esophageal laceration were identified and sutured immediately because the region of stenosis was under the surgeon's direct vision. In two of the three cases of splenal injury, conservative therapy was possible (cauterization and suture); the third case required splenectomy. No deaths occurred in this series.

Late follow-up

Sixty-eight patients were followed-up annually, for 6–10 years (mean 4.9 years) with clinical, radiological and endoscopic examinations. Table 2 shows the results: nine

Table 2. Late follow-up

	No. of cases	%
Asymptomatic	49	71.0
Slight dysphagia (residual stricture)	9	13.2
Recurrence of reflux	11	15.8

Table 3. Late follow-up (68 cases)

	No. of cases		
	Without stenosis: 40	With stenosis: 28	Total: 68
Recurrence of reflux	2 (5.0 %)	9 (32.1 %)	11 (15.8%)

p = 0.05.

patients required postoperative dilatations due to recurrence of stenosis, however, reflux could not be confirmed in these patients. Reflux occurred in 11 cases. This was significantly higher in the group with preoperative stenosis, as illustrated in Table 3. No significant alteration was noted in the length of columnar epithelium compared to preoperative length: before treatment: 5.1 ± 1.9 cm; after treatment: 5.5 ± 2.1 cm, NS.

Eighteen months postoperatively, one of the patients (1.4%) developed carcinoma, an elevated lesion 2 mm in diameter. Recurrence of esophagitis was not observed in this case. The patient was submitted to transhiatal esophagectomy without thoracotomy. The pathological examination revealed adenocarcinoma invading even the muscularis mucosa. The patient is still alive 9 years after surgery.

Conclusion

Partial abdominal fundoplication is a safe procedure without morbidity or mortality. After partial fundoplication, reflux recurred in 15.6% of patients, mainly in those with stenosis. The extension of columnar epithelium remained unchanged after surgery. It is still not clear whether elimination of reflux wards off malignancy.

References

1. Lind JF, Burns CM, MacDougall JT. Physiological repair for hiatus hernia — manometric study. Arch Surg 1965;91:233–237.
2. Nissen R. Gastropexy and "fundoplication" in surgical treatment of hiatal hernia. Am J Dig Dis 1961;6:954–961.
3. Pinotti HW. Esofagectomia subtotal por túnel transmediastinal sem toracotomia. Rev Med Bras 1977;23:395.

Does complete suppression of acidity and alkaline reflux contribute to healing?

W.A. Williamson (Boston)

The notion that complete suppression of acidity and alkaline reflux by total duodenal diversion might contribute to the healing or regression of Barrett's esophagus is an appealing theoretical concept. It has been demonstrated [1–3] that patients with Barrett's esophagus have increased episodes of acid reflux, delayed clearance of acid, and higher basal and stimulated gastric acid secretion compared with patients with uncomplicated gastroesophageal reflux disease. Furthermore, patients with complications of Barrett's esophagus, such as strictures, ulceration, and dysplasia, have more frequent episodes of alkaline reflux according to some investigators [4–6]. Excessive duodenal gastric reflux has also been demonstrated [7] in patients with Barrett's esophagus by hepatobiliary scanning. It would seem plausible, then, that total control of acidity and alkaline reflux might result in regression.

Because standard antireflux procedures should result in a competent barrier to both acid and alkaline reflux, it is appropriate to review the effect of these procedures on regression of Barrett's mucosa. Only 16 cases of partial regression and five cases of complete regression of Barrett's mucosa have been reported [5,8–19] after a standard antireflux procedure in a total of 249 patients (Table 1). Thus, 92% of patients with Barrett's esophagus who have undergone an antireflux procedure have no evidence of regression.

I have recently updated our follow-up data on patients with Barrett's esophagus who have undergone antireflux procedures at the Lahey Clinic over the past 20 years.

Table 1. Standard antireflux procedures and regression of Barrett's esophagus

Author	Year	Patients	Regression	Antireflux procedure
Mangla et al. [8]	1976	4	0	Nissen
Radigan et al. [9]	1977	13	1 complete	Nissen
Brand et al. [10]	1980	10	4 partial	Nissen/Hill
Dooner and Cleator [11]	1982	3	0	Nissen
Ransom et al. [12]	1982	10	4 partial	Nissen
Skinner [13]	1990	12	2 partial 1 complete	Belsey/Nissen
Starnes et al. [14]	1984	8	0	Nissen + partial gastric vagotomy
Harle et al. [15]	1985	13	1 complete	Nissen
Wellinger et al. [16]	1989	39	0	Nissen
DeMeester et al. [5]	1990	35	0	Nissen/Belsey/Collis
Ollyo et al. [17]	1990	40	1 partial	Nissen
Attwood et al. [18]	1992	19	2 complete	Partial anterior fundoplication
Williamson et al. [19]	1990	43	5 partial	Nissen/Belsey/Collis
Total		249	16 partial (6.4%) 5 complete (2%)	

Many of these cases were reported [19] in 1989. Of a total of 51 patients, 43 were available for long-term endoscopic follow-up study, which ranged from 8 months to 20 years with a median of 5.7 years. These patients underwent yearly endoscopic surveillance with biopsy specimens taken every 2 cm. A total of 45 antireflux procedures were performed in these 43 patients.

Endoscopic esophagitis resolved in 34 out of 36 patients (94%). Seven out of nine patients with strictures and dysphagia have had complete relief of symptoms and resolution of the stricture. All five Barrett's ulcers have healed. Antireflux surgery resulted in normalization of lower esophageal sphincter pressures in 29 out of 31 patients (93%) who had both preoperative and postoperative manometry. In all seven patients (16%) who had preoperative and postoperative 24-h pH monitoring, values have reverted to normal. Only five patients (11.6%) had partial regression of Barrett's mucosa, which was endoscopically documented. Partial regression was defined as a 3 cm or greater decrease in the total length of Barrett's mucosa with histologic evidence of regenerating squamous mucosa. In addition, carcinoma developed in Barrett's esophagus in four patients (9.3%) while they were under surveillance after having undergone an antireflux procedure. This is an incidence of one per 75 patient-years of follow-up study.

Many of the reports listed in Table 1 have been criticized because of the lack of accurate mapping of the esophageal mucosa, the lack of postoperative 24-h pH studies to document the efficacy of the antireflux procedure, and the lack of a uniform definition of regression. However, if only studies that use preoperative and postoperative 24-h pH studies and endoscopic criteria for regression are included, only seven of the 91 reported cases of partial regression and four reported cases of complete regression remain (Table 2). Of patients with effective antireflux procedures, 88% had no evidence of regression of Barrett's mucosa.

There are 26 patients with Barrett's esophagus reported in the literature [20,21] who have had total acid suppression and duodenal diversion. These patients have had vagotomy, antrectomy, and Roux-en-Y anastomosis. Of the 26 patients, two had complete regression and five had partial regression; 73% of the patients who had vagotomy, antrectomy, and Roux-en-Y anastomosis with total duodenal diversion have no evidence of regression of Barrett's mucosa. Of interest, however, is the observation [20] that regression may not occur within the first year after the acid

Table 2. Antireflux surgery documented with 24-h pH study and regression of Barrett's mucosa

Author	Year	Patients	Regression	Antireflux procedure
Skinner [13]	1990	12	2 partial 1 complete	Belsey/Nissen
Perniceni et al. [20]	1989	25	5 partial 1 complete	Vagotomy, antrectomy, Roux-en-Y anastomosis
DeMeester et al. [5]	1990	35	0	Nissen/Belsey/Collis
Attwood et al. [18]	1992	19	2 complete	partial antrectomy, fundoplication
Total		91	7 partial (7.7%) 4 complete (4.4%)	

suppression and alkaline diversion procedure. In one of the patients, complete regression occurred 47 months after total duodenal diversion. This may indicate that longer term follow-up evaluation is necessary in these patients to document regression accurately.

Based on the 26 cases reported in the literature, evidence is not sufficient to suggest that total duodenal diversion and acid suppression will result in regression of Barrett's esophagus in the majority of patients. Furthermore, although standard antireflux procedures are effective in treating the complications of Barrett's esophagus, such as strictures and ulcers, they do not consistently result in regression of Barrett's mucosa.

References

1. Stein HJ, Hoeft SF, DeMeester TR. Functional foregut abnormalities in Barrett's esophagus. J Thorac Cardiovasc Surg 1993;105:107—111.
2. Iascone C, DeMeester TR, Little AG, Skinner DB. Barrett's esophagus: functional assessment, proposed pathogenesis, and surgical therapy. Arch Surg 1983;118:543—549.
3. Mulholland MW, Reid BJ, Levine DS, Rubin CE. Elevated gastric acid secretion in patients with Barrett's metaplastic epithelium. Dig Dis Sci 1989;34:1329—1334.
4. Attwood SEA, Ball CS, Barlow AP, Jenkinson L, Norris TL, Watson A. Role of intragastric and intraoesophageal alkalinisation in the genesis of complications in Barrett's columnar-lined lower esophagus. Gut 1993;34:11—15.
5. DeMeester TR, Attwood SE, Smyrk TC, Therkildsen DH, Hinder RA. Surgical therapy in Barrett's esophagus. Ann Surg 1990;212:528—542.
6. Attwood SE, DeMeester TR, Bremner CG, Barlow AP, Hinder RA. Alkaline gastroesophageal reflux: implications in the development of complications in Barrett's columnar-lined lower esophagus. Surgery 1989;106:764—770.
7. Waring JP, Legrand J, Chinichian A, Sanowski RA. Duodenogastric reflux in patients with Barrett's esophagus. Dig Dis Sci 1990;35:759—762.
8. Mangla J, Schenk EA, Desbaillets L, Guarasci G, Kubasik NP, Turner MD. Pepsin secretion, pepsinogen, and gastrin in "Barrett's esophagus": clinical and morphological characteristics. Gastroenterology 1976;70(5/1):669—676.
9. Radigan LR, Glover JL, Shipley FE, Shoemaker RE. Barrett's esophagus. Arch Surg 1977;112:486—491.
10. Brand DL, Ylvisaker JT, Gelfand M, Pope CE II. Regression of columnar esophageal (Barrett's) epithelium after antireflux surgery. N Engl J Med 1980;302:844—848.
11. Dooner J, Cleator IG. Selective management of benign esophageal strictures. Am J Gastroenterol 1982;77:172—177.
12. Ransom JM, Patel GK, Clift SA, Womble NE, Read RC. Extended and limited types of Barrett's esophagus in the adult. Ann Thorac Surg 1982;33:19—27.
13. Skinner DB. Controversies about Barrett's esophagus. Ann Thorac Surg 1990;49:523—524.
14. Starnes VA, Adkins RB, Ballinger JF, Sawyers JL. Barrett's esophagus: a surgical entity. Arch Surg 1984;119:563—567.
15. Harle IA, Finley RJ, Belsheim M, Bondy DC, Booth M, Lloyd D, McDonald JW, Sullivan S, Valberg LS, Watson WC et al. Management of adenocarcinoma in a columnar-lined esophagus. Ann Thorac Surg 1985;40:330—336.
16. Wellinger J, Ollyo JB, Savary M, Fontolliet C, Chapuis G. Le traitement chirurgical de l'endobrachy-oesophage. A propos de 110 cas. Helv Chir Acta 1989;55:695—698.
17. Ollyo JB, Lang F, Fontolliet C, Monnier P, Restellini A, Krayenbuhl M, Savary M. Barrett's oesophagus: regression/disappearance following effective treatment of gastro-oesophageal reflux? Gastroenterology 1990;98:A100.
18. Attwood SEA, Barlow AP, Norris TL, Watson A. Barrett's oesophagus: effect of antireflux surgery on symptom control and development of complications. Br J Surg 1992;79:1050—1053.
19. Williamson WA, Ellis FH Jr, Gibb SP, Shahian DM, Aretz HT. Effect of antireflux operation on Barrett's mucosa. Ann Thorac Surg 1990;49:537—542.
20. Perniceni T, Leymarios J, Molas G et al. L'endobrachyoesophage régresse-t-il après diversion duodénale totale? Gastroenterol Clin Biol 1988;12:709—712.
21. Henrion J, Schapira M, Pourbaix A, Heller FR. Régression complète d'un endobrachyoesophage (oesophage de Barrett) après correction du reflux biliaire chez un malade gastrectomisé. Gastroenterol Clin Biol 1989;13:745—746.

What are the indications for resection in Barrett's esophagus?

I. Cecconello, A. Nasi, B. Zilberstein, H.W. Pinotti
(São Paulo)

In the 1950s, esophageal lesions such as ulcerations or stenoses were promptly resected [1,2]. Starting from the 1960s, most of these cases were managed conservatively through partial or total fundoplication, with or without esophageal dilatations. Currently, esophageal resection for Barrett's esophagus is indicated under the following circumstances:

— presence of extensive and/or severe stenosis difficult to dilate;
— association with esophageal motor disorders (scleroderma, previously operated achalasia), in which treatment by fundoplication improves the esophagitis but leads to increased dysphagia; and
— carcinomatous degeneration.

Upon assessing these indications, distal resections of the esophagus with interposition of a jejunal loop (Merendino's operation) are indicated only in cases in which the stenosis is in the inferior esophagus.

Twenty-four (19.3%) of the 124 cases of Barrett's esophagus treated in our department underwent resection. Transhiatal esophagectomy without thoracotomy was accomplished, followed by gastroplasty with esophagogastric anastomosis at the cervical level, and transposition of the stomach through the esophageal bed [3]. This procedure was employed in 24 cases, as shown in Table 1.

Because of systemic involvement and immunosuppression, and sometimes malnutrition, the surgical risk of patients with scleroderma is high. Two deaths occurred in our series, from pneumonia and pancreatic abscess followed by septic shock and multiple organ failure. Ten patients (7.2%) of the 124 cases of Barrett's esophagus presented cancer. One patient died before treatment was begun, and another during the postoperative period. Of the remaining eight patients, two exhibited superficial carcinoma (survival of 8 and 9 years), and six exhibited advanced lesions (mean survival of 16 months).

The histological examination of the 10 cases is illustrated in Table 2: elevated

Table 1. Esophageal resections

Diagnosis	No. of cases	Fistula	Mortality	Mean extension columumnar epithelium
Adenocarcinoma	9	1	1	9.7 cm
Scleroderma	6	3	2	
Achalasia	7	—	—	4.8 cm
Severe stenosis	2	—	—	
Total	24	4 (16.6%)	3 (12.5%)	

Table 2. Barrett's esophagus with adenocarcinoma (10 cases)

	No. of cases
Well differentiated/tubular (intestinal type)	9
Faveolar tubular (without intestinal metaplasia)	1
Mucocellular/signet ring cell (diffuse type)	—

lesions in epithelium with intestinal metaplasia were present in nine patients. All lesions were located proximal to the transition of columnar and stratified epithelium. Therefore, the location of the lesion depends on the extension of the columnar epithelium.

As mentioned in Table 1, the mean length of epithelial ectopia was significantly higher in patients with carcinomatous degeneration, compared with those without associated neoplasia.

Indications for esophagectomy should be assessed carefully in cases of severe dysplasia, as regression is possible in some cases; in others, it may already be carcinoma. The best management in such cases is a regular evaluation every 3 months made by well-trained endoscopists and pathologists.

After intensive medical treatment of the peptic disease, biopsy samples should be taken, attempting to select areas with small elevated lesions and/or erosions. When available, studies with oncogenetic markers or cellular DNA may be realized.

Conclusion

Resection is indicated in cases of Barrett's esophagus with extensive stricture, severe motility disorders or adenocarcinoma. The median extension of columnar epithelium is significantly higher in cases with carcinoma. Adenocarcinoma is, in 90% of the cases, an elevated lesion of the differentiated type, and is localized over intestinal metaplasia.

References

1. Allison PR, Johnstone AS. The esophagus lined with gastric mucous membrane. Thorax 1953;8:87–101.
2. Paulino F, Cavalcanti AR, Aprigliano F. Úlcera de Barrett. Rev Bras Cir 1960;39:457–462.
3. Pinotti HW. Esofagectomia subtotal por túnel transmediastinal sem toracotomia. Rev Ass Med Bras 1977;23:395.

What are the indications of Saidi's operation?

F. Saidi (Tehran)

The basic concept

The endoesophageal pull-through (EEPT) operation is a method for reconstruction following resection of an esophageal cancer. It is analogous to the transhiatal esophagectomy technique in dispensing with thoracotomy, but differing from it in one major respect: the plane of dissection, instead of proceeding in the mediastinum outside the esophagus, rests within the esophageal wall in its submucosal layer. The thick and supple normal esophageal submucosa permits an easy digital stripping of the mucosal layer, which can then be cored out intact (Fig. 1). Left behind is the denuded esophageal muscular layer which then serves as a distensible conduit through which either the stomach (Fig. 2) or the colon (Fig. 3) can be pulled from the abdomen to the neck.

This approach reduces operative trauma to an absolute minimum, not only because it avoids thoracotomy for upper and lower end esophageal cancers, but also because it sidesteps the risks of excessive bleeding, tracheal injury, chylothorax and even pleural entry, since mediastinal structures are not encroached upon.

Mucosal stripping commences at a tumor-safe margin proximal to a lower-end, or distal to an upper-end esophageal cancer (Fig. 5). Actual tumor resection, whether for palliation or cure, precedes and does not influence reconstruction by the endo-esophageal technique. While thoracotomy can be readily avoided for tumors of the upper and lower ends of the esophagus, mid-esophageal or low-esophageal tumors, whose proximal edge rests at mid-heart level, require a right thoracotomy for staging and complete nodal dissection. In these two latter situations the mucosal dissection starts at the level of the azygos vein, a tumor-safe margin above the tumor (Fig. 3). The muscular tunnel created from within the chest, though short in length, is an effective barrier between the clean intrathoracic and the contaminated cervical surgical fields (Fig. 4).

Anatomically, the esophageal muscular tunnel, with its mucosal layer stripped off, provides the shortest route between the abdomen and the neck. Contrary to expectation, such a muscular tunnel readily stretches to accommodate a pulled-through stomach or colon. Not only will this viable esophageal muscular tube not interfere with swallowing, but it will maintain the transposed stomach or colon well aligned, preventing kinking or redundancy.

Indications

(In decreasing order of applicability:)
1. Cancers of the proximal stomach – Following a curative or palliative total

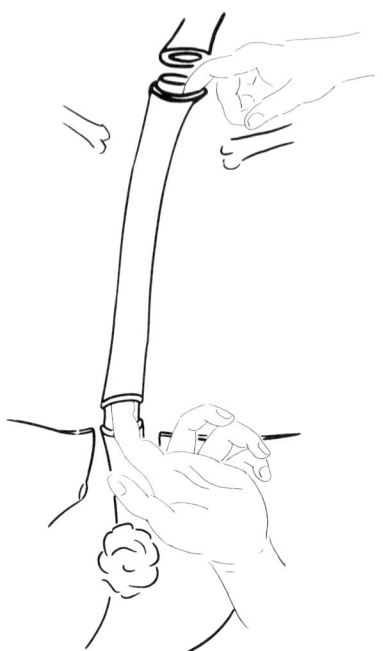 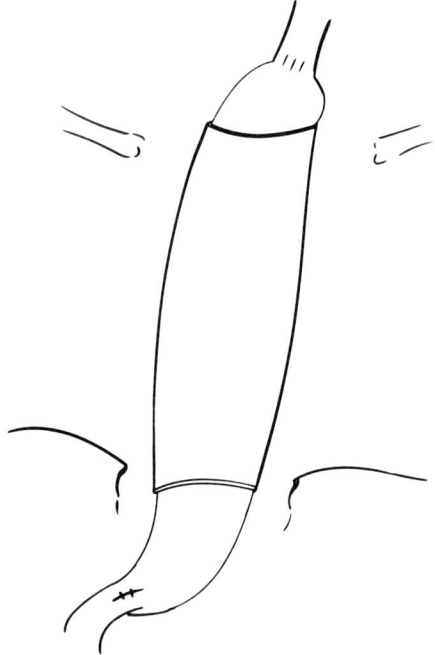

Fig. 1. For small cancers at the cardia, the diaphragmatic hiatus is opened widely and mucosectomy started at a tumor-safe margin proximally. Digital mucosal stripping also begins in the neck. After working with both index fingers simultaneously from above and below in the submucosal layer, the freed-up mucosal layer is transected in the neck. The resected tumor specimen is removed from the abdomen with the attached mucosal sleeve trailing behind out of the muscular layer.

Fig. 2. Same patient as in Fig. 1. Resection has been completed and the mucosal layer has been extracted. A gastric tube has been fashioned from the remaining normal stomach and pulled through the esophageal muscular tunnel to the neck for cervical esophagogastrostomy. Pyloroplasty or pyloromyotomy is optional. This operation is called "EEPT I", having been first performed in ten patients.

gastrectomy, the esophageal mucosa is cored out and a colon loop pulled to the neck providing an adequate gastric reservoir in the least traumatic manner without thoracotomy.

2. Cancers of the cardia and lower esophagus — The tumor area is removed with adequate margins proximally and distally, pulling a gastric tube by the apex of the fundus through the denuded muscular tunnel to the neck for a cervical anastomosis without thoracotomy.

3. Cancers of the cervical esophagus — After total laryngectomy and cervical esophagectomy with or without cervical node dissection, the full length esophageal mucosa is cored out and the whole stomach brought to the neck without a thoracotomy.

4. Cancers of the middle portion of the esophagus — A right thoracotomy is essential for resection under direct vision and to start mucosectomy at a tumor-safe margin proximal to the tumor.

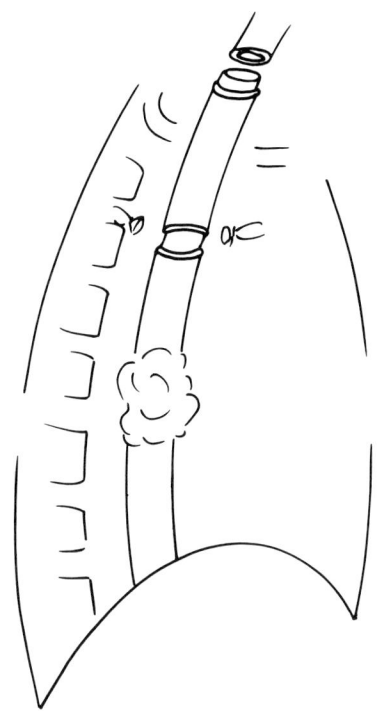
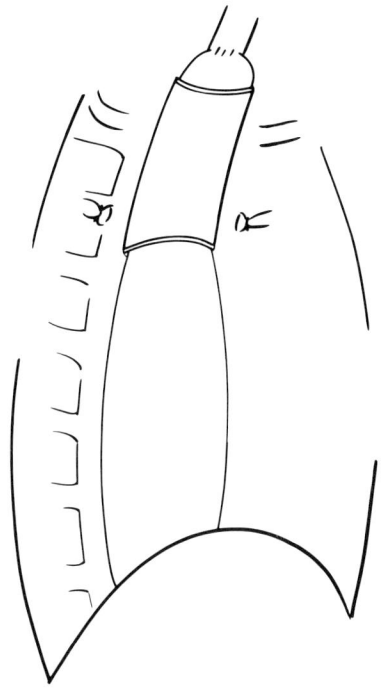

Fig. 3. A mid-esophageal tumor requires a thoracotomy for staging and resection under direct vision. Mucosectomy begins at the level of the divided azygos vein. After mucosal dissection and its transection in the neck, the specimen in the chest with attached short length mucosal sleeve is removed.

Fig. 4. Same patient as in Fig. 3. The whole stomach, mobilized separately through the abdomen either before or after thoracotomy, has been pulled first to the chest and next through the short muscular tunnel into the neck for a cervical esophagostomy. This operation has been called "EEPT II".

Contraindications

1. Cancers of the upper esophagus or thoracic inlet — In these situations not enough length of proximal normal esophagus is available to permit mucosectomy and creation of a muscular tunnel.
2. Pre-existing esophagitis — The submucosal plane has become fibrotic and is usually obliterated, precluding easy mucosectomy.
3. Prior radiotherapy — Same reason as for pre-existing esophagitis.

Technical hints

To begin mucosal dissection either in the abdomen or the neck, the anterior layer of the esophageal muscular layer is first incised down to the mucosal layer, leaving the

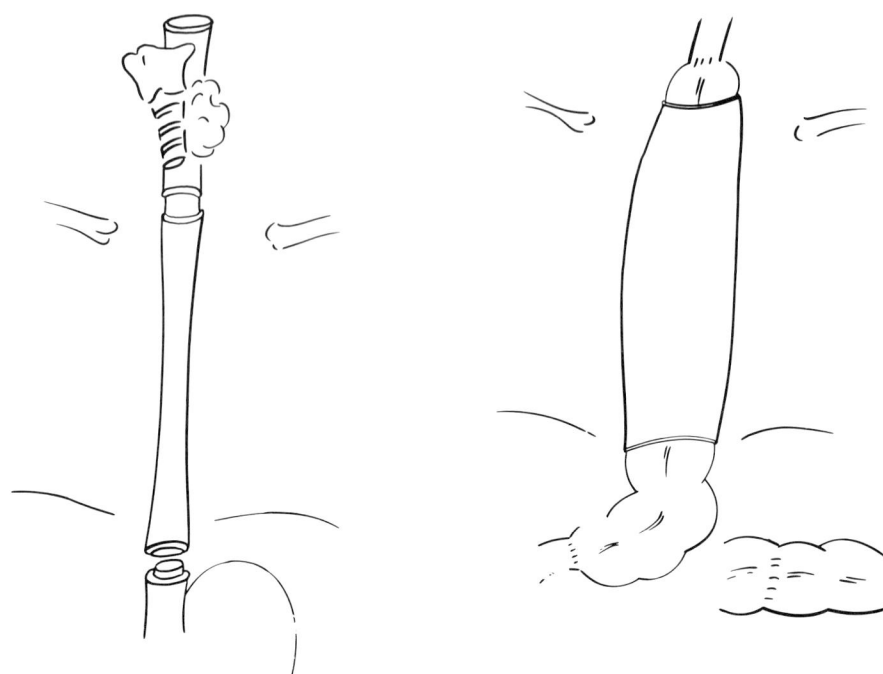

Fig. 5. For cancers of the cervical esophagus a cervical esophagectomy and laryngectomy is required. Mucosal stripping is performed through the neck and abdomen without opening the chest. After transecting the mucosal layer at the gastro-esophageal junction the whole length of esophageal mucosa is extracted through the neck, followed by a pull-through of the whole stomach to the neck for a pharyngogastrostomy. This operation is called "EEPT III".

Fig. 6. For advanced cancers of the proximal stomach, usually nothing less than total gastrectomy can be offered. Esophagojejunostomy has drawbacks. A left colon loop is not only a gastric substitute of ample reservoir capacity, but can be readily pulled through the denuded esophageal muscular tunnel, without opening the chest to the neck for cervical coloesophagostomy. Colo-duodenostomy and colocolostomy re-establishes gastrointestinal continuity. This operation has been called "EEPT IV".

posterior muscle wall temporarily intact to facilitate countertraction. The fingertip is insinuated into the mucosal layer and pushed forward as far as it will go, upwards when working from the abdomen and downwards when dissecting from the neck side. An indwelling nasogastric tube is of help in always keeping the exploring finger in the proper submucosal plane. Digital mucosal stripping must have been completed from both the abdominal and cervical ends before attempting to core out an intact full-length normal esophageal mucosal sleeve [1]. Actual extraction of the mucosal sleeve should never be by force. A steady and gentle pull with a good measure of patience is usually followed by a sudden sensation of a "give", heralding the exit of the full length of the mucosal sleeve.

To avoid entry into the pleural spaces when starting mucosectomy from the abdominal side, the posterior inferior pleural extensions on either side are gently pushed off at the level of the hiatus.

Before attempting pull-through of the mobilized gastric tube or the whole stomach or a colon loop, the denuded esophageal muscular tube, which usually constricts down somewhat, must first be gently dilated digitally: an indwelling nasogastric tube, left behind after extraction of the mucosal sleeve, is grasped in the abdomen and the neck and pulled taut. The surgeon's fingers follow the stretched tube to enter the muscular tunnel from the abdomen and the neck, dilating it gently in a lateral direction [2]. Insertion of feeding jejunostomy is optional.

Mediastinal drainage, either through the abdomen or the neck, is not required. Cervical anastomosis is performed with necessary care to avoid leakage. Occasionally mild to moderate pleural effusion may develop on either side, even if thoracotomy has not been performed, requiring drainage. Oral fluids can be started on the third or fourth postoperative day and advanced to regular diet within a fortnight.

References

1. Saidi F. Ann Surg 1988;207(4):446–454.
2. Saidi F, Behgam Shadmehr M, Khoshnevis-Asl GH. J Thorac Cardiovasc Surg 1991;102(1):43–50.

Follow-up

Is 24-h pH measurement adequate to assess these patients?

T.R. DeMeester, P. Burdiles, H.J. Stein, S.E.A. Attwood
(Los Angeles)

We have shown that Barrett's esophagus is associated with end stage reflux disease characterized by high esophageal acid exposure, gastric hypersecretion, and the loss of esophageal function. Further, 24-h esophageal pH monitoring measured an increase in esophageal exposure to a pH > 7, indicating abnormal esophageal alkaline exposure in addition to the known, increased acid exposure [1] (Fig. 1).

Our studies indicate that the source of the increased esophageal alkaline exposure was duodenal juice refluxed into the stomach and then into the esophagus [3]. Twenty-four hour gastric pH monitoring documented duodenogastric reflux in 42% of the patients with Barrett's esophagus, and half of these had increased esophageal alkaline exposure. Increased esophageal alkaline exposure was never seen in the absence of duodenogastric reflux. It may be that this finding represents the extreme, and that duodenal juice is in the esophagus even when the esophageal pH is less than 7.

To further explore this finding, we evaluated the composition of the refluxed gastric juice in 43 normal volunteers and 52 patients with gastroesophageal reflux disease (GERD) using a newly developed device which allows ambulatory 24-h esophageal aspiration [4]. Compared to normal volunteers, the total bile acid concentration in the reflux aspirates was higher in patients with GERD (p < 0.01), particularly at night (p < 0.01). This occurred only in patients with strictures or Barrett's esophagus (p < 0.01) (Fig. 2).

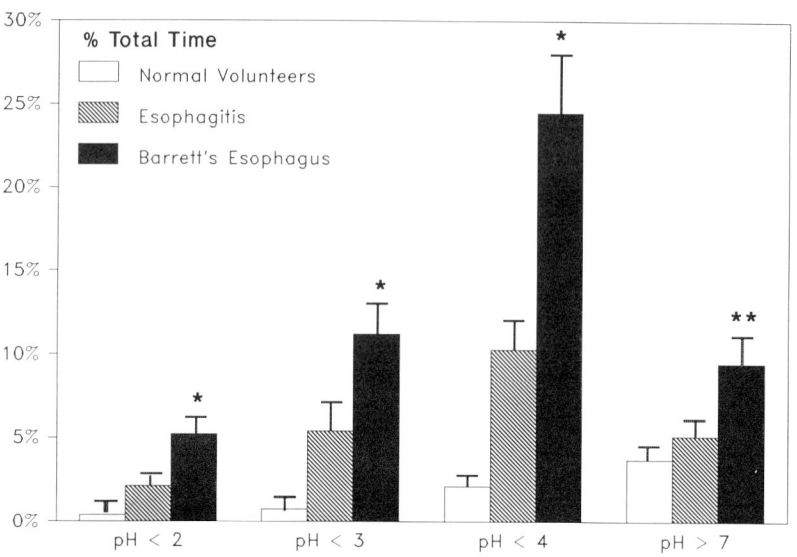

Fig. 1. **Mean** esophageal acid and alkaline exposure on ambulatory 24-h esophageal pH monitoring in normal volunteers, patients with esophagitis, and patients with Barrett's esophagus. *p < 0.01 vs. esophagitis and normal volunteers; **p < 0.05 vs. esophagitis and normal volunteers.

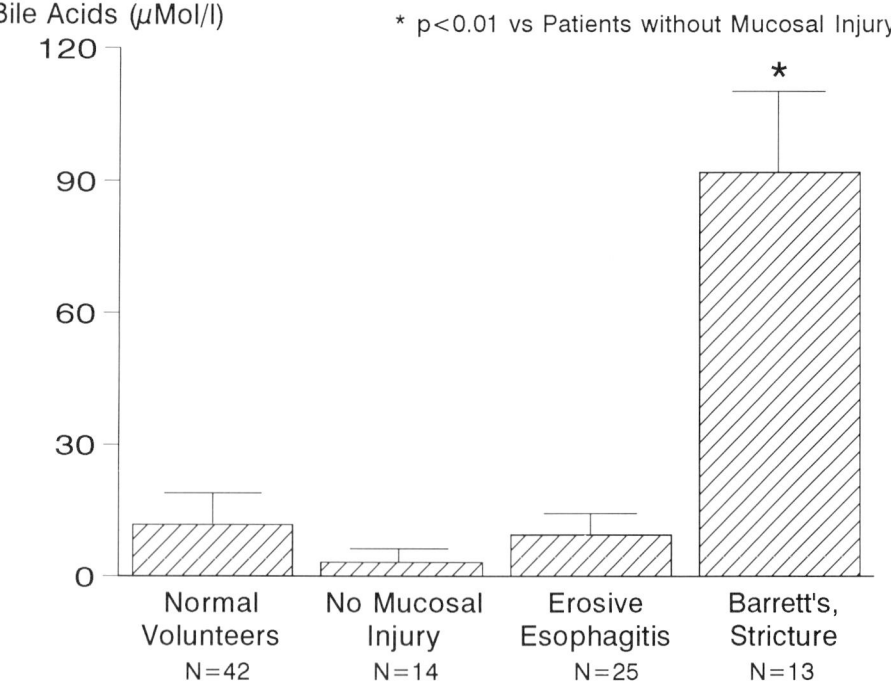

Fig. 2. Total acid bile concentration in esophageal reflux aspirates with various degrees of mucosal injury.

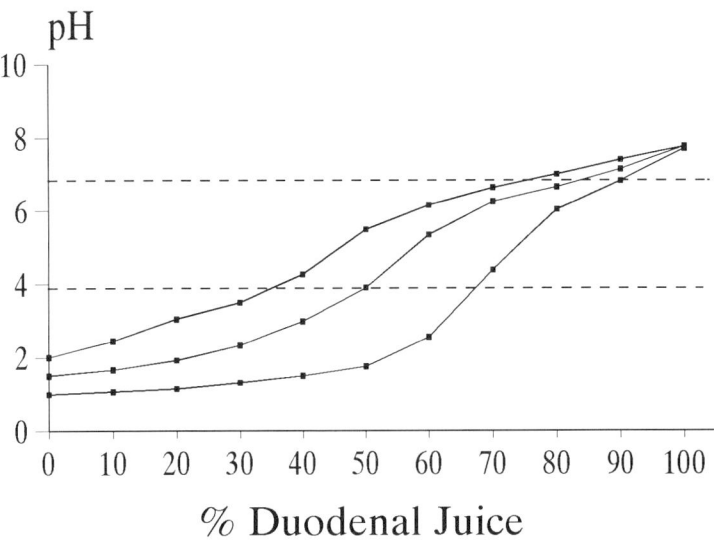

% Duodenal Juice

Dilutions with HCl at pH = 1.0, 1.5 and 2.0

Fig. 3. The pH of gastric juice after various percent dilutions with duodenal juice. Note that dilution with 40–70% duodenal juice can raise the pH of gastric juice, initially measured at 2 or less, to between 4 and 6, the normal pH band of the esophagus. This would make reflux undetectable for pH monitoring.

These data suggest that contamination of the refluxed gastric juice with bile acids occurs in patients with Barrett's esophagus. An increase in the percentage of time that pH was >7 on esophageal pH monitoring in an individual patient suggests biliary reflux. Our data indicate that this usually occurs, but not always, after previous foregut surgery. A normal pH > 7 does not, however, exclude contamination of the refluxed gastric juice with duodenal contents. In a patient with Barrett's esophagus and abnormal duodenogastric reflux, it is possible for reflux to occur through a mechanically defective sphincter, even though the percentage of time the esophageal pH is < 4 is within normal limits. In a recent study we have shown that if gastric juice with a pH of 2 is mixed with 40% duodenal juice, the resulting pH of the material refluxed into the esophagus is above 4 (Fig. 3). Consequently, in the presence of duodenogastric reflux, 24-h pH monitoring may not be adequate to assess the presence of reflux in patients with Barrett's esophagus.

References

1. Stein HJ, Hoeft SF, DeMeester TR. Functional foregut abnormalities in Barrett's esophagus. J Thorac Cardiovasc Surg 1993;105(1):107–111.
2. DeMeester TR, Attwood SEA, Smyrk TC, Therkildsen DH, Hinder RA. Surgical therapy in Barrett's esophagus. Ann Surg 1990;212:528–542.
3. Attwood SEA, Smyrk TC, DeMeester TR, Mirvish SS, Stein HJ, Hinder RA. Duodenoesophageal reflux and the development of esophageal adenocarcinoma in rats. Surgery 1992;111:503–510.

4. Stein HJ, Feussner H, Kauer W, DeMeester TR, Siewert JR. "Alkaline" gastroesophageal reflux — assessment by ambulatory esophageal aspiration and pH monitoring. Am J Surg (in press).

How does Barrett's mucosa heal?

Th.P.J. Hennessy (Dublin)

Barrett's esophagus is a metaplastic epithelial change in which squamous epithelium is replaced by columnar cell epithelium. Robbins and Cotran [1] have defined metaplasia as a *reversible* change in which one adult cell type is replaced by another. Despite the scanty clinical evidence it would seem, therefore, since the condition is alleged to be reversible, that regression of the metaplastic Barrett's epithelium ought to be possible.

Regression of Barrett's epithelium after treatment with omeprazole has been reported by Deviere et al. [2] and Gore et al. [3]. The latter observed both island regression and encroachment of squamous epithelium over the glandular columnar epithelium. This latter form of regression which Skinner [4] also observed in his patients may represent the process by which the new squamous epithelium advances down the esophagus.

Reports of complete regression, however, are rare. In other reports of response to medical treatment, inflammation has subsided and Barrett's ulcers have healed but without evidence of regression.

Antireflux surgery has induced regression in four out of 10 patients reported by Brand [5], and Henrion [6] identified complete regression of columnar epithelium 2.5 years after biliary division. Skinner's patients experienced reversion from dysplastic to nondysplastic epithelium and other patients progressed to regression to squamous epithelium, following antireflux surgery. Nevertheless, several authors reported no regression of metaplastic epithelium after antireflux surgery, and both Williamson [7] and Perniceni [8] concluded that regression of Barrett's epithelium after antireflux surgery was the exception rather than the rule.

Such disparate results are difficult to understand on clinical grounds and both the question of the development of the metaplastic epithelium and its regression are inextricably linked.

Although the derivation of the metaplastic epithelium remains speculative, various suggestions have been put forward. Allison and Johnstone [9] suggested an origin from proximal extension of the columnar epithelium lining the gastroesophageal junction and the cardia. Trier [10] proposed the esophageal mucous glands or embryonic remnants as the source of the ectopic mucosa.

Experimental studies carried out in our department suggest that the metaplastic epithelium is derived from cuboidal cells lining the ducts of the esophageal mucosal glands. In these studies, a fixed sliding hiatus hernia and a Wendel cardioplasty were established in a canine model. A strip of squamous mucosa was then excised from the posterior wall of the lower esophagus proximal to the squamocolumnar junction. A hyperacidity state was then induced by a daily subcutaneous injection of pentagastrin. After 3 months it could be demonstrated that healing of the mucosal defects was by columnar epithelium and that this columnar epithelium arose from the cuboidal cells lining the deeper portion of the esophageal gland ducts.

In the second part of the experiment this columnar epithelium was removed, thus recreating the mucosal defect. The hiatus hernia was then repaired and the cardioplasty reversed. Pentagastrin was discontinued and omeprazole administered. Three months later the mucosal defect had healed largely by columnar epithelium, but on this occasion there were pockets or islands of squamous epithelium present.

The explanation of the different epithelial types involved in the healing of the defect is as follows: the two proximal thirds of these ducts are lined with columnar epithelium and the distal third is lined by squamous epithelium. After stripping off the mucosa the gland ducts are exposed to the surface and luminal contents at varying levels along their length. Where the mucosa has been removed down to the level of the columnar duct lining, attempts at repair will be due to migration of columnar cells from the ducts that will survive in an acid milieu. Where the stripping has been more superficial some squamous duct lining will remain, but attempts at repair by migration of squamous duct cells will fail when reflux is present because the latter will not survive in an acid milieu. However, if the reflux is corrected such migrating squamous cells will give rise to squamous islands. At the junction of the two epithelium types, overlapping can be seen to occur similar to that seen in the clinical situation.

Extrapolating from the experimental to the clinical situation, if the mucosal injury is superficial and squamous duct lining remains, correction of the reflux will allow squamous regression to occur. However, if the mucosal injury has been severe and deep so that no squamous duct lining remains, no regression will be possible even if the reflux is corrected.

The above theory offers an acceptable and logical explanation for island regression, but would not convincingly account for the complete regression reported by some workers. This latter type of regression may be due to distally advancing squamous epithelium growing over the ectopic columnar epithelium in the absence of reflux.

References

1. Robbins SL, Cotran RS. The normal and the adapted cell. In: Robbins SL, Cotran RS (eds) Pathologic Basis of Disease. Philadelphia: W.B. Saunders, 1979;1—21.
2. Devière J, Buset R, Dumonceau JM, Rickaert F, Cremer M. Regression of Barrett's epithelium with omeprazole. N Engl J Med 1989;320:1497—1498.
3. Gore S, Sutton R, Eyre-Brook IA, Gear MWL, Shepherd NA, Wilkinson SP. Regression of columnar epithelium in Barrett's oesophagus with continuous omeprazole. Gut 1990;31:A1191—1192.

4. Skinner DB, Walther BC, Riddell RH, Schmidt H, Iascone C, DeMeester TR. Barrett's esophagus: comparison of benign and malignant cases. Ann Surg 1983;198:554−565.
5. Brand DL, Ylvisaker JT, Gelfand M, Pope CE. Regression of columnar esophageal (Barrett's) epithelium after antireflux surgery. N Engl J Med 1980;302:844−848.
6. Henrion J, Schapira M, Pourbaix A, Heller FR. Régression complète d'un endobrachyoesophage après correction du reflux biliaire chez un malade gastrectomise. Gastroenterol Clin Biol 1989;13:745−746.
7. Williamson WA, Ellis FH, Gibb SP, Shalian DM, Aretz HT. Effect of antireflux operation on Barrett's mucosa. Ann Thorac Surg 1990;49:537−542.
8. Perniceni T, Leymarios J, Molas G et al. Does Barrett's esophagus regress after total duodenal diversion? Gastroenterol Clin Biol 1988;12:709−712.
9. Allison PR, Johnstone AS. The oesophagus lined by gastric mucous membrane. Thorax 1953;8:87−101.
10. Trier JS. Morphology of the epithelium of the distal esophagus in patients with mid-esophageal stricture. Gastroenterology 1970;58:441−461.

What are the histologic criteria that justify claiming the regression of Barrett's esophagus?

J.F. Fléjou (Paris)

Barrett's esophagus is defined as the replacement of the squamous epithelium of the lower esophagus with a metaplastic columnar epithelium (Barrett's mucosa) covering more than 3 cm over the esophagogastric junction. Patients with Barrett's esophagus have an increased risk of esophageal adenocarcinoma of 30 to 125 times as compared to the general population [1]. This risk justifies precise programs of surveillance, with the aim of detecting cancer at an early stage, or especially precancerous dysplasia [2].

Treatments that induce regression and replacement of the metaplastic mucosa with normal squamous epithelium could suppress this risk of cancer. As Barrett's mucosa is a complication of chronic gastroesophageal reflux (GERD), any effective antireflux treatment can theoretically induce the regression of metaplasia; such treatments include drug therapy (antacids, anti-H_2, proton-pump inhibitors) and surgery.

The assessment of regression needs very strict criteria. The diagnosis of Barrett's esophagus is based on endoscopy that shows the characteristic pink columnar mucosa over the esophagogastric junction [2]. In theory, as only manometry is able to locate the lower esophageal sphincter, this technique is mandatory to ascertain the regression of Barrett's mucosa. However, endoscopy with biopsies is now commonly used in routine practice. The biopsies show in Barrett's esophagus a columnar epithelium, either of fundic, cardiac, or "specialized" type; only this latter type is diagnostic of Barrett's mucosa, but it is present in only 80% of the cases [3]. To assert the regression of Barrett's mucosa, endoscopy has to show a decrease in the length of the metaplastic columnar mucosa. After drug therapy, this length can theoretically be assessed by measuring the distance from the incisors to the squamocolumnar junction, keeping in mind the variation of this measurement [4], that has to be compared with the short regression that can be obtained initially. After surgical treatment of GERD, the distance from the incisors to the squamocolumnar junction is increased, making this criterion unusable [5]. Therefore, it is mandatory to have successive multiple biopsy specimens obtained by a "mapping" of the esophagus, with repeated endoscopic examinations performed ideally by the same endoscopist. Only the comparison of specimens obtained at the same site can demonstrate the replacement of the columnar epithelium by squamous epithelium. However, this regression can occur with the development of squamous islands surrounded by columnar epithelium; in such cases, biopsies have to be performed on those islands. The use of an initial endoscopic tattoo with indian ink has been recently proposed [6].

Numerous medical (using anti-H_2) and surgical series have failed to show any regression of Barrett's esophagus under treatment. Among the few surgical reports of regression, most are unreliable due to the methodological problems that have been discussed already [7,8]; only a report by Perniceni et al. demonstrated one case of partial regression after total duodenal diversion that was assessed with a rigorous endoscopic and bioptic protocol [9]. Several medical reports of patients receiving prolonged omeprazole treatment are now available with convincing reports of partial regression of Barrett's esophagus [10−12]. These are, however, preliminary results, not found by other workers [6,13], and there are no data demonstrating a reduction in the cancer risk for the patients involved in such trials. Recent reports presenting regression after laser "ablation" [14,15] and dynamic phototherapy [16] could represent interesting new approaches. In one of the reported cases [15], the regression was assessed by the comparison of one half of Barrett's mucosa treated with laser to the other untreated half.

In conclusion, there is no absolute histological criteria for establishing the regression of Barrett's esophagus. This regression is ascertained using a combination of endoscopic and histological criteria, that require rigorous protocols with repeated systematic mapping of the esophagus.

References

1. Dent J, Bremner CG, Cullen MJ, Haggitt RC, Spechler SJ. Working party report to the world congresses of Gastroenterology, Sydney 1990. Barrett's oesophagus. J Gastroenterol Hepatol 1991;6:1−22

2. Potet F, Fléjou JF, Gervaz E, Paraf F. Adenocarcinomas of the lower oesophagus and the oesophagogastric junction. Sem Diag Pathol 1991;8:126−136.

3. Paull A, Trier JS, Dalton MD, Camp RC, Loeb P, Goyal RK. The histologic spectrum of Barrett's esophagus. N Engl J Med 1976;295:476−480.

4. Kim SL, Waring JP, Spechler SJ et al. Accuracy of esophageal measurements in Barrett's esophagus. Gastroenterology 1993;104:A117.

5. Galmiche JP. Endobrachyoesophage: la régression est-elle possible? La surveillance est-elle justifiée? Gastroenterol Clin Biol 1988;12:705−708.

6. Francis J, Shaffer R, Kadakia S, Carrougher J. Effect of omeprazole on Barrett's epithelium at 3 and 9 months of therapy. Gastroenterology 1993;104:A80.

7. Brand DL, Ylvisaker JT, Gelfand M, Pope CE. Regression of columnar esophageal (Barrett's) epithelium after antireflux surgery. N Engl J Med 1980;302 844−848.

8. Sprung D, Ellis H, Gibb SP. Regression of Barrett's epithelium after antireflux surgery. Am J Gastroenterol 1984;79:A817.

9. Perniceni T, Leymarios J, Molas G. L'endobrachyoesophage régresse-t-il après diversion duodénale totale? Gastroenterol Clin Biol 1988;12:709–712.
10. Devière J, Buset M, Dumonceau J-M, Rickaert F, Cremer M. Regression of Barrett's epithelium with omeprazole. N Engl J Med 1989;320:1497–1498.
11. Gore S, Healey CJ, Sutton R, Sheperd NA, Wilkinson SP. Regression of columnar epithelium in Barrett's oesophagus with omeprazole. Gut 1990;31:A1191.
12. Galmiche J-P, Dumas R, Boyer J et al. Effet de l'omeprazole au long terme sur l'extension de l'endobrachyoesophage. Gastroenterol Clin Biol 1993;17:A43.
13. Bologna S, Blumenkehl M, Schubert TT, Wong D. Barrett's esophagus response to long-term omeprazole therapy. Gastroenterology 1992;102:A2498.
14. Brandt LJ, Kauver DR. Laser-induced transient regression of Barrett's epithelium. Gastrointest Endosc 1992;38:619–622.
15. Sampliner RE, Hixson LJ, Fennerty B, Garewal HS. Regression of Barrett's esophagus by laser ablation in an anacid environment. Dig Dis Sci 1993;38:365–368.
16. Berenson MM, Johnson TD, Markowitz NR, Buchi KN, Samowitz WS. Gastroenterology 1993;104:1686–1691 (abstract).

In which instances is regression of Barrett's esophagus maintained during long-term follow-up?

M. Dei Poli, G. Gasparri (Turin)

The first point is to determine if regression really exists. In literature there are still controversies on this point: Naef and Starnes observed no regression after antireflux surgery; in contrast, Brand, Skinner and Pinotti reported regression after surgery. In our experience, as reported in 1986, the reply to this question is yes.

Seventy-seven patients with Barrett's esophagus were followed from 1980 to 1992. Excluding 18 cases of adenocarcinoma, 59 patients showed columnar epithelium in the esophagus associated with symptoms of reflux. Thirty-one were not operated on and were treated medically; no regression of columnar epithelium in squamous epithelium was seen in this group. Relief of symptoms and ulcer healing were observed in cases treated by anti-H_2, but improvement of stenosis was only seen after treatment with omeprazole. Considering the operated group, 22 Nissen-Rossetti were performed with the same technique, using intraoperative manometry to obtain a LES of 30 ± 4 mmHg, four Belsey-Mark IV, one Lortat-Jacob, one total duodenal diversion. Regression was only observed after Nissen-Rossetti: total in two cases that we prefer not to consider, because of possible endoscopic misinterpretation (pseudoregression because of repositioning the esophagogastric junction can give the appearance of more distal cardias), partial in 12. All these patients were controlled every year by the same group of endoscopists, with endoscopy and biopsy, manometry and 24-h pH-monitoring. The mean period of observation was 7.2 years, with a maximum of 11 years and a minimum of 1 year. If regression appeared, the efficiency of antireflux procedure was always confirmed by manometry and pH-monitoring, as well as by endoscopy and multiple biopsies. This group was composed of eight men and four women, the mean age was 54, the Z-line was preoperatively at 30 cm and the cardias at 37 cm.

In most of the cases with postoperative reflux, regression was not seen. In some others, very few islands of squamous epithelium were found. We almost never observe development of cancer after antireflux procedure: one single patient developed a cancer 12 years after an unsuccessful Nissen.

It is possible to conclude that a successful antireflux procedure can produce partial regression and, if the good results persist, regression of CLE is maintained after very long-term follow-up. Considering ulcer and stenosis, but not regression, our experience shows that a long period of treatment with omeprazole can obtain a healing of this lesion, but not its regression.

What is the proportion of regression of esophagitis and motor disorders of CLE after antireflux surgery?

N.K. Altorki (New York)

The columnar-lined esophagus (CLE) is no longer a medical rarity. The last three decades witnessed a significant increase in the number of new cases of CLE and the prevalence of this disease is estimated at 22 clinically diagnosed cases per 100,000 [1]. Notwithstanding that this increase in prevalence has generally paralleled the widespread use of upper gastrointestinal endoscopy, it is clear that Barrett's esophagus is no longer the rare entity it was once thought to be. The clinical interest in CLE stems directly from its acknowledged premalignant potential [2,3]. Since the initial report by Morson and Belcher of an esophageal adenocarcinoma arising within a columnar-lined esophagus [4], the incidence of Barrett's associated adenocarcinoma has sharply increased and in most major centers in the United States it presently accounts for 30–40% of all esophageal malignancies [5]. This propensity to malignant degeneration inevitably raises issues that pertain to the pathophysiology and pathology of this disorder. This communication attempts to discuss two questions. First, what is the frequency of regression of motor abnormalities after antireflux repair in CLE? Secondly, what is the proportion of regression of esophagitis postoperatively?

Motor disorders and CLE

Several investigators have elegantly demonstrated that CLE is associated with profound disturbances in esophageal motility. These abnormalities in motility involve both the lower esophageal sphincter (LES) as well as the esophageal body. The hallmark of esophageal motility in CLE is a profoundly hypotensive LES. Sphincteric hypotension in CLE was reported by Iascone in 1981 [6] and by other investigators subsequently [7,8], and was noted to be significantly lower than LES pressure in patients with esophagitis. Furthermore, the overall sphincter length and the length of the segment of esophagus exposed to positive intra-abdominal pressure is less than that in control subjects as well as that in patients with uncomplicated gastro-esophageal reflux (GER). Combining sphincter pressure and length as determinants of cardial competence, the prevalence of an incompetent LES in patients with CLE exceeds 90%.

Fewer studies have focused on the abnormalities in motor function of the esophageal body in patients with CLE. Studies utilizing 24-h pH-monitoring in patients with CLE have shown not only an increase in esophageal acid exposure but a markedly impaired clearance function of the esophageal body [6]. Perhaps the characteristically dilated esophagus below a mid-esophageal Barrett's stricture is the radiographic manifestation of the motor abnormality in such instances. Subsequent studies with standard manometry have confirmed that in patients with CLE the mean amplitude of esophageal contractions in the distal half of the esophagus was markedly reduced compared to patients with esophagitis and a corresponding control group [9]. Additionally, patients with CLE had a higher frequency of interrupted (non-propagated) and simultaneous contractions. These latter findings were confirmed by 24-h esophageal motility [10]. CLE patients had a significantly higher frequency of low amplitude and simultaneous contractions when compared to patients with esophagitis and control subjects. These motor disorders of the esophageal body may account for the increased prevalence of dysphagia in patients with nonmalignant CLE.

There is little or no information on the effect of antireflux repairs on motor disturbances of the LES or esophageal body. Williamson reported on preoperative and postoperative LES pressures in 26 out of 37 patients with CLE, who underwent antireflux repair [11]. Normalization of LES pressures occurred in 73% of patients and improvement to at least 10 mmHg occurred in another 19% on immediate postoperative measurements. Unfortunately, there are no reports on the long-term effects of antireflux repairs on LES pressure. The effect of antireflux repairs on motor disorders in the esophageal body are even less well studied, at least partly due to the fact that these disorders have only recently been defined. However, a body of indirect evidence suggests a salutary effect of antireflux repair. Skinner reported on 10 patients with CLE who underwent either a Nissen or Belsey Mark IV repair who submitted to 24-h pH-monitoring 2–7 years postoperatively [12]. Reflux episodes lasting more than 5 min occurred in 3/10 patients postoperatively, compared to 9/10 patients prior to antireflux repair. These findings suggest a restoration of clearance function to the esophageal body once GER is effectively eliminated. Further indirect evidence can be inferred from studies on the postoperative effect of fundoplication in patients with GER without CLE. Gill and associates assessed esophageal manometry before and after fundoplication in a group of 32 patients with GER and compared them with 18 healthy control subjects [13]. Fundoplication resulted in a significant elevation in LES pressure which was not statistically different from LES pressure in the control group. Additionally, after antireflux repair the mean amplitude of esophageal contraction was increased significantly at all levels within the esophagus and approached values seen in healthy controls. Both the duration of contractions and peristaltic velocity approached control values and were significantly improved beyond preoperative levels. The postoperative resolution of manometric abnormalities associated with gastroesophageal reflux disease (GERD) has been reported by other investigators [14] and suggests that the motor dysfunction is a consequence of reflux rather than an initiating factor. One can assume that similar improvement in motor function of the esophageal body and sphincter can occur following antireflux repair for patients with CLE, but the extent of resolution may be influenced by the severity of the preoperative dysfunction. A controlled prospective study would be required to prove this hypothesis.

Esophagitis and CLE

Patients with CLE may have no significant inflammation above the squamocolumnar junction. In the majority of patients the indication for operation is severe reflux symptoms, while the remainder are operated on for Barrett's stricture or rarely for ulcers within the columnar lining itself. Williamson reported resolution of "esophagitis" in 30/37 patients, but did not document the presence and severity of preoperative esophagitis [11]. In that report, 23 patients were operated on for severe reflux symptoms, nine for strictures, four for nonhealing ulcers and one for bleeding. It thus appears that the salient question is not the regression of esophagitis above the squamocolumnar junction (an infrequent event) but rather the regression of the columnar metaplasia which itself may be a measure of esophageal injury.

There is considerable clinical and experimental evidence to support the acquired theory for CLE [6,12]. However, one cannot readily exclude the possibility of a genetic predisposition. The rare but definite occurrence of a familial clustering of patients with CLE lends support to a congenital origin [15]. Importantly, despite the wide prevalence of GERD and endoscopic esophagitis, CLE occurs in only 10–15% of all patients [3]. One should consider GER and CLE to be highly associated disorders without a definite proof of a teleological relationship. It is thus not surprising that regression of the columnar metaplasia is the exception rather than the rule. Most cases of reported regression are partial, and there is as yet no reported case where complete regression occurred after surgical or medical antireflux therapy. Skinner reported a phenomenon whereby the squamous epithelium overgrows areas of columnar metaplasia [12]. However, the fate of the submerged metaplastic epithelium and its premalignant potential remain unknown. The same phenomenon has also been described by Gayet and is said to occur in 25% of patients following adequate reflux control [16]. This phenomenon has not been described by others.

Williamson reported that no patient in his series had complete regression and that 4/37 (11%) had partial regression, defined as regenerating squamous mucosa infiltrating areas of columnar mucosa and accompanied by a decrease of 3 cm or greater in the length of the CLE [11].

The confusion surrounding the issue of regression of CLE stems from the lack of a universal definition of regression and the absence of well controlled studies. Does regression imply a receding squamocolumnar junction or is it the outgrowth of squamous epithelium from squamous islands within the CLE? I believe it to be the latter, particularly since islands of squamous epithelium have been noted in untreated patients with CLE as well as autopsy specimens [1]. In either event, endoscopy in the early postoperative period is mandatory since any of the commonly performed antireflux procedures will likely relocate the cardia caudally into the abdomen and thus alter the preoperative level of the squamocolumnar junction. Naturally, a Collis gastroplasty done in conjunction with an antireflux repair will only add to that confusion. A postoperative endoscopy with accurate mapping of the metaplastic segment would thus serve as an essential postoperative baseline against which one assesses the possibility of regression on follow-up. Additionally, one has to ascertain the adequacy of the newly created antireflux barrier by objective criteria. Neither symptomatology nor manometry should be acceptable criteria for assessing reflux control in patients with CLE. Indeed, the former is notoriously misleading in such patients due to the established acid insensitivity of the metaplastic epithelium, and the latter lacks a one-on-one correlation. Twenty-four-hour pH-monitoring should therefore be done within a few months postoperatively and periodically thereafter. Finally, given the relative infrequency of patients with CLE, especially those coming for operation, a multicenter collaborative study with long-term follow-up is essential for adequately addressing the question of regression.

References

1. Cameron AJ, Zinsmeister AR, Ballard DJ, Carney JA. Prevalence of columnar-lined (Barrett's) esophagus. Gastroenterology 1990;99:918–922.
2. Bozymski EM, Herlihy KJ, Orlando RC. Barrett's esophagus. Ann Intern Med 1982;97:103–107.
3. Naef AP, Savary M, Ozzello L. Columnar-lined lower esophagus, an acquired lesion with malignant predisposition: report on 140 cases of Barrett's esophagus with 12 adenocarcinomas. J Thorac Cardiovasc Surg 1975;70(5):826–835.
4. Morson BC, Belcher JR. Adenocarcinoma of the oesophagus and ectopic gastric mucosa. Br J Cancer 1952;6;127–130.
5. Blot WJ, Devessa SS, Knellen RW, Fraumeni JF Jr. Rising incidence of adenocarcinoma of the esophagus and cardia. JAMA 1991;265(10);1287–1289.
6. Iascone C, DeMeester TR, Little AG, Skinner DB. Barrett's esophagus: functional assessment, proposed pathogenesis, and surgical therapy. Arch Surg 1983;118:543–549.
7. Zaninotto G, DeMeester TR, Schwizer W et al. The lower esophageal sphincter in health and disease. Am J Surg 1988;155; 104–109.
8. Zaninotto G, DeMeester TR, Bremner CG et al. Esophageal function in patients with reflux-induced strictures and its relevance to surgical treatment. Ann Thorac Surg 1989;47:362–370.
9. DeMeester TR, Attwood SEA, Smyrk TC, Therkildsen DH, Hinder RA. Surgical therapy in Barrett's esophagus. Ann Surg 1990;212:528–542.
10. Stein HJ, Hoeft S, DeMeester TR. Functional foregut abnormalities in Barrett's esophagus. J Thorac Cardiovasc Surg 1993;105:107–111.
11. Williamson WA, Ellis FH Jr, Gibb SP, Aretz HT. Effect of antireflux operation on Barrett's mucosa. Ann Thorac Surg 1990;49:537–542.
12. Skinner DB, Walther BC, Riddell RH, Schmidt H, Iascone C, DeMeester TR. Barrett's esophagus: comparison of benign and malignant cases. Ann Surg 1983;198:554–566.

13. Gill RC, Bowes KL, Murphy PD, Kingma YJ. Esophageal motor abnormalities in gastroesophageal reflux and the effects of fundoplication. Gastroenterology 1986;91:364–369.
14. Russell COH, Pope CE, Gannan RM, Allen FD, Velasco N, Hill LD. Does surgery correct esophageal motor dysfunction in gastroesophageal reflux? Ann Surg 1981;194;290–296.
15. Fahmy N, King JF. Barrett's esophagus: an acquired condition with genetic predisposition. Am J Gastroenterol 1993;88: 1262–1265.
16. Gayet B. Barrett's esophagus; VIth International Post Graduate Course on Esophageal Diseases, Albano, Italy, March 22, 1990 (abstract).

Does suppression of reflux protect against subsequent malignant change?

R.E. Sampliner (Tucson)

Barrett's esophagus is recognized as a premalignant lesion — a metaplastic step that can lead to the development of adenocarcinoma of the esophagus. It is important to separate two processes: metaplasia and neoplasia. Metaplasia — Barrett's esophagus of the specialized type — develops as a result of injury to the squamous lining of the esophagus in the setting of gastroesophageal reflux disease (GERD). Neoplasia occurs on the background of this metaplastic process. Dysplasia and ultimately adenocarcinoma of the esophagus develop as a result of cell cycle abnormalities and genomic instability. It would be reasonable to assume that control of GERD may prevent the development or the progression of the *metaplastic* process. However, there is no reason to expect that control of reflux will effect the *neoplastic process*. If profound acid suppression results in complete regression of Barrett's esophagus — which has not been proven to date — then one could assume that neoplasia would not develop.

In the preproton pump inhibitor era, pharmacologic therapy has not had an impressive impact in Barrett's esophagus [1,2]. It is too early to draw a conclusion on the impact of proton pump inhibition. Although there are favorable early reports [3,4], there are other trials that have failed to show a systematic response over a period of 1–2 years of therapy [5,6].

The surgical experience may provide the best evidence that suppression of reflux will fail to protect against subsequent malignant change. In perhaps the best documented case, the patient underwent subtotal resection of Barrett's esophagus with a colonic interposition. Prolonged pH probe recording failed to show abnormal acid exposure yet the patient developed adenocarcinoma in the remnant of Barrett's esophagus [7]. Many other cases of adenocarcinoma of the esophagus after antireflux surgery are scattered in the surgical literature with lesser documentation of ablation of esophageal acid exposure [8–10].

Suppression of reflux has not been proven to protect against malignant change and may not be expected to on a theoretical basis.

References

1. Sampliner RE, Garewal HS, Fennerty MB et al. Lack of impact of therapy on extent of Barrett's esophagus in 67 patients. Dig Dis Sci 1990;35:93—96.
2. Cameron AJ, Lomboy CT. Barrett's esophagus: age, prevalence, and extent of columnar epithelium. Gastroenterology 1992;103:1241—1245.
3. Devière J, Buset M, Dumonceau J-M et al. Regression of Barrett's epithelium with omeprazole. N Engl J Med 1989;320:1497—1498.
4. Gore S, Healey CJ, Sutton R et al. Regression of columnar lined (Barrett's) esophagus with continuous omeprazole therapy. Gastroenterology 1992;102:A75.
5. Sampliner RE, Mackel C, Jennings D et al. Effect of 12 months of a proton pump inhibitor (lansoprazole) on Barrett's esophagus — a randomized trial. Gastroenterology 1992;102:A157.
6. Bologna S, Blumenkehl M, Schubert TT et al. Barrett's esophagus response to long-term omeprazole therapy. Gastrointest Endosc 1992;38:A229.
7. Hamilton SR, Hutcheon DF, Ravitch WJ et al. Adenocarcinoma in Barrett's esophagus after elimination of gastroesophageal reflux. Gastroenterology 1984;86:356—360.
8. Haggitt RC, Tryzelaar J, Ellis FH et al. Adenocarcinoma complicating columnar epithelium-lined (Barrett's) esophagus. Am J Clin Pathol 1978;70:1—5.
9. Cameron AJ, Ott BJ, Payne WS. The incidence of adenocarcinoma in columnar lined (Barrett's) esophagus. N Engl J Med 1985;311:857—859.
10. Williamson WA, Ellis FH, Gibb SP. Effect of antireflux operation on Barrett's mucosa. Ann Thorac Surg 1990;49:537—542.

Is brush cytology an acceptable alternative to endoscopic examination with biopsies in a surveillance program?

M. Schapiro (Los Angeles)

This question presupposes that the techniques of endoscopic biopsy and brush cytology are mutually exclusive which indeed they are not.

Follow-up of patients with Barrett's esophagus requires more than endoscopic surveillance. Histologic surveillance for dysplastic change is the benchmark upon which decisions concerning medical and surgical therapy are made. When the endoscope is in place it is nearly always appropriate to obtain multiple biopsies at interval and target sites now more clearly defined by emerging guidelines [1].

The addition of mucosal brushing in order to obtain cytological material to enable a larger surface area to be sampled in the surveillance program has theoretical advantage, but is not universally carried out or frequently recommended. Mapping studies have shown that dysplasia can involve variable areas of the mucosa. A thorough sampling of the Barrett's mucosa must be carried out in order to adequately survey for dysplasia or carcinoma. The substitution of cytological brushing for biopsy predisposes that a satisfactory cost saving, nonendoscopic procedure is readily available to obtain reliable samples for surveillance.

The reliance on cytological material for a diagnosis of dysplasia has not been the subject of prospective trials. In two retrospective studies, the correlation between biopsy and cytology was good and cytology was shown to be diagnostic in the absence of associated positive biopsy [2,3]. In one of these studies [3], brushings revealed a higher incidence of carcinoma and a higher grade of dysplasia than biopsy. The overall agreement between the two techniques was 72%. These authors have described criteria for the cytological diagnosis of dysplasia, however, their validity has not been confirmed in prospective studies.

Brush cytology is directly dependent upon the cytology rendering. In addition to sampling errors, the diagnosis of significant dysplasia should be made with caution when the characteristic changes do not involve the mucosal surface. The differentiation between reactive change due to inflammation is difficult, and should be correlated with histologic and endoscopic evidence concerning active inflammation. Since carcinoma begins in the crypts, the surface epithelium may be normal when significant dysplasia is present in the crypts.

For these reasons it is not appropriate at this time to recommend the substitution of cytological collection techniques for surveillance of patients with Barrett's esophagus. The two techniques of biopsy and brush cytology are, however, complementary. It does appear that a greater number of cases associated with severe dysplasia or carcinoma will be diagnosed by the combination rather than by either technique alone. It is hoped that newer collection techniques may offer reliable, comfortable, and lower cost screening in this patient population. Prospective trials will be required to determine this.

It is interesting to speculate on the value of such a program for mass screening of patients symptomatic for gastroesophageal reflux disease (GERD), as has been carried out in China [4]. However, there is no evidence that such a program has any clinical merit in developed areas where endoscopy is readily available, or that there would be cost-effective consequences. The suggestion has been made that blind non-endoscopically directed cytology collections performed by paramedical personnel in known Barrett's patients could be substituted for endoscopic surveillance with cost savings [5]. This approach has not been tested, is less direct, and requires some form of naso-esophageal intubation to gather cytologic material. These techniques have for the most part been abandoned due to poor patient acceptance compared to endoscopy with sedation. This discussion will therefore focus on the more usual circumstance of the addition of brush cytology to the program of mucosal biopsy.

When ulcerative and plaque-like lesions are associated with Barrett's mucosa, target biopsy is carried out, frequently with the addition of brush cytology. The intervening Barrett's mucosa should be thoroughly sampled with four-quadrant biopsies carried out at 2 cm intervals [6]. The addition of brush cytology to the intervening mucosa can identify metaplastic epithelium within the tubular esophagus, as there is a good correlation of histological and cytological diagnosis [2].

References

1. American Society for Gastrointestinal Endoscopy. The role of endoscopy in the surveillance of premalignant conditions of the upper gastrointestinal tract. Guidelines for clinical application. Gastrointest Endosc 1988;34:185–205.
2. Robey SS, Hamilton SR, Gupta PK et al. Diagnostic value of cytopathology in Barrett's esophagus and associated carcinoma. Am J Clin Pathol 1988;89:493–498.

3. Geisinger KR, Teot LA, Richter JE. A comparative cytopathologic and histologic study of atypia, dysplasia and adeno-carcinoma in Barrett's esophagus. Cancer 1992;69:8–16.
4. Shu YJ. Cytopathology of the esophaus. An overview of esophageal cytopathology in China. Acta Cytol 1983;27:7–16.
5. Richter JE. Endoscopic surveillance of Barrett's esophagus: another viewpoint. Am J Gastroenterol 1993;88:630–632.
6. Reid BJ, Weinstein WM, Lewin KJ, Haggit RC et al. Endoscopic biopsies diagnose high-grade dysplasia or early operable adenocarcinoma in Barrett's esophagus without grossly recognizable neoplastic lesions. Gastroenterology 1988;94:81–90.

Should colonoscopy be routinely performed during follow-up for Barrett's esophagus?

S.J. Sontag (Hines)

In 1984, we discovered two patients with adenocarcinoma of the colon and concomitant Barrett's esophagus. Because of the possible relationship between colonic cancer and the columnar-lined esophagus, we hypothesized that patients with Barrett's esophagus may have a higher prevalence of colonic cancer than the general population. We therefore studied prospectively [1], all of our patients with Barrett's esophagus by means of colonoscopy.

We performed colonoscopy on 65 patients with Barrett's esophagus (Fig. 1). Overall, 29.2% of the patients with Barrett's had benign colon adenomas, 15.4% had malignant tumors, and 55.4% had no neoplasms. Further statistical analysis was required, however, to appropriately deal with selection bias. After deleting from analysis the two index cases that initially alerted us to the possible relationship, the five patients who had had previous hemicolectomy for colon cancer, and the three patients who had had previous polypectomy for benign adenomas, we were left with 55 patients with Barrett's esophagus at potential risk for colon cancer. In these 55 patients, three had malignant tumors (5.5%) and 16 had benign adenomas (29%). Because we had no adequate control group of patients at risk for colon cancer and because the true prevalence rate of colon cancer in the general population was not known, we could conclude only that the 5.5% prevalence rate that we discovered in patients with Barrett's esophagus appeared elevated above that which would be expected in the general population. An attempted analysis was made, however, and a very conservative estimate of the prevalence rate of colon cancer, based on the age-adjusted incidence, was determined to be 40 new cases of colon cancer per year per 100,000 males of this age; or an incidence of 0.04%. We determined that, even if the prevalence of colon cancer in men of that age group was assumed to be 1% (25 times the incidence), the probability of finding eight or more colon cancers in 63 randomly selected patients (by binomial expansion) was less than one-in-a-million. Even a more conservative approach, utilizing three of 58 patients with Barrett's esophagus, still resulted in a p = 0.02 value, still a statistically significant difference. We suggested that colonoscopy to detect colonic tumors in patients with Barrett's esophagus might be more rewarding than frequent esophagoscopies to detect early esophageal carcinoma in the Barrett's epithelium.

Since our publication, at least four other studies have been published [2–5] (Fig. 2). One of the studies [3] reported a 9% prevalence rate of colon cancer (three out of 32 patients) and a 25% prevalence rate of benign adenomas (eight out of 32 patients). In three studies [2,4,5], no cancers were found in a total of 97 patients.

All five studies had deficiencies: the numbers of patients were small [1–5]; Barrett's was not defined [4]; and the presence of Barrett's was questionable, with seven out of 36 patients having only gastric columnar epithelium [2].

It is quite possible that the positive relationship reported by us was due to a hidden bias and did not represent a true relationship between Barrett's and colon cancer. Indeed, Berkson's fallacy (which states that the interplay of differential admission rates from an underlying population to a study group can result in an artificial association in the study group) may well explain the powerful relationship we reported between Barrett's esophagus and colon cancer [6].

Until the true prevalence of colonic tumors in the general population is known, and until appropriate control groups are studied in larger clinical trials, the true relationship, if any, between Barrett's esophagus and colon cancer will not be known. Until that time, however, the results of our 1985 study should not be used to justify colonoscopy on all patients with Barrett's esophagus.

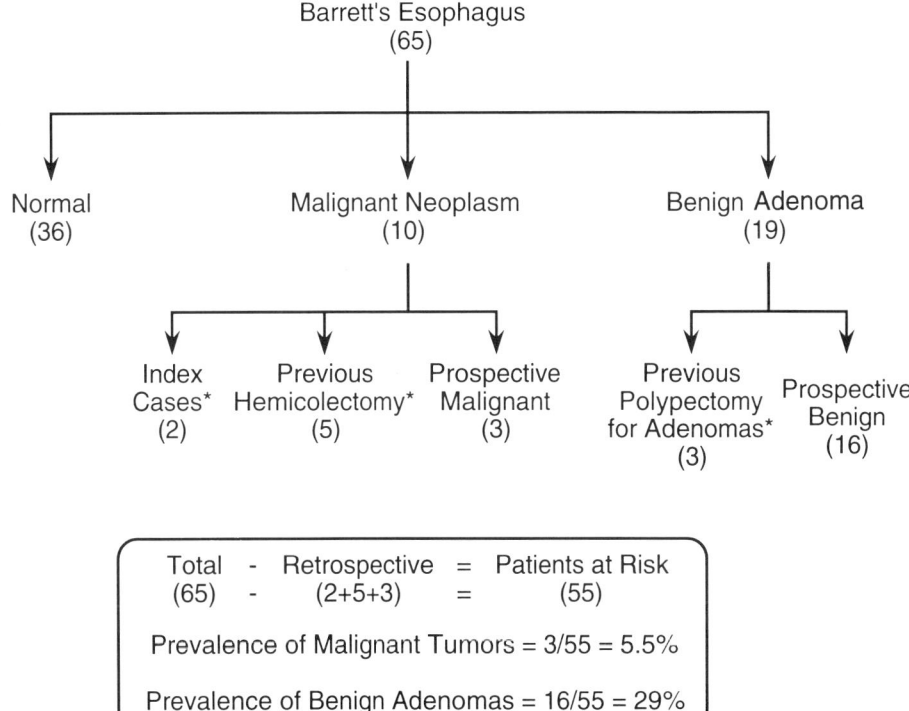

Fig. 1.

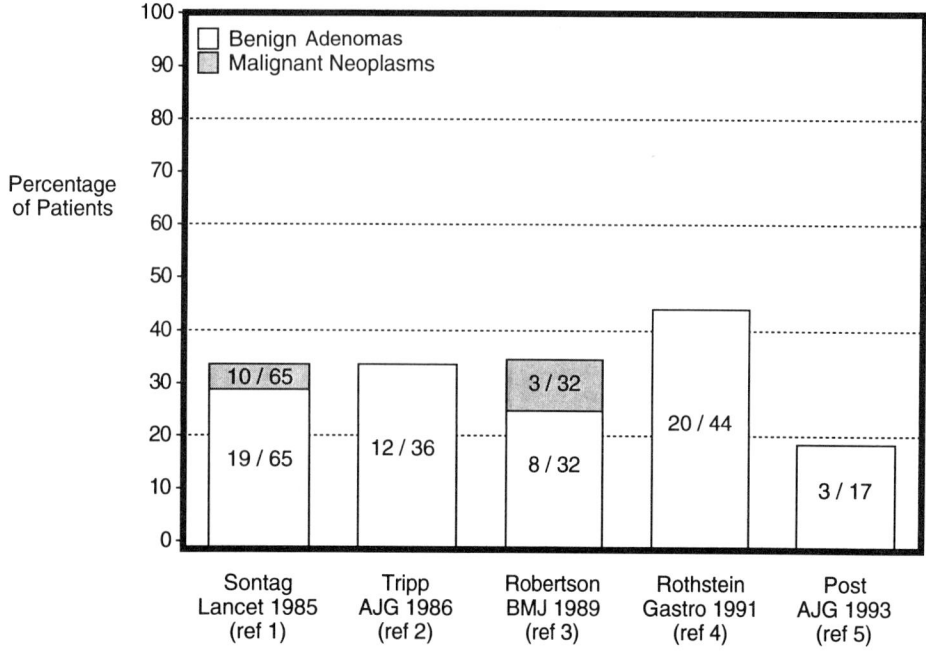

Fig. 2. Prevalence of colon neoplasia in patients with Barrett's esophagus.

A large multicenter study will be needed to determine any true relationship between Barrett's esophagus and colon cancer, if one truly exists.

Conclusions

In 1985, we reported a statistically significant relationship between colon neoplasia and Barrett's esophagus. One subsequent study supports our findings, but three others do not. Until large, well-controlled clinical studies are performed, any relationship between colon neoplasia and Barrett's esophagus should be considered as unproven. We do not recommend colonoscopy in patients, based on the presence of Barrett's esophagus.

References

1. Sontag SJ, Schnell TG, Chejfec G et al. Barrett's oesophagus and colonic tumors. Lancet 1985;1:946–948.
2. Tripp MR, Sampliner RE, Kogan KJ et al. Colorectal neoplasms and Barrett's esophagus. Am J Gastroenterol 1986;81: 1063–1064.
3. Robertson DA, Ayres AC, Smith CC. Screening for colonic cancer in patients with Barrett's oesophagus. Br Med J 1989;298:650.
4. Rothstein RI, Smith RE, Power GC. Barrett's esophagus and colonic neoplasia. Gastroenterology 1991;100(5):A150.
5. Post AB, Achkar E, Carey WD. Prevalence of colonic neoplasia in patients with Barrett's esophagus. Am J Gastroenterol 1993;88(6):877–880.
6. Berkson J. The statistical study of association between smoking and lung cancer. Mayo Clin Proc 1955;30:319–324.

The dysplastic mucosa

The dysplastic mucosa

 ## What factors are involved in effective endoscopic monitoring?

M. Schapiro (Los Angeles)

There must be a standardized approach for the endoscopic examination with biopsies in patients with Barrett's esophagus. This plan needs to provide an accurate description of the metaplastic mucosal zone, an appropriate and consistent plan to obtain histological and cytological material, consideration for the use of chromoendoscopy and an appraisal of the degree and extent of any associated mucosal inflammation.

Metaplastic mucosal zone

Barrett's esophagus is defined by the presence of goblet cell columnar epithelium within the esophagus. The length of the area of squamous epithelium replacement by this metaplastic process (Barrett's zone) is defined by measuring in centimeters the extent of esophageal involvement by this process. The accurate and consistent accomplishment of this determination requires the measurement of the number of centimeters from the incisor teeth to the region of the lower esophageal sphincter (LES) as well as the measurement to the proximally relocated squamo-columnar junction (Z line). Though sniffing and breathing techniques may be utilized to identify more clearly the diaphragmatic pinch, this should not be confused with the LES. It is not always possible to define this area. If the LES region is not evident, the number of centimeters to the tapering off of the gastric folds in the hiatus hernia is used [1]. Aspiration of air from this hiatal hernia segment will make the presence of these folds more prominent.

Following the accurate measurements of these landmarks, the endoscopist must describe the degree of circumferential involvement by the metaplastic epithelium and the amount of squamous mucosa remaining within the Barrett's zone. The distance to plaques, ulcerations and strictures, if present, is recorded and a notation made if irregular mucosal tongues of metaplastic mucosa are present at the upper margin of the zone. When short tongues of columnar epithelium extend upward from the region defined as the LES, it is not possible to determine if this represents a short segment of Barrett's mucosa or an irregular Z line without biopsy and appropriate histologic determination of goblet cells contained within the columnar epithelium.

Histologic and cytologic specimens

A protocol for obtaining biopsies must take into account the variable areas of dysplastic involvement which may occur within the metaplastic zone. If dysplasia is limited in extent, a thorough sampling of the Barrett's mucosa must be carried out in order not to miss small areas of dysplasia or early carcinoma. It is common practice to obtain biopsy specimens with the standard forceps through the 2.8 mm channel of the standard endoscope. More generous samples may be obtained with the "jumbo" pinch biopsy forceps when a large channel "therapeutic" endoscope is available [2]. The entire extent of the Barrett's mucosa should be thoroughly sampled with four-quadrant biopsies carried out at 2 cm intervals [3]. The first specimen should be obtained from the proximal stomach just below the region of the LES in order to be certain that the distal portion of the metaplastic mucosa is evaluated. When ulcerative and plaque-like lesions are associated with Barrett's mucosa target biopsy is carried out frequently with the addition of brush cytology. The final specimens should be obtained from the squamous mucosa at the proximally displaced Z line.

The addition of brush cytology to the intervening mucosa can identify metaplastic epithelium within the tubular esophagus as there is a good correlation of histological and cytological diagnosis [4]. The reliance on this cytological material for a diagnosis of dysplasia has not been the subject of prospective trials. However, in two recent retrospective studies the correlation between biopsy and cytology was good and cytology was shown to be diagnostic in the absence of associated positive biopsy [4,5].

Each of the biopsy specimens must be separately labeled and sent for processing so that if rebiopsy is necessary, the area may be identified and target biopsy obtained. Multiple specimen containers and sufficient paramedical assistance are necessary to accomplish this with accuracy and with a minimum of delay time to the usually sedated patient.

Chromoendoscopy

The Barrett's mucosa is a specialized intestinal metaplasia with goblet cells and, as such, has an increased affinity to take up dyes such as toluidine (or methylene) blue. The technique of direct application of the dye to the mucosa (chromoendoscopy) has been utilized to detect areas of intestinal metaplasia in the stomach [6]. This procedure may be applied to the esophagus for the purpose of performing biopsy on areas demonstrating intense staining. An appropriate acid pH is provided through the application of weak acidic acid. The reaction is akin to the frequently performed histological staining technique utilizing Alcian blue pH 2.5. With this technique intestinal type goblet cells containing acid mucin stain blue, while the normal gastric type columnar cells do not stain. Chromoendoscopy with toluidine blue may be considered when attempts are indicated to try to more precisely localize areas of metaplastic epithelium in cases of a suspected short Barrett's zone. Biopsy here, of areas of mucosa taking up the dye, should demonstrate metaplastic epithelium. Since dysplastic epithelium is frequently associated with a diminution or depletion of goblet cell mucin, the staining characteristics of Barrett's mucosa associated with dysplasia may offer variations that also allow target biopsy to areas of decreased uptake of the blue dye within the Barrett's zone.

Inflammation evaluation

The diagnosis of dysplasia is difficult in the inflamed mucosa. When inflammation is present, particularly when associated with linear tongue-like erosions, biopsies may be impossible to differentiate from reactive change. In these circumstances the patient should receive intense medical treatment, usually with an ATPase pump inhibitor agent, and the procedure rescheduled. The tongue-like mucosal projections may then be differentiated from a normal Z line with biopsy, and areas of dysplasia within the Barrett's zone more reliably diagnosed.

References

1. McClave SA, Boyce HW Jr, Gottfried MR. Early diagnosis of columnar-lined esophagus: a new endoscopic diagnostic criterion. Gastrointest Endosc 1987,33:413—416.
2. McArdle JE, Klaus JL, Randall G, Weinstein WM. Distribution of dysplasias and early invasive carcinoma in Barrett's esophagus. Hum Pathol 1992;23:479—482.
3. Reid BJ, Weinstein WM, Lewin KJ, Haggit RC et al. Endoscopic biopsies diagnose high grade dysplasia or early operable adenocarcinoma in Barrett's esophagus without grossly recognizable neoplastic lesions. Gastroenterology 1988;94:81—90.
4. Robey SS, Hamilton SR, Gupta PK et al. Diagnostic value of cytopathology in Barrett's esophagus and associated carcinoma. Am J Clin Pathol 1988;89:493—498.
5. Geisinger KR, Teot LA, Richter JE. A comparative cytopathologic and histologic study of atypia, dysplasia and adenocarcinoma in Barrett's esophagus. Cancer 1992;69:8—16.
6. Fennerty MB, Sampliner RE, McGee DL et al. Intestinal metaplasia of the stomach: identification by a selective mucosal staining technique. Gastrointest Endosc 1992;38:696—698.

Is alkaline reflux more common in patients with dysplasia?

T.C. Smyrk (Omaha)

I do not know if alkaline reflux is more common in patients with dysplasia. The idea is attractive on theoretical grounds, and there is experimental evidence to support it, but it has not been proven.

Bremner first proposed that bile reflux contributed to ulceration in Barrett's esophagus [1]. Gillen extended the concept to other complications, such as stricture and dysplasia, by showing that 11 patients with complicated Barrett's esophagus had higher postprandial bile acid concentrations than seven patients with uncomplicated Barrett's [2]. Others have argued that bile acids do not reflux into the esophagus and have questioned the validity of the commonly used enzymatic assay for bile acids [3].

More recent studies have used esophageal pH as a marker of alkaline reflux, but there is debate about whether episodic elevations in esophageal pH reflect an effect of refluxed alkaline material or saliva and esophageal secretions. Singh et al. recently presented evidence favoring the latter view [4]. They found esophageal alkalinization during the day, but not at night, suggesting an effect of saliva. Also, simultaneous probes in the stomach and esophagus showed that the esophagus spent more time above pH 7 than the gastric fundus, a result inconsistent, the authors thought, with reflux of alkaline material from stomach to esophagus. Finally, when episodes of gastric alkalinization did occur, there was no corresponding rise in esophageal pH. Attwood, on the other hand, did find a temporal relationship between episodes of esophageal and gastric alkalinization [5]. Two separate studies have shown a correlation between alkaline esophageal pH and complications of Barrett's esophagus, including dysplasia. In the first study, Attwood and others at Creighton University studied 23 consecutive patients with Barrett's esophagus and divided them into two groups, one without complications (11 patients) and one with complications, including stricture (11), ulcer (four) and dysplasia (three) [6]. Esophageal manometry and 24-h esophageal pH monitoring were performed in all patients. Patients with complicated and uncomplicated Barrett's had similar esophageal exposure to pH less than 4, but there was a marked increase in alkaline exposure (as indicated by esophageal pH greater than 7) in the group with complications. Ten of 12 patients with complicated Barrett's esophagus had increased alkaline exposure compared to one of 11 patients without complications. Furthermore, three patients had gastric pH studies suggesting duodenogastric reflux and all three had complicated Barrett's esophagus. Six patients with negative gastric pH studies had no complications of their Barrett's.

More recently, Attwood et al. studied 26 patients in Lancaster, England with Barrett's esophagus [5]. Ten of the 26 had complications, including stricture (eight), ulcer (one) and carcinoma (one). Esophageal alkaline exposure was significantly greater in patients with complications (24% vs. 8%), while esophageal acid exposure was similar in both groups.

The theoretical support for an association between alkaline reflux and dysplasia is 2-fold: First, there is abundant animal evidence that conjugated bile salts and pancreatic enzymes damage esophageal mucosa [7]. Second, bile acids have long been suspected of having a causative role in cancer of the GI tract, particularly the colon [8]. Work with an animal model for esophageal adenocarcinoma indicates that some promoter of carcinogenesis is present in duodenal juice, since exposure of the rat esophagus to duodenal contents increases the tumor yield in carcinogen treated rats [9].

In summary, there is debate about whether duodenal contents reflux into the esophagus and, if reflux occurs, whether there is an adverse effect. The studies of Gillen and Attwood show a statistical association between complications of Barrett's esophagus and presumed markers of duodenogastroesophageal reflux. The number of reported patients with dysplasia is too small to support a conclusion about an association between alkaline reflux and dysplasia. The question is still open and further study is required, particularly until improved methods for documenting duodenogastroesophageal reflux are developed.

References

1. Bremner CG. The columnar-lined (Barrett's) esophagus. Surg Annual 1977;9:103.
2. Gillen P, Kelling P, Byrne PJ et al. Implication of duodenogastric reflux in the pathogenesis of Barrett's oesophagus. Br J Surg 1988;75:540.
3. Mittal RK, Reuben A, Whitney JO, McCallum RW. Do bile acids reflux into the esophagus? Gastroenterology 1987;92: 371.
4. Singh S, Bradley LA, Richter JE. Determinants of oesophageal "alkaline" pH environment in controls in patients with gastroesophageal reflux disease. Gut 1993;34:309.
5. Attwood SEA, Ball CS, Barlow AP et al. Role of intragastric and intraesophageal alkalinisation in the genesis of complications in Barrett's columnar-lined lower esophagus. Gut 1993;34:11.
6. Attwood SEA, DeMeester TR, Bremner CG, Barlow AP, Hinder RA. Alkaline gastroesophageal reflux: implications in the development of complications in Barrett's columnar-lined lower esophagus. Surgery 1989;106:764.
7. Lillemoe KD, Johnson LF, Harmon JW. Alkaline esophagitis: a comparison of the ability of components of gastroduodenal contents to injure the rabbit esophagus. Gastroenterology 1983;85:621.
8. Nagengast FM. Bile acids and colonic carcinogenesis. Scand J Gastroenterol 1988;23:76.
9. Attwood SEA, Smyrk TC, DeMeester TR et al. Duodenoesophageal reflux and the development of esophageal adenocarcinoma in rats. Surgery 1992;111:503.

Where should biopsies be made in a zone of Barrett's esophagus?

A.H. Hölscher (Munich)

To elucidate the early events of cancer development in the columnar cell lined lower esophagus, 13 esophagectomy specimens with early adenocarcinoma (T1) were histopathologically studied and the morphometry of the lesion was performed on a histologic map [1]. Eleven (84.6%) of the 13 early Barrett's carcinomas were contiguous to both the distinctive specialized type of Barrett's mucosa and squamous epithelium. Furthermore, 10 (76.9%) of the 13 tumors had residual squamous islands on the surface. The length of Barrett's esophagus ranged from 1.5—10.2 cm (average: 5.2 cm) and the distance between the tumor center and the esophagogastric junction ranged from 0.8—4.5 cm (average: 2.5 cm). There was a highly significant correlation ($r = 0.79$, $p = 0.0013$) between the length of Barrett's esophagus and the distance between the tumor center and the esophagogastric junction. To further investigate the probable primary site of cancer development in the 13 early Barrett's carcinomas, the distance between the tumor center and the squamocolumnar border, including squamous islands, was measured. This distance was 2 cm or less in all but one of the 13 cases. In the smaller carcinomas, in which the tumor size was 2 cm or less (n = 5) this distance was 0.5 cm or less in all cases. To detect the influence of the tumor size on the distance between the tumor center and the squamocolumnar border, the relationship between the two parameters was assessed. There was a highly significant correlation ($r = 0.91$, $p = 0.00001$) between the tumor size and the distance between the tumor center and the squamocolumnar border. These data suggest that carcinomas in Barrett's esophagus mostly develop at a place very close to the squamocolumnar epithelial border. Therefore, the authors conclude that the primary site of cancer development in Barrett's esophagus is the metaplastic columnar lined area, particularly of the specialized type, within 2 cm of the squamocolumnar epithelial

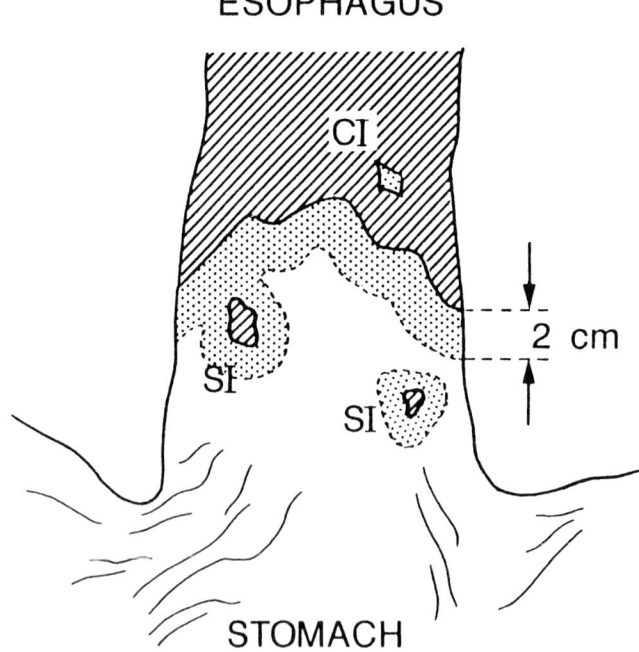

Fig. 1. High risk area of cancer development in Barrett's esophagus (dotted area). Cross-hatched area shows squamous epithelium; blank area shows columnar epithelium island; CI: columnar epithelial island; SI: squamous island. (From [1], with permission).

border, including squamous islands (Fig. 1).

These results certainly have practical implications on the regular endoscopic surveillance of patients with Barrett's esophagus, because the preferable biopsy site should be close to the circumferential squamocolumnar epithelial border and around squamous islands, since early carcinomas mostly develop in these areas [2].

References

1. Nishimaki T, Hölscher AH, Schüler M, Bollschweiler E, Becker K, Siewert JR. Histopathologic characteristics of early adenocarcinoma in Barrett's esophagus. Cancer 1991;68(8):1731−1736.
2. Hölscher AH. Präcancerosen des Gastroösophagealen Überganges. In: Langhans P, Schreiber HW, Häring R, Reding R, Siewert JR, Günther H (eds) Aktuelle Therapie des Cardiacarcinoms. Berlin, Heidelberg, New York, London, Paris, Tokyo: Springer, 1988;34−42.

Can the use of vital staining limit the number of routine biopsies for detecting dysplasia?

E. Brossard, C. Fontolliet, J.-B. Ollyo, P. Monnier
(Lausanne)

Adenocarcinoma is a recognized complication of Barrett's esophagus, as the dysplasia associated with this condition is considered to be a precursor [1,2]. The latent period between diagnosis of Barrett's esophagus and the development of adenocarcinoma can be as long as 15−20 years. For this reason, patients with Barrett's esophagus often undergo regular endoscopic surveillance. In view of the fact that the precancerous changes are usually multifocal and invisible, multiple, serial biopsies are usually recommended. These not only allow detection of foci of dysplasia, but also enable the Barrett's epithelium to be typed. This typing has a direct bearing on patient follow-up. Metaplastic epithelium of specialized type presents the greatest risk of malignant degeneration [3,4]. Endoscopic surveillance in patients with Barrett's esophagus is therefore aimed at checking for the presence of dysplasia. This is difficult to detect as the foci of dysplasia cannot be distinguished from normal columnar mucosa by endoscopic examination. Although vital stains play a determinant role in the early diagnosis of epidermoid carcinomas of the esophagus, they are of no value in patients with columnar mucosal changes of the lower esophagus.

3% Lugol

A 3% Lugol solution stains the glycogen-rich cells of normal malpighian mucosa brown. The glycogen content of these epithelial cells is already greatly diminished at the dysplasic stage [5]. A Lugol solution will therefore negatively stain all areas that may be suspected of early epidermoid cancer (Fig. 1). However, Lugol does not stain the columnar epithelial cells characteristic of Barrett's esophagus. It is used to demarcate the normal esophageal epithelium from Barrett's epithelium but cannot reveal dysplasia.

1% toluidine blue

Toluidine blue is the agent most commonly used for vital staining of the mucosa of the upper gastrointestinal tract. It belongs to the family of thiazine stains that have the property of binding to cellular DNA and RNA.

Its absorption into the tissues is promoted by the structural disorganization of the carcinomatous epithelium [6,7] (Figs. 2 and 3).

The preferential binding of toluidine blue to carcinomatous tissue rather than to

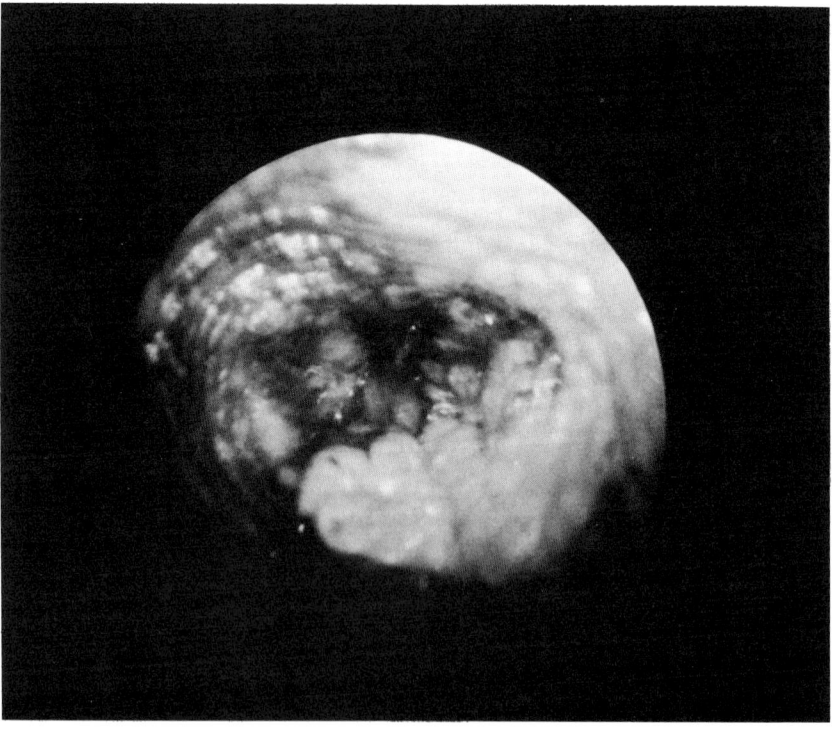

Fig. 1. Where the esophagus is lined with the usual smooth mucosa, the glycogen content of the epithelial cells is already diminished at the dysplasic stage. It can be seen from this endoscopic picture that the area exhibiting early signs of cancerous change is negatively stained by the Lugol solution.

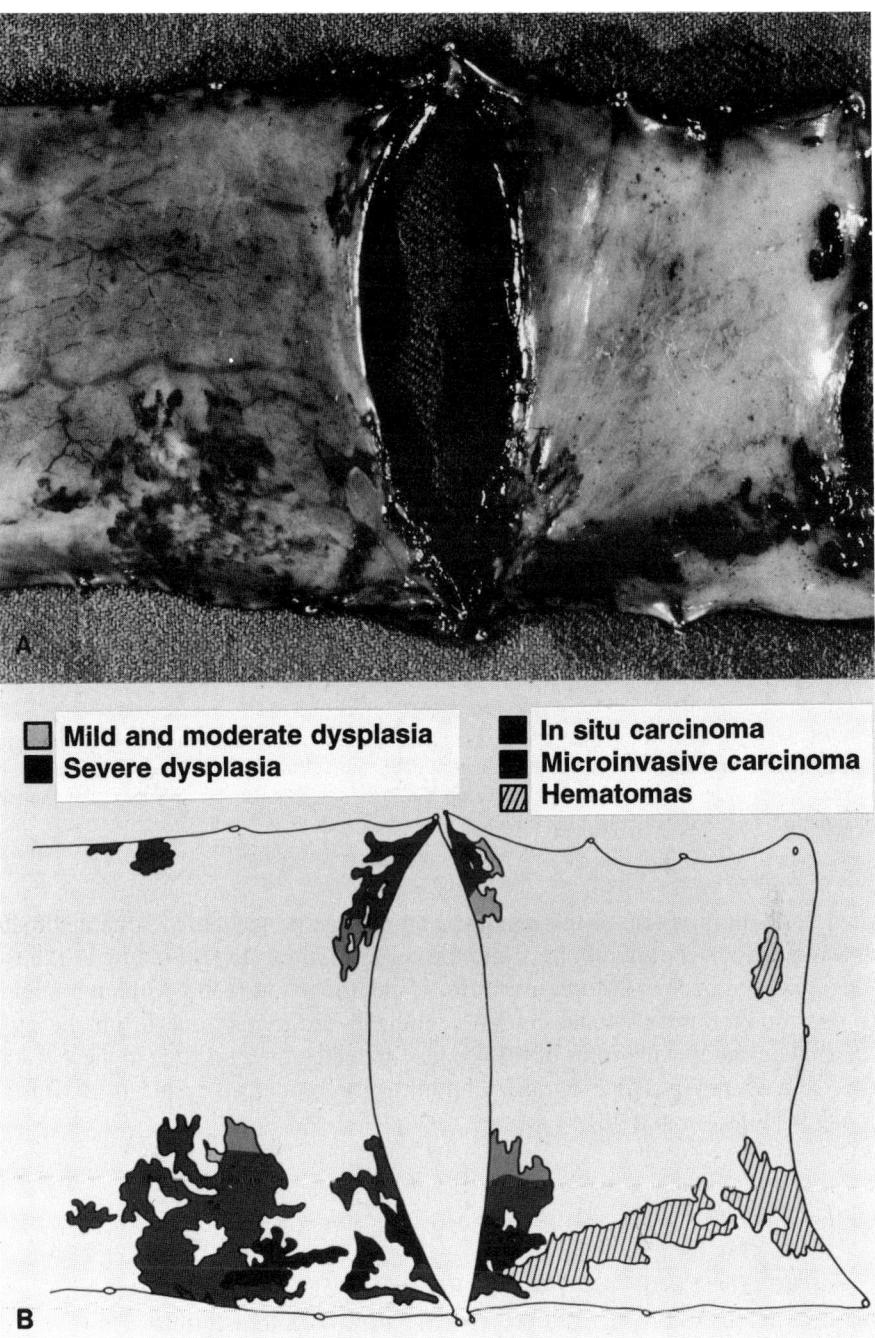

Mild and moderate dysplasia
Severe dysplasia

In situ carcinoma
Microinvasive carcinoma
Hematomas

Fig. 2. A. In this sample of excised esophageal tissue, the topically applied toluidine blue stains early or invasive carcinomatous lesions blue, but leaves the normal epithelium unstained. B. Histological examination of serial sections of the same specimen reveals carcinomatous lesions, ranging from slight dysplasia to microinvasive carcinoma, which have all taken up the blue stain.

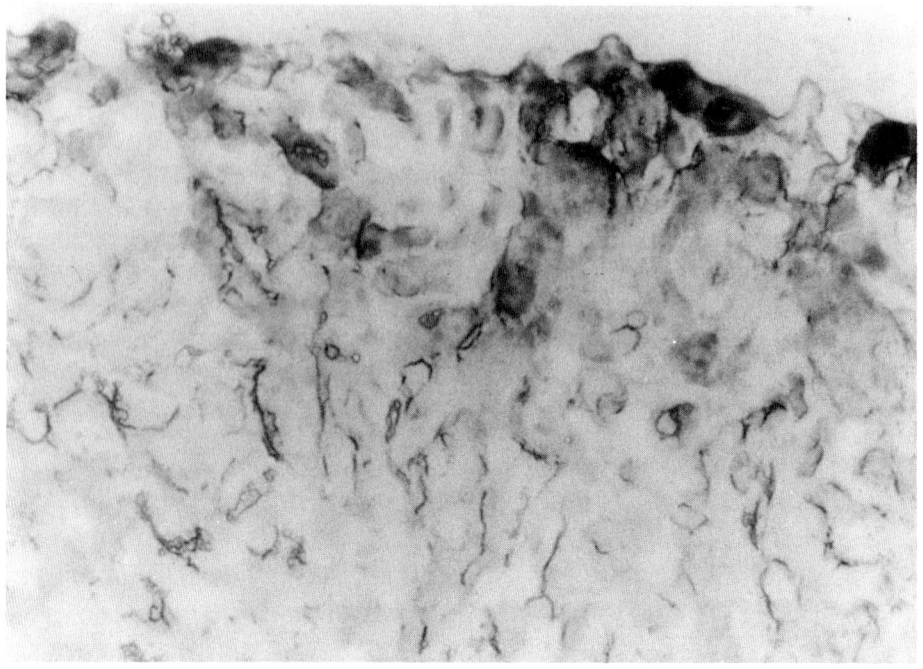

Fig. 3. The mode of action of toluidine blue is demonstrated in this frozen section of a specimen taken from the junction between normal and carcinomatous epithelium. The cells of the normal epithelium have a skeletal appearance as they have not taken up the stain. In contrast, the disrupted carcinomatous epithelium has absorbed and bound the toluidine blue to a depth of 4–5 cell layers.

normal epithelium is due to the increased membrane permeability of carcinomatous cells which allows the stain to pass into the cells. Its intracellular binding is enhanced by the increased nuclear-cytoplasmic ratio of carcinomatous cells. Although toluidine blue does stain Barrett's mucosa, this staining is an artefact due to uptake by the surface mucus and by the folds of the pseudociliated epithelium. Due to these staining artefacts, it is not possible to use toluidine blue to detect dysplasia in Barrett's esophagus (Figs. 4a and 4b).

Conclusion

Vital stains (3% Lugol and 1% toluidine blue) can be used on smooth, normal mucosa to detect and demarcate pre-invasive carcinomatous lesions. However, vital staining cannot be used to detect foci of dysplasia in Barrett's epithelium and is consequently of no help in limiting the number of systematic biopsies required.

At the present time, the only clinical method of detecting these foci of dysplasia involves serial biopsies and brushing of the Barrett's epithelium [8].

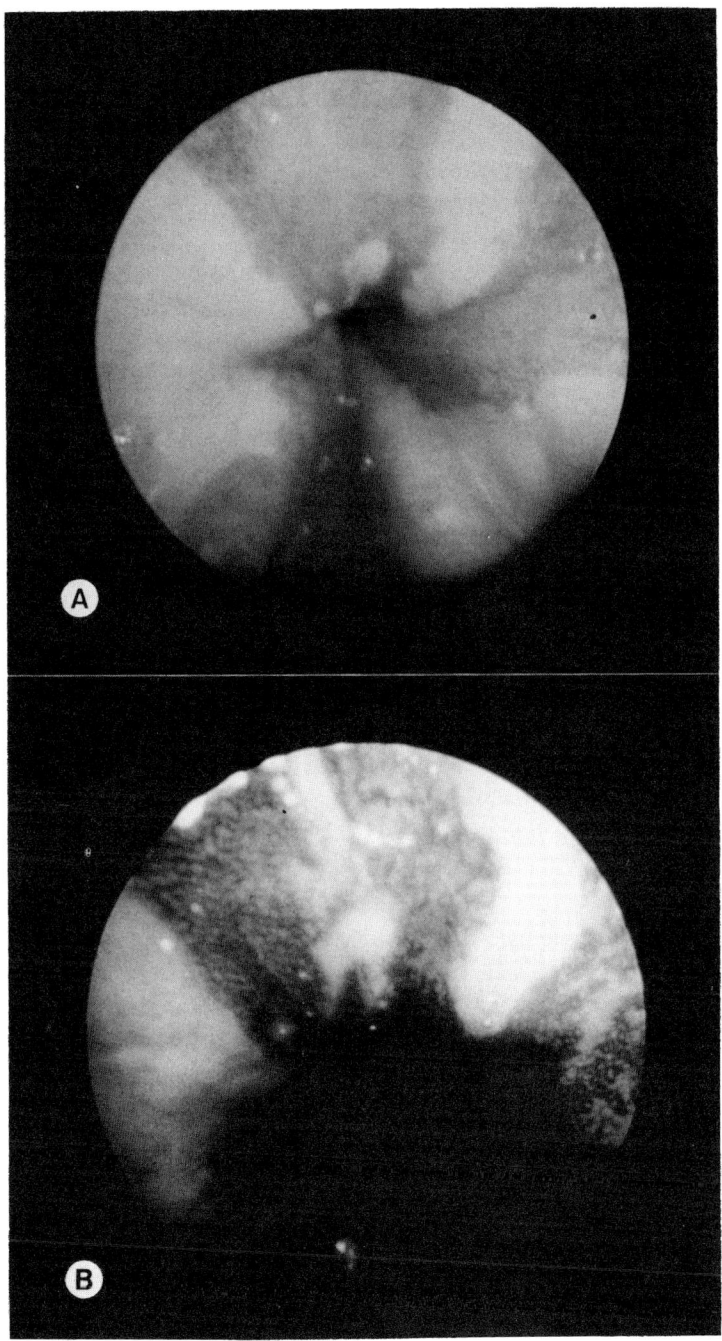

Fig. 4. A. This specimen of type II Barrett's epithelium is known to contain a focus of dysplasia, identified by multiple serial biopsies. B. Staining of the specimen with toluidine blue failed to detect the
known focus of dysplasia. The staining of Barrett's epithelium with toluidine blue is an artefact attributable to uptake of the stain by the mucus and its trapping in the folds of the pseudociliary epithelium.

References

1. Haggitt RC. Adenocarcinoma in Barrett's esophagus: a new epidemy? Hum Pathol 1992;234:475–476.
2. Hameeteman W, Tytgat GNJ, Houthoff HJ, van den Tweel JG. Barrett's esophagus: development of dysplasia and adenocarcinoma. Gastroenterology 1989;96:1249–1256.
3. Monnier Ph, Fontolliet Ch, Savary M, Ollyo JB. Barrett's oesophagus or columnar epithelium of the lower oesophagus. Baillière's Clin Gastroenterol 1987;1(4):769–789.
4. Fontolliet Ch, Monnier Ph, Ollyo JB. Oesophageal dysplasia within the squamous and columnar cell mucosa: histopathological aspects. Acta Endoscopica 1991;21(5):607–615.
5. Mandard AM, Tourneux J, Gignoux M. In situ carcinoma of the esophagus, macroscopic study with particular reference to the Lugol test. Endoscopy 1980;12:51–57.
6. Monnier Ph, Savary M, Pasche Ph. Contribution of toluidine blue to bucco-pharyngo-oesophageal cancerology. Acta Endoscopica 1981;9(4–5):299–315.
7. Fontolliet Ch, Monniet Ph. The histological reliability of vital staining with toluidine blue. Acta Endoscopica 1991; 21(5):617–621.
8. Geisinger KR, Teot LA, Richter JE. A comparative cytopathologic and histologic study of atypia, dysplasia and adenocarcinoma in Barrett's oesophagus. Cancer 1992;69:8–16.

Which histologic methods are best for demonstrating architectural and cytologic details of dysplasia in Barrett's esophagus?

K.R. Geisinger (Winston-Salem)

In order to prevent or reduce deaths from esophageal adenocarcinoma, the disease must be detected in its earliest stages, preferably before it has invaded into the organ's wall [1,2]. This preinvasive, neoplastic stage is glandular dysplasia which has been defined on the basis of specific histomorphologic features. In patients with a columnar-lined esophagus, the morphologic diagnosis of such dysplasia relies on the identification of prominent (i.e., neoplastic) alterations both in the intercellular arrangements or architecture of the epithelial elements and in the constituent cells themselves, especially their nuclei. The histologic preparation of esophageal biopsy specimens requires a series of technical steps, including tissue fixation, specimen orientation, embedding in paraffin, sectioning of paraffin blocks, mounting sections on glass slides and staining. Although most of these steps may be performed by any of several acceptable technical variations, each is important in the quality of the final product for interpretation.

This cascade of technical procedures for the preparation of biopsies has been addressed excellently in a succinct yet eloquent chapter by Haggitt and Rubin [3]. These authors promote, what can be considered, an ideal approach in this setting. First, mucosal biopsies, they argue, should be procured utilizing jumbo forceps. They also claim that properly oriented biopsies are essential to the recognition of dysplasia and recommend that orientation occur immediately after procurement and prior to fixation. Plastic mesh is their preference for the substrate upon which the tissue specimen is placed. Haggitt and Rubin also firmly support the use of Hollande's solution as the best fixative [3]. For embedding, tissue fragments should be placed so that in the next step, sectioning, their long axes are cut through. They frown upon embedding more than two fragments in the same paraffin block. Blocks should be trimmed of excessive paraffin before sectioning so that more sections may be placed on a slide. Then, specimens are step-serial-sectioned a minimum of three levels. Finally, their routine stain consists of a mixture of hematoxylin and eosin, alcian blue and saffron [3].

Unfortunately, even in the cubby holes of academia, we do not live in an ideal world. Several practical problems exist with the above histologic schema. For one, in our experience, it is unusual to find gastroenterologists who use jumbo forceps for esophageal biopsies. The smaller specimens obtained with conventional forceps are much more difficult to orient prior to fixation. It is probably true that Hollande's solution consistently provides crisper nuclear detail than does formalin (Figs. 1–8). However, the former fixative is both more expensive and more difficult for histotechnologists to work with. The cost to my laboratory for one gallon of Hollande's solution is $55, while it is only $3 for the same volume of formalin; that is, it is more than 18 times as expensive. From a technical viewpoint, there are several considerations. Hollande's yellow color needs to be washed out before processing. Picric acid is considered by some to be a dangerous chemical and thus has been banned in its powdered form in several states in the USA. It should be

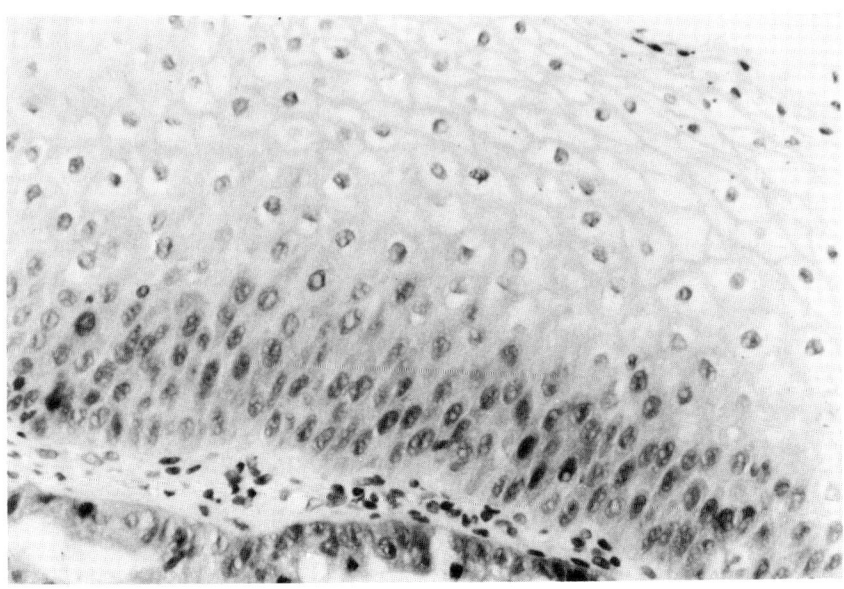

Fig. 1. This squamous mucosa is from a patient with Barrett's esophagus and is fixed in formalin. The chromatin is pale, often with a homogeneous or washed out appearance. A few nuclei appear to have "holes" or pseudoinclusions. Nucleoli are inconspicuous to absent (×100).

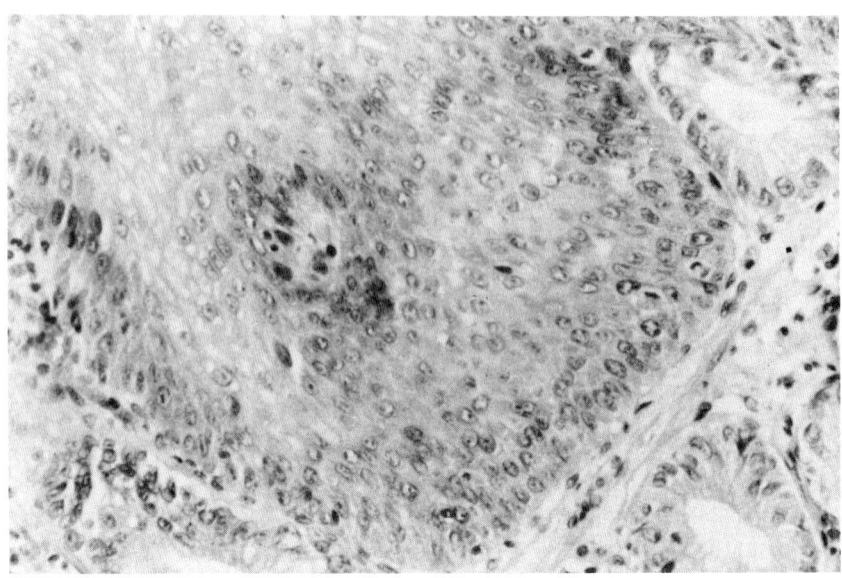

Fig. 2. This is from the same patient and obtained at the same endoscopic session as the tissue in Fig. 1, but it is fixed in Hollande's solution. Distinct chromatin granularity is evident in many nuclei, as are small nucleoli (×100).

mentioned that most published studies which have defined and characterized Barrett's dysplasia have included formalin-fixed tissues. In their thought provoking study of

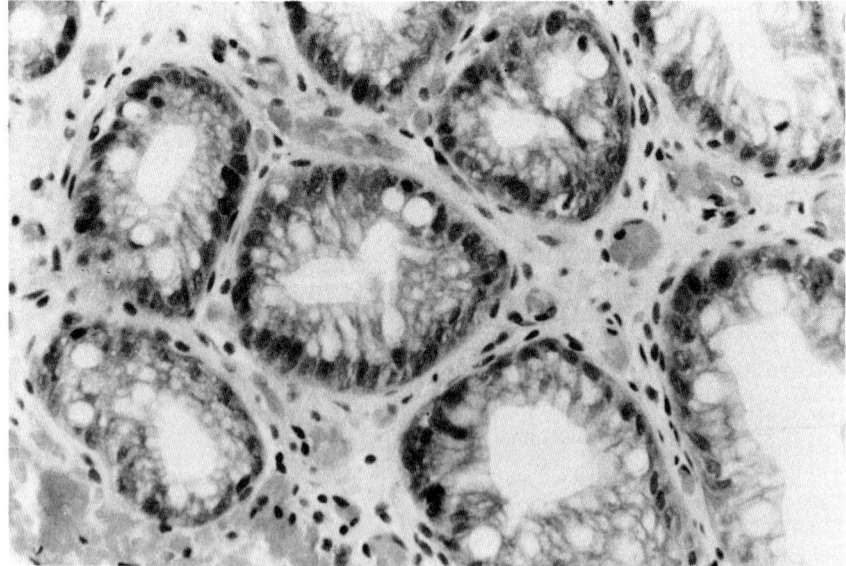

Fig. 3. Barrett's metaplasia with intestinal metaplasia is present in this formalin-fixed biopsy. Most of the epithelial nuclei are vesicular with small nucleoli. Basal polarity is well maintained (×100).

986

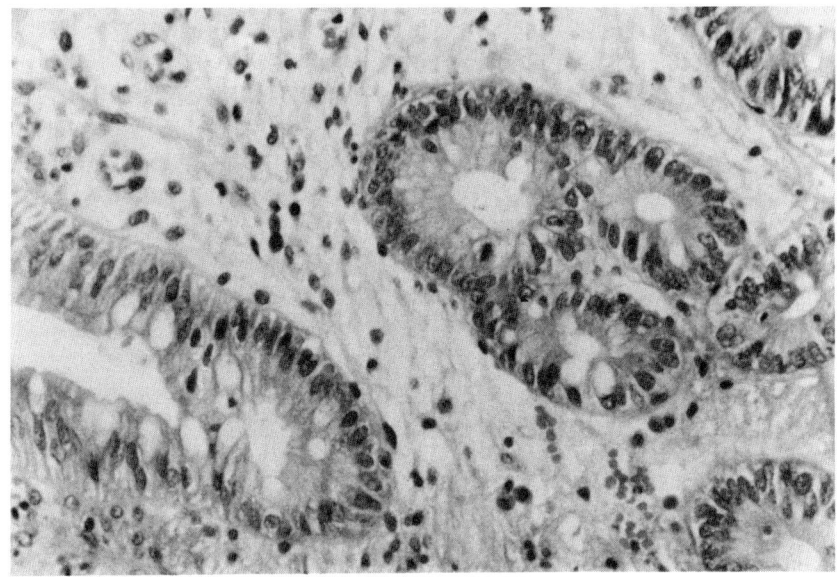

Fig. 4. These glandular elements were from the same patient as in Fig. 3, but were fixed in Hollande's solution. Nuclear membranes and chromatin granularity are more distinct (×100).

biopsies from patients with Barrett's esophagus, Reid et al. [4] stated that specific fixatives did not affect diagnostic reproducibility among pathologists. Step-serial-sections are worthwhile in a search for small focal lesions, but I wonder whether this

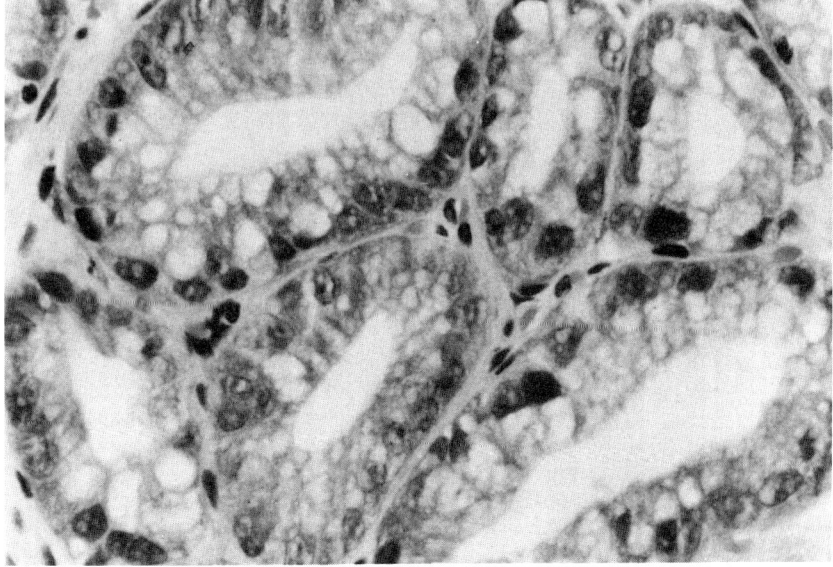

Fig. 5. This benign Barrett's metaplasia was adjacent to an erosion. Nuclei are enlarged, but do not appear hyperchromatic. In many cells, the nucleoplasm has a foamy or bubbly appearance. In a few, distinct vacuoles are evident (×400).

987

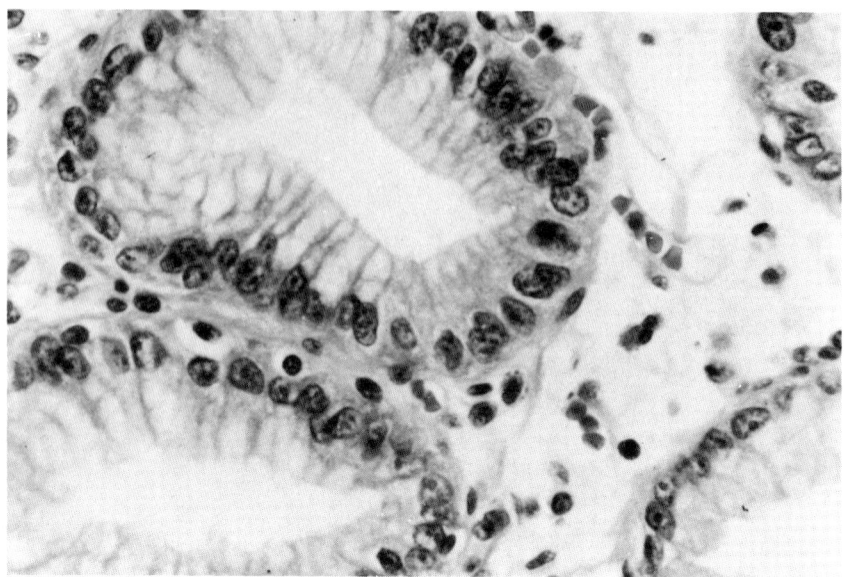

Fig. 6. This is from the same patient as in Fig. 5, but is fixed in Hollande's solution, rather than formalin. The finely granular chromatin and nuclear membranes are more distinct (×400).

applies to the hunt for dysplasia [5]. In my laboratory, step-serial-sections take a technologist an extra 5—10 min per block, compared to simple leveling. The cost of

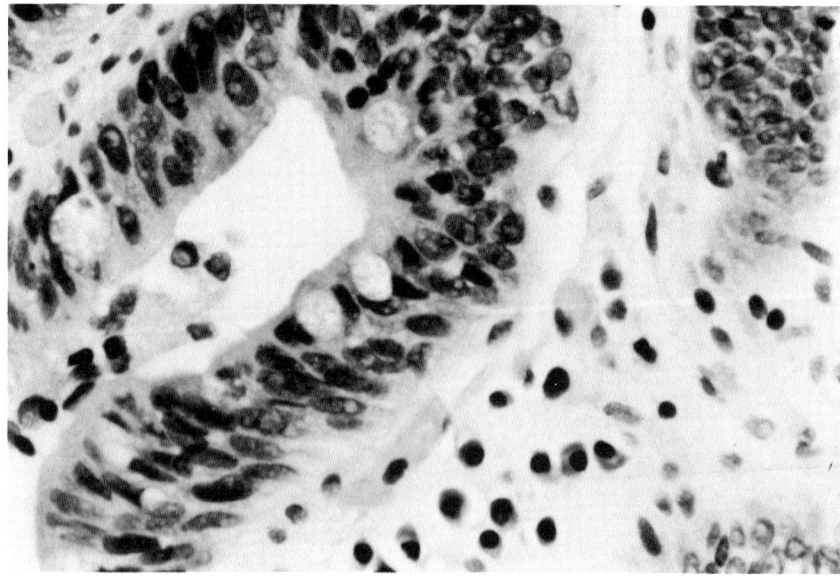

Fig. 7. Dysplastic glandular nuclei in Barrett's esophagus are obviously enlarged, variably elongated and hyperchromatic. In formalin-fixed tissue, the chromatin appears more or less homogeneous and indistinct, as its granularity is not readily apparent. Nucleoli are not easily seen (×400).

988

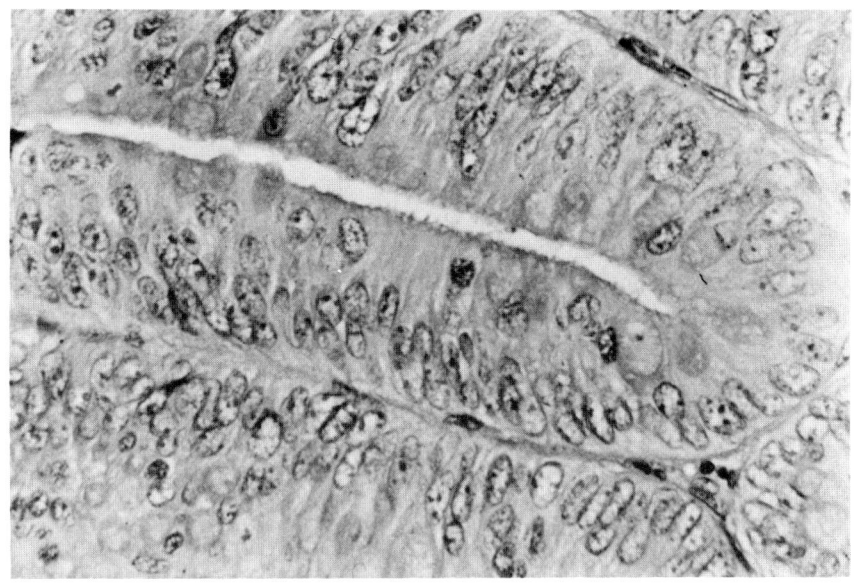

Fig. 8. This is dysplastic glandular tissue fixed in Hollande's solution. Compared to formalin fixation, nuclear membranes are more distinct and chromatin is crisper in appearance. Nucleoli are also more apparent (×400).

special stains needs to be mentioned. For example, an eight ounce bottle of saffron is $72.

I attempted to discover which processing steps are actually performed for esophageal biopsies in the laboratories of experts in this field. I mailed a simple checklist survey to fifty members of the Gastrointestinal Pathology Society in the United States and Canada. At the time of this writing, I had received responses from 42 (84%). Overwhelmingly, formalin is the fixative of choice for esophageal biopsies, being used 80% of the time; one institution uses formalin for adults and Bouin's for pediatric patients. Bouin's and Hollande's fixatives are used by four and three pathologists, respectively. Fifteen responders (36%) claim that biopsies are oriented, most often by a gastrointestinal endoscopy technician (53%), followed by the gastroenterologist (23%). The most commonly used substrate is a filter (60%). With respect to sectioning of esophageal biopsies, the most common procedure followed is step-serial-sectioning at three levels (43%), followed by three simple levels (17%). Most rely on hematoxylin and eosin as their routine stain (83%) with the remainder adding a mucin reaction which always included alcian blue. Finally, 33% of the responding gastrointestinal pathologists stated that their institution had an established formal surveillance program for patients with Barrett's esophagus. Although there was considerable overlap between programs with and without such a procedure, definite trends exist for the more complex or elaborate histologic procedures to be employed by those who are involved in surveillance.

Endoscopic screening programs with multiple biopsies throughout the length of the involved metaplastic segment have proven to be effective in detecting patients with glandular dysplasia or early carcinoma [1,2,6,7]. However, the sensitivity of surveillance is not as high as desired. It also appears that many if not most patients with Barrett's esophagus will never progress to severe dysplasia or invasive tumor. Furthermore, it should be noted that the actual cost per patient can be considerable [6]. Consequently, this has prompted the search for ancillary or additional assays that can be performed on biopsy specimens. One of the most widely examined is the detection of DNA ploidy abnormalities by flow cytometry [8,9]. The Seattle team uses a protocol that quantitates the DNA by flow cytometry of a biopsy from every 2 cm of the involved length of the esophagus [5,8]. They and others have reported aneuploidy occurring not only in most examples of adenocarcinoma and dysplasia, but also in metaplastic mucosa without histologic evidence of neoplasia; both aneuploidy and/or elevated proliferative activity may select a subgroup of patients with a greater risk for cancer [8,10–13]. However, despite these advances, others argue that flow cytometry in this setting is not the end-all answer [14]. For one thing, cost needs to be considered. In one institution that I am familiar with, the total technical and professional fees for a single flow cytometric study of DNA alone is $168.00 and $240.00 for fresh and frozen tissue, respectively. For a more in-depth exam of this situation, let us hypothesize a patient with a 6-cm segment of glandular metaplasia without any gross abnormality endoscopically. This would entail at least three biopsy specimens (several every 2 cm) with flow cytometry on three samples. The total (minimal) cost for histology and flow cytometry would be $746.00; this includes a combined technical and professional charge of $242 for the routine production and evaluation of histologic sections.

The potential use of brushing cytology of the esophagus in surveillance must be considered [15,16]. As has been stated elsewhere in this volume, there are several valuable reasons for a cytologic exam to be incorporated into (or even replace) a screening program, as described above. Most importantly, I believe that cyto-morphologic criteria for glandular dysplasia and carcinoma are reproducible, as witnessed by several publications [15–17]. In addition, ploidy measurements by image (static) cytometry, which has several advantages and disadvantages vis-à-vis flow cytometry, can be performed directly on Feulgen-stained cytologic smears. As brushing samples a much larger surface area of mucosa than do multiple biopsies, only a single ploidy analysis may be adequate [18]. In the same institution mentioned above, the total cost for the evaluation of both conventional esophageal cytology and DNA image analysis is $338.00. Consideration of image rather than flow cytometry on tissue biopsies is also valid [19].

To summarize, an overwhelming consensus as to the single best approach to the diagnosis of Barrett's dysplasia does not yet exist. I suspect that considerable time will elapse before gastroenterologists, medical economists, and pathologists agree on this. It must be admitted that everything we look at under the microscope is an "artifact" and part of this problem is that we grow accustomed to and comfortable with the artifacts generated by our own laboratories.

References

1. Spechler SJ, Goyal RK. Barrett's esophagus. N Engl J Med 1986;315:362—371.
2. Spechler SJ. Endoscopic surveillance for patients with Barrett's esophagus: does the cancer risk justify the practice? Ann Int Med 1987;106:902—904.
3. Haggitt RC, Rubin CE. In: Ming S-C, Goldman H (eds) Endoscopy and endoscopic biopsy in pathology of the gastrointestinal tract. Philadelphia: WB Saunders Co., 1992;37—47.
4. Reid BJ, Haggitt RC, Rubin CE et al. Observer variation in the diagnosis of dysplasia in Barrett's esophagus. Hum Pathol 1988;19:166—178.
5. Surawicz CM. Serial sectioning of a portion of a rectal biopsy detects more focal abnormalities. A prospective study of patients with inflammatory bowel disease. Dig Dis Sci 1982;27:434—436.
6. Achkar E, Carey W. The cost of surveillance for adenocarcinoma complicating Barrett's esophagus. Am J Gastroenterol 1988;83:291—294.
7. Spechler SJ. Barrett's esophagus: what's new and what to do. Am J Gastroenterol 1989;84:220—223.
8. Reid BJ, Haggitt RC, Rubin CE, Rabinovitch PS. Barrett's esophagus. Correlation between flow cytometry and histology in detection of patients at risk for adenocarcinoma. Gastroenterology 1987;93:1—11.
9. Fennerty MB, Sampliner RE. Flow cytometry in Barrett's esophagus: when all is said and done, more is said than done! Am J Gastroenterol 1993;88:319—320.
10. Reid BJ, Blount PL, Rubin CE, Levine DS, Haggitt RC, Rabinovitch PS. Flow cytometric and histological progression to malignancy in Barrett's esophagus: prospective endoscopic surveillance of a cohort. Gastroenterology 1992;102:1212—1219.
11. Flejou JF, Doublet B, Potet F, Metayer J, Hemet J. DNA ploidy in adenocarcinoma of Barrett's esophagus. Ann Pathol 1990;10:161—165.
12. Robaszkiewicz M, Hardy E, Volant A et al. Flow cytometric analysis of cellular DNA content in Barrett's esophagus. A study of 66 cases. Gastroenterol Clin Biol 1991;15:703—710.
13. Robaszkiewicz M, Volant A, Hardy E et al. Demonstration of clonal heterogeneity in adenocarcinomas in Barrett's esophagus by flow cytometric study of cellular DNA content. Gastroenterol Clin Biol 1992;16:540—546.
14. Fennerty MB, Sampliner RE, Way D, Riddell R, Steinbronn K, Garewal HS. Discordance between flow cytometric abnormalities and dysplasia in Barrett's esophagus. Gastroenterology 1989;97:815—820.
15. Wang HH, Doria MI, Purohit-Buch S, Schnell T, Sontag S, Chejfec G. Barrett's esophagus. The cytology of dysplasia in comparison to benign and malignant lesions. Acta Cytol 1992;36:60—64.
16. Geisinger KR, Teot LA, Richter JE. A comparative cytopathologic and histologic study of atypia, dysplasia and adenocarcinoma in Barrett's esophagus. Cancer 1992;69:8—16.
17. Wang HH, Ducatman BS, Thibault S. Cytologic features of premalignant glandular lesions in the upper gastrointestinal tract. Acta Cytol 1991;35:199—203.
18. Teot LA, Accettullo LM, Geisinger KR. Barrett's esophagus: the complementarity of endoscopic cytologic brushings and biopsies and DNA ploidy by image analysis. Acta Cytol 1992;36:624.
19. James PD, Atkinson M. Value of DNA image cytometry in the prediction of malignant change in Barrett's esophagus. Gut 1989;30:899—905.

What is the definition of dysplasia, as it applies to Barrett's mucosa?

R.H. Riddell (Hamilton)

The definition of dysplasia in Barrett's esophagus is that first developed for use in dysplasia in ulcerative colitis [1]. Dysplasia is defined as an unequivocal neoplastic alteration of the epithelium. It should be stressed that such dysplastic epithelium not only may be a marker or precursor of carcinoma, but may itself be malignant and associated with direct invasion into the underlying tissue. Using this definition all biopsies can be classified as negative, indefinite or positive for dysplasia by asking two questions:

1. Is the biopsy unequivocally negative for dysplasia?
2. Is the biopsy unequivocally dysplastic?

By definition, if the answer to both of these questions is "no" then one is dealing with mucosa that is indefinite for dysplasia.

Further, if required, dysplasia can itself be subdivided objectively into high grade and low grade depending on the position of the nuclei within the cell. In low grade dysplasia nuclei are largely confined to the basal halves of the cell, whereas in high grade dysplasia they regularly reach the upper part of the cell. While it is advised that the worst area of the biopsy be used for grading, the qualifying adjectives largely and regularly provide a subjective component and a potential area for inter-observer disagreement between pathologists. Nevertheless, interobserver agreement between pathologists has been tested and been shown to be quite good [2], with approximately 85% agreement in distinguishing high grade from other forms of dysplasia. If one bears in mind that a spectrum of changes is being observed, one expects a normal distribution curve for the results of many pathologists examining a single slide. In low grade dysplasia there is the potential for overlap between high grade dysplasia at one end and indefinite for dysplasia at the other, depending on the breadth of the distribution curve. The hope is that areas of overlap with adjacent grades in the spectrum do not occur; however, this is an unrealistic expectation. Some slides can be deliberately selected that straddle different parts of the grading spectrum; unselected biopsies can clearly do the same.

Perhaps the most important feature that disagreements have is their implication on patient management. The criterion for therapeutic intervention is usually intramucosal or invasive carcinoma. It might be expected that there would be no disagreement between pathologists regarding these diagnoses. Surprisingly, in one study agreement for intramucosal carcinoma was reached in only 87% of cases [2].

Clearly there are other problem areas. One is in recognizing features of active repair at the cytological level, which to the untrained eye can resemble dysplasia. A second is that repair can also lead to glandular proliferation producing a back-to-back or gland within gland appearance that can also be in carcinoma in situ (CIS), although without the typical cytological features accompanying carcinoma in situ. Nevertheless the potential for misreading CIS as reactive changes can be appreciated.

This definition of dysplasia has several direct implications that are imperative to understand. The most important of these is that dysplasia of any grade can give rise directly to an invasive carcinoma. Initially this flies in the face of traditional teaching that invasion occurs on a background of dysplasia that goes successively from low to high grade, which includes carcinoma in situ, from which invasion occurs. However, the fact that invasion can occur directly from low grade dysplasia is an intrinsic part of the definition and, although relatively uncommon, is known to occur in virtually all organs. In deliberately choosing to follow any grade of dysplasia, one must be aware firstly that a lesion is being followed that has the potential to give rise directly to an invasive carcinoma and secondly that carcinomas in Barrett's epithelium are frequently invisible endoscopically, being found either incidentally on random biopsy or in erection carried out for dysplasia [3]. Nevertheless, there has been an unconfirmed report that multiple large particle biopsies can take the guesswork out of this clinical situation. That is, if sufficient biopsies are taken then the presence of intramucosal or invasive carcinoma can be detected histologically, so that unexpected carcinoma is not found incidentally in resected specimens [4].

References

1. Riddell RH, Goldman H, Ransohoff DE et al. Dysplasia in inflammatory bowel disease: standardized classification with provisional clinical implications. Human Pathol 1983;14:931—968.
2. Reid BJ, Haggitt RC, Rubin CE et al. Observer variation in the diagnosis of Barrett's esophagus. Human Pathol 1988; 19:166—178.
3. Reid BJ, Weinstein WM, Lewin KJ et al. Endoscopic biopsy can detect high-grade dysplasia or early adenocarcinoma in Barrett's esophagus without grossly recognizable neoplastic lesions. Gastroenterology 1988;94:81—90.
4. Levine DS, Haggitt RC, Blount PL et al. An endoscopic biopsy protocol can differentiate high-grade dysplasia from early adenocarcinoma in Barrett's esophagus. Gastroenterology 1993;105:40—50.

Is there a great variation in histologic grading of dysplastic mucosa among highly-experienced gastrointestinal pathologists?

K. Geboes (Leuven)

Dysplasia is a term used in various subspecialties of medicine including gynecology, urology, radiology and gastroenterology for the description of macroscopic and microscopic lesions. It is originally an ancient Greek word which means "malforma-tion", or "a morphologic structure which is different from what normally is expected". As such it can indicate either a congenital or an acquired malformation, and it is still used with this meaning for macroscopic and radiological lesions. For microscopic and pathological lesions "dysplasia" has various significations. It can indicate a "malformation" or a lesion having a relation to malignancy. An example of the former is the term "angiodysplasia" which was used for vascular lesions, especially of the colon. A more appropriate term for this condition is "vascular ectasia" [1].

From these considerations it is clear that at present no general definition of dysplasia is available. The lack of such a definition for a term which is so commonly used is responsible for many misunderstandings and a great deal of confusion. The purpose of the present review is to explain the term "dysplasia" as it is used in gastrointestinal pathology and to indicate some differences, rather than to present a new classification or to indicate one single meaning for the word. We will, however, indicate the most appropriate definition as it is now currently used, while other definitions are still available and are not necessarily wrong. It is therefore extremely important that the pathologist and the clinicians working closely together are aware of the meaning of the term, and when using it do so in complete understanding of each other.

In gastrointestinal pathology the use of the term "dysplasia" is mainly limited to microscopic epithelial and nonepithelial lesions related to malignancy. The various epithelia of the gastrointestinal tract in which dysplastic lesions are described have different characteristics and a different microenvironment. The esophagus is covered by a multilayered squamous epithelium, which may be replaced by a metaplastic columnar epithelium. The colon is lined by a columnar epithelium. In the stomach the glandular compartment of the epithelium is much more developed than in the other segments. However, because of these differences the criteria for the diagnosis of dysplasia and, more important, the consequences of the finding of dysplasia differ according to organs.

Definition of dysplasia

The term "dysplasia" has been introduced in gastrointestinal pathology in studies on gastrointestinal cancer. It was defined as "a process of disordered cell growth" [2], "epithelial atypia or alteration" or "excessive abnormal proliferation of the gastric epithelium". The lesions are subdivided into several categories and usually a distinction is made between mild, moderate and severe or grade I, grade II and grade III [3,4]. Clinical and experimental studies have shown that mild and moderate degrees or grade I and II dysplasia, as used in the classifications of Ming [2] and Oehlert [3], are probably clinically insignificant and largely reactive or regenerative in nature [5,6].

The fact that regenerative alterations of columnar epithelia may be mistaken for dysplasia is not strange because all cells in regenerative epithelia show signs of cell growth and proliferation, including larger nuclei, basophilia of the cytoplasm and architectural changes.

Therefore, because of the obvious differences in behavior between regenerative and degenerative epithelial alterations, there was a need for a more precise definition of dysplasia. This was introduced in 1983, when an international group studying dysplasia in ulcerative colitis defined dysplasia as: "epithelial changes, lesions or alterations that are unequivocally neoplastic", thus excluding all reactive (regenerative) changes and equivocal changes [7]. A similar definition has been introduced for dysplasia in Barrett's esophagus [8,9]. The evaluation of the neoplastic nature of the lesions is based on light microscopic observations (cytological and architectural alterations). More sophisticated methods such as immunohistochemistry using specific markers (Ki67, recognizing a nuclear antigen expressed in all phases of the cell cycle, PCNA — proliferating cell nuclear antigens — and others), or flow cytometry, may help in the future to identify the neoplastic nature more precisely. Furthermore, for the esophagus it must be remembered that Barrett's mucosa is a metaplastic mucosa that is quite different from the colonic mucosa from which colitic carcinomas arise.

994

Dysplastic lesions have been identified in the whole gastrointestinal tract. Yet the classifications that have been proposed and that are used in the various segments of the gastrointestinal tract are not entirely similar. Roughly, we can state that for simple colorectal adenomas and for the stomach, the lesions are subdivided into mild, moderate and severe [10], and that in the earlier studies concerning the stomach, dysplasia is not always unequivocally neoplastic [5].

In Barrett's esophagus the lesions are classified into negative, indefinite or positive for dysplasia. The latter is subdivided into low grade and high grade [8,9]. (Figs. 1 and 2). Yet other classifications have been used and have appeared in the literature. Hamilton classified dysplasia in columnar cell lined esophagus into three grades: low, intermediate and high, similar to an international classification of gastric dysplasia, although the intermediate grade can be included in the high-grade category [8,11]. Schmidt and coworkers used two types of dysplasia: low grade and high grade, based upon the appearance and position (basal or apical) of the nuclei. For each grade of dysplasia these authors also describe two types [12]. In general most authors also include carcinoma in situ or intraepithelial carcinoma in the high-grade dysplasia category [9].

If we compare these classifications and regard dysplasia as unequivocally

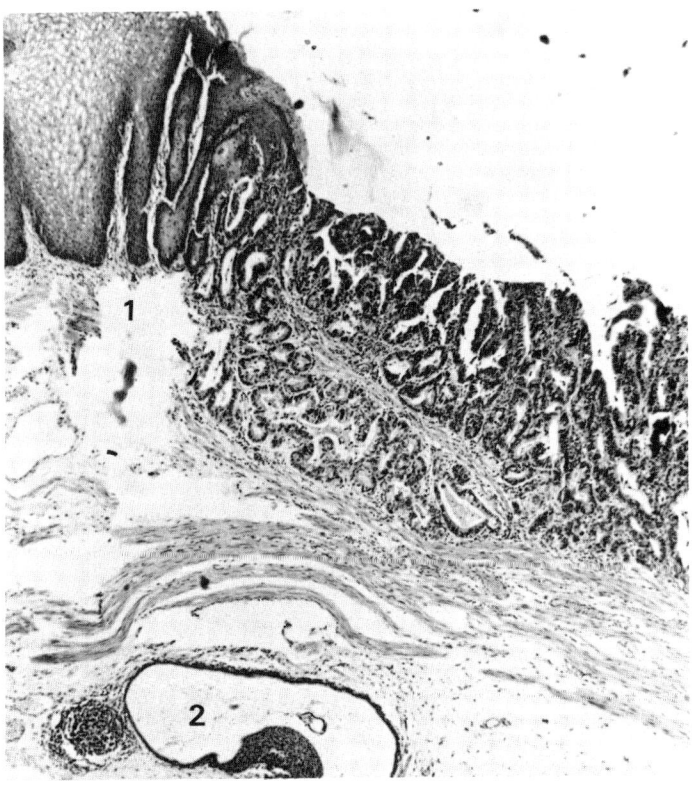

Fig. 1. High-grade dysplasia in Barrett's mucosa: on the left squamous epithelium (1). The columnar epithelium is diffusely dysplastic (with areas of minimal invasion). A dilated tubular duct of an esophageal gland is present in the submucosa (2) (H.E. × 50).

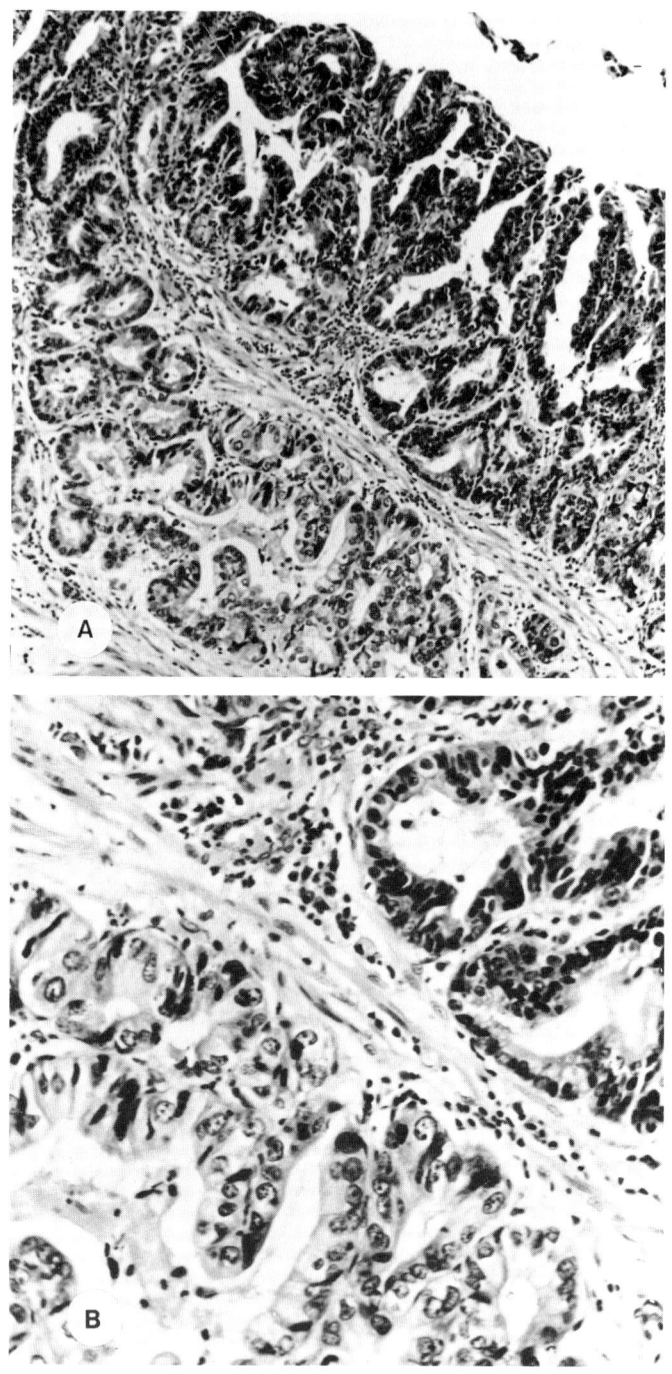

Fig. 2. Higher magnification of Fig. 1 showing the dysplastic nature of the surface and glandular epithelium characterized by enlarged nuclei with loss of polarity and striking cytological abnormalities (A: H.E. × 125; B: H.E. × 200).

neoplastic, it appears that low-grade dysplasia in Barrett is equivalent to forms of mild dysplasia in the stomach, while high-grade dysplasia equals moderate and severe dysplasia. The moderate or intermediate grade is not classically used for Barrett's esophagus.

The fact that different classifications are available, the incorrect use of words and the lack of a proper definition, rather than differences in opinion, are often the cause of confusion. Misunderstandings can thus be avoided by using proper terminology in a specific setting and by defining exactly the meaning of terms.

Interobserver and intraobserver variation in the classification of dysplasia

The microscopic diagnosis of dysplasia is based upon the identification of cytological and architectural criteria. According to most authors cytological criteria are superior to disorganized architecture and more important for the classification of the lesions as low grade or high grade.

Although not clearly established, various studies show that, in specimens from patients operated for high-grade dysplasia, a carcinoma is frequently already present. Therefore, it seems that the criteria used to distinguish low grade from high grade are adequate. On the other hand, some studies have shown a discordance between histologic dysplasia and the finding of aneuploidy on flow cytometry. Flow cytometry might identify other subgroups at risk, and the microscopic evaluation of the presence of dysplasia might not be the best or the only good technique for the early identification of cancer [13].

Another problem is to see whether pathologists of equal experience assess dysplasia reliably. We must realize that as such the alterations characteristic for dysplasia may present interpretative problems for the pathologists. Clearly, this is a very important issue, because if clinicians will decide esophagectomies on the basis of pathology reports they need to be confident of the ability of the pathologists to diagnose dysplasia.

This problem has been studied extensively and it appears that:
— indefinite and low-grade dysplasia are difficult to distinguish and there may be classification problems. An interobserver agreement of 70% can be reached [14,15].
— the interobserver and intraobserver (the same pathologist seeing the same biopsy at a different moment) agreement is good for high-grade dysplasia. An inter-observer agreement of 87% was reached for high-grade dysplasia [14,15].
— similar results are obtained by experienced pathologists and by pathologists of different specific or general interest.
— the terminology used in reporting the lesions may be different (low grade or mild, high grade or severe, three categories or two) but, if a good agreement is made on terminology, no major difference of opinion exists among pathologists for the classification, especially not for the high-grade lesions.

References

1. Boley S, Brandt LJ. Vascular ectasias of the colon. Dig Dis Sci 1986;31: 26S–42S.
2. Ming SCH, Bajtai A, Correa P. Gastric dysplasia: significance and pathologic criteria. Cancer 1984;54:1794–1801.
3. Oehlert W, Keller P, Henke M, Strauch M. Die dysplasien der Magenschleimhaut. Dtsch Med Wochenschr 1975;100: 1950–1956.
4. Sipponen P. Gastric dysplasia. In: Williams GT (ed) Gastrointestinal Pathology. Berlin: Springer Verlag, 1990;61–76.
5. Farini R, Farinati F, Leandro G. Gastric epithelial dysplasia in relapsing and nonrelapsing gastric ulcer. Am J Gastroenterol 1982;77:844–853.
6. Farinati F, Cardin F, Di Mario F. Follow-up in gastric dysplasia patients. Am J Surg Pathol 1989;13:173–174.
7. Riddell RH, Goldman H, Ransohoff D, Appelman HD, Fenoglio CM, Haggitt RC, Ahren C, Correa P, Hamilton SR, Morson BC, Sommers SC, Yardley JH. Dysplasia in inflammatory bowel disease. Hum Pathol 1983;14:931–967.
8. Hamilton SR. Reflux esophagitis and Barrett's esophagus. In: Goldman H, Appelman HD, Kaufman N (eds) Gastrointestinal Pathology. Baltimore: Williams & Wilkins, 1990;11–68.
9. Potet F, Duchatelle V. Barrett's Oesophagus. In: Williams GT (ed) Current Topics in Gastrointestinal Pathology. Berlin: Springer Verlag, 1990;43–60.
10. Pascal RR. Consistency in the terminology of colorectal dysplasia. Hum Pathol 1988;19:1249–1250.
11. Hamilton SR, Smith RRL. The relationship between columnar epithelial dysplasia and invasive carcinoma arising in Barrett's esophagus. Am J Clin Pathol 1987;87:301–312.
12. Schmidt HG, Riddell RH, Walther BC, Skinner DB, Riemann JF. Dysplasia in Barrett's esophagus. J Cancer Res Clin Oncol 1985;110:145–152.
13. Fennerty MB, Sampliner RE, Way D, Riddell RH, Steinbronn K, Garewal HS. Discordance between flow cytometric abnormalities and dysplasia in Barrett's esophagus. Gastroenterology 1989;97:815–820.
14. Reid BJ, Haggitt RC, Rubin CE, Roth G, Surawicz CM, Van Belle G, Lewin K, Weinstein WM, Antonioli DA, Goldman H, MacDonald W, Owen D. Criteria for dysplasia in Barrett's esophagus: a cooperative consensus study. Gastroenterology 1987;88:1552.
15. Reid BJ, Haggitt RC, Rubin CE, Roth G, Surawicz CM. Observer variation in the diagnosis of dysplasia in Barrett's esophagus. Hum Pathol 1988;19:166–178.

S.R. Hamilton (Baltimore)

Adenocarcinoma arising in columnar-lined mucosa is a well-known complication of Barrett's esophagus (columnar epithelial replacement of previously squamous-lined esophageal mucosa, usually due to chronic gastroesophageal reflux). Mortality in patients presenting with symptomatic Barrett's adenocarcinoma is high. Therefore, the strategy of surveying patients with known Barrett's esophagus for preinvasive neoplasia in the form of columnar epithelial dysplasia (intraepithelial neoplasia) and for early adenocarcinoma is currently recommended in patients who are suitable surgical candidates for esophagectomy. In the absence of proven efficacious endoscopic ablation procedures or pharmacologic agents effective against dysplasia, prophylactic esophagectomy is the currently available treatment. Esophagectomy is recommended for Barrett patients with dysplasia severe enough to warrant major concern about synchronous or metachronous adenocarcinoma, although the natural history of the dysplasia-carcinoma sequence is not yet well defined in large numbers of patients. Esophagectomy carries the risk of serious morbidity and mortality even

998

in the hands of the expert esophageal surgical teams who should be entrusted with the prophylactic procedure. Therefore, accurate histopathologic interpretation of dysplasia in endoscopic biopsy specimens and brush cytology specimens of Barrett's mucosa is of great concern, because of the implications for patient management.

Dysplasia is identified histopathologically on the basis of abnormalities in mucosal architecture, epithelial morphology and cytology. The histopathology of columnar epithelial dysplasia in Barrett's mucosa is impressively heterogeneous. In addition, dysplasia can be difficult to distinguish from reactive columnar epithelial changes due to the effects of ongoing gastroesophageal reflux. Intraobserver and interobserver variation in the interpretation of the spectrum of dysplasia is therefore expected.

The most useful classification schemes for communication among gastroenterologists, esophageal surgeons and pathologists regarding dysplasia in Barrett's mucosa employ modifications of the scheme developed for dysplasia in idiopathic inflammatory bowel disease. As shown in Table 1, the findings are classified into negative for dysplasia, indefinite for dysplasia and positive for dysplasia.

The negative category indicates no concern for dysplasia in the specimens. The indefinite category is used for abnormalities which are of concern, but not interpreted as diagnostic of dysplasia, usually due to inflammation or artifact complicating interpretation, but also due to uncertainty about the interpretation of the findings. This category can be subdivided into probably negative, of unknown significance, and probably positive for the pathologist to express the level of concern [1]. In the positive for dysplasia category, three grades were used by the group (low-, intermediate- and high-grade dysplasia) to classify the severity of the dysplasia. This approach is based on the study of features of dysplasia associated with invasive adenocarcinoma, in order to establish criteria [1]. Some investigators use three grades analogous to gastric dysplasia [2]. Other groups use two grades (low- and high-grade) with criteria adapted from colonic dysplasia in idiopathic inflammatory bowel disease [3] (Table 1). The two-grade system permits greater observer agreement, but cases at the low end of the high-grade dysplasia spectrum in Barrett's mucosa, using colonic criteria for idiopathic inflammatory bowel disease, have a relatively infrequent association with synchronous adenocarcinoma.

In the clinical application of dysplasia classification, two decision points are

Table 1. Classification schemes for dysplasia in Barrett's mucosa

Three grades of dysplasia [1]	Two grades of dysplasia [2]
Negative for dysplasia	Negative for dysplasia
Indefinite for dysplasia	Indefinite for dysplasia
Probably negative	
Of unknown significance	
Probably positive	
Positive for dysplasia	Positive for dysplasia
Low-grade	Low-grade
Intermediate-grade	High-grade
High-grade	
Adenocarcinoma	Adenocarcinoma

important: the interface between indefinite for dysplasia vs. negative for dysplasia, which may influence frequency of follow-up, and the interface between high-grade dysplasia vs. low-grade/intermediate-grade dysplasia, which will influence consideration of prophylactic esophagectomy. One study addressed the agreement among eight experienced gastrointestinal pathologists in the diagnosis of dysplasia, with two grades in the positive for dysplasia category [4]. A slide set of 71 sections, including biopsy and resection specimens, was chosen to include some especially difficult cases. Interobserver agreement of 85 and 87% was found in two successive rounds of evaluation comparing the combined category of high-grade dysplasia and intermucosal carcinoma against the combined category of low-grade dysplasia, indefinite for dysplasia and negative for dysplasia. At the other end of the spectrum, interobserver agreement was 71 and 72% in the two rounds when negative for dysplasia was compared against the combined category of indefinite for dysplasia, positive for dysplasia and intermucosal adenocarcinoma.

All diagnostic tests have inherent variability. In ideal circumstances, variation is reduced to a minimum. The study described above demonstrates that there is acceptable reproducibility of classification at the two clinically important decision points in the hands of experienced gastrointestinal pathologists. The level of agreement is better than that for preinvasive breast disease evaluated by experienced breast pathologists [5].

No marker which improves on dysplasia as an indicator of risk of adenocarcinoma is yet available. Such markers may never become available, because the diverse molecular, genetic and biochemical pathways which provide potential markers are all associated with the same morphologic endpoint (i.e., dysplasia and ultimately adenocarcinoma). Furthermore, dysplasia appears to be related to accumulated molecular abnormalities of various types, as evidenced by the heterogeneity of results in studies published thus far. For example, abnormalities in p53 occur in a subset of Barrett's adenocarcinomas, but certainly not all cases [6,7]. Thus, none of the currently identified genetic abnormalities are absolutely associated with neoplasia, and furthermore neoplasia is not uniformly associated with any of the genetic abnormalities. Although important for investigational studies of the pathogenesis of dysplasia and carcinoma, the individual genes and biochemical pathways seem unlikely to provide markers with clinical utility exceeding dysplasia itself.

In conclusion, variability in the grading of dysplasia in Barrett's mucosa by gastrointestinal pathologists occurs at an acceptable level for satisfactory clinical management. Given the rarity of patients with dysplasia in Barrett's esophagus and the high stakes for the patient being considered for prophylactic esophagectomy, surgical management in centers with a highly experienced esophageal surgery team and gastrointestinal pathologist, who has reviewed the biopsy specimens, is prudent.

References

1. Hamilton SR, Smith RRL. The relationship between columnar epithelial dysplasia and invasive adenocarcinoma in Barrett's esophagus. Am J Clin Pathol 1987;87:301–312.

2. Morson BC, Sobin LH, Grundmann E, Johansen A, Nagayo T, Serck-Hanssen A. Precancerous conditions and epithelial dysplasia in the stomach. J Clin Pathol 1980;33:711—721.
3. Riddell RH, Goldman H, Rensohoff DF et al. Dysplasia in inflammatory bowel disease. Standardized classification with provisional clinical applications. Hum Pathol 1983;14:931—968.
4. Reid BJ, Haggitt RC, Rubin CE et al. Observer variation in the diagnosis of dysplasia in Barrett's esophagus. Hum Pathol 1988;19:166—178.
5. Schnitt SJ, Connolly JL, Tavassoli FA et al. Interobserver reproducibility in the diagnosis of ductal proliferative breast lesions using standardized criteria. Am J Surg Pathol 1992;16:1133—1143.
6. Flejou JF, Potet F, Muzeau F et al. Overexpression of p53 protein in Barrett's syndrome with malignant transformation. J Clin Pathol 1993;46:330—333.
7. Blount PL, Ramel S, Raskind WH et al. 17p allelic deletions and p53 protein overexpression in Barrett's adenocarcinoma. Cancer Res 1991;51;5482—5486.

Are there any histologic features of high-grade dysplasia which make this diagnosis equivocal?

M.D. Diebold (Reims)

The diagnosis of high-grade dysplasia in Barrett's mucosa is based upon the combination of architectural and cytologic criteria. Potential diagnostic problems concern each end of the spectrum of high-grade dysplasic lesions. At one end of the spectrum the diagnosis depends on the assessment of cytologic abnormalities and especially of nuclear alterations.

The signification of cytologic prominent abnormalities associated with a heavy inflammatory infiltrate may be questionable. The lack of true stratification, the normal or decreased nuclear-cytoplasmic ratio associated with cytoplasmic clarification and polymorphs within the epithelium, are in favor of inflammation related lesions. Nevertheless, dysplastic changes and inflammation lesions can coexist. Of the utmost importance for the diagnosis of high-grade dysplasia are polymorphism and hyperchromatism of the nuclei and loss of nuclear polarity. At the other end of the lesion spectrum is the distinction between high-grade dysplasia and infiltrating adenocarcinoma. The cytologic criteria are indiscriminative and the differential diagnosis is based upon the integrity of basement membrane in high-grade dysplasia and invasion in infiltrating adenocarcinoma.

In Barrett's mucosa, misleading features are realized by pseudo-invasion of lamina propria, muscularis mucosae and submucosa. Among them, crowding and infolding of dysplastic glands must be differentiated from cribriform or back-to-back pattern of adenocarcinoma. The bottoms of tortuous dysplastic glands may appear on some sections as isolated nests of atypical infiltrating cells. Another pattern of architectural distortion in Barrett's mucosa is represented by dysplastic gland entrapment in hyperplastic and disorganized fibers of the muscularis mucosae ascending upwards into the lamina propria. Glandular cysts, of unknown signification, are frequent in

Barrett's mucosa; they may be lined partially or totally by a dysplastic epithelium and should not be mistaken for an invasive adenocarcinoma.

The pathologist should be familiar with this range of changes. These potential pitfalls also emphasize the necessity of a rigorous histopathological examination.

The best conditions for diagnosis include numerous and large biopsy samples (eventually obtained by aspiration-section technique) and adequate orientation before embedding.

Serial-step sectioning allows better understanding of the architectural distortion of glands, unmasking isolated atypical cells, if any, originating from an underlying or neighboring adenocarcinoma.

 L. Le Bodic (Nantes)

Dysplasia refers to various cellular and architectural defects of the intraepithelial topography resulting from abnormal proliferative activity. These defects may be considered as the usual, but not ineluctable, phase in transition from a normal to a cancerous cell. Thus, two types of problems are involved: the diagnosis and exact grading of dysplasia as well as the therapeutic strategy to be employed.

Dysplastic alterations occur in cells (differentiation defects with secretion loss or abnormalities; anisocytosis and anisokaryosis; atypical mitoses) and tissues (architectural disorganization). None of these defects are specific, and their association and severity can vary in the same biopsy specimen.

A distinction should be made between two esophageal forms which raise different problems: dysplasia of the esophageal mucosa and Barrett's esophagus.

Dysplasia of the esophageal mucosa

It has been investigated in two types of studies: the Asiatic approach is based on cytological data without endoscopy, and the Western approach on biopsies obtained during endoscopy. The correlations between cytological and histopathological classifications have not been documented. Mukada et al. [1] proposed three grades for this dysplasia: slight, moderate and severe. The severe form is characterized by defects involving the entire mucous membrane. However, microinvasive carcinoma is indicated when the chorion is involved.

The diagnosis of severe dysplasia in esophageal mucosa may be uncertain. When there is intense inflammation with ulceration, the presence of tumescent and atypical endothelial cells in neoformative capillaries within regenerative granulation tissue may prove misleading. Cytological abnormalities related to viral infections (herpes, cytomegalovirus) are sometimes quite marked, wrongly suggesting dysplasia. There is also the possibility of pseudoepitheliomatous epithelial hyperplasia with dyskeratosis in the case of Abrikosoff's tumor. Finally, the poor quality of a shredded specimen can make interpretation difficult, especially if the lesions are not uniformly distributed.

Barrett's esophagus

In Barrett's esophagus, or glandular mucosa of the endobrachyesophagus (EBE), the prevalence of dysplasia is estimated to be 10% in the absence and 80% in the presence of associated cancer [2–4]. In Riddell's classification, which is generally used, moderate or low-grade dysplasia (LGD) is characterized by basophilic cells with large, rounded hyperchromatic nuclei; pseudostratification features, with nuclei occupying only the lower half of cells which appear to be compressed; and reduced cell secretion. In addition to these LGD abnormalities, severe or high-grade dysplasia (HGD) is characterized by an increased nucleocytoplasmic ratio as well as nuclear defects, with pseudostratification of nuclei along the entire cell layer, mucosecretion defects and architectural abnormalities (disorganized, proliferative and ramified crypts, with occasional luminal epithelial vegetation), but without involvement of the basement membrane and the chorion. Although it is not absolutely certain that HGD will always progress to cancer, it has been demonstrated that HGD is frequently present within the year preceding cancer diagnosis [3,5].

In 11 series totaling 438 patients, dysplasia was present in 10% of cases, with HGD occurring in only 2% of simple EBE without visible carcinoma, whereas the mean incidence in 16 published series of EBE complicated by carcinoma was 78% (59–100%), 79% of which were HGD [6]. The problem is one of reproducibility and thus of the reliability of the diagnosis reached by the pathologist. In a retrospective study based on 37 biopsies examined by four pathologists [6], total diagnostic concordance was found for 20 (54%), 16 (80%) of which concerned HGD. When these 37 biopsies were reviewed simultaneously by the interpreters, diagnostic concordance was reached for 34 (92%), and two discordances concerned LGD and HGD.

Improvement in diagnostic concordance depends on a good definition of histopathological criteria. It is likely that concordance is lower for pathologists not often required to interpret dysplasias, particularly in an inflammatory context. The persistence of gastroesophageal reflux seems to play a role in the worsening of dysplastic lesions [2], although therapeutic control of this reflux does not eliminate the risk of dysplasia and carcinoma.

In cases of Barrett's esophagus, personal factors can condition interpretation of dysplastic lesions, especially for the differentiation of nondysplastic from dysplastic (or slightly dysplastic) mucosa, particularly in an inflammatory context. We are not concerned here with techniques currently under evaluation which may prove useful for the diagnosis of dysplasia or for histopathological prognosis (flow cytometry, mucus alterations, nucleolar organizers, etc.). Results have been disappointing for some of these techniques and are still preliminary for others.

It can therefore be concluded that it is essential to have a precise definition of the criteria of dysplasia in order to provide for reinterpretation by an experienced pathologist and examination of new biopsy specimens in case of doubt.

References

1. Mukada T, Sato E, Sasano N. Comparative studies on dysplasia of oesophageal epithelium in four prefectures of Japan, with reference to risk of carcinoma. Tohoku J Exp Med 1976;119:51–63.
2. Skinner DB, Walther BC, Riddell R, Schmidt H. Barrett's oesophagus: comparison of benign and malignant cases. Ann Surg 1983;198:554–566.
3. Hameeteman W, Tytgat GNJ, Houthoff HJ, van den Tweel JG. Barrett's oesophagus: development of dysplasia and adenocarcinoma. Gastroenterology 1989;96:1249–1256.
4. Pateron D, Flejou JF. Dysplasies sévères de l'oesophage: quelle attitude adopter? Gastroenterol Clin Biol 1991; 15:509–511.
5. Gayet B. Barrett's adenocarcinoma. VIIth National Congress on Surgery, Lisbon, 1987 (abstract).
6. Sagan C. Dysplasies sur endobrachyoesophage. Concordance diagnostique entre pathologistes. Thesis, Nantes, 1992.

Are there histological criteria that are capable of distinguishing high-grade dysplasia with biologic potential of invasion from high-grade dysplasia without invasive potential?

R.H. Riddell (Hamilton)

What this question really asks is whether there is any evidence that the traditional gold standard of histology can be replaced using other techniques. The short answer to this question is, at present, NO. However, as data accumulate which looks more closely at, and uses as its gold standard, the morphological spectrum of changes from nondysplastic through to high-grade dysplasia, a series of changes occurs in the following:
1. An increase in the amount of epithelial nuclear DNA (aneuploidy).
2. An increase in the proportion of cells entering the G_1, S and G_2 part of the cell cycle, resulting in an increased mitotic rate.
3. The expression of oncogenes and their products.
4. Chromosomal abnormalities.
5. Mucin changes.
6. Nuclear organizer regions.

All of these are discussed elsewhere in this book and what follows is a brief summary. The bottom line is that while it is clear that a sequence of changes tends to occur in any patient as this spectrum is travelled, and that there are overall broad correlations, the single best predictor of invasion remains high-grade dysplasia. Let us examine some of these.

Aneuploidy

There is evidence that aneuploidy precedes or accompanies both dysplasia and invasion [1], although the total number of cancers and background mucosa examined to date is relatively small. However, measurement of aneuploidy is dependent on a flow cytometer, or equivalent, to measure the amount of nuclear DNA and the ability to take biopsies of adequate size with sufficient tissue to carry out the procedure reliably. The easiest way to achieve this is using large (e.g., 9 mm open) biopsy forceps for both histology and flow cytometry. However, cell image analysis can be carried out on thick paraffin embedded sections, but counts many fewer cells. If available, this procedure has several implications. The first is that provided multiple biopsies are evaluated, then patients with no aneuploidy are very unlikely to have dysplasia or invasive carcinoma. The real question is whether, because of this, aneuploidy can be used to stratify patients into those without aneuploidy, who could be screened much less frequently than those with aneuploidy. For example, every 2 or even 3 years compared with those with aneuploidy who might be endoscoped annually or even more frequently if aneuploidy is widespread. To date no studies are known that have actually used aneuploidy in this way. Interestingly not all tumors in Barrett's esophagus (BE) are aneuploid; there has been a modest number of cancers not arising on a background of aneuploidy [2]; if confirmed this policy will need to be revised. There appears to be no role for aneuploidy in the decision for surgical resection.

Proportion of cells entering the G_1, S and G_2 part of the cell cycle

While it is difficult to measure each part of the cell cycle independently, the availability of flow cytometry, which allows measurement of the proportion of cells in S-phase and G_2M, and antibodies such as Ki-67 which allows assessment of cells not in the G_0 part of the cell cycle. One study assessing all of these parameters in the same patient cohort found that, compared with normal controls from the gastric fundus and cardia, patients with Barrett's esophagus had an increased proportion of cells in the non-G_0 part of the cell cycle [3]. Increased S-phase was particularly found in those patients with higher grades of dysplasia or carcinoma and aneuploidy. They concluded that neoplastic progression in BE was associated with at least three types of cell cycle abnormalities, including mobilization from G_0 to G_1, loss of control of the G_1/S phase transition and accumulation of cells in G_2.

Molecular markers

A variety of oncogenes or their products have been examined in BE. The question is whether any of these are markers of increased risk of having or developing invasive carcinoma, independent of other markers such as dysplasia or even aneuploidy. Many of these are found in nondysplastic BE with a variable increase as dysplasia and cancer are sampled. The frequency varies markedly depending on the method used. Follow-up studies have shown the following changes:

p53. This is a chromosome 17 gene product that is not detectable in the normal or if there is an allelic deletion, however, mis-sense mutations are associated with a product having an increased half-life which is therefore detectable immunocytochemically. It is variably (5–75%) present in BE without dysplasia and in about the same number of patients with dysplasia or carcinoma [4,5]. For example, it was found in 50% of carcinomas in one series [6] and 67% in another [7]. In some studies there was a correlation with the degree of dysplasia [8].

Ras. This was found in 40% of nondysplastic mucosa and 56% of high-grade dysplasia [9].

Fos. This was found in 20% nondysplastic and 44% of high-grade dysplasia [9].

Myc. This was found in 60% nondysplastic and 78% of high-grade dysplasia [9].

c-erb 2. This tends to be present in intestinal cancers and, in the small proportion of patients examined, tends to portend a poor prognosis [10–12].

There currently appears to be little role for molecular markers in the decision tree of patients with BE at risk for carcinoma.

Chromosomal abnormalities

A variety of deletions have been described in Barrett's cancers including p53 (v.s.), the adenomatous polyposis gene (APC), the MCC, Retinoblastoma and DCC genes [4,13–17]. Deletions of the Y chromosome have also been reported [18].

Mucins

BE frequently stains with acidic (intestinal) type mucins and sulfated (colonic) mucins are frequently present, particularly in patients with carcinoma [19–21]. Consequently, related lectins, including peanut and sialosyl-Tn, are also frequently present [21]. However, these parameters have neither the sensitivity nor specificity to be of value in determining patients at high risk of developing carcinoma.

Nuclear organizer regions

These are genes that code for ribosomal RNA and are located on the achrosomal chromosomes 13-15, 21 and 22, and are demonstrated by a silver staining technique. In Barrett's mucosa, their number is increased in dysplastic mucosa, but there is no distinction between high- and low-grade dysplasia, while they are also seen in reactive changes. This technique is therefore unlikely to be of value [22].

References

1. Reid BJ, Blount PL, Rubin CE, Levine DS, Haggitt RC, Rabinovitch PS. Flow cytometric and histological progression to malignancy in Barrett's esophagus: prospective endoscopic surveillance of a cohort. Gastroenterology 1992;102:1212–1219.
2. Menke-Pluymers MBE, Hop WCJ, Mulder AH, Tilanus HW. The role of DNA-ploidy, stage and grade as prognostic factors in the survival of patients with Barrett's adenocarcinoma. Gastroenterology 1993;104:A428.
3. Reid BJ, Sanchez CA, Blount PL, Levine DS. Barrett's esophagus: cell cycle abnormalities in advancing stages of neoplastic progression. Gastroenterology 1993;105:119–129.
4. Ramel S, Reid BJ, Sanchez CA et al. Evaluation of p53 protein expression in Barrett's esophagus by two-parameter flow cytometry. Gastroenterology 1992;102:1220–1228.
5. Gray MR, Thomas DM, Kingsnorth AN, Hall PA. p53 immunocytochemistry in metaplastic and Barrett's esophagus. Gastroenterology 1993;104:A91.
6. Audrezet MP, Robaszkiewicz M, Mercier B, Nousbaum JB, Guillermit H, Ferec C. Screening for TP53 gene mutations in esophageal carcinomas. Gastroenterology 1993;104:A386.
7. Fléjou J-F, Muzeau F, LePelletrier F, Paraf F, Hénin D, Potet F. Overexpression of p53 protein in carcinomas of the esophagus and stomach. Gastroenterology 1993;104:A400.
8. Krishadath KK, Mulder AH, Tilanus HW. p53 protein overexpression in Barrett's adenocarcinoma and Barrett's esophagus in paraffin embedded tissue. Gastroenterology 1993;104:A1045.
9. McGuigan J, Gibbons JRP. Differential oncogene expression in the development of Barrett's neoplasia. Gastroenterology 1993;104:A178.
10. Jankowski J, Coghill G, Hopwood D, Wormsley KG. Oncogenes and onco-suppresser gene in adenocarcinoma of the esophagus. Gut 1992;33:1033–1038.
11. Fléjou J-F, Paraf F, Muzeau F, Hénin D, Jothy S, Potet F. c-erb B2 oncogene expression and prognosis in Barrett's adenocarcinoma. Gastroenterology 1993;104:A400.
12. Gramlich T, Grossl L, Fritsch C, Gansler T. c-erb B-2 proto-oncogene expression and amplification in Barrett's adenocarcinoma. Gastroenterology 1993;104:A407.
13. Blount PL, Ramel S, Raskind WH et al. 17p alletic deletions and p53 protein overexpression in Barrett's adenocarcinoma. Cancer Res 1991;51:5482–5486.
14. Meltzer SJ, Yin J, Huang J et al. Reduction to homozygosity involving p53 in esophageal cancers demonstrated by the polymerase chain reaction. Proc Nat Acad Sci USA 1991;88:4976–4980.
15. Boynton RF, Blount PL, Yin J et al. Loss of heterozygosity involving the APC and MCC genetic loci in the majority of human esophageal cancers. Proc Nat Acad Sci USA 1992;89:3385–3388.
16. Boynton RF, Huang Y, Blount PL et al. Frequent loss of heterozygosity at the retinoblastoma locus in human esophageal cancers. Cancer Res 1991;51:5766–5769.
17. Huang Y, Boynton RF, Blount PL et al. Loss of heterozygosity involves multiple tumor suppresser genes in human esophageal cancers. Cancer Res 1992;52:6525–6530.
18. Krishadath KK, Tilanus HW, Mulder AH, van Dekken H. Detection of numerical chromosomal aberrations in Barrett's adenocarcinoma and Barrett's esophagus by non-isotopic in situ hybridization to tumour sections. Gastroenterology 1993;104:A1045.
19. Rothery GA, Patterson JE, Stoddard CJ, Day DW. Histological and histochemical changes in the columnar-lined (Barrett's oesophagus). Gut 1986;27:1062–1068.
20. Lapertosa G, Baracchini P, Fulcheri E et al. Mucin histochemical analysis in the interpretation of Barrett's esophagus. Am J Clin Pathol 1992;98:61–66.
21. Itzkowitz SH, Kahn E, Auerbach M, Stiel L, Gerardi F, McKinley M. Sialosyl-Tn (STn) antigen: a potential marker of malignant transformation in Barrett's esophagus. Gastroenterology 1993;104: A412.
22. Burke AP, Sobin LH, Shekitka KM, Avallone FA. Correlation of nuclear organizer regions and glandular dysplasia in the stomach and esophagus. Mod Pathol 1990;3:357–360.

S.R. Hamilton (Baltimore)

Are there histological criteria which are capable of distinguishing high-grade dysplasia with the biologic potential of invasion from high-grade dysplasia without invasive potential?. The answer to this question in a word, is "NO". Dysplasia is unequivocably neoplastic epithelial proliferation [1], i.e., intraepithelial neoplasia, and is recognized in Barrett's mucosa on the basis of histopathologic abnormalities of mucosal architecture, epithelial morphology and cytology [2,3]. The continuous spectrum of dysplasia is categorized artificially into discrete grades to permit the pathologist to communicate the severity of the abnormalities. Grading is important in the management of patients because the more severe the dysplasia the higher the likelihood of synchronous and metachromous invasive adenocarcinoma. However, because sampling plays a role in the apparent relationship between dysplasia and adenocarcinoma, especially in biopsy specimens, the precise relationship in an individual patient is often subject to uncertainty. For example, endoscopic biopsies may be too superficial to include areas of adenocarcinoma in the submucosa and even in the mucosa itself an area of cancer may not be sampled. Columnar epithelial dysplasia in Barrett's mucosa may differ morphologically from adenocarcinoma only in lacking identifiable invasion. Furthermore, the neoplastic process does not need to proceed through the phase identifiable histopathologically as high-grade dysplasia in order to have invasion. In other words, invasion can occur in areas of dysplasia less severe than that categorized as high-grade dysplasia. The consequence of the lack of histopathologic criteria capable of distinguishing dysplasia with malignant potential, or more importantly dysplasia without invasive potential, is the necessity to consider prophylactic esophagectomy. Whether or not markers capable of predicting invasive behavior can ultimately be identified remains to be seen.

References

1. Riddell RH, Goldman H, Ransohoff DF et al. Dysplasia in inflammatory bowel disease. Standardized classification with provisional clinical applications. Hum Pathol 1993;14:931–968.
2. Hamilton SR, Smith RRL. The relationship between columnar epithelial dysplasia and invasive adenocarcinoma arising in Barrett's esophagus. Am J Clin Pathol 1987;87:301–312.
3. Reid BJ, Haggitt RC, Rubin CE et al. Observer variation in the diagnosis of dysplasia in Barrett's esophagus. Hum Pathol 1988;19:166–178.

Is intense medical therapy necessary before taking biopsies for dysplasia?

M.F. Dixon (Leeds)

The answer to this question is patently, "no". Biopsies taken from actively inflamed or ulcerated mucosa will usually exhibit reactive or regenerative epithelial changes, but these can generally be distinguished from dysplasia. In a minority of cases the appearances may be equivocal and biopsy after a period of medical therapy will frequently resolve the diagnostic problem. However, these circumstances are not sufficiently common to militate against pretreatment biopsies.

As with other questions concerning dysplasia, the problems centre on the definition of dysplasia and the expertise of the observer. If we regard dysplasia as an unequivocal neoplastic alteration of the epithelium which has characteristic cytological and architectural features, then it is clearly possible to recognize high-grade dysplasia even in the presence of active inflammation and ulceration. Difficulties arise when less experienced observers misinterpret simple regenerative hyperplasia and reactive changes as "dysplasia". Under such circumstances dysplasia (usually designated "low grade") will be overdiagnosed and the patient subjected to unnecessary repeat biopsies and anxiety.

Even more serious is the failure to recognize bizarre regenerative changes in epithelium at the margins of an ulcer, and the subsequent receipt of a "negative" esophagectomy specimen. Pathologists should always have a high threshold for the diagnosis of dysplasia and malignancy if such errors are to be avoided. Where the findings are in any way equivocal (i.e., indefinite for dysplasia), then it is certainly prudent to advocate rebiopsy after a course of medical therapy, but these circumstances should not dictate a general rule. Furthermore, all patients with Barrett's esophagus should undergo regular surveillance with multiple biopsies. Patients showing equivocal changes can be "flagged", so that future biopsies are compared with previous biopsies and the finding of progression or regression will determine clinical management.

What is the definition of "indefinite for dysplasia" in Barrett's mucosa?

W.V. Bogomoletz (Reims)

Dysplasia occurs in patients with Barrett's esophagus (BE), either extensively or focally and with or without associated adenocarcinoma. Dysplasia is considered as a precursor of adenocarcinoma arising in BE [1,2]. Moreover, dysplasia in BE has been defined as an unequivocal neoplastic alteration [3].

In recent years, dysplasia in BE has been graded by many experts according to a system similar to that used for grading dysplasia in inflammatory bowel disease [4]. This system comprises three major categories: negative for dysplasia (including inflammatory and regenerative changes), indefinite for dysplasia and positive for dysplasia, the latter being subdivided into a low grade and a high grade [4].

The indefinite for dysplasia category includes all mucosal changes in which it is not possible to decide whether these changes are inflammatory or regenerative in nature, or constitute genuine neoplastic lesions. The inference is that a diagnosis of indefinite for dysplasia should be restricted to cases in which the changes are too marked for negative, but not sufficient for dysplasia. At the other end of the scale, however, it may be difficult to differentiate between the indefinite for dysplasia category and low-grade dysplasia [5].

In practical terms, a diagnosis of indefinite for dysplasia is an unsatisfactory situation. The pathologist should certainly ask for further biopsies and the endoscopist should be encouraged to take them.

References

1. Spechler SJ, Goyal RK. Barrett's esophagus. N Engl J Med 1986;315:362–371.
2. Potet F, Duchatelle V. Barrett's oesophagus. In: Williams GT (ed) Gastrointestinal Pathology. Current Topics in Pathology No.81. Berlin: Springer Verlag, 1990;43–60.
3. Riddell RH. Dysplasia and regression in Barrett's epithelium. In: Spechler SJ, Goyal RK (eds) Barrett's Esophagus. New York: Elsevier, 1985;143–152.
4. Schmidt HG, Riddell RH, Walther B, Skinner DB, Riemann JF. Dysplasia in Barrett's esophagus. J Cancer Res Clin Oncol 1985;110:145–152.
5. Reid BJ, Haggitt RC, Rubin CE et al. Observer variation in the diagnosis of dysplasia in Barrett's esophagus. Hum Pathol 1988;19:166–178.

Can medical treatment lead to regression of dysplasia?

R.E. Sampliner (Tucson)

Although "intensive medical treatment" is recommended for patients with Barrett's esophagus and dysplasia demonstrated by biopsy [1], there is little data to substantiate the natural history of dysplasia, let alone its response to therapy. Two major caveats have to be kept in mind when evaluating data on regression of dysplasia:
1. The adequacy of biopsy sampling and the problem of sampling error; and
2. The issue of observer variability — even in the presence of high-grade dysplasia, the interobserver agreement is only in the 85—87% range [2].

Hameeteman et al. reported 50 patients with Barrett's esophagus actively treated when reflux esophagitis was seen at endoscopy. Treatment consisted of H_2-receptor antagonists, omeprazole and six patients underwent antireflux surgery. In spite of this therapy of active inflammatory disease, five patients progressed from negative or low-grade dysplasia to carcinoma and 13 patients either developed or continued to have dysplasia [3]. High-grade dysplasia without progression was present in two patients for 36 and 44 months.

Reid et al. described a prospective endoscopic surveillance of 62 patients with Barrett's esophagus. Although the therapy of these patients is not described, four out of nine patients with high-grade dysplasia remained stable, histologically, over an 11—20-month interval. In addition, four out of 20 patients with indefinite or low-grade dysplasia subsequently did not have dysplasia during follow-up [4].

In conclusion, data are lacking which indicate that medical therapy leads to regression or stabilization of dysplasia in Barrett's esophagus. Due to the relative infrequency of dysplasia, multicenter studies with standardized observations and central pathology readings will be necessary to define the natural history of dysplasia and the response to therapy.

References

1. Spechler SJ, Goyal RK. Barrett's esophagus. N Engl J Med 1986;315:362—371.
2. Reid BJ, Haggitt RC, Rubin CE et al. Observer variation in the diagnosis of dysplasia in Darrett's esophagus. Hum Pathol 1988;19:166—178.
3. Hameeteman W, Tytgat GNJ, Houthoff HJ et al. Barrett's esophagus: development of dysplasia and adenocarcinoma. Gastroenterology 1989;96:1249—1256.
4. Reid BJ, Blount PL, Rubin CE et al. Flow-cytometric and histologic progression to malignancy in Barrett's esophagus: prospective endoscopic surveillance of a cohort. Gastroenterology 1992;102:1212—1219.

Is it possible to demonstrate the impact of antireflux surgery on dysplastic changes of the mucosa?

T.C. Smyrk (Omaha)

Do sampling errors adversely effect our ability to monitor mucosal changes following antireflux surgery? The same question can be asked about follow-up of any therapy and the answer is more than a matter of academic curiosity. If regression or stabilization of dysplasia in Barrett's esophagus cannot be adequately documented, how can different modes of treatment be compared? Also, if progression cannot be documented, can the clinician and patient be comfortable choosing conservative treatment for a high-risk condition such as Barrett's esophagus with high-grade dysplasia?

Some sense of the difficulty in monitoring posttreatment changes in dysplasia can be gained by examining efforts to follow posttreatment changes in the length of Barrett's esophagus. Hassall and Weinstein recently reviewed previous reports claiming regression of Barrett's esophagus and found that all suffered from some deficiencies, such as poor identification of esophageal landmarks, inadequate pre- and posttreatment histology and inadequate documentation (i.e., pH studies) of therapeutic efficacy [1]. When dysplasia is added to the equation, with its usual absence of gross changes and its dependence on subjective histologic interpretation, the problem becomes even more complex.

That complexity is reflected in prevailing attitudes about high-grade dysplasia in Barrett's esophagus. Due to fear that high-grade dysplasia might progress to advanced invasive carcinoma during follow-up or that high-grade dysplasia might be accompanied by undiagnosed adenocarcinoma at presentation, esophagectomy has been recommended in that setting [2]. Recent work from the University of Washington suggests that observation can be a safe option [3]. Levine et al. presented 22 patients followed with prospective endoscopic surveillance for Barrett's esophagus with high-grade dysplasia. There was no mortality from adenocarcinoma not diagnosed at an early stage (compared to an operative mortality of 14%). The authors argue that high-grade dysplasia alone does not necessarily require surgical resection.

The experience of the UW group can be applied to the question under consideration: Yes, it is possible to demonstrate the impact of antireflux surgery on dysplasia, provided the physician and the patient are willing to follow a rigorous biopsy protocol. Any attempt to monitor dysplastic Barrett's esophagus, following any type of treatment, must include the following:

1. Minimize the number of endoscopists involved in follow-up for better standardization.
2. Document the linear extent of Barrett's mucosa, based on accepted esophageal landmarks such as the Z line or the top of the LES.
3. Take multiple biopsies at each endoscopy in a systematic fashion.

The UW group recommends four quadrant biopsies taken every 1–2 cm over the entire length of Barrett's esophagus. In addition, multiple biopsies should be taken from sites at which high-grade dysplasia has been documented previously.

It can be hoped that improvements in adjunctive methods such as DNA analysis by flow cytometry will soon provide useful information in this setting. There may even come a day when areas of high-grade dysplasia can be labeled in vivo to allow endoscopic visualization. Until then, surveillance of high-grade dysplasia and assessment of posttreatment changes will depend on a carefully followed biopsy protocol and close co-operation between endoscopist and pathologist.

References

1. Hassall E, Weinstein WM. Partial regression of childhood Barrett's esophagus after fundal plication. Am J Gastroenterol 1992;87:1506.
2. Hamilton SR, Smith RRL. The relationship between columnar epithelial dysplasia and invasive adenocarcinoma arising in Barrett's esophagus. Am J Clin Pathol 1987;87:301–312.
3. Levine DS, Haggitt RC, Blount PL et al. An endoscopic biopsy protocol can differentiate high-grade dysplasia from early adenocarcinoma in Barrett's esophagus. Gastroenterology 1993;105:40–50.

Can dysplasia in Barrett's esophagus regress?

K.J. Lewin (Los Angeles)

It is estimated that about 10% of patients who have chronic gastroesophageal reflux will develop Barrett's esophagus. Of these about 10% will go on to develop dysplasia and carcinoma.

The relationship of dysplasia to carcinoma is based on a number of studies. Firstly, all studies indicate that high-grade dysplasia is almost invariably found in association with adenocarcinoma in Barrett's esophagus and that the high-grade dysplasia in turn is associated with regions of lesser grades of dysplasia. Secondly, some patients with Barrett's esophagus followed by serial endoscopy appear to progress from Barrett's to low-grade dysplasia, to high-grade dysplasia and then on to cancer. However, it should be stressed that the progression of Barrett's esophagus to carcinoma is not inevitable and that even when dysplasia develops, it commonly does not progress further. Furthermore, there are some reports of regression of dysplasia.

Flow cytometric studies in patients with Barrett's esophagus with and without dysplasia and/or carcinoma, have shown that neoplastic progression is associated with a process of genomic instability that generates abnormal clones of cells, some of which have aneuploid or increased G_2/tetraploid DNA contents. Thus, the development of dysplasia is not the result of a single event, but a process of clonal evolution resulting in progressive loss of proliferative control [1].

There have been sporadic reports of the regression of dysplasia in Barrett's esophagus [2,3]. Since the development of dysplasia is the result of genomic instability and progressive genetic changes, it is hard to visualize regression of this process. To me it seems more likely that, if dysplasia truly disappears, it may in fact be due to progression of the clonal process to a point of nonviability (i.e., necrosis) rather than to malignancy. However, there may be simpler answers to this apparent regression namely:

1. The histologic changes diagnosed as dysplasia were in fact reactive atypia rather than true dysplasia.
2. Dysplasia is still present, but not detectable endoscopically.
3. Dysplasia has been entirely removed on biopsy.

References

1. Reid BJ. Barrett's esophagus and esophageal adenocarcinoma. Gastroenterol Clin North Am 1991;20:817–834.
2. Riddell RH. Dysplasia and regression in Barrett's esophagus. In: Spechler SJ, Goyal RK (eds) Barrett's Esophagus. Pathophysiology, Diagnosis and Management. New York: Elsevier 1984;143–152.
3. Schnell T, Sontag S, Chejfec G et al. High grade dysplasia in Barrett's esophagus: a report of experience with 43 patients. Gastroenterology 1989;96:A452 (abstract).

Can low-grade dysplasia progress to adenocarcinoma?

K. Geboes, N. Ectors (Leuven)

Dysplasia occurring in Barrett's esophagus is usually subdivided into two categories: low-grade and high-grade dysplasia. An "intermediate" grade has been proposed by Hamilton. Specimens classified as intermediate-grade and high-grade in his scheme are included in the high-grade category of the schemes with two grades [1] (Fig. 1).

The answer to the above question therefore depends upon the definition and classification used for dysplasia in Barrett's esophagus. The classification dividing dysplasia into mild, moderate and severe is based on principles similar to those used for gastric dysplasia [2]. Several arguments are in favor for such an approach: the metaplastic Barrett's mucosa is more like gastric than colonic mucosa. Microscopically, gastric carcinomas are quite different from colonic carcinomas and gastric

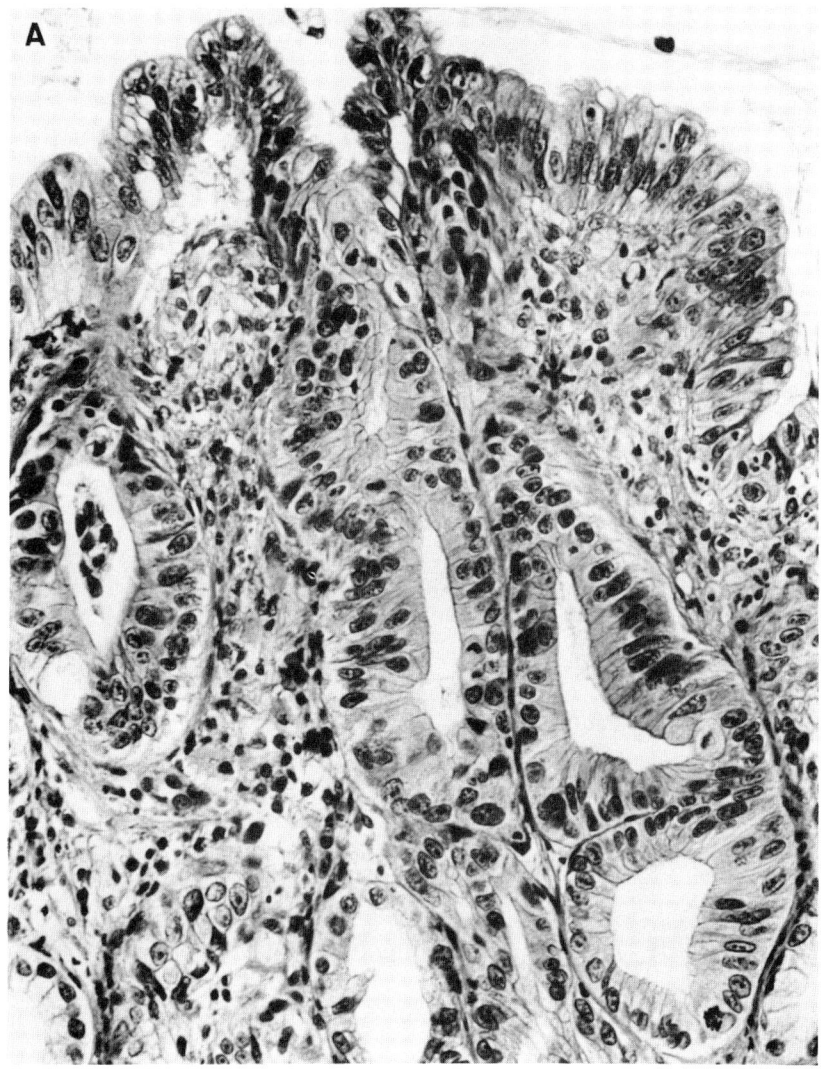

Fig. 1A. Intermediate grade dysplasia in Barrett's mucosa may be classified as a subset or can (according to some classifications) be classified into high-grade dysplasia.

dysplasia and the closely related, if not identical, Barrett's dysplasia is quite different from colonic dysplasia. In most studies reported in the literature, the classification used for Barrett's esophagus is, however, now subdivided into two grades based on the original classification introduced for inflammatory bowel diseases and eventually modified [3,4]. The first reason for this is the fact that classification schemes using only two grades have less intra- and interobserver variation [1,4]. They may, however, reflect the malignant potential of Barrett's dysplasia less reliably. A second reason lies in the major difference between dysplasia in the stomach and dysplasia in the esophagus. This difference is not whether dysplasia can or will progress to

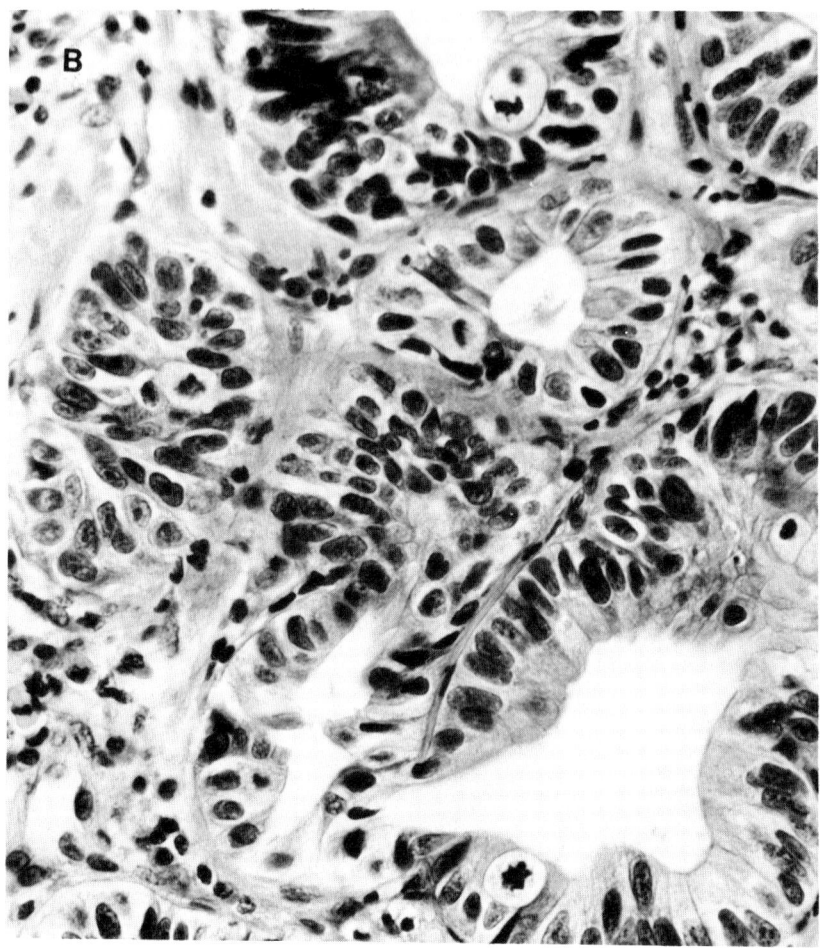

Fig. 1B. High-grade dysplasia may be found simultaneously in the same biopsy with less severe forms of esophagitis (H.E. × 125).

carcinoma or not. Lesions defined as unequivocally neoplastic will most probably progress given time. The major difference between the stomach and esophagus is that adenocarcinomas arising in intestinalization and proceeding through dysplasia are more aggressive in the esophagus, because of its microenvironment and because of anatomical and microanatomical differences.

Moderate dysplasia and adenocarcinoma

The question whether moderate dysplasia can progress could thus have several answers. One answer could be that moderate dysplasia must be considered as severe and that the term "moderate" must not be used. Yet it is clear that the evolution of

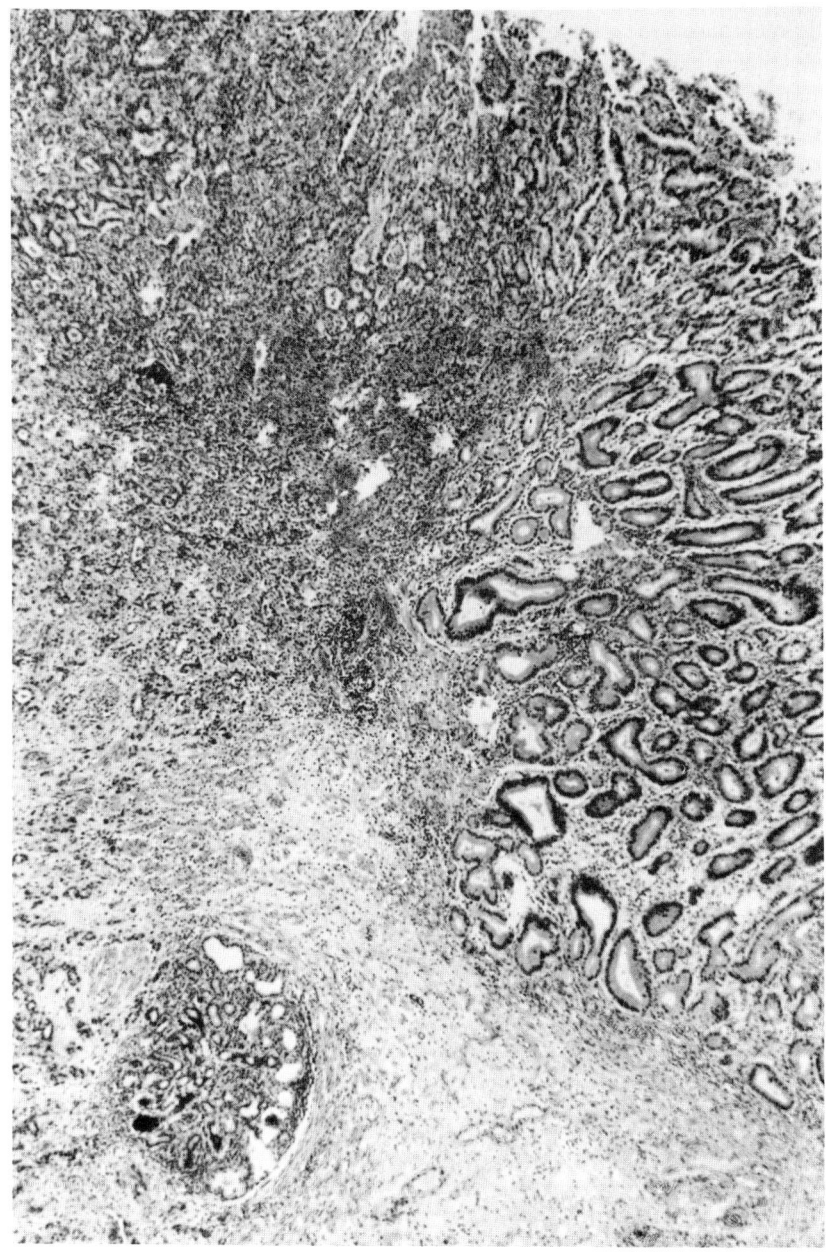

Fig. 2. Undifferentiatcd carcinoma (on the left) in Barrett's metaplasia with low-grade (according to the classification based on the principles outlined for inflammatory bowel diseases) or moderate type dysplasia on the right. In the submucosa an esophageal gland can be observed (H.E. × 40).

dysplasia in different patients shows considerable variations. Therefore, we will try to provide some indications.

Low-grade dysplasia is considered more aggressive in Barrett's metaplasia than in gastric metaplasia [5]. However, in a study comparing patients with Barrett's and gastric dysplasia it was shown that low-grade dysplasia progression to carcinoma is low in both groups [5].

A progression of low-grade into high-grade dysplasia and carcinoma has been documented anecdotally in the literature [6], although the time-lapse between these two findings may be highly variable (1.5–4 years) [2]. In most cases reported in the literature, high-grade dysplasia is already associated with invasive carcinoma when the diagnosis is made [6].

For high-grade dysplasia (including the "intermediate grade" according to the classification of Hamilton, or the "moderate" grade according to a classification following the principles outlined for the stomach) a progression into carcinoma has been demonstrated. Here too, the time-lapse shows considerable variation. High-grade dysplasia has been found for as long as 3.5 years without evidence of carcinomatous degeneration [2]. Obviously proper sampling is needed for an accurate evaluation of the grade of dysplasia.

So, in conclusion, we can state that dysplasia can progress into high grade and carcinoma, and that moderate dysplasia, defined as an unequivocally neoplastic lesion, can progress into adenocarcinoma (Fig. 2).

References

1. Hamilton SR. Reflux esophagitis and Barrett's esophagus. In: Goldman H, Appelman HD, Kaufman N (eds) Gastrointestinal Pathology. Baltimore: Williams & Wilkins, 1990;11–68.
2. Hameeteman W. Columnar-lined esophagus. MD Thesis 1989, Amsterdam.
3. Riddell RH, Goldman H, Ransohoff D, Appelman HD, Fenoglio CM, Haggitt RC, Ahren C, Correa P, Hamilton SR, Morson BC, Sommers SC, Yardley JH. Dysplasia in inflammatory bowel disease. Hum Pathol 1983;14:931–967.
4. Reid BJ, Haggitt RC, Rubin CE, Roth G, Surawicz CM. Observer variation in the diagnosis of dysplasia in Barrett's esophagus. Hum Pathol 1988;19:166–178.
5. Burke AP, Sobin LH, Shekitka KM, Helwig EB. Dysplasia of the stomach and Barrett's esophagus: a follow-up study. Mod Pathol 1991;4:336–341.
6. Lee RG. Dysplasia in Barrett's esophagus. Am J Surg Pathol 1985;9:845–852.

Must the opinion of two pathologists be obtained before deciding on the treatment of high-grade dysplasia?

K.J. Lewin (Los Angeles)

This question has great clinical relevance, because the management of patients with Barrett's esophagus varies depending upon whether it is simple Barrett's or Barrett's with low-grade dysplasia or with high-grade dysplasia. Thus, Barrett's patients with low-grade dysplasia will have more frequent surveillance endoscopies and biopsies; whereas esophagectomy is indicated for some patients with high-grade dysplasia.

In a multicenter study by a group of experienced gastrointestinal pathologists, the interobserver agreement in the diagnosis of dysplasia in Barrett's esophagus was about 85% in high-grade dysplasia and intramucosal carcinoma. However, interobserver agreement was substantially lower in recognizing lesser grades of biopsy abnormality. For example, there was only 72% agreement in the diagnosis of biopsies negative for dysplasia. Interobserver agreement in the diagnosis of indefinite dysplasia or low-grade dysplasia was even lower [1]. It is probable that these discrepancies in interobserver agreement would be even greater amongst pathologists who rarely see cases of Barrett's with dysplasia. It should be noted that the problems in interobserver agreement, with respect to dysplasia, are not unique to the esophagus and have been described in other sites such as the colon in ulcerative colitis [2,3].

To overcome the problems associated with interobserver discrepancies, the following recommendations have been proposed:

1. Obtaining additional and adequate biopsy samples. It has been found that taking additional biopsies frequently resolves the histologic problems [4,5]. (It should be stressed that it is critical to adequately sample the esophagus, starting in the cardia and proceeding proximally until the normal squamous mucosa is reached.)
2. Consultation with a pathologist who has experience with cases of dysplasia in Barrett's esophagus.
3. Flow cytometric studies for the detection of aneuploidy [5,6].

This may be particularly valuable in those cases where there is difficulty distinguishing low-grade dysplasia from reactive changes. It has been shown that patients with aneuploidy are more likely to develop high-grade dysplasia and carcinoma than those without aneuploidy. However, presently these techniques are only available in a few laboratories.

The question of second opinion in high-grade dysplasia may become moot since more and more centers are no longer automatically performing esophagectomy for high-grade dysplasia. This is because not all cases progress to carcinoma and also because of the mortality rate of esophagectomy which is between 10–15%. Furthermore, it has been found that patients with early carcinoma can be picked up by surveillance and can still be cured of their disease if it is confined to the mucosa [5,7]. Thus, the treatment of high-grade dysplasia will not differ significantly from the other forms of dysplasia.

References

1. Reid BJ, Haggitt RC, Rubin CE et al. Observer variation in the diagnosis of dysplasia in Barrett's esophagus. Hum Pathol 1988;19:166–178.
2. Riddell RH, Goldman H, Ransohoff DR et al. Dysplasia in inflammatory bowel disease: Standardized classification with provisional clinical applications. Hum Pathol 1983;11:931–967.
3. Dixon MF, Brown LJR, Gilmour HM et al. Observer variation in the assessment of dysplasia in ulcerative colitis. Histopathology 1988;13:385–397.
4. Rubin CE, Haggitt RC, Levine DS. Endoscopic mucosal biopsy. In: Yamada T, Alpers DH, Owyang C, Silverstein FE (eds) Textbook of Gastroenterology. Philadelphia: Lippincott, 1991:2479–2523.

5. Levine DS, Haggitt RC, Blount PL, Rabinovitch PS, Rusch VW, Reid BJ. An endoscopic biopsy protocol can differentiate high-grade dysplasia from early adenocarcinoma in Barrett's esophagus. Gastroenterology 1993;105:40—50.
6. Reid BJ. Barrrett's esophagus and esophageal adenocarcinoma. Gastroenterol Clin North Am 1991;20:817—834.
7. Reid BJ, Weinstein WM, Lewin KJ et al. Endoscopic biopsy can detect high-grade dysplasia or early adenocarcinoma in Barrett's esophagus without grossly recognizable neoplastic lesions. Gastroenterology 1988;94:81—90.

Is high-grade dysplasia an indication for esophagectomy?

H. Obertop (Amsterdam)

Dysplasia of the mucosa is an unequivocal neoplastic alteration that is found in about 10% of the patients with a Barrett's columnar-lined esophagus (CLE) without presence of visible carcinoma [1]. Dysplastic mucosa in CLE is most frequently classified as low-grade, whereas high-grade dysplasia is very unusual [1]. However, the true incidence of dysplasia is not known. The risk of cancer development in CLE is estimated to be 30—40 fold increase above that in the general population [2,3]. The incidence of esophageal adenocarcinoma in patients with CLE varies between one per 46 to one per 441 patient-years follow-up [3—5]. To detect one case of adenocarcinoma, about one hundred patients with CLE should undergo esophagoscopy [6]. It is known that almost only those patients with dysplasia progress to adenocarcinoma [7]. Furthermore, dysplasia is found adjacent to adenocarcinoma in CLE in 68—91% [8,9] and high-grade dysplasia in 50—84% [10,11] of the patients undergoing esophagectomy for Barrett's carcinoma. Thus, dysplasia is generally accepted as a precursor of invasive cancer [2]. High-grade dysplasia and carcinoma in situ, which are indistinguishable histologically, indicate that invasive cancer is imminent [12]. In fact, high-grade dysplasia is the most important marker to identify patients with a high risk of developing or having Barrett's carcinoma. Other markers, such as flow-cytometric abnormalities [13] and the prevalence of p53 overexpression [14], are inferior in that respect, but may play a role in identification of a subset of patients who merit frequent endoscopic surveillance.

Should we then perform esophagectomy for high-grade dysplasia?

Proponents of this approach advise that, when high-grade dysplasia is diagnosed, excision of all the esophagus which is lined by columnar epithelium should be taken into consideration [1,11,12,15,16]. The most convincing reasons are:
1. Invasive adenocarcinoma is found in the resection specimens of 42% of the patients undergoing esophagectomy for high-grade dysplasia [11,15—19] (Table 1).

1020

Table 1. Prophylactic esophagectomy for high-grade dysplasia in CLE. Postoperative mortality, coexisting invasive carcinoma and tumor stage

Author	Year	No. of patients	Postoperative mortality	No. of patients with coexisting invasive carcinoma	Tumor stage
Hamilton [11]	1987	5	0	3	T_1:2 T_2:1
Reid [17]	1988	4	1	0	$-^a$
DeMeester [18]	1990	2	0	1	T_1(?):1
Altorki [16]	1991	9	0	4	T_1:3 T_4:1
Pera [15]	1992	18	0	9	StI:6 StIIA:2 StIIB:1
Obertop [19]	1993	4	0	2	T_1:2
Total		42	1 (2.4%)	19 (45%)	

[a]Data not given.

2. Long-term survival after esophagectomy for high-grade dysplasia is 100% and lower for invasive cancer, even when resected in an early stage [15,20,21] (Table 2).
3. Postoperative mortality can be low [11,15–19] (Table 1) in patients with high-grade dysplasia who are in a good nutritional state and do not otherwise suffer from the sequelae of cancer.

Opponents of this approach advise performing esophagectomy only when unquestionable (invasive) carcinoma has been detected [4,17]. The following reasons for this attitude can be put forward:

1. Mortality and morbidity are high after esophagectomy. Postoperative mortality that has been reported to be as high as 29% before 1980 [22] decreased to 13% 10 years later [23]. Although mortality can be lower than 5% in experienced hands [20] and with increasing experience [24], the tumor stage does not seem to play a role [23].
2. When multiple biopsies of CLE are taken and this is repeated frequently during follow-up, invasive cancer can probably be excluded, as reported by Reid et al. [17] (Table 1).

Table 2. Five-year survival after esophagectomy for high-grade dysplasia/carcinoma in situ and early-stage invasive cancer in CLE

Author	Year	High-grade dysplasia		Early cancer		
		n	%	n	Stage	%
Streitz [20]	1991	4	100	10	StI	85.7
Pera [15]	1992	9	100	9	StI–IIB	35.7
Menke Pluymers [21]	1993	$-^a$	$-^a$	12	$T_{is}-T_1$	~60

[a]Data not given.

1021

3. Since CLE occurs more frequently in males in their sixties with a history of smoking and alcohol abuse [3], a higher operative risk can be expected.

What operation should be performed when esophagectomy is selected for the treatment of high-grade dysplasia?

All columnar-lined epithelium should be resected to prevent tumor recurrence in residual dysplastic mucosa. At least in seven patients selected from the literature [8,20,25,26] invasive carcinoma has been documented after incomplete esophagectomy for dysplastic mucosa. Therefore, a total esophagectomy is advised, preferably through the transhiatal route to lower postoperative mortality and morbidity. A cervical esophagogastrostomy or esophagocolostomy can be performed [26]. In cases of doubt about the completeness of resection, frozen sections of the proximal margin can be examined during the operation for the presence of columnar-lined epithelium.

Conclusions

Based on the literature and our own experience, the approach as suggested by Hamilton and Smith [11] is strongly supported (i.e., that "prophylactic esophagectomy is indicated in a patient with persistent high-grade dysplasia in esophageal biopsy specimens of Barrett's mucosa if the patient is likely to tolerate the resection"). When all of the columnar-lined epithelium has been removed, the chance of (recurrent) esophageal cancer will be extremely low.

References

1. Streitz JM, Williamson WA, Ellis FH. Current concepts concerning the nature and treatment of Barrett's esophagus and its complications. Ann Thorac Surg 1992;54:586–591.
2. DeMeester TR. Barrett's esophagus. Surgery 1993;113:239–241.
3. Spechler SJ, Goyal RK. Barrett's esophagus. N Engl J Med 1986;315:362–371.
4. Hameeteman W, Tytgat GNJ, Houthoff HJ, van den Tweel JG. Barrett's esophagus: development of dysplasia and adenocarcinoma. Gastroenterology 1989;96:1249–1256.
5. van der Veen AH, Dees J, Blankensteijn JD, van Blankenstein M. Adenocarcinoma in Barrett's oesophagus: an overrated risk. Gut 1989;30:14–18.
6. Williamson WA, Ellis FH, Gibb SP, Shahian DM, Aretz HTh, Heatley GJ, Watkins E. Barrett's esophagus: prevalence and incidence of adenocarcinoma. Arch Int Med 1991;151:2212–2216.
7. Miros M, Kerlin P, Walker N. Only patients with dysplasia progress to adenocarcinoma in Barrett's oesophagus. Gut 1991;32:1441–1446.
8. Harle IA, Finley RJ, Belsheim M, Bondy DC, Booth M, Lloyd D, McDonald JWD, Sullivan S, Valberg LS, Watson WC, Frei JV, Slinger R, Troster M, Meads GE, Duff JH. Management of adenocarcinoma in a columnar-lined esophagus. Ann Thorac Surg 1985;40:330–336.
9. Kalish RJ, Clancy PE, Orringer MB, Appelman HD. Clinical, epidemiologic and morphologic comparison between adenocarcinomas arising in Barrett's esophageal mucosa and in the gastric cardia. Gastroenterology 1984;86:461–467.
10. Duhaylongsod FG, Wolfe WG. Barrett's esophagus and adenocarcinoma of the esophagus and gastroesophageal junction. J Thorac Cardiovasc Surg 1991;102:36–42.
11. Hamilton SR, Smith RRL. The relationship between columnar epithelial dysplasia and invasive adenocarcinoma arising in Barrett's esophagus. Am J Clin Pathol 1987;87:301–312.
12. Atkinson M. Barrett's oesophagus — to screen or not to screen? Gut 1989;30:2–5.
13. Reid BJ, Blount PL, Rubin CE, Levine DS, Haggitt RC, Rabinovitch PS. Flow-cytometric and histological progression to

malignancy in Barrett's esophagus: prospective endoscopic surveillance of a cohort. Gastroenterology 1992;102:1212—1219.

14. Ramel S, Reid BJ, Sanchez CA, Blount PL, Levine DS, Neshat K, Haggitt RC, Dean PJ, Thor K, Rabinovitch PS. Evaluation of p53 protein expression in Barrett's esophagus by two-parameter flow cytometry. Gastroenterology 1992;102:1220—1228.

15. Pera M, Trastek VF, Carpenter HA, Allen MS, Deschamps C, Pairolero PC. Barrett's esophagus with high-grade dysplasia: an indication for esophagectomy? Ann Thorac Surg 1992;54:199—204.

16. Altorki NK, Sunagawa M, Little AG, Skinner DB. High-grade dysplasia in the columnar-lined esophagus. Am J Surg 1991; 161:97—100.

17. Reid BJ, Weinstein WM, Lewin KJ, Haggitt RC, VanDeventer G, DenBesten L, Rubin CE. Endoscopic biopsy can detect high-grade dysplasia or early adenocarcinoma in Barrett's esophagus without grossly recognizable neoplastic lesions. Gastroenterology 1988;94:81—90.

18. DeMeester TR, Attwood SEA, Smyrk TC, Therkildsen DH, Hinder RA. Surgical therapy in Barrett's esophagus. Ann Surg 1990;212:528—542.

19. Obertop H, Poen H, Kooijman CD. Carcinoom in een vroeg stadium in de Barrett-oesofagus; toevallige vondst of speurwerk? Ned Tijdschr Geneeskd 1993;137:436—439.

20. Streitz JM, Ellis FH, Gibb SP et al. Adenocarcinoma in Barrett's esophagus. Ann Surg 1991;213:122—125.

21. Menke-Pluymers MBE, Schoute NW, Mulder AH, Hop WCJ, Blankenstein van M, Tilanus HW. Outcome of surgical treatment of adenocarcinoma in Barrett's oesophagus. Gut 1992;33:1454—1458.

22. Earlam R, Cunha-Melo JR. Oesophageal squamous cell carcinoma: I. A critical review of surgery. Br J Surg 1980;67: 381—390.

23. Müller JM, Erasmi H, Stelzner M, Zieren U, Pichlmaier H. Surgical therapy of oesophageal carcinoma. Br J Surg 1990; 77:845—857.

24. Eeftinck Schattenkerk M, Obertop H, Mud HJ, Eijkenboom WMH, van Andel JG, van Houten H. Survival after resection for carcinoma of the oesophagus. Br J Surg 1987;74:165—168.

25. Sanfey H, Hamilton SR, Smith RRL, Cameron JL. Carcinoma arising in Barrett's esophagus. Surg Gynecol Obstet 1985; 161:570—574.

26. Rosenberg JC, Budev H, Edwards RC, Singal S, Steiger Z, Sundareson AS. Analysis of adenocarcinoma in Barrett's esophagus utilizing a staging system. Cancer 1985;55:1353—1360.

How often are invasive carcinomas discovered in specimens resected for high-grade dysplasia alone?

V.F. Trastek (Rochester, Minnesota)

The association of adenocarcinoma with Barrett's disease was first reported by Morson and Belcher in 1952 [1]. Numerous patients are affected by reflux esophagitis, less by Barrett's metaplasia, and an even smaller group by adenocarcinoma. Despite this, adenocarcinoma has increased in incidence especially during the past 2 decades [2]. Hamilton has suggested that high-grade dysplasia is a marker of associated invasive carcinoma [3]. The natural history of this process is not completely understood, and consequently, management of patients with only high-grade dysplasia by endoscopic biopsy remains unanswered and controversial. Esophagectomy has been recommended, whereas others have proposed surveillance if no evidence of concomitant invasive carcinoma is present [4—6].

Whether esophagectomy is a reasonable recommendation for patients with only high-grade dysplasia will depend on how many patients have invasive carcinoma at the time of initial resection and the rate at which it develops, if it is not resected. The mortality and morbidity of the operation must also be considered. Obviously, the goal is to prevent malignancy or at least discover it at an early stage.

We initially reported 19 patients who had high-grade dysplasia without preoperative evidence of invasive carcinoma [7]. Eighteen of these patients underwent resection without operative mortality. Nine patients (50%) had invasive carcinoma which was postsurgical stage I in six patients, stage IIA in two and stage IIB in one. The remaining nine patients had high-grade dysplasia only (stage 0). Median follow-up was 34 months. Recurrent cancer developed in two patients. Overall 5-year survival was 66.7%.

Over the ensuing year since this report, we have seen another 23 patients with high-grade dysplasia. Twenty-two of these patients have undergone resection and eight patients (36%) had invasive carcinoma [8]. Combining the two groups (42 patients, 40 resections), 17 patients (43%) had invasive adenocarcinoma following resection. Overall 5-year survival was 69.4%. There continues to be no operative deaths.

Patients with an increased risk of invasive carcinoma included those with abnormalities found at the time of endoscopy (small nodules, narrowing, and ulceration) and those with high-grade dysplasia diagnosed at the time of the initial endoscopy (nonsurveillance group). Of the 14 patients with normal endoscopies, 12 were found to have high-grade dysplasia only (stage 0) and only one had invasive disease (stage I). One patient is still under continued observation. Of the 28 patients with abnormal endoscopic appearance, 11 were found to have high-grade dysplasia only (stage 0), 16 patients had invasive disease with nine stage I, four stage-IIA and IIB and three stage III. One patient is still under continued observation. We found that of the 25 patients in the surveillance group, 14 were stage 0, eight stage I, one stage III and two were still being followed. In contrast, of the 17 patients in the nonsurveillance group, nine patients were stage 0, two stage I, four stage IIA and IIB and two stage III.

The importance of surveillance cannot be overstated. It is an extremely valuable technique to discover progression of normal Barrett's metaplasia to high-grade dysplasia or invasive carcinoma. We continue to recommend yearly surveillance with four-quadrant biopsies every 2 cm for all patients found to have Barrett's mucosa.

We have noted a decreasing rate of invasive carcinoma in our studies. The initial rate of 50% in the first group of 18 patients decreased to 36% in the second group of 22 patients, with an overall combined rate of 43%. Obviously, improvement in determining "high-risk" Barrett's mucosa is important and needed.

We currently recommend esophagectomy for patients with high-grade dysplasia documented by endoscopic biopsy and confirmed by one of the two pathologists who reads all of the Barrett's disease slides at our institution. (The importance of a consistent pathologist in helping to make this diagnosis cannot be stressed enough.) The discovery of disease at an earlier stage has yielded a survival of 69.4% at 5 years. Hopefully, in the future, the ability to better define high-risk Barrett's mucosa will be available. Continued work on the pathophysiology of Barrett's disease is extremely important.

References

1. Morson BC, Belcher JR. Adenocarcinoma of the oesophagus and ectopic gastric mucosa. Br J Cancer 1952;6:127–130.
2. Pera M, Cameron AJ, Trastek VF, Carpenter HA, Zinsmeister AR, Ballard DJ. Esophageal adenocarcinoma: a population-based study of its incidence and the role of Barrett's esophagus. Gastroenterology 1991;100:A394 (abstract).
3. Hamilton SR, Smith RRL. The relationship between columnar epithelial dysplasia and invasive adenocarcinoma arising in Barrett's esophagus. Am J Clin Pathol 1987;87:301–312.
4. Altorki NK, Sunagawa M, Little AG et al. High-grade dysplasia in the columnar-lined esophagus. Am J Surg 1991;161: 97–100.
5. DeMeester TR, Attwood SE, Smyrk TC et al. Surgical therapy in Barrett's esophagus. Ann Surg 1990;212:528–542.
6. Reid BJ, Weinstein WM, Lewin KJ et al. Endoscopic biopsy can detect HGD or early adenocarcinoma in Barrett's esophagus without grossly recognizable neoplastic lesions. Gastroenterology 1988;94:81–90.
7. Pera M, Trastek VF, Carpenter HA, Allen MS, Deschamps C, Pairolero PC. Barrett's esophagus with high-grade dysplasia: an indication for esophagectomy? Ann Thorac Surg 1992;54:199–204.
8. Trastek VF, Pera M, Pairolero PC, Carpenter HA, Allen MS, Deschamps C. High-grade dysplasia in Barrett's esophagus: role of surveillance and resection (presented at the 19th Annual Meeting of the Western Thoracic Surgical Association, June 23–26, 1993, Carlsbad, California).

Is dysplasia an essential intermediate stage before adenocarcinoma?

R.H. Riddell (Hamilton)

To the best of our knowledge the answer to this is *yes*. However, in Barrett's epithelium (BE) this is based on the assumption that by at least one definition BE contains intestinalized mucosa, and that this goes through two traditional pathways of dysplasia known as type I and type II dysplasia before becoming invasive [1]. Type I is the traditional adenomatous pathway as seen throughout the gastrointestinal tract in any adenoma, with enlarged, hyperchromatic stratified ovoid nuclei. Type II differs in that the nuclei are enlarged and regularly hyperchromatic, but are larger, frequently occupying the whole basal half of the cell, more pleomorphic, varying in size and shape, and not overlapping or stratifying as seen in type I dysplasia. This type of dysplasia tends to give rise to some of the more poorly differentiated tumors. Type II dysplasia is more difficult to recognize morphologically, but is so frequently accompanied by type I dysplasia that this is not an important clinical problem. To the best of our knowledge because *all* cancers in BE are associated with either or both of these pathways, then the answer to this question remains yes.

Theoretically, one can always ask questions such as "does one always find dysplasia in patients with BE and cancer?" to which the answer is no. However, one does not always find BE adjacent to all adenocarcinomas of the lower esophagus, particularly if the presentation is symptomatic and the tumor is large. Under these circumstances we tend to accept that the tumor destroyed all evidence of a pre-existing or coexisting condition. However, like the adenomatous edge of carcinomas in the large bowel, the smaller the tumor, the more frequently one finds evidence of dysplasia, to the point that it can be mapped out. Cynics can of course argue that such patients are selected because of the presence of dysplasia and BE, and that, in patients presenting for the first time with clinical symptoms of carcinoma, we do not always know the basis on which the tumor developed, with which one can sometimes only agree if there is no evidence of dysplasia in the adjacent mucosa.

A second potential point of argument is whether, because we define patients at risk from BE by the presence of intestinal metaplasia, patients without this feature are still at risk of developing adenocarcinoma, that is, if one accepts the definition of "3 cm or more of glandular epithelium" (irrespective of type) as the defining characteristic of BE. This situation would likely result in patients developing carcinomas of the so-called diffuse type of gastric cancer (most gastric cancers being broadly divisible into intestinal and diffuse using the Lauren classification). While this is quite possible, diffuse type cardiac cancers associated with unequivocal long-standing gastroesophageal reflux disease are rare, but this study has not yet been carried out. However, it should be pointed out that the preinvasive lesion of diffuse gastric carcinoma in the stomach (and hence cardia) is very poorly documented with only scant descriptions [2]; these are not currently likely diagnosable on biopsies. This is therefore a theoretical risk, but even if it occurs it is likely not a major factor in carcinogenesis in Barrett's esophagus.

References

1. Schmidt HG, Riddell RH, Walther BC, Skinner DB, Riemann JF. Dysplasia in Barrett's esophagus. J Cancer Res Clin Oncol 1985;110:145–152.
2. Ghandur-Mneymneh L, Paz J, Roldan E, Cassady J. Dysplasia of nonmetaplastic gastric mucosa; a proposal for its classification and its possible relationship to diffuse-type gastric carcinoma. Am J Surg Pathol 1988;12:96–114.

Is the surface extent of the dysplastic zone related to the development of adenocarcinoma?

T.C. Smyrk (Omaha)

Intuitively, one would suspect that adenocarcinoma is more likely to develop in Barrett's esophagus with extensive high-grade dysplasia than in Barrett's esophagus with focal high-grade dysplasia, just as invasive carcinoma is found more often in large colorectal adenomas than in small adenomas. Invasive cancer of any site probably results from progressive accumulation of genetic alterations, leading to loss of normal growth control mechanisms and there is ample evidence that this paradigm applies to adenocarcinoma arising in Barrett's esophagus. Several investigators, for example, have shown that the proliferative compartment of specialized columnar epithelium is expanded and disordered [1,2]. Abnormal p53 immunoreactivity has been described in Barrett's esophagus, both with and without dysplasia, and may be an early event in the malignant degeneration of Barrett's esophagus [3,4]. Ras, Fos and Myc oncoproteins are all found in the specialized columnar epithelium of Barrett's esophagus and are found more frequently in epithelium with high-grade dysplasia [5]. Investigators from the University of Washington have used flow cytometry and cytogenetics to demonstrate that clones of abnormal cells arise in Barrett's esophagus, expanding in some patients to cover large areas of mucosa [6,7]. Presumably, investigators will soon identify a set of acquired mutations necessary for the development of esophageal adenocarcinoma, as Vogelstein et al. have done for colorectal cancer [8]. Indeed, allelic deletions of tumor suppressor genes, including APC, MCC and DCC have been described in Barrett's adenocarcinoma [9–11]. If high-grade dysplasia results from the accumulation of several mutations and requires just one or two additional mutations to acquire the capacity for invasion, it follows that the greater the area of high-grade dysplasia, the greater the chance for the critical mutations to occur.

The speculation above is neither supported nor refuted by clinical evidence. Retrospective descriptions of Barrett's esophagus with adenocarcinoma do not generally quantify the surface extent of dysplasia. One exception is the classic description of Barrett's esophagus by Thompson et al. [12]. They categorized the dysplasia in eight cases of resected Barrett's esophagus, as focal or multifocal. Six patients had multifocal dysplasia and two had focal dysplasia. Five of the former had associated tumors compared to one of the latter. Our own review of 25 patients undergoing resection for adenocarcinoma in Barrett's esophagus described low-grade dysplasia in every specimen and high-grade dysplasia in thirteen specimens, but did not mention the extent of dysplastic change [13]. I have reviewed the material and found seven specimens with extensive high-grade dysplasia and six with focal high-grade dysplasia (unpublished data). Retrospective studies cannot really answer the question; the data above tell us only that adenocarcinoma may occur in both settings — focal dysplasia and extensive dysplasia. The question can really only be answered by a long-term prospective study in which patients are followed with an endoscopic biopsy protocol, as proposed by the University of Washington group [14]. No such study, to my knowledge, has been published.

In summary, while there is a theoretical basis for assuming a positive correlation between the surface area of dysplasia and the risk of adenocarcinoma, there is no evidence supporting that assumption. The question is not without practical import, given the uncertainty about management of patients with high-grade dysplasia. If a patient has high-grade dysplasia in multiple biopsies, should he be given more consideration for esophagectomy than the patient with high-grade dysplasia in only one biopsy? I do not think so; there is no rationale for allowing the surface extent of dysplasia to influence patient management. It does not appear that efforts to quantify the surface extent of dysplasia will ease the difficult task of managing Barrett's esophagus with high-grade dysplasia. As more is learned about the specific genetic alterations that accompany progression from dysplasia to carcinoma, identification of these abnormalities will play a much stronger role in the decision making process.

References

1. Gray MR, Hall PA, Nash J et al. Epithelial proliferation in Barrett's esophagus by proliferating cell nuclear antigen immunolocalization. Gastroenterology 1992;103:1769.
2. Smyrk TC. Cellular proliferation in Barrett's esophagus. Mod Pathol 1993;6:52A.
3. Gray MR, Thomas DM, Kingsnorth AN et al. p53 immunocytochemistry in metaplastic and dysplastic Barrett's esophagus. Gastroenterology 1993;104:891.
4. Ramel S, Reid BJ, Sanchez CA et al. Evaluation of p53 protein expression in Barrett's esophagus by two-parameter flow cytometry. Gastroenterology 1992;102:1220–1228.
5. Ritchie AJ, Johnston C, McGuigan J, Gibbons JRP. Differential oncogene expression in the development of Barrett's neoplasia. Gastroenterology 1993;104:8178.
6. Rabinovitch PS, Reid BJ, Haggitt RC, Norwood TH, Rubin CE. Progression to cancer in Barrett's esophagus is associated with genomic instability. Lab Invest 1988;60:65–71.
7. Raskind WH, Norwood T, Levine DS et al. Persistent clonal areas and clonal expansion in Barrett's esophagus. Cancer Res 1992;52:2496.
8. Vogelstein B, Fearon ER, Hamilton SR et al. Genetic alterations during colorectal tumor development. N Engl J Med 1988; 319:525.
9. Blount PL, Ramel S, Raskind WH et al. 17p allelic deletions and p53 protein overexpression in Barrett's adenocarcinoma. Cancer Res 1991;51:5482.
10. Boynton RF, Blount PL, Yin J et al. Loss of heterozygosity involving the APC and MCC genetic loci occurs in the majority of human esophageal cancers. Proc Natl Acad Sci USA 1992;89:3385.
11. Huang Y, Boynton RF, Blount PL et al. Loss of heterozygosity involves multiple tumor suppressor genes in human esophageal cancers. Cancer Res 1992;52:6525.
12. Thompson JJ, Zinsser KR, Enterline HT. Barrett's metaplasia and adenocarcinoma of the esophagus and gastroesophageal junction. Hum Pathol 1983;14:42.
13. DeMeester TR, Attwood SEA, Smyrk TC, Therkildsen DH, Hinder RA. Surgical therapy in Barrett's esophagus. Ann Surg 1990;212:528.
14. Levine DS, Haggitt RC, Blount PL et al. An endoscopic biopsy protocol can differentiate high-grade dysplasia from early adenocarcinoma in Barrett's esophagus. Gastroenterology 1993;105:40.

How can one define a subpopulation most at risk of degeneration?

R.W. McCallum (Charlottesville)

Barrett's esophagus and its related complications have received increased attention in recent years as adenocarcinoma of the esophagus has become one of the fastest growing gastrointestinal malignancies. Compared to the incidence of esophageal cancer in the general population, the incidence of cancer occurring in patients with Barrett's is reported to be 30–125 times greater [1,2]. Previous studies have stressed the importance of dysplastic changes from the columnar metaplasia, in that they are felt to be possible precancerous conditions. Dysplasia occurs in 10% of patients with Barrett's. These dysplastic changes primarily occur in specialized intestinal-type epithelium (82%), but also may be found in fundic-type epithelium (50%) [3]. High grade dysplastic lesions are frequently found accompanying invasive carcinoma and are felt to be a precursor to adenoma carcinoma formation. Dysplastic Barrett's metaplasia has been shown to coexist with adenocarcinoma in 80–100% of cases [4]. This dysplasia-carcinoma sequence has alluded investigators as to why this occurs; however, it is shown that patients appear to progress from Barrett's specialized metaplasia to a low-grade dysplasia and subsequently to high-grade dysplasia and possibly adenocarcinoma. Studies have shown that carcinoma is found in up to 50% of cases with resected specimens, even though there is no evidence of preoperative cancer [5,6]. Much attention has been focused on the actual mechanism by which this dysplasia occurs as well as progresses; however, few factors have been elucidated.

Genetic instability is often cited as an occurrence which is seen with dysplastic progression in Barrett's epithelium. Numerous studies have shown that genetic instability, manifested by abnormal DNA content (aneuploidy) and/or cell cycle abnormalities, correlated with the histological diagnosis of dysplasia or carcinoma in Barrett's esophagus [7–9]. Rabinovitch showed a gradual progression in the actual number of anaplastic cells found in Barrett's metaplasia progressing to dysplasia and subsequent adenocarcinoma [10]. This study suggests that one is at high risk for malignancy or its subsequent development, if found to have multiple aneuploidy population in contrast to the usual 1–2 aneuploidy cell line seen in other types of malignancies.

Further studies looking at genetic causes for progression of dysplasia have shown an increase in S-phase fraction in cellular development as well as an increase in G_2/tetraploid fractions, both of which are associated with increased aneuploidy, high-grade dysplasia and adenocarcinoma development [11]. This abnormality in the G_2 phase leads to improper repair of damaged cells, resulting in tetraploidal cell formation, which may be the precursor to aneuploidy cell lines. Chromosomal abnormalities have also been found in patients with Barrett's dysplasia, where trisomy 5 and 7, structural chromosomal translocation and rearrangements and loss of the Y chromosome. This genetic instability is thought to result in tumor propagation by selection of new malignant clones which are thought to be characterized by a loss of proliferative control and the assumption of malignant behavior.

The role of environmental factors in the progression of dysplasia to the development of adenocarcinoma is poorly understood. Tobacco and alcohol have been studied extensively in their role as an etiological agent for Barrett's esophagus. However, few studies have addressed their effect on dysplastic Barrett's or the development of Barrett's malignancy [12–14]. Levi looked at 30 histologically confirmed cases of adenocarcinoma and 140 cases of Barrett's without malignancy. Results from this study suggested that alcohol and tobacco consumption are not important determinants in the risk of adenocarcinoma from Barrett's esophagus. In a study done by Williamson et al. [15], alcohol and tobacco consumption was equally prevalent in groups of patients with benign and malignant Barrett's. Skinner et al. found an association with smoking, but not alcohol, in patients with adenocarcinoma associated with Barrett's esophagus [12].

Chronic esophagitis, presumably from persistence of reflux disease has been speculated as the cause of the development of adenocarcinoma from Barrett's dysplasia. The presence of reflux or hiatal hernia has been found to have varying results in the subsequent occurrence of Barrett's carcinoma. Williamson minimized their role in the development of adenocarcinoma in Barrett's patients, as he found that heartburn and regurgitation were more frequently seen in patients with benign Barrett's esophagitis when compared to patients with carcinoma, and that 48% (30 out of 63) patients with Barrett's malignancy had no history of pyrosis [15]. Smith supported this lack of association, as he found a substantial number of patients with Barrett's esophagitis and adenocarcinoma with no symptoms of GERD at the time of presentation of the carcinoma [13]. This fact is further supported by the persistent development of adenocarcinoma after antireflux surgery that prevents further GERD occurrence. Other studies, such as those done by Haggitt, showed a much stronger association, with 10 out of 12 patients progressing to Barrett's adenocarcinoma having symptoms of reflux or hiatal hernia [2]. The extent of Barrett's is not significantly different from those with benign or malignant disease.

Much is yet to be learned regarding dysplasia carcinoma progression seen in Barrett's esophagus. Other than genetic changes found to occur with the progression of dysplasia, little is known about the actual mechanism allowing dysplasia to transform into adenocarcinoma or those triggers which propagate this occurrence. Until this is more clearly understood and we develop markers which allow one to detect high-grade dysplasia in adenocarcinoma at the earliest stages, aggressive therapy and surveillance will need to be mandated as the standard of care in Barrett's esophagitis.

References

1. Cameron AJ, Ott BJ, Payne WS. The incidence of adenocarcinoma and columnar-lined (Barrett's esophagus). N Engl J Med 1985;313:857–859.
2. Haggitt RC, Tryzelaar J, Ellis FH et al. Adenocarcinoma complicating columnar epithelium-lined (Barrett's) esophagus. Am J Clin Pathol 1978;70:1–5.
3. Hameeteman W, Tytgat GNJ, Houthoff HJ et al. Barrett's esophagus: development of dysplasia in adenocarcinoma. Gastroenterology 1989;96:1249–1256.
4. Hamilton SR, Smith RRL. The relationship between columnar epithelium dysplasia and invasive adenocarcinoma arising in Barrett's esophagus. Am J Clin Pathol 1987;87:301–312.
5. Payne WS, Trastek VF, Papiehler JM et al. Current technique for the surgical management of malignant lesions in the thoracic esophagus and cardia. Mayo Clin Proc 1986;61:564.
6. Reid BJ. Barrett's esophagus and esophageal adenocarcinoma. Gastroenterol Clin North Am 1991;20:817–833.
7. Reid BJ, Blount PL, Rubin CE et al. Predictions of progression to malignancy in Barrett's esophagus: Endoscopic, histologic and flow cytometric follow-up of a cohort. Gastroenterology 1990;98:A305 (abstract).
8. Reid BJ et al. Flow cytometric and histologic progression to malignancy in Barrett's esophagus. Prospective endoscopic surveillance of a cohort. Gastroenterology 1992;102:1212–1219.
9. Reid BJ, Haggit RC, Rubin CE et al. Barrett's esophagus flow cytometry complements histology in detection of patients at risk for adenocarcinoma. Gastroenterology 1987;93:1.
10. Rabinovitch PS et al. Progression to cancer in Barrett's esophagus is associated with genomic instability. Lab Invest 1988;60:65–71.

11. Schnell T, Sontag S, Chejfec G et al. High grade dysplasia in BE: a report of experience with 43 patients. Gastroenterology 1989;96:A452 (abstract).
12. Skinner DB, Walther BC, Riddell RH et al. Barrett's esophagus: comparison of benign and malignant cases. Ann Surg 1983; 198:554—556.
13. Smith RRL et al. The spectrum of carcinoma arising in Barrett's esophagus. Am J Surg Pathol 1984;8:563.
14. Thompson JJ, Zinsser KR, Interline HT. Barrett's metaplasia and adenocarcinoma of the esophagus and GE junction. Hum Pathol 1983;14:42—61.
15. Williamson WA et al. Barrett's esophagus: prevalence and incidence of adenocarcinoma. Arch Int Med 1991;151:2212—2216.

Markers

What is the predictive value of sulfomucins for concomitant high-grade dysplasia in Barrett's mucosa?

F. Potet (Paris)

Modifications in cellular differentiation are often described in precancerous lesions. In Barrett's mucosa dysplasia and carcinoma are only diagnosed in specialized mucosa, a particular type of incomplete intestinal metaplasia (IM). The other observed types are junctional type, which resembles normal cardiac epithelium, and gastric fundic type, which resembles gastric body epithelium. These two latter epithelia are of the same type as the contiguous gastric epithelium and their mucus secretion is similar to the gastric mucus secreting cells (i.e., neutral mucins).

The specialized IM type exhibits an abnormal differentiation, and consequently, an abnormal mucus secretion; the epithelium is characterized by a mucus secretion similar to that of IM of the stomach: goblet cells containing sialo- and/or sulfomucins, columnar cells secreting or not secreting neutral or acid mucins. Usual histochemical techniques easily show the three kinds of mucus secretion, neutral, sialo- and sulfomucins. Other histochemical reactions permit to distinguish O- and N-acetylated sialomucins.

Jass and Filipe [1] described in the stomach an incompletely differentiated variant of intestinal metaplasia secreting sulfomucins. This Type III IM has been shown in several studies to be associated with the presence of gastric carcinoma. Jass [2] has reported a similar association between this variant of IM and a well differentiated

1033

adenocarcinoma arising in Barrett's mucosa, and he suggested that the presence of this type of IM in esophageal biopsies may serve as an important marker for identification of a subgroup of patients at risk of developing Barrett's adenocarcinoma. In a prospective study on biopsy material [3], we studied 38 patients with symptoms of reflux esophagitis and Barrett's esophagus. We found 58% of type III IM secreting sulfomucins.

Our results, as well as those of other studies, show a high incidence of type III in Barrett's mucosa and suggests two questions:
— May the presence of the variant of IM secreting sulfomucins serve as a marker to identify a high-risk group for the Barrett's adenocarcinoma?
— What relationship could be found between the mucus modifications and the dysplastic lesions?

The incidence of type III IM in the literature seems too high [4,5], as was also the case in our study aimed to define a high risk population. Other studies in the literature try to refine the interpretation of their histochemical studies. Haggitt et al. [6] showed the importance of measuring the predominance of sulfomucins in the IM; out of 152 biopsy specimens they found their presence in about 42% of cases, but the predominance of sulfomucins in only 4.5%. They conclude that the presence of sulfomucins has a good sensitivity (82%), but a poor specificity (39%); the predominance of sulfomucins has a poor sensitivity (9%), but a good specificity (94%). Consequently, the presence of sulfomucins is a poor marker of high risk, but their predominance seems to be a good marker for surveying a high-risk population of Barrett's esophagus.

Lapertosa et al. [7] studied 111 biopsy series from Barrett's mucosa. Out of these 111 Barrett's mucosa, 46 showed an incomplete IM with presence of sulfomucins. In all of these cases with incomplete IM, they found a complete loss of O-acetylated sialomucins. On the contrary, in two-thirds of cases with complete IM, without sulfomucins, goblet cells contained O-acetylated sialomucins. For these authors, the reduction or the loss of O-acetylated sialomucins might indicate relative tissue immaturity, which could represent an early sign of neoplastic dedifferentiation or dysplasia. This loss indicates more profound phenotypic changes related to prolonged and persistent stimuli and thus more prone to evolve into a malignant condition.

What is the relationship between mucin modification and dysplasia? Two papers try to answer this question. However, one of the difficulties is analyzing the mucosecretion when the mucosa is dysplastic, because of the important diminution of the mucin secretion, and particularly a complete loss of mucosecretion in the case of high-grade dysplasia. Haggitt et al. and Lapertosa et al. [6,7] observed a thin film of sulfomucins on surface glycocalyx in high-grade cases. Besides this, Lapertosa et al. [7] found in all six cases with low-grade dysplasia a loss of mucins in the cytoplasm of the goblet cells with a prevalence of sulfomucins over sialomucins and an absence of O-acetylated sialomucins.

In conclusion, the presence of sulfomucins could not be considered as a specific marker of precancerous condition. On the contrary, the predominance of sulfomucins, and probably the loss of O-acetylated sialomucins observed in Barrett's mucosa, seem to be a good marker of dysplasia, and consequently of precancerous lesions. These modifications are important to detect and permit the careful survey of these patients.

References

1. Jass JR, Filipe I. A variant of intestinal metaplasia associated with gastric carcinoma: a histochemical study. Histopathology 1979;3:191–195.
2. Jass JR. Mucin histochemistry of the columnar epithelium of the oesophagus: a retrospective study. J Clin Pathol 1981; 34:866–870.
3. Peuchmaur M, Potet F, Goldfain D. Mucin histochemistry of the columnar epithelium of the oesophagus (Barrett's oesophagus): a prospective study. J Clin Pathol 1984;37:607–610.
4. Lee RG. Mucins in Barrett's esophagus: a histochemical study. Am J Clin Pathol 1984;81:500–503.
5. Rothery GA, Patterson JE, Stoddard CJ, Day DW. Histological and histochemical changes in the columnar lined (Barrett's) oesophagus. Gut 1986;27:1062–1068.
6. Haggitt RC, Reid BJ, Rabinovitch PS, Rubin CE. Barrett's esophagus. Correlation between mucin histochemistry, flow cytometry and histologic diagnosis for predicting increased cancer risk. Am J Pathol 1988;131:53–61.
7. Lapertosa G, Baracchini P, Fulcheri E, and the Operative Group for the Study of Esophageal Precancer. Mucin histochemical analysis in the interpretation of esophageal precancer. Am J Clin Pathol 1992;98:61–66.

What is the significance of ornithine-decarboxylase dosage?

R.E. Sampliner (Tucson)

Ornithine decarboxylase (ODC) is the first and usually rate limiting step in polyamine metabolism. Polyamines play a central role in cellular growth and differentiation. An important role in carcinogenesis has been attributed to ODC and the polyamine pathway based on *in vitro* and animal model studies. This enzyme is currently being studied for its potential to serve as an intermediate marker for cancer risk. ODC levels have been shown to be elevated in other premalignant conditions – familial adenomatous polyposis of the colon.

Increased ornithine decarboxylase levels have been documented in patients with the specialized columnar type of Barrett's epithelium and, more recently, with intestinal metaplasia of the stomach. In our study, patients with previously recognized Barrett's esophagus had adjacent biopsies of Barrett's epithelium taken for histologic evaluation and for ODC determination. ODC activity in Barrett's epithelium was 0.13 μ/mg protein compared to either adjacent (0.02 μ/mg protein) or small intestinal epithelium (0.02 μ/mg protein) [1,2]. In a preliminary study of Barrett's esophagus patients with and without dysplasia, ornithine decarboxylase activity was greater in dysplastic mucosa (1.6 μ/mg protein in four patients vs. 0.19 μ/mg protein in 11 patients negative or indefinite for dysplasia) [3].

When measuring ODC as well as other marker analyses on whole biopsies, such as flow cytometry, epithelial cells are not specifically targeted. The entire biopsy is processed for the assay, therefore, the result may reflect any cellular component present. In the above cited study there was no correlation between ODC activity and the presence or absence of histologic inflammation [3]. The degree of inflammation in specimens with and without dysplasia did not differ.

Polyamine levels have also been evaluated in Barrett's esophagus. Despite an increased ODC activity, putrescine and spermidine levels were not different in Barrett's gastric and small intestinal mucosa. Spermine levels in gastric mucosa were significantly higher than in Barrett's (4.88 nmol/mg protein vs. 2.95 nmol/mg). There was no relationship between total polyamine content and ODC activity or between spermidine/spermine ratios and ODC activity [1]. In another study the content of putrescine increased from gastric fundus to fundic Barrett's, to specialized Barrett's, to dysplasia and adenocarcinoma. However, only adenocarcinoma showed a significant difference from gastric fundus or fundic Barrett's [4]. Mucosal spermine, spermidine and total polyamine values were greater in the gastric fundus than in fundic, specialized and dysplastic Barrett's. The implication of this study is that mucosal polyamines are not useful as markers of dysplasia.

The biologic basis for elevated ODC activity in metaplastic mucosa is not known. However, it may be a potential marker for the increased cancer risk and therefore serve as a surrogate or intermediate endpoint in cancer prevention trials. Polyamines have not been documented to be elevated in metaplasia or dysplasia. Further delineation of a clinical role for ODC, as is true for any marker, will require prospective evaluation in the context of a clinical trial, involving a defined follow-up protocol.

References

1. Garewal HS, Gerner EW, Sampliner RE et al. Ornithine decarboxylase and polyamine levels in columnar upper gastrointestinal mucosa in patients with Barrett's esophagus. Cancer Res 1988;48:3288–3291.
2. Fennerty MB, Garewal HS, Ramsey L et al. Demonstration of a field defect in gastric preneoplasia by ornithine decarboxylase activity but not by BrdU labeling index. Gastroenterology 1993;104:A399.
3. Garewal HS, Sampliner RE, Gerner EW et al. Ornithine decarboxylase activity in Barrett's esophagus: a potential marker for dysplasia. Gastroenterology 1988;94:819–821.
4. Gray MR, Wallace HM, Goulding H et al. Mucosal polyamine metabolism in the columnar lined esophagus. Gut 1993;34: 584–587.

Is there a common reactive epitope between colonic and Barrett's epithelia?

K.M. Das, I. Prasad, S. Garla, P. Amenta (New Brunswick)

Objective

Barrett's epithelium arises as a complication of chronic reflux esophagitis and predisposes patients to esophageal carcinoma [1–2]. We explored an immunocyto-chemical detection of this condition using a novel monoclonal antibody specifically reactive to colonic epithelial cells.

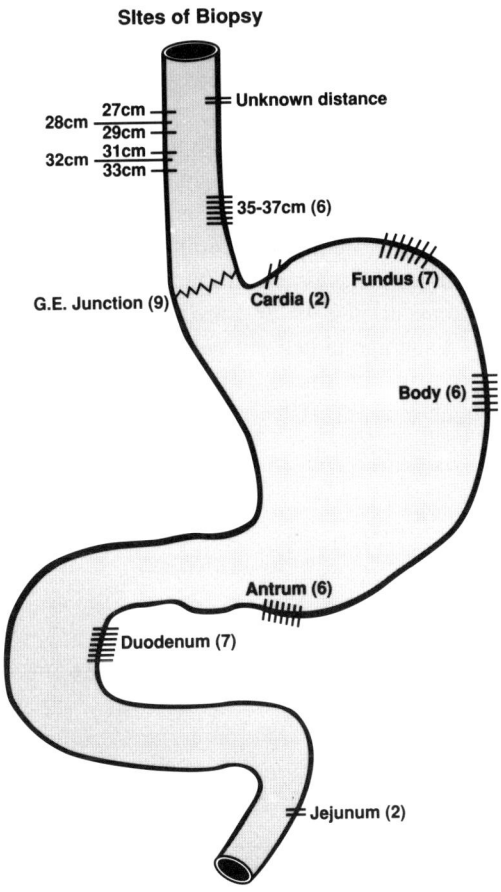

Fig. 1. Sites of biopsy taken prospectively from the esophagus, stomach, duodenum and jejunum from patients with acid reflux syndrome.

Design, Methods and Materials

The murine monoclonal antibody (moAb), $7E_{12}H_{12}$ (IgM isotype) was developed against a colonic epithelial protein which reacts specifically to colon epithelium and not with any other parts of the gastrointestinal tract [3]. A total of 114 tissue specimens from esophagus, stomach, duodenum and jejunum were examined by the immunocytochemical method described by us [3]. Twenty-two biopsy specimens were taken from 22 patients with benign Barrett's epithelium (specialized columnar type) and 12 specimens were obtained from 12 patients with adenocarcinoma arising in Barrett's epithelium. Fourteen specimens were obtained from patients with active esophagitis (7 from gastroesophageal junction, 7 from distal esophagus) and 13 with esophageal squamous cell carcinoma. Additional esophageal specimens included 14 from normal esophagus, proximal to the squamocolumnar junction, and nine from normal gastroesophageal (GE) junctional mucosa. Thirty normal tissue specimens were also obtained from various sites of the stomach (cardia-2, fundus-7, body-6, antrum-6, duodenum-7 and jejunum-2) (Fig. 1).

Results

Twenty-one of 22 (95%) benign Barrett's epithelium specimens reacted with the $7E_{12}H_{12}$ moAb. However, all other tissues including squamous epithelium of the esophagus (Fig. 2), GE junctional mucosa and mucosal epithelium from various parts of the stomach, duodenum and jejunum did not react with the moAb. Twelve of 12 (100%) adenocarcinomas arising from Barrett's epithelium reacted with $7E_{12}H_{12}$ moAb. None of the 13 squamous cell carcinoma of the esophagus reacted with the moAb. Two of 14 biopsy specimens from active esophagitis without a clinical diagnosis of Barrett's epithelium, also reacted with $7E_{12}H_{12}$ moAb.

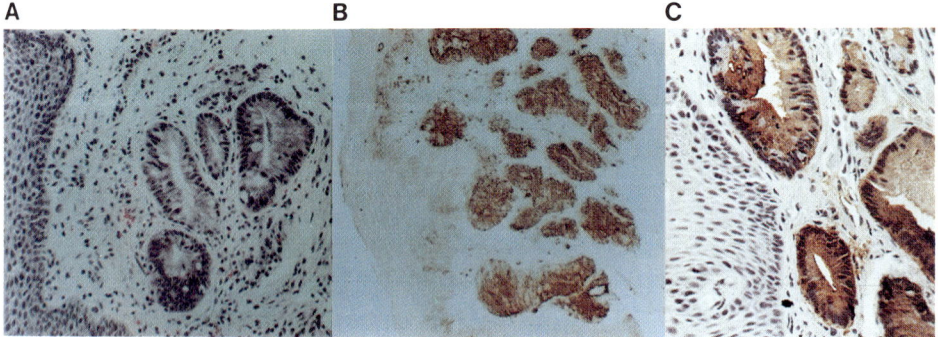

Fig. 2. Endoscopic biopsy of Barrett's epithelium from two patients taken at 25 cm (A and B) and at 30 cm (C) from the incisor teeth, having morphology of specialized columnar type. The reactivity (brownish staining) of $7E_{12}H_{12}$ moAb is evident in the specialized columnar epithelial cells. The staining is mainly cytoplasmic. Original magnification for A: 40×, for B: 20×, and for C: 60×; hematoxylin counterstain. Note that squamous epithelium of the esophagus did not react with $7E_{12}H_{12}$ moAb.

Conclusions

These data indicate that there is a common reactive epitope shared between specialized Barrett's epithelium and colonic epithelium. The results may provide an important clue regarding the origin of specialized Barrett's epithelium. The high incidence of reactivity and specificity of $7E_{12}H_{12}$ moAb to Barrett's epithelium and adenocarcinoma of the esophagus may aid in the diagnosis of these conditions. Further studies are also needed to examine the timing of appearance of the immunoreactivity in patients with chronic reflux esophagitis.

References

1. Spechler SJ, Goyal RK. Barrett's esophagus. N Engl J Med 1986;315:362–371.
2. Haggitt RC, Dean PJ. Adenocarcinoma in Barrett's epithelium. In: Spechler SJ, Goyal RK (eds) Barrett's Esophagus: Pathophysiology, Diagnosis and Management. New York: Elsevier Science Publishers 1985:153–166.
3. Das KM, Vecchi M, Sakamaki S. The production and characterization of monoclonal antibodies to the human colonic antigen associating with ulcerative colitis: cellular localization of the antigen by using the monoclonal antibody. J Immunol 1987;139:77–84.

Are allelic lesions of the p53 gene associated with malignant change?

S. Ramel, K. Thor (Stockholm)

Mutation of the p53 gene, located on chromosome 17p, is one of the most common genetic events found in human cancer [1–4]. Initially the gene was regarded as an oncogene, but it is now known to be a tumor suppressor gene with effects on the regulation of the cell cycle. Recent research has shown that the p53 gene acts as a cell-cycle checkpoint, taking effect on the G1 phase of the cell cycle [5]. The intranuclear concentration of p53 protein is low in normal quiescent cells and increases slightly as a response to entry into the cell cycle [6,7]. A greater increase of the protein is seen as an effect of either DNA damage or as an effect of mutations within the p53 gene itself [4,8]. Overexpression of wild-type p53 results in a G1 arrest or cell death (apoptosis) [5,9]. Studies show that inactivation of the p53 gene by complex with DNA tumor virus proteins, such as the Simian virus 40 (SV40) large T antigen and E6 protein from human papilloma virus, inhibits p53-mediated transactivation and thereby acts to inhibit the tumor suppression effect of wild-type p53 [10]. One of the main roles of checkpoint proteins is to maintain the fidelity of the cell division mechanism and even though the p53 gene plays an important role in cell cycle control it is not, however, essential for normal cell development. In a recent study in transgenic mice constructed with a null allele of p53, the mice developed normally, but were prone to developing different tumors at an early age [11]. One definition of checkpoint proteins is that they are not essential to the viability of the cell, they act through a negative feed-back on the progression through the cell cycle and they enhance the fidelity of the cell division mechanism. The p53 gene fulfills all of these criteria.

Barrett's esophagus is a condition where the normal squamous epithelium is replaced with a metaplastic columnar epithelium of the tubular esophagus as a result of chronic gastroesophageal reflux and predisposes for the development of adenocarcinoma of the esophagus [12,13].

Unfortunately, most esophageal adenocarcinomas are detected at a late stage when they are not curable and most of the patients will die of their disease [14]. The incidence of Barrett's adenocarcinoma is increasing rapidly in the western countries at the present time [15]. Fortunately, however, the group of patients with Barrett's esophagus is well defined and there is a possibility to detect these patients, because of their symptoms of gastroesophageal reflux. A prospective study was performed on 100 consecutive patients with symptoms of gastroesophageal reflux disease (GERD) who were referred for upper GI-endoscopy. Biopsies from the esophagus were evaluated histologically in all patients and 15 were found to have Barrett's esophagus, eight of them were not recognized macroscopically, because of severe esophagitis and short segments of columnar metaplasia (unpublished data). Several studies have shown the benefit of surveillance programs in patients with Barrett's esophagus for the early detection of Barrett's adenocarcinoma [16–18]. Histologic evaluation, however, is not sufficient to detect patients at high risk of cancer development. There is a good agreement in the diagnosis of high-grade dysplasia, but the intraobserver variation in the diagnosis of lesser degrees of dysplasia limits the usefulness of histology in endoscopic biopsy surveillance [19]. Furthermore, only a subset of patients with histological abnormalities will progress to cancer; other patients remain stable or will even regress [16].

The neoplastic progression from metaplasia to adenocarcinoma in Barrett's esophagus is associated with increased genomic instability leading to gross changes in the DNA content or ploidy of the cell [20–22]. During the neoplastic progression, further genomic instability leads to the development of multiple aneuploid cell populations of which one will develop into cancer [20]. Although aneuploidy and the presence of multiple aneuploid cell populations within the columnar epithelium is predictive of a high risk of cancer development, it is a late event in the neoplastic pathway. Equally important and detectable at earlier stages of neoplastic progression is the increase in S- and G2-phase fractions of the cell cycle. The advantage of flow cytometry is, besides recognizing gross DNA changes, that the S- and G2-phases of the cell cycle and p53 protein expression can be determined and analyzed, and patients with cell cycle abnormalities or p53 overexpression can be selected and put on surveillance at shorter intervals.

Lesions on chromosome 17p in Barrett's esophagus and adenocarcinoma

To evaluate p53 protein expression in Barrett's esophagus and Barrett's adenocarcinoma we have developed a two-parameter flow cytometric assay that can be performed on endoscopic biopsies collected during routine endoscopic surveillance. The data acquired include DNA content, the percentage of cells within different cell cycle compartments and p53 protein expression simultaneously detected on the same cell nuclei. It is, therefore, possible to correlate changes in DNA content with cell cycle abnormalities such as increased S- and G2-phases and p53 protein expression [23]. We evaluated 60 patients with Barrett's esophagus and adenocarcinoma and, as control tissue, we analyzed 20 biopsies from normal fundic gland mucosa, representing normal columnar epithelium from the upper GI-tract. Fifteen of the patients had adenocarcinoma of the tubular esophagus, 21 patients had Barrett's esophagus without dysplasia and 24 patients had Barrett's esophagus with different degrees of histologically detectable dysplasia (Table 1). None of the fundic gland biopsies had aneuploid cell populations or p53 overexpression. One of 21 patients with metaplasia without dysplasia, two of 13 with dysplasia in the indefinite or low-grade dysplasia range, five of 11 with high-grade dysplasia, and eight of 15 with Barrett's adenocarcinoma had p53 protein overexpression (Table 1 and Fig. 1). The results indicate that mutations occur within the p53 gene in high-grade dysplasia and in adenocarcinoma. It also indicates that a few patients without dysplasia or with lesser degrees of dysplasia have p53 overexpression. This may be due to either mutations of the p53 gene itself or it may indicate more general DNA damage in the affected cells. Further investigations are ongoing to determine if patients with p53 protein overexpression are those who later develop adenocarcinoma.

Allelic deletions of one p53 allele is a common event in the mutational pattern of the p53 gene in neoplastic progression. The sequence with two normal alleles, allelic loss and finally point mutation of the remaining allele has been postulated [24]. To investigate the occurrence of allelic loss of the p53 gene in Barrett's adenocarcinoma and p53 protein overexpression, we analyzed 13 adenocarcinomas of the tubular esophagus with restriction fragment length polymorphism (RFLP) analysis to detect allelic deletions of chromosome 17p. Cell nuclei for RFLP were sorted on a cell sorter for aneuploidy to avoid contamination with normal diploid stromal cells. Simultaneously, two-parameter flow cytometric analysis for the detection of p53 protein overexpression was performed [25]. Fifteen aneuploid and one tetraploid cell population from the 13 tumors were analyzed. Twelve of 13 patients (92%) had 17p

Table 1. p53 expression in Barrett's esophagus and adenocarcinoma

Tissue	No. of patients	No. with p53 overexpression
Fundic gland mucosa	20	0 (0%)
Metaplasia	21	1 (5%)
Indefinite/low-grade dysplasia	13	2 (15%)
High-grade dysplasia	11	5 (45%)
Adenocarcinoma	15	8 (53%)

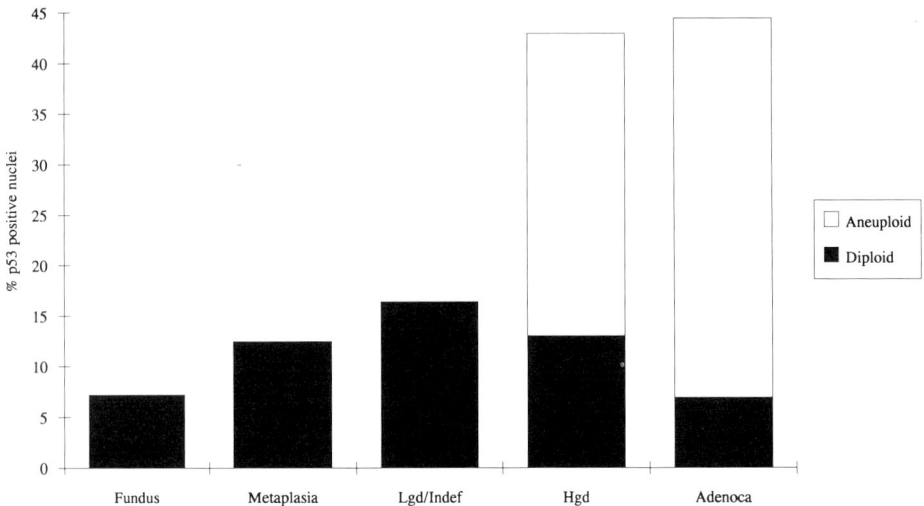

Fig. 1. Graph showing the percentage of cells with p53 protein overexpression. p53 protein expression increases in diploid cell populations in metaplasia without dysplasia and in metaplasia with dysplasia in the indefinite/low-grade dysplasia range compared to fundic gland mucosa. The p53 overexpression in diploid cells with high-grade dysplasia may be neoplastic, but still diploid. In adenocarcinoma most neoplastic cells are aneuploid. Note that the diploid cells have the same p53 protein expression as fundic gland mucosa indicating that they represent normal diploid stromal cells.

allelic deletions and eight of 13 tumors (62%) had p53 protein overexpression. Eight of the 12 tumors (67%) with 17p allelic deletions also had p53 protein overexpression. The results indicate that the prevalence of 17p allelic deletions and p53 protein overexpression is high in Barrett's adenocarcinoma and that p53 overexpression is associated with allelic deletions of chromosome 17p.

Discussion

The prognosis for patients presenting with symptoms of Barrett's adenocarcinoma is dismal [14]. We will not change the outcome of the disease if we do not change our strategy in dealing with patients with Barrett's esophagus, such that early detection of neoplastic change can be recognized and the patients offered surgical treatment at an early stage of the disease. Biopsies from the esophagus should be taken in patients with symptoms of chronic gastroesophageal disease to detect the presence of Barrett's columnar metaplasia. With our two-parameter flow cytometric method for the analysis of endoscopic biopsies, we are able to simultaneously detect cell cycle abnormalities, the presence of aneuploidy and p53 overexpression. The analysis is rapid and many biopsies can be analyzed within a short time which makes the method useful in a clinical setting. This gives us the opportunity to select patients with Barrett's esophagus having cell cycle abnormalities or p53 protein overexpression that are in need of surveillance at short intervals. With this strategy we are able to detect malignant lesions at an early and curable stage. We would also recommend a patient with Barrett's esophagus and high-grade dysplasia, multiple aneuploid cell populations and p53 protein overexpression an esophagectomy if the procedure is not contraindicated by the patient's general medical condition. We believe that this surveillance strategy may change the dismal outcome of adenocarcinoma in Barrett's esophagus.

References

1. Baker SJ, Fearon ER, Nigro JM, Hamilton SR, Preisinger AC, Jessup JM, VanTuinen P, Ledbetter DH, Barker DF, Nakamura Y, White R, Vogelstein B. Chromosome 17 deletions and p53 mutations in colorectal carcinomas. Science 1989; 244:217−221.
2. Nigro JM, Baker SJ, Preisinger AC, Jessup JM, Hostetter R, Cleary K, Bigner SH, Davidson N, Baylin S, Devilee P, Glover T, Collins FS, Weston A, Modali R, Harris CC, Vogelstein B. Mutations in the p53 gene occur in diverse human tumor types. Nature 1989;342:705−708.
3. Hollstein MC, Metcalf RA, Welsh JA, Montesano R, Harris CC. Frequent mutation of the p53 gene in human esophageal cancer. Proc Natl Acad Sci USA 1990;87:9958−9961.
4. Levine AJ, Momand J, Finlay CA. The p53 tumor suppressor gene. Nature 1991;351:453−456.
5. Martinez J, Georgeoff I, Martinez J, Levine AJ. Cellular localization and cell cycle regulation by a temperature-sensitive p53 protein. Genes Devel 1991;5:151−159.
6. Mercer WE, Baserga R. Expression of the p53 protein during the cell cycle of human peripheral blood lymphocytes. Exp Cell Res 1985;160:31−46.
7. Levine AJ. Tumor suppressor genes. Bioessays 1990;12:60−66.
8. Davidoff AM, Humphrey PA, Iglehart JD, Marks JR. Genetic basis for p53 overexpression in human breast cancer. Proc Natl Acad Sci USA 1991;88:5006−5101.
9. Shaw P, Bovey R, Tardy S, Sahli R, Sordat B, Costa J. Induction of apoptosis by wild-type p53 in a human colon tumor-derived cell line. Proc Natl Acad Sci USA 1992;89:4495−4499.
10. Mietz JA, Unger T, Huibregste JM, Howley PM. The transcriptional transactivation function of wild-type p53 is inhibited by SV40 large T-antigen and by HPV-16 E6 oncoprotein. EMBO J 1992;11:5013−5020.
11. Donehower LA, Harvey M, Slagle BL, McArthur MJ, Montgomery CA, Butel JS, Bradley A. Mice deficient for p53 are developmentally normal but susceptible to spontaneous tumors. Nature 1992;356:215−221.
12. Sjogren RW, Johnson LF. Barrett's esophagus: a review. Am J Med 1983;74:313−321.
13. Reid BJ, Weinstein WM. Barrett's esophagus and adenocarcinoma. Ann Rev Med 1987;38:477−492.
14. Skinner DB, Walther BC, Riddell RH, Schmidt H, Iascone C, DeMeester TR. Barrett's esophagus. Comparison of benign and malignant cases. Ann Surg 1983;198:554−566.
15. Blot WJ, Devesa SS, Kneller RW, Fraumeni JF. Rising incidence of adenocarcinoma of the esophagus and gastric cardia. JAMA 1991;265:1287−1289.
16. Reid BJ, Weinstein WM, Lewin KJ, Haggitt RC, Van Deventer G, DenBesten L, Rubin CE. Endoscopic biopsy can detect high-grade dysplasia or early adenocarcinoma in Barrett's esophagus without grossly recognizable neoplastic lesions. Gastroenterology 1988;94:81−90.
17. Robertson CS, Mayberry JF, Nicholson DA, James PD, Atkinson M. Value of endoscopic surveillance in the detection of neoplastic change in Barrett's oesophagus. Br J Surg 1988;75:760−763.
18. Spechler SJ Endoscopic surveillance for patients with Barrett's esophagus: Does the cancer risk justify the practice? Ann Int Med 1987;106:902−904.
19. Reid BJ, Haggitt RC, Rubin CE, Roth G, Surawicz CM, VanBelle G, Lewin KJ, Weinstein WM, Antonioli DA, Goldman H, MacDonald W, Owen D. Observer variation in the diagnosis of dysplasia in Barrett's esophagus. Hum Pathol 1988;19:166−178.
20. Reid BJ, Haggitt RC, Rubin CE, Rabinovitch PS. Barrett's esophagus. Correlation between flow cytometry and histology in detection of patients at risk for adenocarcinoma. Gastroenterology 1987;93:1−11.
21. Rabinovitch PS, Reid BJ, Haggitt RC, Norwood TH, Rubin CE. Progression to cancer in Barrett's esophagus is associated with genomic instability. Lab Invest 1988;60:65−71.
22. Blount PL, Rabinovitch PS, Reid BJ. DNA content flow cytometry, and neoplastic progression in the gastrointestinal tract. In: Eastwood GL (ed) Premalignant conditions of the gastrointestinal tract: Pathogenesis, diagnosis, and management. New York: Elsevier Science Publishers, 1989:55−77.
23. Ramel S, Reid BJ, Sanchez CA, Blount PL, Levine DS, Neshat K, Haggitt RC, Dean PJ, Thor K, Rabinovitch PS. Evaluation of p53 protein expression in Barrett's esophagus by two parameter flow cytometry. Gastroenterology 1992;102:1220−1228.

24. Baker SJ, Preisinger AC, Jessup JM, Paraskeva C, Markowitz S, Willson JKV, Hamilton S, Vogelstein B. p53 gene mutations occur in combination with 17p allelic deletions as late events in colorectal tumorigenesis. Cancer Res 1990; 50:7717–7722.
25. Blount PL, Ramel S, Raskind WH, Haggitt RC, Sanchez CA, Dean PJ, Rabinovitch PS, Reid BJ. 17p allelic deletions and p53 overexpression in Barrett's adenocarcinoma. Cancer Res 1991;51:5482–5486.

What is the value of karyotypic (chromosome 7 or 5) or EGFR (epidermal growth factor receptor) changes in predicting malignant transformation of Barrett's mucosa?

S.R. Hamilton (Baltimore)

Columnar epithelial dysplasia (intraepithelial neoplasia) and adenocarcinoma are well known complications of Barrett's esophagus. Patients presenting with symptomatic Barrett's adenocarcinoma have poor prognosis. As a consequence, intervention in the neoplastic process at an earlier phase, in order to attempt to improve the outcome, is desirable. Various markers are under investigation in the dysplasia-adenocarcinoma sequence in Barrett's esophagus.

In 1990, a case of Barrett's esophagus with trisomy 7 on cytogenetic analysis and overexpression by ligand binding assay of epidermal growth factor receptor (EGFR), which resides on chromosome 7, was reported [1]. Trisomy 5 was also identified in a subset of examined metaphases in the case. Eight additional patients in the report had normal karyotypes in their Barrett's mucosa. Alterations in total DNA content by flow cytometry or image analysis, which reflect increased numbers of chromosomes, have been reported in several studies of patients with Barrett's esophagus [2,3]. By contrast, in another study [4], 7/10 cytogenetically evaluable specimens of Barrett's mucosa had clonal loss of the Y chromosome. In four patients with high-grade dysplasia or adenocarcinoma, cytogenetic abnormalities were evident in Barrett's mucosa as well as in the neoplasms [5]. These alterations included trisomy 3 and 8 in Barrett's mucosa without dysplasia in one patient.

As is evident, the cytogenetics of Barrett's mucosa have not been evaluated in large numbers of patients. At the present time, however, there is no good evidence to suggest that specific karyotypic abnormalities can predict malignant transformation in Barrett's mucosa. If data are generated subsequently, the technique of fluorescent in situ hybridization with chromosome-specific probes could eventually be useful so that standard cytogenetic studies with their inherent vagaries may not be needed.

In addition to the single case [1] with overexpression of EGFR and trisomy 7, a recent flow cytometric analysis of 21 consecutive patients with Barrett's esophagus and seven with adenocarcinoma of the esophagus, showed that the percentage of cells labeled with anti-EGFR antibody was higher as compared to normal gastric mucosa in three of five patients whose Barrett's mucosa had dysplasia [6,7]. All seven esophageal adenocarcinomas had increased epidermal growth factor, transforming growth factor α, EGFR and proliferating cell nuclear antigen expression as compared to normal gastric mucosa. Overexpression of EGFR has also been found in Barrett's mucosa by immunohistochemistry [8]. Study of additional patients will be needed to determine the clinical utility, if any, of analysis of growth regulatory peptides and their receptors in predicting malignant transformation of Barrett's mucosa.

References

1. Garewal HS, Meltzer P, Trent JM, Prabhala R, Sampliner RE, Korc M. Epidermal growth factor receptor overexpression and trisomy 7 in a case of Barrett's esophagus. Dig Dis Sci 1990;9:1115–1120.
2. Garewal HS, Sampliner RE, Fennerty MB. Flow cytometry in Barrett's esophagus – what have we learned so far? Dig Dis Sci 1991;36:548–552.
3. James PD, Atkinson M. Value of DNA image cytometry in the prediction of malignant changes in Barrett's esophagus. Gut 1989;30:899–905.
4. Garewal HS, Sampliner RE, Liu Y, Trent JM. Chromosomal rearrangements in Barrett's esophagus. A premalignant lesion of esophageal carcinoma. Cancer Genet Cytogenet 1989;42:281–296.
5. Raskind WH, Norwood T, Levine DS, Haggitt RC et al. Persistent clonal areas and clonal expansion in Barrett's esophagus. Cancer Res 1992;52:2946–2950.
6. Jankowski J, Hopwood D, Wormsley KG. Flow-cytometric analysis of growth-regulatory peptides and their receptors in oesophagus and Barrett's oesophageal adenocarcinoma. Scand J Gastroenterol 1992;27:147–154.
7. Jankowski J, Hopwood D, Pringle R, Wormsley KG. Increased expression of epidermal growth factor receptor in Barrett's esophagus associated with alkaline reflux: a putative model for carcinogenesis. Am J Gastroenterol 1993;88:402.
8. Poller DN, Steele JC, Morrell K. Epidermal growth factor receptor expression in Barrett's esophagus. Arch Pathol Lab Med 1992;116:1226–1227.

Does flow cytometry provide any information about the genomic changes during carcinogenesis in the mucosa in CLE?

M. Robaszkiewicz (Brest)

Barrett's esophagus is a condition in which the normal stratified squamous epithelium of the distal esophagus is replaced by a metaplastic columnar epithelium. Barrett's metaplasia develops as a complication of chronic gastroesophageal reflux and pre-disposes to the development of esophageal adenocarcinoma [1]. Adenocarcinomas arising in Barrett's mucosa are generally far advanced at the time of diagnosis. Extension through the esophageal wall and lymph node metastasis are noted in most patients, and the prognosis for such advanced cases is dismal. The goal of endoscopic surveillance for patients with Barrett's esophagus is to detect esophageal neoplasm in an early, presymptomatic stage when cure is still feasible. Currently, the most effective screening method appears to examine for dysplasia with multiple closely-spaced biopsies.

Adenocarcinomas arising in Barrett's esophagus generally evolve through a series of progressively severe dysplastic changes. Prospective follow-up studies support the concept of a sequential progression of dysplasia to carcinoma. In these studies, an increase in severity of dysplasia is reported in patients who ultimately develop carcinoma [2,3]. Therefore, dysplasia is widely regarded as the precursor of adenocarcinoma in Barrett's esophagus. Unfortunately, dysplasia falls far short of being an ideal biomarker of malignant potential in Barrett's mucosa for several reasons: first, there is the substantial problem of biopsy sampling errors, because of the patchy distribution of dysplasia. Next, the histologic interpretation of dysplasia is largely a subjective skill. Whereas there is good interobserver agreement in the diagnosis of high-grade dysplasia, there can be considerable disagreement among experienced pathologists in the diagnosis of lesser degrees of dysplasia, particularly when attempting to distinguish low-grade dysplasia from reactive and regenerative changes [4]. Finally, the natural history of dysplasia is not perfectly clear, neither the frequency nor speed with which the dysplasia progresses to invasive cancer are known.

There have been many investigations into various potential markers that may be more sensitive predictors of heightened risk for development of malignancy. Nuclear DNA content analysis by flow cytometry has been applied to Barrett's esophagus by several investigators [5–8]. Flow cytometry provides rapid nuclear DNA content evaluation and cell cycle analysis. In this technique, a suspension of cell nuclei prepared from tissue specimens is treated with a fluorescent dye that binds stoichiometrically to DNA. The stained nuclei are passed through a flow cytometer in which the DNA-bound fluorochrome is excited by laser irradiation. The intensity of the fluorescence emitted by each nucleus represents an estimate of its DNA content. The data are collected by fluorescence detectors and expressed as a DNA histogram. DNA content flow cytometry can identify aneuploid cell populations and can provide information on the fractions of the cell population present in different phases of the cell cycle.

Reid et al. [5] have reported a good concordance between dysplasia and DNA aneuploidy or increased G2/tetraploid fraction. Quite similar results were observed in a recent study, in which we evaluated 497 biopsies from 66 patients with Barrett's esophagus [8]. Of 35 patients with specialized metaplastic epithelium negative for dysplasia, all had diploid DNA content, whereas all of the six patients with high-grade dysplasia, or cancer had DNA aneuploidy or increased G2/tetraploid fraction. These flow cytometric abnormalities were found in 10 out of 25 patients whose biopsies were classified as indefinite for dysplasia or low-grade dysplasia. The two other studies report a lower number of patients [6,7]. The results reported by Fennerty are discordant with the two previous studies: of 73 nondysplastic biopsy specimens, eight were aneuploid and 15 had increased G2M fraction, whereas among 13 dysplastic biopsies, only two were aneuploid and two had increased G2M fraction [7].

1046

Making comparisons of results between these series is difficult, because each group expresses data differently (by patient or by biopsy) or uses a different histologic classification system. Nevertheless, two studies report an increased prevalence of aneuploidy with high-grade dysplasia or cancer [5,8]. These flow cytometric abnormalities are undetectable by conventional histologic techniques. They are associated with a process of genomic instability that generates abnormal clones of cells in specialized metaplasia. This genomic instability is present in a subset of patients who have aneuploidy in the absence of high-grade dysplasia or carcinoma. Infrequently, aneuploidy can be detected in patients with Barrett's specialized metaplasia negative for dysplasia [5]. The relationship of aneuploidy to genomic instability has been established in some patients by cytogenetic analysis which confirmed karyotypic abnormalities corresponding to DNA content abnormalities [9]. The meaning of increased G2M fractions is less clear. Some of these abnormalities appear to be the result of an increased proportion of cells in the G2 interval, whereas others seem to be due to tetraploid or near-tetraploid aneuploid populations [5]. An increased G2 fraction may be evidence of cells attempting to repair DNA damage that occurs during replication (S phase) [10]. If repair is incomplete, these cells are at high risk of developing mutations and chromosome rearrangement. Tetraploid cells may be the precursors of aneuploid clones that develop as a result of nondisjunctions or deletions, which are common during carcinogenesis.

The analysis of the distribution of aneuploid clones in Barrett's mucosa can provide information on the mechanisms of neoplastic progression in Barrett's esophagus. In all cases, the aneuploid clones are confined to the metaplastic mucosa; biopsy specimens taken from normal gastric and esophageal squamous epithelium are always diploid. Some aneuploid clones of cells can spread over large regions of columnar epithelium. In some patients, multiple aneuploid populations may be detected by flow cytometry. Two studies have analyzed the spatial distribution of flow cytometric abnormalities in esophagectomy specimens from patients with Barrett's adenocarcinomas. In the study of Rabinovitch et al. [11], 12 of the 14 esophagectomy specimens had multiple aneuploid clones in the cancer and the surrounding mucosa. In a similar study, we compared the spatial distribution of nuclear DNA content with histologic findings in Barrett's mucosa [12]. All six tumors were aneuploid. Each adenocarcinoma, apart from the most advanced, seemed to arise from a single clone of aneuploid or near-tetraploid cells which was found in all biopsy specimens taken from the tumor. Multiple aneuploid populations were seen in the larger tumors. In all cases, one or several aneuploid populations were detected in the mucosa surrounding the carcinoma. Some areas were characterized by the same DNA index as in the tumor, others contained distinct aneuploid cell populations. The spatial distributions of aneuploid clones and dysplastic areas were not perfectly superimposed and this may provide an additional clue for the potential utility of flow cytometry in assessing the risk of neoplastic progression in Barrett's mucosa.

The results of these studies suggest that some patients with Barrett's esophagus develop an acquired genomic instability that generates an abnormal clone of cells. This clone can spread to involve large regions of esophageal mucosa. With continued genomic instability, multiple aneuploid subclones may evolve, one of which may acquire a malignant phenotype and the capacity of invasion. With continued genomic instability, other subclones may evolve in the cancer leading to tumor cell heterogeneity.

There are some available data suggesting that the combination of histology and flow cytometry could probably identify patients who might be candidates for more intensive endoscopic surveillance. However, the clinical significance of flow cytometric abnormalities will only be established by long-term follow-up studies.

Reid et al. [3] have recently reported the results of a prospective histologic and flow-cytometric surveillance of 62 patients with Barrett's esophagus evaluated for a mean interval of 34 months. In this study, nine of 13 patients who showed aneuploidy or increased G2/tetraploid fraction in their initial flow cytometric analysis developed high-grade dysplasia or adenocarcinoma during follow-up, whereas none of the 49 patients without these abnormalities progressed to high-grade dysplasia or cancer. Neoplastic progression was characterized by the development of multiple aneuploid population of cells and by progressive histological abnormalities. Increased G2/tetraploid fractions were early findings in most of the patients who subsequently progressed. This study indicates that the combination of histological and flow cytometric evaluation of endoscopic biopsy specimens can be useful in managing the cancer risk in patients with Barrett's esophagus. Nevertheless, these results need to be confirmed by other studies before flow cytometry is applied to routine clinical investigation.

In conclusion, flow cytometry appears to be a promising technique for managing the risk of neoplastic progression in patients with Barrett's esophagus. It will probably provide valuable information to define optimal follow-up intervals for endoscopic evaluation of Barrett's metaplasia by selecting patients who merit more intensive surveillance.

References

1. Spechler SJ, Goyal RK. Barrett's esophagus. N Engl J Med 1986;315:362–371.
2. Hameeteman W, Tytgat GNJ, Houthoff HJ, van den Tweel JG. Barrett's esophagus: development of dysplasia and adenocarcinoma. Gastroenterology 1989;96:1249–1256.
3. Reid BJ, Blount PL, Rubin CE, Levine DS, Haggitt RC, Rabinovitch PS. Flow cytometric and histological progression to malignancy in Barrett's esophagus: prospective endoscopic surveillance of a cohort. Gastroenterology 1992;102:1212–1219.
4. Reid BJ, Haggitt RC, Rubin CE et al. Observer variation in the diagnosis of dysplasia in Barrett's esophagus. Hum Pathol 1988;19:166–178.
5. Reid BJ, Haggitt RC, Rubin CE, Rabinovitch PS. Barrett's esophagus. Correlation between flow cytometry and histology in detection of patients at risk for adenocarcinoma. Gastroenterology 1987;93:1–11.
6. McKinley MJ, Budman DR, Grueneberg D, Bronzo RL, Weissman GS, Kahn E. DNA content in Barrett's esophagus and esophageal malignancy. Am J Gastroenterol 1987;82:1012–1015.
7. Fennerty MB, Sampliner RE, Way D, Riddell R, Steinbronn K, Garewal HS. Discordance between flow cytometric abnormalities and dysplasia in Barrett's esophagus. Gastroenterology 1989;97:815–820.
8. Robaszkiewicz M, Hardy E, Volant A et al. Analyse du contenu cellulaire en ADN par cytométrie en flux dans les endobrachyoesophages: étude de 66 cas. Gastroenterol Clin Biol 1991;15:703–710.
9. Raskind WH, Norwood T, Levine DS et al. Persistent clonal areas and clonal expansion in Barrett's esophagus. Cancer Res 1992;52:2946–2950.
10. Hartwell LH, Weinert TA. Checkpoints: controls that ensure the order of cell cycle events. Science 1989;246:629–634.
11. Rabinovitch PS, Reid BJ, Haggitt RC et al. Progression to cancer in Barrett's esophagus is associated with genomic instability. Lab Invest 1988;60:65–71.
12. Robaszkiewicz M, Volant A, Hardy E et al. Mise en évidence d'une hétérogénéité clonale au niveau des adénocarcinomes sur endobrachyoesophage par l'étude cytofluorométrique du contenu cellulaire en ADN. Gastroenterol Clin Biol 1992;16:540–546.

What is the relationship between aneuploidy, dysplasia, and cancer?
What is the implication of the finding of aneuploidy on a single occasion in a patient with Barrett's epithelium?

H.S. Garewal (Tucson)

There are two main objectives, that are best considered separately, to the use of flow cytometry for measurement of cellular DNA content in Barrett's mucosal biopsies. The clinical objective is to develop better prognostic and cancer risk markers than the current "standard" of dysplasia. The biologic objective is to enhance our understanding of the carcinogenesis process as it occurs in Barrett's mucosa. It is helpful to keep these distinct goals in mind when evaluating the results and conclusions of reported studies, particularly in the context of seeking answers to the above questions. Observations of importance in understanding the biology of the transformation process may or may not be of clinical significance to the care of patients.

Aneuploidy, the presence of an abnormal amount of DNA per cell, is the most significant abnormality detected by flow cytometry in this setting. Although some investigators have recommended the use of quantitative measurements of phases of the cell cycle, such as the tetraploid G_2/M and S-phase, this approach has severe limitations since the observed fraction (percent) will depend on the number of nonepithelial, normal, diploid stromal and inflammatory cells that will always be present in the specimen in varying numbers [1–3]. Consequently, we and other have found it impossible to establish this as a criterion for abnormality. The following discussion will therefore deal with aneuploidy only.

Clinically, the presence or absence of dysplasia, particularly high-grade dysplasia, remains the most useful and widely applied criterion in monitoring Barrett's patients for cancer risk assessment and appropriate intervention [4]. Its limitations are well known (i.e., interobserver variability in readings and sampling problems). Nevertheless, any method that is proposed to improve the accuracy and reliability of surveillance endoscopies must be clinically significantly better than assessment of dysplasia to warrant routine use. As discussed below, at present the available data do not support such a conclusion for aneuploidy and, therefore, flow cytometry remains a research tool.

Aneuploidy and dysplasia are clearly discordant in Barrett's esophagus. Although an initial report suggested a 100% incidence of aneuploidy in Barrett's adenocarcinoma and a 100% correlation of aneuploidy and/or increased G_2 phase with dysplasia [3], reports from several groups have now confirmed that aneuploidy and dysplasia are more commonly discordant, rather than concordant findings, in agreement with our initial study [2,5,6]. In fact, aneuploidy is more commonly encountered than definite dysplasia, being found in nondysplastic epithelium as well as specimens with the more uncertain readings of indefinite or low-grade dysplasia.

The clinical importance of a single aneuploid clone found in one biopsy remains doubtful. There are very few published reports of serial flow cytometric analyses on subjects in whom a single aneuploid clone is detected. In our own experience, most such single aneuploid clones occur in the setting of no or indefinite/low-grade dysplasia and are often undetectable in future examinations [1]. Furthermore, failure to demonstrate aneuploidy on repeated examinations has been uniformly associated with a benign course. In contrast, repeated findings of aneuploidy, or the detection of multiple aneuploid clones, have a closer association with high-grade dysplasia and cancer [1,6]. In the recent report by Reid et al. the clinical significance of aneuploidy was evaluated prospectively [6]. Patients demonstrating aneuploidy, usually with multiple clones, went on to develop high-grade dysplasia and/or cancer.

From the clinical standpoint, the important question is whether flow cytometry added anything to the care of patients. The studies reported thus far have failed to clearly demonstrate any clinical gain. In the prospective study mentioned earlier, although the authors attempt to present a more positive conclusion, close scrutiny of the results reveals that every patient developing cancer showed the usual sequence of increasing dysplasia, with high-grade dysplasia being detected prior to the cancer [6]. Consequently, all such cancer cases would have been picked up by the histologic progression, as is routinely done, in the absence of flow cytometry data.

Is the converse true? In other words, if no aneuploidy is detected, does this confer a no or lower-risk status than that ascertained by histology alone? Although intuitively appealing, leading to recent statements to the effect that "aneuploidy-negative and dysplasia-free patients develop no cancers", the key issue is whether being aneuploidy-free adds anything to being dysplasia-free. Much larger trials than those currently published would be required to answer this question with any level of confidence.

From the clinical standpoint, therefore, the contribution of flow cytometry to surveillance and cancer risk assessment remains to be proven. It appears that patients with repeated findings of aneuploidy on sequential examinations, and probably those with multiple aneuploid clones, are at a higher risk of malignancy. Since aneuploidy, just like dysplasia, has a patchy distribution, repeated demonstration or detection of multiple clones probably indicates large areas of involved mucosa. However, these are almost always the same patients in whom definite dysplastic changes, usually high-grade are detected. Consequently, the added value of flow cytometry to clinical decision making becomes questionable.

From a biologic standpoint, however, these findings are of considerable interest, in that they demonstrate the genetic instability which precedes tumor formation in many tissues. The lack of significance of finding a single aneuploid clone on one occasion could reflect sampling or may actually represent disappearance of the clone. Since even cancers can regress spontaneously, why should this not be possible with a more benign, but aneuploid clone? Only those aneuploid clones will persist that have a sustained growth advantage, possibly conferred by the accumulation of more genetic damage that leads to histologic dysplasia and multiple aneuploidies.

Table 2.

At entry	No. of patients	Developed adenocarcinoma
DYS – , AN –	22	0
DYS – , AN +	11	0
DYS + , AN –	4	0
DYS + , AN +	1	1

Note: DYS = dysplasia; AN = aneuploidy.

years. One patient with both high-grade dysplasia and aneuploidy on biopsies had carcinoma in situ in the surgical resection specimen.

Herman et al. [8] (Table 2) followed 38 patients with CLE for a mean of 4.0 years. One patient with both high-grade dysplasia and aneuploidy developed adenocarcinoma on follow-up.

Reid et al. [9] (Table 3) followed 62 patients with CLE for a mean of 34 months. Flow cytometric abnormality was defined as aneuploidy or increased tetraploidy. Five patients developed adenocarcinoma. In all five, flow cytometry was abnormal on entry to the study. The initial histology showed high-grade dysplasia in two of the five cases, low-grade dysplasia in two and CLE without dysplasia in one. However, these last three cases all developed high-grade dysplasia after the entry to the study, but before the appearance of carcinoma.

Seven of 49 patients whose flow cytometry was negative on entering this study developed flow cytometric abnormalities later, but none of these developed carcinoma.

The data from these studies indicate that abnormal flow cytometry and dysplasia are both markers for the subsequent development of adenocarcinoma in patients with CLE. However, these two markers have a limited degree of independence. All seven patients developing adenocarcinoma in the three series, previously had abnormal flow cytometry, but all seven also had high-grade dysplasia either at the time of entering their study or later. Flow cytometric analysis of DNA is a useful research tool, but the additional information it provides when histology is already available seems insufficient to consider it as a routine investigation in the monitoring of CLE at the present time. This recommendation is in agreement with the opinion expressed in three editorial reviews of the subject [7,10,11].

Table 3.

At entry	No. of patients	Developed adenocarcinoma
Flow CYT +	13	5
Flow CYT –	49	0
DYS, high grade	3	2
DYS, low grade/indefinite	20	2
DYS –	39	1

Note: CYT = cytometry; DYS = dysplasia.

References

1. Williamson WA, Ellis FH, Gibb SP et al. Barrett's esophagus. Prevalence and incidence of adenocarcinoma. Arch Int Med 1991;151:2212—2216.
2. Spechler SJ. Endoscopic surveillance for patients with Barrett's esophagus: does the cancer risk justify the practice? Ann Int Med 1987;106:902—904.
3. Robertson CS, Mayberry JF, Nicholson DA et al. Value of endoscopic surveillance in the detection of neoplastic change in Barrett's esophagus. Br J Surg 1988;75:760—763.
4. Streitz JM, Ellis FH, Gibb SP et al. Adenocarcinoma in Barrett's esophagus. Ann Surg 1991;213:122—125.
5. Reid BJ, Haggitt RC, Rubin CE et al. Observer variation in the diagnosis of dysplasia in Barrett's esophagus. Hum Pathol 1988;19:166—178.
6. Fennerty MB, Sampliner RE, Way D et al. Discordance between flow cytometric abnormalities and dysplasia in Barrett's esophagus. Gastroenterology 1989;97:815—820.
7. Garewal HS, Sampliner RE, Fennerty MB. Flow cytometry in Barrett's esophagus. What have we learned so far? Dig Dis Sci 1991;36:548—551.
8. Herman RD, McKinely MJ, Bronzo RL et al. Flow cytometry and Barrett's esophagus (letter). Dig Dis Sci 1992;37:635.
9. Reid BJ, Blount PL, Rubin CE et al. Flow-cytometric and histological progression to malignancy in Barrett's esophagus: prospective endoscopic surveillance of a cohort. Gastroenterology 1992;102:1212—1219.
10. Ahnen DJ. Flow cytometric analysis of deoxyribonucleic acid content in the gastrointestinal tract. Gastroenterology 1987;93:197—199.
11. Cameron AJ. Barrett's esophagus and adenocarcinoma: from the family to the gene. Gastroenterology 1992;102:1421—1424.

Is image analysis a viable alternative approach to flow cytometry in assaying nuclear DNA content and pattern?

H.S. Garewal (Tucson)

Detection of "aneuploidy" by histologic evaluation or quantitation of nuclear material (i.e., DNA) is of considerable interest, because it allows the observer to study the cells of interest, since epithelial or glandular cells can be identified and their nuclear DNA assessed. At our center, we attempted to develop histologic criteria for nuclear shape and size, to be applied to routine hematoxylin-eosin stained specimens to try and correlate these with the presence or absence of aneuploidy detected by flow cytometry (Fennerty MB, Riddell RH, Sampliner RE, Garewal HS, unpublished results). These criteria were tested in a blinded comparison on a set of 25 biopsies, in which flow cytometry results and histologic sections were available. Flow cytometric aneuploidy was present in nine specimens, six of which were considered "aneuploid" by the histologic criteria. The pathology readings in these six were: two high-grade, one indefinite and three negative for dysplasia. Of the 16 cases with normal flow cytometry 12 were normal by the histologic criteria, while four were read as "aneuploid". Interestingly, the pathology readings of the latter four were: one high grade, two low grade and one indefinite for dysplasia. The 12 that were aneuploidy negative by flow cytometry and by histologic criteria had: one high grade, one indefinite and 10 negative for dysplasia. Overall there was concordance between flow cytometry and the histologic criteria in 18 of the 25 biopsies (72%).

A more sophisticated approach uses image cytometry on Feulgen stained sections. The DNA content of epithelial cells is quantitated by comparing it with diploid lymphocytes, using automated systems available for this purpose. In this manner, aneuploid cells can be defined as those whose DNA content differs from diploid cells by an arbitrary amount. James and Atkinson have reported techniques for the application of this approach to Barrett's esophagus [1]. As can be expected, there are numerous technical problems with this approach, not the least of which is development and testing of criteria for abnormality. Once again, the critical issue relating to clinical significance is demonstration of improvement over the use of dysplasia. Studies with this objective have not been reported.

Reference

1. James PD, Atkinson M. Value of DNA image cytometry in the prediction of malignant change in Barrett's esophagus. Gut 1989;30:899–905.

In the light of cost-assessment of the disorder, does the risk of adenocarcinoma justify regular endoscopic monitoring of a patient with Barrett's esophagus?

S.J. Spechler (Boston)

Patients with Barrett's esophagus develop esophageal adenocarcinoma at the rate of approximately 0.8% per year [1]. Consequently, regular endoscopic surveillance has been recommended for patients who have a columnar cell-lined esophagus, with the goal of detecting esophageal neoplasia in an early, curable stage [2]. The American Cancer Society has identified four criteria by which to evaluate cancer surveillance procedures [3]:
1. There should be good evidence that the procedure is effective in reducing cancer morbidity or mortality;
2. The medical benefits should outweigh the risks;
3. The cost should be reasonable; and
4. The procedure should be practical and feasible.

Judged by these criteria, endoscopic surveillance for patients with Barrett's esophagus remains a controversial practice.

There is no proof that endoscopic surveillance reduces the morbidity or mortality from esophageal cancer in patients with Barrett's esophagus. Indeed, the number of patients and duration of follow-up necessary for a study to demonstrate that endoscopic surveillance significantly affects cancer mortality are so great that such a study is impractical [4]. Nevertheless, the rationale that endoscopic surveillance can detect curable neoplasia seems reasonable and indirect evidence strongly supports the practice. In one recent investigation, for example, survival after resection for adenocarcinoma in Barrett's esophagus was far better in patients who had the cancer detected by endoscopic surveillance than in patients who presented initially with symptoms of esophageal cancer [5].

Patients who are too old or too infirm to undergo esophageal resection for cancer should not have endoscopic surveillance. Therefore, endoscopic surveillance is limited to otherwise healthy individuals with Barrett's esophagus. The risks of elective esophagoscopy in such patients is virtually negligible [6]. Therefore, virtually any reduction in esophageal cancer mortality resulting from endoscopic surveillance would outweigh the risks.

Cost is the major drawback to endoscopic surveillance for Barrett's esophagus. One recent report has estimated the direct cost of annual endoscopic surveillance at approximately $62,000 for every cancer discovered [7]. Presumably, a program of every-other-year surveillance would cost considerably less. Although this price is substantial, there are no clear guidelines by which to determine if the cost of endoscopic surveillance is reasonable compared to its expected benefits.

Finally, endoscopic services are widely available and therefore endoscopic surveillance is a procedure that is both practical and feasible. For a physician to withhold this potentially life-saving procedure either because of financial concerns or because efficacy has yet to be proved, seems inappropriate.

References

1. Spechler SJ. Epidemiology and natural history of gastro-oesophageal reflux disease. Digestion 1992;51(suppl 1):24–29.
2. Dent J, Bremner CG, Collen MJ, Haggitt RC, Spechler SJ. Working party report to the World Congresses of Gastroenterology, Sydney 1990. Barrett's oesophagus. J Gastroenterol Hepatol 1991;6:1–22.
3. American Cancer Society. Guidelines for the cancer-related checkup: recommendations and rationale. CA 1980;30:194–240.
4. Spechler SJ. Endoscopic surveillance for patients with Barrett's esophagus: does the cancer risk justify the practice? Ann Int Med 1987;106:902–904.
5. Streitz JM Jr, Andrews CW Jr, Ellis FH Jr. Endoscopic surveillance of Barrett's esophagus. Does it help? J Thorac Cardiovasc Surg 1993:105:383–388.
6. Goy JA, Herold E, Jenkins PJ, Colman JC, Russell DM. "Open-access" endoscopy for general practitioners: experience of a private gastrointestinal clinic. Med J Aust 1986;144:71–74.
7. Achkar E, Carey W. The cost of surveillance for adenocarcinoma complicating Barrett's esophagus. Am J Gastroenterol 1988;83:291–294.

The adenocarcinomatous mucosa

The adenocarcinomatous mucosa

 The incidence of adenocarcinoma of the esophagus is currently increasing and accounts for 50% of esophageal carcinomas in some series

L. Bernstein (Los Angeles)

During the 1970s and 1980s incidence rates of esophageal adenocarcinoma in the United States (US) [1—4] and United Kingdom (UK) [4] increased dramatically. These population-based trends have confirmed the increase in the frequency of esophageal adenocarcinomas reported in clinically-based series [5—8]. A similar, although smaller increase in incidence rates of adenocarcinomas of the gastric cardia has also been documented [1,4], again confirming clinical reports [9,10]. In sharp contrast to these patterns, during the same time period, incidence rates of distal gastric carcinomas have remained constant or declined [1,4] and rates of squamous cell carcinoma of the esophagus have remained fairly constant [1,3].

Data derived from clinical series and population-based cancer registries can be used concurrently to assess anatomic subsite and morphologic trends in esophageal and gastric cancer. Although clinical series allow for uniform histologic review and subsite classification, they generally represent a biased subset of patients and do not permit determination as to whether observed increases in one subtype of cancer are absolute or relative increases, or even an artifact of changing referral patterns. As population-based cancer registry data include all cancers diagnosed in a geographically defined population, they can be used to evaluate relative changes in frequency of a subgroup of cancers (in a fashion similar to that of clinical series), as well as to investigate absolute increases in incidence. One drawback of registry data is that morphologic diagnostic criteria may not be uniformly applied as diagnoses are made by community pathologists. Subsite determination is based on medical and pathology reports reviewed by medical records technicians or tumor registrars. Furthermore, except in special circumstances, there is no uniform review of morphology or subsite. Thus, with temporal improvements in diagnostic techniques, such as the increased use of endoscopy, an observed increase in incidence rates may be artifactual.

Incidence patterns

The percentages shown in Table 1 illustrate the dramatic increase in the frequency of adenocarcinoma of the esophagus relative to all esophageal carcinomas over the past 3 decades. Bosch and colleagues [5] summarized data for clinical series published prior to 1979. These series indicated that prior to 1975 the proportion of true esophageal adenocarcinomas (with no involvement of the cardia) ranged from 0.2–7% (composite: 2.3%). The more recent data of Wang and colleagues suggest that, by the 1980s, more than 34% of esophageal cancer patients had adenocarcinomas and that within the lower esophagus 60% were adenocarcinomas [7].

Table 1. Relative frequency of adenocarcinoma of the esophagus in clinical series and population-based cancer registries

Type of series	First author and year	Time period	Percentage of adenocarcinomas
Clinical	Bosch, 1979	prior to 1975	4.0
		prior to 1975	2.4[a,b]
	Levine, 1984	1979–1982	19.1
	Wang, 1986	1975–1982	34.3[b]
	Hesketh, 1989	1980–1986	30.9
		1980-1986	17.9[b]
Cancer registry[c]	Bosch, 1979	prior to 1976	7.7[a]
	Yang, 1988	1973–1982	16.4
	Hesketh, 1989	1982–1984	26.6
	Powell, 1990	1967–1971	8.0[d]
		1977–1981	19.8[d]
	Blot, 1991	1984–1987	34[e]
	Los Angeles	1972–1978	15.8[e]
	County	1979–1982	23.6[e]
	(current study)	1983–1986	26.6[e]
		1987–1990	43.2[e]

[a]Composite based on several studies; [b]true esophageal adenocarcinoma, no involvement of the cardia or gastroesophageal junction; [c]based on incident cases ascertained by population-based cancer registries; [d]based on cases with known histology; [e]restricted to white male cases.

The relative percentages of esophageal adenocarcinomas from population-based cancer registries are similar to those from clinical series. Our own data derived from the Los Angeles County (USA) population-based cancer registry indicate that adenocarcinomas now comprise 43% of esophageal carcinomas (Table 1).

Data from population-based cancer registries reflect a marked increase in the incidence rates of esophageal adenocarcinoma during the 1970s and 1980s in the US and UK (Table 2). Blot and colleagues have estimated that incidence rates increased nearly 10% per year among white men in the US between 1976 and 1987, twice the rate observed among white women [1]. In Los Angeles County a 10% annual increase in the incidence rates of white males between 1972 and 1990 was also observed; however, the rate of increase among white females (19% per year) was substantially higher. Comparable increases in the incidence rates of esophageal adenocarcinoma among black men have been observed in Los Angeles County (data not shown) and elsewhere in the US [1], although overall black men have only one third to one fourth the risk of white men.

The subsite distribution of adenocarcinomas of the esophagus differs from that of squamous cell carcinomas. More than 80% of adenocarcinomas, but only 30% of

Table 2. Trends in age-adjusted incidence rates of esophageal adenocarcinoma per 100,000 population

First author year	Location of registry	Time period	Age-adjusted incidence rate			
Powell, 1990	United Kingdom[a]	1967–1971		0.18		
		1972–1976		0.37		
		1977–1981		0.63		
Blot, 1991	United States[b]	1976–1979	M:	0.92	F:	0.15
		1980–1983		1.30		0.18
		1984–1987		1.90		0.20
Zheng, 1992	United States[c]	1970–1974	M:	0.6	F:	0.1
		1975–1979		0.9		0.2
		1980–1984		1.5		0.3
		1985–1989		2.7		0.4
Pera, 1993	United States[d]	1935–1971	E:	0.13	GE:	0.25
		1974–1989		0.74		1.34
Current study	United States[e]	1972–1978	M:	0.58	F:	0.06
		1979–1982		1.12		0.18
		1983–1986		1.46		0.21
		1987–1990		1.72		0.32

[a]West Midlands — males and females combined, rates are adjusted to the World Standard Population; [b]nine SEER (Surveillance, Epidemiology and End Results) registries — rates are for whites and were estimated from graphs, rates are adjusted to the 1970 US population; M = males, F = females; [c]Connecticut — rates are for whites and were adjusted to the 1970 US population; M = males, F = females; [d]Olmstead County, Minnesota — E = esophageal adenocarcinomas and GE = adenocarcinomas of the gastroesophageal junction; [e]Los Angeles County, California — rates are for non-Hispanic whites and are adjusted to the 1970 US population; M = males, F = females.

squamous cell carcinomas occur in the lower third of the esophagus [1,7,8]. Forty to 50% of squamous cell esophageal carcinomas are found in the middle third.

Increases in the relative frequency and incidence rates of adenocarcinomas of the gastric cardia have also occurred over the past 3 decades, although these increases are of a lower magnitude than those observed for esophageal adenocarcinomas. In two clinical series, one from the US [9] and the other from Greece [10], the relative frequencies indicate that the proportion of adenocarcinomas of the cardia has doubled. In contrast, incidence rates in the UK increased only 60% from the late 1960s to the late 1970s [4] (Table 3). Furthermore, the increase in incidence in the US has been even more modest, with only a 27% increase among white men and a 50% increase among white women from the mid-1970s to the mid-1980s [1]. Although black men in the US are only half as likely as white men to be diagnosed with adenocarcinoma of the gastric cardia, their incidence rates have also shown modest increases [1]. In Los Angeles County, no increase in the incidence of cardia tumors among women has been observed.

As illustrated in Fig. 1, the incidence rates of distal stomach tumors have remained relatively constant among white males in Los Angeles County over the past 2 decades and incidence rates of squamous cell carcinoma of the esophagus began to decline only recently, probably as a result of a decline in the number of cigarette smokers. These observations are consistent with those reported for other cancer registries in the US [1]. In the UK, there has actually been an increase in the incidence of stomach tumors occurring at other single sites [4]. Population-based cancer registries have recorded substantial decreases in the incidence rates of stomach tumors with unspecified subsites (Fig. 1) [1,4].

Table 3. Trends in age-adjusted incidence rates of adenocarcinoma of the gastric cardia per 100,000 population

First author year	Location of registry	Time period	Age-adjusted incidence rate		
Powell, 1990	United Kingdom[a]	1967-1971		1.25	
		1972-1976		1.51	
		1977-1981		2.01	
Blot, 1991	United States[b]	1976-1979	M: 2.6	F:	0.4
		1980-1983	2.8		0.6
		1984-1987	3.3		0.6
Current study	United States[c]	1972-1978	M: 2.58	F:	0.51
		1979-1982	2.81		0.45
		1983-1986	3.00		0.59
		1987-1990	2.90		0.46

[a]West Midlands — males and females combined, rates are adjusted to the World Standard Population; [b]nine SEER (Surveillance, Epidemiology and End Results) registries — rates are for whites and were estimated from graphs, rates adjusted to the 1970 US population, M = males, F = females; [c]Los Angeles County, California — rates are for non-Hispanic whites and adjusted to the 1970 US population, M = males, F = females.

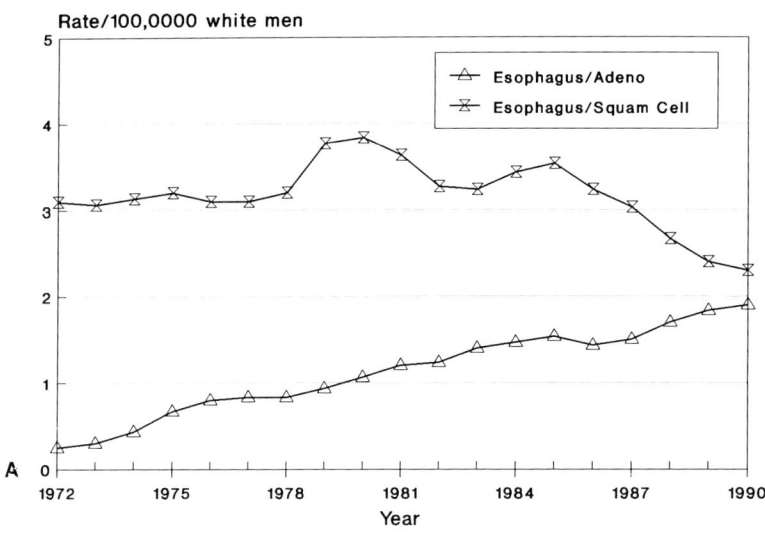

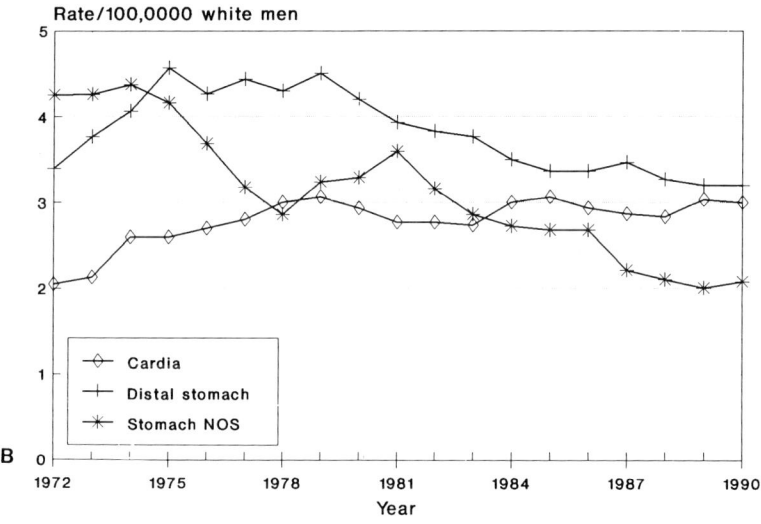

Fig. 1. Secular trends in the age-adjusted incidence rates of carcinomas of the esophagus and stomach of non-Hispanic white males in Los Angeles County, 1972–1990. A) Adenocarcinoma and squamous cell carcinoma of the esophagus. B) Adenocarcinoma of the cardia, other single sites of the stomach and sites not otherwise specified (NOS).

Other characteristics

The similarity of demographic characteristics of persons diagnosed with adenocarcinomas of the esophagus and gastric cardia further distinguishes these tumors from those occurring at other subsites of the stomach and from squamous cell carcinomas of the esophagus. The male-to-female incidence rate ratio ranges from 6—10 for esophageal adenocarcinomas and from 5—7 for adenocarcinomas of the gastric cardia (Tables 1 and 2). This contrasts with a male-to-female rate ratio of 2 for distal gastric tumors and 2—4 for squamous cell carcinomas of the esophagus [1,4]. Although white males have only one third to one half the risk of black males for tumors of the distal stomach, their incidence rates of cardia tumors are 2 times greater than those of blacks [1]. The range of differences is even greater for the esophagus. Black males have 4—5 times the risk of squamous cell carcinoma of the esophagus, but only one third to one fourth the risk of esophageal adenocarcinoma [1].

British patients diagnosed with adenocarcinoma of the esophagus are of a higher social class standing than those diagnosed with squamous cell carcinomas [4]. Similar trends have been noted among whites in Los Angeles County. Furthermore, in Los Angeles County whites diagnosed with adenocarcinomas of the cardia have higher social class standing than those with tumors of the distal stomach or stomach tumors in which no subsite is specified. Although there has been a dramatic decline in these nonspecific gastric adenocarcinomas, the social class distribution has remained constant, suggesting that better classification of subsite would account for only a small part of the increase in incidence of cardia tumors.

Summary

The major question regarding the marked increase in esophageal adenocarcinomas is whether it reflects a true increase, or is an artifact of changing subsite classification or improved histologic diagnosis. As incidence rates of squamous cell carcinoma of the esophagus among whites have remained relatively constant over the time period that adenocarcinoma rates have increased, improved histologic diagnosis is not a likely explanation. The increasing use of endoscopy, which allows determination of the precise location of many tumors near the gastroesophageal junction, may have shifted classification from the cardia to the esophagus. However, if this were the sole reason for the increase in esophageal adenocarcinomas, it is unlikely that concomitant increases in gastric cardia tumors would have been observed. Furthermore, there has been little or no change in the incidence rates of distal stomach tumors. Although incidence rates of gastric tumors with no subsite specified have declined substantially, patients diagnosed with these tumors are similar demographically to those with distal stomach tumors and not to those with adenocarcinomas of the gastric cardia or esophagus. Based on their data from nine US cancer registries, Blot and colleagues estimated that only 25% of the increase in incidence of cardia tumors observed between 1976 and 1987, could be attributed to improved specification of subsite [1]. Therefore, it seems reasonable to conclude that a substantial portion of the increase in incidence of esophageal adenocarcinomas, as well as a small increase in incidence of cardia tumors, is real.

References

1. Blot WJ, Devesa SS, Kneller RW, Fraumeni JF. Rising incidence of adenocarcinoma of the esophagus and gastric cardia. JAMA 1991;265:1287–1289.
2. Pera M, Cameron AJ, Trastek VF et al. Increasing incidence of adenocarcinoma of the esophagus and esophagogastric junction. Gastroenterology 1993;104:510–513.
3. Zheng T, Mayne ST, Holford TR et al. Time trend and age-period-cohort effects on incidence of esophageal cancer in Connecticut 1935–89. Cancer Cause Control 1992;3:481–492.
4. Powell J, McConkey CC. Increasing incidence of adenocarcinoma of the gastric cardia and adjacent sites. Br J Cancer 1990;59:440–443.
5. Bosch A, Frias Z, Caldwell WL. Adenocarcinoma of the esophagus. Cancer 1979;43:1557–1561.
6. Levine MS, Caroline D, Thompson JJ et al. Adenocarcinoma of the esophagus: relationship to Barrett mucosa. Radiology 1984;150:304–309.
7. Wang HH, Antonioli DA, Goldman H. Comparative features of esophageal and gastric adenocarcinomas: recent changes in type and frequency. Hum Pathol 1986;17:482–487.
8. Hesketh PJ, Clapp W, Doos WG, Spechler SJ. The increasing frequency of adenocarcinoma of the esophagus. Cancer 1989;64:526–530.
9. Kalish RJ, Clancy PE, Orringer MB, Appelman HD. Clinical, epidemiologic, and morphologic comparison between adenocarcinomas arising in Barrett's esophageal mucosa and in the gastric cardia. Gastroenterology 1984;86:461–467.
10. Golematis B, Tzardis P, Hatzikostas P et al. Changing pattern of distribution of carcinoma of the stomach. Br J Surg 1990;77:63–64.
11. Yang PC, Davis S. Incidence of cancer of the esophagus in the US by histologic type. Cancer 1988;61:612–617.

What is the current status of investigations on the role of drugs and dietary changes?

L. Bernstein (Los Angeles)

The incidence rates for adenocarcinoma of the esophagus are rapidly rising, and it is likely that some environmental risk factors for these cancers are also increasing. Currently two major case-control studies are being conducted in the United States (US) to determine factors that may account for this changing incidence.

A collaborative study sponsored by the National Cancer Institute began data collection in April 1993 in three areas of the US (Connecticut and selected counties in New Jersey and Washington). It is expected that interviews will be completed with 234 patients with esophageal adenocarcinomas, 329 with adenocarcinomas of the gastric cardia, 269 with other stomach tumors and 255 with squamous cell tumors of the esophagus. An equal number of nondiseased control subjects will be interviewed.

Our study in Los Angeles County (which has more than 9 million residents) began data collection in February 1993. Interviews are expected to be completed with 151 patients newly diagnosed with esophageal adenocarcinoma, 258 with adenocarcinomas of the gastric cardia and 273 with other stomach tumors. Control subjects will be individually matched to the cases with regard to sex, race-ethnicity, age and neighborhood of residence with two controls matched to each of the esophageal adenocarcinoma cases.

Both studies are designed to evaluate and contrast possible risk factors for adeno-carcinomas of the esophagus and gastric cardia, as well as those occurring in the distal stomach. Potential risk factors being evaluated include the use of drugs for the treatment of conditions of the duodenum, stomach and esophagus, the existence of these conditions themselves, the use of other drugs, tobacco and alcohol consumption, dietary intake, other characteristics of food consumption and occupational exposures.

Histamine (H2) receptor antagonists (blockers)

H2-blockers have become widely used in the US since the late 1970s as a preferred treatment for duodenal and gastric ulcers, esophageal reflux and other benign conditions of the stomach, esophagus and duodenum. There are several mechanisms whereby H2-blockers might contribute to carcinogenesis of the gastric cardia and esophagus.

Under normal gastric conditions, when alkaline bile is refluxed through the pyloric sphincter into the gastric lumen, it is immediately neutralized by the normally low intragastric pH. In the presence of H2-blockers, however, gastric pH is elevated and neutralization does not occur. The resulting exposure of the mucosal surface of the gastric cardia and lower esophagus to alkaline duodenal refluxate may contribute to cancer development at these sites [1].

Use of H2-blockers may result in higher amounts of gastric colonization by nitrate-reducing bacteria, thereby increasing intragastric levels of carcinogenic nitrosamines. Furthermore, two H2-blockers, cimetidine and ranitidine, are themselves nitrosated under acidic conditions [2,3]. Cimetidine also influences cytochrome P450 enzymes that regulate the metabolism of drugs and other compounds and may inhibit the clearance of cytotoxic agents [4].

Antacids are widely used for gastrointestinal disorders, and may also lead to an alkaline pH in the stomach. It is not known whether these frequently used agents are related to development of gastroesophageal adenocarcinomas, but because they may also promote bacterial colonization of the stomach they are being investigated in the two studies.

The issues involved in assessing the risk associated with use of H2-blockers and other antacids is complex. Conditions for which these drugs may be prescribed are also potential risk factors for adenocarcinomas of the esophagus and gastric cardia. It is also possible that some users of these drugs had early gastric cancer when the drugs were prescribed. Because of this, detailed medical histories are being collected and radiological, endoscopic and surgical reports on all cases in our case-control study in Los Angeles are being reviewed.

Other drugs

Other drugs such as tetracycline, chlorpheniramine, chlorpromazine, tolazamide, cyclizine, ethambutol and chlordiazepoxide lower gastric acidity and, like H2-blockers, create conditions which may favor duodenal reflux to the gastric cardia and lower esophagus. Drugs that cause esophageal injury, "pill esophagitis" or gastritis may also play a role in the etiology of esophageal adenocarcinoma.

Nonsteroidal anti-inflammatory drugs (NSAID) including aspirin have been associated with benign esophageal stricture. They also act as irritants to the gastric mucosa. Increased cell division may occur during the process of repair of the damaged tissue resulting eventually in neoplastic transformation [5]. There is also some evidence that the continued use of NSAIDs impairs the healing of gastric ulcers by H2-blockers [6]. Although NSAIDs have not been previously evaluated as a gastric cancer risk factor, any effect on risk would be important as they are so frequently used to treat a wide variety of specific and nonspecific symptoms. Drugs that reduce lower esophageal sphincter pressure (LESP) including calcium-channel blockers, β adrenergic agonists, α adrenergic antagonists, anticholinergics, theophylline, diazepam, nitroglycerin and dopamine may be involved in the pathogenesis of esophageal adenocarcinoma. The degree to which this reduction in LESP promotes gastroesophageal reflux (GER) is unknown.

Associated medical conditions

Patients diagnosed with Barrett's esophagus have a high risk of esophageal adenocarcinoma. A number of medical conditions and symptoms, including a history of chronic reflux symptoms, esophagitis, hiatal hernia and duodenal ulcer have been reported in clinical series to be more prevalent among patients with adenocarcinomas of the esophagus and cardia than among patients with more distal gastric tumors or squamous cell carcinoma of the esophagus. Conditions associated with low gastric acidity, such as pernicious anemia and achlorhydria, have been associated with increased risk of gastric cancer.

Diet

A number of dietary factors are thought to be involved in the etiology of stomach cancer, particularly precursors of N-nitroso compounds, salt, fresh fruits and vegetables. The precursors of N-nitroso compounds that are most often investigated for stomach cancer derive from dietary sources [7,8]. Foods rich in nitrate or nitrite and their derivatives which can form N-nitroso compounds include bacon and other cured meats, fish, green vegetables and cooked proteins. Studies have suggested that a diet high in salt (which may act as an irritant to the stomach mucosa) increases the risk of gastric cancer. On the other hand, fresh vegetables and fruits, rich in vitamin C and allium vegetables, as well as wheat bran, which may act as a nitrite scavenger, may protect against stomach cancer by blocking production of nitrosamines.

Other characteristics of diet may also be important determinants of the risk for adenocarcinomas of the esophagus and cardia. These include meal size and frequency, consumption of foods that decrease LESP (fats, chocolate, alcohol, coffee, tea) and consumption of acidic foods (citric juices, tomato products).

Tobacco and alcohol

Cigarette smoking and alcohol abuse are known risk factors for squamous cell esophageal cancer [9] and both may cause esophagitis. Condensation products from tobacco smoke may have an irritant effect on the esophagus and gastric mucosa. Tobacco smoke also has a wide range of effects on gastrointestinal physiology which include slowing gastric emptying, altering acid secretion, inducing duodenogastric and GER and impairing the healing and increasing rates of recurrence of duodenal ulcer [10–13]. All of these conditions may in turn contribute to the risk of esophageal and cardia adenocarcinomas.

Tobacco smoke is another source of N-nitroso compounds. In fact, the levels of N-nitroso compounds in both mainstream and sidestream (second-hand) smoke may be hundreds of times greater than the concentrations in foods.

Occupation

Finally, because adenocarcinomas of the esophagus and gastric cardia occur significantly more frequent among men than among women, it is possible that occupational factors play a role. Some studies have suggested that the risk of stomach cancer is associated with exposure to dusty environments [14]. Two previous studies indicated that metal dust might play a role in the development of cancer of the cardia [15] and lower esophagus [16]. It is possible that these dusts serve as irritants to the gastric epithelium.

References

1. Attwood SEA, Smyrk TC, DeMeester TR et al. Duodenoesophageal reflux and the development of esophageal adenocarcinoma in rats. Surgery 1992;111:502–510.
2. Ichinotsubo D, MacKinnon EA, Liu C et al. Mutagenicity of nitrosated cimetidines. Carcinogenesis 1981;2:261–264.
3. De Flora S, Bennicelli C, Camoirano A et al. Genotoxicity of nitrosated ranitidine. Carcinogenesis 1983;4:255–260.
4. Alberts DS, Liddi NM, Plegia PM et al. Lack of ranitidine effects on cyclophosphamide bone marrow toxicity or metabolism: a placebo-controlled clinical trial. J Natl Cancer Inst 1991;83:1739–1743.
5. Preston-Martin S, Pike MC, Ross RK et al. Increased cell division as a cause of human cancer. Cancer Res 1990;50:7415–7421.
6. Walan A, Bader JP, Classen M et al. Effect of omeprazole and ranitidine on ulcer healing and relapse rates in patients with benign gastric ulcer. N Engl J Med 1989;320:69–75.
7. Mirvish SS. The etiology of gastric cancer: intragastric nitrosamide formation and other theories. J Natl Cancer Inst 1983;71:629–647.
8. Howson CP, Hirayama T, Wynder EL. The decline in gastric cancer: epidemiology of an unplanned triumph. Epidemiol Rev 1986;8:1–27.
9. International Agency for Research on Cancer. Monographs on the evaluation of the carcinogenic risk of chemicals to humans. Tobacco smoking. vol 38. Lyon, France: IARC, 1986.
10. Johnson RD, Horowitz M, Maddox AF et al. Cigarette smoking and rate of gastric emptying: effect on alcohol absorption. Br Med J 1991;302:20–23.
11. Murthy SNS, Dinoso VP, Clearfield HR, Chey WY. Simultaneous measurement of basal pancreatic, gastric acid secretion,

plasma gastrin and secretion during smoking. Gastroenterology 1977;73:758–761.

12. Muller-Lissner SA. Bile reflux is increased in cigarette smokers. Gastroenterology 1986;90:1205–1209.

13. McCarthy DM. Smoking ulcers — time to quit. N Engl J Med 1984;311;726–728.

14. Borss JDJ, Viadana E, Houten L. Occupational cancer in men exposed to dust and other environmental hazards. Arch Environ Health 1978;33:300–307.

15. Wu-Williams A, Yu MC, Mack TM. Life-style, workplace and stomach cancer by subsite in young men of Los Angeles County. Cancer Res 1990;50:2569–2576.

16. Yu MC, Garabrant DH, Peters JM, Mack TM. Tobacco, alcohol, diet, occupation and carcinoma of the esophagus. Cancer Res 1988;48;3843–3848.

Experimental columnar metaplasia in the canine esophagus has demonstrated columnar cells capable of producing morphological differences in mucin distribution

R.J.S. Thomas (Melbourne)

Columnar-epithelium lined esophagus (CLE) has been demonstrated to show changes in mucin histochemistry compared with the normal columnar epithelium of the gastroesophageal junction. Where intestinal metaplasia is seen in CLE, sulfur mucins have been demonstrated. There may be minimal amounts of sulfur mucins occasionally seen in cardiac glands of the normal gastroesophageal junction [1]. The significance of these mucin histochemistry changes is the indication of the true metaplastic change in CLE compared with normal gastric mucosa.

The question posed is directed towards the characteristics of experimentally-induced CLE in the canine model. If changes in mucin histochemistry can be demonstrated in this type of mucosa it reinforces the value of the experimental model as being reflective of the human CLE condition.

Review

The literature on experimental Barrett's esophagus as produced in the canine model is limited. Bremner et al. showed that after destruction of the lower esophageal mucosa, and in the presence of gastroesophageal reflux and gastric hypersecretion, re-epithelialization of the denuded segment of squamous epithelium by columnar mucus secreting cells took place. Destruction of the epithelium without induced reflux was followed by a return of squamous epithelium to the denuded area. They postulated that the columnar-lined epithelium arrived by "creeping substitution" from columnar cells of gastric or junctional origin [2].

Gillen et al., from Dr Hennessy's group, published an elegant study which confirmed the replacement of a denuded segment of lower esophageal mucosa with columnar epithelium in a situation where reflux was induced by a Wendel cardioplasty and acid reflux was augmented by the use of pentagastrin [3]. A group of animals also had a cholecystogastrostomy performed to induce bile reflux.

This group denuded a separate ring of mucosa in the esophagus which was isolated from the gastric cardia epithelium by a strip of squamous epithelium. This prevented "creeping substitution". Columnar epithelium grew in this situation where there was both reflux and acid present, with acid suppression or no reflux the defects healed by squamous epithelium alone.

They were able to demonstrate anatomically that re-epithelialization seemed to be occurring from the neck of glands where ulceration persisted.

They demonstrated regenerated columnar epithelium with occasional goblet and parietal cells, but *pseudo-absorptive cells*, seen in specialized intestinal-type Barrett's epithelium in man, were not seen. Periodic acid-Schiff and Alcian blue staining demonstrated morphological differences in the mucin distribution in the experimental epithelium and cardiac mucosa. Neutral mucin was present throughout the supra-nuclear region in experimental columnar epithelium, in contrast to the gastric epithelium where its distribution was in the apical portion of the cell.

Thus this study does show that experimentally-induced columnar epithelium regeneration has goblet cells with mucin production, but the mucin was situated in a different area of the cell compared with the normal gastric mucosa. It also demonstrated regenerating columnar epithelium from cells lining esophageal gland ducts.

Other workers have demonstrated that Barrett's mucosa can be induced by similar methods and squamous epithelium overgrowth will occur with endoscopic laser ablation of the CLE and inhibition of acid reflux.

Conclusion

The canine experimental models do demonstrate the development of CLE after esophageal mucosal injury in the situation where gastric hypersecretion and esophageal reflux are induced. Mucin histochemistry indicates that the cells being produced are morphologically and anatomically different than that seen in normal gastric mucosa. It has been demonstrated that regenerating columnar epithelium develops from the esophageal gland ducts [2]. It should be noted that in the dog there are very prominent esophageal glands lying in the submucosal setting.

It is postulated that the damage to the epithelium exposes stem cells in the esophageal gland ducts to luminal reflux. These cells may be multi-possessed and built to differentiate in a variety of ways, accounting for the different cell types and histological appearance seen in Barrett's epithelium in man.

The conclusion is that the demonstration of goblet cells, parietal cells and variations in mucin distribution in the canine model, supports the concept of the metaplastic nature of Barrett's epithelium in man, and its possible origin from the submucosal esophageal gland.

References

1. Peuchmaur M, Potet F, Goldfain D. Mucin histochemistry of the columnar epithelium of the oesophasus (Barrett's oesophagus): a prospective biopsy study. J Clin Pathol 1984;37:607–610.
2. Bremner CG, Lynch VP, Ellis FH. Barrett's esophagus: congenital or acquired? An experimental study of esophageal mucosal regeneration in the dog. Surgery 1970;68:209–216.
3. Gillen P, Keeling P, Byrne P, West A, Hennessy T. Experimental columnar metaplasia in the canine oesophasus. Br J Surg 1988;75:113–115.

Is there an animal model for CLE and esophageal adenocarcinoma?

T.C. Smyrk (Omaha)

An animal model for esophageal adenocarcinoma has been developed by Pera and Cardesa [1]. The authors used the nitrosamine 2,6-dimethylnitrosomorpholine (DMNM) in conjunction with esophagojejunostomy to produce adenocarcinoma in the esophagus of Sprague-Dawley rats. DMNM is known to produce squamous tumors of the rat esophagus. Pera and co-workers divided the gastroesophageal junction and performed an end-to-side esophagojejunostomy to produce chronic reflux esophagitis. These experimental conditions produced adenocarcinoma in 23 of the 62 animals. Rats exposed to carcinogen alone developed squamous papillomas and squamous carcinomas, but no adenocarcinomas.

Our initial work with the model confirmed and extended the results of Pera [2]. We added a gastroesophageal reflux group (by performing esophagogastroplasty) to the duodenoesophageal reflux group (esophagoduodenostomy) and nonoperated controls. Surgically induced duodenoesophageal reflux doubled the frequency of malignant tumors in carcinogen-treated rats compared to the gastroesophageal reflux group and nonoperated controls. Nine of the 26 (34%) animals in the esophago-duodenostomy plus carcinogen group developed adenocarcinoma; none of the animals with esophagogastroplasty or no operation had an adenocarcinoma. Surprisingly, one animal (of 14) subjected to duodenoesophageal anastomosis without exposure to DMNM also developed adenocarcinoma of the esophagus.

Clark et al. used the animal model to study the effect of diet on tumor production [3]. Among 111 rats given esophagoduodenostomy and nitrosamine, 63 (57%) developed carcinoma; 42% of the carcinomas were adenocarcinoma. The number of rats bearing tumors was higher in animals that had a high fat diet compared to rats on controlled diet, calorie restricted diet and chow diet. As in our study, one rat subjected to esophagoduodenostomy developed malignancy in the absence of exposure to carcinogen. In this case, the tumor was a squamous cell carcinoma.

Pera described areas of columnar metaplasia in 11 animals after esophagojejunostomy (seven in the noncarcinogen group and four in the carcinogen group). Recognizing columnar metaplasia is difficult in this model, since the esophagus is anastomosed to small intestinal epithelium and surgically induced scar makes the anastomosis irregular. In our first set of experiments, several animals appeared to have columnar lining of the esophagus, but we did not comment on the fact, because the diagnosis was equivocal. In Clark's study, a number of animals clearly had columnar epithelium above the esophagoduodenal anastomosis. Four of 39 (10%) animals given esophagoduodenostomy without carcinogen and 14 of 111 (13%) of animals with operation plus carcinogen had specialized columnar epithelium of the esophagus. There was no dysplastic change in the columnar epithelium.

In summary, the animal model of Pera and Cardesa provides an excellent setting in which to study adenocarcinoma of the distal esophagus. We believe that the same model also produces metaplastic columnar-lined esophagus. Two animals subjected to esophagoduodenostomy developed malignancy of the distal esophagus in the absence of exposure to carcinogen. If confirmed, this finding offers exciting possibilities for studying the pathogenesis of esophageal carcinoma.

References

1. Pera M, Cardesa A, Bombi JA et al. Influence of esophagojejunostomy on the induction of adenocarcinoma of the distal esophagus in Sprague-Dawley rats by subcutaneous injection of 2,6-dimethylnitrosomorpholine. Cancer Res 1989;49:6803.
2. Attwood SEA, Smyrk TC, DeMeester TR et al. Duodenoesophageal reflux and the development of esophageal adenocarcinoma in rats. Surgery 1992;111:502–510.
3. Clark GWD, Smyrk TC, Mirvish SS et al. The effect of gastroduodenal juice and dietary fat on the development of Barrett's esophagus and esophageal neoplasia: an experimental rat model. Ann Surg Oncol 1994;1:252–261.

Can any conclusion be drawn from increased expression of EGFR (epidermal growth factor receptor) in gastric and esophageal adenocarcinomas?

A. Yasui (Shizuoka)

Epidermal growth factor (EGF) is a polypeptide of 53 amino acids which is secreted from submaxillary glands, Brunner's glands in the duodenum, Paneth cells of the small intestine and other exocrine glands, including the pancreas. Epidermal growth factor receptor (EGFR) is a transmembrane glycoprotein with intrinsic tyrosine kinase activity. The esophageal squamous epithelium normally has 20,000–200,000 EGFR per cell. By binding to the receptor, EGF exerts protean actions (i.e., wound healing, cellular proliferation differentiation and oncogenesis) in the gastrointestinal tract. EGF also increases epithelial proliferation throughout the gastrointestinal tract and in other squamous epithelia, including the skin.

Since the v-erbB oncogene of the avian erythroblastosis virus has been reported to code a product homologous to a portion of the EGFR [1], the EGFR gene has been known as the c-erbB-1, a proto-oncogene related to the v-erbB oncogene. Amplification and overexpression of EGFR gene has been detected in human esophageal squamous cell carcinoma [2].

Yasui et al. [3] reported that EGF positive tumor cells were detected in 29% of 130 advanced gastric carcinomas, and EGFR immunoactivity was observed in 33%. A good correlation was demonstrated between the synchronous expression of EGF and EGFR and the tumor staging. The incidence of EGF positive cells was significantly higher in metastatic tumors than in primary tumors. Patients with a synchronous expression of EGF and EGFR had a far poorer prognosis than those without, which suggested that EGF and EGFR would be potential metastatic or prognostic markers for gastric carcinoma and play a role in tumor progression.

The direct measurement of EGFR in gastric carcinoma has been reported by several authors: Pfeiffer et al. [4] measured EGFR by (^{125}I) EGF-binding assays in 15 gastric carcinomas. A comparison of pairs of gastric mucosa and carcinomas showed an increase of EGFR in nine of 15 carcinomas (60%), no change in three and a decrease in two carcinomas. EGF activity was only increased in two of 22 carcinomas. These data were consistent with the immunohistochemical studies, in respect of a relative overexpression of EGFR in a fraction of gastric carcinomas, but do not support increased production of EGF by tumors. Another study [5] showed relatively higher affinity of EGFR in five of six gastric carcinoma cell lines, but the number of EGFR on these cell lines was smaller and had no correlation with their histologic types.

Recently, Jankowski et al. [6] studied 30 Barrett's esophagus specimens immunohistochemically, and showed that the "intestinal type" of Barrett's mucosa had the greatest expression of EGFR compared with other types of Barrett's metaplasia, and that adenocarcinomas in the Barrett's mucosa also overexpressed EGFR, compared with normal gastric mucosa. The same results were shown by flow-cytometric analysis, which was developed to assess the percentage of cells expressing EGFR [7].

Expression of EGFR was also demonstrated in normal small intestinal epithelium and intestinal metaplasia of the stomach [8]. Increased expression of EGFR may merely represent a regeneration after injury to the esophageal mucosa from gastroesophageal reflux. Overexpression of EGFR in intestinal metaplastic Barrett's epithelium may represent a nonneoplastic regenerative phenomenon, as seen at other sites within the gastrointestinal tract [9]. In gastric carcinoma higher levels of EGFR positive staining were also found in the intestinal type of carcinoma [10].

However, Jankowski's finding of overexpression of both ligand and receptor in a stepwise increase from fundic-type Barrett's mucosa through intestinal-type Barrett's mucosa to high dysplasia and Barrett's adenocarcinoma by both immunohisto-chemistry and flow-cytometric analysis, which is more quantitative than the former, may indicate that those changes of EGFR are not only regenerative, but proliferative as seen in oncogenic responses. In addition, they recently assessed the immunohisto-chemical expression of a number of oncogenes in both Barrett's metaplasia and Barrett's adenocarcinoma: 50% of Barrett's adenocarcinomas expressed identifiable p53 protein mutations, 80% of Barrett's metaplastic epithelium and all Barrett's adenocarcinomas overexpressed c-erbB-2 oncogene protein [11].

In conclusion, at the present time, the demonstration of EGF and EGFR in advanced gastric adenocarcinoma may have a prognostic as well as a diagnostic potential. In the esophageal mucosa, the detection of an increased expression of both EGF and EGFR may indicate a neoplastic change. Further investigation by measuring the receptor directly in both gastric and esophageal adenocarcinomas is necessary, and the study of gene mutation on EGFR gene [12] is also indicated to ascertain the mechanism of malignant change in Barrett's esophagus.

References

1. Ullrich A, Coussens L, Hayflick JS et al. Human epidermal growth factor and aberrant expression of the amplified gene in A431 epidermoid carcinoma cells. Nature 1984;309:418−425.
2. Hunts J, Ueda M, Ozawa S et al. Hyperproduction and gene amplification of epidermal growth factor receptor in squamous cell carcinomas. Jpn J Cancer Res 1985;76:663−666.
3. Yasui W, Hata J, Yokozaki H et al. Interaction between epidermal growth factor and its receptor in progression of human gastric carcinoma. Int J Cancer 1988;41:211−217.
4. Pfeiffer A, Rothbauer E, Wiebecke B et al. Increased epidermal growth factors in gastric carcinomas. Gastroenterology 1990;98:961−967.
5. Ochiai A, Takanashi A, Takeura N et al. Effect of human epidermal growth factor on cell growth and its receptor in human gastric carcinoma cell lines. Jpn J Oncol 1988;18:15−25.
6. Jankowski J, McMenemin R, Hopwood D et al. Abnormal expression of growth regulatory factors in Barrett's oesophagus. Clin Sci 1991;81:663−668.
7. Jankowski J, Hopwood D, Wormsley KG. Flow-cytometric analysis of growth regulatory peptides and their receptors in Barrett's oesophagus and oesophageal adenocarcinoma. Scand J Gastroenterol 1992;27:147−154.
8. Leimoine NR, Jain S, Silvestre F et al. Amplification and overexpression of EGF receptor and c-erbB-2 proto-oncogenes in human stomach cancer. Br J Cancer 1991;64:79−83.
9. Poller DN, Steel RJC, Morrell K. Epidermal growth factor receptor expression in Barrett's esophagus. Arch Pathol Lab Med 1992;116:1226−1227.
10. Nasim MM, Ahnen D, Thomas DM et al. Expression of transforming factor alpha, epidermal growth factor receptor and proliferating cell nuclear antigen in gastric carcinoma. Int J Oncol 1993;22:191−196.
11. Jankowski J. Flow-cytometric assessment of regulatory peptides in Barrett's mucosa. Gastroenterology 1992;103:1121.
12. Selva E, Raden DL, Davis RJ. Mitogen-activated protein kinase stimulation by a tyrosine kinase-negative epidermal growth factor receptor. J Biol Chem 1993;263:2250−2254.

Could the accumulation of free radicals explain the development of tumoral forms of Barrett's esophagus by their effect on nucleic acids?

M. Mathonnet, A. Gainant, P. Cubertafond (Limoges)

Characteristics of cancer arising from Barrett's esophagus

Barrett's esophagus results when squamous epithelium of the esophagus is replaced by columnar epithelium similar to that found in the stomach. It is most often a consequence of esophageal mucosal irritation from gastric acid that occurs during chronic gastroesophageal reflux. Since there is an associated risk of malignant degeneration, certain authors consider it a premalignant lesion. Indeed, when present, the risk of developing an adenocarcinoma is multiplied 30 to 125 times [1,2]. Malignant degeneration occurs in 10% of patients with Barrett's esophagus [2–5]. Metaplasia develops over a mean period of 1 year [6], after which the condition appears to be stationary. Next, dysplastic changes occur and progress from mild, moderate and severe dysplasia, to finally carcinoma [2,7–9]. Adenocarcinoma only develops from high-grade dysplasia [2,9]. The mean age of onset in patients with Barrett's esophagus and those who subsequently develop carcinoma is respectively 40 and 63 years. This implies that a mean interval of 20 years is required for carcinoma to develop from Barrett's esophagus [6]. When there is high-grade dysplasia, it develops in 2.6 to 4.5 years [9].

Dysplasia is characterized by architectural and cytologic alterations [1] which progress to frank carcinomatous changes, making it difficult to histologically differentiate severe dysplasia from carcinoma in situ.

A quantitative study of dysplastic cells using flow cytometry has revealed important abnormalities of DNA characterized by the presence of aneuploidy. The prevalence of aneuploidy, cell fractions with the G2 interval of the cell cycle, and the DNA synthetic (S) phase increase with the degree of dysplasia [3,10]. Genomic instability which results can give rise to a cancer cell [3]. A clonal cell population originates from a progenitor cell that has been genetically altered [11].

A qualitative study of DNA from aneuploid cell population of adenocarcinoma arising in Barrett's epithelium has frequently shown the loss of one allele from the short arm of chromosome 17, which is the site of gene p53, and increased expression of this protein [10,12].

Gene mutations are of clonal origin [3,12]. Clones of cancer cells arising in Barrett's epithelium are characterized by trisomy of chromosomes 5 and 7, structural rearrangement [t(3;6) (q21;p23)] and loss of the Y chromosome [3,13].

Among the factors responsible for carcinogenesis, free radicals play a preponderant role.

Free radicals

A free radical is a molecular fragment or atom whose outer orbit lacks an electron, or conversely, possesses excess electrons. It is highly reactive and unstable, with a very short half-life [14,15]. As soon as it is formed, it seeks out an electron in its environment with which it can pair up, thus creating new free radicals. Once initiated, this chain reaction is difficult to control and highly destructive [16]. Cell respiration, which produces energy in the form of ATP and water, is a natural source of free radicals: at normal oxygen concentration 95% of molecular oxygen undergoes tetravalent reduction during Kreb's cycle and reaction with cytochrome oxydases in microsomes; the remaining 5% of the molecular oxygen undergoes univalent reduction with the addition of one electron. This pathway, catalyzed by metal salts (iron, copper, nickel), leads to free radicals formation, superoxide anion radical, hydrogen peroxide and hydroxyl radicals [17]. Multiple biological oxidation reactions produce free radicals [18] (Table 1).

Under normal conditions, free radical production is quantitatively low and constantly inactivated by the natural defense systems that are present in the cell which also has the ability to enzymatically repair DNA damage caused by free radicals [18] (Table 2).

Many pathologic conditions lead to excessive free radical production that surpass the cell's natural defense mechanisms [16]. Inflammation causes a respiratory burst in polymorphonuclear leukocytes (PMNs), with an increase in oxygen consumption and the production of free radicals. An activated PMN produces 10^6 mol of superoxide anion radicals [19]. With chronic inflammation, a vicious cycle develops where superoxide anion radical production stimulates the catabolism of arachidonic acid which induces the production or the stimulation of chemotactic substances that attract phagocytic cells and destroy healthy cells [20,21]. In vivo, these phagocytic cells are activated by carcinogens, xenobiotics, ionizing radiation, the tar of cigarette smoke, pesticides such as paraquat, certain medications, antibiotics derived from quinones and chemotherapeutic agents [18]. Vitamin A or E deficiency, fatty acid metabolism, the induction of oxidizing enzymes or the inhibition of antioxidant

Table 1. Normal processes that produce free radicals [18]

1 — Normal cell respiration
2 — Metabolism of xenobiotics
    — microsomal electron transport by cytochromes p450 and b5
    — peroxidatic oxidation
3 — Activation of phagocytic cells by natural stimuli
    — peripheral blood PMNs, basophils and monocytes
    — tissue macrophages
    — Kupfer cells (liver)
    — Clara cells (lung)
4 — Biosynthetic and biodegrading processes
    — arachidonic acid and fatty acid metabolism
    — fatty acid CoA oxidases, urate oxidases, D-amino oxidases
    — tyrosine peroxidase

Table 2. Normal antioxidant and repair defenses [18]

1 — Antioxidant enzymes
      — superoxide dismutase
      — catalase
      — GSH peroxidase, GSH reductase, GSH-S-transferase
2 — Antioxidant proteins
      — ceruloplasmin
      — transferrin
      — lactoferrin
      — albumin
      — haptoglobin
3 — Antioxidant low molecular weight substances
      — GSH, NAD(P)H
      — ascorbate, urate
      — α-tocopherol, β-carotene
4 — DNA repair enzymes
      — glycosylases
      — endonucleases
      — poly(ADP)ribose transferase

enzymes are also a pathologic source of free radicals [18].

In tissue, undestroyed free radicals break down mucopolysaccharides and collagen in the extracellular space and oxidize polyunsaturated fatty acid in cell and mitochondrial membranes and intracellular enzymes and nucleic acids inside cells.

Action of free radicals on nucleic acids

Only hydrogen peroxide can cross nuclear membranes [18]. This molecule is stable when reduced metal ions are absent, however, it can destroy nucleic bases that have reducing agents (iron or copper ions). The effect of free radicals on nucleic acids has been demonstrated on isolated DNA, isolated cell and tissue.

In the presence of tumors promoters (TPA [12-O-tetradecanoyl-phorbol-13-acetate], benzo(a)pyrene, chromium, nickel, cigarette tar), human PMN or macrophage DNA undergoes breakage, causing hereditary genetic abnormalities [22]. These tumor promoters have both a direct and indirect effect on DNA that is time- and dose-dependent [18]. In vivo, after introduction of a tumor promoter, the cell's inflammatory response induced free-radical production and oxidation of DNA bases. Cell regeneration incorporated the DNA abnormalities, causing genetic mutations. An agent's carcinogenic effect depends on its ability to activate circulating leukocytes and stimulate free radical production by epidermal cells, and not the ability of leukocytes to infiltrate the dermis.

The use of antioxidant substances decreases the level of peroxides and the carcinogenicity of tumor promoters [18].

In man, the nucleic acid oxidation is demonstrated in leukocytes in women at high risk for breast cancer [23], in cells from intraductal breast carcinomas [18] and in patients with systemic lupus erythematous [18].

The carcinogenic effect of free radicals

Free radicals play an active role in the three stages of carcinogenesis: during initiation, they act as a carcinogenic agent, inducing genetic mutations in DNA bases; during promotion the genetic mutation becomes transmissible, a clone of cells appears; during propagation the cancer appears followed by metastatic spread [18].

Free radicals are mutagenic. They cleave DNA, oxidize nucleic acids and are a source of translocations (t16:18) with abnormal karyotypes in chromosomes 13 and 22 [24]. The expression of genes that are normally involved in growth and cell differentiation (expression that is rapid and transitory) is enhanced by free radicals [18].

The carcinogenic effect of free radicals has been demonstrated in patients with the immunodeficiency syndrome, acute or chronic myeloid leukemia, and other cancers [18].

Free radicals and Barrett's esophagus

At the present time, due to the rarity of Barrett's esophagus and the difficulty dosing nucleic acids, it has not been possible to demonstrate that free radicals are implicated in the development of carcinoma from Barrett's esophagus. Indirect evidence of free radical involvement, however, is found in all stages: DNA cleavage, gene mutations and prolongation of the G2 phase of DNA repair are found in cells of adenocarcinoma; these changes are found to a lesser degree in the dysplastic cells of Barrett's esophagus. Free radicals produced by PMNs continually activated by chronic esophageal reflux, probably represent a cause of malignant degeneration.

Although the dosage of free radicals remains problematic, improvement of new methods to detect nucleic acids and their derivatives [25] will open new perspectives in the prognosis and treatment of Barrett's esophagus.

References

1. Streitz JM, Williamson WA, Ellis FH. Current concepts concerning the nature and treatment of Barrett's esophagus and complications. Ann Thorac Surg 1992;54:586–591.
2. Haggitt RC. Adenocarcinoma in Barrett's esophagus: a new epidemic?. Hum Pathol 1992;23:475–476.
3. Reid BJ. Barrett's esophagus and esophageal adenocarcinoma. Gastroenterol Clin North Am 1991;20:817–834.
4. Michel CH, Launoy G, Maurel J, Auvray S, Segol Ph, Gignoux M. Adénocarcinomes sur endobrachyoesophage. J Chir (Paris) 1992;129:187–190.
5. Garewal HS, Sampliner RE. Barrett's esophagus: a model premalignant lesion for adenocarcinoma. Prev Med 1989;8: 749–756.
6. Cameron AJ, Lomboy CT. Barrett's esophagus: age, prevalence, and extent of columnar epithelium. Gastroenterology 1992; 103:1241–1245.
7. Wang HH, Ducatman BS, Thibault S. Cytologic features of premalignant glandular lesions in the upper gastrointestinal tract. Acta Cytol 1991;35:199–203.
8. Jaskiewicz K. Oesophageal carcinoma: cytopathology and nutritional aspects in aetiology. Anticancer Res 1989;9:1847–1852.
9. Miros M, Kerlin P, Walker N. Only patients with dysplasia progress to adecarcinoma in Barrett's oesophagus. Gut 1991; 32:1441–1446.
10. Robasziewicz M, Volant A, Hardy E, Nousbaum LB, Calament G, Cauvin M et al. Mise en évidence d'une hétérogénéité clonale au niveau des adénocarcinomes sur endobrachyoesophage par l'etude cytofluorométrique du contenu cellulaire en ADN. Gastroenterol Clin Biol 1992;16:540–546.
11. Nowell PC. Mechanisms of tumor progression. Cancer Res 1986;46:2303–2307.

12. Casson AG, Mukhopadhyay T, Cleary KR, Ro JY, Levin B, Roth JA. p53 gene mutations in Barrett's epithelium and esophageal cancer. Cancer Res 1991;51:4495—4499.
13. Garewal HS, Sampliner RE, Liu Y, Trent JM. Chromosomal rearrangements in Barrett's esophagus a premalignant lesion in esophageal adenocarcinoma. Cancer Genet 1989;42:281—286.
14. Sava P, Blondeau C, Cubertafond P, Magnin P. Radicaux libres et pathologie digestive. Gastroenterol Clin Biol 1988;12: 1—8.
15. Maquart FX. Biochimie dynamique. Maloine, Paris, 1987.
16. Emerit J, Michelson AM. Les radicaux libres en médecine et biologie. Sem Hôp Paris 1982;45:2670—2675.
17. Menashe P, Grousset C, Gauduel Y, Mouas C, Piwnica A. Les piégeurs de radicaux libres dans la protection myocardique en chirurgie cardiaque. Ann Cardiol Angéiol 1986;35(no. 7 bis):447—452.
18. Frenkel K. Carcinogen-mediated oxidant formation and oxidative DNA damage. Pharmacol Ther 1992;53:127—166.
19. Segal AW, Allison AC. Oxygen consumption by stimulated human neutrophils in oxygen free radicals and tissue damage. Ciba Foundation Symposium 1979;65:205—225.
20. Maccord JM. Superoxide and inflammation: a mechanism for the anti-inflammatory activity of superoxide dismutase. Acta Physiol Scand 1980;(suppl 492):25.
21. Delmaestro RF, Thaw HH. Free radicals as mediators of tissue injury. Acta Physiol Scand 1980;(suppl 492):43—57.
22. Birnboim HC. Factors which affect DNA strand breakage in human leukocytes exposed to a tumor promoter phoroblamyristate acetate. Can J Physiol Pharmacol 1982;60:1359—1366.
23. Correa P. Epidemiological correlation between diet and cancer frequency. Cancer Res 1981;41:3685—3689.
24. Weitberg AB, Corvese D. Translocation of chromosome 16 and 18 in oxygen radical transformed human fibroblasts. Biochem Biophys Res Commun 1990;169:70—74.
25. Cadet J, Anselmino C, Douky T, Voituriez L. Photochemistry of nucleic acids in cells. J Photochem Photobiol B Biol 1992;15:277—298.

Does the presence of LIMA (large intestine mucin antigen) or SIMA (small intestine mucin antigen) and acid mucins suggest that adenocarcinomas with or without CLE arise from a common cell type?

R.J.S. Thomas (Melbourne)

This question is directed towards the problem of the cell of origin of adenocarcinomas in the lower esophagus and cardia. The relationship between adenocarcinoma of the gastric cardia (GC) and of columnar lined esophagus (CLE) is unclear. If all adenocarcinomas from this region arise from a common cell type, it might be expected that the clinical features of the patients and the biological features of the tumors would be similar. Characteristically, CLE contains different cell types, depending on the histological pattern present.

Mucin glycoproteins are potential markers of differentiation. Classified by histochemical means, they divide into neutral mucins and acid mucins, with acid mucins being further subdivided into sialo mucins and sulphur mucins. The distribution of mucins within the normal gastrointestinal tract shows a characteristic pattern with specific mucins being present in particular areas of the gastrointestinal tract [1]. Many other mucins can be defined by the reduction of monoclonal antibodies to extracts of gastrointestinal mucosal tissue or tumors. Two such mucin antigens have been defined as LIMA (large intestine mucin antigen) and SIMA (small intestine mucin antigen) [2]. Mucins are heterogenous, for example, cell lines give rise to specific mucins and up to six variances of LIMA have been demonstrated [3]. These variances are site specific and changes can be demonstrated with inflammation in the region of benign tumors and cancers, and they can be used as an indicator of a change in epithelium.

In a study designed to address the question posed above, mucin characteristics were used in an attempt to define the type of cells present in the adenocarcinoma. This study was carried out by comparing the expressions of mucins and adenocarcinomas arising in CLE with those arising at the gastric cardia, and then to determine if these tumors exhibited a similar heterogeneity of mucin expression. Clinicopathological features and survival were also compared [4].

The comparison of the clinical features revealed no difference between the two tumors, that is, carcinoma arising in Barrett's esophagus (n = 12) and carcinoma arising at the gastric cardia (n = 55). The median age, sex, presence of a smoking history and resectability were not significantly different between the two groups (Mann-Witney test).

The pathological features including tumor size, positivity of node and the degree of differentiation of the tumor were also not significantly different between the two groups.

Examination of the tissue histochemistry revealed that neutral mucins, acid mucins, SIMA and LIMA were all expressed in equal amounts in both groups of tumors. In general, SIMA was only expressed in half the tumors and almost all tumors expressed LIMA, acid and neutral mucins.

The appearance of LIMA, SIMA and acid mucins in both groups suggested that these tumors arise from a common cell type and the heterogeneity in mucin production within the tumors suggests that this cell may in fact be a multipotential stem cell capable of producing malignant cells of different phenotypes. It should be noted that acid mucins, SIMA and LIMA are uncommon in normal esophagogastric mucosa. Once neoplasia has developed, all three of these mucins are often present.

Conclusions

Thus the answer to the question posed is that, on the basis of the histochemistry of the mucin expression in the tumors present, it is possible that there is a common cell type origin of adenocarcinomas arising from the gastric cardia or from CLE.

References

1. Filipe MI. Mucins in the human gastrointestinal epithelium: a review. Invest Cell Pathol 1979;2:195–216.
2. Ma J, De Boer W, Nayman J. Intestinal mucinous substances in gastric intestinal metaplasia and carcinoma studied by immunofluorescence. Cancer 1982;49:1664–1667.

3. Pilbrow SJ, Hartzog PJ, Pinczower GD, Linnane AW. Expression of large intestinal mucin antigen (LIMA) epitopes in the normal and neoplastic gastrointestinal tract. J Pathol 1993;169:361–373.
4. Gregory P, Bhathal P, Abbott M, Thomas R, Morstyn G. Clinical and pathologic similarity between adenocarcinoma of Barrett's esophagus and gastric cardia. Diseases of the Esophagus 1989;II(3):191–195.

How can the incidence of carcinoma in Barrett's esophagus be satisfactorily assessed?
— What are the shortcomings of the different incidence studies?

S.J. Spechler (Boston)

The incidence of cancer in a population is estimated by identifying a group of cancer-free individuals, and then following those individuals to observe the frequency of cancer development in a specified period of time. Studies which have provided data on the incidence of adenocarcinoma in Barrett's esophagus are summarized in Table 1 [1–8]. All of these studies suffer from one or more deficiencies which might affect the accuracy of the estimates on cancer incidence.

All of these studies are primarily retrospective analyses in which cancer incidence was estimated by reviewing the records of patients who had no adenocarcinoma noted on initial endoscopic examination. Ideally, incidence data should be collected prospectively using standardized protocols for identifying cancer in the study subjects.

The definition of Barrett's esophagus varied among studies and usually required an arbitrary extent of columnar epithelium in the distal esophagus to establish the diagnosis (e.g., ≥3 cm). Patients with short-segment Barrett's esophagus were often excluded by this criterion and therefore little is known about the cancer risk for patients with short segments of columnar epithelium lining the distal esophagus.

Table 1. Incidence of adenocarcinoma in Barrett's esophagus

Reference	Total patients	Cancers developed	Follow-up (patient-years)	Cancers per patient-years
Hameeteman [1]	50	5	260	1/52
Ovaska [2]	32	3	166	1/55
Robertson [3]	56	3	168	1/56
Williamson [4]	176	5	497	1/99
Achkar [5]	62	1	166	1/166
Van der Veen [6]	166	4	681	1/170
Spechler [7]	105	2	350	1/175
Cameron [8]	104	2	882	1/441

Furthermore, some studies did not require the presence of specialized columnar epithelium, the epithelial type most often associated with adenocarcinoma. The inclusion of many patients without specialized columnar epithelium could result in underestimation of the true cancer incidence rate for Barrett's esophagus.

Finally, the total number of patients included in these studies was relatively small, as was the duration of follow-up. Consequently, few patients in any study developed esophageal cancer. These features have profound effects on the estimate of cancer incidence. In the study by Achkar et al., for example, if two patients had developed cancer instead of only one, then the estimate of cancer incidence would have changed from one cancer per 166 patient years, to one cancer per 88 patient years.

To eliminate these shortcomings, future studies on cancer incidence in Barrett's esophagus ideally should be large, long-term, prospective investigations which utilize clearly-defined diagnostic criteria and endoscopic biopsy protocols.

References

1. Hameeteman W, Tytgat GNJ, Houthoff HJ, Van den Tweel JG. Barrett's esophagus: development of dysplasia and adenocarcinoma. Gastroenterology 1989;96:1249–1256.
2. Ovasaka J, Miettinen M, Kivilaakso E. Adenocarcinoma arising in Barrett's esophagus. Dig Dis Sci 1989;34:1336–1339.
3. Robertson CS, Mayberry JF, Nicholson DA, James PD, Atkinson M. Value of endoscopic surveillance in the detection of neoplastic change in Barrett's oesophagus. Br J Surg 1988;75:760–763.
4. Williamson WA, Ellis FH Jr, Gibb SP, Shahian DM, Aretz HT, Heatley GJ, Watkins E Jr. Barrett's esophagus: prevalence and incidence of adenocarcinoma. Arch Int Med 1991;151:2212–2216.
5. Achkar E, Carey W. The cost of surveillance for adenocarcinoma complicating Barrett's esophagus. Am J Gastroenterol 1988;83:291–294.
6. Van der Veen AH, Dees J, Blankenstein JD, Van Blankenstein M. Adenocarcinoma in Barrett's oesophagus: an overrated risk. Gut 1989;30:14–18.
7. Spechler SJ, Robbins AH, Rubins HB, Vincent ME, Heeren T, Doos WG, Colton T, Schimmel EM. Adenocarcinoma and Barrett's esophagus. An overrated risk? Gastroenterology 1984;87:927–933.
8. Cameron AJ, Ott BJ, Payne WS. The incidence of adenocarcinoma in the columnar-lined (Barrett's) esophagus. N Engl J Med 1985;313:857–859.

What are the radiologic appearances of Barrett's carcinoma?

M.S. Levine (Philadelphia)

Despite its frequency, Barrett's esophagus would not be important if it were a benign entity. However, there is considerable evidence that it is a premalignant condition associated with a significantly increased risk of developing esophageal adenocarcinoma. It is widely believed that adenocarcinoma evolves through a sequence of progressively severe epithelial dysplasia, eventually leading to the development of invasive carcinoma [3,7,8]. In various studies, the prevalence of adenocarcinoma in patients with Barrett's esophagus has ranged from 2.4—46.5%, with an overall prevalence of about 15%. Prevalence data may exaggerate the risk of cancer, as most patients with Barrett's esophagus do not seek medical attention until they develop complications such as ulcers, strictures or malignancy. Nevertheless, prospective studies have found that the annual incidence of malignant transformation in Barrett's esophagus is 1—2% and that the overall risk of developing esophageal adenocarcinoma may be 125 times greater than that in the general population [2]. Thus, most investigators accept the need for routine endoscopic surveillance of patients with known Barrett's esophagus.

Like squamous cell carcinoma of the esophagus, most adenocarcinomas diagnosed radiographically are advanced lesions with an extremely poor 5-year survival. Although most patients with early adenocarcinomas in Barrett's esophagus are asymptomatic, some may have melena, guaiac-positive stool, or iron-deficiency anemia due to low-grade bleeding from the friable surface of the tumor. Other patients may seek medical attention because of their underlying gastroesophageal reflux disease (GERD), so that these lesions may be detected fortuitously in patients with reflux symptoms. Finally, early adenocarcinomas may be discovered on routine surveillance of asymptomatic patients with known Barrett's esophagus.

Frequency

Primary adenocarcinoma of the esophagus has traditionally been considered a rare lesion, accounting for only 1—4% of all esophageal cancers. As most adenocarcinomas in the esophagus involve the gastroesophageal junction or proximal portion of the stomach, they have been generally classified as primary gastric carcinomas secondarily invading the lower end of the esophagus. However, it has been well documented that esophageal adenocarcinomas may spread distally to involve the gastric cardia or fundus. Virtually all of these tumors have been found to arise on a background of Barrett's mucosa in the esophagus. When these cases are included, adenocarcinoma comprises 5—20% of all esophageal cancers [1,5,6]. Nevertheless, many questions remain about the risk of malignant degeneration in Barrett's esophagus and the appropriate long term management of patients with this condition.

Radiographic findings

Early adenocarcinoma

Like squamous cell carcinomas, early adenocarcinomas in Barrett's esophagus may appear radiographically as plaque-like lesions or as flat, sessile polyps [6]. Sessile or pedunculated polyps in the distal esophagus may also represent adenomatous polyps in Barrett's mucosa with or without foci of invasive carcinoma. In patients with peptic strictures, the earliest manifestation of a developing adenocarcinoma may be a localized area of flattening or stiffening in one wall of the stricture (Fig. 1) [6]. Other patients may have superficial spreading cancers with diffuse nodularity of the

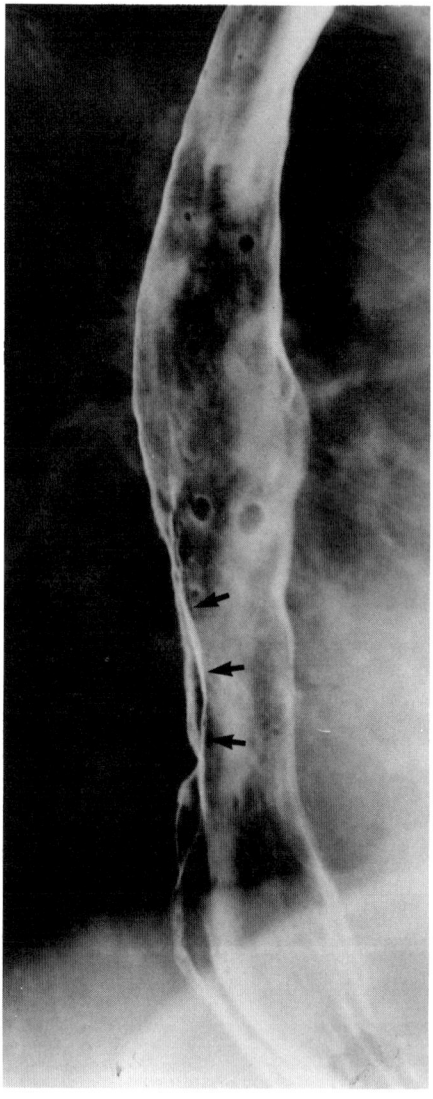 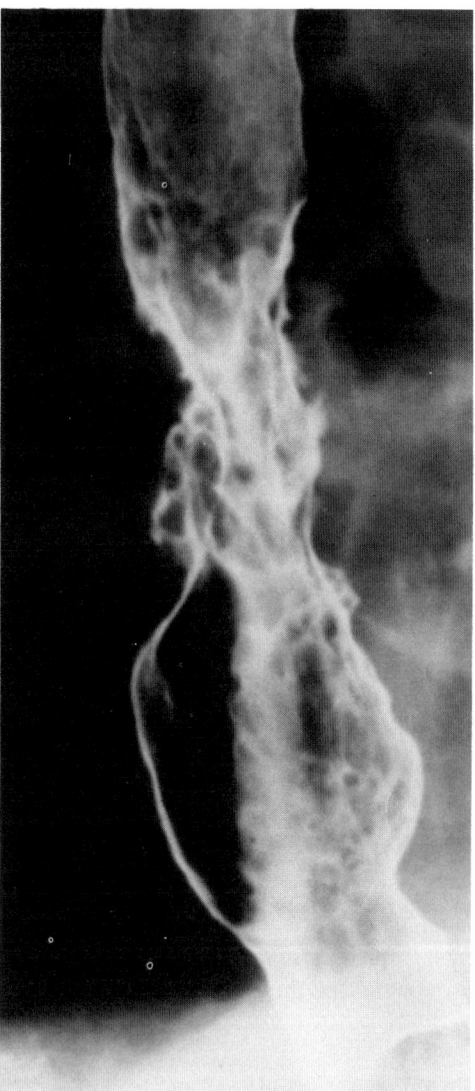

Fig. 1. Early adenocarcinoma in Barrett's esophagus. A relatively long peptic stricture is seen in the distal esophagus, with slight flattening and irregularity of one wall of the stricture (arrows). At surgery this patient was found to have an early adenocarcinoma arising in Barrett's mucosa. (The rounded filling defects are air bubbles.)

Fig. 2. Infiltrating adenocarcinoma in Barrett's esophagus. An advanced carcinoma is present in the distal esophagus. Note how the lesion causes irregular luminal narrowing with mucosal ulceration and relatively abrupt proximal and distal borders.

mucosa, but no focal lesion. Although early cancers are classically small lesions, some patients with early adenocarcinomas may have relatively large polypoid masses that are indistinguishable radiographically from advanced esophageal carcinomas.

Most early adenocarcinomas in Barrett's esophagus reported in the radiologic literature have been discovered fortuitously during radiologic evaluation of patients with reflux symptoms. However, asymptomatic lesions could also be detected by radiologic surveillance of patients with known Barrett's esophagus. In my opinion, an optimal screening program for these patients might therefore alternate double contrast esophagography and endoscopy at 6-month intervals in the hope of detecting malignant change in Barrett's esophagus at the earliest possible stage.

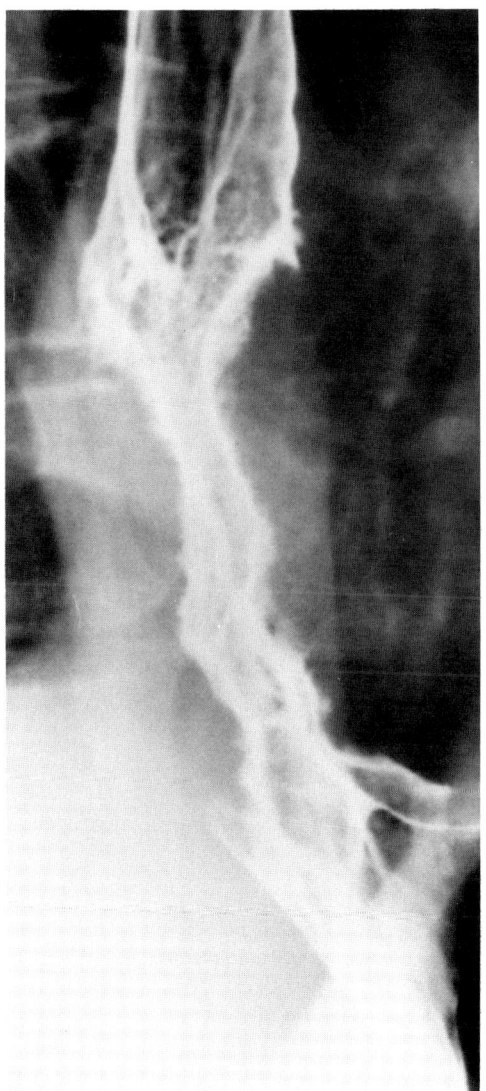

Fig. 3. Infiltrating adenocarcinoma in Barrett's esophagus. This lesion is causing marked luminal narrowing and involves a long vertical segment of the esophagus. Long, infiltrating lesions in the distal esophagus are often found to be adenocarcinomas.

Advanced adenocarcinoma

Advanced esophageal adenocarcinomas usually appear radiographically as infiltrating lesions with irregular luminal narrowing, nodularity or ulceration of the mucosa and abrupt, asymmetric borders (Fig. 2) [1,5,6]. In general, these lesions cannot be distinguished radiographically from squamous cell carcinomas. However, esophageal adenocarcinomas tend to involve a longer vertical segment of the esophagus than squamous cell carcinomas, so that the presence of an unusually long, infiltrating

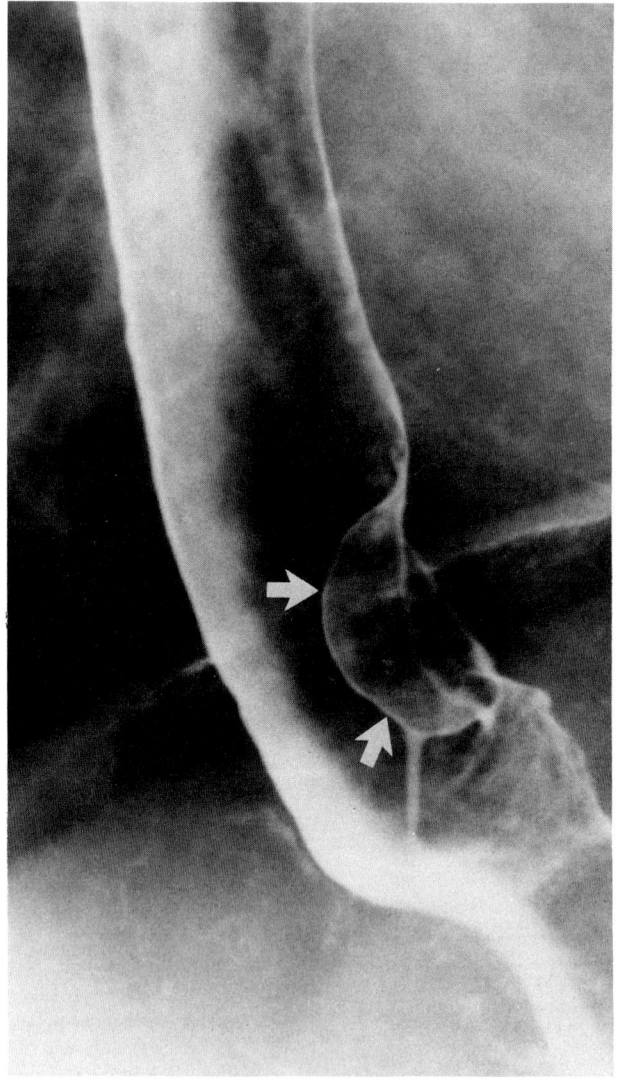

Fig. 4. Polypoid adenocarcinoma in Barrett's esophagus. A discrete polypoid mass (arrows) is present in the distal esophagus.

lesion should suggest the possibility of adenocarcinoma (Fig. 3) [1].

Less frequently, these tumors may appear as polypoid intraluminal masses (Fig. 4) or as primary ulcerative lesions with a meniscoid ulcer surrounded by a narrow ridge of tumor (Fig. 5). Occasionally, these lesions may have a varicoid appearance due to submucosal spread of the tumor (Fig. 6). Similar findings may be present in patients with squamous cell carcinomas. However, many patients with adenocarcinomas arising in Barrett's esophagus have associated hiatal hernias or gastroesophageal reflux. They may also have reflux esophagitis, a mid or distal esophageal stricture or a reticular pattern of the mucosa. Thus, the possibility of adenocarcinoma should be

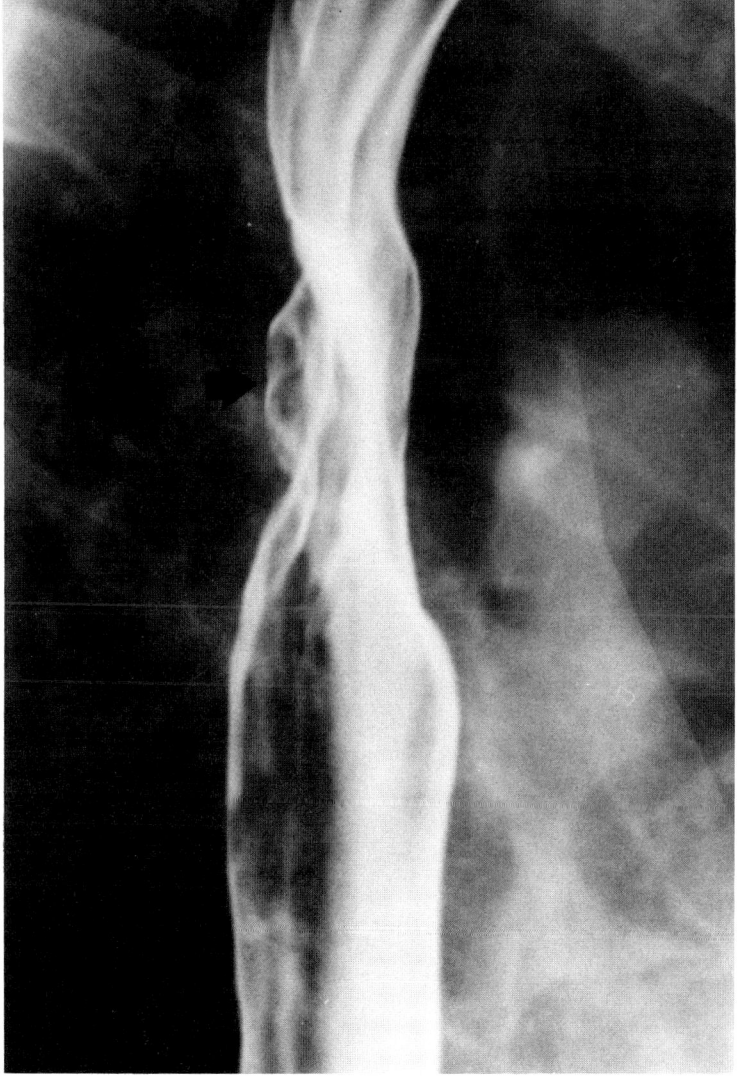

Fig. 5. Ulcerative adenocarcinoma in Barrett's esophagus. A relatively flat, meniscoid ulcer (arrow) is present in the midesophagus with an adjacent rim of tumor.

considered in any patient with esophageal cancer who has other clinical or radiologic signs of GERD.

When adenocarcinomas are located in the distal esophagus, they have a marked tendency to invade the gastric cardia or fundus [6]. Gastric involvement may be manifested radiographically by a polypoid or ulcerated mass in the fundus. In other patients, these tumors may cause obliteration of the normal anatomic landmarks at the cardia and irregular areas of ulceration without a discrete mass. The findings may be quite subtle, so that optimal double contrast views of the gastric cardia and fundus are required to demonstrate these lesions. In general, esophageal adenocarcinomas invading the gastric cardia or fundus cannot be distinguished radiographically from carcinomas of the cardia or fundus invading the distal esophagus [4]. However,

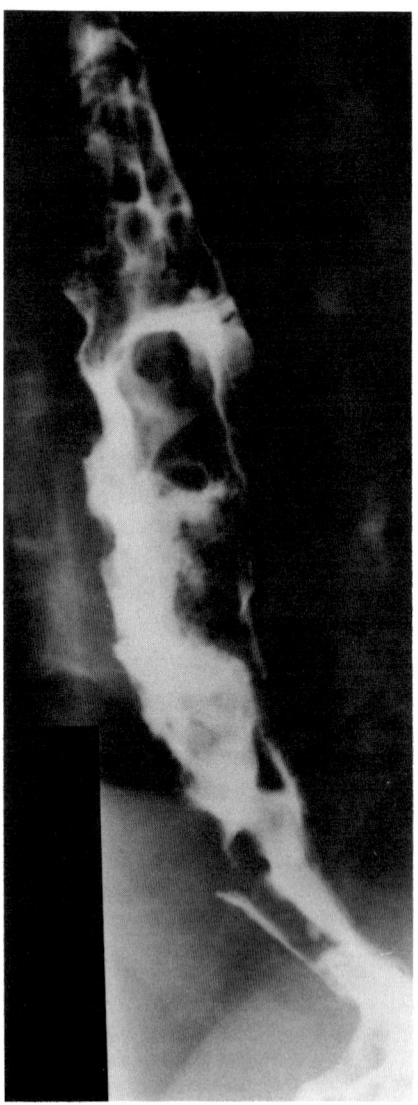

Fig. 6. Varicoid adenocarcinoma in Barrett's esophagus. Large submucosal defects are present in the distal third of the esophagus, resembling varices. This appearance results from submucosal spread of tumor.

esophageal adenocarcinomas usually have a greater degree of esophageal involvement in relation to that of the stomach, whereas gastric or cardiac carcinomas have a greater degree of fundal involvement. A significant history of GERD should also suggest the correct diagnosis.

References

1. Agha FP. Barrett carcinoma of the esophagus: clinical and radiographic analysis of 34 cases. AJR 1985;145:41–46.
2. Cameron AJ, Ott BJ, Payne WS. The incidence of adenocarcinoma in the columnar-lined (Barrett's) esophagus. N Engl J Med 1985;313:857–859.
3. Hameeteman W, Tytgat GNJ, Houthoff HJ et al. Barrett's esophagus: development of dysplasia and adenocarcinoma. Gastroenterology 1989;96:1249–1256.
4. Kalish RJ, Clancy PE, Orringer MB et al. Clinical, epidemiologic, and morphologic comparison between adenocarcinomas arising in Barrett's esophageal mucosa and in the gastric cardia. Gastroenterology 1984;86:461–467.
5. Keen SJ, Dodd GD, Smith JL. Adenocarcinoma arising in Barrett's esophagus: pathologic and radiologic features. Mt Sinai J Med 1984;51:442–450.
6. Levine MS, Caroline D, Thompson JJ et al. Adenocarcinoma of the esophagus: relationship to Barrett's mucosa. Radiology 1984;150:305–309.
7. Spechler SJ, Goyal RK. Barrett's esophagus. N Engl J Med 1986;315:362–371.
8. Thompson JJ, Zinsser KR, Enterline HT. Barrett's metaplasia and adenocarcinoma of the esophagus and gastroesophageal junction. Hum Pathol 1983;14:42–61.

What is the endoscopic aspect of early Barrett's cancer?

G.N.J. Tytgat (Netherlands)

Columnar metaplasia is the single most important risk factor for esophageal adenocarcinoma [1]. Genuine dysplasia represents a neoplastic alteration of the columnar epithelium and is widely regarded as the precursor of invasive malignancy [2]. In patients found to have high-grade dysplasia with no apparent tumor mass on endoscopy, approximately one third already has invasive cancer [3]. Endoscopic surveillance for carcinoma in columnar metaplasia is performed largely to discover dysplasia with the rationale that resection of the dysplastic epithelium may prevent the progression to incurable disease or to discover malignancy at an early curable stage [4].

A columnar-lined esophagus is generally recognized as a precancerous condition. The annual incidence of adenocarcinoma in patients who develop malignancy after the columnar-lined esophagus has been diagnosed varies from 1 in 152–441 patient years, which is a 30–40-fold increased risk as compared with the general population [2,5–9]. About half of the malignancies discovered in the surveillance studies recognized at a stage of early or superficial cancer.

Moreover, half of these malignancies are almost invisible endoscopically and are only discovered through routine endoscopic biopsies. Most important in all surveillance studies is the discovery of severe dysplasia as a precancerous marker of malignant degeneration. Besides random biopsies endoscopists should pay special attention to tiny areas with a rough appearance or surface unevenness, areas of discoloration, areas of slight elevation and any mucosal erosive or ulcerative defect [10]. High-grade dysplasia is so frequently associated with adenocarcinoma that its detection in a biopsy specimen makes repeat endoscopy with multiple biopsies mandatory to rule out a coexisting carcinoma. A sequence from mild- or low-grade dysplasia to severe- or high-grade dysplasia with progression to carcinoma has been demonstrated in sequential biopsies [11].

Endoscopic detection of dysplasia

The endoscopic identification of dysplasia may be problematic. Occasionally, dysplastic areas may be visible as whitish plaques, although most often such plaques consist of innocent-looking areas of mucosal thickening. Occasionally, dysplasia may be discovered in areas that appear inflamed or disclose increased vascularity. Dysplasia may also be present in areas that appear as shallow depressions of the mucosal surface or as slight villiform elevations. In general, however, no peculiar endoscopic features permit a distinction between dysplastic and nondysplastic mucosa as the mucosa has an innocuous appearance. Whether in vivo staining with toluidine blue is truly helpful clinically in detecting areas of severe dysplasia suitable for targeted biopsy, is questionable [11].

Definition of early superficial malignancy

There are several definitions of "early" esophageal malignancy in the literature. Most commonly early malignancy is defined as a cancer that is confined to the mucosa and submucosa, with no evidence of lymph node metastasis. Others accept the presence of lymph node metastasis [12].

Endoscopic appearance of early malignancy

In line with the Japanese tradition, early or superficial esophageal malignancy is subdivided in three main macroscopic subtypes according to the difference in height in relation to the noncancerous epithelial surface adjacent to the tumor:

type I   elevated or protruded type (high ≥ 3 mm in height; low ≤ 3 mm in height);
type II   superficial flat type;
type III   depressed or excavated type.

Their gross appearance is schematically illustrated in Fig. 1 [12]. A common appearance of early cancer is that of a circumscribed polypoid or protruded lesion.

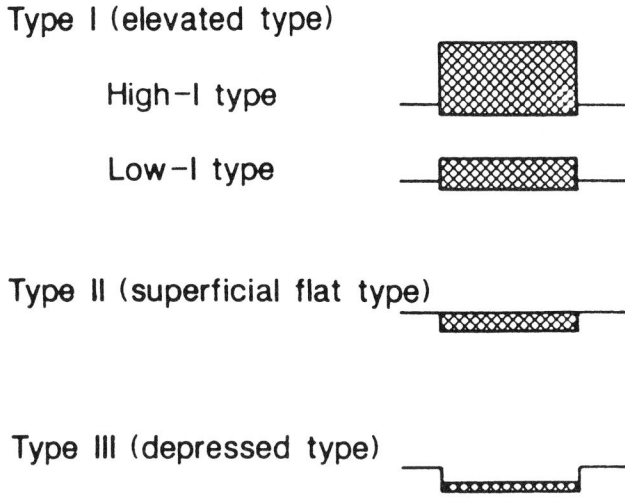

Type I (elevated type)

High-I type

Low-I type

Type II (superficial flat type)

Type III (depressed type)

Fig. 1. Gross classification of early Barrett's carcinoma [12].

Furthermore, early malignancy may appear as a plaque-like lesion in which the cancerous area appears slightly elevated with a granular coarse nobby surface. The cancerous area may also appear as a slightly depressed area with grey erosive spots against a reddish background. Occasionally, early malignancy presents as an innocent-looking "Barrett-type" ulcer. The columnar epithelium surrounding the ulcer may be "heaped up" and somewhat polypoid, but this is not always so.

Early Barrett cancer may also be presented as a combination of roughened wart-like thickening with superimposed irregular ulceration. Not uncommonly, the only visible abnormality is either a circumscribed area of altered pliability, or a circumscribed patch of mucosal discoloration. Early cancer is called occult when almost no endoscopic abnormalities are visible.

It is essential that multiple biopsies be taken at various levels within the columnar segment to establish the spread of the malignancy. If only severe dysplasia is found, biopsies should be repeated, as severe dysplasia is often associated with (early) malignancy [2,13,14].

Concluding remarks

There is still a controversy with respect to the diagnosis of early adenocarcinoma in esophageal columnar metaplasia. Theoretically early cancer should be defined as a T1 (Tis) cancer, with maximum depth of involvement into the submucosa with or without lymph node metastasis. The main problem for esophageal cancer relates to the fact that lymph node metastasis is common in case of submucosal invasion, but rare in case of intraepithelial or mucosal cancer. Some investigators therefore feel that early esophageal cancer should be limited to the mucosa. Again, it would be desirable to have uniform guidelines. The gross appearance of early columnar metaplasia-associated adenocarcinoma is of particular clinical importance because it directly concerns the early detection. Grossly three types (elevated, flat, depressed) should be distinguished. Type I, especially when higher than 3 mm is the easiest to detect because of the conspicuous protuberant configuration. Type II is considered to be the most difficult to detect because of its superficial flat appearance. The gross diagnosis relies entirely on the detection of sometimes subtle changes of surface architecture or changes in color. Type III discovery is of an intermediate degree of difficulty.

References

1. Haggitt RC. Adenocarcinoma in Barrett's esophagus: a new epidemic? Hum Pathol 1992;23:475–476.
2. Hameeteman W, Tytgat GNJ, Houthoff HJ, van den Tweel JG. Barrett's esophagus: development of dysplasia and adenocarcinoma. Gastroenterology 1989;96:1249–1256.
3. Altorki NH, Sunagawa M, Little AG, Skinner DB. High-grade dysplasia in the columnar-lined esophagus. Am J Surg 1991;161:97–100.
4. Spechler SJ. Endoscopic surveillance for patients with Barrett esophagus: does the cancer risk justify the practice? Ann Int Med 1987;106:902–904.
5. Hameeteman W, Den Hartog Jager FCA, Tio TL, Tytgat GNJ. Early adenocarcinoma of the esophagus. In: Siewert JR, Holscher AH (eds) Diseases of the Esophagus. Berlin: Springer, 1987;555–558.
6. Cameron AJ, Ott BJ, Payne WS. The incidence of adenocarcinoma in the columnar-lined (Barrett's) esophagus. N Engl J Med 1985;313:857–859.
7. Spechler SJ, Robbins AH, Rubins HB, Vincent ME, Heeren T, Doos WG, Colton T, Scimmel EM. Adenocarcinoma and Barrett's esophagus. An overrated risk? Gastroenterology 1984;87:927–933.
8. Sprung DJ, Ellis FH, Gibb SP. Incidence of adenocarcinoma in Barrett's esophagus. Am J Gastroenterol 1984;79:817A.
9. Tytgat GNJ, Hameeteman W. The neoplastic potential of columnar-lined (Barrett's) esophagus. World J Surg 1992;16: 308–312.
10. Tytgat GNJ, Hameeteman W, Onstenk R, Schotborg R. The spectrum of columnar-lined esophagus — Barrett's esophagus. Endoscopy 1989;21:177–185.
11. Chobanian SJ, Cattau EL Jr, Winters C Jr, Johnson DA, Van Ness MM, Miremadi A, Horwitz SL, Colcher H. In vivo staining with toluidine blue as an adjunct to the endoscopic detection of Barrett's esophagus. Gastrointest Endosc 1987;33:99.
12. Nishimaki T, Hölscher A, Schüler M et al. Histopathologic characteristics of early adenocarcinoma in Barrett's esophagus. Cancer 1991;68:1731–1736.
13. Reid BJ, Weinstein WM, Lewin KJ, Haggitt RC, Van Deventer G, DenBesten L, Rubin CE. Endoscopic biopsy can detect high-grade dysplasia or early-adenocarcinoma in Barrett's esophagus without grossly recognizable neoplastic lesions. Gastroenterology 1988;94:81.
14. Reid BJ, Haggitt RC, Rubin CE, Roth G, Surawicz CM, Van Belle G, Lewin KJ, Weinstein WM, Antonioli DA, Goldman H, MacDonald W, Owen D. Observer variation in the diagnosis of dysplasia in Barrett's esophagus. Hum Pathol 1988; 19:166–178.

Is an initial multifocal or diffuse appearance characteristic of adenocarcinoma in CLE?

J.A. Roth (Houston)

Columnar lined esophagus and p53 mutations

Adenocarcinoma of the esophagus is increasing in incidence [1]. It is frequently associated with the replacement of the squamous epithelial lining of the lower esophagus with columnar epithelium, a condition commonly called columnar lined esophagus (CLE) or Barrett's esophagus. Patients with CLE have a 50-fold increase in adenocarcinoma incidence. Although CLE is common, occurring in 10% of patients with esophageal reflux, only a small percentage of individuals with the condition will develop cancer. The question of the multifocal or unifocal nature of adenocarcinoma arising in CLE can be analyzed at both the cellular and the molecular level. Specific markers which are associated with the development of malignancy in CLE would be useful clinically. Markers currently in use, such as dysplasia, are not always reliable for predicting the development of malignancy. Therefore, it would be helpful to identify markers that would predict which patients with CLE will develop esophageal cancer. If such prediction were possible, esophagectomy could be done before the development of invasive cancer in high-risk patients and it would be curative. Once invasive esophageal cancer develops, less than 10% of patients are cured. Genetic abnormalities could also be targets for prevention and therapy strategies.

Genetic markers in CLE

The p53 gene has been proposed as a possible marker for predicting malignant change in CLE [2]. The p53 gene encodes a 375 amino acid phosphoprotein that can form complexes with host proteins such as large-T antigen and E1B. Missense mutations are the most common gene mutation yet identified for human cancers. The mechanism of p53 transformation is controversial. The wildtype p53 gene may directly suppress or indirectly activate genes that suppress uncontrolled cell growth. The wildtype p53 is dominant over the mutant form and thus will suppress the transformed phenotype [3,4]. Absence of the wildtype p53 or inactivation of wildtype p53 may, therefore, contribute to transformation. However, some studies indicate the presence of the mutant p53 may be necessary for full expression of the transforming potential of the gene. The presence of the mutant p53 gene can confer a growth advantage to some cells [4,5].

Mutations of p53 are common in a wide spectrum of tumors [6]. Two types of mutations occur: transitions in which a purine is substituted for a purine or pyrimidine for a pyrimidine and a transversion in which a purine is substituted for pyrimidine or vice versa [7]. Transversions have been identified in association with carcinogens such as benzo[a]pyrene. Transitions which have a predilection for CpG dinucleotides (frequently having 5-methylcytosine residues) are indicative of the spontaneous mutation rate.

Mutations in the p53 gene are frequent in esophageal cancers [8—12]. Mutations have been detected in cancers from high incidence regions including Uruguay, Normandy (France), Japan and China. Deletions in chromosome 17p which is the locus for p53 and loss of a p53 allele have also been reported [13,14].

Specimens of CLE epithelium were analyzed for p53 mutations by Casson and co-workers [2]. Unlike the ras family of oncogenes where mutations occur in two "hot spots", mutations of p53 occur in multiple sites throughout the open reading frame. Fortunately, most mutations are limited to a region highly conserved among species that spans exons 5 to 8 [7]. Thus, it is impractical to directly sequence the PCR products for large numbers of samples. The approach we used was to screen the conserved region of p53 for mutations using single-strand conformation polymorphism (SSCP) analysis. PCR-SSCP is a powerful approach for qualitative analysis of the DNA. The method is based on the observation that the electrophoretic mobility of a DNA molecule through a neutral polyacrylamide gel can be altered by the size and shape of the DNA molecule. Under nondenaturating conditions, single stranded DNA has a folded structure that is determined by intramolecular interaction related to its base sequence. The single stranded DNA with a base substitution has a different folded structure than that of the wild type sequences. As a result, the mutated single stranded DNA shows a mobility difference in a polyacrylamide gel. Since the introduction of the technique for detection of polymorphism in the human gene, it has become widely used [15]. This property of the DNA molecule has been utilized to identify the gene mutations in a variety of genetic abnormalities. Mutations in the p53 gene were identified in CLE epithelium associated with adenocarcinoma. The mutations were C:A→T:G transitions and they resulted in amino acid substitutions. In an ongoing prospective study, mutations were found in three out of five patients with CLE metaplasia and a coexisting adenocarcinoma (Table 1). Mutations in p53 were less frequent in specimens from CLE metaplasia with no evidence of cancer (5/17, 29%). Allelic deletions of 17p and p53 protein overexpression have been reported for adenocarcinoma associated with CLE epithelium [16]. Mutations in the p53 gene appear to be independent of the development of dysplasia (Table 1).

CLE may develop large areas of clonal proliferation of the epithelium which can be documented by cytogenetic markers [17]. The p53 mutations detected in CLE also appeared to be clonal with the same mutation present in epithelium from multiple

Table 1. Incidence of p53 mutations in DNA extracted from Barrett's epithelium. Mutations were identified using single strand conformation polymorphism analysis of polymerase chain reaction amplified DNA. Primers were used for p53 exons 5 to 8 as described previously [2]

	Cancer absent	Cancer present
Metaplasia	5/17 (29%)	3/5 (60%) (3/8 cancers)
Dysplasia	0/9 (0%)	2/11 (18%) (1/8 cancers)

sites of CLE [2]. This suggests that in some cases the p53 mutation, or other genetic abnormality, leads to a selective clonal growth advantage resulting in tumor formation. In other cases the presence of p53 mutations indicates genetic instability in the epithelium with a nonmutant clone eventually forming the tumor. Thus, the identification of p53 mutations in CLE epithelium may be an independent marker for the risk of developing esophageal cancer. Multiple clones which can be distinguished on the basis of ploidy have also been identified in CLE from individual patients [18].

The pathologic findings following surgical resection in patients with adenocarcinoma associated with CLE and adenocarcinoma without CLE were compared for the presence of multifocal carcinomas. Twenty-nine consecutive patients at the M.D. Anderson Cancer Center from 1987 to 1991 had resection of adenocarcinoma associated with CLE. Only one of the 29 patients had a second primary focus of adenocarcinoma. Of 50 adenocarcinomas without CLE resected during the same time, one primary tumor of the gastroesophageal junction was associated with a second primary adenocarcinoma in the stomach.

It is likely that an adenocarcinoma in CLE develops from a highly proliferative clone of CLE. Multiple distinct clonal populations can exist with the potential for malignant progression. These pathological and molecular observations would lead one to expect a significant incidence of multifocal carcinogenesis. However, virtually all patients, with rare exceptions, in our experience present with a single focus of adenocarcinoma.

Acknowledgements

This study was partially supported by grants from the National Cancer Institute and National Institute of Health (RO1 CA45187) [J.A.R.]; the National Cancer Institute Training Grant (CA09611) [J.A.R.]; by gifts to the Division of Surgery from Tenneco and Exxon for the Core Lab Facility; by the M.D. Anderson Cancer Center Support Core Grant (CA16672); and by a grant from the Mathers Foundation.

References

1. Blot WJ, Devesa SS, Kneller RW, Fraumeni JF Jr. Rising incidence of adenocarcinoma of the esophagus and gastric cardia. JAMA 1991;265(10):1287–1289.
2. Casson AG, Mukhopadhyay T, Cleary KR, Ro JY, Levin B, Roth JA. p53 gene mutations in Barrett's epithelium and esophageal cancer. Cancer Res 1991;51:4495–4499.
3. Baker SJ, Markowitz S, Fearson ER, Villson JKV, Vogelstein B. Suppression of human colorectal carcinoma cell growth by wild-type p53. Science 1990;249:912–915.
4. Chen P-L, Chen Y, Bookstein R, Lee W-H. Genetic mechanisms of tumor suppression by the human p53 gene. Science 1990;250:1576–1580.
5. Hinds P, Finlay C, Levine AJ. Mutation is required to activate the p53 gene for cooperation with the ras oncogene and transformation. J Virol 1989;63(2):739–746.
6. Nigro JM, Baker SJ, Preisinger AC et al. Mutations in the p53 gene occur in diverse human tumor types. Nature 1989; 342:705–708.
7. Hollstein M, Sidransky D, Vogelstein B, Harris CC. p53 mutations in human cancers. Science 1991;253:49–53.
8. Imazeki F, Omata M, Nose H, Ohto M, Isono K. p53 gene mutations in gastric and esophageal cancers. Gastroenterology 1992;103:892–896.
9. Hollstein MC, Metcalf RA, Welsh JA, Montesano R, Harris CC. Frequent mutation of the p53 gene in human esophageal cancer. Proc Natl Acad Sci USA 1990;87:9958–9961.

10. Bennett WP, Hollstein MC, He A et al. Archival analysis of p53 genetic and protein alterations in Chinese esophageal cancer. Oncogene 1991;6:1779–1784.
11. Hollstein MC, Peri L, Mandard AM et al. Genetic analysis of human esophageal tumors from two high incidence geographic areas: frequent p53 base substitutions and absence of ras mutations. Cancer Res 1991;51:4102–4106.
12. Tamura G, Maesawa C, Suzuki Y, Satodate R, Ishida K, Saito K. p53-gene mutations in esophageal cancer detected by polymerase chain reaction single-strand conformation polymorphism analysis. Jpn J Cancer Res 1992;83:559–562.
13. Wagata T, Ishizaki K, Imamura M, Shimada Y, Ikenaga M, Tobe T. Deletion of 17p and amplification of the int-2 gene in esophageal carcinomas. Cancer Res 1991;51:2113–2117.
14. Meltzer SJ, Yin J, Huang Y et al. Reduction to homozygosity involving p53 in esophageal cancers demonstrated by the polymerase chain reaction. Proc Natl Acad Sci USA 1991;88:4976–4980.
15. Orita M, Iwahana H, Kanazawa H, Hayashi K, Sekiya T. Detection of polymorphisms of human DNA by gel electrophoresis as single-strand conformation polymorphisms. Proc Natl Acad Sci USA 1989;86:2766–2770.
16. Blount PL, Ramel S, Raskind WH et al. 17 allelic deletions and p53 protein overexpression in Barrett's adenocarcinoma. Cancer Res 1991;51:5482–5486.
17. Raskind WH, Norwood T, Levine DS, Haggitt RC, Rabinovitch PS, Reid BJ. Persistent clonal areas and clonal expression in Barrett's esophagus. Cancer Res 1992;52:2946–2950.
18. Reid BJ, Blount PL, Rubin CE, Levine DS, Haggitt RC, Rabinovitch PS. Flow-cytometric and histological progression to malignancy in Barrett's esophagus: prospective endoscopic surveillance of a cohort. Gastroenterology 1992;102:1212–1219.

How useful is cytology in the diagnosis of carcinoma in CLE?

K.R. Geisinger (Winston-Salem)

The premalignant nature of Barrett's metaplasia is now widely recognized, as the overwhelming majority of adenocarcinomas of the esophagus arise on a background of pre-existing benign glandular metaplasia [1]. This has prompted the development of surveillance programs to detect early carcinomas and glandular dysplasia in order to improve the otherwise dismal prognosis for patients with this tumor. Unfortunately, in many patients adenocarcinoma continues to be advanced at the time of initial diagnosis of esophageal disease.

A recent edition of Webster's Dictionary defines "useful" as an adjective meaning "of particular advantage" [2]. From this perspective, it is believed that brushing cytology is quite useful in patients with Barrett's esophagus including for the identification of adenocarcinoma. This opinion derives from the several advantages that exfoliative cytology offers vis-à-vis tissue biopsy.

In several major centers, surveillance protocols include procurement of two or more biopsies for every 2 cm or so along the entire length of the metaplastic segment [3]. It is well recognized that glandular dysplasia and even early carcinoma may appear endoscopically indistinguishable from pure metaplasia. Yet, only a small proportion of the entire Barrett's mucosa is evaluated by this approach. The major advantage of cytology is that the brush may theoretically contact the entire mucosal surface [4]. Thus, the surface area sampled for cytology is considerably greater than with multiple biopsies, increasing the likelihood of finding morphologically abnormal cells, which, of course, is the goal of surveillance screening. In addition, as stated by Wang et al., the brushing procedure has a proclivity to sample selectively epithelial cells with reduced intercellular cohesion [5]. It has been our experience that dysplastic and frankly malignant cells are dyshesive relative to normal or metaplastic elements lining the gastrointestinal tract, and thus are more apt to appear in cytologic smears [4]. Tissue biopsy specimens do not appear to be privileged to possess this property.

Brushing the mucosa is less traumatic to the patient than are forceps biopsies and thus may be more acceptable to all concerned. Furthermore, there are clinical situations, e.g., thrombocytopenia, in which a biopsy should not be performed, yet brushing may proceed safely.

The need to maintain or reduce medical costs has never been greater than today [6,7]. Purely from the charges secondary to the pathologic examination of endoscopically-obtained material, surveillance programs with their numerous biopsies are expensive. At my institution, the combined technical and professional fee for a single esophageal biopsy is over $141. A series of such specimens could generate a total charge of astronomical proportions. On the other hand, the total bill for the processing, screening and pathologic examination of a cytologic preparation from the entire abnormal mucosa is $163. Nothing more needs to be said about this advantage.

As mentioned by Wang and her colleagues, esophageal brushings may be processed and examined rapidly [8]. In my institution, diagnostic cytology reports are often issued approximately 20 h before the corresponding esophageal biopsy diagnosis. Although this factor may not be very important, especially in surveillance programs, it should still be noted.

Of course, to be truly useful, brushing cytology must add significantly to the morphologic diagnosis of cancer and dysplasia which may be achieved by histologic examination of biopsy specimens, which I believe remains the diagnostic gold standard (Fig. 1—7). Webster's Dictionary defines complementary as "something that completes or perfects" [2]. I contend that cytology and biopsy are complementary in detecting metaplasia, dysplasia and neoplasia in the esophagus. Although the literature is somewhat garbled, there is no doubt that published reports support this belief [5,8—11]. One problem with the interpretation of some of these published accounts, is that cellular material is often combined from the stomach and the esophagus into series of upper gastrointestinal tract specimens. In some reports, one can at least distinguish the carcinomas into those including the esophagus, gastroesophageal junction and cardia and thus exclude more distally occurring gastric tumors. As the biology of esophageal and cardiac adenocarcinomas appear to overlap, this scenario is not exceptionally important [12—14]. Very few periodical publications deal solely with cytology from patients with Barrett's esophagus [8,9,11].

The first sizeable manuscript dedicated to the cytomorphology of the columnar lined esophagus was that of Robey et al. [9]. This work involved about 66 patients with glandular epithelium identified in either or both specimens of concurrently obtained biopsies and brushings. Barrett's esophagus was diagnosed in both members of only 54% of the specimen pairs; it was identified in the brushings alone in 32% of the pairs and in biopsies alone in the remaining 14%. Eight specimens contained

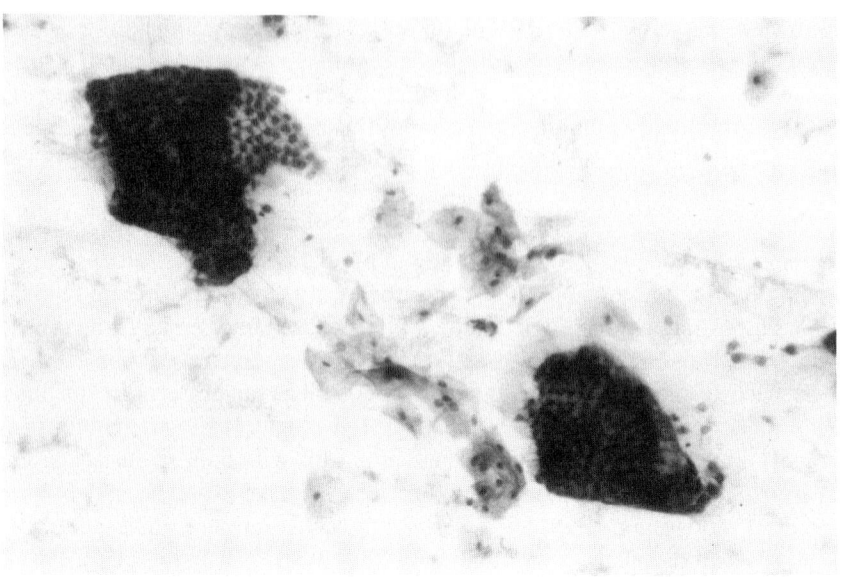

Fig. 1. In brushings of benign Barrett's epithelium, the smears are characterized by the presence of large, sharply delineated epithelial cellular aggregates. The borders of these sheets and aggregates are sharp and smooth. This is a reflection of the maintenance of normal intercellular cohesion. The smear background is relatively clean (× 40).

carcinomas (one was squamous in type) and two had dysplasia. Biopsies and brushings were essentially equally and highly sensitive for their detection. We also reported a similar series of 66 endoscopically-obtained specimen pairs from 42 consecutive patients with Barrett's esophagus [11]. With one exception, Barrett's epithelium was found in both brushings and biopsies of all specimen pairs. Adenocarcinoma and glandular dysplasia were identified in 10 and seven of the biopsy specimens, respectively, whereas carcinoma and dysplasia were diagnosed in 14 and 4, respectively, of the concurrently obtained brushing specimens. All 18 of the latter specimens were eventually followed by esophageal resections which contained either invasive adenocarcinomas or multifocal severe dysplasia. Nine of the remaining brushing specimens were interpreted as inconclusive or suspicious, that is, we were unable to distinguish a marked reparative, but benign process from true dysplasia. These patients have had a clinically benign follow-up. Thus, I admit that, in my hands, this distinction at times may be very difficult or impossible [11]. Similarly, using histologic methods, the separation of benign metaplasia from low grade dysplasia may be problematic, even for experts [15].

From a different perspective, the Johns Hopkins group also presented a series of 18 cytologic specimens which were evaluated morphologically, because their concurrently obtained biopsies contained an esophageal adenocarcinoma [10]. A cytologic diagnosis of frank adenocarcinoma could be rendered in 15 of the cytologic specimens, with the remaining three labeled as suspicious for malignancy. These authors showed that adenocarcinoma can be reliably identified in smears using

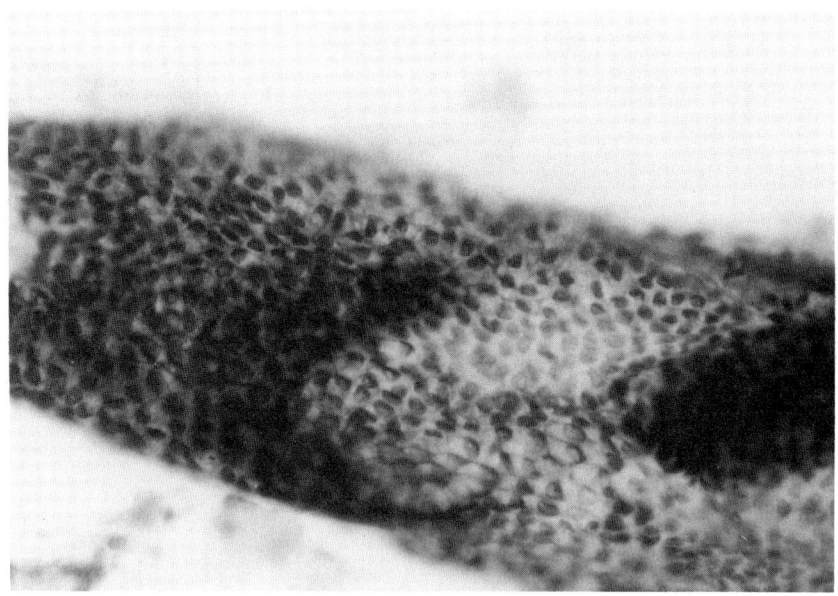

Fig. 2. Within the benign metaplastic aggregates, the cells are characterized by round to slightly oval nuclei with delicate regular nuclear membranes, very finely granular and evenly distributed chromatin, and small and often inconspicuous nucleoli. Cells are approximately equally distant from one another, a reflection of the normal polarity being maintained (× 100).

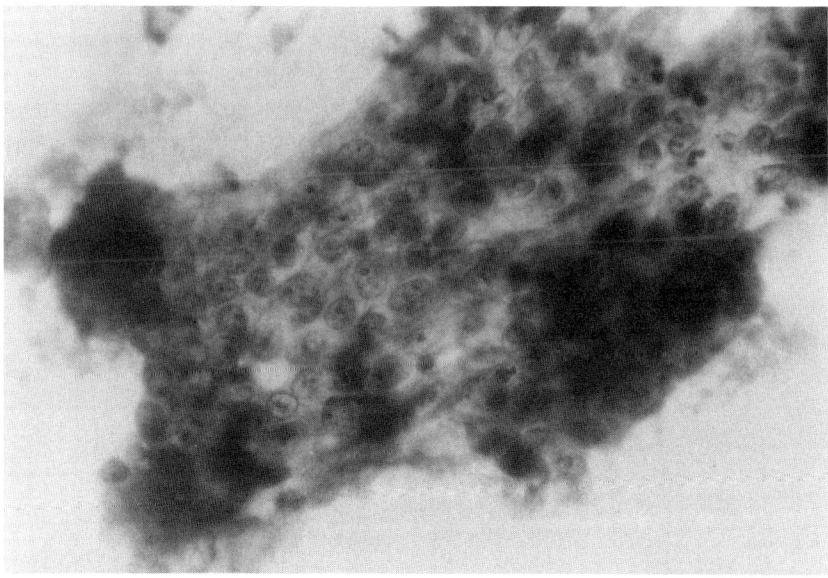

Fig. 3. With benign reparative atypia, there may be an enlargement of the nuclei resulting in an accentuation of the nuclear to cytoplasmic ratios and a relative crowding of the nuclei. However, the nuclei are uniform from cell to cell and do not demonstrate true piling-up or prominent overlapping. Nucleoli are evident (× 400).

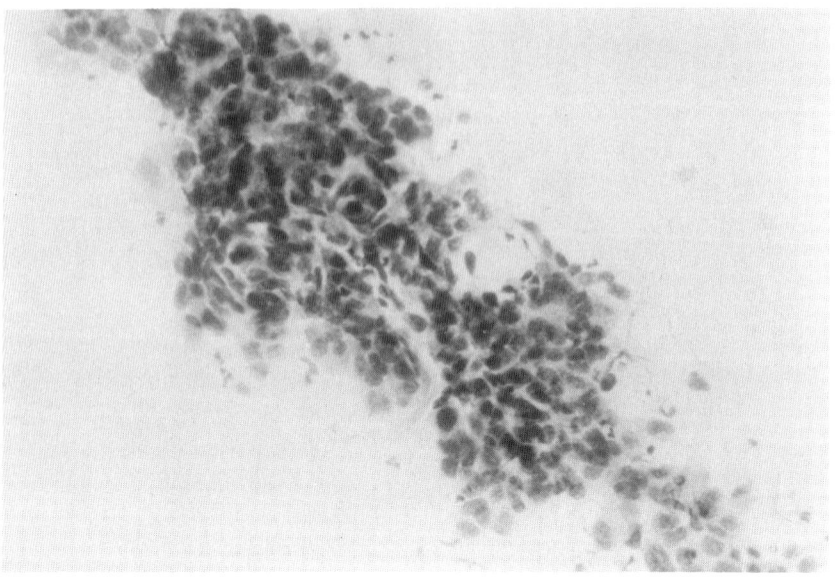

Fig. 4. This is a sizeable fragment of dysplastic glandular elements. The border of the aggregate is irregular with a serrated appearance. The abnormal cells have enlarged and obviously hyperchromatic nuclei. Although the cells in the lower right corner are arranged in a monolayer, elsewhere they are piled up on one another. Intact abnormal cells isolated from the aggregate are distinctly absent (× 100).

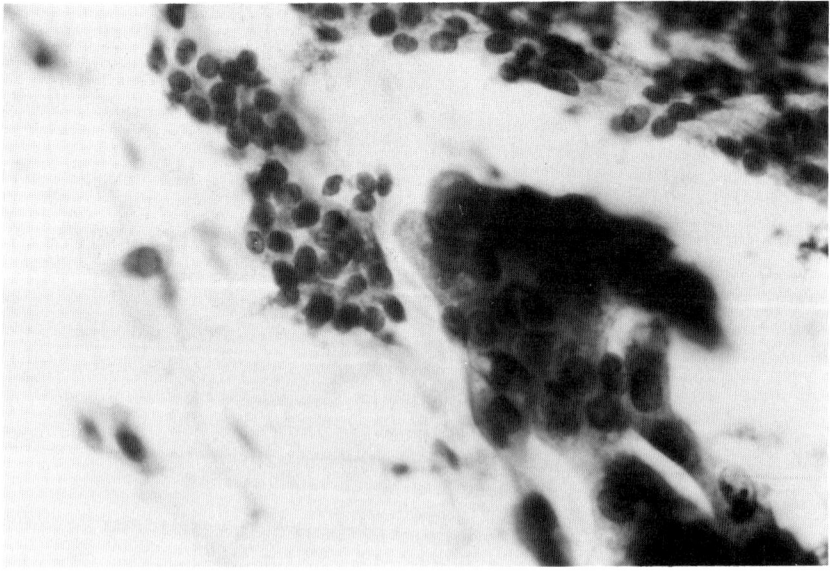

Fig. 5. Dysplastic glandular elements are present in a cohesive aggregate which is adjacent to a sheet of benign glandular metaplastic cells. The dysplastic cells and their nuclei are greatly increased in size (× 100).

1100

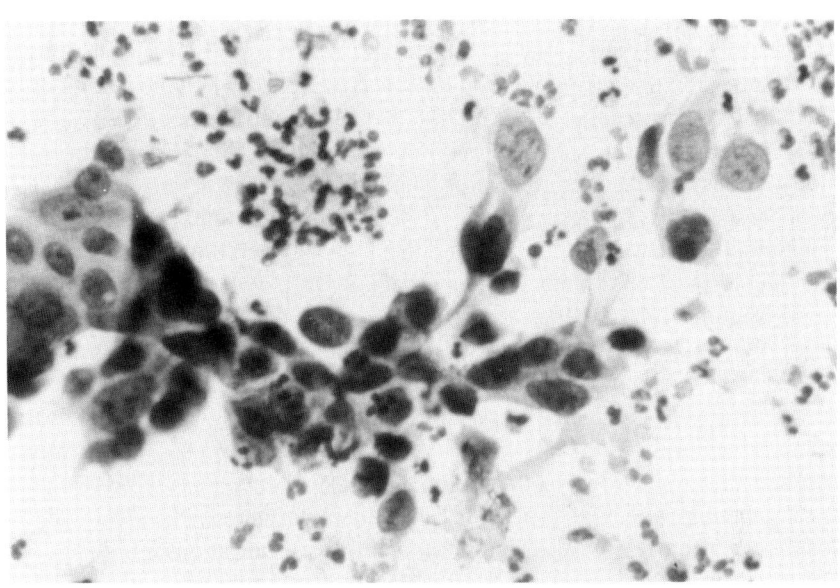

Fig. 6. Dispersion of individual malignant cells from the larger mass of adenocarcinoma is readily apparent. This accounts for the frayed irregular edges that are apparent at very low (scanning) magnifications. Neutrophils are plentiful (× 400).

standard cytomorphologic features of malignant cells [10]. Cusso et al. studied 83 patients with adenocarcinomas involving the esophagus and perijunctional region

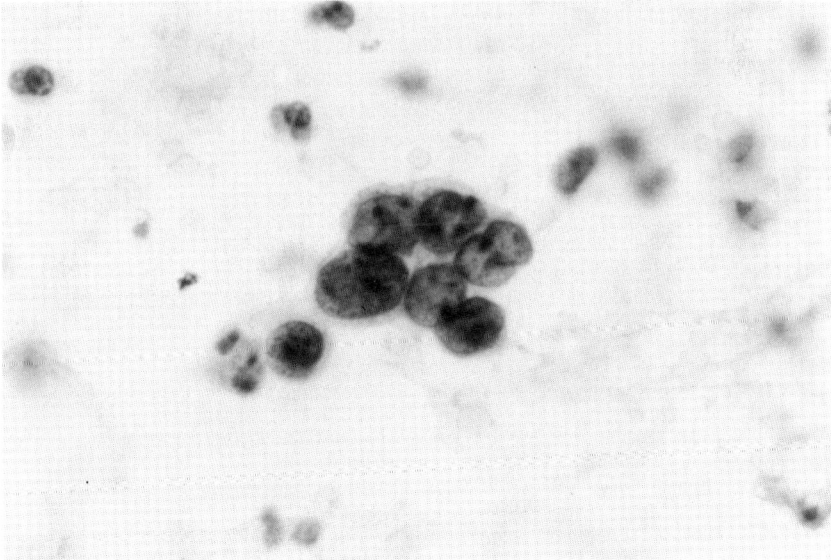

Fig. 7. Adenocarcinoma cells have high nuclear to cytoplasmic ratios, thick irregular membranes and hyperchromatic chromatin. Macronucleoli are not well developed. The latter are not essential for a diagnosis of adenocarcinoma. Histologically, this tumor was high grade (poorly differentiated) (× 400).

[16]. Cytology was positive in 88%, while biopsies were positive in 86%. However, in a subset of their patients, one specimen type was positive for carcinoma while the other was not. The diagnostic yield of 95% was achieved when the results of biopsies and brushings were combined. Similarly, Kobayashi et al. reported a series of 173 cancers (some of them were primary in the cardia) [17]. Diagnostic yields for cytology, biopsy and both procedures combined were 84%, 77% and 88% of the patients, respectively. These results, I believe, prove that cytologic criteria for adenocarcinoma are well established and that cytology and biopsy are complementary for the diagnosis of this tumor. This is especially true when the esophageal lumen is stenosed by tumor [4,16–19].

From the point of view of surveillance, the cytologic diagnosis of glandular dysplasia is also certainly significant. It is important (and interesting) that three independent groups published very similar cytomorphologic criteria for Barrett's-associated dysplasia within less than 1 year of each other [5,8,11]. All three groups determined that reductions in intercellular cohesion and polarity were the keys in separating benign, reactive processes, as seen in inflamed and ulcerated Barrett's mucosa, from true dysplasia. This combination of aberrations produces cytologic smears with relatively small and irregularly contoured, often three-dimensional cellular aggregates. Within the latter, a haphazard array of atypical glandular cells with crowded, molded and overlapped hyperchromatic nuclei are present. Solitary intact morphologically abnormal cells are relatively sparse. From our own experience, as well as that portrayed in the literature, I believe that most cytologic specimens which are recognizable as dysplasia are histologically high grade. Adenocarcinomas, on the other hand, show a much greater loss of cohesion, resulting in a large proportion of individually dispersed malignant cells. Thus, with adequate experience, I believe that benign and malignant (dysplasia and carcinoma) cytologic smears can be distinguished in the majority of instances.

References

1. Spechler SJ, Goyal RK. Barrett's esophagus. N Engl J Med 1986;315:362–371.
2. Webster's II New Riverside Dictionary. Berkley Books, New York, 1984.
3. Haggitt RC. Adenocarcinoma in Barrett's esophagus: a new epidemic? Hum Pathol 1992;23:475–476.
4. Geisinger KR, Wang HH, Ducatman BS, Teot LA. Gastrointestinal cytology. Clin Lab Med 1991;11:403–441.
5. Wang HH, Ducatman BS, Thibault S. Cytologic features of premalignant glandular lesions in the upper gastrointestinal tract. Acta Cytol 1991;35:199–203.
6. Spechler SJ. Endoscopic surveillance for patients with Barrett's esophagus: does the cancer risk justify the practice? Ann Int Med 1987;106:902–904.
7. Achkar E, Carey W. The cost of surveillance for adenocarcinoma complicating Barrett's esophagus. Am J Gastroenterol 1988;83:291–294.
8. Wang HH, Doria MI, Purohit-Buch S, Schnell T, Sontag S, Chejfec G. Barrett's esophagus. The cytology of dysplasia in comparison to benign and malignant lesions. Acta Cytol 1992;36:60–64.
9. Robey SS, Hamilton SR, Gupta PK, Erozan YS. Diagnostic value of cytopathology in Barrett's esophagus and associated carcinoma. Am J Clin Pathol 1988;89:493–498.
10. Shurbaji MS, Erozan YS. The cytopathologic diagnosis of esophageal adenocarcinoma. Acta Cytol 1991;35:189–194.
11. Geisinger KR, Teot LA, Richter JE. A comparative cytopathologic and histologic study of atypia, dysplasia, and adeno-carcinoma in Barrett's esophagus. Cancer 1992;69:8–16.
12. Kalish RJ, Clancy PE, Orringer MB, Appelman HD. Clinical, epidemiologic, and morphologic comparison between adeno-carcinomas arising in Barrett's esophageal mucosa and in the gastric cardia. Gastroenterology 1984;86:461–467.
13. MacDonald WC, MacDonald JB. Adenocarcinoma of the esophagus and/or gastric cardia. Cancer 1987;60:1094–1098.

14. Hamilton SR, Smith RRL, Cameron JL. Prevalence and characteristics of Barrett's esophagus in patients with adenocarcinoma of the esophagus or esophagogastric junction. Hum Pathol 1988;19:942—948.
15. Reid BJ, Haggitt RC, Rubin CE, Roth G, Surawicz CM, VanBelle G, Lewin K, Weinstein WM, Antonioli DA, Goldman H, MacDonald W, Owen D. Observer variation in the diagnosis of dysplasia in Barrett's esophagus. Hum Pathol 1988; 19:166—178.
16. Cussó X, Monés-Xiol J, Vilardell F. Endoscopic cytology of cancer of the esophagus and cardia: a long-term evaluation. Gastrointest Endosc 1989;35:321—323.
17. Kobayashi S, Kasugai T. Brushing cytology for the diagnosis of gastric cancer involving the cardia or the lower esophagus. Acta Cytol 1978;22:155—157.
18. Witzel L, Halter F, Grétillat, Scheurer U, Keller M. Evaluation of specific value of endoscopic biopsies and brush cytology for malignancies of the esophagus and stomach. Gut 1976;17:375—377.
19. Kasugai T, Kobayashi S, Kuno N. Endoscopic cytology of the esophagus, stomach and pancreas. Acta Cytol 1978;22: 327—330.

What are the minimal criteria for the biopsy diagnosis of well-differentiated adenocarcinomas?

H.D. Appelman (Ann Arbor)

In Barrett's mucosa, the columnar epithelium undergoes a sequence of changes, beginning with the original metaplastic epithelium, which, although it is obviously not normal, we nevertheless regard as the equivalent of normal baseline epithelium. Within some components of this baseline Barrett's epithelium, possibly the intermediate columnar cells in the specialized epithelium, the progressive dysplasias evolve, beginning with the low grades and progressing to the high. These cytologic changes include gradually intensifying increases in nuclear size relative to cell volume, nuclear and cellular pleomorphism, nuclear hyperchromatism and number and complexity of mitoses. The highest dysplastic grade has the cytologic features of carcinomatous epithelium, but it is an in situ lesion and therefore incapable of invasion and metastasis. As a result, we have a choice of name for these highest grade dysplastic epithelia. We can recognize their lack of growth potential beyond the epithelium and call them high-grade dysplasias. In contrast we can concentrate on their cytologic resemblance to cancer cells and call them adenocarcinomas in situ. For this discussion, the designation adenocarcinoma will be reserved for neoplastic epithelium that has invaded beyond the normal basement membrane of the Barrett's mucosa and into the lamina propria. Therefore, the question really becomes one of establishing the minimal criteria for the diagnosis of invasion by well differentiated neoplastic columnar epithelium.

Minimal invasion is always difficult to identify. The invading islands, nests or tubules of esophageal carcinomas, particularly squamous carcinomas, are sometimes accompanied by a change in the stroma from normal lamina propria to desmoplasia, as is almost the rule for invading colonic cancers. However, this is not the rule in the esophagus. In fact, most early invasion of esophageal carcinomas, especially adenocarcinomas, has no desmoplastic stroma. Therefore, we must depend upon other features than the stroma for the diagnosis of invasion. The two most helpful morphologic clues are: 1) compromise of the lamina propria and 2) finding tubules between smooth muscle fibers of the muscularis mucosae. The compromise of the lamina propria occurs when the dysplastic tubules are crowded together with little intervening stroma, comparable to the "back-to-back" arrangement seen in early invading endometrial cancers. As long as the configuration of the tubules conforms to their configuration in Barrett's mucosa, including the architectural adenoma-like changes of dysplastic Barrett's mucosa, then invasion is not present, or at least it cannot be diagnosed.

The finding of one or more well-differentiated, but clearly dysplastic, tubules between fibers of the muscularis mucosae is another manifestation of beginning invasion, because the muscularis mucosae is almost always separate from the epithelial elements in Barrett's mucosa. The major problem with this feature is prolapsed mucosa, in which slips of hyperplastic muscularis mucosae extend perpendicularly into the base of the mucosa between the basal tubules, appearing to trap such tubules, so that they resemble invasive carcinoma. Fortunately, prolapse is very rare in Barrett's mucosa, so this is not likely to be a problem.

Does adenocarcinoma accompanying high-grade dysplasia have a particular tendency to metastasis?

T.C. Smyrk (Omaha)

The behavior of adenocarcinoma of the distal esophagus is not altered by the presence of Barrett's esophagus, nor does the presence of high-grade dysplasia confer special behavior. Several large series have shown no difference in tumor stage between adenocarcinoma associated with Barrett's mucosa and other adenocarcinomas of the gastroesophageal junction [1,2]. More recently, Potet et al. reviewed their experience with 51 adenocarcinomas arising in Barrett's esophagus and 61 patients with adenocarcinoma of the gastroesophageal junction [3]. The frequency of lymph node involvement was 77% in the former group and 89% in the latter. Studies of early adenocarcinoma are particularly revealing with regard to the potential for metastatic spread of tumors arising in Barrett's mucosa. De Baecque described 12 early adenocarcinomas arising in Barrett's, four confined to the mucosa and eight extending to submucosa [4]. Only one patient had lymph node metastases and that patient had only one positive lymph node. Our own experiences is similar [5]. Among five patients who had esophagectomy for intramucosal carcinoma, none had lymph node metastases. Seven patients had tumors confined to the esophageal wall; five of these had lymph node metastases, but in four of the five patients the tumor invaded into the muscularis propria. There was no correlation between the presence of high-grade dysplasia and the presence of lymph node metastases, suggesting that Barrett's esophagus with high-grade dysplasia does not develop metastases with an unusually high frequency or at an unusually early point. The experience of the University of Washington group with a prospective endoscopic surveillance program bears this out [6]. Among 14 patients who presented with high-grade dysplasia and were followed for more than a year, two progressed to early adenocarcinoma and underwent surgery. Neither had evidence of metastases at the time of surgery. Thus, fear of early metastases should not prompt esophagectomy for high-grade dysplasia.

References

1. Kalish RJ, Clancy PE, Oringer MB, Appelman HD. Clinical, epidemiologic and morphologic comparison between adenocarcinomas arising in Barrett's esophageal mucosa and in the gastric cardia. Gastroenterol 1984;86:461–467.
2. Wang HH, Antonioli DA, Goldman H. Comparative features of esophageal and gastric adenocarcinomas: recent changes in type and frequency. Hum Pathol 1986;17:482.
3. Potet F, Flejou JF, Gervaz H, Paraf F. Adenocarcinoma of the lower esophagus and the esophagogastric junction. Sem Diagn Pathol 1991;8:126.
4. De Baecque C, Potet F, Molas G et al. Superficial adenocarcinoma of the esophagus arising in Barrett's mucosa with dysplasia: a clinical pathological study of twelve patients. Histopathology 1990;16:213.
5. DeMeester TR, Attwood SEA, Smyrk TC, Therkildsen DH, Hinder RA. Surgical therapy in Barrett's esophagus. Ann Surg 1990;212:528.
6. Levine DS, Haggitt RC, Blount PL et al. An endoscopic biopsy protocol can differentiate high-grade dysplasia from early adenocarcinoma in Barrett's esophagus. Gastroenterology 1993;105:40.

Does the finding of aneuploidy as opposed to diploidy on flow cytometry indicate a different prognosis for adenocarcinoma of the esophagus?

M. Robaszkiewicz (Brest)

Flow cytometry is a technique for cell analysis that allows simultaneous investigation of several parameters in a large number of cells in a very short time. It is commonly used in oncology to quantify the DNA content of tumor cells.

Adenocarcinomas of the esophagus mainly develop on a metaplastic mucosa. Their prognosis is usually poor and the 5-year survival rates are globally low, as most of these tumors are diagnosed late [1–3]. The many cases of cancer associated with

Barrett's esophagus have demonstrated the prognostic value of the spread of the tumor to the parietal tissues and lymph nodes. The better prognosis of the superficial forms has been confirmed by several studies [4–6].

Two studies evaluated the DNA of the cells in cancers associated with Barrett's esophagus. Fléjou et al. carried out a retrospective study of 23 specimens provided by esophagectomy for adenocarcinoma [7]. Analysis of DNA content was carried out on material that was fixed and embedded in paraffin. Sixteen of the 23 tumors examined (70%) were DNA-aneuploid. Of the seven DNA-diploid tumors, six were intramural, whereas 14 of the 16 DNA-aneuploid tumors had attained the adventitia. Spread to the lymph nodes was also more frequent for the DNA-aneuploid tumors. The number of cases was too small to allow statistical comparison of survival for the DNA-aneuploid and DNA-diploid forms. However, the prognosis appeared to be better for the DNA-diploid forms than for the DNA-aneuploid forms, since six of the seven patients with a DNA-diploid tumor were still alive 15–52 months after the operation, whereas 11 of the 16 with a DNA-aneuploid tumor had died; the other five patients were still alive 12–18 months after the operation. Schneeberger et al. also carried out a retrospective study of 75 adenocarcinomas of the cardia, of which 28 were associated with Barrett's mucosa [8]. DNA-aneuploidy was found in 81% of cases and in 86% of the cancers associated with Barrett's esophagus. The DNA-aneuploid tumors were more frequently associated with lymph node metastases than were the DNA-diploid tumors. Over the study population as a whole, global survival and recurrence-free survival were better for the DNA-diploid tumors than for the DNA-aneuploid tumors, but the difference was only significant for recurrence-free survival. Multivariate analysis indicated that survival and the risk of local recurrence were influenced by spread of the tumor to the lymph nodes, depth of wall penetration, and the degree of differentiation of the tumor. DNA-ploidy had no independent prognostic value.

In these retrospective studies carried out with fixed material, the frequency of DNA-aneuploidy appears to be lower than that reported in other studies conducted with fresh or frozen material. In the study performed by Rabinovitch et al., the 14 adenocarcinomas examined were all DNA-aneuploid [9], as were the tumors examined in our own study [10]. In addition, Levine et al., who examined 20 superficial cancers restricted to the mucosa or submucosa, found 90% of the tumors to be DNA-aneuploid or to have a high G2M/tetraploid fraction [11]. These results are in conflict with those obtained by Fléjou, who found that only two of the eight tumors that did not spread further than the muscular coat (24%) were DNA-aneuploid [7]. This disagreement may be accounted for in part by the number of samples analyzed per tumor, and the methods used to prepare the nuclei. When interpreting the results of flow cytometric studies it is important to take into account the technique used, the quality of the material and the number of biopsies examined. Studies carried out with fresh or frozen material are likely to be more reliable than those carried out with fixed material.

In conclusion therefore, the majority of studies show that the prevalence of DNA-aneuploidy is greater for adenocarcinomas associated with Barrett's esophagus than for other types of cancers. There are no objective data that allow the DNA content to be given a prognostic value in Barrett's adenocarcinomas. The prognostic value of DNA-aneuploidy and its independence from other criteria can only be evaluated by multifactorial statistical analysis of a large number of cases followed up over a long period of time. The genomic instability that predisposes to the development of DNA-aneuploid clones of cells appears to be an early event in the neoplastic progression of Barrett's mucosa [13]. This cytometric criterion cannot distinguish high-grade dysplasia from intermucosal or submucosal carcinomas [11], and it is unlikely that it has any influence on the prognosis of Barrett's adenocarcinomas. In patients with Barrett's esophagus, flow cytometry appears to be principally useful and promising in helping to identify those who are at high risk of malignant transformation among patients without dysplasia, or with only moderate dysplasia.

References

1. Naef AP, Savary M, Ozzello L et al. Columnar lined lower esophagus: an acquired lesion with malignant predisposition. Report of 140 cases of Barrett's esophagus with 12 adenocarcinoma. J Thorac Cardiovasc Surg 1975;70:826−835.
2. Skinner DB. En block resection for neoplasms of the esophagus and the cardia. J Thorac Cardiovasc Surg 1983;85:59−70.
3. Sanfey H, Hamilton SR, Smith RRL et al. Carcinoma arising in Barrett's esophagus. Surg Gynecol Obstet 1985;161:570−574.
4. DeMeester TR, Attwood SEA, Smyrk TC et al. Surgical therapy in Barrett's esophagus. Ann Surg 1990:212:528−540.
5. De Baecque C, Potet F, Molas G et al. Superficial adenocarcinoma of the esophagus arising in Barrett's mucosa with dysplasia. Histopathology 1990;16:213−220.
6. Streitz JM, Ellis FH, Gibb SP et al. Adenocarcinoma in Barrett's esophagus: a clinicopathologic study of 65 cases. Ann Surg 1991;213:122−125.
7. Fléjou JF, Doublet B, Potet F et al. Etude de l'ADN-ploïdie dans les adénocarcinomes sur endobrachyoesophage. Ann Pathol 1990;10:161−165.
8. Schneeberger AL, Finley RJ, Troster M et al. The prognostic significance of tumor ploidy and pathology in adenocarcinoma of the esophagogastric junction. Cancer 1990;65:1206−1210.
9. Rabinovitch PS, Reid BJ, Haggitt RC et al. Progression to cancer in Barrett's esophagus is associated with genomic instability. Lab Invest 1988;60:65−71.
10. Robaszkiewicz M, Volant A, Hardy E et al. Mise en évidence d'une hétérogénéité clonale au niveau des adénocarcinomes sur endobrachyoesophage par l'étude cytofluorométrique du contenu cellulaire en ADN. Gastroenterol Clin Biol 1992;16:540−546.
11. Levine DS, Haggitt RC, Blount PL et al. An endoscopic biopsy protocol can differentiate high-grade dysplasia from early adenocarcinoma in Barrett's esophagus. Gastroenterology 1993;105:40−50.
12. Shankey TV, Rabinovitch PS, Bagwell B et al. Guidelines for implementation of clinical DNA cytometry. Cytometry 1993; 14:472−477.
13. Reid BJ, Blount PL, Rubin CE et al. Flow cytometric and histological progression to malignancy in Barrett's esophagus: prospective endoscopic surveillance of a cohort. Gastroenterology 1992;102:1212−1219.

What is the histologic differential diagnosis for Barrett's carcinoma?

H.D. Appelman (Ann Arbor)

The carcinomas that arise in Barrett's mucosa are adenocarcinomas, but they have the entire range of differentiation, from very well differentiated which produces outstanding tubular or glandular structures to miserable differentiated which produces no tubules, but grows as solid masses of various types or as single undifferentiated cells diffusely infiltrating the esophageal wall. However, as long as the carcinoma, no matter its degree of differentiation 1) arises within the esophagus, 2) has a patch of Barrett's mucosa at its margin which, in turn, 3) contains a dysplastic focus, then the diagnosis of Barrett's carcinoma is assured, and for all practical purposes there is no differential diagnosis. When the three conditions listed above are not met, then other carcinomas become part of a differential diagnosis, such as:

1. carcinoma arising from the gastric cardia (cardiac carcinoma) which are histologically indistinguishable from Barrett's carcinomas, probably because they arise from the same type of precursors [1,2];
2. adenosquamous carcinoma arising from squamous cell in situ neoplasia in the esophagus [3];
3. endocrine/neuroendocrine or oat cell carcinoma primary in the esophagus [1];
4. poorly differentiated squamous cell carcinomas, especially the basaloid squamous variant which grows in cords that may superficially resemble poorly formed tubules of an adenocarcinoma [4]; and
5. metastatic neoplasms, especially carcinomas from breast, lung and melanomas, which can mimic carcinomas histologically.

Much of the morphology of these tumors are discussed and illustrated in the papers from the O.E.S.O. pathology symposium. Therefore, this discussion will be brief.

Cardiac cancer are separated from Barrett's cancer by site of origin. The bulk of the tumor is situated below the cardioesophageal junction, although cardiac carcinomas often extend into the lower esophagus. There is no Barrett's mucosa at its proximal margin. About 10% of all adenocarcinomas arising in the region of the junction obliterate the junction and do not have Barrett's mucosa above them or dysplasia in cardia below them. These we refer to as "junctional" carcinomas, thereby admitting our ignorance of their site of origin.

Squamous-derived adenosquamous carcinomas may look like comparable carcinomas arising in Barrett's mucosa, so the only way to tell them apart is to find the in situ component, whether dysplastic Barrett's mucosa or in situ high grade squamous intraepithelial neoplasia or dysplasia.

Endocrine malignancies, including oat cell carcinomas, are distinguished by their characteristic cellular constituents and/or by their endocrine markers, such as chromogranin, neuron-specific enolase or synaptophysin, all of which are demonstrated by immunohistochemical technics.

The poorly differentiated squamous variants probably pose the biggest differential diagnostic headache, because they can look very much like equally poorly differentiated adenocarcinomas. Experienced gastrointestinal pathologists probably can tell them apart. For less experienced pathologists, finding the in situ component, the dysplastic Barrett's or the dysplastic squamous, is the best determinant.

Finally, metastatic tumors produce different gross lesions than do primary carcinomas. They tend to be intramural and spread in an expansile fashion, so that there may be only a small mucosal lesion, such as ulcer, while there is a large expansile mass below this.

References

1. Appelman HD, Kalish RJ, Clancy PE, Orringer MB. Distinguishing features of adenocarcinoma in Barrett's esophagus and in the gastric cardia. In: Spechler SJ, Goyal RK (eds) Barrett's Esophagus: Pathophysiology, Diagnosis and Management. New York: Elsevier, 1985;167—187.
2. Kalish RJ, Clancy PE, Orringer MB, Appelman HD. Clinical, epidemiologic, and morphologic comparison between adenocarcinomas arising in Barrett's esophageal mucosa and in the gastric cardia. Gastroenterology 1984;86:461—467.
3. Kuwano H, Ueo H, Sugimachi K, Inokuchi K, Toyoshima S, Enjoji M. Glandular or mucin-secreting components in squamous cell carcinoma of the esophagus. Cancer 1985;56:514—518.
4. Epstein JI, Sears DL, Tucker RS, Eagan JW Jr. Carcinoma of the esophagus with adenoid cystic differentiation. Cancer 1984;53:1131—1136.

Do all adenocarcinomas of the esophagus arise in Barrett's mucosa?

J.H. Peters, G.W.B. Clark, T.R. DeMeester (Los Angeles)

The incidence of esophageal adenocarcinoma is rising faster than any other solid tumor in the United States and Great Britain [1—3]. In many referral centers adenocarcinoma, once an uncommon malignancy, represents up to 50—90% of patients referred for esophagectomy. The reasons for this striking increase in the incidence of esophageal adenocarcinoma are unclear. The most important etiologic factor in the development of primary adenocarcinoma of the esophagus is a metaplastic columnar lined or Barrett's esophagus, which occurs as a complication in approximately 10% of patients with gastroesophageal reflux disease (GERD) [4]. The incidence of adenocarcinoma in a patient with Barrett's esophagus has been estimated between 1/56 to 1/441 patient years [5]. Although this risk appears to be small, it is at least 30—40 times that expected for a similar population without Barrett's esophagus. This risk is similar to the risk for developing cancer of the lung in a person with a 20 pack-year history of smoking.

Do all adenocarcinoma's of the esophagus arise in Barrett's mucosa? Perhaps. There are three lines of evidence that suggest that this may be so, epidemiologic similarities, physiologic characteristics and histologic findings.

Epidemiologic evidence

Squamous carcinoma accounts for the majority of esophageal carcinomas worldwide. The epidemiologic characteristics of esophageal squamous carcinoma are in striking contrast to that of adenocarcinoma. In the United States squamous carcinoma occurs most commonly in black male smokers, often with a history of heavy alcohol use. In areas where there is a particularly high incidence, environmental factors may play a role.

This epidemiologic pattern is quite different than that seen in esophageal adenocarcinoma. Esophageal adenocarcinomas almost always arise in areas of Barrett's metaplasia, usually in specialized intestinal type mucosa, and predominantly affect elderly white males who often have a history of heavy smoking. Barrett's metaplasia is accepted as a complication of GERD and links this common disease to one of the most lethal carcinomas. The pathogenesis of the remainder of esophageal adenocarcinomas, usually located at the gastroesophageal junction, is less clear, but characteristics of tumors at this site are strikingly similar to Barrett's cancers and are rising in a parallel fashion (Fig. 1) [6]. Both occur with peak incidence in the seventh decade of life. Both have a markedly male predominance. Ninety three percent of patients with esophageal adenocarcinoma with or without Barrett's metaplasia were male (Table 1). Over half of both groups had a history of smoking. Barrett's cancers have a somewhat higher incidence GER symptoms. Seventy five percent of patients with adenocarcinoma arising in Barrett's metaplasia had a history of GERD while only 39% of non-Barrett's cancer patients did. These similar epidemiologic characteristics, coupled with the markedly differing epidemiology of squamous cell carcinoma, suggest a common etiology for Barrett's and non-Barrett's tumors.

Physiologic evidence

Barrett's esophagus is now accepted to be the result of severe GERD. Ninety percent of patients have a mechanically defective lower esophageal sphincter and 93% having abnormal esophageal acid exposure on pH monitoring [7].

In order to convincingly postulate that all esophageal adenocarcinomas arise within Barrett's mucosa, the existence of premalignant short segment Barrett's must be accepted [8]. Many tumors of the gastroesophageal junction probably originate from short segments of Barrett's, but the tumors quickly overgrow these short segments of change making it impossible to determine the source of the tumor from the resected specimen. If this is true then the association between chronic GERD and adenocarcinoma may be higher than generally appreciated. Physiologic similarities between short- and long-segment Barrett's suggest that this might be the case.

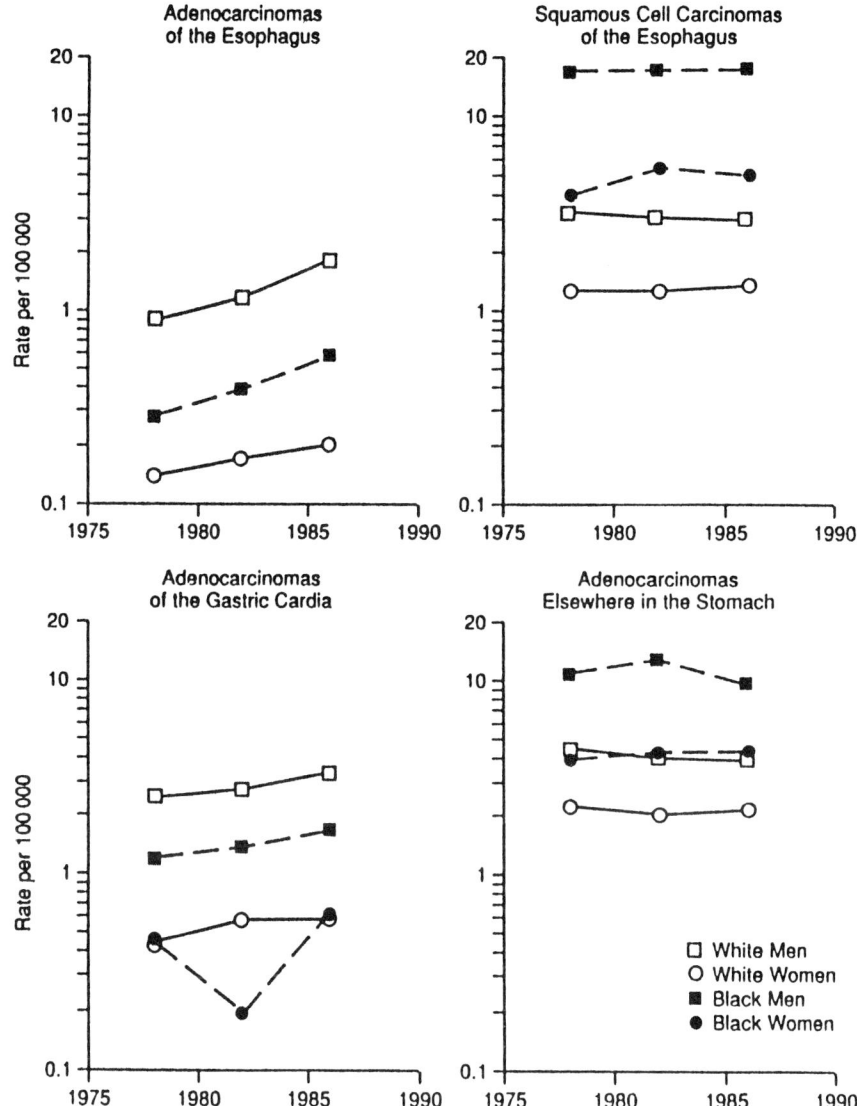

Fig. 1. Trends in age-adjusted incidence rates of esophageal and stomach cancers by histology and anatomic site, sex and race, showing a rise in the incidence of both adenocarcinoma of the esophagus and gastric cardia, suggesting that factors responsible for the development of these concerns may be similar. With permission from [2].

We investigated hypothesis that patients with short segments of Barrett's esophagus, measuring 3 cm or less, but with specialized intestinal columnar metaplasia on biopsy, have similar pathophysiological abnormalities to patients with more extensive Barrett's change, including the propensity for complications and in particular the development of malignancy [9].

Table 1. Epidemiologic characteristics of patients with esophageal adenocarcinoma, with and without Barrett's metaplasia

Characteristic	Barrett's (n = 51)	Non-Barrett's (n = 28)
% White males	92%	93%
Smoking history	80%	68%
History of GERD	75%	39%

Short segments of Barrett's esophagus (≤3 cm) were detected in 20 patients who presented to our laboratory. These patients had a high prevalence of a mechanically defective lower esophagal sphincter (LES) and were shown to have abnormal esophageal acid exposure on esophageal pH testing, the same physiologic abnormalities as were identified in patients with more extensive Barrett's metaplasia (Fig. 2). Furthermore, patients with short segments of Barrett's metaplasia had poor esophageal body motility which affected more than 4/5 of the esophageal length, despite the fact that the length of Barrett's was restricted to several centimeters, emphasizing the severity of the reflux disease. The extent of the pathophysiological abnormalities in patients with short segment Barrett's were graded in between those of the patients with esophagitis and those of the patients with extended Barrett's. This suggests that short-segment disease occurs at an earlier stage of disease compared to patients with extended Barrett's esophagus. The prevalence of complications was similar in patients with short-segment Barrett's and patients with extended Barrett's (Fig. 3). Complica-

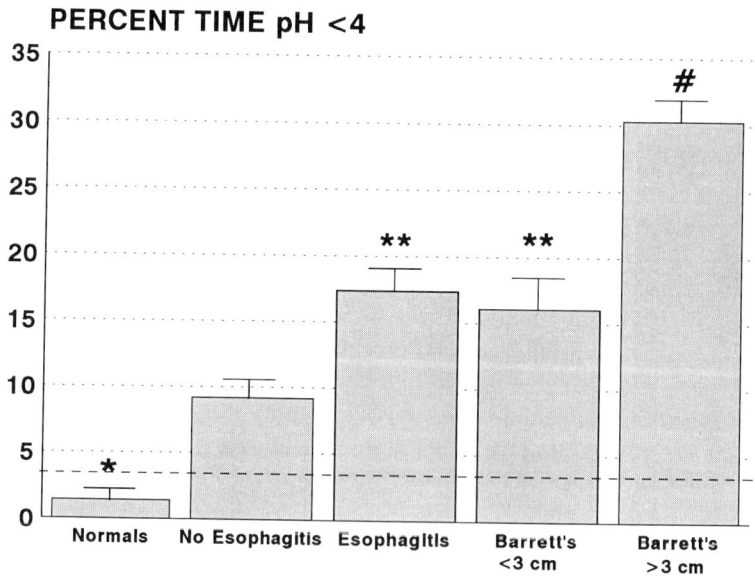

Fig. 2. Percent of the total time the esophageal pH was below 4 in each of the study groups.
* = significant difference between the groups (Kruscal Wallis, χ^2 = 129.9, df, p < 0.01). ** = significant difference vs. normals and no esophagitis (Mann Whitney, p < 0.01 and p < 0.05, respectively).
# = significantly different to no esophagitis, esophagitis and short segment Barrett's groups (Mann Whitney, all p < 0.01).

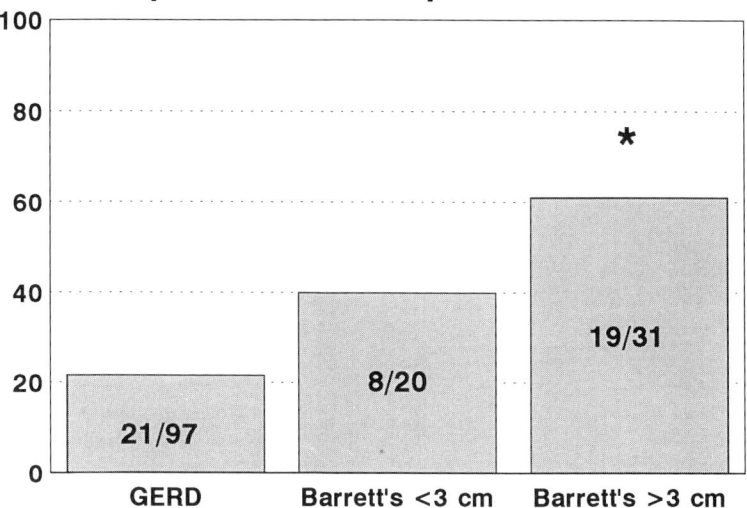

% of patients with complications

Fig. 3. Prevalence of complications in the GERD group vs. the prevalence in each of the Barrett's groups. * = p < 0.01 vs. GERD (Fisher's exact test).

tions occurred in 40% of patients with short segments of Barrett's including stricture and more importantly dysplasia. Two of our patients underwent esophagectomy for high-grade dysplasia in segments of Barrett's measuring ≤3 cm in length which were located at the gastroesophageal junction.

In a series of patients with small noncircumferential Barrett's adenocarcinomas (measuring ≤3 cm long, many of whom had intramucosal carcinomas), 25% had adenocarcinomas arising in Barrett's mucosa which was estimated to be ≤3 cm in length (Table 2). High-grade dysplasia was present in the Barrett's segment in all of these tumors suggesting that the Barrett's was the source of these tumors.

The results of this study indicate that all lengths of specialized intestinal metaplasia are associated with GERD, and that short segments of Barrett's have a potential for complications and adenocarcinoma formation. When specialized intestinal metaplasia is present, even in a single biopsy, the endoscopist can confidently make the diagnosis of Barrett's esophagus. The 3-cm rule for the diagnosis of Barrett's esophagus may no longer be appropriate in the presence of specialized intestinal columnar metaplasia. Patients with short segment Barrett's esophagus should be considered at risk for malignancy and should be offered endoscopic surveillance.

Histologic evidence

Although only 40% of patients with esophageal adenocarcinoma have Barrett's metaplasia detected on preoperative endoscopy, careful histologic examination

Table 2. Endoscopic and histological characteristics in patients with small Barrett's adenocarcinomas

Patient number	Endoscopic length of tumor (cm)[a]	Endoscopic length of Barrett's (cm)[b]	Appearance of Barrett's	Dysplastic Barrett's on histology
1	2	microscopic		High grade
2	3	microscopic		High grade
3	1	1	Circumferential	High grade
4	3	2	Tongue	High grade
5	None	5	Circumferential	High grade
6	3	5	Circumferential	High grade
7	1	6	Circumferential	No
8	1	6	Circumferential	High grade
9	1	7	Circumferential	High grade
10	None	7	Circumferential	High grade
11	3	8	Circumferential	High grade
12	None	9	Circumferential	High grade
13	None	10	Circumferential	High grade
14	2	10	Circumferential	High grade
15	3	11	Circumferential	Low grade
16	2	12	Circumferential	No

[a]None refers to invasive intramucosal carcinomas, detected histologically in the absence of any obvious mucosal abnormality.
[b]In two tumors there was no Barrett's mucosa seen endoscopically but specialized intestinal metaplasia was present at the margins of the tumor on histology.

demonstrates associated Barrett's changes in 65–75% of patients. In addition, esophageal adenocarcinoma occurs almost exclusively at or near the gastroesophageal junction, particularly in patients with no evidence of Barrett's mucosa. Why should this be so if GER plays no role in its development? Hamilton and Cameron carefully reviewed the specimens of 61 patients with esophageal adenocarcinoma (39 Barrett's, 22 non-Barrett's) [10]. In nearly all patients, the tumor was close to, or included, the gastroesophageal junction. The mean length from the center of the tumor to the gastroesophageal junction was 20 mm in Barrett's cancers and 1 mm in non-Barrett's adenocarcinoma's. The propensity of esophageal adenocarcinoma to arise in close apposition to the gastroesophageal junction, particularly so when Barrett's changes are not seen, supports the concept that all esophageal adenocarcinoma's arise within Barrett's metaplastic changes.

Summary

Esophageal adenocarcinoma has replaced squamous cell cancer as the predominant histologic type in most Western countries. Several lines of evidence suggest that the majority, if not all, esophageal adenocarcinoma arises within Barrett's esophagus. Seventy percent of esophageal adenocarcinoma arises in conjunction with Barrett's metaplastic changes. The epidemiologic features of esophageal adenocarcinoma are in striking contrast to those of squamous cell cancer and appear similar with or without Barrett's mucosal changes. Short segment Barrett's metaplasia does occur, has similar physiologic characteristics to longer segment disease and can result in malignancy. Finally, careful histologic examination demonstrates the majority of esophageal adenocarcinoma to arise at or near the gastroesophageal junction. Taken together these data strongly suggest that GER and Barrett's metaplasia play a role in most instances of esophageal adenocarcinoma.

References

1. Hesketh PJ, Clapp RW, Doos WG, Spechler SJ. The increasing frequency of adenocarcinoma of the esophagus. Cancer 1989;64:526–530.
2. Blot WJ, Devesa SS, Kneller RW, Fraumeni JF. Rising incidence of adenocarcinoma of the esophagus and gastric cardia. JAMA 1991;265(10):1287–1289.
3. Pera M, Cameron AJ, Trastek VF, Carpenter HA, Zinmeister AR. Increasing incidence of adenocarcinoma of the esophagus and esophagogastric junction. Gastroenterology 1993;104:510–513.
4. Cameron AJ, Lomboy CT. Barrett's esophagus: age, prevalence, and extent of columnar epithelium. Gastroenterology 1992;103:1241–1245.
5. Williamson WA, Ellis FH, Gibb SP et al. Barrett's esophagus: prevalence and incidence of adenocarcinoma. Arch Int Med 1991;151:2212–2216.
6. Duhaylongsod FG, Wolfe WG. Barrett's esophagus and adenocarcinoma of the esophagus and gastroesophageal junction. J Thorac Cardiovasc Surg 1992;102:36–42.
7. Iascone C, DeMeester TR, Little AG, Skinner DB. Barrett's esophagus. Functional assessment, proposed pathogenesis and surgical therapy. Arch Surg 1993;118:543–549.
8. Schnell TG, Sontag SJ, Chejfec G. Adenocarcinoma arising in tongues or short segment Barrett's esophagus. Dig Dis Sci 1992;37:137–143.
9. Clark GB, Smyrk TC, Hoeft SF, Burdiles P, Dreuw B, Crookes PF, Peters JH, DeMeester TR. Is the length of Barrett's mucosa related to prevalence of complications and adenocarcinoma in Barrett's esophagus. Gastroenterology 1993;104(4):A393.
10. Hamilton SR, Smith RR, Cameron JL. Prevalence and characteristics of Barrett esophagus in patients with adenocarcinoma of the esophagus or esophagogastric junction. Hum Pathol 1988;19:942–948.

Does the identical specific chromosomal rearrangements recently identified in adenocarcinomas of gastric and esophageal origin suggest that these tumors are biologically related?
What is the clinical value of oncogene amplification and protein overexpression?

Y. Nabeya, N.K. Altorki, A.P. Albino (New York)

Among adenocarcinomas of esophageal and gastric origin, cancers arising from the esophagus, gastroesophageal (GE) junction and proximal stomach (cardia) have been reported to be increasing in incidence in the United States, while cancer incidence elsewhere in the stomach is steady or in slight decline [1]. In addition, stage for stage, even after curative resections, the prognosis for patients with proximal (esophagus, GE junction and cardia) tumors is poor compared with that of patients with distal (gastric body and antrum) tumors [2]. These clinical observations suggest the existence of biological differences between proximal and distal tumors. Furthermore, these data raise the question of whether esophageal cancer and cardia cancer (i.e., proximal tumors), share molecular characteristics which result in a worse clinical outcome, characteristics that are not shared by distal tumors. Techniques in cell biology, molecular genetics and molecular biology have advanced so much that it is now possible to use these methodologies to more precisely define the molecular basis of esophageal and gastric cancers and apply this knowledge to better understand the development and clinical outcome of these neoplasms. In this brief summary two independent, but related questions, will be addressed: firstly, does the identical specific chromosomal rearrangements recently identified in adenocarcinomas of esophageal and gastric origin suggest that these tumors are biologically related? Secondly, what is the clinical value of oncogene amplification and protein over-expression?

The normal gastric mucosa is lined by columnar epithelial cells which populate the adenocarcinoma upon malignant transformation. In contrast, the normal esophagus is lined by squamous epithelium from which adenocarcinoma could not arise directly. Most esophageal and GE junction adenocarcinomas appear to arise from Barrett's esophagus, where damaged squamous cells are replaced by columnar cells which proliferate to form an abnormal epithelium with histologic features of both gastric and intestinal mucosae [3]. Specific or nonrandom cytogenetic changes have been shown to correlate with tumor histology and clinical behavior in a number of tumor systems. Moreover, these changes have identified chromosomal sites of gene derangement of significance, to tumor etiology and progression and have targeted sites for molecular analyses. No specific or nonrandom chromosomal abnormalities have yet been identified in esophageal or gastric adenocarcinomas. However, we have recently identified gene amplification in the form of homogeneously staining regions (HSRs) and double minute chromosomes (DMs), and determined that rearrangements involving the region 11p13-15 are a frequent abnormality in adenocarcinomas developing in the lower esophageal, GE junction and gastric regions [4]. Pathologically, these tumors are closely related, to the extent that adenocarcinomas of the lower esophagus and GE junction develop in Barrett's metaplasia where the squamous epithelium of the esophagus is replaced by glandular epithelium. Thus, our cytogenetic data suggest that the tumors arising at all these sites are biologically related. Genetic changes affecting the 11p13-15 region have been previously associated with several types of solid tumors (e.g., Wilms' tumor, hepatoblastoma and rhabdomyosarcoma [5], carcinoma of the bladder [6] and carcinoma of the breast [7]). These types of changes may involve loss of a suppressor gene function. Moreover, because this common chromosomal rearrangement at 11p13-15 was not observed in premalignant Barrett's esophagus [8], it may be more relevant to the development of frank cancers of esophageal and gastric origin rather than to initiation events. However, the frequent occurrence of isochrome 5p and rearrangements involving the 3p14-23 regions in esophageal and gastric cancers found in this study [4] is consistent with findings in other adenocarcinomas, such as those developing in the kidney, lung and breast [9] and may reflect critical defects in the evolution of these cancer types. The c-*ras* Ha-1 proto-oncogene is localized to band 11p15, and enhanced expression of the Ha-*ras* gene has been found in gastric adenocarcinomas compared with benign lesions [10]. This suggests that transformation of gastric mucosa is associated with overexpression of the *ras* gene protein. However, since no significant difference has been shown in the incidence of mutated *ras* genes between proximal and distal tumors [11], consistent gene rearrangements in the region of the *ras* gene may cause a deregulation of this gene. An earlier study demonstrated a significantly higher incidence of DNA aneuploidy in proximal cancers than in distal gastric cancers and a worse disease-free survival of patients with aneuploid tumors [12]. Thus, these data suggest a more rapid accumulation of genetic defects in proximal tumors, and imply that while adenocarcinomas of the lower esophagus, GE junction and proximal and distal stomach may share a common genetic origin, the necessary alterations required for a fully developed cancer at these sites may differ. The higher frequency of genetic derangement in proximal cancers may be due to additional defects in the mechanisms that monitor DNA damage and effect repair in this subset of cancers which do not arise or are mitigated by other genes in distal cancers. Further experimentation should elucidate the molecular basis for the increase in proximal cancers of the esophagus and gastric cardia, and determine whether these cancers have a common origin with adenocarcinomas of the distal stomach.

In addition to potential clinical significance of chromosomal rearrangements, the presence of DMs in 45% of esophageal and gastric adenocarcinomas suggests frequent gene amplification. Double minute chromosomes as well as HSRs have been noted occasionally in esophageal and gastric tumors [8,13,14]. Concomitant with the development of DMs and HSRs regions is the amplification of proto-oncogenes. This appears to be a common event in adenocarcinomas arising at many anatomical sites and suggests that this is an important mechanism of tumor progression. Accordingly, a number of studies have detected amplifications of several proto-oncogenes in gastric adenocarcinomas including c-*myc* [15,16], c-*yes*-1 [17], *int*-2/*hst*-1 [18], c-*erb*B [19], c-*met* [20] and HER-2/*neu* (c-*erb*B-2) [20]. However, direct evidence for the consistent, and thus direct, involvement of any known oncogene, growth factor, regulatory element or other type of gene in the pathogenesis of adenocarcinomas of the esophagus and stomach is still lacking. Moreover, there is no clear correlation between increases in the gene dosages of proto-oncogenes and tumor development. Despite this paucity of information, genetic alterations, such as amplifications, are thought to represent a critical, if as yet undefined, perturbation in the malignant process.

Studies in a number of other solid tumors indicate that various types of genetic alterations, including amplifications, may have valuable clinical applications. For example, amplification of HER-2/*neu* has been shown to be associated with aggressive behavior of breast carcinomas [21]. HER-2/*neu* may be one gene which has a significant role in the biology of gastric cancer, since HER-2/*neu* is overexpressed in 8—12% of gastric cancers with several instances of gene rearrangements [20], and appears to be a potential prognostic indicator in the development of gastric cancer [22].

In an ongoing study designed to determine if the observed clinical differences between proximal and distal gastric cancers are due to defined genetic abnormalities such as gene amplification, we evaluated HER-2/*neu* in adenocarcinomas of GE junction and stomach. In this study, we noticed that HER-2/*neu* gene amplification (from 16—24 fold) was found in 10% of distal tumors, but not in any proximal tumor (unpublished data). However, no correlation was found between gene amplification and histological type. In contrast, another study has observed that amplification and overexpression of HER-2/*neu* may be associated with well-differentiated (or intestinal type) gastric adenocarcinoma [23]. Thus, although no specific chromosomal re-arrangements involving 17q21 (the location of the HER-2/*neu* gene) have been reported in esophageal and gastric adenocarcinomas, amplification of this gene may define a subset of distal tumors. The reason and clinical significance of this specific amplification of HER-2/*neu* gene in distal tumors, however, is still unclear. There is speculation that HER-2/*neu* rearrangements may be involved in the genesis or progression of distal gastric cancers. These cancers are frequently accompanied by atrophic gastritis and intestinal metaplasia with aging that may, therefore, be a region of the stomach predisposed to develop adenocarcinomas. This is in contrast to GE junction where chronic excessive GE reflux may have an implication for the devel-opment of adenocarcinomas around this anatomical site, especially in Barrett's epi-thelium [3]. That is, it is possible that differences in progenitor cells or cellular milieu as well as exposure to different carcinogens could cause the specific HER-2/*neu* amplification in distal tumors, although these differences would not account for the divergence in clinical outcomes.

At present, the proto-oncogene most frequently implicated in gastric cancer may be c-*met* gene. The c-*met* gene was initially identified in human osteosarcoma cell line transformed in vitro by N-methyl-N'-nitro-N-nitrosoguanidine (MNNG) [24]. Since MNNG is a potent carcinogen which can induce gastric tumors in experimental animals [25], it is of interest to reveal a possible role of the c-*met* gene in gastric carcinogenesis. A recent study showed good correlation between c-*met* amplification and clinical stage or patient prognosis [26]. However, no specific chromosomal defects (e.g., rearrangements, DMs, HSRs, etc.) of 7q31 (the location of c-*met*) have been found to account for c-*met* gene amplification in esophageal and gastric adenocarcinomas. A c-*met* 6.0-kilobase (kb) mRNA transcript expressed in gastric cancer was reported to be linked with tumor staging, lymph node metastasis and depth of tumor invasion [26]. An additional defect involving this gene has been noted in gastritis as well as gastric cancer [27]. This defect involves a rearrangement that places the translocated promoter region (tpr) of an unknown gene located on chromosome 1p to the proximal region of the c-*met* gene. This rearrangement causes the expression of a novel *tpr-met* 5.0-kb transcript in gastritis as well as gastric cancer [27]. While the biological significance of these observations are still unclear, these results do suggest that amplifications and rearrangements of the c-*met* proto-oncogene may play a role at an early stage of gastric carcinogenesis and could, therefore, be a useful predictive marker.

Other types of genetic alterations occurring in esophageal and gastric adenocarcinomas may involve dysfunction of tumor suppressor genes (e.g., the p53 gene). Mutations and allelic deletions of the p53 gene, which is located at chromosome 17p13, have been found in a variety of human neoplasms and are among the most common defects in human cancers [28]. Although p53 mutations and 17p deletions may play an important role in carcinogenesis of the esophagus [29] and stomach [30], no good correlation has been reported between the disruption of this gene and clinical parameters such as histological grade or primary site. Thus, the clinical significance of p53 mutations and 17p alterations in esophageal and gastric cancers is not clear. One interesting report has detected p53 mutations in esophageal epithelium in five out of 12 patients with Barrett's esophagus and coexisting adenocarcinoma, whereas no mutations were found in 10 patients with Barrett's esophagus, but with no concomitant cancer [31]. Cancers arising in Barrett's epithelium with a mutant p53 did not contain p53 mutations corresponding to those found in the Barrett's epithelium [32]. These results suggest that p53 mutations in premalignant Barrett's esophagus may reflect a generalized genetic instability (possibly a "field cancerization" effect) and susceptibility to malignant change and that p53 mutations in Barrett's epithelium may be of predictive value for the risk of developing esophageal cancer. Another possibility is that p53 mutations are necessary for the progression of premalignant to malignant cells. Moreover, these data also suggest that cells with p53 mutations may be more at risk for accumulating lethal types of DNA or cellular damage and thus do not survive in Barrett's epithelium. From this point of view, p53 mutations might occur as a response to various stresses, including chronic GE reflux, and may therefore, be a result rather than a cause of genetic damage in carcinogenesis of Barrett's cancer.

In summary, the linkage of genetic alterations with specific neoplasms has been accelerating [33]. The determination of specific alterations would clearly be advantageous in designing novel therapies and in screening high-risk populations. However, convincing evidence for the association of a specific genetic defect in the development of esophageal and gastric adenocarcinomas is still lacking. Despite this caveat, some genetic alterations could be useful if their incidence is found to be significantly higher in cancer lesions than corresponding normal tissue. Such common genetic or chromosomal defects could represent an underlying etiologic event in adenocarcinomas. If specific genetic alterations were found in esophageal and gastric cancers, their detection would be useful for determining several clinical parameters (e.g., the risk of metastasis or developing a second cancer), the likelihood of response to specific chemotherapeutic agents, etc. [31]. It is expected that, with further study, the evolution of esophageal and gastric adenocarcinoma can, like colorectal tumors, be correlated with specific genetic defects that occur in a temporal manner. The identification of these defects would be of immense value in understanding cancers of the esophagus and stomach, which world-wide are among the most common cancers in humans.

References

1. Blot WJ et al. Rising incidence of adenocarcinoma of the esophagus and gastric cardia. JAMA 1991;265:1287—1289.
2. Fein R et al. Adenocarcinoma of the esophagus and gastroesophageal junction: Prognostic factors and results of therapy. Cancer 1985;56:2512—2518.
3. DeMeester TR. Barrett's esophagus. Surgery 1993;113:239—241.
4. Rodriguez E et al. 11p13-15 is a specific region of chromosomal rearrangement in gastric and esophageal adenocarcinomas. Cancer Res 1990;50:6410—6416.
5. Koufos A et al. Loss of heterozygosity in three embryonal tumors suggests a common pathogenic mechanism. Nature 1985; 316:330—334.
6. Fearon ER et al. Loss of genes on the short arm of chromosome 11 in bladder cancer. Nature 1985;318:377—380.
7. Theillet C et al. Loss of a c-H-*ras*-1 allele and aggressive human primary breast carcinomas. Cancer Res 1986;46:4776—4781.
8. Garewal HS et al. Chromosomal rearrangements in Barrett's esophagus: A premalignant lesion of esophageal adenocarcinoma. Cancer Genet Cytogenet 1989;42:281—296.
9. Chaganti RSK et al. In: Cossman J (ed) Molecular Genetics and the Diagnosis of Cancer. New York: Elsevier Science Publishers, 1992.
10. Nakajima K et al. Immunohistochemical study of *ras* p21 expression in human gastric cancers and benign lesions. Oncology 1989;46:260—265.
11. Nanus DM et al. Infrequent point mutations of *ras* oncogenes in gastric cancers. Gastroenterology 1990;98:955—960.
12. Nanus DM et al. Flow cytometry as a predictive indicator in patients with operable gastric cancer. J Clin Oncol 1989;7: 1105—1112.
13. Ferti-Passantonopoulou AD et al. Common cytogenetic findings in gastric cancer. Cancer Genet Cytogenet 1987;24:63—73.
14. Young GP et al. The genetics, epidemiology and early detection of gastrointestinal cancers. Curr Opin Oncol 1992;4: 728—735.
15. Shibuya M et al. Amplification and expression of a cellular oncogene (c-*myc*) in human gastric adenocarcinoma cells. Mol Cell Biol 1985;5:414—418.
16. Koda T et al. C-*myc* gene amplification in primary stomach cancer. Jpn J Cancer Res 1985;76:551—554.
17. Seiki T et al. Amplification of c-*yes*-1-oncogene in a primary human gastric cancer. Jpn J Cancer Res 1985;76:907—910.
18. Yoshida MC et al. Human HST/(HSTF1) gene maps to chromosome band 11q13 and coamplifies with the INT2 gene in human cancer. Proc Natl Acad Sci USA 1988;85:4861—4864.
19. Yoshida K et al. Amplification of epidermal growth factor receptor (EGFR) gene and oncogenes in gastric carcinomas. Virchows Arch 1989;57:285—290.
20. Houldsworth J et al. Gene amplification in gastric and esophageal adenocarcinomas. Cancer Res 1990;50:6417—6422.
21. Slamon DJ et al. Studies of the HER-2/*neu* proto-oncogene in human breast and ovarian cancer. Science 1989;244:707—712.
22. Jain S et al. c-*erb*B-2 proto-oncogene expression and its relationship to survival in gastric carcinoma: An immunohistochemical study on archival material. Int J Cancer 1991;48:668—671.
23. Kameda T et al. Expression of ERBB2 in human gastric carcinomas: Relationship between p185[ERBB2] expression and the gene amplification. Cancer Res 1991;50:8002—8009.
24. Cooper CS et al. Molecular cloning of a new transforming gene from a chemically transformed human cell line. Nature 1984;311:29—33.
25. Sugimura T et al. Tumor production in glandular stomach of rat by N-methyl-N'-nitro-N-nitrosoguanidine. Nature 1967; 216:943—944.
26. Kuniyasu H et al. Gene alteration and mRNA expression of c-*met* gene in human gastric carcinomas. Jpn Res Soc Gastroenterol Carcino 1992;4:19—25.
27. Soman NR et al. The *tpr-met* oncogenic rearrangement is present and expressed in human gastric carcinoma and precursor lesions. Proc Natl Acad Sci USA 1991;88:4892—4896.
28. Nigro JM et al. Mutations in the p53 gene occur in diverse human tumor types. Nature 1989;342:705—708.
29. Blount PL et al. 17p allelic deletions and p53 protein overexpression in Barrett's adenocarcinoma. Cancer Res 1991;51: 5482—5486.
30. Matozaki T et al. p53 gene mutations in human gastric cancer: Wild-type p53 but not mutant p53 suppresses growth of human gastric cancer cells. Cancer Res 1992;52:4335—4341.
31. Roth JA. Molecular surgery for cancer. Arch Surg 1992;127:1298—1302.
32. Casson AG et al. p53 gene mutations in Barrett's epithelium and esophageal cancer. Cancer Res 1991;51:4495—4499.
33. Marx J. New colon cancer gene discovered. Science 1993;260:751—752.

Does squamous cell carcinoma complicate Barrett's mucosa?

S.R. Hamilton (Baltimore)

Barrett's esophagus is a well-known premalignant condition for adenocarcinoma of the esophagus. In addition, however, squamous carcinoma of the esophagus has been reported in patients with Barrett's esophagus [1–6]. These cancers are typically located in the native squamous-lined esophageal mucosa proximal to the Barrett-lined segment, rather than within the columnar-lined region. Adenosquamous carcinoma has also been associated with Barrett's esophagus [7–9]. Of note, this subset of adenocarcinoma is typically within the Barrett-lined segment, rather than proximal to it, as is the case for "pure" squamous carcinomas.

In our series, squamous carcinoma represented 2% of Barrett-associated esophageal carcinomas over a 7-year period [1]. All eight cases reported in the literature [1–6] occurred in white men, representing a dramatic demographic difference from squamous carcinoma of the esophagus which is the most common in nonwhite patients in the United States. A common theme of the reported patients with squamous carcinoma in association with Barrett's esophagus is alcohol and tobacco usage along with neoplasia in other portions of the upper gastrointestinal tract.

The implications of the association of squamous carcinoma of the esophagus with Barrett's mucosa are uncertain at present since these tumors are infrequent. Due to the increased risk of esophageal adenocarcinoma, many authors recommend endoscopic surveillance of Barrett's mucosa. Biopsy of the squamous-lined segment proximal to the Barrett's mucosa can be accomplished at the time of surveillance. In addition, the association of alcoholic beverage and tobacco usage with neoplasia in patients with Barrett's esophagus suggests that cessation should be strongly recommended.

References

1. Rosengard A, Hamilton SR. Squamous carcinoma of the esophagus in patients with Barrett's esophagus. Mod Pathol 1989;2:2.
2. Allan NK, Weitzner S, Scott I., Khalil KG. Adenocarcinoma arising in Barrett's esophagus with synchronous squamous cell carcinoma of the esophagus. Southern Med J 1986;79:1036.
3. Burke EL, Sturm J, Williamson D. The diagnosis of microscopic carcinoma of the esophagus. Dig Dis Sci 1978;23:148.
4. Resano CH, Cabrera N, Gonzalez Cueto D, Sanchez Basso AE, Rubio HH. Double early epidermoid carcinoma of the esophagus in columnar epithelium. Endoscopy 1985;17:73.
5. Sheahan DG, Berman MA. Barrett's mucosa with multiple carcinomas of the esophagus and oral cavity. J Clin Gastroenterol 1986;8:103.
6. Tamura H, Schulman SA. Barrett-type esophagus associated with squamous carcinoma. Chest 1971;59:330.
7. Banner BF, Memoli VA, Warren WH, Gould VE. Carcinoma with multidirectional differentiation arising in Barrett's esophagus. Ultrastruct Path 1983;4:205.
8. Pascal RR, Clearfield HR. Mucoepidermoid (adenosquamous) carcinoma arising in Barrett's esophagus. Dig Dis Sci 1987;32:428.
9. Haggitt RC, Dean PJ. Adenocarcinoma in Barrett's epithelium. In: Spechler SJ, Goyal RK (eds) Barrett's Esophagus: Pathophysiology, Diagnosis, and Management. New York: Elsevier Science Publishers, 1985;153.

What are the characteristic differences between adenocarcinoma arising in CLE and squamous cell carcinoma of the esophagus?

A.H. Hölscher, E. Bollschweiler, J.R. Siewert (Munich)

In a series of 505 patients with resected esophageal carcinomas, we saw 302 squamous cell carcinomas (SC) (59.8%) and 203 adenocarcinomas (AC) (40.2%). The ratio of male to female was quite similar with 7:1 for squamous cell carcinomas and 8:1 for adenocarcinomas. The patients with squamous cell carcinomas, however, were in the median about 7 years younger than those with adenocarcinomas (SC: 52.9 (32–80) years; AC: 60.1 (29–82) years).

The localization of the esophageal cancers showed the usual distribution with all adenocarcinomas located in the infrabifurcal part of the esophagus whereas the squamous cell carcinomas showed 7% in the cervical part, 24% suprabifurcal, 21% *ad bifurcationem* and 51% infrabifurcal.

The histologic grading of the esophageal carcinomas was quite similar for squamous cell or adenocarcinomas (G1: 9.6 vs. 7.2%, G2: 45.4 vs. 47.8%, G3: 34.9 vs. 39.9%, G4: 10.1 vs. 5.1%). The postoperative T-category demonstrated more advanced T-stages for resected adenocarcinomas. The stage pT1 was found in 17% for SC and 13.5% for AC whereas stage pT2 amounted to 18.5% in SC and AC in 30.7%. The most striking difference was concerning the pT3-stage with 51% for SC and 30.1% for AC. In pT4-stages there were 13.5% for SC and 25.7% for AC. The comparison of the postoperative N-category between SC and AC is difficult because it is questionable if the UICC-classification of 1987 for squamous cell carcinoma of the esophagus should also be applied for adenocarcinoma of the distal esophagus. If one uses the pN-classification of gastric cancer for the adenocarcinoma of the distal esophagus, as we do for the adenocarcinoma of the gastroesophageal junction, the results are as follows: SC had 39% NO and AC 27.3%, whereas pN1-stage was found in 45.5% for SC and 34.1% for AC. 15.5% of the SC were classified as pM1 LYMPH, that means distal lymph node metastases and 38.6% of the AC-patients had a pN2-status. Concerning distant organ metastases (M1), like liver etc., the distribution was 6.3% for SC vs. 14.2% for AC.

If the alcohol consumption is compared between patients with squamous cell carcinoma and those with adenocarcinoma, there were more patients with high alcohol intake in the group of squamous cell carcinoma patients than in the group of adenocarcinoma patients (normal alcohol intake SC 21%, AC 34%; medium intake SC 55%, AC 56%; high intake SC 24%, AC 10%).

The long-term prognosis after resection of squamous cell carcinoma (transthoracic enbloc-resection) or adenocarcinoma (transmediastinal esophagectomy), was not significantly different. The 5-year survival rate for the series of 302 patients with resected squamous cell carcinomas was 22% vs. 28% for the patients with resected adenocarcinoma (n = 203). This slight, but not significant difference in survival between the two whole series, is due to a significant difference in the prognosis concerning the T 1-stage. Patients with Tl-adenocarcinoma (n = 27) had a significantly (p < 0.05) better prognosis than those patients with a T1-squamous cell carcinoma (n = 51) of the esophagus (78 vs. 53% 5-year survival rate) [1].

Reference

1. Hölscher AH, Bollschweiler E, Schüler M, Tachibana M, Nakamura T, Siewert JR. Early esophageal cancer: prognostic advantage of a adeno- compared to squamous cell carcinomas. Proceedings of the 5th International Congress of the International Society for Diseases of the Esophagus, Kyoto 1992;95.

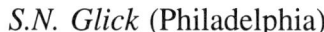 *S.N. Glick* (Philadelphia)

Malignant epithelial neoplasms of the hollow gastrointestinal viscera have a limited number of morphologic manifestations. Any combination of intraluminal polypoid growth, ulceration or narrowing of the lumen involving a length of approximately 3–6 cm and with abrupt transition to the adjacent uninvolved segments, is the rule. These tumors are predominantly adenocarcinomas with the exception of the esophagus, where the mucosa is lined by squamous cells. However, exposure to gastroesophageal reflux (GER) predisposes the latter to columnar metaplasia (Barrett's esophagus) in some patients and these individuals are at risk for the development of adenocarcinoma in the transformed tissue [1–5]. Indeed, almost all cases (with rare exceptions) of adenocarcinoma of the esophagus result from this pathogenetic pathway [6]. Furthermore, recent data suggests that adenocarcinoma represents over 1/3 of cancers of the esophagus and that the importance of this entity has been under-emphasized [2,4].

The diagnosis of adenocarcinoma arising in CLE is based upon the recovery of tissue through endoscopic biopsy. Thus a prospective specific histologic diagnosis based upon epidemiologic and radiologic information has little impact on patient management in most cases. However, they provide an improved understanding with regard to the significance of this process and in some cases contribute to the overall outcome. There are several diagnostic dilemmas that can be clarified. A high probability of adenocarcinoma of the esophagus can be suggested, with a distinction made between both squamous carcinoma of the esophagus and gastric carcinoma extending into the esophagus. Of greater importance is the ability to recognize radiologic features which suggest malignant neoplasm as opposed to, or superimposed upon, a benign peptic stricture. On occasion, endoscopy, even with biopsy and brushing, can be misleading.

From an epidemiologic perspective, Barrett's adenocarcinoma occurs predominantly in white males [1]. This relationship is not well understood. Conversely, squamous cell carcinoma is common in black males and has a high association with a history of alcohol ingestion and smoking. While there has been no evidence to link drinking with adenocarcinoma there have been conflicting reports concerning the influence of smoking [1]. Although a number of patients with adenocarcinoma in CLE will have a history of reflux symptoms, in as many as 50% such complaints cannot be elicited.

On barium esophagram, the most consistent feature of adenocarcinoma is the location of the lesion (Fig. 1A,B). A personal review of 23 cases of adenocarcinoma of the esophagus revealed 20 of the lesions having the epicenter (midpoint) within the lower 6–8 cm of the esophagus. Furthermore, during this same period there were

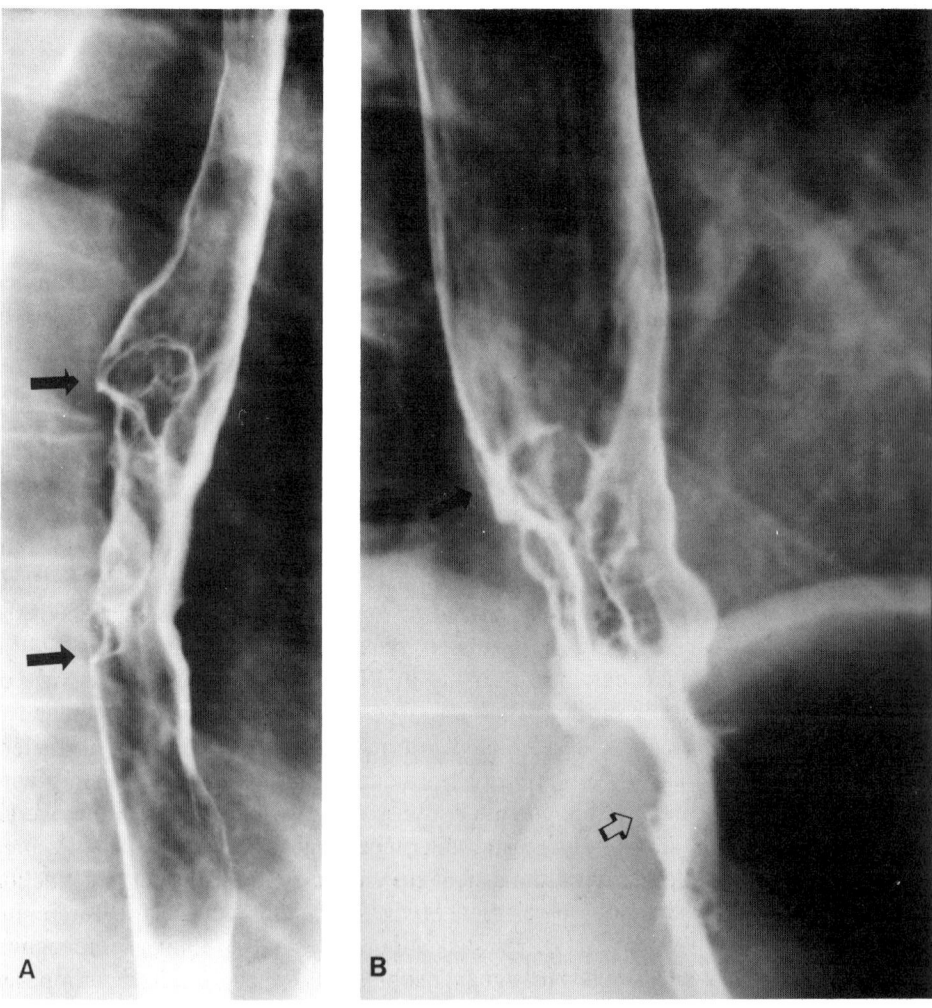

Fig. 1. A) Typical squamous cell carcinoma (arrows) appearing as lobulated plaque in the midesophagus. B) Adenocarcinoma in CLE with its superior component located in the distal 6 cm of the esophagus (black arrow) and its distal limit at the gastroesophageal junction (open arrow).

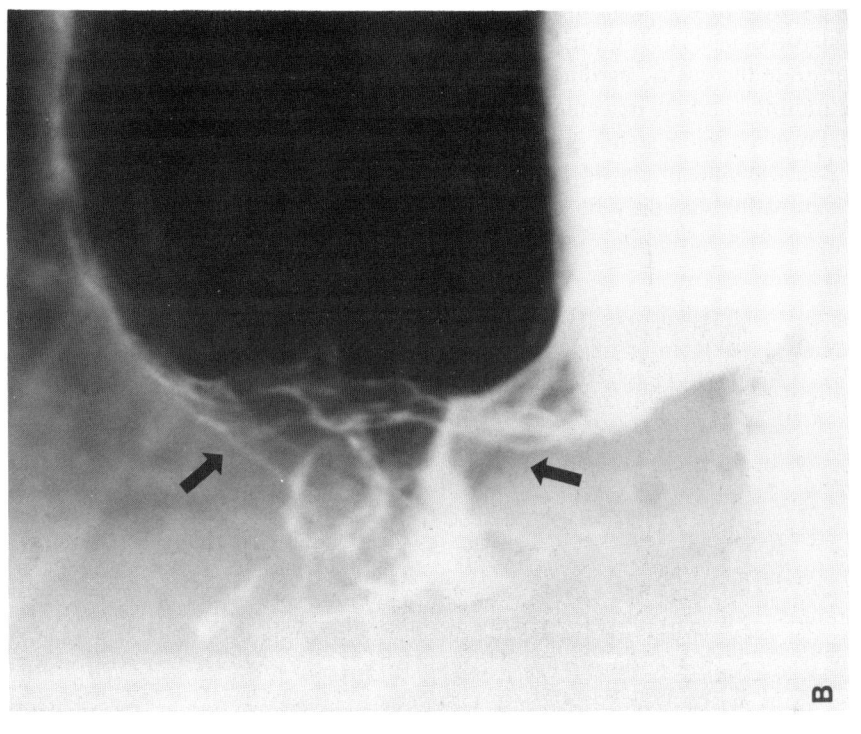

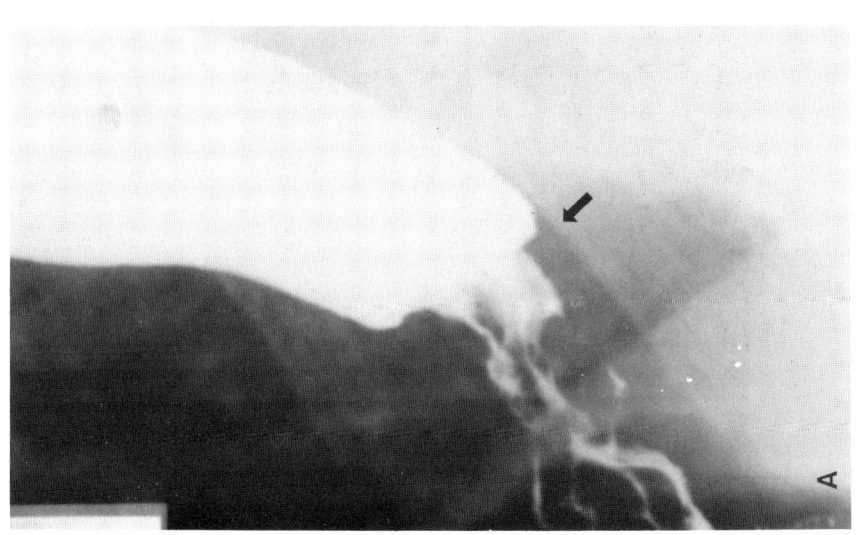

Fig. 2. A) Adenocarcinoma in CLE. Annular infiltrative lesion in the distal esophagus. B) Extension into the gastric cardia (arrows). Involvement of the stomach is minimal.

only two instances of squamous cell carcinoma arising in this segment. This is consistent with the proposed pathogenesis, as adenocarcinoma in CLE tends to arise within 2 cm of the histologic squamocolumnar junction and the transition is seldom higher than 8 cm from the anatomic gastroesophageal junction. In distinction from esophageal involvement from gastric adenocarcinoma, a minority of the tumors in CLE will infiltrate the gastric cardia, but as a rule the abnormalities identified in the stomach are minimal and the epicenter of the lesion will suggest an esophageal origin (Fig. 2A,B). From a clinical standpoint, this differential is probably of little relevance, although it is always beneficial to know the extent of a primary gastric tumor. At times this information can only be assessed by radiology, as the endoscope cannot

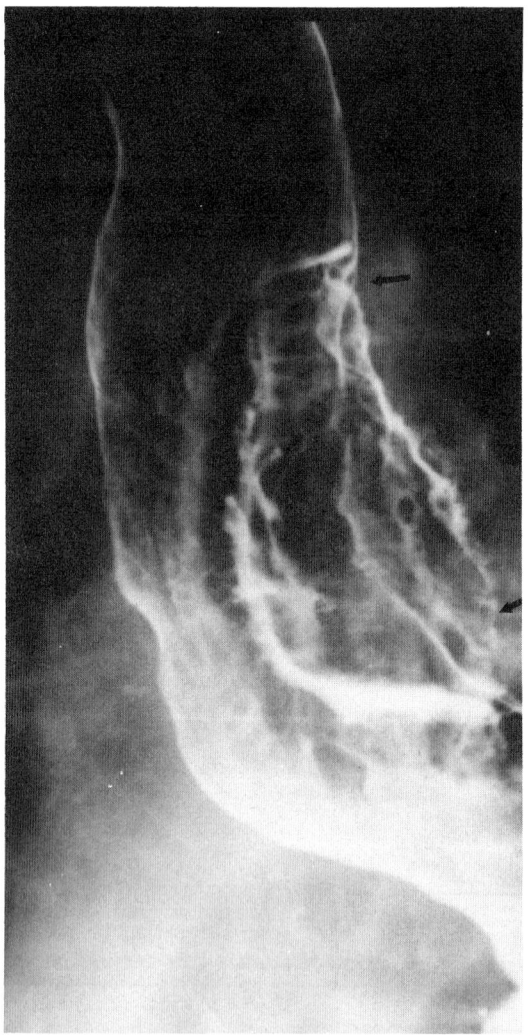

Fig. 3. Adenocarcinoma in CLE. Plaque-like appearance confined to one wall in distal esophagus (arrows). The lower esophagus is patulous and the adjacent mucosa demonstrates a reticular pattern.

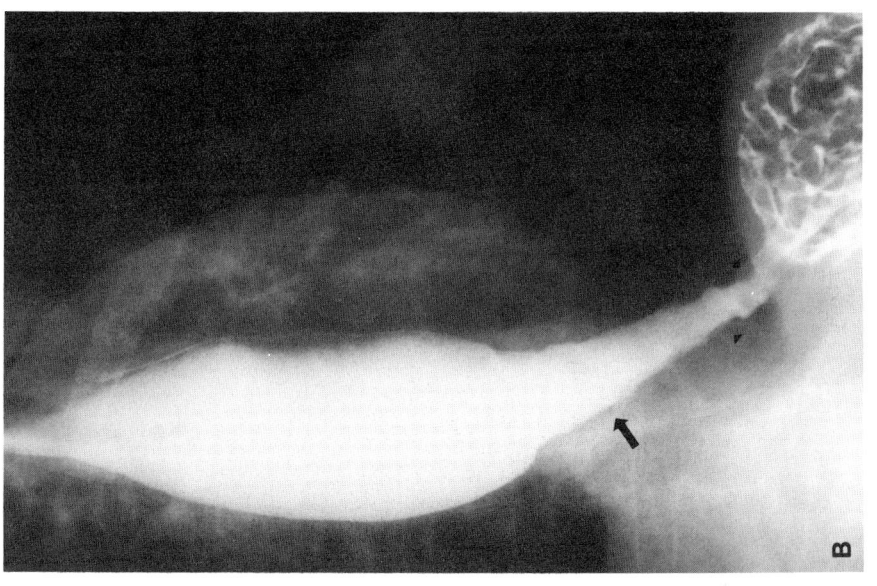

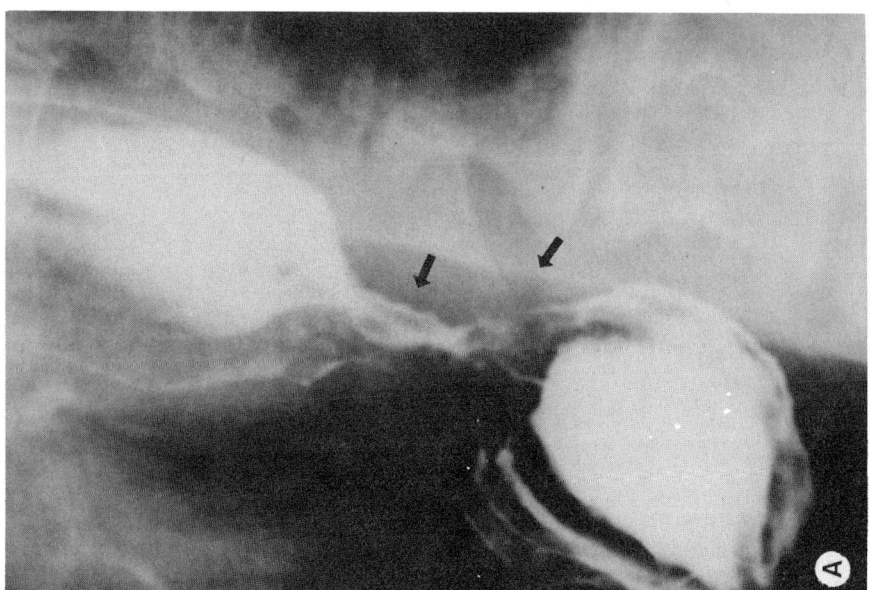

Fig. 4. A) Peptic stricture with malignant degeneration. Asymmetric narrowing with rounded mass effect and spiculatal contour (arrows). B) Peptic stricture with malignant degeneration. Long benign appearing stenosis (large arrow) with subtle nodular scalloping (small arrows) along mucosal surface.

transverse a high-grade stenosis, or the invasion is predominantly submucosal.

As stated previously, there usually is nothing specific with regard to the morphologic appearance of these epithelial neoplasms [7]. However, there are a few trends that should be recognized. Squamous cell carcinoma has a tendency to be circumferential while adenocarcinoma in CLE is, in the vast majority, confined to one wall (Fig. 3). The major exception is when adenocarcinoma is superimposed within a peptic stricture. The features that suggest neoplasm in this setting are: discrete mucosal nodules within the stenosis; numerous irregular barium spiculations within the stenosis (representing superficial ulceration and/or barium collecting between smaller nodules); submucosal defects within the stricture; and asymmetric transition with the normal lumen (proximally and/or distally) (Fig. 4A,B). Not only is the mass

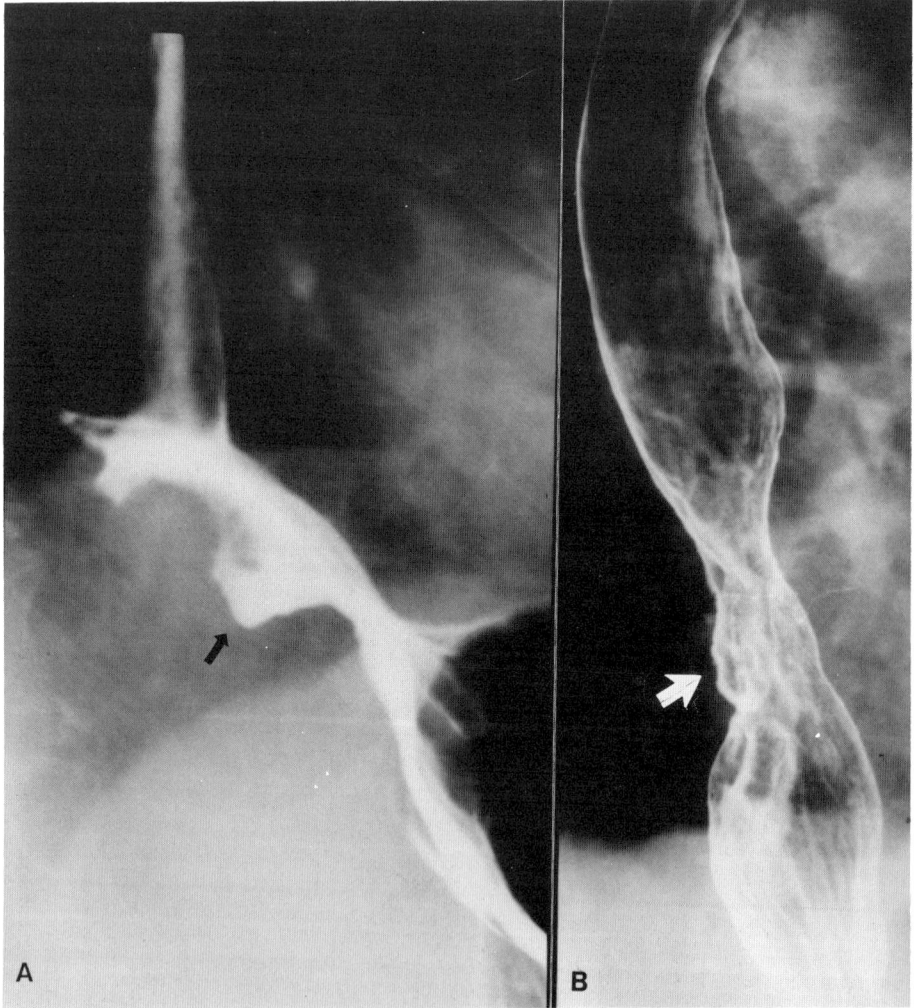

Fig. 5. A) Adenocarcinoma in CLE. Large mass in distal esophagus with deep central ulceration (arrow). B) Adenocarcinoma in CLE. Ulcerated mass (arrow) within benign peptic stricture just superior to a hiatal hernia.

in adenocarcinoma usually on one wall, but in the majority, a deep central ulcer crater surrounded by tumor can be demonstrated (Fig. 5A,B). This may be related to its columnar origin with behavioral characteristics more consistent with gastric adenocarcinoma. Such an appearance is uncommon in squamous cell carcinoma, so that when a lesion with these features is identified closer to the midesophagus, the possibility of adenocarcinoma increases. It has been suggested [7] that the involvement of a longer length segment of the esophagus with an infiltrative or varicoid appearance may be more typical of adenocarcinoma (Fig. 6A,B). While this does occur (and possibly in some, reflects the presence of a long peptic stricture), in my experience, it also may be seen in squamous cell carcinoma and neither the frequency nor the specificity is sufficient for reliable differentiation.

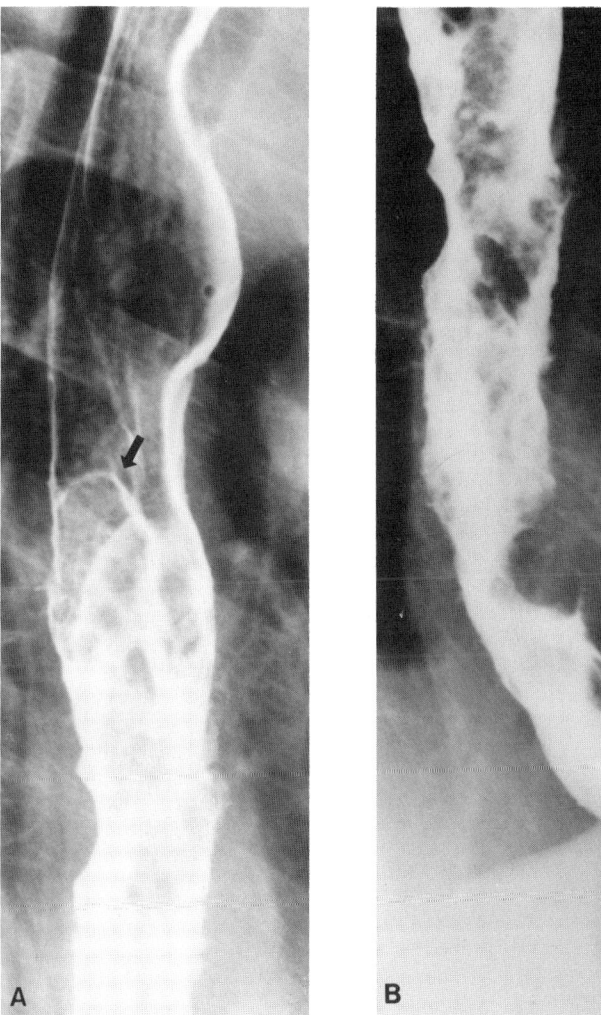
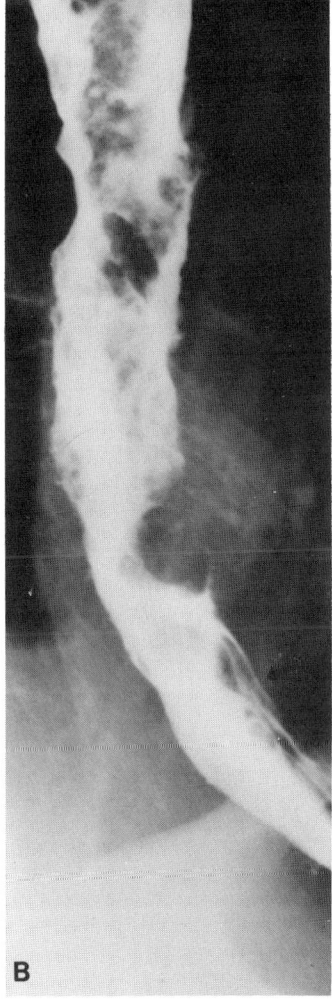

Fig. 6. A) Extensive varicoid adenocarcinoma. Proximal margin (arrow) is at the level of the tracheal bifurcation. B) The lesion extends to the distal esophagus. It has been postulated that this appearance is suggestive of adenocarcinoma.

On occasion, ancillary observations on barium study may predict a malignant appearing lesion to be adenocarcinoma. A large hiatal hernia, massive repeated GER, a wide patulous lower esophageal sphincter (LES) (>4 cm) and specific findings that suggest Barrett's esophagus (e.g., reticular mucosal pattern and midesophageal stricture) are included in this group [5].

One specific scenario should be mentioned. The previous discussion has focused upon cases of advanced adenocarcinoma. However, as patients with reflux symptoms undergo radiologic evaluation more frequently than those with squamous carcinoma (symptoms are usually late) the likelihood of detecting earlier lesions is increased [8].

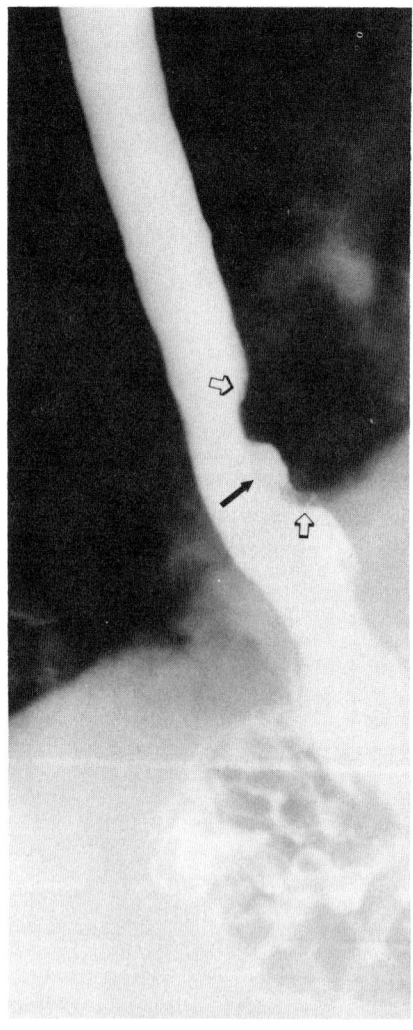

Fig. 7. Early adenocarcinoma. Small mass (open arrows) with central ulcer (arrow) in the distal esophagus. This was detected during work-up of reflux symptoms. The lesion was confined to the submucosa and the lymph nodes were normal.

The presence of any slight asymmetric narrowing or contour defect (i.e., flattening or mural elevation) or nodular or polypoidal mucosal excrescences should heighten the index of suspicion (Fig. 7). Any discrete ulcer should also be approached cautiously. Even when initial endoscopy and biopsy are not confirmatory, such alterations should be aggressively pursued.

In summary, in most cases the radiologic distinction between adenocarcinoma in CLE and squamous cell carcinoma can be readily made on the basis of a distal location, particularly in a white male. The presence of a history of reflux symptoms provides further support. With more proximal tumors, a deep discrete ulcer may also help differentiate. However, the major value of barium radiology involves those instances of malignant degeneration within a peptic stricture, determining the presence and extent of gastric involvement and, most importantly, subtle alterations which may predict an early and more curable lesion.

References

1. Menke-Pluymers MBE, Hop WCJ, Dees J et al. Risk factors for the development of an adenocarcinoma in columnar-lined (Barrett's) esophagus. Cancer 1993;72:1155–1158.
2. Pera M, Cameron AJ, Trastek VF et al. Increasing incidence of adenocarcinoma of the esophagus and esophagogastric junction. Gastroenterology 1993;104:510–513.
3. Duhaylongsod FG, Wolfe WG. Barrett's esophagus and adenocarcinoma of the esophagus and gastroesophageal junction. J Thorac Cardiovasc Surg 1992;102:36–42.
4. Haggitt RC. Adenocarcinoma in Barrett's esophagus: a new epidemic. Hum Pathol 1992;23:475–476 (editorial).
5. Glick SN, Teplick SK, Amenta PS. The radiologic diagnosis of Barrett esophagus: importance of mucosal surface abnormalities on air-contrast barium studies. AJR 1991;157:951–954.
6. Levine MS, Caroline D, Thompson JJ et al. Adenocarcinoma of the esophagus: relationship to Barrett's mucosa. Radiology 1984;150:305–309.
7. Agha FP. Barrett's carcinoma of the esophagus: clinical and radiographic analysis of 34 cases. AJR 1985;145:41–46.
8. Levine MS, Dillon EC, Saul SH et al. Early esophageal cancer. AJR 1986;146:507–512.

What are the indications of laser therapy for esophageal cancer?

R. Lambert (Lyons)

Tissular photocoagulation vs. tissular photoablation

Phototherapy (i.e., the therapeutic use of photons) covers a large field of heterogeneous procedures from UV therapy, to external high-voltage radiation therapy; such procedures are applied to tumoral or nontumoral diseases. The present report is restricted to the achievement of tumor destruction with photons emitted by laser sources. Laser sources emit a beam of coherent light: photons synchronized in wave length, emission and direction in space. A high density of energy characterizes the laser beam. In the esophageal lumen the laser beam is transmitted through a flexible quartz fiber introduced through the channel of the fiberscope. The therapeutic effect is expected from tissular absorption of the photons and depends on the wave length, the total amount of energy delivered (joules), the power of emission (Watts) and the energy density (joules/cm^2).

The absorption of the photon beam results in an increased temperature (above 60°C) and cytotoxic effects, when the power is over 5 Watts; this is a thermal procedure of photodestruction. Photocoagulation includes the following effects: blood coagulation, hemostasis and tissue destruction without volatilization through protein denaturation. Photoablation includes tissue carbonization and volatilization and may also achieve tissue section.

The tissue absorption of a weak power laser beam (approximately 1 Watt) does not increase the temperature significantly (2–3°C); therefore, cytotoxic effects require photobiologic reactions such as being mediated through a photosensitizer; this is a nonthermal procedure of photodestruction.

Laser sources adapted to phototherapy in oncology

The CO_2 laser source is of no practical value in endoscopy. Indeed, the infrared wave length (10,000 nm) is not transported through a quartz fiber. The Nd YAG crystal, emitting in the near infrared (1,064 nm), is the elective laser source adapted to the effective thermal destruction of tumors without hemorrhage. It should be used in the power range of 30–80 Watts; the emission may be continuous or by pulses. The Dye laser tuned at 630 nm is adapted to nonthermal laser photodestruction with the hematoporphyrin derivative photosensitizer. The reference instrument combines a dye laser circulating rhodamine and an argon laser used as an energy pump. Synthetic photosensitizers, currently on trial, are excited at slightly higher wave lengths requiring other dyes and a tunable laser. Diode lasers will probably be used in place of dye lasers in the near future.

Indications of thermal Nd YAG laser photodestruction

The objective of thermal laser photodestruction is palliation of dysphagia through lumen recanalization of the esophagus. This concerns all adenocarcinoma at the cardia, obstructing the lower esophagus and adenocarcinoma in a columnar lined esophagus (Barrett's esophagus).

Best results are obtained when the tumor is protruding, exophytic, noninfiltrant and noncircumferential; the relief of dysphagia is then almost complete and obtained just after the session. In transmural, circumferential and stenotic tumors, the results are poor; the lumen is not enlarged or the dysphagia relieved. Therefore, an alternative procedure of palliation should be proposed, such as placement of an expansive metal stent.

Therefore, indications of laser photoablation in esophageal adenocarcinoma are proposed, following a careful endoscopic analysis of the morphology of the tumor when there is contraindication to surgical resection (T3, N$^+$ tumor, associated metastases, old age, associated diseases, etc.).

The laser session is performed under sedation and is eventually combined to dilation. The fiberscope is introduced distally to the tumor and irradiation is performed in the retrograde mode to prevent perforation. Sessions must be repeated at 6–12 weeks intervals, depending on the rapidity of tumor regrowth. The average duration of palliation is under 6 months and in around 10% of patients, the relief is prolonged up to 1 year. The major complication is perforation; at the level of the lower esophagus it may result in mediastino-pleural and/or peritoneal complications. Perforation is favored by the angulation at the cardia and may concern either the tumor or the normal digestive wall. Treatment requires immediate placement of an aspiration sonde, parenteral nutrition and large spectrum antibiotics. Stenting or surgical treatment are not recommended.

Indications of nonthermal laser photodynamic therapy

Indications are restricted to endoscopic treatment with a curative objective of small adenocarcinomas at the cardia or in the columnar lined esophagus. They are considered as an alternative to endoscopic strip biopsy [1]. We obtained good results in such tumors, with a complete tumor response rate of 94% at 6 months, the recurrence rate (between 12–18 months) was 65% and the 5-year survival rate was 31%, while the disease specific survival rate increased to 80%. A few recent reports in the literature concern the treatment of adenocarcinomas in a Barrett's esophagus [3,4].

The endoscopic treatment may be proposed as an alternative to surgical resection only in patients at risk for surgery and with superficial tumor invasion, staged as T1 N0 at echoendoscopy.

Recent data demonstrate that, after laser destruction of the columnar epithelium in the esophagus, repair occurs as a squamous epithelium [5–7] if an antacid environment is ensured (prolonged administration of a proton pump inhibitor). Destruction of the nondysplastic columnar epithelium is possible using a Nd YAG laser. While there is convincing evidence of regeneration, the efficacy of the procedure on a large surface is questionable. On the other hand, nonthermal photodynamic therapy is adapted to the elective destruction of areas of dysplasia; the procedure should be preferred to surveillance.

References

1. Inoue H, Endo M, Takeshita K et al. Endoscopic resection of early-stage esophageal cancer. Surg Endosc 1991;5:59–62.
2. Lambert R, Sibille A, Souquet JC et al. Results of photodynamic therapy in upper gastrointestinal cancer. In: Spinelli P, DaFante M, Marchesini R (eds) Photodynamic Therapy and Biomedical Lasers. Amsterdam: Elsevier Science Publishers 1992;256–261.
3. Heier SK, Rothman K, Heier LM et al. Final results of a randomized trial: photodynamic therapy vs. Nd:Yag Laser therapy. Gastroenterology 1993;104:A408.

4. Overholt B, Panjehpour M, Tefftellar RN, Rose M. Photodynamic therapy for treatment of early adenocarcinoma in Barrett's esophagus. Gastrointest Endosc 1993;39:73—76.
5. Brandt LJ, Kauver DR. Laser induced transient regression of Barrett's epithelium. Gastrointest Endosc 1992;38:619—622.
6. Laukka MA, Wang KK, Cameron AJ et al. The use of photodynamic therapy in the treatment of Barrett's esophagus: Preliminary results. Gastrointest Endosc 1993;39:291.
7. Sampliner RE, Hixson LJ, Fennerty B, Garewal HS. Regression of Barrett's esophagus by laser ablation in an antacid environment. Dig Dis Sci 1993;38:365—368.

What can be expected from the use of Protoporphyrins?

R. Lambert (Lyons)

Nonthermal effects of photosensitizing agents in oncology

In oncology, photobiologic reactions concern the detection and the treatment of neoplasia at its early stages. A natural endogenous, or synthetic exogenous, photosensitizer agent when present in the tissue submitted to irradiation, will absorb energy, therefore generating photobiologic reactions. The specific application to oncology is based upon a higher fixation of the photosensitizer in neoplastic vs. nonneoplastic tissue [1—4]. The higher fixation is observed in most neoplastic tissues, on malignant cells and on the lamina propria; therefore glandular neoplasia as well as squamous cell neoplasia is concerned. As yet, most clinical studies concern porphyrins as photosensitizers. The activating photons are produced by laser monochromatic sources; irradiation does not result in a significant increase in tissue temperature.

Applications to diagnosis are based upon an excited status of the photosensitizer resulting in the emission of a fluorescence spectrum, this is achieved when the tissue is irradiated with UV photons (in the range 300—400 nm) such as emitted by a nitrogen or a krypton laser source. The emission spectrum of fluorescence (range 600—700 nm) may be recorded, amplified and eventually submitted to spectrometric analysis; however, this requires a sophisticated and costly instrumentation and, as yet, there is no clinical relevance. Laser-induced autofluorescence of the glandular mucosa in humans [5] was studied without prior injection of a fluorophore; the normal and neoplastic mucosa display different patterns at spectroscopy. A potential application to the Barrett's mucosa has been suggested.

Applications to treatment are based upon the excited status of the photosensitizer absorbing photons emitted in its absorption spectrum (green to red). This is achieved by a laser beam at 630 nm. A dye laser circulating rhodamine and pumped by an argon laser is the usual instrumentation. The energy absorbed by the photosensitizer agent is transferred to oxygen in tissue; oxygen is then transformed in an excited state, the singlet oxygen. The latter molecule is the agent of tissue destruction. Specificity in destruction depends upon the specific higher fixation of the photosensitizer in the tumor and the geometry of irradiation. The latter includes wave length of the photon beam, tissue penetration at this wave length and quantitative factors expressed in power density per cm^2 of irradiated surface.

Biological photosensitizers

Most studies concern the porphyrins and their derivatives. Indeed, endogenous porphyrins are present in most tissues and display a photobiologic activity. A hematoporphyrin derivative, still heterogeneous in chromatography, has been prepared and commercialized; the dihematoporphyrin ether (Photofrin II from QLT) is a more purified form, used as reference in most studies. Synthetic analogues of porphyrins have been prepared; among them the benzoporphyrin from QLT is in a phase I/II trial; other molecules include the porphyrin isomer tetrapropylporphyrin and the monomethyl ether hematoporphyrin.

Other agents have been proposed and tested in experimental or clinical trials; they consist of chlorins, pheophorbides, chlorophils and sulfonated phthalocyanines.

The hematoporphyrin derivative: efficacy and limits

The dihematoporphyrin ether (Photofrin II from QLT) has been adopted in most trials. The emission fluorescence spectrum is obtained following irradiation at the 405 nm wave length (krypton laser); the transfer of energy to oxygen in tissue, the basis of cytotoxicity, is achieved following irradiation at 630 nm with a dye laser. The specific action on tumors is based on a rather low gradient of concentration in the tumor vs. normal tissue: a T/N of around two is obtained after an interval of 48–72 h. Indeed the ratio results from different kinetics of the photosensitizer in both type of tissues. The prolonged presence of Photofrin in the skin at a low concentration is a major drawback requiring complete prevention of direct exposure to sunlight for 1 month. The agent is injected intravenously at a dose of 2 mg/kg.

The second generation photosensitizers: perspectives

Synthetic photosensitizers demonstrate a considerably increased efficacy/safety ratio. This results from a higher ratio of concentration in tumoral vs. normal tissue, reaching six to eight and an increased clearance of the agent, shortening the interval between injection and irradiation (around 24 h) and shortening the period of cutaneous sensitization from 48–72 h. These parameters altogether characterize the benzoporphyrin developed by QLT, Vancouver and the phthalocyanine developed by CIBA. The respective wave length ensuring excitation of the photosensitizer and energy transfer to oxygen is 690 nm for benzoporphyrin and 675 nm for phthalo-cyanine. Therefore, an adjustment of the dye laser source will be required.

Potential applications of endogenous porphyrins in oncology

The precursor, 5-aminolevulinic acid, is a substrate for porphyrin synthesis. Malignant and regenerating tissues display a higher capacity to synthesize porphyrins, due to an increased porphobilinogen deaminase activity. Experimental data [6] point to a potential application in the treatment of liver metastases. The model was a syngenic transplantable colon adenocarcinoma implanted in the liver of rats. In animals fed with 5-aminolevulinic acid, porphyrin concentration increased in liver metastases with an increased concentration ratio of four, when comparing the tumor to the normal liver. The clinical relevance and application to treatment of metastases from esophageal adenocarcinoma is of course still speculative.

Conclusions

Natural porphyrins, as first generation photosensitizers, demonstrated efficacy in the curative endoscopic treatment at an early stage in both types of esophageal cancer: squamous-cell cancer and adenocarcinoma. Application to palliation of advanced cancer is not recommended. The phase I/II trials on synthetic second generation photosensitizers confirm increased efficacy vs. decreased side effects, as compared to natural porphyrins. A significant role of photobiologic reactions in the treatment and/or diagnosis of esophageal adenocarcinoma at an early stage depends upon commercialization of new synthetic photosensitizers, such as benzoporphyrins or phthalocyanines.

References

1. Spinelli P, Dal Fante M, Marchesini R. Photodynamic Therapy and Biomedical Lasers, vol 1. Amsterdam: Excerpta Medica, 1992.
2. Kessel D, Dougherty TJ (eds) Porphyrin Photosensitization, vol 1. New York: Plenum Press Publishers, 1983.
3. Doiron DR, Gomer CJ (eds) Porphyrin Localization and Treatment of Tumors, vol 1. New York; Alan R. Liss Inc. Publishers, 1984.
4. Bock D, Harnet S (eds) Photosensitizing Compounds: their Chemistry, Biology, Clinical Use, vol 1. Ciba Foundation Symposium 146. New York: John Wiley and Sons, 1989.
5. Kappadia CR, Cutruzollo FW, O'Brian KM, Stetz ML et al. Laser induced fluorescence spectroscopy of human colonic mucosa. Detection of adenomatous transformation. Gastroenterology 1990;99:150–157.
6. Van Hillegersberg R, Van den Berg JWO, Kort WJ, Terpstra OT, Wilson JHP. Selective accumulation of endogenously produced porphyrins in a liver metastasis model in rats. Gastroenterology 1993;103:647–651.

How should the intraoperative staging to switch from curative to palliative procedure be conducted?

M. Endo (Tokyo)

A total of 1707 cases of esophageal cancer were resected in our hospital between 1965 and 1992. Adenocarcinoma was observed in 62 cases (3.6%). Of these 62, six arose in Barrett's esophagus, five arose in esophageal mucus gland and one in ectopic gastric mucosa. The histologic origin could not be determined definitely in most cases, because they were large and advanced.

Intraoperative findings requiring a switch to a palliative procedure were as follows:
1. unremovable T4 cancer or unresectable lymph node invading vital organs;
2. extensive lymph nodes metastases; particularly preaortic retroperitoneal lymph nodes;
3. peritoneal dissemination.

For T4 cancer cases, combined resection of the left lobe of liver, diaphragm, lung or distal pancreas was frequently carried out. Two cases of combined partial resection of the descending aorta for squamous cell carcinoma of the lower esophagus were performed, however, no such experience was noted in adenocarcinoma. Conventionally palliative procedures such as intubation, laser therapy, by-pass operation, were performed. A curved prosthesis for esophagocardiac junctional cancers was developed.

Peritoneal dissemination was a most important problem for esophagocardial cancer. Peritoneal dissemination occurred frequently in poorly differentiated adenocarcinoma and could not be detected before an operation.

Lower esophagectomy and total or subtotal proximal gastrectomy without sufficient lymph node dissection was performed, and a catheter was placed in the pelvic cavity. Intraperitoneal infusion chemotherapy with 5FU and CDDP using an implantable reservoir was commenced immediately after the operation.

In cases with lymphatic invasion in the esophagus, total gastrectomy and transhiatal esophagectomy or left transthoracic esophagectomy, were usually performed avoiding palliative resection.

What is gained from mediastinal nodal clearance during surgical resection of adenocarcinoma arising in CLE?

T.R. DeMeester, J.A. Hagen, J.H. Peters, G.W.B. Clark
(Los Angeles)

Current strategies for treatment of esophageal carcinoma limit the role of surgery to removing the primary tumor, with the hope that adjuvant therapy will increase cure rates by destroying systemic disease. This approach emphasizes the concept of biological predetermination; that is, the outcome of treatment in esophageal cancer is determined at the time of diagnosis, and that surgical therapy aimed at removing lymph nodes in addition to the primary tumor is not helpful. Lymph node metastases are considered simply markers of systemic disease. Based on this concept is the belief that removal of the primary tumor by transhiatal esophagogastrectomy results in the same survival as a more extensive en bloc resection. This attitude, if in error, could be detrimental in the treatment of early adenocarcinomas arising in Barrett's mucosa, as the prevalence of metastatic lymph nodes in patients with intramucosal adenocarcinomas approaches 30%. To determine which procedure, transhiatal esophagogastrectomy or extended en bloc esophagogastrectomy with mediastinal lymphadenectomy, has a better outcome, we compared the survival of patients with early cancer of the distal esophagus and cardias who had one or the other procedure by the same surgeon [1].

The decision regarding the procedure performed was made as follows: patients with early lesions on preoperative clinical and intraoperative surgical evaluation, who were under the age of 75 and who were free of significant cardiovascular or pulmonary disease, underwent extended en bloc esophagogastrectomy (n = 30). Transhiatal esophagogastrectomy was performed in patients with early lesions, if they were over the age of 75 or had significant cardiac or pulmonary disease (n = 16).

The specimens were examined with respect to the known prognostic indicators, that is, the extent of esophageal wall penetration and the presence of more than four lymph node metastases [2]. Early lesions were defined as those in which the tumor was limited to the esophageal mucosa or muscle layers, with four or fewer lymph node metastases [3].

All hospital survivors were followed at 3-month intervals for the first 3 years, then every 6 months with routine laboratory studies, a chest X-ray and a chest and abdominal CT scan. All surviving patients were either seen in person or contacted for follow-up by telephone within 3 months prior to preparation of the manuscript. The median follow-up time of surviving patients was 14 months, with a range of 1–108 months.

Comparison of continuous variables was performed using the Student's *t*-test. Fisher's exact test was used for comparison of proportions. Survival probabilities were calculated, according to the method of Kaplan-Meier. Hospital deaths were included in all calculations of survival. Comparisons of survival between groups was performed using the log-rank method of Mantel-Cox.

Since the depth of tumor penetration of the esophageal wall and the number of metastatic lymph nodes are the most important independent variables affecting survival, survival based upon the method of resection was compared in patients with intramural tumors and those with ≤4 metastatic lymph nodes (Figs. 1 and 2). There was a clear survival advantage associated with en bloc esophagogastrectomy in patients with tumors limited to the esophageal wall ($X2 = 4.45$, $p < 0.05$). The validity of this observation is underscored, in that the proportion of patients with ≤4 involved nodes was similar in both groups (9/9 transhiatal esophagogastrectomy (THE) vs. 10/13 en bloc esophagogastrectomy (EBE), $p = 0.54$). Comparison of survival in patients with ≤4 metastatic nodes also demonstrated a significant advantage for en bloc esophagogastrectomy ($X2 = 9.38$, $p < 0.005$). The validity of this observation was similarly underscored in that the proportion of tumors limited to the esophageal wall was similar in both groups (9/27 THE vs. 10/21 EBE, $p = 0.38$).

When just patients with early lesions, that is with tumors limited to the esophageal wall and no more than four lymph node metastases were compared, a clear survival advantage was observed following en bloc esophagogastrectomy where the 5-year

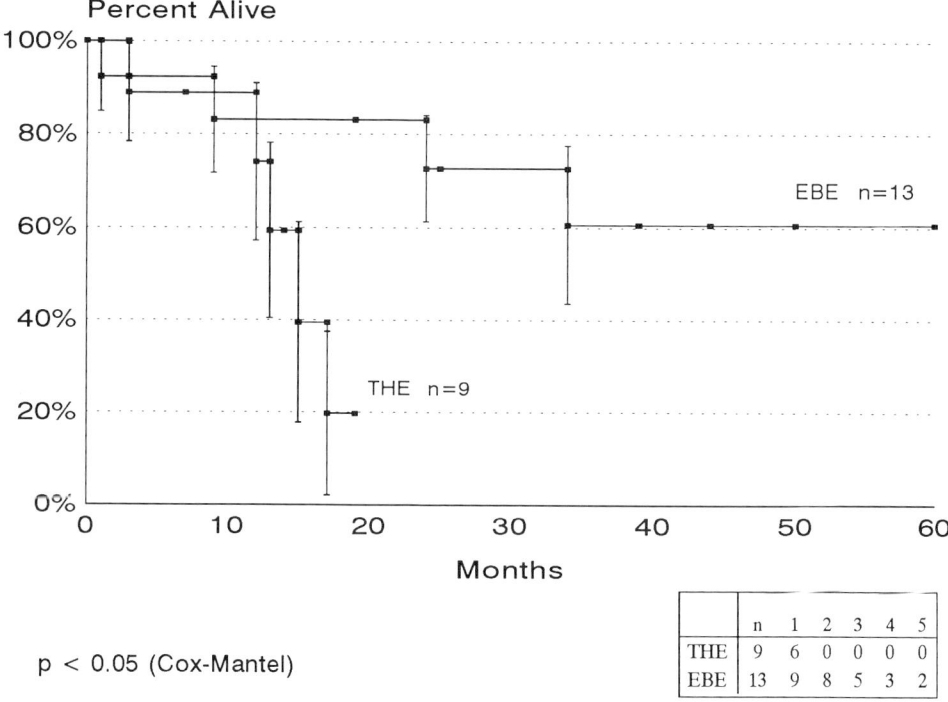

	n	1	2	3	4	5
THE	9	6	0	0	0	0
EBE	13	9	8	5	3	2

p < 0.05 (Cox-Mantel)

Fig. 1. Survival probabilities calculated by the method of Kaplan-Meier, according to the type of procedure performed in patients staged with intramural tumors. EBE = en bloc esophagogastrectomy. THE = transhiatal esophagogastrectomy.

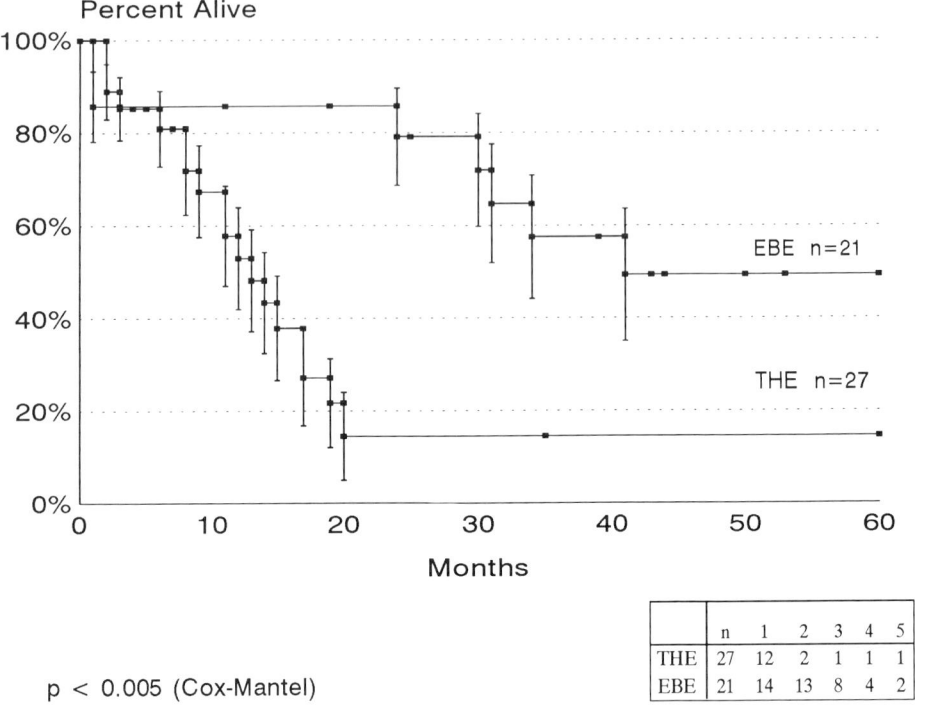

	n	1	2	3	4	5
THE	27	12	2	1	1	1
EBE	21	14	13	8	4	2

p < 0.005 (Cox-Mantel)

Fig. 2. Survival probabilities calculated by the method of Kaplan-Meier, according to the type of procedure performed in patients staged with ≤4 lymph node metastases. EBE = en bloc esophagogastrectomy. THE = transhiatal esophagogastrectomy.

survival was 75% (Fig. 3). The validity of this observation is underscored, in that the pathologic stage of the two groups of patients was similar (Table 1).

The argument could be made that the above results can be explained by a staging bias, that is, there was less accurate lymph node staging in the patients who had a transhiatal resection. Since a similar abdominal lymph node dissection was performed in both procedures, the relationship between abdominal and thoracic lymph node pathology was used in patients following an en bloc resection, to support the adequacy of staging thoracic nodes in patients having a transhiatal resection. Only one of the 22 patients who had ≤4 nodal metastases in the abdomen following en bloc esophagogastrectomy had evidence of lymph node metastases in the thoracic node dissection. This would strongly indicate that, when a thorough abdominal lymph node dissection reveals four or fewer involved nodes, the thoracic nodes are free of metastases, and that the staging of early disease in patients following a transhiatal resection is dependable.

We also investigated the possibility that the above results can be explained on the basis that patients undergoing transhiatal resection were older, near the end of their life span, and would be more likely to die from physiologic causes rather than recurrent tumor. This did not appear to be so, in that the hospital mortality for each

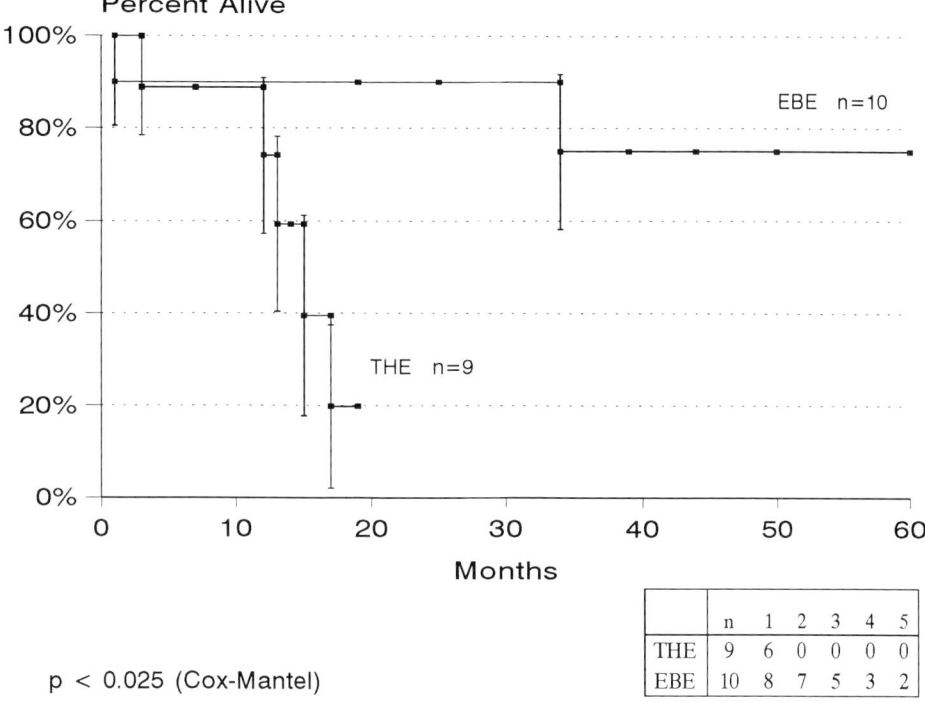

	n	1	2	3	4	5
THE	9	6	0	0	0	0
EBE	10	8	7	5	3	2

p < 0.025 (Cox-Mantel)

Fig. 3. Survival probabilities calculated by Kaplan-Meier method, according to type of procedure performed in patients with early disease at time of pathologic classification of removed specimen. EBE = en bloc esophagogastrectomy, THE = transhiatal esophagogastrectomy.

procedure was similar (THE = 12.8%, EBE = 10%, p = 1.0) and the analysis of deaths occurring during the follow-up period showed that all patients, irrespective of the surgical procedure, died with recurrent disease.

This study shows that for early cancers of the lower esophagus and cardia, en bloc esophagogastrectomy results in significantly better survival than transhiatal esophagogastrectomy. This finding cannot be explained by a bias in the stage of disease resected, a difference in operative mortality or death from nontumor causes.

Table 1.

Groups	WNM classification[a]	No. of patients	
		THE	EBE
Early	W0N0	1	1
	W0N1	0	0
	W1N0	5	5
	W1N1	3	4
Total		9	10

[a]See reference [3].

Rather, it appears to be due to the type of operation performed. The procedure which focused on removal of the primary tumors (THE) is inferior in outcome to the procedure which removes the regional nodes in addition to the primary tumor (EBE).

There are several possible explanations for the failure of a transhiatal resection to achieve the results obtained with an en bloc resection in favorably staged patients. First, is the potential to disseminate tumor cells at the time of the blunt dissection of the thoracic esophagus. Second, is accepting an inadequate distal tumor margin because of efforts to preserve a full length of the stomach in order to reestablish gastrointestinal continuity with a cervical esophagogastrostomy. This can result in the development of recurrent disease along the gastric suture line [4]. Third, is the transfer of unrecognized perigastric metastatic nodes into the thorax with the gastric pull-up. Fourth, is the possibility that the transhiatal dissection leaves residual nodal metastasis in the mediastinum. An en bloc esophagogastrectomy effectively eliminates all of these potential causes of recurrence.

On the basis of this experience, we would conclude that survival, following surgical removal of a carcinoma arising in the distal esophagus or cardia, is dependent upon the method of resection. Patients with early lesions (i.e., tumors limited to the esophageal wall with four or less nodes involved) have significantly better survival after extended en bloc resection.

References

1. Hagen JA, Peters JH, DeMeester TR. Superiority of extended en bloc esophagogastrectomy for carcinoma of the lower esophagus and cardia. J Thorac Cardiovasc Surg 1993;(in press).
2. Skinner DB, Dowlatshahi KD, DeMeester TR. Potentially curable cancer of the esophagus. Cancer 1982;50:2571–2575.
3. Skinner DB, Ferguson MK, Soriano A, Little AG, Staszak VM. Selection of operation for esophageal cancer based on staging. Ann Surg 1986;204(4):391–401.
4. Wong J. Esophageal resection for cancer: the rationale of current practice. Am J Surg 1987;153:18–24.

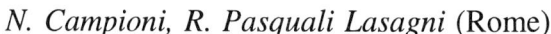

N. Campioni, R. Pasquali Lasagni (Rome)

Columnar-lined esophagus is defined as a condition in which the distal tubular esophagus is lined with columnar-type epithelium, regardless of the presence or the absence of a hiatus hernia [1]. There are two theories about the etiology of this condition: the former (i.e., the congenital theory) states that a remnant of the columnar epithelium persists from the fetal to the adult esophagus, and the more recent (i.e., the acquired theory), which is most accepted: this hypothesis states that injured squamous epithelium adapts to chronic injury by undergoing destruction and subsequent metaplastic changes to become columnar epithelium, which is more acid resistant. The metaplastic epithelium has the potential to undergo dysplasia and eventually become an adenocarcinoma [2].

Malignant columnar-lined esophagus is defined as the condition in which adenocarcinoma occurs above the anatomical gastroesophageal junction, and arises from columnar epithelium lining the distal tubular esophagus [3].

Adenocarcinoma arising in the lower esophagus and cardia does not meet this condition, and therefore, theoretically must be distinguished from the previous [4].

Along with Duhaylongsod [5], we think that adenocarcinoma of the lower esophagus and cardia is not often classified as CLE adenocarcinoma for the following reasons: the tumor is presumed to be of gastric origin; there is failure to suspect or search for Barrett's mucosa; advanced esophageal or gastroesophageal cancer obliterates all remnants of Barrett's mucosa; and unresectable cancer is not being subjected to further pathologic review.

Especially for the two latter factors, we do not believe that the prognosis of Barrett's adenocarcinoma is better than the non-Barrett's adenocarcinoma arising into the lower esophagus and cardia.

The differences, reported from many authors between prognosis for Barrett's and non-Barrett's adenocarcinoma, should be ascribed to the different average stages being lower in the Barrett's, because of the surveillance to which these patients are subjected to, and higher in the remnant adenocarcinomas, in which diagnosis is late and often made at a very advanced stage; analysis of the results concerning stages generally shows no statistical differences [5].

For these reasons we prefer to group altogether the adenocarcinomas of the lower esophagus and of the cardia.

Furthermore, a distinction between adenocarcinoma with major spreading towards the esophagus or towards the stomach, taking into account the maximum tumor thickness and the Z line, is possible, but it seems not to influence the surgical strategies.

In fact, in an a recent study reporting the results of a 2-year national surveillance on the surgical treatment of adenocarcinoma in the gastroesophageal junction in selected Italian Hospitals, only 20% of patients with major esophageal spreading underwent esophageal dissection by thoracotomy, while the remaining 80% underwent transhiatal limited esophagectomy [6].

An analysis of data reported to the recent 5th ISDE Congress shows a parity between transthoracotomic and transhiatal esophagectomy, both in terms of prevalence and in terms of results [7] (Table 1).

As regards the role of lymphadenectomy, the data reported from the majority of the authors show that mediastinal lymphadenectomy play more of a staging role than a "curative" role.

In fact, long-term survival after "blunt", or transhiatal, esophageal dissection is not different from that achieved with transthoracic dissection. The only specific prognostic factor is the stage of disease. Nevertheless, a right staging is achieved only when all the nodal sites are explored. It is well known that the extravisceral lymph stream of the esophagus goes preferentially toward the abdomen, and that the submucosal lymph stream undoubtedly goes up, but sometimes it is possible to find

Table 1.

Author	THE	TTE	Results
Hagen	24	29	TTE > THE (for limited disease)
Zilberstein	35	32	TTE = THE
Hölscher	101	20	TTE = THE
Aikou	3	51	TTE > THE (for limited disease)
Roher	46	41	TTE = THE
Riemenschneider	16	19	No long-term results, TTE > THE

Note: THE = trans-hiatal-esophagectomy; TTE = trans-thoracic-esophagectomy.

"jump" mediastinal nodal involvement at a distance from the tumor. For this reason, in the case of adenocarcinoma of the cardia, when the general condition of the patient enables us, a left thoracotomy followed by a left subcostal laparotomy is performed, without changing the position the patient. This way allows to explore all the mediastinal and all the abdominal nodal sites, in order to achieve the best staging and a better control of the operatory field. This answers the primary question: the only gain from mediastinal node clearing is in staging.

References

1. Naef AP et al. Columnar-lined lower esophagus: an acquired lesion with malignant predisposition. J Thorac Cardiovasc Surg 1975;75:826.
2. Kalish RJ et al. Clinical, epidemiologic, and morphologic comparison between adenocarcinomas arising in Barrett's esophageal mucosa and in gastric cardia. Gastroenterology 1984;86:461.
3. Skinner DB et al. Barrett's esophagus: comparison of benign and malignant cases. Ann Surg 1983;198:554.
4. Streitz JM Jr et al. Adenocarcinoma in Barrett's Esophagus. Ann Surg 1991;213(2):122.
5. Duhaylondsod FG et al. Barrett's esophagus and adenocarcinoma of the esophagus and gastroesophageal junction. J Thorac Cardiovasc Surg 1991;102:36.
6. Campioni N. Il cancro del cardias. In: Santoro E, Garofalo A, Scutari F (eds) Il cancro dello stomaco negli ospedali italiani. Roma: Edizioni Scientifiche Romane, 1989.
7. 5th World Congress of the International Society for Diseases of the Esophagus. Kyoto, Japan. Book of Abstracts, 1992.

What are the advantages of using the colon rather than the stomach for esophageal reconstruction?

T.R. DeMeester, S. Johnson (Los Angeles)

The first successful resection of the thoracic esophagus for carcinoma was performed by Torek near the turn of the century in a patient with esophageal carcinoma [1]. Gastrointestinal continuity was established via an external "rubber tube" between a cervical esophagostomy and gastrostomy. The patient survived for 13 years and was able to swallow food, provided it was chewed to almost a liquid state. Immediate reconstruction of the gastrointestinal tract after an esophagectomy with an esophago-gastrostomy did not occur until the mid 1930s.

In malignant disease, esophageal resection is performed to cure early or to palliate advanced disease. The indications in benign disease are less well defined and symptom-driven. Usually the patient's esophageal function has deteriorated to the point where there is persistent dysphagia, crippling odynophagia or chronic aspiration.

A successful outcome is more dependent on the ability to re-establish gastrointestinal continuity than on the technique of resection. Options for esophageal replacement include gastric advancement, colon or jejunal interposition and free jejunal graft. In some situations combinations of these are necessary. Surgical technique must be flawless, as the consequences of errors are logarithmic rather than additive. A functional result is dependent upon attention to detail before, during and after surgery.

Indications

Esophagectomy with replacement for benign disease is indicated in patients whose esophageal function — namely, bolus transport from the oral pharynx to the stomach — has been destroyed by a primary disease process or multiple previous esophageal procedures. Fibrosis of the esophagus can obstruct the lumen or destroy its normal function such that motility becomes disorganized, contraction amplitudes decrease or becomes absent altogether. These end-stage abnormalities can result from chemical, infectious or drug induced injury; chronic reflux disease; iatrogenic or traumatic injury; motor disorders such as achalasia; or connective tissue disease such as scleroderma. The end stage of these diseases destroy the function of the esophageal body so that esophageal replacement becomes necessary. It is not uncommon with these abnormalities to have a superimposed drug induced injury resulting from entrapment of swallowed medication. The local dissolution of the medication can cause additional injury with panmural fibrosis which is resistant to dilatation and requires resection for relief. A not uncommon pathway to esophageal resection is a history of multiple previous antireflux procedures. Each redo surgery of the esophagus causes further damage with additional loss of function. The blood supply to the organ is reduced with each successive mobilization, and ischemic necrosis can occur. Experience has taught that a successful outcome after three previous procedures is unlikely, and that the need for a 4th procedure is a signal for esophageal resection with replacement.

Patient assessment

The perception of dysphagia by the patient is a balance between the severity of the underlying etiology producing the difficulty and the patient's adjustment to that difficulty by the alteration in his eating habits. Consequently, any complaint of dysphagia that does not have an assessment of the patient's dietary history is of little value. Information must be obtained as to whether the patient experiences pain, choking or vomits with eating; whether he is the last to finish; whether he needs to take liquids with the meal; whether he has ever interrupted a social meal to go to the rest room to regurgitate; and whether he has been admitted on an emergency basis for food impaction. These assessments reflect the individual's response to dysphagia and are important in determining the severity of the complaint.

Endoscopy typically shows extensive stricturing, retained food within the esophagus or a massively dilated, tortuous esophagus. Particular attention should be made to determine the proximal extent of disease, as it is preferable to retain as much proximal esophagus as possible. This allows the anastomosis to be made below the thoracic inlet and aids in bolus transport. In patients with caustic injury the proximal anastomotic site must be selected wisely as pharyngeal and hypopharyngeal structures can be damaged. A video esophagram and pharyngeal laryngoscopy are of invaluable help in selecting the site. The video esophagram is also useful in assessing the pharyngeal phase of swallowing which is often otherwise difficult to evaluate.

Severe esophageal motility disorders necessitating esophagectomy typically reveal absent or low amplitude contractions on manometry. More than 50% of contractions are interrupted or dropped, implying severe intrinsic disease within the esophageal body. Scarring of the distal esophageal sphincter may be revealed by unyielding high pressure. Twenty-four hour pH monitoring may show prolonged acid exposure to the distal esophagus due to its inability to effectively clear acid.

Patients undergoing esophageal replacement for benign disease who are candidates for colon interposition should undergo colonoscopy before surgery to rule out occult neoplasms, diffuse colitis or severe diverticular disease. A mesenteric arteriogram should be obtained to assess variations in the blood supply of the colon, as well as identify potentially flow-limiting atherosclerotic lesions. It can also aid in selecting the optimal segment of colon to be used for interposition. Tests should also be done to assess the patient's physiologic condition. An FEV_1 of less than 1.5 l or ejection fraction less than 40% indicate little cardiopulmonary reserve [2,3]. Sequential procedures (i.e., esophageal resection followed by replacement) should be considered in these patients. Likewise, decreased oral intake before surgery may result in poor wound healing and immune dysfunction [4,5]. Improving nutritional reserve in these patients, by placement of a feeding jejunostomy tube several weeks prior to undergoing resection and replacement, can improve the outcome.

General principles in choosing a substitute

Prior to surgery the choice of an esophageal substitute, as well as the extent of resection, should be carefully planned. Resected segments can only be adequately replaced by living viscus (i.e., stomach, jejunum or colon). Normal esophagus is superior to any potential substitute in its ability to transport a bolus from the mouth to the stomach. As a consequence, maximal preservation of proximal normal eso-phagus will aid in preservation of function. The choice of the esophageal substitute is based on the adequacy of its blood supply, its freedom from intrinsic disease and the length of resected esophagus that it is capable of bridging. If the patient has had previous gastric surgery, the length of stomach available for esophageal replacement may be compromised. Likewise, extensive diverticular disease, colitis or diffuse atherosclerotic disease, which tends to affect the blood supply to the colon more often than the stomach, may prohibit the use of the colon. The choice of substitute in relation to the patient's age and overall prognosis is an important consideration, since patients with good overall long-term expectant survival will require grafts with maximal function and durability. The general indications for the use of the colon are: 1) stomach is not available; 2) reconstruction after curative resection of tumor in distal esophagus or cardia; 3) use of substernal route; or 4) replacement must last for the majority of a lifetime.

The jejunum is a more dynamic graft and contributes to bolus transport, whereas the stomach and colon function primarily as a passive conduit. Of the three, the colon provides the longest graft, followed by the stomach and jejunum. The stomach can usually reach to the neck, so long as the amount of lesser curve resected does not interfere with the blood supply to the fundus. Mobilization of the duodenum is necessary to allow the fundus of the stomach to be advanced into the neck. Previous pancreatitis or a history of prior upper abdominal surgeries may preclude the surgeon's ability to obtain this amount of length on the gastric pedicle. Similarly, the jejunum can usually reach only to the inferior border of the pulmonary hilum and rarely beyond that, due to the architecture of its blood supply [6]. It functions well for distal interpositions between the midesophagus and gastric antrum, but does not provide the reservoir capacity of the colon. As the anastomosis is within the chest, a thoracoabdominal approach is necessary. A free jejunal graft anastomosed to the internal mammary vessels may become necessary if the amount of colon or stomach available is unable to bridge a gap.

The choice of replacement will affect the number of anastomoses performed, as well as the magnitude of the operation. A colon or jejunal interposition demands added technical expertise. In general, increasing the number of anastomoses will increase the hazards of the procedure, both in terms of operating time and postoperative morbidity. Use of the stomach requires only one anastomosis, whereas the colon or jejunum requires three. Consequently, the stomach is preferred as the esophageal replacement in terms of anastomotic complications and ease of operation. The route in which to place the esophageal substitute (e.g., substernal vs. posterior mediastinal) must be considered. A history of previous mediastinitis may preclude safe tunneling through the posterior mediastinum; likewise, a previous coronary bypass may require placement of the graft in the posterior mediastinum. In any case, the graft should be placed isoperistaltic without redundancy to avoid subsequent dilation and stasis.

Esophageal resection

The management of a damaged esophagus is problematic. If the native diseased esophagus is left in place, continued ulceration from gastroesophageal reflux (GER) can occur. This ulceration can be severe due to the absence of the buffering capacity of saliva, leading to erosion into major vessels with hemorrhage. Leaving a damaged esophagus in place can also result in a mediastinal cyst which can potentially become the source of mediastinal abscesses later in life. On the other hand, to remove the esophagus requires an extensive dissection in the presence of marked periesophagitis and has a significant morbidity. On the other hand, a benefit of leaving the esophagus in place is preservation of the vagus nerves and better postoperative gastric function. Most experienced surgeons, however, recommend that the damaged esophagus be removed unless the operative risk is too high.

The thoracic esophagus can be approached transthoracically or transhiatally. A transhiatal esophagectomy can often be performed with minimal morbidity and is the desired approach. A thoracotomy is indicated when there is mediastinal scarring or a massively dilated esophagus with enlarged vessels, both of which make the transhiatal approach dangerous. The decision to proceed with thoracotomy is also based on coexisting diseases (e.g., empyema) and whether an intrathoracic anastomosis is planned. As the esophagus lies to the right of the aortic arch, a right thoracotomy provides superior exposure when performing a total esophagectomy. Likewise, a left thoracoabdominal incision allows access to the distal esophagus and stomach when performing distal jejunal interpositions. Reconstruction can be performed immediately or delayed, depending upon the stability of the patient and the presence of ongoing sepsis. If delayed reconstruction is favored, a feeding jejunostomy and cervical end esophagostomy is performed.

Use of the colon

The use of long segments of colon, either for replacement or bypass of all or part of the thoracic esophagus, was introduced independently by Kelling [7] and Vulliet [8] in 1911. It was not until the late 1940s, however, after the advent of powerful antibiotics, did use of the colon as an esophageal substitute become popular. Since that time the colon has earned the reputation as a well-functioning and durable esophageal substitute. The success of using the colon as an esophageal substitute is critically dependent on the adequacy of its blood supply and its ability to transport food effectively from the pharynx to the stomach. As a consequence, seemingly minor judgmental or technical errors can result in poor outcome.

The colon graft can come from the right side where it is based on the middle colic artery and vein, or from the left side based on the inferior mesenteric artery and inferior mesenteric, sigmoidal and hemorrhoidal veins [9]. The left colon is preferred, because of its better size match, thicker wall and more dependable blood supply (Fig. 1A,B). The marginal artery is in close proximity to the left colonic wall which makes it less likely to limit the length of the graft. The graft can traverse the chest in the posterior mediastinum or in the substernal position. The right colon is a second choice, because its length is shorter and blood supply less dependable. It can be used when there is a fixed left colon mesentery, stenosis of the inferior mesenteric artery or extensive diverticular disease of the left colon.

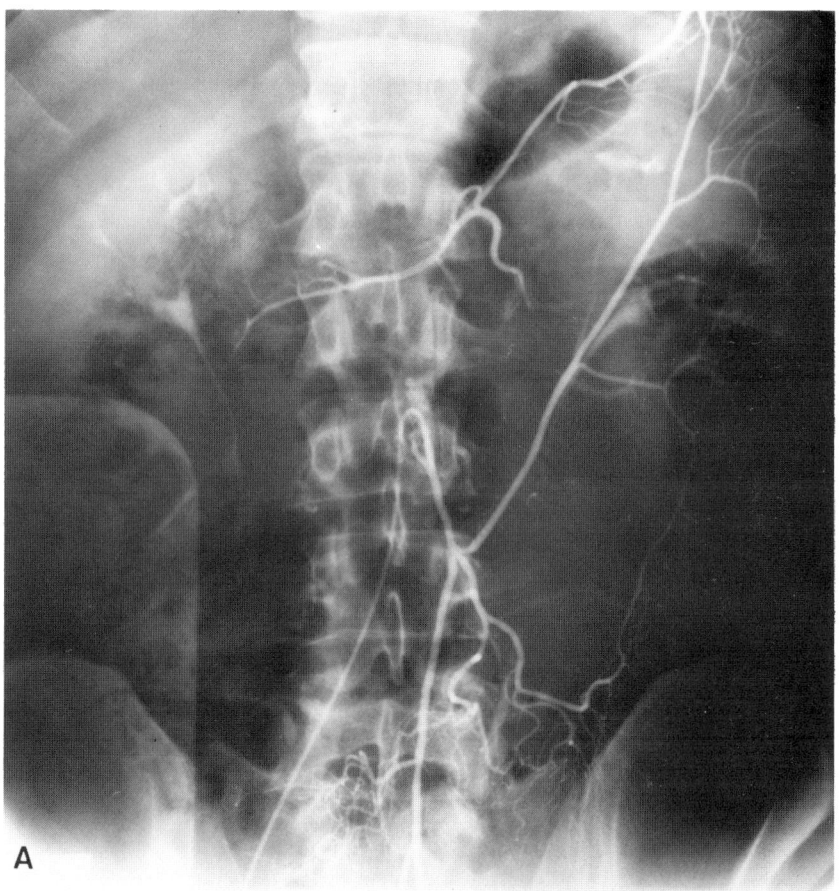

Fig. 1A. Angiogram showing a selective injection of the inferior mesenteric artery to illustrate the arterial supply to the left colon via the ascending branch of the left colic artery and the marginal branch.

Gastric advancement vs. colon interposition for esophageal replacement in benign disease

No pretense should be made that the intrathoracic stomach or colon functions as well as the native normal esophagus. A gastric advancement is without doubt the best esophageal replacement when esophagectomy is performed for palliative reasons and long-term survival is not likely. There is, however, controversy over whether colon or stomach is the better long-term substitute for the esophagus in patients with benign disease. Those who prefer the stomach admit that an intrathoracic stomach is a poor long-term substitute [10,11]. Although technically easier to perform, the gastric advancement is frequently associated with postprandial symptoms. Most patients experience discomfort during or shortly after eating. The most common of these symptoms is a postprandial pressure sensation and early satiety, probably related to

1149

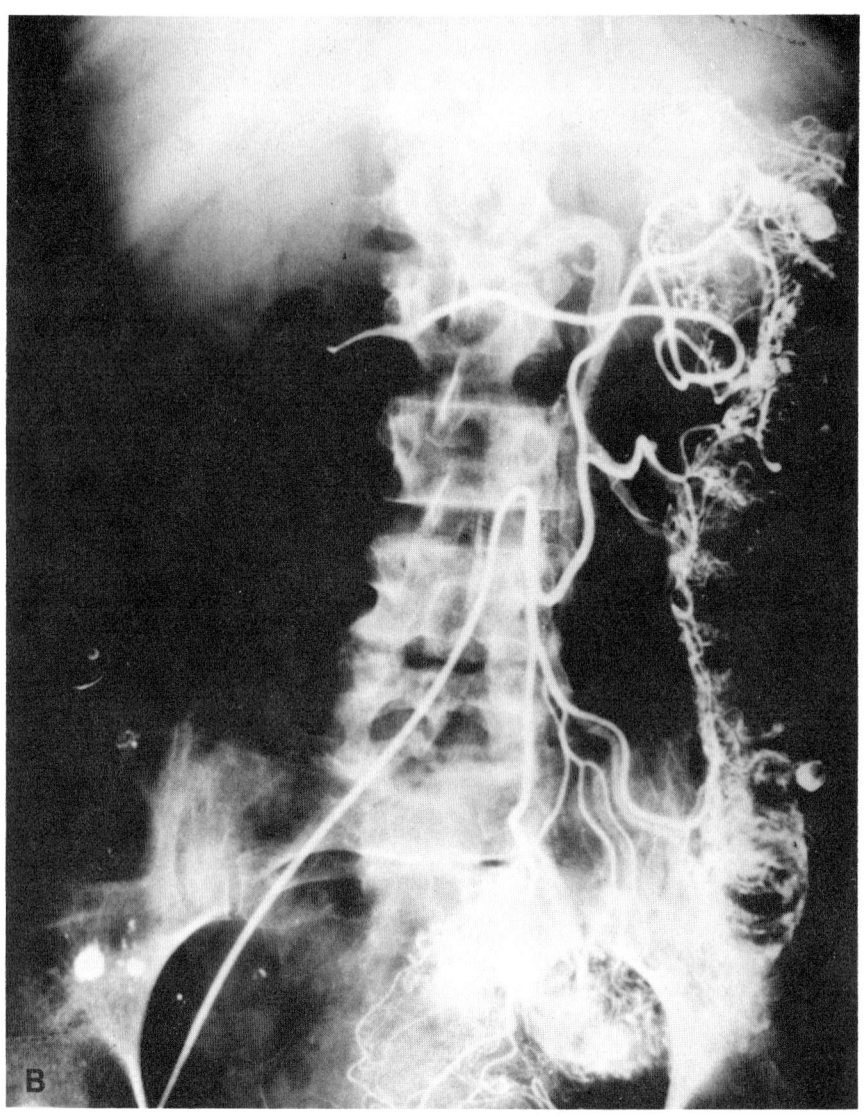

Fig. 1B. Angiogram showing a selective injection of the inferior mesenteric artery to illustrate its venous drainage via the inferior mesenteric vein and superior hemorrhoidal veins.

loss of the gastric reservoir. These symptoms are less common when the colon is used as the esophageal substitute, probably because the distal third of the stomach is retained within the abdomen and the interposed colon functions as additional reservoir.

Dysphagia requiring dilatation is more frequent when the stomach is used as the esophageal replacement. In a study by Orringer and Stirling [11] there was a 61% incidence of dysphagia among 87 patients who had undergone esophageal replacement using the stomach for benign disease; two-thirds of these patients required

1150

immediate dilatation postoperatively and one fourth had persistent dysphagia requiring home dilatation. In comparison, there was only an 18% incidence of dysphagia among 92 patients who had undergone colon interposition for both benign and malignant disease. This was more a sensation of early filling rather than difficulty swallowing. Only 4% required dilatations and in all of these patients the dysphagia was permanently relieved by revising the stenotic anastomosis [9]. Similarly, Isolauri et al. [12] reported on 248 patients with colon interpositions and noted a 24% incidence of dysphagia 12 months after the operation. When it did occur, the most common cause in this series was recurrent mediastinal tumor.

Another consequence of transposing the stomach into the chest is the development of postoperative duodenogastric reflux [11]. Following a gastric advancement, the pylorus lies at the level of the esophageal hiatus and a distinct pressure gradient develops between the intrathoracic gastric and intra-abdominal duodenal lumens. Unless the pyloric valve is extremely efficient, the pressure differential will encourage reflux of duodenal contents into the stomach. Adding a pyloroplasty may worsen the problem. Duodenogastric reflux is less likely to occur following colonic interposition, since the pylorus and duodenum are retained within their natural position and there is sufficient intra-abdominal colon compressed by the positive intra-abdominal pressure.

In benign disease, the late development of proximal esophagitis, stenosis and Barrett's esophagus is more common with an esophagogastric anastomosis made within the chest. For this reason alone an intrathoracic esophagogastrostomy should be abandoned, even in cases of malignant disease. On the contrary, the interposed colon functions to protect the remaining esophagus from refluxed gastric juice. This may be related to both its mucous production and its intra-abdominal segment which is subjected to positive intra-abdominal pressures.

Although there is general acceptance of the concept that an esophagogastric anastomosis in the neck results in less postoperative esophagitis and stricture formation than one performed within the chest, reflux esophagitis following a cervical anastomosis does occur. Patients undergoing a cervical esophagogastrostomy for benign disease may develop problems associated with the anastomosis in the fourth or fifth postoperative year. This may be severe enough to require anastomotic revision. This is less likely to develop in patients who have had a colon interposition for esophageal replacement. Consequently, in patients with benign disease a colon interposition is usually preferred to obviate the late problems associated with a cervical esophagogastrostomy. In addition, the colon gives excellent long-term results and appears to undergo little if any histologic changes once placed in the chest as an esophageal substitute [13]. In a long-term study by Kelly, 20 out of 23 children who had undergone colon interposition for esophageal replacement had excellent radiological and functional results at a mean follow-up of 12.8 years [14].

Composite grafts

In some patients it may be impossible to use the colon or stomach to fully bridge the gap necessary to restore gastrointestinal continuity. In others, it may become necessary to partially resect or revise colon grafts, due to immediate ischemic or late functional failure. In these situations, composite grafts consisting of various combinations of native esophagus, colon, stomach and/or jejunum can be constructed. This may become necessary in adult patients who as children underwent antiperistaltic colon interpositions. In these patients graft dilatation typically develops over time leading to stasis, regurgitation, repeated aspiration and eventual pulmonary complications. A colon revision may be necessary with placement of a jejunal interposition between the revised colon graft and distal gastric antrum. This can be done in the posterior mediastinum via a thoracoabdominal incision or in the substernal space via median sternotomy. This gives excellent results since the jejunum is actively involved in peristalsis and the stomach, which is usually not vagotomized, retains its reservoir function. Likewise, a free pedicled jejunal graft may be used to bridge a gap between a short colon graft distally and native esophagus proximally [15]. It may also be necessary to use it when both the stomach and colon are partially or completely absent because of previous surgery, contain intrinsic disease or are compromised with respect to overall length for any reason. In these patients, the pedicled artery and vein are anastomosed via microsurgical techniques usually to the internal mammary vessels.

References

1. Torek F. The first successful case of resection of the thoracic portion of the esophagus for carcinoma. Surg Gynecol Obstet 1913;16:614–617.
2. Diener CF, Burrows B. Further observations on the course and prognosis of chronic obstructive lung disease. Am Rev Respir Dis 1975;111:719–724.
3. Boucher CA, Brewster DC, Darling RC et al. Determination of cardiac risk by dipyridamole-thallium imaging before peripheral vascular surgery. N Engl J Med 1985;312:389–394.
4. Heatly RV, Lewis MH, Williams RHP. Preoperative intravenous feeding: a controlled trial. Postgrad J Med 1979;55: 541–545.
5. Piccone VA, Ahmed N, Crossberg S et al. Esophagogastrectomy for carcinoma of the esophagus. Ann Thorac Surg 1979; 28:369–377.
6. Foker JE, Ring WE, Varco RL. Technique of jejunal interposition for esophageal replacement. J Thorac Cardiovasc Surg 1982;83:928–933.
7. Kelling G. Oesophagoplastik mit Hilfe des Querkolon. Zent Bl Chir 1911;38:1209–1212.
8. Vulliet H. De l'oesophagoplastie des diverses modifications. Sem Med 1911;31:529–534.
9. DeMeester TR, Johansson KE, Franze I et al. Indications, surgical technique, and long-term functional results of colon interposition or bypass. Ann Surg 1988;208:460–474.
10. Hölsher AH, Butterman H, Siewert JR. Function of the intrathoracic stomach. World J Surg 1988;12:835–844.
11. Orringer MB, Stirling MC. Cervical esophagogastric anastomosis for benign disease: functional results. J Thorac Cardiovasc Surg 1988;96:887–893.
12. Isolauri J, Markkula H, Antio V. Colon interposition in the treatment of carcinoma of the esophagus and gastric cardia. Ann Thorac Surg 1987;43:420–424.
13. Isolauri J, Helen H, Markkula H. Colon interposition for esophageal disease: histologic findings of colonic mucosa after a follow-up of 5 months to 15 years. Am J Gastroenterol 1991;86:277–280.
14. Kelly JP, Shackelford GD, Roper CL. Esophageal replacement with colon in children: functional results and long-term growth. Ann Thorac Surg 1983;36:634–643.
15. McDonough JJ, Gluckman JL. Microvascular reconstruction of the pharyngoesophagus with free jejunal graft. Microsurgery 1988;9:116–127.

Operability and resectability rates are higher in adenocarcinomas arising in CLE than in other types of esophageal cancer, but is late survival higher?

R. Bardini, M. Asolati, L. Bonavina, A. Ruol, A. Peracchia (Padua)

It seems that we are just now becoming aware of the Barrett's adenocarcinoma and focusing on it, because many aspects remain controversial, even if many articles on the topic have been already published.

The incidence, that is the risk, of the development of an adenocarcinoma in the columnar-lined esophagus during a follow-up interval is not yet defined, as the estimated risk varies from 30—125 times more than in the general population [1—6]. Prevalence varies from 2.5—46% [1,2] reflecting perhaps referral patterns rather than true prevalence. Most of the series reporting on adenocarcinoma and Barrett's esophagus are retrospective, and the diagnosis of the adenocarcinoma on Barrett's esophagus is made on the presence of the columnar mucosa inside the tumor. Therefore, we should be able to distinguish in these retrospective series, firstly between the adenocarcinoma arising in a limited columnar lined esophagus from that arising in a real Barrett's esophagus (lower esophagus circumferentially lined by columnar epithelium for a distance of 3 cm or more above the gastroesophageal junction), and secondly from the adenocarcinoma of the cardia. It is very difficult to achieve this result when in presence of a large tumor. The considerations on operability and resectability rate differ widely depending on whether patients are considered retrospectively or prospectively.

When the patients are considered retrospectively and the diagnosis of adenocarcinoma on a Barrett's esophagus is made on the operative specimen, the operability and resectability rate is the same as for other cancers located in same esophageal tract. We have to remember that in the majority of cases this cancer is located in the lower esophagus, and also for the epidermoid cancers of this area, that the resectability rate is higher when compared to the cancers located in the upper esophagus.

When the patients are considered prospectively (patients under endoscopic surveillance, because of the presence of a Barrett's esophagus), the cancer is diagnosed very early, and the resectability rate can reach 100%, as stated by Streitz [7] and Nishimaki [8].

Operability rate depends on the general conditions, associated diseases (lung, heart, liver and kidney functions) and it has nothing to do with the kind of histologic cancer. As far as late survival is concerned, there are very few papers comparing the late survival of Barrett's adenocarcinoma and other types of esophageal cancers when the stage of the disease is taken into consideration. Moreover, the comparison should be made between the different cancers arising in the same esophageal tract, as a statistical difference in the survival exists between an epidermoid cancer located in the upper esophagus and one located in the lower third [9]. However, there is no difference in late survival between Barrett's adenocarcinoma and the other types of esophageal cancers, as clearly demonstrated by Streitz [7]. The 5-year survival rate after resection was in fact 23.7% for Barrett's adenocarcinoma; 22.4% for adeno-carcinoma of the cardia and 17.3% for epidermoid esophageal cancers without any statistical difference.

In our experience, (unpublished data) the 5-year survival rate after curative resection for disease stage 0, 1 and 2, operative mortality included, was as depicted in Table 1.

Table 1. Five-year survival rate after curative resection for stages 0, 1 and 2

Barrett's adenocarcinoma (29 cases)	51.9%
Cardia adenocarcinoma (160 cases)	51.8%
Epidermoid cancer (lower esophagus) (77 cases)	45.9%

These data confirm that there is no difference in late survival between the different cancers of the esophagus when the stage of the disease is correctly compared. In fact, in our experience, the overall 5-year survival of Barrett's adenocarcinoma (41.9%) was higher than that of cardia adenocarcinoma (26.6%), but this result was due to the higher percentage of early cases in Barrett's adenocarcinoma (75.9%) compared to those in cardia adenocarcinoma (36.9%).

In conclusion, all esophageal cancers have a bad prognosis, and only early diagnosis can improve late survival.

References

1. Spechler SJ, Robbins AH, Rubins HB et al. Adenocarcinoma in Barrett's esophagus: an overrated risk? Gastroenterology 1984;87:927—933.
2. Cameron AJ, Zinsmeister AR, Ballard DJ, Carney JA. Prevalence of columnar-lined (Barrett's) esophagus: comparison of population-based clinical and autopsy findings. Gastroenterology 1990;99:918—922.
3. Robertons CS, Mayberry JF, Nicholson DA, James PD, Atkinson M. Value of endoscopic surveillance in the detection of the neoplastic change in Barrett's esophagus. Br J Surg 1988;75:760—763.
4. Achkar E, Carey W, Hall G et al. The clinical features and biological behavior of adenocarcinoma of the esophagus complicating Barrett's esophagus. In: Abstracts: International Esophageal Week Grafelfing, West Germany: Demeter Verlag, 1986;94.
5. Hameeteman W, Tytgat GNJ, Houthoff HJ, van den Tweel JG. Barrett's esophagus: development of dysplasia and adeno-carcinoma. Gastroenterology 1989;96:1249—1256.
6. Van der Veen AH, Dees J, Blankesteijn JD, Van Blankenstein M. Adenocarcinoma in Barrett's esophagus: an overrated risk. Gut 1989;30:14—18.
7. Streitz JM Jr, Ellis FH Jr, Gibb SP, Balogh K, Watkins E Jr. Adenocarcinoma in Barrett's esophagus: a clinicopathologic study of 65 cases. Ann Surg 1991;213:122—125.
8. Nishimaki T, Holscher AH, Schuler M, Bollschweiler E, Becker K, Siewert R. Histopathologic characteristics of early adenocarcinoma in Barrett's esophagus. Cancer 1991;68:1731—1736.
9. Bardini R, Castoro C, Sorrentino P, Ruol A, Borelli P, Ruffatto A, Tremolada C, Peracchia A. Prognostic factors for squamous cell carcinoma of the thoracic esophagus after curative resection. In: Ferguson MK, Little AG, Skinner DB (eds) Diseases of the Esophagus: Malignant Diseases, vol 1. Mount Kisco, NY: Futura Publishing Company, 1990;219—228.

Concluding Remarks

Tous les livres précédents de l'O.E.S.O. comportaient, sur leur dernière page, quelques lignes signées de la main de notre Président d'Honneur, et mon Maître durant de longues et précieuses années, Jean-Louis Lortat-Jacob.

Depuis sa triste disparition, dans cette continuité affectueuse que je n'ai jamais cessé de lui manifester, la structure de l'O.E.S.O. a subi une modification essentielle: pour assumer la responsabilité de Président d'Honneur, j'ai fait appel à deux amis, deux personnalités dominantes chacune dans leur spécialité, et qui synthétisent bien le caractère *polydisciplinaire* qui a, depuis sa création, été le vrai moteur de l'O.E.S.O.

D'un côté, un grand nom de la gastro-entérologie, Guido Tytgat,
de l'autre, l'un des très grands de la chirurgie mondiale, qui fait partie de ces "chirurgiens qui pensent", Tom DeMeester.

Et pour rendre encore plus évidente l'originalité de l'O.E.S.O., nous avons décidé de mettre en place un *Comité Scientifique Permanent* de 80 personnalités, venant de 19 pays.

C'est ainsi, par ces particularités, qu'O.E.S.O., représente aujourd'hui une structure de référence véritablement unique, réunissant
dans un même groupe,
au plus haut niveau mondial,
venant des cinq parties du monde,
la plupart des spécialistes les plus prestigieux représentant 18 disciplines*, tous voués à la recherche clinique et fondamentale portant sur *un seul organe*: l'oesophage.

*

Les travaux nombreux actuellement en cours de réalisation témoignent de l'enthousiasme de tous ceux qui sont montés dans le train polydisciplinaire O.E.S.O., et les Congrès triennaux, même s'ils sont consacrés à un thème unique, continueront d'en faire le point exhaustif.

Le prochain Congrès, celui de 1996, se déroulera lui aussi dans le même environnement prestigieux du siège de l'U.N.E.S.C.O. à Paris. Il traitera de façon aussi encyclopédique que possible les problèmes posés aujourd'hui par la *"Jonction oesophago-gastrique"*, en restant fidèle à la formule originale et efficace de 'réponses ponctuelles à une symphonie de questions brèves' dont parle Tom DeMeester dans sa préface.

*

*Physiologie — Radiologie — Endoscopie — Gastro-entérologie — Nutrition — Pharmacologie — Biochimie — Anesthésiologie — Chirurgie — Coelio-chirurgie — Oto-rhino-laryngologie — Pédiatrie — Anatomo-pathologie — Biologie moléculaire — Oncologie — Economie de la Santé -Epidémiologie et Statistiques.

All the preceding books of O.E.S.O. concluded by several lines written by our President of Honor, and my teacher during many long and valuable years, Jean-Louis Lortat-Jacob.

Since he passed away, and to prolong the affectionate respect I have always had for him, O.E.S.O. has undergone an essential modification: to fulfill the role of President of Honor, I have called on two friends, two foremost personalities, each in his own area of specialization, and who clearly synthetize the unique and very distinct *polydisciplinary nature* which has been since the beginning, the true driving force of the group.

On the one hand, a renowned authority in gastroenterology, Guido Tytgat.

On the other hand, a prominent and globaly known, "thinking surgeon", Tom DeMeester.

And to further emphasize the originality of O.E.S.O., we have set up a *Permanent Scientific Committee*, comprising 80 specialists from 19 countries.

This has come to make O.E.S.O. what it is today, a unique referential structure, bringing together:

> in one single group;
> at the highest level;
> coming from the four corners of the globe;
> a great majority of the most prestigious specialists representing 18 different disciplines*.

all devoted to clinical and fundamental research, focused *on one and only one organ*: the esophagus.

*

The numerous experimental and multicenter clinical studies, currently underway, bear witness to the collective enthusiasm of all those who have boarded the O.E.S.O. polydisciplinary train, and the triennial Congresses, although concentrated on only one theme, will, however, address all their relating subjects.

The next Meeting, in 1996, will also take place in the same prestigious setting of the U.N.E.S.C.O. headquarters in Paris. It will, as thoroughly as possible, explore the problems posed today by the gastroesophageal junction, following the same original format of "pithy answers to a symphony of questions", referred to by Tom DeMeester in the preface to this book.

*

Physiology — Radiology — Endoscopy — Gastroenterology — Nutrition — Pharmacology — Biochemistry — Anesthesiology — Surgery — Endoscopic Surgery — Otolaryngology — Pediatrics — Pathology — Molecular Biology — Oncology — Health Economics — Epidemiology and Statistical Evaluation.

Nous pouvons tous mesurer aujourd'hui cet élan qui existe dans l'O.E.S.O., et s'amplifie régulièrement d'année en année.

J'espère que le lecteur de cet ouvrage, même s'il n'a fait que le parcourir, en aura retiré, çà et là, le détail utile qu'il lui importait de préciser, l'opinion structurée qu'il retiendra et fera sienne, ou encore la question imprévue qui aura suscité en lui d'autres fructueuses interrogations.

Là, le but des éditeurs de cet ouvrage aura été atteint, pleinement.

Robert Giuli

All of us today, can witness the keen energy that exists within O.E.S.O. and continues to steadily grow year by year.

I personally hope that the reader of this volume, even after having only browsed through it, will have unearthed, here or there, the needed detail sought after, the borrowed opinion that will be adopted as one's own, or even the unsuspected question that will incite further fruitful reflection.

If this be the case, the aim of the editors of this book will have been achieved, fully.

Robert Giuli, MD, FACS
Professor of Surgery
Scientific Director of O.E.S.O.

Index of Authors

Subject Index

1168

Reflux and mucosa

Wound healing 276

Endoscopy

Antisecretory agents

Prokinetic agents

Long-term treatments

1181

Indications for surgery

Hill operation

THE CYLINDRIC MUCOSA

1192

Mucosa and radiology

Mucosa and histology

THE DYSPLASTIC MUCOSA

Markers

THE ADENOCARCINOMATOUS MUCOSA

Previous books of OESO

— Cancer of the Esophagus. Answers to 135 questions. R. Giuli Ed., Maloine S.A. Publ. Paris (1984), 426 pages.

— Benign Lesions of the Esophagus and Cancer. Answers to 210 questions. R. Giuli, R.W. McCallum Eds., Springer Verlag, Heidelberg (1989), 901 pages.

— Primary Motility Disorders of the Esophagus. 450 questions - 450 answers. R. Giuli, R.W. McCallum, D.B. Skinner Eds., John Libbey Eurotext, Paris, London (1991), 1217 pages.